ICD·10·PCS

International Classification of Diseases
10th Revision

Procedure Coding System

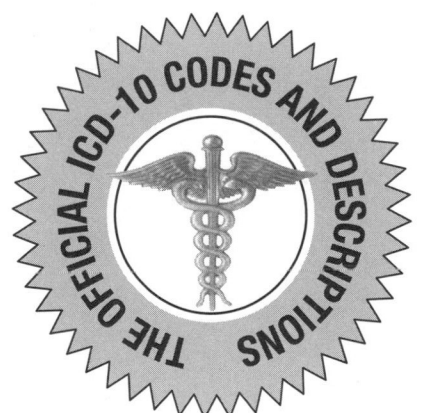

THE OFFICIAL ICD-10 CODES AND DESCRIPTIONS

2017

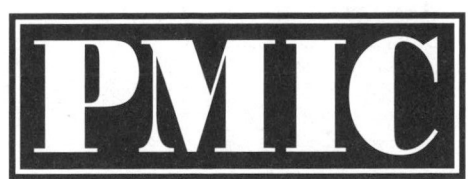

ISBN: 978-1-943009-52-7 (Print book)
        978-1-943009-55-8 (Electronic book)

Practice Management Information Corporation (PMIC)
4727 Wilshire Boulevard
Los Angeles, California 90010
http://www.pmiconline.com

Printed in the United States of America

On October 1, 2015, a key element of the data foundation of the United States' health care system underwent a major transformation…the transition from the decades-old Ninth Edition of the International Classification of Diseases (ICD-9) set of diagnosis and inpatient procedure codes to the far more contemporary, vastly larger, and much more detailed Tenth Edition of those code sets—or ICD-10—used by most developed countries throughout the world. The transition had a major impact on any person or entity recording health care information containing a diagnosis and/or inpatient procedure code.

All "covered entities"—as defined by the Health Insurance Portability and Accountability Act of 1996 (HIPAA)—were required to adopt ICD-10 codes for use in all HIPAA transactions with dates of service on or after the October 1, 2015 compliance date. for HIPAA inpatient claims, ICD-10 diagnosis and procedure codes are required for all inpatient stays with discharge dates on or after October 1, 2015.

This edition of ICD-10-PCS includes all official codes, descriptions and guidelines. A new edition is available approximately mid-September of each year. New editions may be purchased from:

ICD-10-PCS CHANGES HIGHLIGHTS

- In the Medical and Surgical section, root operation definitions for the root operations Control and Creation revised
- In the Extracorporeal Therapies section, new root operation Perfusion created
- ICD-10-PCS guidelines revised in response to public comment and internal review
- Code conversion table, new file available for ICD-10-PCS

SUMMARY OF CHANGES

Total Codes 2016	71,974
New Codes	3,827
Revised Titles	491
Deleted Codes	12
Total Codes 2017	**75,789**

Practice Management Information Corporation
4727 Wilshire Boulevard
Los Angeles, CA 90010
1-800-MED-SHOP
http://pmiconline.com

DISCLAIMER

This publication is designed to offer basic information regarding the ICD-10 coding system. The information presented is based upon extensive review of existing literature and the experience and interpretations of the author. Though all of the information has been carefully researched and checked for accuracy and completeness, neither the authors nor the publisher accepts any responsibility or liability with regard to errors, omissions, misuse or misinterpretation.

CONTENTS

TERMINOLOGY

Acute Conditions – The medical conditions characterized by sudden onset, severe change, and/or short duration.

Additional Diagnosis – The secondary diagnosis code used, if available, to provide a more complete picture of the primary diagnosis.

Alteration -- Modifying the anatomic structure of a body part without affecting the function of the body part

Applied mapping – Distillation of a reference mapping to conform to the needs of a particular application (e.g., data quality, research).

Approach (5th character) – Defines the technique used to reach the site of the procedure.

Backward mapping – mapping that proceeds from a newer code set to an older code set, for example from ICD-10-CM to ICD-9-CM.

Bilateral – For bilateral sites, the final character of the codes in the ICD-10-CM indicates laterality. An unspecified side code is also provided should the side not be identified in the medical record. If no bilateral code is provided and the condition is bilateral, assign separate codes for both the left and right side.

Body Part or Region (4th character) – Defines the specific anatomical site where the procedure is performed.

Body System (2nd character) – Defines the general physiological system on which the procedure is performed or anatomical region where the procedure is performed.

Bypass -- Altering the route of passage of the contents of a tubular body part.

Category – The three-digit diagnosis code classifications that broadly define each condition (e.g., 250 for diabetes mellitus).

Centers for Disease Control and Prevention (CDC) – A federal health data organization that helps maintain several code sets included in the HIPAA standards, including the ICD-9-CM codes.

Centers for Medicare & Medicaid Services (CMS) – The federal agency that runs the Medicare program. In addition, CMS works with the States to run the Medicaid program. CMS works to make sure that the beneficiaries in these programs are able to get high quality healthcare.

Change -- Taking out or off a device from a body part and putting back an identical or similar device in or on the same body part without cutting or puncturing the skin or a mucous membrane

Character – One of the seven components that comprise an ICD-10-PCS procedure code.

Chronic Conditions – Medical conditions characterized by long duration, frequent recurrence over a long period of time, and/or slow progression over time.

Cluster – in a combination entry, one instance where a code is chosen from each of the choice lists in the target system entry, that when combined satisfies the equivalent meaning of the corresponding code in the source system

Combination Codes – A single code used to classify any of the following: two diagnoses; a diagnosis with an associated secondary process (manifestation); or a diagnosis with an associated complication.

Control -- Stopping, or attempting to stop, postprocedural bleeding.

Conventions of ICD-10 – The general rules for use of the classification independent of guidelines. These conventions are incorporated within the Index and Tabular of the ICD-10-CM as instructional notes.

Creation -- Making a new genital structure that does not take over the function of a body part.

Crosswalk/mapping – A new test is determined to be similar to an existing test, multiple existing test codes, or a portion of an existing test code. The new test code is then assigned to the related existing local fee schedule amounts and resulting national limitation amount. In some instances, a test may only equate to a portion of a test, and, in those instances, payment at an appropriate percentage of the payment for the existing test is assigned.

Destruction -- Physical eradication of all or a portion of a body part by the direct use of energy, force or a destructive agent.

Detachment -- Cutting off all or a portion of the upper or lower extremities.

Dilation -- Expanding an orifice or the lumen of a tubular body part.

Division -- Cutting into a body part without draining fluids and/or gases from the body part in order to separate or transect a body part.

Drainage -- Taking or letting out fluids and/or gases from a body part.

Excision -- Cutting out or off, without replacement, a portion of a body part.

External (approach) -- Procedures performed directly on the skin or mucous membrane and procedures performed indirectly by the application of external force through the skin or mucous membrane.

Extirpation -- Taking or cutting out solid matter from a body part.

Extraction -- Pulling or stripping out or off all or a portion of a body part by the use of force.

Federal Register – The "Federal Register" is the official daily publication for rules, proposed rules and notices of federal agencies and organizations, as well as Executive Orders and other Presidential documents.

Forward mapping – mapping that proceeds from an older code set to a newer code set, for example from ICD-9-CM Volume 3 to ICD-10-PCS.

Fragmentation -- Breaking solid matter in a body part into pieces.

Fusion -- Joining together portions of an articular body part rendering the articular body part immobile.

GEMs - This reference mapping attempts to include all valid relationships between the codes in the ICD-9-CM diagnosis classification and the ICD-10-CM diagnosis classification.

General Equivalence Map (GEM) – reference mapping that attempts to include all valid relationships between the codes in the ICD-9- CM diagnosis classification and the ICD-10-CM diagnosis classification

Health Insurance Portability & Accountability Act (HIPAA) – A law passed in 1996 which is also sometimes called the "Kassebaum-Kennedy" law. This law expands healthcare coverage for patients who have lost or changed jobs, or have pre-existing conditions. HIPAA does not replace the states' roles as primary regulators of insurance.

HIPAA 4010 – The original healthcare transactions version of HIPAA (officially known as Version 004010 of the ASC X12 transaction implementation guides) named as part of HIPAA's Electronic Transaction Standards regulation. Version 4010 was required to be used by HIPAA covered healthcare entities by Oct. 16, 2003.

HIPAA 5010 – Required by Jan. 1, 2012 to be the new version of the HIPAA healthcare transactions. Officially known as Version 005010 of the ASC X12 transaction Technical Report Type 3. This new version was required as a result of Department of Health and Human Services (HHS) final rules published on Jan. 6, 2009.

ICD-10 – The mortality and morbidity classification coding system implemented by WHO in 1993 to replace ICD-9.

ICD-10-CM – The updated version of the clinical modification coding set defined by the National Center for Health Statistics that will replace ICD-9-CM on Oct. 1, 2013.

ICD-10-PCS – The updated procedural coding system defined by CMS that will replace Volume 3 of ICD-9-CM for hospital inpatient services.

ICD-9 – The mortality and morbidity classification coding system that is currently used throughout most of the world, including the United States. The ICD-9 classification of death and disease is based a series of classifications systems first adopted in 1893.

ICD-9-CM – The "clinical modification" to the ICD-9 code set that is currently used in America to report medical diagnoses. The "Clinical Modification" refers to the base WHO defined ICD-9 code set that has been defined for use in United State by the National Center for Health Statistics (NCHS) division of the Centers for Disease Control (CDC).

ICD-9-PCS – The procedural coding system currently used in America primarily for hospital inpatient services. It is contained in Volume 3 of ICD-9-CM.

Index (to diseases) – The ICD-10-CM is divided into the Alphabetic Index, an alphabetical list of terms and their corresponding code, and the Tabular List, a chronological list of codes divided into chapters based on body system or condition. The Alphabetic Index consists of the following parts: the Index of Diseases and Injury, the Index of External Causes of Injury, the Table of Neoplasms and the Table of Drugs and Chemicals.

Insertion -- Putting in a nonbiological device that monitors, assists, performs or prevents a physiological function but does not physically take the place of a body part.

Inspection -- Visually and/or manually exploring a body part.

International Classification of Diseases (ICD) – A medical code set maintained by the World Health Organization (WHO). The primary purpose of this code set is to classify both causes of death or mortality and diseases or morbidity. A U.S. extension, known as ICD-CM, "Clinical Modification," is maintained by the NCHS within the CDC to more precisely define ICD use in the U.S.

Manifestation Codes – Certain conditions have both an underlying etiology and multiple body system manifestations due to the underlying etiology. For such conditions, the ICD-10-CM has a coding convention that requires the underlying condition be sequenced first followed by the manifestation. Wherever such a combination exists, there is a "use additional code" note at the etiology code, and a "code first" note at the manifestation code. These instructional notes indicate the proper sequencing order of the codes, etiology followed by manifestation.

Map -- Locating the route of passage of electrical impulses and/or locating functional areas in a body part.

Medical Necessity – Services or supplies that: are proper and needed for the diagnosis or treatment of a medical condition; are provided for the diagnosis, direct care, and treatment of a medical condition; meet the standards of good medical practice in the local area; and are not mainly for the convenience of the patient or doctor.

Morbidity – Term refers to the disease rate or number of cases of a particular disease in a given age range, gender, occupation, or other relevant population based grouping.

Mortality –Term refers to the death rate reflected by the population in a given region, age range, or other relevant statistical grouping

National Center for Health Statistics (NCHS) – A federal organization within the CDC that collects, analyzes, and distributes healthcare statistics. The NCHS helps maintain the ICD-CM codes.

No Map Flag – attribute in a GEM that when turned on indicates that a code in the source system is not linked to any code in the target system .

Occlusion -- Completely closing an orifice or the lumen of a tubular body part.

Open (approach) -- Cutting through the skin or mucous membrane and any other body layers necessary to expose the site of the procedure.

Percutaneous (approach) -- Entry, by puncture or minor incision, of instrumentation through the skin or mucous membrane and any other body layers necessary to reach the site of the procedure.

Percutaneous Endoscopic (approach) -- Entry, by puncture or minor incision, of instrumentation through the skin or mucous membrane and any other body layers necessary to reach and visualize the site of the procedure.

Principle Diagnosis – First-listed/primary diagnosis code. The code sequenced first on a medical record defines the primary reason for the encounter as determined at the end of the encounter.

Procedure – The complete specification of the ICD-10-PCS seven characters.

Reattachment -- Putting back in or on all or a portion of a separated body part to its normal location or other suitable location.

Release -- Freeing a body part from an abnormal physical constraint by cutting or by use of force.

Removal -- Taking out or off a device from a body part.

Repair -- Restoring, to the extent possible, a body part to its normal anatomic structure and function.

Replacement -- Putting in or on biological or synthetic material that physically takes the place and/or function of all or a portion of a body part.

Reposition -- Moving to its normal location, or other suitable location, all or a portion of a body part.

Resection -- Cutting out or off, without replacement, all of a body part.

Restriction -- Partially closing an orifice or the lumen of a tubular body part.

Reverse lookup – using a GEM by looking up a target system code to see all the codes in the source system that translate to it.

Revision -- Correcting, to the extent possible, a portion of a malfunctioning device or the position of a displaced device.

Root Operation/Type (3rd character) – Defines the objective of the procedure.

Section (1st character) – Defines the general type of procedure.

Sequelae – A late effect is the residual effect (condition produced) after the acute phase of an illness or injury has terminated. There is no time limit on when a late effect code can be used. The residual may be apparent early, such as in cerebral infarction, or it may occur months or years later, such as that due to a previous injury.

Signs/Symptoms – Codes that describe symptoms and signs, as opposed to diagnoses, are acceptable for reporting purposes when a related definitive diagnosis has not been established (confirmed) by the provider.

Source system -- code set of origin in the mapping; the set being mapped 'from'

Supplement -- Putting in or on biological or synthetic material that physically reinforces and/or augments the function of a portion of a body part

Tabular List – It is essential to use both the Alphabetic Index and Tabular List when locating and assigning a code. The Alphabetic Index does not always provide the full code. Selection of the full code, including laterality and any applicable 7th character can only be done in the Tabular List. A dash (-) at the end of an Alphabetic Index entry indicates that additional characters are required. Even if a dash is not included at the Alphabetic Index entry, it is necessary to refer to the Tabular List to verify that no 7th character is required.

Target system – destination code set in the mapping; the set being mapped 'to'.

Transfer -- Moving, without taking out, all or a portion of a body part to another location to take over the function of all or a portion of a body part.

Transplantation -- Putting in or on all or a portion of a living body part taken from another individual or animal to physically take the place and/or function of all or a portion of a similar body part.

Uniform Hospital Discharge Data Set (UHDDS) – The UHDDS definitions are used by hospitals to report inpatient data elements in a standardized manner. These data elements and their definitions can be found in the July 31, 1985, Federal Register (Vol. 50, No, 147), pp. 31038-40.

Value – Individual units defined for each character of ICD-10-PCS and represented by a number or letter.

Via Natural or Artificial Opening (approach) -- Entry of instrumentation through a natural or artificial external opening to reach the site of the procedure.

Via Natural or Artificial Opening Endoscopic (approach) -- Entry of instrumentation through a natural or artificial external opening to reach and visualize the site of the procedure.

Via Natural or Artificial Opening With Percutaneous Endoscopic Assistance (approach) -- Entry of instrumentation through a natural or artificial external opening and entry, by puncture or minor incision, of instrumentation through the skin or mucous membrane and any other body layers necessary to aid in the performance of the procedure.

Volume I – The detailed, tabular list of diagnosis codes in the ICD-9-CM manual.

Volume II – The alphabetical index to diseases in the ICD-9-CM diagnosis coding manual.

Volume III – The ICD-9/ICD-10 list of procedure codes, used in inpatient settings.

World Health Organization (WHO) – An organization that maintains the International Classification of Diseases (ICD) medical code set.

INTRODUCTION TO ICD-10-PCS

The International Classification Of Diseases Tenth Revision Procedure Coding System (ICD-10-PCS) was created to accompany the World Health Organization's (WHO) ICD-10 diagnosis classification. The new procedure coding system was developed to replace ICD-9-CM procedure codes for reporting inpatient procedures.

Unlike the ICD-9-CM classification, ICD-10-PCS was designed to enable each code to have a standard structure and be very descriptive, and yet flexible enough to accommodate future needs. Information about the structure, organization, and application of ICD-10-PCS codes, along with reference material for coding with ICD-10-PCS, is provided in this manual.

WHAT IS ICD-10-PCS?

The **I**nternational **C**lassification of **D**isease tenth revision **P**rocedure **C**oding **S**ystem (**ICD-10-PCS**) is a system of medical classification used for procedural codes used to collect data, determine payment, and support the electronic health record for all inpatient procedures performed in the United States. On October 1, 2015, ICD-10-PCS replaced ICD-9-CM Volume 3 as the reporting system for procedure codes in the inpatient environment.

The World Health Organization has maintained the International Classification of Diseases (ICD) for recording cause of death since 1893. It has updated the ICD periodically to reflect new discoveries in epidemiology and changes in medical understanding of disease.

The International Classification of Diseases Tenth Revision (ICD-10), published in 1992, is the latest revision of the ICD. The WHO authorized the National Center for Health Statistics (NCHS) to develop a clinical modification of ICD-10 for use in the United States. This version of ICD-10 is called ICD-10-CM. ICD-10-CM is intended to replace the previous U.S. clinical modification, ICD-9-CM, that has been in use since 1979. ICD-9-CM contains a procedure classification; ICD-10-CM does not.

The Centers for Medicare and Medicaid Services, the agency responsible for maintaining the inpatient procedure code set in the U.S., contracted with 3M Health Information Systems in 1993 to design and then develop a procedure classification system to replace Volume 3 of ICD-9-CM. ICD-10-PCS is the result. ICD-10-PCS was initially released in 1998. It has been updated annually since that time.

ICD-9-CM VOLUME 3 COMPARED TO ICD-10-PCS

With ICD-10 implementation, the U.S. clinical modification of the ICD will not include a procedure classification based on the same principles of organization as the diagnosis classification. Instead, a separate procedure coding system has been developed to meet the rigorous and varied demands that are made of coded data in the healthcare industry. This represents a significant step toward building a health information infrastructure that functions optimally in the electronic age.

The following table highlights basic differences between ICD-9-CM Volume 3 and ICD-10-PCS.

ICD-9-CM VOLUME 3	ICD-10-PCS
Follows ICD structure (designed for diagnosis coding)	Designed/developed to meet healthcare needs for a procedure code system
Codes available as a fixed/finite set in list form	Codes constructed from flexible code components (values) using tables
Codes are numeric	Codes are alphanumeric
Codes are 3 through 4 digits long	All codes are seven characters long

ICD-10-PCS CODE STRUCTURE

Undergirding ICD-10-PCS is a logical, consistent structure that informs the system as a whole, down to the level of a single code. This means that the process of constructing codes in ICD-10-PCS is also logical and consistent: individual letters and numbers, called "values," are selected in sequence to occupy the seven spaces of the code, called "characters."

CHARACTERS

All codes in ICD-10-PCS are seven characters long. Each character in the seven-character code represents an aspect of the procedure, as shown in the following diagram of characters from the main section of ICD-10-PCS, called Medical and Surgical.

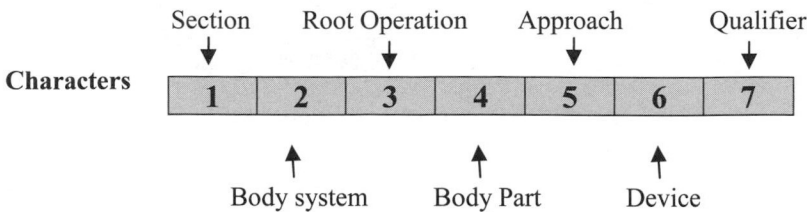

An ICD-10-PCS code is best understood as the result of a process rather than as an isolated, fixed quantity. The process consists of assigning values from among the valid choices for that part of the system, according to the rules governing the construction of codes.

VALUES

One of 34 possible values can be assigned to each character in a code: the numbers 0 through 9 and the alphabet (except I and O, because they are easily confused with the numbers 1 and 0). A finished code looks like the example below.

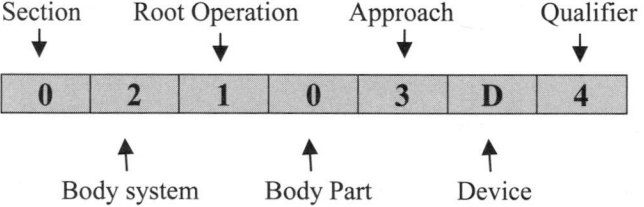

This code is derived by choosing a specific value for each of the seven characters. Based on details about the procedure performed, values for each character specifying the section, body system, root operation, body part, approach, device, and qualifier are assigned.

Because the definition of each character is a function of its physical position in the code, the same value placed in a different position in the code means something different. The value 0 in the first character means something different than 0 in the second character, or 0 in the third character, and so on.

CODE STRUCTURE: MEDICAL AND SURGICAL SECTION

The following pages define each character using the code 0LB50ZZ, "Excision of right lower arm and wrist tendon, open approach" as an example. This example comes from the Medical and Surgical section of ICD-10-PCS.

CHARACTER 1: SECTION

The first character in the code determines the broad procedure category, or section, where the code is found. In this example, the section is Medical and Surgical. 0 is the value that represents Medical and Surgical in the first character. The sample code looks like this so far:

Character 1 Section	Character 2 Body System	Character 3 Root Operation	Character 4 Body Part	Character 5 Approach	Character 6 Device	Character 7 Qualifier
Medical and Surgical						
0						

CHARACTER 2: BODY SYSTEM

The second character defines the body system—the general physiological system or anatomical region involved. Examples of body systems include Lower Arteries, Central Nervous System, and Respiratory System. In this example, the body system is Tendons, represented by the value L.

Character 1 Section	Character 2 Body System	Character 3 Root Operation	Character 4 Body Part	Character 5 Approach	Character 6 Device	Character 7 Qualifier
Medical and Surgical	Tendons					
0	L					

CHARACTER 3: ROOT OPERATION

The third character defines the root operation, or the objective of the procedure. Some examples of root operations are Bypass, Drainage, and Reattachment. In the sample code below, the root operation is Excision. When used in the third character of the code, the value B represents Excision.

Character 1 Section	Character 2 Body System	Character 3 Root Operation	Character 4 Body Part	Character 5 Approach	Character 6 Device	Character 7 Qualifier
Medical and Surgical	Tendons	Excision				.
0	L	B				

CHARACTER 4: BODY PART

The fourth character defines the body part, or specific anatomical site where the procedure was performed. The body system (second character) provides only a general indication of the procedure site. The body part and body system values together provide a precise description of the procedure site.

Examples of body parts are Kidney, Tonsils, and Thymus. In this example, the body part value is 5, Lower Arm and Wrist, Right. when the second character is L, the value 5 when used in the fourth character of the code represents the right lower arm and wrist tendon.

Character 1 Section	Character 2 Body System	Character 3 Root Operation	Character 4 Body Part	Character 5 Approach	Character 6 Device	Character 7 Qualifier
Medical and Surgical	Tendons	Excision	Lower Arm and Wrist, Right			‘
0	L	B	5			

CHARACTER 5: APPROACH

The fifth character defines the approach, or the technique used to reach the procedure site. Seven different approach values are used in the Medical and Surgical section to define the approach. Examples of approaches include Open and Percutaneous Endoscopic.

In the sample code below, the approach is Open and is represented by the value 0.

Character 1 Section	Character 2 Body System	Character 3 Root Operation	Character 4 Body Part	Character 5 Approach	Character 6 Device	Character 7 Qualifier
Medical And Surgical	Tendons	Excision	Lower Arm And Wrist, Right	Open		
0	L	B	5	0		

CHARACTER 6: DEVICE

Depending on the procedure performed, there may or may not be a device left in place at the end of the procedure. The sixth character defines the device. Device values fall into four basic categories:

- Grafts and Prostheses
- Implants
- Simple or Mechanical Appliances
- Electronic Appliances

In this example, there is no device used in the procedure. The value Z is used to represent NO DEVICE, as shown below.

Character 1 Section	Character 2 Body System	Character 3 Root Operation	Character 4 Body Part	Character 5 Approach	Character 6 Device	Character 7 Qualifier
Medical And Surgical	Tendons	Excision	Lower Arm And Wrist, Right	Open	No Device	
0	**L**	**B**	**5**	**0**	**Z**	

CHARACTER 7: QUALIFIER

The seventh character defines a qualifier for the code. A qualifier specifies an additional attribute of the procedure, if applicable.

Examples of qualifiers include Diagnostic and Stereotactic. Qualifier choices vary depending on the previous values selected. in this example, there is no specific qualifier applicable to this procedure, so the value is No Qualifier, represented by the letter Z.

Character 1 Section	Character 2 Body System	Character 3 Root Operation	Character 4 Body Part	Character 5 Approach	Character 6 Device	Character 7 Qualifier
Medical And Surgical	Tendons	Excision	Lower Arm And Wrist, Right	Open	No Device	No Qualifier
0	**L**	**B**	**5**	**0**	**Z**	**Z**

0LB50ZZ is the complete specification of the procedure "Excision of right lower arm and wrist tendon, open approach."

ICD-10-PCS SYSTEM ORGANIZATION

ICD-10-PCS is composed of 16 sections, represented by the numbers 0 through 9 and the letters B through D and F. The broad procedure categories contained in these sections range from surgical procedures to substance abuse treatment.

- Medical and Surgical
- Obstetrics
- Placement
- Administration
- Measurement and Monitoring
- Extracorporeal Assistance and Performance
- Extracorporeal Therapies
- Osteopathic
- Other Procedures
- Chiropractic
- Imaging
- Nuclear Medicine
- Radiation Oncology
- Physical Rehabilitation and Diagnostic Audiology
- Mental Health

- Substance Abuse Treatment

MEDICAL AND SURGICAL SECTION

The first section, Medical and Surgical, contains the great majority of procedures typically reported in an inpatient setting. As shown in the previous section discussing ICD-10-PCS code structure, all procedure codes in the Medical and Surgical section begin with the section value 0.

	Character 2 Body System	Character 3 Root Operation	Character 4 Body Part	Character 5 Approach	Character 6 Device	Character 7 Qualifier
Medical and Surgical	Tendons	Excision	Lower arm and Wrist, right	Open	No device	No qualifier
0	**L**	**B**	**5**	**0**	**Z**	**Z**

Sections 1 through 9 of ICD-10-PCS comprise the Medical and Surgical-related sections. These sections include obstetrical procedures, administration of substances, measurement and monitoring of body functions, and extracorporeal therapies, as listed in the table below.

Section Value	Description
1	Obstetrics
2	Placement
3	Administration
4	Measurement and Monitoring
5	Extracorporeal Assistance and Performance
6	Extracorporeal Therapies
7	Osteopathic
8	Other Procedures
9	Chiropractic

In sections 1 and 2, all seven characters define the same aspects of the procedure as in the Medical and Surgical section.

Codes in sections 3 through 9 are structured for the most part like their counterparts in the Medical and Surgical section, with a few exceptions. For example, in sections 5 and 6, the fifth character is defined as duration instead of approach, as in this code for intra-aortic balloon pump (IABP):

	Character 2 Body System	Character 3 Root Operation	Character 4 Body system	Character 5 Duration	Character 6 Function	Character 7 Qualifier
Extracorporeal Assist. And Performance	Physiological Systems	Assistance	Cardiac	Continuous	Output	Balloon Pump
5	**A**	**0**	**2**	**2**	**1**	**0**

Additional differences include these uses of the sixth character:

- Section 3 defines the sixth character as substance.
- Sections 4 and 5 define the sixth character as function.
- Sections 7 through 9 define the sixth character as method.

ANCILLARY SECTIONS

Sections B through D and F through H comprise the ancillary sections of ICD-10-PCS. These six sections include imaging procedures, nuclear medicine, and substance abuse treatment, as listed in the following table.

Section Value	Description
B	Imaging
C	Nuclear Medicine
D	Radiation Therapy

F	Physical Rehabilitation and Diagnostic Audiology
G	Mental Health
H	Substance Abuse Treatment

The definitions of some characters in the ancillary sections differs from that seen in previous sections. In the Imaging section, the third character is defined as type, and the fifth and sixth characters define contrast and contrast/qualifier respectively, as in the CT scan example below.

Character 1 Section	Character 2 Body System	Character 3 Type	Character 4 Body Part	Character 5 Contrast	Character 6 Qualifier	Character 7 Qualifier
Imaging	Central Nervous	Computerized Tomography	Brain	High Osmolar	Unenhanced and Enhanced	None
B	**0**	**2**	**0**	**0**	**0**	**Z**

Additional differences include:

- Section C defines the fifth character as radionuclide.
- Section D defines the fifth character as modality qualifier and the sixth character as isotope.
- Section F defines the fifth character as type qualifier and the sixth character as equipment.

TABLES

The complete ICD-10-PCS is presented in three parts: the Tables, the Index, and the List of Codes.

The Tables are organized in a series, beginning with section 0, Medical and Surgical, and body system 0, Central Nervous, and proceeding in numerical order. Sections 0 through 9 are followed by sections B through D and F through H. The same convention is followed within each table for the second through the seventh characters—numeric values in order first, followed by alphabetical values in order.

The following examples use the Medical and Surgical section to describe the organization and format of the ICD-10-PCS Tables.

The Medical and Surgical section (first character 0) is organized by its 31 body system values. Each body system subdivision in the Medical and Surgical section contains tables that list the valid root operations for that body system. These are the root operation tables that form the system. These tables provide the valid choices of values available to construct a code.

The root operation tables consist of four columns and a varying number of rows, as in the following example of the root operation Bypass, in the Central Nervous body system.

Four columns contain the applicable values for characters 4 through 7, given the values in characters 1 through 3.

Section	0	Medical And Surgical

Section   **0**   **Medical And Surgical**
Body System   **0**   **Central Nervous**
Operation   **1**   **Bypass:** Altering the route of passage of the contents of a tubular body part (Root operation)

Body Part (Character 4)	Approach (Character 5)	Device (Character 6)	Qualifier (Character 7)
6 Cerebral Ventricle	**0** Open	**7** Autologous Tissue Substitute **J** Synthetic Substitute **K** Nonautologous Tissue Substitute	**0** Nasopharynx **1** Mastoid Sinus **2** Atrium **3** Blood Vessel **4** Pleural Cavity **5** Intestine **6** Peritoneal Cavity **7** Urinary Tract **8** Bone Marrow **B** Cerebral Cisterns
U Spinal Canal	**0** Open	**7** Autologous Tissue Substitute **J** Synthetic Substitute **K** Nonautologous Tissue Substitute	**4** Pleural Cavity **6** Peritoneal Cavity **7** Urinary Tract **9** Fallopian Tube

A table may be separated into rows to specify the valid choices of values in characters 4 through 7. A code built using values from more than one row of a table is not a valid code.

ALPHABETIC INDEX

The ICD-10-PCS Index can be used to access the Tables. The Index mirrors the structure of the Tables, so it follows a consistent pattern of organization and use of hierarchies.

The Index is organized as an alphabetic lookup. Two types of main terms are listed in the Index:

- Based on the value of the third character
- Common procedure terms

MAIN TERMS

For the medical and surgical and related sections, the root operation values are used as main terms in the index. in other sections, the values representing the general type of procedure performed, such as nuclear medicine or imaging type, are listed as main terms.

For the medical and surgical and related sections, values such as excision, bypass, and transplantation are included as main terms in the index. the applicable body system entries are listed beneath the main term, and refer to a specific table. for the ancillary sections, values such as fluoroscopy and positron emission tomography are listed as main terms.

In the example below, the index entry "bypass" refers to the medical and surgical section tables for all applicable body systems, including anatomical regions and central nervous system.

Bypass
    by Body System
        Anatomical Regions 0W1....
            Central Nervous System 001....

The body system listings may be followed by entries for specific body parts, as in the excerpt below. In the root operations CHANGE, INSERTION, REMOVAL, and REVISION, the device entries follow the body system listings.

    by Body Part
        Artery
            Aorta, Abdominal 0410...
            Aorta, Thoracic 021W...
            Axillary 031....
            Brachial 031....
            Common Carotid 031....

COMMON PROCEDURE TERMS

The second type of term listed in the Index uses procedure names, such as "appendectomy" or "fundoplication." These entries are listed as main terms, and refer to a table or tables from which a valid code can be constructed, as shown in the following example.

Cholecystectomy

-   see Excision, Hepatobiliary System & Pancreas 0FB....
-   see Resection, Hepatobiliary System & Pancreas 0FT....

DEFINITIONS

The ICD-10-PCS Definitions contain the official definitions of ICD-10-PCS values in characters 3 through 7 of the seven-character code, and may also provide additional explanation or examples. The definitions are arranged in section order and designate the section and the character within the section being defined.

The Medical and Surgical section body part value definitions refer from the body part value to corresponding anatomical terms. The Medical and Surgical section device definitions refer from the device value to corresponding device terms or manufacturer's names. The Substance value definitions in the Administration section refer from the substance value to a common substance name or manufacturer's substance name. These definitions are also sorted by common term and listed separately as the Body Part Key, Device Key, and Substance Key respectively.

The ICD-10-PCS Device Aggregation Table contains entries that correlate a specific ICD-10-PCS device value with a general device value to be used in tables containing only general device values.

LIST OF CODES

The ICD-10-PCS List of Codes is a resource that displays all valid codes in alphanumeric order. Each entry begins with the seven-character code, followed by the full text description. The code descriptions are generated using rules that produce standardized, complete, and easy-to-read code descriptions.

ICD-10-PCS DESIGN

ICD-10-PCS is fundamentally different from ICD-9-CM in its structure, organization, and capabilities. It was designed and developed to adhere to recommendations made by the National Committee on Vital and Health Statistics (NCVHS). It also incorporates input from a wide range of organizations, individual physicians, healthcare professionals, and researchers.

Several structural attributes were recommended for a new procedure coding system. These attributes include

- Multiaxial structure
- Completeness
- Expandability

MULTIAXIAL STRUCTURE

The key attribute that provides the framework for all other structural attributes is multiaxial code structure. Multiaxial code structure makes it possible for the ICD-10-PCS to be complete, expandable, and to provide a high degree of flexibility and functionality. ICD-10-PCS codes are composed of seven characters. Each character represents a category of information that can be specified about the procedure performed. A character defines both the category of information and its physical position in the code.

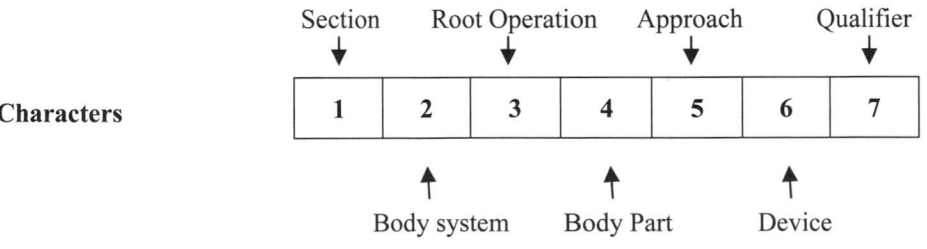

A character's position can be understood as a semi-independent axis of classification that allows different specific values to be inserted into that space, and whose physical position remains stable. Within a defined code range, a character retains the general meaning that it confers on any value in that position. For example, the fifth character retains the general meaning "approach" in sections 0 through 4 and 7 through 9 of the system. Any specific value in the fifth character will define a specific approach, such as Open.

Each group of values for a character contains all of the valid choices in relation to the other characters of the code, giving the system completeness. in the fifth character, for example, each significantly distinct approach is assigned its own approach value and all applicable approach values are included to represent the possible versions of a procedure.

Each group of values for a character can be added to as needed, giving the system expandability. if a significantly distinct approach is used to perform procedures, a new approach value can be added to the system.

Each group of values is confined to its own character, giving ICD-10-PCS a stable, predictable readability across a wide range of codes. In sections 0 through 4 and 7 through 9 of the system, for example, the fifth character always represents the approach.

ICD-10-PCS' multiaxial structure houses its capacity for completeness, expandability, and flexibility, giving it a high degree of functionality for multiple uses.

COMPLETENESS

Completeness is considered a key structural attribute for a new procedure coding system. The specific recommendation for completeness includes these characteristics:

- A unique code is available for each significantly different procedure.
- Each code retains its unique definition. Codes are not reused.

In Volume 3 of ICD-9-CM, procedures performed on many different body parts using different approaches or devices may be assigned to the same procedure code. In ICD-10-PCS, a unique code can be constructed for every significantly different procedure.

Within each section, a character defines a consistent component of a code, and contains all applicable values for that character. The values define individual expressions (open, percutaneous) of the character's general meaning (approach) that are then used to construct unique procedure codes.

Because all approaches by which a procedure is performed are assigned a separate approach value in the system, every procedure which uses a different approach will have its own unique code. This is true of the other characters as well. The same procedure performed on a different body part has its own unique code, the same procedure performed using a different device has its own unique code, and so on.

In the case of the coronary artery bypass graft (CABG), ICD-9-CM contains a total of nine codes to describe different versions of the procedure. These codes specify the version based on one aspect of the procedure, and the aspect defined is not consistent for all nine codes. Four of the codes specify the number of coronary arteries bypassed, four specify the source of the new blood flow, and one is an "unspecified" choice.

By contrast, ICD-10-PCS components can be combined to produce 34 unique codes defining all significantly different versions of the comparable CABG procedure. All 34 codes specify the same four aspects of the procedure: the number of coronary artery sites bypassed, i.e., the approach to the procedure site, the type of graft if used, and the origin of the bypass (source of the new blood flow). The differences are summarized in the table below.

ICD-9-CM VOLUME 3 CODE & DESCRIPTION		ICD-10-PCS CODE & DESCRIPTION	
36.11	Aortocoronary bypass of one coronary artery (1of 4)	0 2 1 0 0 9 W	Bypass coronary artery, one site to aorta with autologous venous tissue, open approach(1 of 8)
36.15	Single internal mammary- coronary artery bypass (1of 2)	0 2 1 0 0 Z 8	Bypass coronary artery, one site to right internal mammary, open approach (1 of 16)
36.17	Abdominal-coronary artery bypass (1 of 2)	0 2 1 0 0 A F	Bypass coronary artery, one site to abdominal artery with autologous arterial tissue, open approach (1 of 10)
36.10	Aortocoronary bypass for heart revascularization, not otherwise specified (1of 1)	No Equivalent	ICD-10-PCS codes all contain a minimum level of specificity

UNIQUE DEFINITIONS

Because ICD-10-PCS codes are constructed of individual values rather than lists of fixed codes and text descriptions, the unique, stable definition of a code in the system is retained. New values may be added to the system to represent a specific new approach or device or qualifier, but whole codes by design cannot be given new meanings and reused.

EXPANDABILITY

Expandability was also recommended as a key structural attribute. The specific recommendation for expandability includes these characteristics:

* Accommodate new procedures and technologies
* Add new codes without disrupting the existing structure

ICD-10-PCS is designed to be easily updated as new codes are required for new procedures and new techniques. Changes to ICD-10-PCS can all be made within the existing structure, because whole codes are not added. Instead, one of two possible changes is made to the system:

* A new value for a character is added as needed to the system.
* An existing value for a character is added to a table(s) in the system.

ICD-10-PCS UPDATE: PICVA

An example of how the updating of ICD-10-PCS works can be seen in the coronary artery bypass procedure called Percutaneous In-situ Coronary Venous Arterialization (PICVA). This procedure is no more invasive than a percutaneous coronary angioplasty, but achieves the benefits of a bypass procedure by placing a specialized stent into the diseased coronary artery, through its wall into the adjacent coronary vein, and diverting blood flow through the stent into the artery past the blockage.

ICD-10-PCS was updated in 2004 to include an appropriate range of codes for the PICVA procedure (16 possible codes). This was accomplished simply by adding another row to the relevant table (as shown in the example below) containing two approach values for the non-invasive approach, two device values for the possible types of stent, and a single qualifier defining the coronary vein as the source of the new blood flow, as in the example below.

SECTION	0	MEDICAL AND SURGICAL	
BODY SYSTEM	2	HEART AND GREAT VESSELS	
OPERATION	1	BYPASS: Altering the route of passage of the contents of a tubular body part	
Body Part (Character 4)	Approach (Character 5)	Device (Character 6)	Qualifier (Character 7)
0 Coronary Artery, One Site 1 Coronary Artery, Two Sites 2 Coronary Artery, Three Sites 4 Coronary Artery, Four or More Sites	3 Percutaneous 4 Percutaneous Endoscopic	4 Drug-eluting Intraluminal Device D Intraluminal Device	D Coronary Vein

STRUCTURAL INTEGRITY

As shown in the previous example, ICD-10-PCS can be easily expanded without disrupting the structure of the system.

In the PICVA example, one new value—the qualifier value Coronary Vein—was added to the system to effect this change. All other values in the new row are existing values used to create unique, new codes.

This type of updating can be replicated anywhere in the system when a change is required. ICD-10-PCS allows unique new codes to be added to the system because values for the seven characters that make up a code can be combined as needed. The system can evolve as medical technology and clinical practice evolve, without disrupting the ICD-10-PCS structure.

ICD-10-PCS ADDITIONAL CHARACTERISTICS

ICD-10-PCS possesses several additional characteristics in response to government and industry recommendations. These characteristics are

- Standardized terminology within the coding system
- Standardized level of specificity
- No diagnostic information
- No explicit "not otherwise specified" (NOS) code options
- Limited use of "not elsewhere classified" (NEC) code options

STANDARDIZED TERMINOLOGY

Words commonly used in clinical vocabularies may have multiple meanings. This can cause confusion and result in inaccurate data. ICD-10-PCS is standardized and self-contained. Characters and values used in the system are defined in the system.

For example, the word "excision" is used to describe a wide variety of surgical procedures. In ICD-10-PCS, the word "excision" describes a single, precise surgical objective, defined as "Cutting out or off, without replacement, a portion of a body part."

NO EPONYMS OR COMMON PROCEDURE NAMES

The terminology used in ICD-10-PCS is standardized to provide precise and stable definitions of all procedures performed. This standardized terminology is used in all ICD-10-PCS code descriptions.

As a result, ICD-10-PCS code descriptions do not include eponyms or common procedure names. Two examples from ICD-9-CM are 22.61, "Excision of lesion of maxillary sinus with Caldwell-Luc approach," and 51.10, "Endoscopic retrograde cholangiopancreatography [ERCP]." In ICD-10-PCS, physicians' names are not included in a code description, nor are procedures identified by common terms or acronyms such as appendectomy or CABG. Instead, such procedures are coded to the root operation that accurately identifies the objective of the procedure.

The procedures described in the preceding paragraph by ICD-9-CM codes are coded in ICD-10-PCS according to the root operation that matches the objective of the procedure. Here the ICD-10-PCS equivalents would be Excision and Inspection respectively. By relying on the universal objectives defined in root operations rather than eponyms or specific procedure titles that change or become obsolete, ICD-10-PCS preserves the capacity to define past, present, and future procedures accurately using stable terminology in the form of characters and values.

NO COMBINATION CODES

With rare exceptions, ICD-10-PCS does not define multiple procedures with one code. This is to preserve standardized terminology and consistency across the system. Procedures that are typically performed together but are distinct procedures may be defined by a single "combination code" in ICD-9-CM. An example of a combination code in ICD-9-CM is 28.3, "Tonsillectomy with adenoidectomy."

A procedure that meets the reporting criteria for a separate procedure is coded separately in ICD-10-PCS. This allows the system to respond to changes in technology and medical practice with the maximum degree of stability and flexibility.

STANDARDIZED LEVEL OF SPECIFICITY

In ICD-9-CM, one code with its description and includes notes may encompass a vast number of procedure variations while another code defines a single specific procedure. ICD-10-PCS provides a standardized level of specificity for each code, so that each code represents a single procedure variation.

The ICD-9-CM code 39.31, "Suture of artery," does not specify the artery, whereas the code range 38.40 through 38.49, "Resection of artery with replacement," provides a fourth-digit subclassification for specifying the artery by anatomical region (thoracic, abdominal, etc.).

In ICD-10-PCS, the codes identifying all artery suture and artery replacement procedures possess the same degree of specificity. The ICD-9-CM examples above coded to their ICD-10-PCS equivalents would use the same artery body part values in all codes identifying the respective procedures.

In general, ICD-10-PCS code descriptions are much more specific than their ICD-9-CM counterparts, but sometimes an ICD-10-PCS code description is actually less specific. In most cases this is because the ICD-9-CM code contains diagnosis information. The standardized level of code specificity in ICD-10-PCS cannot always take account of these fluctuations in ICD-9-CM level of specificity. Instead, ICD-10-PCS provides a standardized level of specificity that can be predicted across the system.

DIAGNOSIS INFORMATION EXCLUDED

Another key feature of ICD-10-PCS is that information pertaining to a diagnosis is excluded from the code descriptions.

ICD-9-CM often contains information about the diagnosis in its procedure codes. Adding diagnosis information limits the flexibility and functionality of a procedure coding system. It has the effect of placing a code "off limits" because the diagnosis in the medical record does not match the diagnosis in the procedure code description. The code cannot be used even though the procedural part of the code description precisely matches the procedure performed.

Diagnosis information is not contained in any ICD-10-PCS code. The diagnosis codes, not the procedure codes, will specify the reason the procedure is performed.

NOS CODE OPTIONS RESTRICTED

ICD-9-CM often designates codes as "unspecified" or "not otherwise specified" codes. By contrast, the standardized level of specificity designed into ICD-10-PCS restricts the use of broadly applicable NOS or unspecified code options in the system. A minimal level of specificity is required to construct a valid code.

In ICD-10-PCS, each character defines information about the procedure and all seven characters must contain a specific value obtained from a single row of a table to build a valid code. Even values such as the sixth-character value Z, No Device and the seventh-character value Z, No Qualifier, provide important information about the procedure performed.

LIMITED NEC CODE OPTIONS

ICD-9-CM often designates codes as "not elsewhere classified" or "other specified" versions of a procedure throughout the code set. NEC options are also provided in ICD-10-PCS, but only for specific, limited use.

In the Medical and Surgical section, two significant "not elsewhere classified" options are the root operation value Q, Repair and the device value Y, Other Device.

The root operation Repair is a true NEC value. It is used only when the procedure performed is not one of the other root operations in the Medical and Surgical section.

Other Device, on the other hand, is intended to be used to temporarily define new devices that do not have a specific value assigned, until one can be added to the system. No categories of medical or surgical devices are permanently classified to Other Device.

ICD-10-PCS APPLICATIONS

ICD-10-PCS code structure results in qualities that optimize the performance of the system in electronic applications, and maximize the usefulness of the coded healthcare data. These qualities include:

- Optimal search capability
- Consistent character definitions
- Consistent values wherever possible
- Code readability

Some have argued that, in the world of the electronic health record, the classification system as we know it is outmoded, that classification doesn't matter because a computer is able to find a code with equal ease whether the code has been generated at random or is part of a classification scheme. While this may be true from an IT perspective, assignment of randomly generated code numbers makes it impossible to aggregate data according to related ranges of codes. This is a critical capability for providers, payers, and researchers to make meaningful use of the data.

OPTIMAL SEARCH CAPABILITY

ICD-10-PCS is designed for maximum versatility in the ability to aggregate coded data. Values belonging to the same character as defined in a section or sections can be easily compared, since they occupy the same position in a code. This provides a high degree of flexibility and functionality for data mining.

For example, the body part value 6, Stomach, retains its meaning for all codes in the Medical and Surgical section that define procedures performed on the stomach. Because the body part value is dependent for its meaning on the body system in which it is found, the body system value D, Gastrointestinal, must also be included in the search.

A person wishing to examine data regarding all medical and surgical procedures performed on the stomach could do so simply by searching the code range below.

0D*6***

CONSISTENT CHARACTERS AND VALUES

In the previous example, the value 6 means Stomach only when the body system value is D, Gastrointestinal. In many other cases, values retain their meaning across a much broader range of codes. This provides consistency and readability.

For example, the value 0 in the fifth character defines the approach Open and the value 3 in the fifth character defines the approach Percutaneous across sections 0 through 4 and 7 through 9, where applicable. As a result, all open and percutaneous procedures represented by codes in sections 0-4 and 7-9 can be compared based on a single character—approach—by conducting a query on the code ranges below.

[0 through 4,7 through 9]***0** vs. [0 through 4,7through 9]***3**

Searches can be progressively refined by adding specific values. For example, one could search on a body system value or range of body system values, plus a body part value or range of body part values, plus a root operation value or range of root operation values.

To refine the search above, one could add the body system value for Gastrointestinal and the body part value for Stomach to limit the search to open vs. percutaneous procedures performed on the stomach:

0D*60** vs. 0D*63"

To refine the search even further and limit the comparison to open and percutaneous biopsies of the stomach, one could add the third-character value for the root operation Excision and the seventh-character qualifier Diagnostic, as below.

0DB60*X vs. 0DB63*X

Stability of characters and values across vast ranges of codes provides the maximum degree of functionality and flexibility for the collection and analysis of data. The search capabilities demonstrated above function equally well for all uses of healthcare data: investigating quality of care, resource utilization, risk management, conducting research, determining reimbursement, and many others.

Because the character definition is consistent, and only the individual values assigned to that character differ as needed, meaningful comparisons of data over time can be conducted across a virtually infinite range of procedures.

CODE READABILITY

ICD-10-PCS resembles a language in the sense that it is made up of semi-independent values combined by following the rules of the system, much the way a sentence is formed by combining words and following the rules of grammar and syntax. As with words in their context, the meaning of any single value is a combination of its position in the code and any preceding values on which it may be dependent.

For example, in the Medical and Surgical section, a body part value is always dependent for its meaning on the body system in which it is found. It cannot stand alone as a letter or a number and be meaningful. A fourth-character value of 6 by itself can mean 31 different things, but a fourth-character value of 6 in the context of a second-character value of D means one thing only—Stomach.

On the other hand, a root operation value is not dependent on any character but the section for its meaning, and identifies a single consistent objective wherever the third character is defined as root operation. For example, the third-character value T identifies the root operation Resection in both the Medical and Surgical and Obstetrics sections.

The approach value also identifies a single consistent approach wherever the fifth character is defined as approach. The fifth-character value 3 identifies the approach Percutaneous in the Medical and Surgical section, the Obstetrics section, the Administration section, and others.

The sixth-character device value or seventh-character qualifier value identifies the same device or qualifier in the context of the body system where it is found. Although there may be consistencies across body systems or within whole sections, this is not true in all cases.

Values in their designated context have a precise meaning, like words in a language. As seen in the code example which began this chapter, 0LB50ZZ represents the text description of the specific procedure "Excision of right lower arm and wrist tendon, open approach." Since ICD-10-PCS values in context have a single, precise meaning, a complete, valid code can be read and understood without its accompanying text description, much like one would read a sentence.

ICD-10-PCS PROCEDURES IN THE MEDICAL AND SURGICAL SECTION

This chapter provides reference material for the root operations in the Medical and Surgical section of ICD-10-PCS. The vast majority of codes reported in an inpatient setting are found in this section.

First, a table presents all root operations in the Medical and Surgical section, organized into logical groups. Following the table are definitions of each root operation, presented in the order shown in the table. Material on each root operation includes

- Definition, explanation, and examples of the root operation
- Coding notes as needed
- A representative procedure excerpt for each root operation, followed by the correct code for the procedure. The code is provided in table excerpt format, along with explanatory notes as needed.
- Coding exercises that provide example procedures and their corresponding ICD-10-PCS codes, with explanatory notes as needed

ROOT OPERATION GROUPS

The Medical and Surgical root operations are divided into groups that share similar attributes. These groups, and the root operations in each, are listed in the table below. Subsequent pages of this chapter provide a definition of each root operation in a group.

Root Operation	What Operation Does	Objective Of Procedure	Procedure Site	Example
Excision	Takes out some/all of a body part	Cutting out/off without replacement	Some of a body part	Breast lumpectomy
Resection	Takes out some/all of a body part	Cutting out/off without replacement	All of a body part	Total mastectomy
Detachment	Takes out some/all of a body part	Cutting out/off without replacement	Extremity only, any level	Amputation above elbow
Destruction	Takes out some/all of a body part	Eradicating without replacement	Some/all of a body part	Fulguration of endometrium
Extraction	Takes out some/all of a body part	Pulling out or off without replacement	Some/all of a body part	Suction D & C
Drainage	Takes out solids/fluids/ gases from a body part	Taking/letting out fluids/ gases	Within a body part	Incision and Drainage
Extirpation	Takes out solids/fluids/ gases from a body part	Taking/cutting out solid matter	Within a body part	Thrombectomy
Fragmentation	Takes out solids/fluids/ gases from a body part	Breaking solid matter into pieces	Within a body part	Lithotripsy
Division	Involves cutting or separation only	Cutting into/separating a body part	Within a body part	Neurotomy
Release	Involves cutting or separation only	Freeing a body part from constraint	Around a body part	Adhesiolysis
Transplantation	Puts in/puts back or move some/all of a body part	Putting in a living body part from a person/animal	Some/all of a body part	Kidney transplant
Reattachment	Puts in/puts back or move some/all of a body part	Putting back a detached body part	Some/all of a body part	Reattach severed finger
Transfer	Puts in/puts back or move some/all of a body part	Moving, to function for a similar body part	Some/all of a body part	Skin transfer flap
Reposition	Puts in/puts back or move some/all of a body part	Moving, to normal or other suitable location	Some/all of a body part	Move undescended testicle
Restriction	Alters the diameter/route of a tubular body part	Partially closing orifice/ lumen	Tubular body part	Gastroesophageal fundoplication
Occlusion	Alters the diameter/route of a tubular body part	Completely closing orifice/ lumen	Tubular body part	Fallopian tube ligation
Dilation	Alters the diameter/route of a tubular body part	Expanding orifice/lumen	Tubular body part	Percutaneous transluminal coronary angioplasty (PTCA)

Root Operation	What Operation Does	Objective Of Procedure	Procedure Site	Example
Bypass	Alters the diameter/route of a tubular body part	Altering route of passage	Tubular body part	Coronary artery bypass graft (CABG)
Insertion	Always involve a device	Putting in non-biological device	In/on a body part	Central line insertion
Replacement	Always involve a device	Putting in device that replaces a body part	Some/all of a body part	Total hip replacement
Supplement	Always involve a device	Putting in device that reinforces or augments a body part	In/on a body part	Abdominal wall herniorrhaphy using mesh
Change	Always involve a device	Exchanging device w/out cutting/puncturing	In/on a body part	Drainage tube change
Removal	Always involve a device	Taking out device	In/on a body part	Central line removal
Revision	Always involve a device	Correcting a malfunctioning/displaced device	In/on a body part	Revision of pacemaker insertion
Inspection	Involves examination only	Visual/manual exploration	Some/all of a body part	Diagnostic cystoscopy
Map	Involves examination only	Locating electrical impulses/functional areas	Brain/cardiac conduction mechanism	Cardiac mapping
Repair	Includes other repairs	Restoring body part to its normal structure	Some/all of a body part	Suture laceration
Control	Includes other repairs	Stopping/attempting to stop postprocedural bleed	Anatomical region	Post-prostatectomy bleeding
Fusion	Includes other objectives	Rendering joint immobile	Joint	Spinal fusion
Alteration	Includes other objectives	Modifying body part for cosmetic purposes without affecting function	Some/all of a body part	Face lift
Creation	Includes other objectives	Making new structure for sex change operation	Perineum	Artificial vagina/ penis

ROOT OPERATIONS THAT TAKE OUT SOME OR ALL OF A BODY PART

Five root operations represent procedures for taking out or otherwise eradicating some or all of a body part. These root operations are listed in the table below and described in detail in the pages that follow.

Root Operation	Objective of Procedure	Site of Procedure	Example
Excision	Cutting out/off without replacement	Some of a body part	Breast lumpectomy
Resection	Cutting out/off without replacement	All of a body part	Total mastectomy
Detachment	Cutting out/off without replacement	Extremity only, any level	Amputation above elbow
Destruction	Eradicating without replacement	Some/all of a body part	Fulguration of endometrium
Extraction	Pulling out or off without replacement	Some/all of a body part	Suction D&C

EXCISION—ROOT OPERATION B

Excision	Definition	Cutting out or off, without replacement, a portion of a body part
B	Explanation	The qualifier Diagnostic is used to identify excision procedures that are biopsies
	Examples	Partial nephrectomy, liver biopsy

Excision is coded when a portion of a body part is cut out or off using a sharp instrument. All root operations that employ cutting to accomplish the objective allow the use of any sharp instrument, including but not limited to

- Scalpel
- Wire
- Scissors
- Bone saw
- Electrocautery tip

CODING NOTE	**BONE MARROW AND ENDOMETRIAL BIOPSIES** are not coded to the root operation excision. They are coded to Extraction, with the qualifier Diagnostic.

Example: Excision of sebaceous cyst (right buttock)

...the patient was brought in the room and placed on the table in jack knife, prone position and a spinal block was used for anesthesia. She was prepped and draped in the usual sterile manner. A digital rectal examination was performed and we did not notice any communication between mass and rectum. The mass was palpated and a radial transverse incision was made over the mass.

Using blunt and sharp dissection the top of the mass was identified and shown to be a sebaceous cyst. The sebaceous cyst was freed from the surrounding tissue using blunt dissection. The entire cyst was removed. Hemostasis was obtained and the skin was closed using 5-0 Dexon interrupted sutures...

Character 1 Section	Character 2 Body System	Character 3 Root Operation	Character 4 Body Part	Character 5 Approach	Character 6 Device	Character 7 Qualifier
Medical and Surgical	Skin	Excision	Buttock	External	No Device	No Qualifier
0	**H**	**B**	**8**	**X**	**Z**	**Z**

RESECTION—ROOT OPERATION T

Resection	Definition	Cutting out or off, without replacement, all of a body part
T	Explanation	N/A
	Examples	Total nephrectomy, total lobectomy of lung

Resection is similar to Excision, except Resection includes all of a body part, or any subdivision of a body part that has its own body part value in ICD-10-PCS, while Excision includes only a portion of a body part.

CODING NOTE	**LYMPH NODES.** When an entire lymph node chain is cut out, the appropriate root operation is Resection. When a lymph node(s) is cut out, the root operation is Excision.

Example: Right hemicolectomy

...a vertical midline incision was used to enter the abdominal cavity. There was noted to be a mass in the region of the cecum. The mass was easily mobilized and it was felt that a right hemicolectomy was indicated. The right colon was mobilized by incising the white line of Toldt and reflecting colon medially. The loose tissue was taken down bluntly with a hand and adhesions were taken down sharply.

The colon was mobilized to the left end up to the level of the hepatic flexure. The mesentery was incised sharply with a knife and down to the level of the root of the mesentery. The mesentery of the right colon and the distal ileum was then taken down between Kelly's and tied with 2-0 silk, down to the level of the takeoff vessels.

After removing the right colon specimen off the field, a primary anastomosis was planned...

Character 1 Section	Character 2 Body System	Character 3 Root Operation	Character 4 Body Part	Character 5 Approach	Character 6 Device	Character 7 Qualifier
Medical and Surgical	Gastro-intestinal system	Resection	Large Intestine, Right	Open	No Device	No Qualifier
0	**D**	**T**	**F**	**0**	**Z**	**Z**

CODING NOTE	**ANASTOMOTIC TECHNIQUE.** Adjunct information about the anastomotic technique used to *technique* complete a colectomy procedure (e.g., side to end) is not specified in ICD-10-PCS. Only the specific Excision or Resection code is assigned.

DETACHMENT—ROOT OPERATION 6

Detachment represents a narrow range of procedures; it is used exclusively for amputation procedures.

Detachment 6	Definition	Cutting off all or part of the upper or lower extremities
	Explanation	The body part value is the site of the detachment, with a qualifier if applicable to further specify the level where the extremity was detached
	Examples	Below knee amputation, disarticulation of shoulder

Detachment procedure codes are found only in body systems X Anatomical Regions, Upper Extremities and Y Anatomical Regions, Lower Extremities, because amputations are performed on the extremities, across overlapping body layers, and so could not be coded to a specific musculoskeletal body system such as the bones or joints.

Detachment Qualifiers

The specific qualifiers used for Detachment are dependent on the body part value in the upper and lower extremities body systems. The table below defines the meaning of the qualifiers used in both the upper and lower extremities.

Body Part	Qualifier Value	Definition
Upper arm and upper leg	1	High: Amputation at the proximal portion of the shaft of the humerus or femur
	2	Mid: Amputation at the middle portion of the shaft of the humerus or femur
	3	Low: Amputation at the distal portion of the shaft of the humerus or femur
Hand and foot		Complete: Amputation through the carpometacarpal joint of the hand, or through the tarsal-metatarsal joint of the foot
		Partial: Amputation anywhere along the shaft or head of the metacarpal bone of the hand, or of the metatarsal bone of the foot
	0	Complete
	4	Complete 1st Ray
	5	Complete 2nd Ray
	6	Complete 3rd Ray
	7	Complete 4th Ray
	8	Complete 5th Ray
	9	Partial 1st Ray
	B	Partial 2nd Ray
	C	Partial 3rd Ray
	D	Partial 4th Ray
	F	Partial 5th Ray
Thumb, finger, or toe	0	Complete: Amputation at the metacarpophalangeal/metatarsal-phalangeal joint
	1	High: Amputation anywhere along the proximal phalanx
	2	Mid: Amputation through the proximal interphalangeal joint or anywhere along the middle phalanx
	3	Low: Amputation through the distal interphalangeal joint or anywhere along the distal phalanx

Example: Fifth toe ray amputation

...a semi-elliptical incision was made around the base of the left toe with a #15 blade without difficulty. Careful sharp dissection was made down to the bone, and care was taken to avoid the fourth toe's neurovascular bundle. There was obvious osteomyelitis of the proximal phalanx of the fifth toe and the toe itself was disarticulated, the proximal head of the fifth lower extremity metatarsal, without difficulty. Specimens were sent to pathology for culture and examination. Next, both sharp and blunt dissection were used to adequately expose the head of the fifth metatarsal, and this was done without difficulty. A small rongeur was then used to remove the head of the fifth metatarsal, and soft spongy bone was felt beneath this area.

Examination of the patient's x-rays revealed that there was an area of cortical lucency at the base of the head of the fifth metatarsal, and the decision was made to extend the amputation to the midshaft of the fifth metatarsal, and this was done without difficulty using a rongeur. The wound was then flushed with normal saline, and bleeding viable tissue was observed throughout the wound. There was adequate flap coverage of the remaining fifth metatarsal...

Character 1 Section	Character 2 Body System	Character 3 Root Operation	Character 4 Body Part	Character 5 Approach	Character 6 Device	Character 7 Qualifier
Medical and Surgical	Lower Extremities	Detachment	Foot, Left	Open	No Device	Partial 5th Ray
0	**Y**	**6**	**N**	**0**	**Z**	**f**

CODING NOTE	QUALIFIER VALUE. The surgeon uses the word "toe" to describe the amputation, but the operative report says he extends the amputation to the midshaft of the fifth metatarsal, which is the foot, so the qualifier is Partial 5th Ray.

DESTRUCTION—ROOT OPERATION 5

Destruction 5	Definition	Physical eradication of all or a portion of a body part by the direct use of energy, force or a destructive agent
	Explanation	None of the body part is physically taken out
	Examples	Fulguration of rectal polyp, cautery of skin lesion

Destruction "takes out" a body part in the sense that it obliterates the body part so it is no longer there. This root operation defines a broad range of common procedures, since it can be used anywhere in the body to treat a variety of conditions, including:

- Skin and genital warts
- Nasal and colon polyps
- Esophageal varices
- Endometrial implants
- Nerve lesions

> ### Example: Radiofrequency coagulation of the trigeminal nerve
> *...The right cheek was infiltrated dermally with Xylocaine, and a small nick in the skin 2.5 cm lateral to the corner of the mouth was performed with an 18 gauge needle. The radiofrequency needle with 2 mm exposed tip was then introduced using the known anatomical landmarks and under lateral fluoroscopy guidance into the foramen ovale.*
>
> *Confirmation of the placement of the needle was done by the patient grimacing to pain and by the lateral x-ray. The first treatment, 90 seconds in length, was administered with the tip of the needle 3 mm below the clival line at a temperature of 75 degrees C.*
>
> *The needle was then advanced further to the mid clival line and another treatment of similar strength and duration was also administered. Finally the third and last treatment was administered with the tip of the needle about 3 cm above the line. The needle was removed. The patient tolerated the procedure well...*

Character 1 Section	Character 2 Body System	Character 3 Root Operation	Character 4 Body Part	Character 5 Approach	Character 6 Device	Character 7 Qualifier
Medical And Surgical	Central Nervous	Destruction	Trigeminal Nerve	Percutaneous	No Device	No Qualifier
0	0	5	K	3	Z	Z

CODING NOTE	APPROACH VALUE. The small nick in the skin does not constitute an open approach. it was made to accommodate the radiofrequency needle. The needle was advanced all the way to the operative site, so the correct approach value is Percutaneous.

EXTRACTION—ROOT OPERATION D

Extraction D	Definition	Pulling or stripping out or off all or a portion of a body part by the use of force
	Explanation	The qualifier Diagnostic is used to identify extraction procedures that are biopsies
	Examples	Dilation and curettage, vein stripping

Extraction is coded when the method employed to take out the body part is pulling or stripping. Minor cutting, such as that used in vein stripping procedures, is included in Extraction if the objective of the procedure is nevertheless met by pulling or stripping. As with all applicable ICD-10-PCS codes, cutting used to reach the procedure site is specified in the approach value.

Character 1 Section	Character 2 Body System	Character 3 Root Operation	Character 4 Body Part	Character 5 Approach	Character 6 Device	Character 7 Qualifier
Medical and Surgical	Female Reproductive	Extraction	Endometrium	Via Natural/ Artificial Opening	No Device	Diagnostic
0	**U**	**D**	**B**	**7**	**Z**	**X**

ROOT OPERATIONS THAT TAKE OUT SOLIDS/FLUIDS/GASES FROM A BODY PART

The table below lists the root operations that take out solids, fluids, or gases from a body part. Each is described in detail in the pages that follow.

Root Operation	Objective of Procedure	Site of Procedure	Example
Drainage	Taking/letting out fluids/gases	Within a body part	Incision and drainage
Extirpation	Taking/cutting out solid matter	Within a body part	Thrombectomy
Fragmentation	Breaking solid matter into pieces	Within a body part	Lithotripsy

DRAINAGE---ROOT OPERATION 9

Drainage	Definition	Taking or letting out fluids and/or gases from a body part
9	Explanation	The qualifier Diagnostic is used to identify drainage procedures that are biopsies
	Examples	Thoracentesis, incision and drainage

The root operation Drainage is coded for both diagnostic and therapeutic drainage procedures. When drainage is accomplished by putting in a catheter, the device value Drainage Device is coded in the sixth character.

> ### Example: Urinary nephrostomy catheter placement
> *...using fluoroscopy and sterile technique a needle was placed through the skin into a markedly dilated right renal collecting system. Guidewire was inserted and an 8 French locking catheter was positioned with the dilated right renal pelvis. It was attached to a bag and immediate drainage of urine was evident...*

Character 1 Section	Character 2 Body System	Character 3 Root Operation	Character 4 Body Part	Character 5 Approach	Character 6 Device	Character 7 Qualifier
Medical and Surgical	Urinary	Drainage	Kidney Pelvis, Right	Percutaneous	Drainage Device	No Qualifier
0	**T**	**9**	**3**	**3**	**0**	**Z**

ROOT OPERATIONS THAT TAKE OUT SOLIDS/FLUIDS/GASES FROM A BODY PART

EXTIRPATION—ROOT OPERATION C

Extirpation	Definition	Taking or cutting out solid matter from a body part
C	Explanation	The solid matter may be an abnormal byproduct of a biological function or a foreign body; it may be imbedded in a body part or in the lumen of a tubular body part. The solid matter may or may not have been previously broken into pieces.
	Examples	Thrombectomy, endarterectomy, choledocholithotomy

Extirpation represents a range of procedures where the body part itself is not the focus of the procedure. Instead, the objective is to remove solid material such as a foreign body, thrombus, or calculus from the body part.

Example: De-clotting of AV dialysis graft

...the right upper extremity was properly prepped and draped. Local anesthesia was used to explore the graft. A transverse incision in the previous site of the incision, 1 cm below the elbow crease, was performed. The venous limb of the graft was dissected free up to the venous anastomosis. A small incision on the graft was performed. Then a 3 Fogarty catheter was passed on the venous side. The cephalic vein was found obstructed, not on the anastomotic site, but about 4 cm proximal to the anastomosis. A large number of clots were extracted. After the embolectomy a good back flow from the venous side was obtained. Then the embolectomy was performed throughout the limb on the arterial side. More clots were extracted and a good arterial flow was obtained. The procedure was concluded, closing the incision on the graft with 6-0prolene...

Character 1 Section	Character 2 Body System	Character 3 Root Operation	Character 4 Body Part	Character 5 Approach	Character 6 Device	Character 7 Qualifier
Medical and Surgical	Upper Veins	Extirpation	Cephalic Vein, Right	Open	No Device	No Qualifier
0	**5**	**C**	**D**	**0**	**Z**	**Z**

CODING NOTE	**BODY PART VALUE.** Do not code separate body parts based on the words "venous side" and "arterial side" in the procedure report. They refer to the two ends of the cephalic vein used to create the fistula.

FRAGMENTATION—ROOT OPERATION F

Fragmentation **F**	Definition	Breaking solid matter in a body part into pieces
	Explanation	The Physical force (e.g., manual, ultrasonic) applied directly or indirectly is used to break the solid matter into pieces. The solid matter may be an abnormal byproduct of a biological function or a foreign body. The pieces of solid matter are not taken out.
	Examples	Extracorporeal shockwave lithotripsy, transurethral lithotripsy

Fragmentation is coded for procedures to break up, but not remove, solid material such as a calculus or foreign body. This root operation includes both direct and extracorporeal Fragmentation procedures.

Example: ESWL of left kidney

With the patient having been identified, under satisfactory IV sedation and using the MFL 1000for extracorporeal shock wave lithotripsy, 1000 shocks were delivered to the stone in the lower pole of the left kidney, and 800 shocks were delivered to the stone in the upper pole of the same, with change in shape and density of the stone indicating fragmentation. The patient tolerated the procedure well...

Character 1 Section	Character 2 Body System	Character 3 Root Operation	Character 4 Body Part	Character 5 Approach	Character 6 Device	Character 7 Qualifier
Medical and Surgical	Urinary	Fragment.	Kidney Pelvis, Left	External	No Device	No Qualifier
0	**T**	**F**	**4**	**X**	**Z**	**Z**

ROOT OPERATIONS INVOLVING CUTTING OR SEPARATION ONLY

The following root operations represent procedures that cut or separate a body part. These root operations are listed below and described in detail in the pages that follow.

Root Operation	Objective of Procedure	Site of Procedure	Example
Division	Cutting into/separating a body part	Within a body part	Neurotomy
Release	Freeing a body part from constraint	Around a body part	Adhesiolysis

DIVISION---ROOT OPERATION 8

Division	Definition	Cutting into a body part without draining fluids and/or gases from the body part in order to separate or transect a body part
8	Explanation	All or a portion of the body part is separated into two or more portions
	Examples	Spinal cordotomy, osteotomy

The root operation Division is coded when the objective of the procedure is to cut into, transect, or otherwise separate all or a portion of a body part. When the objective is to cut or separate the area around a body part, the attachments to a body part, or between subdivisions of a body part that are causing abnormal constraint, then the root operation Release is coded instead.

Example: *Anal sphincterotomy*

Manual examination of the rectum and anus was done, and examination showed that the patient has an anterior anal fissure. For that reason, lateral sphincterotomy was done at the 3 o'clock position using the closed approach, dividing only the internal sphincter using the 11 blade...

Character 1 Section	Character 2 Body System	Character 3 Root operation	Character 4 Body Part	Character 5 Approach	Character 6 Device	Character 7 Qualifier
Medical and Surgical	Gastro-intestinal System	Division	Anal Sphincter	Percutaneous	No Device	No Qualifier
0	**D**	**8**	**R**	**3**	**Z**	**Z**

CODING NOTE	**APPROACH VALUE.** This is coded to the Percutaneous approach, because the procedure report says that the sphincterotomy was done using the closed approach, dividing only the internal sphincter.

RELEASE—ROOT OPERATION N

Release	Definition	Freeing a body part from an abnormal physical constraint by cutting or by use of force
N	Explanation	Some of the restraining tissue may be taken out but none of the body part is taken out
	Examples	Adhesiolysis, carpal tunnel release

The objective of procedures represented in the root operation Release is to free a body part from abnormal constraint. Release procedures are coded to the body part being freed. The procedure can be performed on the area around a body part, on the attachments to a body part, or between subdivisions of a body part that are causing the abnormal constraint.

Example: *Release of median nerve*

...the right arm was scrubbed with Betadine and prepped and draped in the usual sterile fashion. A well-padded tourniquet was fixed to the right proximal arm but not inflated until after draping. After draping, the right arm was exsanguinated with a combination of elevation and an Esmarch bandage, placing a sponge in the palm. The tourniquet was inflated to 250.

A transverse incision was made at the level of the proximal wrist crease between the palmaris longus and the flexor carpi ulnaris sharply through the skin with a knife, and subcutaneous tissue was dissected by blunt spreading. The volar fascia was identified and a transverse incision was made sharply with a knife. The flat synovial retractor was pushed through the underneath of the transverse carpal ligament, removing synovium from beneath the ligament. The entire carpal tunnel and the fat pad distally was visualized. The blade was inserted into the carpal tunnel, was elevated at the distal edge of the transverse carpal ligament, and was pulled proximally, spreading and cutting through the transverse carpal ligament.

It was visualized that the entire median nerve had been released, and that configuration of the end of the transverse carpal ligament was a rectangle, denoting that both the deep and the superficial fibers had been cut. The wound was then copiously irrigated with saline...

Character 1 Section	Character 2 Body System	Character 3 Root Operation	Character 4 Body Part	Character 5 Approach	Character 6 Device	Character 7 Qualifier
Medical and Surgical	Peripheral Nervous	Release	Median Nerve	Open	No Device	No Qualifier
0	1	N	5	0	Z	Z

CODING NOTE	BODY PART VALUE. The body part value assigned is the structure released and not the structure cut to obtain the release, where the two differ. The transverse carpal ligament was cut to release the median nerve and not for its own sake.

ROOT OPERATIONS THAT PUT IN/PUT BACK OR MOVE SOME/ALL OF A BODY PART

The following root operations represent procedures that put in/put back or move some/all of a body part. These root operations are listed below and described in detail in the pages that follow.

Root Operation	Objective of Procedure	Site of Procedure	Example
Transplantation	Putting in a living body part from a person/ animal	Some/all of a body part	Kidney transplant
Reattachment	Putting back a detached body part	Some/all of a body part	Reattach finger
Transfer	Moving a body part to function for a similar body part	Some/all of a body part	Skin transfer flap
Reposition	Moving a body part to normal or other suitable location	Some/all of a body part	Move undescended testicle

TRANSPLANTATION---ROOT OPERATION Y

Transplantation Y	Definition	Putting in or on all or a portion of a living body part taken from another individual or animal to physically take the place and/or function of all or a portion of a similar body part
	Explanation	The native body part may or may not be taken out, and the transplanted body part may take over all or a portion of its function
	Examples	Kidney transplant, heart transplant

A small number of procedures is represented in the root operation Transplantation and includes only the body parts currently being transplanted. Qualifier values specify the genetic compatibility of the body part transplanted.

Example: Right kidney transplant (syngeneic)

...the abdomen was sterilely prepped and draped in the usual fashion and incision in the right flank, the Gibson technique, performed. In doing so the right pelvis was entered and Book- Walter retractor appropriately positioned to provide exposure of the external iliac artery and vein.

The artery was placed on vessel loop retraction. We then proceeded with the kidney transplant, and the kidney which was trimmed on the back table was brought into the field. The right renal vein was cut short without reconstruction of the inferior vena cava, and single ureter was identified. Kidney was brought up in an ice chest and an end-to-end anastomosis was performed in the usual fashion with 5-0 Prolene between donor renal vein and external iliac vein on the right.

The long renal artery was brought into view, and end-to-side anastomosis performed in the usual fashion with 5-0 Prolene.

We then turned our attention to performing the neoureterocystostomy after appropriate positioning of the graft and evaluation of the vessels.

After the anastomosis was completed there was no evidence of leak. A Blake drain was brought out through a stab incision and the tip of the drain placed near the neoureterocystostomy and both wounds were closed. The infrainguinal wound was closed with running 3-0 Vicryl and the kidney transplant wound was closed with 1 PDS...

Character 1 Section	Character 2 Body System	Character 3 Root Operation	Character 4 Body Part	Character 5 Approach	Character 6 Device	Character 7 Qualifier
Medical and Surgical	Urinary	Transplant.	Kidney, Right	Open	No Device	Syngeneic
0	**T**	**Y**	**0**	**0**	**Z**	**1**

CODING **NOTE**	**BONE MARROW TRANSPLANT.** Bone marrow transplant procedures are coded in section 3 Transplant Administration to the root operation 2 Transfusion.

REATTACHMENT---ROOT OPERATION M

Reattachment **M**	Definition	Putting back in or on all or a portion of a separated body part to its normal location or other suitable location
	Explanation	Vascular circulation and nervous pathways may or may not be reestablished
	Examples	Reattachment of hand, reattachment of avulsed kidney

Procedures coded to Reattachment include putting back a body part that has been cut off or avulsed. Nerves and blood vessels may or may not be reconnected in a Reattachment procedure.

> ## *Example: Complex reattachment, left index finger*
> *A sharp debridement of grossly contaminated tissue was carried out. It was noted that the extensor mechanism distal to the PIP joint had been lost. There were circumferential lacerations about the finger, save for a cutaneous bridge and ulnar vascular pedicle present at the PIP level.*
>
> *Nonviable bony fragments were removed and then the distal portion of the PIP joint was reshaped with removal of cartilage using double- rongeurs. It was noted that the fractures through the proximal phalanx extended longitudinally. Stabilization was then carried out, with 0.062 K-wire brought down through the distal finger, out through the fingertip, and then back into the proximal phalanx centrally.*
>
> *The A2 pulley was restored, using figure of eight interrupted sutures of 4 and 5-0 Vicryl, reapproximating the flexor tendons. The extensor mechanisms and tendons were repaired using 4 and 5-0 Vicryl, and anchored to the periosteum on the middle phalanx. A digital nerve was then carried out on the radial aspect of the digit at the PIP joint level using interrupted sutures of 9-0 Ethilon beneath the microscope.*
>
> *At this point, the skin was trimmed, removing skin margins, and then multiple lacerations were closed with 5-0 Prolene...*

Character 1 Section	Character 2 Body System	Character 3 Root Operation	Character 4 Body Part	Character 5 Approach	Character 6 Device	Character 7 Qualifier
Medical and Surgical	Upper Extremities	Reattachment	Index Finger, Left	Open	No Device	No Qualifier
0	**X**	**M**	**P**	**0**	**Z**	**Z**

TRANSFER---ROOT OPERATION X

Transfer **X**	Definition	Moving, without taking out, all or a portion of a body part to another location to take over the function of all or a portion of a body part
	Explanation	The body part transferred remains connected to its vascular and nervous supply
	Examples	Tendon transfer, skin pedicle flap transfer

The root operation Transfer is used to represent procedures where a body part is moved to another location without disrupting its vascular and nervous supply. In the body systems that classify the subcutaneous tissue, fascia and muscle body parts, qualifiers can be used to specify when more than one tissue layer was used in the transfer procedure, such as a musculocutaneous flap transfer.

Example: *Fasciocutaneous flap from scalp to cheek*

...development of the plane of dissection was completed into the superficial temporal fascia. Development of subgaleal dissection posteriorly was then completed, a distance of 7-8 cm, with hemo- stasis by electrocautery. The flaps were advanced to the cheek defect and secured with 2-0 inverted PDS sutures and3-0 inverted Monocryl...

Character 1 Section	Character 2 Body System	Character 3 Root Operation	Character 4 Body Part	Character 5 Approach	Character 6 Device	Character 7 Qualifier
Medical and Surgical	Subcut Tissue and Fascia	Transfer	Scalp	Open	No Device	Skin, Subcut And Fascia
0	J	X	0	0	Z	C

CODING NOTE	**BODY SYSTEM VALUE.** The body system value describes the deepest tissue layer in the flap. The qualifier can be used to describe the other tissue layers, if any, being transferred. For procedures involving transfer of tissue layers such as skin, fascia and muscle, the procedure is coded to the body system value that describes the deepest tissue layer in the flap. When the tissue transferred is composed of more than one tissue layer, the qualifier can be used to describe the other tissue layers, if any, being transferred. For transfer procedures classified to other body systems such as peripheral nervous system, the body part value specifies the body part that is the source of the transfer ("from"). Where qualifiers are available, they specify the destination of the transfer ("to").

REPOSITION---ROOT OPERATION S

Reposition S	Definition	Moving to its normal location or other suitable location all or a portion of a body part
	Explanation	The body part is moved to a new location from an abnormal location, or from a normal location where it is not functioning correctly. The body part may or may not be cut out or off to be moved to the new location
	Examples	Reposition of undescended testicle, fracture reduction

Reposition represents procedures for moving a body part to a new location. The range of Reposition procedures includes moving a body part to its normal location, or moving a body part to a new location to enhance its ability to function.

Example: *Reposition of undescended right testicle from pelvic region to scrotum*

...Following satisfactory induction of general anesthesia, an incision was made in the inguinal region and dissection carried down to the pelvic cavity, where the right testis was located and mobilized. The spermatic cord was located and freed from surrounding tissue, and its length judged to be sufficient. A one centimeter incision was made in the scrotum and a pouch created in the usual fashion. The right testicle was mobilized down through the inguinal canal into the scrotum, and stitched in place. Meticulous hemostasis was obtained, and the incisions closed in layers...

Character 1 Section	Character 2 Body System	Character 3 Root Operation	Character 4 Body Part	Character 5 Approach	Character 6 Device	Character 7 Qualifier
Medical and Surgical	Male Reproductive	Reposition	Testis, Right	Open	No Device	No Qualifier
0	V	S	9	0	Z	Z

ROOT OPERATIONS THAT ALTER THE DIAMETER/ROUTE OF A TUBULAR BODY PART

The following root operations represent procedures that alter the diameter or route of a tubular body part. Tubular body parts are defined in ICD-10-PCS as those hollow body parts that provide a route of passage for solids, liquids, or gases. They include the cardiovascular system, and body parts such as those contained in the gastrointestinal tract, genitourinary tract, biliary tract, and respiratory tract. These root operations are listed below and described in detail in the pages that follow.

Root Operation	Objective of Procedure	Site of Procedure	Example
Restriction	Partially closing orifice/ lumen	Tubular body part	Gastroesophageal fundoplication
Occlusion	Completely closing orifice/ lumen	Tubular body part	Fallopian tube ligation

| Dilation | Expanding orifice/lumen | Tubular body part | Percutaneous transluminal coronary angioplasty (PTCA) |
| Bypass | Altering route of passage | Tubular body part | Coronary artery bypass graft (CABG) |

RESTRICTION—ROOT OPERATION V

Restriction	Definition	Partially closing an orifice or the lumen of a tubular body part
V	Explanation	The orifice can be a natural orifice or an artificially created orifice
	Examples	Esophagogastric fundoplication, cervical cerclage

The root operation Restriction is coded when the objective of the procedure is to narrow the diameter of a tubular body part or orifice. Restriction includes both intraluminal or extraluminal methods for narrowing the diameter.

> ### Example: Laparoscopic gastroesophageal fundoplication
> ....Insufflation was accomplished through a 5 infraumbilical incision. Five separate 5 mm ports were placed under direct visualization other than the initial port. Laparoscopy revealed a large hiatal hernia. Electrocautery was used to free up adhesions from the hernia sac to the stomach.
>
> Next, the fundus which had been mobilized was brought down into the stomach and it was felt there was enough mobilization to perform a fundoplication. A generous loose fundoplication was then performed by wrapping the fundus around the esophagus. Interrupted 0 Ethibond sutures were used to secure the stomach in this fashion.
>
> There was generally good hemostasis throughout the case. All instruments were removed and ports closed.

Character 1 Section	Character 2 Body System	Character 3 Root Operation	Character 4 Body Part	Character 5 Approach	Character 6 Device	Character 7 Qualifier
Medical And Surgical	Gastro-intestinal System	Restriction	Esophago-gastric Junction	Percutaneous Endoscopic	No Device	No Qualifier
0	**D**	**V**	**4**	**4**	**Z**	**Z**

OCCLUSION—ROOT OPERATION L

Occlusion	Definition	Completely closing an orifice or the lumen of a tubular body part
L	Explanation	The orifice can be a natural orifice or an artificially created orifice
	Examples	Fallopian tube ligation, ligation of inferior vena cava

The root operation Occlusion is coded when the objective of the procedure is to close off a tubular body part or orifice. Occlusion includes both intraluminal or extraluminal methods of closing off the body part. Division of the tubular body part prior to closing it is an integral part of the Occlusion procedure.

> ### Example: Uterine artery embolization
> ... catheter was advanced over a 0.18 Terumo gold guidewire and advanced several centimeters super selectively into the left uterine artery. Contrast injection was performed here, confirming filling of the uterine artery and subsequent opacification of large vascular structures in the uterus compatible with uterine fibroids.
>
> A syringe and a half of 500-700 micron biospheres was then instilled slowly through the catheter, and at the conclusion of this infusion there was cessation of flow through the uterine artery.
>
> The catheter was then removed and hemostasis achieved...

Character 1 Section	Character 2 Body System	Character 3 Root Operation	Character 4 Body Part	Character 5 Approach	Character 6 Device	Character 7 Qualifier
Medical And Surgical	Lower Arteries	Occlusion	Internal Iliac Artery, Left	Percutaneous	Intraluminal Device	Uterine Artery, Left
0	**4**	**L**	**F**	**3**	**D**	**U**

DILATION—ROOT OPERATION 7

Dilation	Definition	Expanding an orifice or the lumen of a tubular body part
7	Explanation	The orifice can be a natural orifice or an artificially created orifice. Accomplished by stretching a tubular body part using intraluminal pressure or by cutting part of the orifice or wall of the tubular body part
	Examples	Percutaneous transluminal angioplasty, pyloromyotomy

The root operation Dilation is coded when the objective of the procedure is to enlarge the diameter of a tubular body part or orifice. Dilation includes both intraluminal or extraluminal methods of enlarging the diameter. A device placed to maintain the new diameter is an integral part of the Dilation procedure, and is coded to a sixth-character device value in the Dilation procedure code.

Example: PTCA of left anterior descending

...under 1% Lidocaine local anesthesia, the right femoral artery was entered by the Seldinger technique and a 7French sheath was placed. A Judkins left guiding catheter was advanced to the left coronary ostium and using a .014 Entree wire and a 2.5 x 30 mm Panther balloon, it was easily placed across the lesion in the left anterior descending.

The balloon was inflated times two for five minutes for up to 9 atmospheres. Angiography demonstrated an excellent result...

Character 1 Section	Character 2 Body System	Character 3 Root Operation	Character 4 Body Part	Character 5 Approach	Character 6 Device	Character 7 Qualifier
Medical and Surgical	Heart and Great Vessels	Dilation	Coronary Art., One Site	Percutaneous	No Device	No Qualifier
0	**2**	**7**	**0**	**3**	**Z**	**Z**

BYPASS—ROOT OPERATION 1

Bypass	Definition	Altering the route of passage of the contents of a tubular body part
1	Explanation	Rerouting contents of a body part to a downstream area of the normal route, to a similar route and body part, or to an abnormal route and dissimilar body part. Includes one or more anastomoses, with or without the use of a device
	Examples	Coronary artery bypass, colostomy formation

Bypass is coded when the objective of the procedure is to reroute the contents of a tubular body part. The range of Bypass procedures includes normal routes such as those made in coronary artery bypass procedures, and abnormal routes such as those made in colostomy formation procedures.

Example: Aorto-bifemoral bypass graft

...the patient was prepped and draped, and groin incisions were opened. The common femoral vein and its branches were isolated and Teflon tapes were placed around the vessels.

The aorta and iliacs were mobilized. Bleeding points were controlled with electrocautery and Liga clips. Tapes were placed around the vessel, the vessel measured, and the aorta was found to be 12 mm. A 12 x 7 bifurcated microvelour graft was then preclotted with the patient's own blood.

An end-to-end anastomosis was made on the aorta and the graft using a running suture of 2-0 Prolene. The limbs were taken down through tunnels noting that the ureters were anterior, and at this point an end-to-side anastomosis was made between the graft and the femoral arteries with running suture of 4-0 Prolene.

The inguinal incisions were closed.

Character 1 Section	Character 2 Body System	Character 3 Root Operation	Character 4 Body Part	Character 5 Approach	Character 6 Device	Character 7 Qualifier
Medical And Surgical	Lower Arteries	Bypass	Abdominal Aorta	Open	Synthetic Substitute	Bilat Femoral Arteries
0	**4**	**1**	**0**	**0**	**J**	**K**

ROOT OPERATIONS THAT ALWAYS INVOLVE A DEVICE

The table below lists the root operations that always involve a device. Each is described in detail in the pages that follow.

Root Operation	Objective of Procedure	Site of Procedure	Example
Insertion	Putting in non-biological device	In/on a body part	Central line insertion
Replacement	Putting in device that replaces a body part	Some/all of a body part	Total hip replacement
Supplement	Putting in device that reinforces or augments a body part	In/on a body part	Abdominal wall herniorrhaphy using mesh
Change	Exchanging device w/out cutting/ puncturing	In/on a body part	Drainage tube change
Removal	Taking out device	In/on a body part	Central line removal
Revision	Correcting a malfunctioning/ displaced device	In/on a body part	Revision of pacemaker insertion

INSERTION---ROOT OPERATION H

Insertion **H**	Definition	Putting in a non-biological device that monitors, assists, performs or prevents a physiological function but does not physically take the place of a body part
	Explanation	N/A
	Examples	Insertion of radioactive implant, insertion of central venous catheter

The root operation Insertion represents those procedures where the sole objective is to put in a device without doing anything else to a body part. Procedures typical of those coded to Insertion include putting in a vascular catheter, a pacemaker lead, or a tissue expander.

> ### Example: Placement of totally implanted central venous access device
>
> *...the right chest and neck were prepped and draped in the usual manner and 10 cc's of 1% Lidocaine were injected in the right infraclavicular area.*
>
> *The right subclavian vein was then punctured and a wire was passed through the needle into the superior vena cava. This was documented by fluoroscopy. Introducer kit was introduced into the subclavian vein and the Port-a-cath was placed through the introducer and by fluoroscopy was placed down to the superior vena cava.*
>
> *The pocket was then made over the right pectoralis major muscle, superior to the breast, and the Port-a-cath reservoir was placed into this pocket and tacked down with #0 Prolene sutures.*
>
> *The catheter was then tunneled through a subcutaneous tunnel to this receptacle. Hemostasis was achieved and the subcutaneous tissue closed...*

Character 1 Section	Character 2 Body System	Character 3 Root Operation	Character 4 Body Part	Character 5 Approach	Character 6 Device	Character 7 Qualifier
Medical and Surgical	Subcut Tissue and Fascia	Insertion	Chest	Percutaneous	Vascular Access Device	No Qualifier
0	**J**	**H**	**6**	**3**	**X**	**Z**

Character 1 Section	Character 2 Body System	Character 3 Root Operation	Character 4 Body Part	Character 5 Approach	Character 6 Device	Character 7 Qualifier
Medical and Surgical	Heart and Great Vessels	Insertion	Superior Vena Cava	Percutaneous	Infusion Device	No Qualifier
0	**2**	**H**	**V**	**3**	**3**	**Z**

CODING **NOTE**	**Imaging Guidance.** Imaging guidance done to assist in the performance of a procedure can be coded separately in the Imaging section, if desired (Section B)..

REPLACEMENT---ROOT OPERATION R

Replacement R	Definition	Putting in or on biological or synthetic material that physically takes the place and/or function of all or a portion of a body part
	Explanation	The body part may have been taken out or replaced, or may be taken out, physically eradicated, or rendered nonfunctional during the Replacement procedure. A Removal procedure is coded for taking out the device used in a previous replacement procedure.
	Examples	Total hip replacement, bone graft, free skin graft

The objective of procedures coded to the root operation Replacement is to put in a device that takes the place of some or all of a body part. Replacement encompasses a wide range of procedures, from joint replacements to grafts of all kinds.

Example: Prosthetic lens implantation

...a superior peritomy was made on the left eye and adequate hemostasis was achieved using eraser cautery. A posterior one-half thickness groove was placed posterior to the blue line. This was beveled forward toward clear cornea.

The anterior chamber was entered at the 11:30position with a blade. The eye was filled with viscoelastic substance. A can-opener type capsulotomy was performed with a cystotome. Hydrodissection was carried out and the lens was rocked gently with a cystotome to loosen it from the cortex.

The wound was then opened with corneal scleral scissors. The lens was prolapsed in the anterior chamber and removed. The anterior chamber was then temporarily closed with 8-0 Vicryl sutures and cortical clean-up was performed.

One of the sutures was removed and a posterior chamber intraocular lens (Alcon model MZ50BD) was inspected, rinsed, and placed into a capsular bag. Miochol was then instilled into the anterior chamber. The conjunctiva was pulled over the incision and cauterized into place...

Character 1 Section	Character 2 Body System	Character 3 Root Operation	Character 4 Body Part	Character 5 Approach	Character 6 Device	Character 7 Qualifier
Medical And Surgical	Eye	Replacement	Lens, Left	Percutaneous	Synthetic Substitute	No Qualifier
0	**8**	**R**	**K**	**3**	**J**	**Z**

SUPPLEMENT---ROOT OPERATION U

Supplement U	Definition	Putting in or on biologic or synthetic material that physically reinforces and/ or augments the function a portion of a body part
	Explanation	The biological material is non-living, or is living and from the same individual. The body part may have been previously replaced, and the Supplement procedure is performed to physically reinforce and/or augment the function of the replaced body part.
	Examples	Herniorrhaphy using mesh, free nerve graft, mitral valve ring annuloplasty, put a new acetabular liner in a previous hip replacement

The objective of procedures coded to the root operation Supplement is to put in a device that reinforces or augments the functions of some or all of a body part. The body part may have been taken out during a previous procedure, but is not taken out as part of the Supplement procedure. Supplement includes a wide range of procedures, from hernia repairs using mesh reinforcement to heart valve annuloplasties and grafts such as nerve grafts that supplement but do not physically take the place of the existing body part.

Example: Posterior colporrhaphy with Gynemesh

...attention was then turned to the posterior wall. Two Allis clamps were placed at the mucocutaneous junction in the region of the fourchette, and another clamp was placed at the apex of the rectocele.

The tissue between the distal clamps and the fourchette was excised, and carefully measured so that the introitus would be a 3-finger introitus The posterior vaginal mucosa was then incised in the midline by sharp and blunt dissection. The mucosa was then dissected to the level at the Allis clamp at the apex of the rectocele, and dissected with blunt and sharp dissection from the underlying tissue. The rectocele was then imbricated using mattress sutures of 2-0 Vicryl, and the area of the levator ani reinforced with Gynemesh.

Two sutures of 2-0 Vicryl were taken in the levator ani muscle, the excess posterior vaginal mucosa excised, and then closed with interrupted sutures of 2-0 Vicryl.

The perineal muscles were then approximated in the midline in layers, using 2-0 Vicryl, after which the perineal skin was approximated using interrupted sutures of 2-0 Vicryl...

Character 1 Section	Character 2 Body System	Character 3 Root Operation	Character 4 Body Part	Character 5 Approach	Character 6 Device	Character 7 Qualifier
Medical and Surgical	Subcutaneous Tissue and Fascia	Supplement	Pelvic Region	Open	Synthetic Substitute	No Qualifier
0	**J**	**U**	**C**	**0**	**J**	**Z**

CHANGE---ROOT OPERATION 2

Change **2**	Definition	Taking out or off a device from a body part and putting back an identical or similar device in or on the same body part without cutting or puncturing the skin or a mucous membrane
	Explanation	All Change procedures are coded using the approach External
	Examples	Urinary catheter change, gastrostomy tube change

The root operation Change represents only those procedures where a similar device is exchanged without making a new incision or puncture. Typical Change procedures include exchange of drainage devices and feeding devices.

CODING NOTE	**CHANGE.** In the root operation Change, general body part values are used when the specific body part value is not in the table

Example: Percutaneous endoscopic gastrostomy (PEG) tube exchange

Character 1 Section	Character 2 Body System	Character 3 Root Operation	Character 4 Body Part	Character 5 Approach	Character 6 Device	Character 7 Qualifier
Medical and Surgical	Gastro-intestinal System	Change	Upper Intestinal Tract	External	Feeding Device	No Qualifier
0	**D**	**2**	**0**	**X**	**U**	**Z**

REMOVAL—ROOT OPERATION P

Removal **P**	Definition	Taking out or off a device from a body part
	Explanation	If a device is taken out and a similar device put in without cutting or puncturing the skin or mucous membrane, the procedure is coded to the root operation Change. Otherwise, the procedure for taking out a device is coded to the root operation Removal.
	Examples	Drainage tube removal, cardiac pacemaker removal

Removal represents a much broader range of procedures than those for removing the devices contained in the root operation Insertion. A procedure to remove a device is coded to Removal if it is not an integral part of another root operation, and regardless of the approach or the original root operation by which the device was put in.

CODING NOTE	**REMOVAL.** In the root operation Removal, general body part values are used when the specific body part value is not in the table.

Example: Removal of right forearm external fixator

...the right upper extremity was prepped and draped in a sterile fashion. A tourniquet was placed at 250 mm of pressure.

The external fixator was removed using the appropriate wrench. The four pins in the ulna were then removed manually, as well as with the drill. The wounds were irrigated with antibiotic solution and a sterile dressing applied...

Character 1 Section	Character 2 Body System	Character 3 Root Operation	Character 4 Body Part	Character 5 Approach	Character 6 Device	Character 7 Qualifier
Medical and Surgical	Upper Bones	Removal	Ulna, Right	External	External Fixation	No Qualifier
0	**P**	**P**	**K**	**X**	**5**	**Z**

ROOT OPERATIONS THAT ALWAYS INVOLVE A DEVICE

REVISION—ROOT OPERATION W

Revision **W**	Definition	Correcting, to the extent possible, a portion of a malfunctioning device or the position of a displaced device
	Explanation	Revision can include correcting a malfunctioning device by taking out and/or putting in part of the device
	Examples	Adjustment of pacemaker lead, adjustment of hip prosthesis

Revision is coded when the objective of the procedure is to correct the position or function of a previously placed device, without taking the entire device out and putting a whole new device in its place. A complete re-do of a procedure is coded to the root operation performed.

CODING NOTE	**REVISION.** In the root operation Revision, general body part values are used when the specific body part value is not in the table.

Example: Revision of artificial anal sphincter

...Proceeding through a suprapubic incision, this was then extended after injecting local anesthetic, thereby exposing the underlying tubing, which was then delivered through the suprapubic region.

Meticulous hemostasis was achieved using electrocautery. At that point the pump device was then repositioned in the left lower quadrant abdominal wall region. The tubing was reinserted using dilators, and the skin reapproximated using 2-0 Vicryl sutures. Sterile dressing was then applied...

Character 1 Section	Character 2 Body System	Character 3 Root Operation	Character 4 Body Part	Character 5 Approach	Character 6 Device	Character 7 Qualifier
Medical and Surgical	Gastrointestinal System	Revision	Anus	Open	Artificial Sphincter	No Qualifier
0	**D**	**W**	**Q**	**0**	**L**	**Z**

ROOT OPERATIONS INVOLVING EXAMINATION ONLY

The table below lists the root operations that involve examination of a body part. Each is described in detail in the pages that follow.

Root operation	Objective of Procedure	Site of Procedure	Example
Inspection	Visual/manual exploration	Some/all of a body part	Diagnostic cystoscopy
Map	Location electrical impulses/ functional areas	Brain/cardiac conduction mechanism	Cardiac mapping

INSPECTION—ROOT OPERATION J

Inspection	Definition	Visually and/or Manually Exploring A Body Part
J	Explanation	Visual Exploration May Be Performed With Or Without Optical Instrumentation. Manual Exploration May Be Performed Directly Or Through Intervening Body Layers
	Examples	Diagnostic Arthroscopy, Exploratory Laparotomy

The root operation Inspection represents procedures where the sole objective is to examine a body part. Procedures that are discontinued without any other root operation being performed are also coded to Inspection.

Example: Diagnostic colposcopy with examination of cervix
...Colposcopy was done which revealed pseudo-white areas at 2 o'clock and 6o'clock on the cervix, with abnormal cells and irregular white borders noted on both...

Character 1 Section	Character 2 Body System	Character 3 Root Operation	Character 4 Body Part	Character 5 Approach	Character 6 Device	Character 7 Qualifier
Medical And Surgical	Female Reproductive	Inspection	Uterus And Cervix	Via Natural/ Artificial Opening Endo	No Device	No Qualifier
0	**U**	**J**	**D**	**8**	**Z**	**Z**

MAP---ROOT OPERATION K

Map	Definition	Locating the route of passage of electrical impulses and/or locating functional areas in a body part
K	Explanation	Applicable only to the cardiac conduction mechanism and the central nervous system
	Examples	Cardiac mapping, cortical mapping

Mapping represents a very narrow range of procedures. Procedures include only cardiac mapping and cortical mapping.

Example: Cardiac mapping
. ..under sterile technique arterial sheath was placed in the right femoral artery. The electrical catheter was advanced up the aorta and into the left atrium under fluoroscopic guidance and mapping commenced. After adequate recordings were obtained the catheter was withdrawn and hemostasis achieved with manual pressure on the right femoral artery...

Character 1 Section	Character 2 Body System	Character 3 Root Operation	Character 4 Body Part	Character 5 Approach	Character 6 Device	Character 7 Qualifier
Medical and Surgical	Heart & Great Vessels	Map	Conduction Mechanism	Percutaneous	No Device	No Qualifier
0	**2**	**K**	**8**	**3**	**Z**	**Z**

ROOT OPERATIONS THAT DEFINE OTHER REPAIRS

The table below lists the root operations that define other repairs. CONTROL describes the effort to locate and stop

Root Operation	Objective of Procedure	Site of Procedure	Example
Control	Stopping/attempting to stop postprocedural bleed	Anatomical region	Post-prostatectomy bleeding control
Repair	Restoring body part to its normal structure	Some/all of a body part	Suture laceration

postprocedural hemorrhage. Repair is described in detail in the pages that follow.

CONTROL---ROOT OPERATION 3

Control	Definition	Stopping, or attempting to stop, postprocedural bleeding
3	Explanation	The site of the bleeding is coded as an anatomical region and not to a specific body part
	Examples	Control of post-prostatectomy hemorrhage, control of post-tonsillectomy hemorrhage

CONTROL is used to represent a small range of procedures performed to treat postprocedural bleeding. If performing Bypass, Detachment, Excision, Extraction, Reposition, Replacement, or Resection is required to stop the bleeding, then Control is not coded separately.

CODING NOTE	CONTROL includes irrigation or evacuation of hematoma done at the operative site. Both irrigation and evacuation may be necessary to clear the operative field and effectively stop the bleeding.

Example: Re-opening of laparotomy site with ligation of arterial bleeder

Character 1 Section	Character 2 Body System	Character 3 Root Operation	Character 4 Body Part	Character 5 Approach	Character 6 Device	Character 7 Qualifier
Medical and Surgical	Anatomical Regions, Gen.	Control	Peritoneal Cavity	Open	No Device	No Qualifier
0	**W**	**3**	**g**	**0**	**Z**	**Z**

REPAIR—ROOT OPERATION Q

Repair Q	Definition	Restoring, to the extent possible, a body part to its normal anatomic structure and function
	Explanation	Used only when the method to accomplish the repair is not one of the other root operations
	Examples	Herniorrhaphy, suture of laceration

The root operation Repair represents a broad range of procedures for restoring the anatomic structure of a body part such as suture of lacerations. Repair also functions as the "not elsewhere classified (NEC)" root operation, to be used when the procedure performed does not meet the definition of one of the other root operations. Fixation devices are included for procedures to repair the bones and joints.

Example: Left open inguinal herniorrhaphy

...an incision in the left groin extending on the skin from the internal to the external inguinal ring was made. The external oblique aponeurosis was exposed.

The hernia sac was then ligated at the internal ring with non-dissolving sutures. A hernia repair was then performed. The internal oblique fascia was sutured in interrupted stitches to the ilio-pubic fascia. The spermatic cord was then returned to its anatomical position.

The external oblique aponeurosis was then repaired in interrupted sutures. Complete hemostasis was obtained, and the skin closed...

Character 1 Section	Character 2 Body System	Character 3 Root Operation	Character 4 Body Part	Character 5 Approach	Character 6 Device	Character 7 Qualifier
Medical and Surgical	Lower Extremities	Repair	Inguinal Region, Left	Open	No Device	No Qualifier
0	**Y**	**Q**	**6**	**0**	**Z**	**Z**

ROOT OPERATIONS THAT DEFINE OTHER OBJECTIVES

The last three root operations in the Medical and Surgical section, Fusion, Alteration, and Creation, describe procedures performed for three distinct reasons. Beyond that they have little in common. A Fusion procedure puts a dysfunctional joint out of service rather than restoring function to the joint. Alteration encompasses a whole range of procedures that share only the fact that they are done to improve the way the patient looks. Creation represents only two very specific sex change operations.

Root operation	Objective of procedure	Site of procedure	Example
Fusion	Rendering joint immobile	Joint	Spinal fusion
Alteration	Modifying body part for cosmetic purposes without affecting function	Some/all of a body part	Face lift
Creation	Making new structure for sex change operation	Perineum	Artificial vagina/penis

FUSION---ROOT OPERATION G

Fusion G	Definition	Joining together portions of an articular body part rendering the articular body part immobile
	Explanation	The body part is joined together by fixation device, bone graft, or other means
	Examples	Spinal fusion, ankle arthrodesis

A limited range of procedures is represented in the root operation Fusion, because fusion procedures are by definition only performed on the joints. Qualifier values are used to specify whether a vertebral joint fusion uses an anterior or posterior approach, and whether the anterior or posterior column of the spine is fused.

> ### Example: Anterior cervical fusion C-2 through C-4 with bone bank graft
> ...after skull tong traction was applied, incision was made in the left neck, and Gardner retractors placed to separate the intervertebral muscles at the C-2 through C-4 levels.
>
> Using the drill, a trough was incised on the anterior surface of the C-2 vertebra, and the C-2/C-3 space evacuated with a rongeur, and the accompanying cartilage removed. This procedure was then repeated at the C-3/C-4 level.
>
> Bone bank patella strut graft was trimmed with a saw and fashioned to fit the C-2/C-3 interspace. After adequate adjustments in the size and shape had been made, the graft was tapped securely into place. The procedure was repeated for the C-3/C-4 level.
>
> X-rays revealed good alignment and final position. Traction was gradually decreased to maintain position. Retractors were removed and the fascia was reapproximated with 0 Vicryl...

Character 1 Section	Character 2 Body System	Character 3 Root Operation	Character 4 Body part	Character 5 Approach	Character 6 Device	Character 7 Qualifier
Medical and Surgical	Upper Joints	Fusion	Cervical Joint, 2 or More	OPEN	Nonautologous Tissue Substance	Ant Approach Ant Column
0	**R**	**G**	**2**	**0**	**K**	**0**

ALTERATION---ROOT OPERATION 0

Alteration 0	Definition	Modifying the natural anatomic structure of a body part without affecting the function of the body part
	Explanation	Principal purpose is to improve appearance
	Examples	Face lift, breast augmentation

Alteration is coded for all procedures performed solely to improve appearance. All methods, approaches, and devices used for the objective of improving appearance are coded here.

CODING NOTE	**ALTERATION.** Because some surgical procedures can be performed for either medical or cosmetic purposes, coding for Alteration requires diagnostic confirmation that the surgery is in fact performed to improve appearance.

> ### Example: Cosmetic blepharoplasty
> ...attention was turned to the redundant upper eyelid skin. The ellipse of skin as marked preoperatively was excised bilaterally. The medial and lateral fat compartments were open bilaterally. The medial compartment had severe fatty excess and periorbital fat herniation. This was resected. The lateral fat compartment was opened and the lateral fat tailored as well. Subdermal closure was performed with interrupted 3-0 sutures bilaterally. The skin was closed.

Character 1 Section	Character 2 Body System	Character 3 Root Operation	Character 4 Body Part	Character 5 Approach	Character 6 Device	Character 7 Qualifier
Medical And Surgical	Eye	Alteration	Upper Eyelid, Left	Open	No Device	No Qualifier
0	**8**	**0**	**P**	**0**	**Z**	**Z**

Character 1 Section	Character 2 Body System	Character 3 Root Operation	Character 4 Body Part	Character 5 Approach	Character 6 Device	Character 7 Qualifier
Medical And Surgical	Eye	Alteration	Upper Eyelid, Right	Open	No Device	No Qualifier
0	8	0	N	0	Z	Z

CREATION---ROOT OPERATION 4

Creation 4	Definition	Making a new genital structure that does not physically take the place of a body part
	Explanation	Used only for sex change operations
	Examples	Creation of vagina in a male, creation of penis in a female

Creation is used to represent a very narrow range of procedures. Only the procedures performed for sex change operations are included here.

CODING NOTE	HARVESTING AUTOGRAFT TISSUE. If a separate procedure is performed to harvest autograft tissue, it is coded to the appropriate root operation in addition to the primary procedure.

Example: Creating a vagina in a male patient using autograft

Character 1 Section	Character 2 Body System	Character 3 Root Operation	Character 4 Body Part	Character 5 Approach	Character 6 Device	Character 7 Qualifier
Medical and Surgical	Anatomical Regions, Gen.	Creation	Perineum, Male	Open	Autologous Tissue Subst.	Vagina
0	W	4	M	0	7	0

ICD-10-PCS PROCEDURES IN THE MEDICAL AND SURGICAL-RELATED SECTIONS

This chapter provides reference material for procedure codes in sections 1 through 9 of ICD-10-PCS. These nine sections define procedures related to the Medical and Surgical section. Codes in these sections contain characters not previously defined, such as substance, function, and method.

First, a table is provided, listing the sections in order. Following the table, reference material is provided for each section, and includes

- General description of the section
- A table listing each root operation in the section, with its corresponding definition
- Coding notes as needed
- Representative examples of procedures coded in that section, in table excerpt format, with explanatory notes as needed
- Coding exercises that provide example procedures and their corresponding ICD-10-PCS codes, with explanatory notes as needed

LIST OF MEDICAL AND SURGICAL-RELATED SECTIONS OF ICD-10-PCS

Nine additional sections of ICD-10-PCS include procedures related to the Medical and Surgical section, such as obstetrical procedures, administration of substances, and extracorporeal procedures.

Section Value	Description
1	Obstetrics
2	Placement
3	Administration
4	Measurement and Monitoring
5	Extracorporeal Assistance and Performance
6	Extracorporeal Therapies
7	Osteopathic
8	Other Procedures
9	Chiropractic

OBSTETRICS—SECTION 1

The Obstetrics section follows the same conventions established in the Medical and Surgical section, with all seven characters retaining the same meaning, as shown in this example of a low forceps extraction.

Character 1 Section	Character 2 Body System	Character 3 Root Operation	Character 4 Body Part	Character 5 Approach	Character 6 Device	Character 7 Qualifier
Obstetrics	Pregnancy	Extraction	Products of Conception	Via Nat./Artificial Opening	No Device	Low Forceps
1	**0**	**D**	**0**	**7**	**Z**	**3**

ROOT OPERATIONS

There are twelve root operations in the Obstetrics section. Ten of these are also found in the Medical and Surgical section.

The two root operations unique to Obstetrics are defined below.

Value	Description	Definition
A	Abortion	Artificially terminating a pregnancy
E	Delivery	Assisting the passage of the products of conception from the genital canal

CODING NOTE	**ABORTION** is subdivided according to whether an additional device such as a laminaria or abortifacient is used, or whether the abortion was performed by mechanical means. If either a laminaria or abortifacient is used, then the approach is Via Natural or Artificial Opening. All other abortion procedures are those done by mechanical means (the products of conception are physically removed using instrumentation), and the device value is Z, No Device.

Example: Transvaginal abortion using vacuum aspiration technique

Character 1 Section	Character 2 Body System	Character 3 Root Operation	Character 4 Body Part	Character 5 Approach	Character 6 Device	Character 7 Qualifier
Obstetrics	Pregnancy	Abortion	Products Of Conception	Via Nat/Artificial Opening	No Device	Vacuum
1	**0**	**A**	**0**	**7**	**Z**	**6**

CODING NOTE	**DELIVERY** applies only to manually-assisted, vaginal delivery and is defined as assisting the passage of the products of conception from the genital canal. Cesarean deliveries are coded in this section to the root operation Extraction.

Example: Manually-assisted delivery

Character 1 Section	Character 2 Body System	Character 3 Root Operation	Character 4 Body Part	Character 5 Approach	Character 6 Device	Character 7 Qualifier
Obstetrics	Pregnancy	Delivery	Products Of Conception	External	No Device	No Qualifier
1	**0**	**E**	**0**	**X**	**Z**	**Z**

PLACEMENT—SECTION 2

The Placement section follows the same conventions established in the Medical and Surgical section, with all seven characters retaining the same meaning, as in the example of cast change on the right forearm below.

Character 1 Section	Character 2 Body System	Character 3 Root Operation	Character 4 Body Part	Character 5 Approach	Character 6 Device	Character 7 Qualifier
Placement	Anatomical Regions	Change	Lower Arm, Right	External	Cast	No Qualifier
2	**W**	**0**	**C**	**X**	**2**	**Z**

ROOT OPERATIONS

The root operations in the Placement section include only those procedures performed without making an incision or a puncture.

Value	Description	Definition
0	Change	Taking out or off a device from a body region and putting back an identical or similar device in or on the same body region without cutting or puncturing the skin or a mucous membrane
1	Compression	Putting pressure on a body region
2	Dressing	Putting material on a body region for protection
3	Immobilization	Limiting or preventing motion of a body region
4	Packing	Putting material in a body region
5	Removal	Taking out or off a device from a body region
6	Traction	Exerting a pulling force on a body region in a distal direction

Example: Change of vaginal packing

Character 1 Section	Character 2 Body System	Character 3 Root Operation	Character 4 Body Part	Character 5 Approach	Character 6 Device	Character 7
Placement	Anatomical Orifices	Change	Female Genital Tract	External	Packing Material	No Qualifier
2	**Y**	**0**	**4**	**X**	**5**	**Z**

Example: Placement of pressure dressing on abdominal wall

	Character 2 Body System	Character 3 Root operation	Character 4 Body Region	Character 5 Approach	Character 6 Device	Character 7 Qualifier
Placement	Anatomical Regions	Compression	Abdominal Wall	External	Pressure Dressing	No Qualifier
2	**W**	**1**	**3**	**X**	**6**	**Z**

Example: Application of sterile dressing to head wound

Character 1 Section	Character 2 Body System	Character 3 Root operation	Character 4 Body Region	Character 5 Approach	Character 6 Device	Character 7 Qualifier
Placement	Anatomical Regions	Dressing	Head	External	Bandage	No Qualifier
2	**W**	**2**	**0**	**X**	**4**	**Z**

CODING NOTE	**IMMOBILIZATION:** The procedures to fit a device, such as splints and braces, as described in F0DZ6EZ and F0DZ7EZ, apply only to the rehabilitation setting. splints and braces placed in other inpatient settings are coded to Immobilization, table 2X3 in the Placement section.

Example: Placement of splint on left finger

	Character 2 Body System	Character 3 Root operation	Character 4 Body Region	Character 5 Approach	Character 6 Device	Character 7 Qualifier
Placement	Anatomical Regions	Immobilization	Finger, Left	External	Splint	No Qualifier
2	**W**	**3**	**K**	**X**	**1**	**Z**

Example: Placement of nasal packing

Character 1 Section	Character 2 Body System	Character 3 Root operation	Character 4 Body Region	Character 5 Approach	Character 6 Device	Character 7 Qualifier
Placement	Anatomical Orifices	Packing	Nasal	External	Packing Material	No Qualifier
2	**Y**	**4**	**1**	**X**	**5**	**Z**

Example: Removal of cast from right lower leg

Character 1 Section	Character 2 Body System	Character 3 Root operation	Character 4 Body Region	Character 5 Approach	Character 6 Device	Character 7 Qualifier
Placement	Anatomical Regions	Removal	Lower Leg, Right	External	Cast	No Qualifier
2	**W**	**5**	**Q**	**X**	**2**	**Z**

CODING NOTE	**TRACTION** in this section includes only the task performed using a mechanical traction apparatus. Manual traction performed by a physical therapist is coded to Manual Therapy Techniques in section F, Physical Rehabilitation and Diagnostic Audiology.

Example: Lumbar traction using motorized split-traction table

Character 1 Section	Character 2 Body System	Character 3 Root Operation	Character 4 Body Part	Character 5 Approach	Character 6 Device	Character 7 Qualifier
Placement	Anatomical Regions	Traction	Back	External	Traction Apparatus	No Qualifier
2	**W**	**6**	**5**	**X**	**0**	**Z**

ADMINISTRATION—SECTION 3

The Administration section includes infusions, injections, and transfusions, as well as other related procedures, such as irrigation and tattooing. All codes in this section define procedures where a diagnostic or therapeutic substance is given to the patient, as in the platelet transfusion example below.

Character 1 Section	Character 2 Body System	Character 3 Root Operation	Character 4 Body System	Character 5 Approach	Character 6 Substance	Character 7 Qualifier
Administration	Circulatory	Transfusion	Central Vein	Percutaneous	Platelets	Non-autologous
3	**0**	**2**	**4**	**3**	**R**	**1**

ROOT OPERATIONS

Root operations in this section are classified according to the broad category of substance administered. If the substance given is a blood product or a cleansing substance, then the procedure is coded to Transfusion and Irrigation respectively. All the other substances administered, such as anti-neoplastic substances, are coded to the root operation Introduction.

Value	Description	Definition
0	Introduction	Putting in or on a therapeutic, diagnostic, nutritional, physiological, or prophylactic substance except blood or blood products
1	Irrigation	Putting in or on a cleansing substance
2	Transfusion	Putting in blood or blood products

Example: Nerve block injection to median nerve

Character 1 Section	Character 2 Body System	Character 3 Root operation	Character 4 Body System	Character 5 Approach	Character 6 Substance	Character 7 Qualifier
Administration	Phys. Sys. & Anat. Regions	Introduction	Peripheral Nerves	Percutaneous	Regional Anesthetic	No Qualifier
3	**E**	**0**	**T**	**3**	**C**	**Z**

Example: Flushing of eye

Character 1 Section	Character 2 Body System	Character 3 Root operation	Character 4 Body System	Character 5 Approach	Character 6 Substance	Character 7 Qualifier
Administration	Phys. Sys. & Anat. Regions	Irrigation	Eye	External	Irrigating Substance	No Qualifier
3	**E**	**1**	**C**	**X**	**8**	**Z**

Example: Transfusion of cell saver red cells into central venous line

Character 1 Section	Character 2 Body System	Character 3 Root operation	Character 4 Body System	Character 5 Approach	Character 6 Substance	Character 7 Qualifier
Administration	Circulatory	Transfusion	Central Vein	Percutaneous	Red Blood Cells	Autologous
3	**0**	**2**	**4**	**3**	**N**	**0**

MEASUREMENT AND MONITORING—SECTION 4

There are two root operations in this section, and they differ in only one respect: Measurement defines one procedure and Monitoring defines a series of procedures.

ROOT OPERATIONS

Measurement describes a single level taken, while Monitoring describes a series of levels obtained at intervals. For example,

- A single temperature reading is considered Measurement.
- Temperature taken every half hour for 8 hours is considered Monitoring. Instead of defining a device, the sixth character defines the physiological or physical function being tested.

Value	Description	Definition
0	Measurement	Determining the level of a physiological or physical function at a point in time
1	Monitoring	Determining the level of a physiological or physical function repetitively over a period of time

Example: External electrocardiogram (EKG), single reading

Character 1 Section	Character 2 Body System	Character 3 Root Operation	Character 4 Body System	Character 5 Approach	Character 6 Function	Character 7 Qualifier
Measurement & Monitoring	Physiological Systems	Measurement	Cardiac	External	Electrical Activity	No Qualifier
4	A	0	2	X	4	Z

Example: Urinary pressure monitoring

Character 1 Section	Character 2 Body System	Character 3 Root operation	Character 4 Body System	Character 5 Approach	Character 6 Device	Character 7 Qualifier
Measurement & Monitoring	Physiological Systems	Monitoring	Urinary	Via Nat./Artificial Opening	Pressure	No Qualifier
4	A	1	D	7	B	Z

EXTRACORPOREAL ASSISTANCE AND PERFORMANCE— SECTION 5

This section includes procedures performed in a critical care setting, such as mechanical ventilation and cardioversion. It also includes other procedures, such as hemodialysis and hyper- baric oxygen treatment. These procedures all use equipment to support a physiological function in some way, whether it is breathing, circulating the blood, or restoring the natural rhythm of the heart.

The fifth and sixth characters in this section define duration and function respectively. These characters describe the duration of the procedure and the body function being acted upon, rather than the approach and device used.

Root operations

Assistance and Performance are two variations of the same kinds of procedures, varying only in the degree of control exercised over the physiological function.

Value	Description	Definition
0	Assistance	Taking over a portion of a physiological function by extracorporeal means
1	Performance	Completely taking over a physiological function by extracorporeal means
2	Restoration	Returning, or attempting to return, a physiological function to its original state by extracorporeal means

CODING NOTE	ASSISTANCE defines procedures that support a physiological function but do not take complete control of it, such as intra-aortic balloon pump to support cardiac output and hyperbaric oxygen treatment.

Example: Hyperbaric oxygenation of wound

Character 1 Section	Character 2 Body System	Character 3 Root Operation	Character 4 Body System	Character 5 Duration	Character 6 Function	Character 7 Qualifier
Extracorporeal Assistance & Performance	Physiological Systems	Assistance	Circulatory	Intermittent	Oxygenation	Hyperbaric
5	A	0	5	1	2	

CODING NOTE	**PERFORMANCE** defines procedures where complete control is exercised over a physiological function, such as total mechanical ventilation, cardiac pacing, and cardiopulmonary bypass.

Example: Cardiopulmonary bypass in conjunction with CABG

Character 1 Section	Character 2 Body System	Character 3 Root Operation	Character 4 Body System	Character 5 Duration	Character 6 Function	Character 7 Qualifier
Extracorporeal Assistance & Performance	Physiological Systems	Performance	Cardiac	Continuous	Output	No Qualifier
5	A	1	2	2	1	Z

CODING NOTE	**RESTORATION** defines only external cardioversion and defibrillation procedures. Failed cardioversion procedures are also included in the definition of Restoration, and are coded the same as successful procedures.

Example: Attempted cardiac defibrillation, unsuccessful

Character 1 Section	Character 2 Body System	Character 3 Root Operation	Character 4 Body System	Character 5 Duration	Character 6 Function	Character 7 Qualifier
Extracorporeal Assist. And Performance	Physiological Systems	Restoration	Cardiac	Single	Rhythm	No Qualifier
5	A	2	2	0	4	Z

EXTRACORPOREAL THERAPIES—SECTION 6

Section 6, Extracorporeal Therapies, describes other extracorporeal procedures that are not defined by Assistance and Performance in section 5 *(see page 3 16)*. Examples are bili-lite phototherapy, apheresis, and whole body hypothermia.

The second character contains a single general body system choice, Physiological Systems, as in the phototherapy example below. The sixth character is defined as a qualifier, but contains no specific qualifier values. The seventh-character qualifier identifies various blood components separated out in pheresis procedures.

Character 1 Section	Character 2 Body System	Character 3 Root Operation	Character 4 Body System	Character 5 Duration	Character 6 Function	Character 7 Qualifier
Extracorporeal Therapies	Physiological Systems	Phototherapy	Skin	Single	No Qualifier	No Qualifier
6	A	6	0	0	Z	Z

ROOT OPERATIONS

The meaning of each root operation is consistent with the term as used in the medical community. Decompression and Hyperthermia have a more specialized meaning. All are defined in the table below.

Value	Description	Definition
0	Atmospheric Control	Extracorporeal control of atmospheric pressure and composition
1	Decompression	Extracorporeal elimination of undissolved gas from body fluids
2	Electromagnetic Therapy	Extracorporeal treatment by electromagnetic rays
3	Hyperthermia	Extracorporeal raising of body temperature
4	Hypothermia	Extracorporeal lowering of body temperature
5	Pheresis	Extracorporeal separation of blood products
6	Phototherapy	Extracorporeal treatment by light rays
7	ultrasound Therapy	Extracorporeal treatment by ultrasound
8	Ultraviolet Light Therapy	Extracorporeal treatment by ultraviolet light
9	Shock Wave Therapy	Extracorporeal treatment by shock waves

CODING NOTE	DECOMPRESSION describes a single type of procedure—treatment for decompression sickness (the bends) in a hyperbaric chamber.

Example: Hyperbaric decompression treatment, single

Character 1 Body System	Character 2 Root Operation	Character 3 Body System	Character 4 Duration	Character 5 Qualifier	Character 6 Qualifier	Character 7 Qualifier
Extracorporeal Therapies	Physiological Systems	Decompression	Circulatory	Single	No Qualifier	No Qualifier
6	A	1	5	0	Z	Z

CODING NOTE	HYPERTHERMIA is used both to treat temperature imbalance, and as an adjunct radiation treatment for cancer. When performed to treat temperature imbalance, the procedure is coded to this section. When performed for cancer treatment, whole-body hyperthermia is classified as a modality qualifier in section D, Radiation Oncology.

Example: Whole body hypothermia treatment for temperature imbalance, series

	Character 2 Body System	Character 3 Root Operation	Character 4 Body System	Character 5 Duration	Character 6 Qualifier	Character 7 Qualifier
Extracorporeal Therapies	Physiological Systems	Hypothermia	None	Multiple	No Qualifier	No Qualifier
6	A	4	Z	1	Z	Z

CODING NOTE	PHERESIS is used in medical practice for two main purposes: to treat diseases where too much of a blood component is produced, such as leukemia, or to remove a blood product such as platelets from a donor, for transfusion into a patient who needs them.

Example: Therapeutic leukapheresis, single treatment

Character 1 Section	Character 2 Body System	Character 3 Root Operation	Character 4 Body System	Character 5 Duration	Character 6 Qualifier	Character 7 Qualifier
Extracorporeal Therapies	Physiological Systems	Pheresis	Circulatory	Single	No Qualifier	Leukocytes
6	A	5	5	0	Z	1

Example: Phototherapy of circulatory system, series treatment

Character 1 Section	Character 2 Body System	Character 3 Root Operation	Character 4 Body System	Character 5 Duration	Character 6 Qualifier	Character 7 Qualifier
Extracorporeal Therapies	Physiological Systems	Phototherapy	Circulatory	Multiple	No Qualifier	No Qualifier
6	A	6	5	1	Z	Z

CODING NOTE	**PHOTOTHERAPY** to the circulatory system means exposing the blood to light rays outside the body, using a machine that recirculates the blood and returns it to the body after phototherapy.

Example: Ultraviolet Light Phototherapy, Series Treatment

Character 1 Section	Character 2 Body System	Character 3 Root Operation	Character 4 Body System	Character 5 Duration	Character 6 Qualifier	Character 7 Qualifier
Extracorporeal Therapies	Physiological Systems	UV Light Phototherapy	Skin	Multiple	No Qualifier	No Qualifier
6	A	8	0	1	Z	Z

OSTEOPATHIC—SECTION 7

Section 7, Osteopathic, is one of the smallest sections in ICD-10-PCS. There is a single body system, Anatomical Regions, and a single root operation, Treatment.

The sixth-character methods such as Lymphatic Pump and Fascial Release are not explicitly defined in ICD-10-PCS, and rely on the standard definitions as used in this specialty.

Value	Description	Definition
0	Treatment	Manual treatment to eliminate or alleviate somatic dysfunction and related disorders

Example: Fascial release of abdomen, osteopathic treatment

Character 1 Section	Character 2 Body System	Character 3 Operation	Character 4 Body Region	Character 5 Approach	Character 6 Method	Character 7 Qualifier
Osteopathic	Anatomical Regions	Treatment	Abdomen	External	Fascial Release	No Qualifier
7	W	0	9	X	1	Z

Example: General osteopathic mobilization of legs

Character 1 Section	Character 2 Body System	Character 3 Operation	Character 4 Body Region	Character 5 Approach	Character 6 Method	Character 7
Osteopathic	Anatomical Regions	Treatment	Lower Extremities	External	General Mobilization	No Qualifier
7	W	0	6	X	2	Z

OTHER PROCEDURES—SECTION 8

The Other Procedures section contains codes for procedures not included in the other medical and surgical-related sections A single root operation, Other Procedures, is defined below.

Value	Description	Definition
0	Other Procedures	Methodologies which attempt to remediate or cure a disorder or disease

There are relatively few procedure codes in this section, for nontraditional, whole body therapies including acupuncture and meditation. There is also a code for the fertilization portion of an in-vitro fertilization procedure.

Example: Acupuncture

Character 1 Section	Character 2 Body System	Character 3 Root Operation	Character 4 Body Region	Character 5 Approach	Character 6 Method	Character 7 Qualifier
Other Procedures	Phys. Sys. & Anat. Regions	Other Procedures	Integumentary Sys. & Breast	Percutaneous	Acupuncture	No Qualifier
8	E	0	H	3	0	Z

Example: Yoga therapy

Character 1 Section	Character 2 Body System	Character 3 Root Operation	Character 4 Body Region	Character 5 Approach	Character 6 Method	Character 7 Qualifier
Other Procedures	Phys. Sys. & Anat. Regions	Other Procedures	None	External	Other Method	Yoga Therapy
8	**E**	**0**	**Z**	**X**	**Y**	**4**

CHIROPRACTIC—SECTION 9

The Chiropractic section consists of a single body system, Anatomical Regions, and a single root operation, Manipulation, defined below.

Value	Description	Definition
B	Manipulation	Manual procedure that involves a directed thrust to move a joint past the physiological range of motion, without exceeding the anatomical limit

Example: Chiropractic treatment of cervical spine, short lever specific contact

Character 1 Section	Character 2 Body System	Character 3 Root Operation	Character 4 Body Region	Character 5 Approach	Character 6 Method	Character 7 Qualifier
Chiropractic	Anatomical Regions	Manipulation	Cervical	External	Short Lever Sp. Contact	No Qualifier
9	**W**	**B**	**1**	**X**	**H**	**Z**

Example: Non-manual chiropractic manipulation of pelvis

Character 1 Section	Character 2 Body System	Character 3 Root Operation	Character 4 Body Region	Character 5 Approach	Character 6 Method	Character 7 Qualifier
Chiropractic	Anatomical Regions	Manipulation	Pelvis	External	Non-Manual	No Qualifier
9	**W**	**B**	**5**	**X**	**B**	**Z**

PROCEDURES IN THE ANCILLARY SECTIONS

This section provides reference material for procedure codes in the six ancillary sections of ICD-10-PCS (B through D, F through H). Codes in these sections contain characters not previously defined, such as contrast, modality qualifier and equipment.

First, a table is provided, listing the sections in order. Following the table, reference material is provided for each section, and includes

- General description of the section
- A table listing each root type in the section, with its corresponding definition (sections B, C and F only)
- Coding notes as needed
- Representative examples of procedures coded in that section, in table excerpt format, with explanatory notes as needed
- Coding exercises that provide example procedures and their corresponding ICD-10-PCS codes, with explanatory notes as needed

LIST OF ANCILLARY SECTIONS IN ICD-10-PCS

Six ancillary sections of ICD-10-PCS include procedures such as imaging, radiation oncology, and rehabilitation.

Section Value	Description
B	Imaging
C	Nuclear Medicine
D	Radiation Oncology
F	Physical Rehabilitation and Diagnostic Audiology
G	Mental Health
H	Substance Abuse Treatment

IMAGING—SECTION B

Imaging follows the same conventions established in the Medical and Surgical section (*see chapter* 2), for the section, body system, and body part characters. However, the third and fourth characters introduce definitions not used in previous sections.

- Third character defines procedure by root type, instead of root operation.
- Fifth character defines contrast if used.
- Sixth character is a qualifier that specifies an image taken without contrast followed by one with contrast.
- Seventh character is a qualifier that is not specified in this section.

ROOT TYPES

The Imaging root types are defined in the following table.

Value	Description	Definition
0	Plain Radiography	Planar display of an image developed from the capture of external ionizing radiation on photographic or photoconductive plate
1	Fluoroscopy	Single plane or bi-plane real time display of an image developed from the capture of external ionizing radiation on a fluorescent screen. The image may also be stored by either digital or analog means
2	Computerized Tomography (CT scan)	Computer reformatted digital display of multiplanar images developed from the capture of multiple exposures of external ionizing radiation
3	Magnetic Resonance Imaging (MRI)	Computer reformatted digital display of multiplanar images developed from the capture of radio-frequency signals emitted by nuclei in a body site excited within a magnetic field
4	Ultrasonography	Real time display of images of anatomy or flow information developed from the capture of reflected and attenuated high frequency sound waves

Example: X-ray of right clavicle, limited study

Character 1 Section	Character 2 Body System	Character 3 Root Type	Character 4 Body Part	Character 5 Contrast	Character 6 Qualifier	Character 7 Qualifier
Imaging	Non-axial Upper Bones	Plain Radiography	Clavicle, Right	None	None	None
B	**P**	**0**	**4**	**Z**	**Z**	**Z**

Example: Fluoroscopy of renal dialysis shunt using CO2 contrast

Character 1 Section	Character 2 Body System	Character 3 Root Type	Character 4 Body Part	Character 5 Contrast	Character 6 Qualifier	Character 7 Qualifier
Imaging	Veins	Fluoroscopy	Dialysis Shunt/Fistula	Other Contrast	None	None
B	**5**	**1**	**W**	**Y**	**Z**	**Z**

Example: CT of brain without contrast followed by high osmolar contrast

Character 1 Section	Character 2 Body System	Character 3 Root Type	Character 4 Body Part	Character 5 Contrast	Character 6 Qualifier	Character 7 Qualifier
Imaging	Central Nervous	Computerized Tomography	Brain	High Osmolar	Unenhanced and Enhanced	None
B	**0**	**2**	**0**	**0**	**0**	**Z**

Example: MRI of liver using Gadoteridol

Character 1 Section	Character 2 Body System	Character 3 Root Type	Character 4 Body Part	Character 5 Contrast	Character 6 Qualifier	Character 7 Qualifier
Imaging	Hepatobiliary & Pancreas	Magnetic Resonance Imaging	Liver	Other Contrast	None	None
B	**F**	**3**	**5**	**Y**	**Z**	**Z**

Example: Ultrasound of prostate gland

Character 1 Section	Character 2 Body System	Character 3 Root Type	Character 4 Body Part	Character 5 Contrast	Character 6 Qualifier	Character 7 Qualifier
Imaging	Male Reproductive	Ultrasonography	Prostate and Seminal Vesicles	None	None	None
B	**V**	**4**	**9**	**Z**	**Z**	**Z**

NUCLEAR MEDICINE—SECTION C

Nuclear Medicine is organized like the Imaging section *(see page 4.5)*. The only significant difference is that the fifth character defines the radionuclide instead of the contrast material used in the procedure, as described below.

- The fifth character specifies the radionuclide, the radiation source used in the procedure. Choices are applicable for the root procedure type.
- The sixth and seventh characters are qualifiers, and are not specified in this section.

ROOT TYPES

The third character classifies the procedure by root type instead of by root operation.

Value	Description	Definition
1	Planar Nuclear Medicine Imaging	Introduction of radioactive materials into the body for single plane display of images developed from the capture of radioactive emissions
2	Tomographic (Tomo) Nuclear Medicine Imaging	Introduction of radioactive materials into the body for three-dimensional display of images developed from the capture of radioactive emissions
3	Positron Emission Tomography (PET)	Introduction of radioactive materials into the body for three-dimensional display of images developed from the simultaneous capture, 180 degrees apart, of radioactive emissions
4	Nonimaging Nuclear Medicine Uptake	Introduction of radioactive materials into the body for measurements of organ function, from the detection of radioactive emissions
5	Nonimaging Nuclear Medicine Probe	Introduction of radioactive materials into the body for the study of distribution and fate of certain substances by the detection of radioactive emissions from an external source
6	Nonimaging Nuclear medicine Assay	Introduction of radioactive materials into the body for the study of body fluids and blood elements, by the detection of radioactive emissions
7	Systemic Nuclear Medicine Therapy	Introduction of unsealed radioactive materials into the body for treatment

Example: Adenosine sestamibi (technetium) planar scan of heart muscle at rest

Character 1 Section	Character 2 Body System	Character 3 Root Type	Character 4 Body Part	Character 5 Radionuclide	Character 6 Qualifier.	Character 7 Qualifier
Nuclear Medicine	Heart	Planar Nuclear Imaging	Myocardium	Technetium 99m	None	None
C	**2**	**1**	**G**	**1**	**Z**	**Z**

Example: Technetium tomo scan of liver

Character 1 Section	Character 2 Body System	Character 3 Root Type	Character 4 Body Part	Character 5 Radionuclide	Character 6 Qualifier	Character 7 Qualifier
Nuclear Medicine	Hepatobiliary And Pancreas	Tomo Nuclear Imaging	Liver	Technetium 99M	None	None
C	**F**	**2**	**5**	**1**	**Z**	**Z**

RADIATION ONCOLOGY—SECTION D

Radiation Oncology contains the radiation procedures performed for cancer treatment. Character meanings are described below.

- Third character defines root type, which is the basic modality.
- Fifth character further specifies treatment modality.
- Sixth character defines the radioactive isotope used, if applicable.
- Seventh character is a qualifier, and is not specified in this section.

ROOT TYPE

The third character defines the treatment modality as root type.

Examples are Brachytherapy and Stereotactic Radiosurgery. Four different root types are used in this section, as listed in the table below.

Value	Description
0	Beam Radiation
1	Brachytherapy
2	Stereotactic Radiosurgery
Y	Other Radiation

Example: LDR Brachytherapy of cervix using Iridium 192

Character 1 Section	Character 2 Body System	Character 3 Root Type	Character 4 Body part	Character 5 Modal. Qualifier	Character 6 isotope	Character 7 Qualifier
Radiation Oncology	Female Reproductive	Brachytherapy	Cervix	LDR Brachy-therapy	Iridium 192	None
D	**U**	**1**	**1**	**B**	**8**	**Z**

Example: Intraoperative radiation therapy (IORT) of bladder

Character 1 Section	Character 2 Body Sys	Character 3 Root Type	Character 4 Body part	Character 5 Modal. Qualifier	Character 6 isotope	Character 7 Qualifier
Radiation Oncology	Urinary System	Other Radiation	Bladder	IORT	None	None
D	**T**	**Y**	**2**	**C**	**Z**	**Z**

PHYSICAL REHABILITATION AND DIAGNOSTIC AUDIOLOGY—SECTION F

Physical Rehabilitation and Diagnostic Audiology contains character definitions unlike the other sections in ICD-10-PCS. The following table defines the special character definitions:

- Second character is a section qualifier that specifies whether the procedure is a rehabilitation or diagnostic audiology procedure.
- Third character defines the general procedure root type.
- Fourth character defines the body system and body region combined, where applicable
- Fifth character further specifies the procedure type.
- Sixth character specifies the equipment used, if any.

ROOT TYPES

This section uses the third character to classify procedures into 14 root types. They are defined in the table below.

Value	Description	Definition
0	Speech Assessment	Measurement of speech and related functions
1	Motor and/or Nerve Function Assessment	Measurement of motor, nerve, and related functions
2	Activities of Daily Living Assessment	Measurement of functional level for activities of daily living
3	Hearing Assessment	Measurement of hearing and related functions
4	Hearing Aid Assessment	Measurement of the appropriateness and/or effectiveness of a hearing device
5	Vestibular Assessment	Measurement of the vestibular system and related functions
6	Speech Treatment	Application of techniques to improve, augment, or compensate for speech and related functional impairment
7	Motor Treatment	Exercise or activities to increase or facilitate motor function
8	Activities of Daily Living Treatment	Exercise or activities to facilitate functional competence for activities of daily living
9	Hearing Treatment	Application of techniques to improve, augment, or compensate for hearing and related functional impairment
B	Hearing Aid Treatment	Application of techniques to improve the communication abilities of individuals with cochlear implant
C	Vestibular Treatment	Application of techniques to improve, augment, or compensate for vestibular and related functional impairment
D	Device Fitting	Fitting of a device designed to facilitate or support achievement of a higher level of function
F	Caregiver Training	Training in activities to support patient's optimal level of function

CODING NOTE	TREATMENT procedures include swallowing dysfunction exercises, bathing and showering techniques, wound management, gait training, and a host of activities typically associated with rehabilitation.

Example: Wound care treatment of left calf ulcer using pulsatile lavage

Character 1 Section	Character 2 Section Qualifier	Character 3 Root Type	Character 4 Body System & Region	Character 5 Type Qualifier	Character 6 Equipment	Character 7 Qualifier
Rehabilitation & Diagnostic Audiology	Rehabilitation	Activities Of Daily Living Treatment	Musculoskeletal Lower Extremity	Wound Management	Physical Agents	None
F	0	8	L	5	B	Z

CODING NOTE	ASSESSMENTS are further classified into more than 100 different tests or methods. The majority of these focus on the faculties of hearing and speech, but others focus on various aspects of body function, and on the patient's quality of life, such as muscle performance, neuromotor development, and reintegration skills.

Example: Articulation and phonology assessment using spectrograph

Character 1 Section	Character 2 Section Qualifier	Character 3 Root Type	Character 4 Body System & Region	Character 5 Type Qualifier	Character 6 Equipment	Character 7 Qualifier
Rehabilitation & Diagnostic Audiology	Rehabilitation	Speech Assessment	None	Articulation/ Phonology	Speech Analysis	None
F	0	0	Z	9	Q	Z

CODING NOTE	DEVICE FITTING. The fifth character used in Device Fitting describes the device being fitted rather than the method used to fit the device. Detailed descriptions of the devices are provided in the reference materials, the table specific to Device Fitting.

Example: Individual fitting of moveable brace, right knee

Character 1 Section	Character 2 Section Qualifier	Character 3 Root Type	Character 4 Body System & Region	Character 5 Type Qualifier	Character 6 Equipment	Character 7 Qualifier
Rehabilitation & Diagnostic Audiology	Rehabilitation	Device Fitting	None	Dynamic Orthosis	Orthosis	None
F	0	D	Z	6	E	Z

CODING NOTE	CAREGIVER TRAINING is divided into eighteen different broad subjects taught to help a caregiver provide proper patient care.

Example: Caregiver training in feeding, no special equipment used

Character 1 Section	Character 2 Section Qualifier	Character 3 Root Type	Character 4 Body System & Region	Character 5 Type Qualifier	Character 6 Equipment	Character 7 Qualifier
Rehabilitation & Diagnostic Audiology	Rehabilitation	Caregiver Training	None	Feeding and Eating	None	None
F	0	F	Z	2	Z	Z

MENTAL HEALTH—SECTION G

Mental Health contains specific values in the third and fourth characters to describe mental health procedures. The remaining characters function as placeholders only. Character meanings are described below.

- Third character describes the mental health procedure root type.
- Fourth character further specifies the procedure type as needed.
- Second, fifth, sixth, and seventh characters do not convey specific information about the procedure. The value Z functions as a placeholder in these characters.

ROOT TYPE

The third character describes the mental health root type. There are 11 root type values in this section, as listed in the table below.

Value	Description
1	Psychological Tests
2	Crisis Intervention
5	Individual Psychotherapy
6	Counseling
7	Family Psychotherapy
B	Electroconvulsive Therapy
C	Biofeedback
F	Hypnosis
G	Narcosynthesis
H	Group Therapy
J	Light Therapy

Example: Galvanic skin response (GSR) biofeedback

Character 1 Section	Character 2 Body System	Character 3 Root Type	Character 4 Type Qualifier	Character 5 Qualifier	Character 6 Qualifier	Character 7 Qualifier
Mental Health	None	Biofeedback	Other Biofeedback	None	None	None
G	**Z**	**C**	**9**	**Z**	**Z**	**Z**

SUBSTANCE ABUSE TREATMENT—SECTION H

Substance Abuse Treatment is structured like a smaller version of the Mental Health section. Character meanings are described below.

- Third character describes the root type.
- Fourth character is a qualifier that further classifies the root type
- Second, fifth, sixth, and seventh characters do not convey specific information about the procedure. The value Z functions as a placeholder in these characters.

ROOT TYPES

There are seven different root type values classified in this section, as listed in the following table.

Value	Description
2	Detoxification Services
3	Individual Counseling
4	Group Counseling
5	Individual Psychotherapy
6	Family Counseling
8	Medication Management
9	Pharmacotherapy

Example: Pharmacotherapy treatment with Antabuse for alcohol addiction

Character 1 Section	Character 2 Body System	Character 3 Root Type	Character 4 Type Qualifier	Character 5 Qualifier	Character 6 Qualifier	Character 7 Qualifier
Substance Abuse Treatment	None	Pharmaco-therapy	Antabuse	None	None	None
H	**Z**	**9**	**3**	**Z**	**Z**	**Z**

NEW TECHNOLOGY–SECTION X

Section X New Technology is the section in ICD-10-PCS for codes that uniquely identify procedures requested via the New Technology Application Process, and for codes that capture new technologies not currently classified in ICD-10-PCS.

This section may include codes for medical and surgical procedures, medical and surgical- related procedures, or ancillary procedures designated as new technology.

In section X, the seven characters are defined as follows:

- First character: section (X)
- Second character: body system
- Third character: operation
- Fourth character: body part
- Fifth character: approach
- Sixth character: device/substance/technology
- Seventh character: new technology group

The New Technology section includes infusions of new technology drugs, and can potentially include a wide range of other new technology medical, surgical and ancillary procedures. The example below is for infusion of a new technology drug.

Example: New Technology

Character 1 Section	Character 2 Body System	Character 3 Root Type	Character 4 Type Qualifier	Character 5 Qualifier	Character 6 Qualifier	Character 7 Qualifier
New Technology	Anatomical Regions	Introduction	Central Vein	Percutaneous	Ceftazidime-Avibactam Anti-infective	New Technology Group 1
X	**W**	**0**	**4**	**3**	**2**	**1**

CODING NOTE	**Seventh Character New Technology Group.** In ICD-10-PCS, the type of information specified in the seventh character is called the qualifier, and the information specified depends on the section. In this section, the seventh character is used exclusively to indicate the new technology group. The New Technology Group is a number or letter that changes each year that new technology codes are added to the system. For example, Section X codes added for the first year have the seventh character value 1, New Technology Group 1, and the next year that Section X codes are added have the seventh character value 2 New Technology Group 2, and so on. Changing the seventh character New Technology Group to a unique value every year that there are new codes in this section allows the ICD-10-PCS to "recycle" the values in the third, fourth, and sixth characters as needed. This avoids the creation of duplicate codes, because the root operation, body part and device/substance/technology values can specify a different meaning with every new technology group, if needed. Having a unique value for the New Technology Group maximizes the flexibility and capacity of section X over its lifespan, and allows it to evolve as medical technology evolves.

BODY SYSTEM VALUES

Second character body systems in this section do not change from year to year. They are a fixed set of values that combine the uses of body system, body region, and physiological system as specified in other sections in ICD-10-PCS. As a result, the second character body system values are broader values. This allows body part values to be as general or specific as they need to be to efficiently represent the body part applicable to a new technology.

ROOT OPERATIONS

Third character root operations in this section use the same root operation values as their counterparts in other sections of ICD-10-PCS. The example above uses the root operation value Introduction. This root operation has the same definition as its counterpart in section 3 of ICD-10-PCS, as given below.

- 0 – Introduction: Putting in or on a therapeutic, diagnostic, nutritional, physiological, or prophylactic substance except blood or blood products

BODY PART VALUES

Fourth character body part values in this section use the same body part values as their closest counterparts in other sections of ICD-10-PCS. The example above uses the body part value 4 Central Vein. This is its closest counterpart in section 3 of ICD-10-PCS.

DEVICE/SUBSTANCE/TECHNOLOGY VALUES

In this section, the sixth character contains a general description of the key feature of the new technology. The example above uses the device/substance/technology value 2 Ceftazidime-Avibactam Anti-infective.

ICD-10-PCS ROOT OPERATIONS AND APPROACHES

This section contains reference tables listing the root operations and approaches used in the Medical and Surgical section. The first table includes the definition of each root operation, with explanation and examples. The second table includes the definition of each approach.

The root operations are listed by name in alphabetical order. The approaches are listed by approach value, in numeric order followed by alphabetical order. For the full ICD-10-PCS definitions, please refer to the Definitions portion of the ICD-10 Procedure Coding System.

ROOT OPERATIONS		
Alteration	Definition	Modifying the anatomic structure of a body part without affecting the function of the body part
	Explanation	Principal purpose is to improve appearance
	Examples	Face lift, breast augmentation
Bypass	Definition	Altering the route of passage of the contents of a tubular body part
	Explanation	Rerouting contents of a body part to a downstream area of the normal route, to a similar route and body part, or to an abnormal route and dissimilar body part. Includes one or more anastomoses, with or without the use of a device
	Examples	Coronary artery bypass, colostomy formation
Change	Definition	Taking out or off a device from a body part and putting back an identical or similar device in or on the same body part without cutting or puncturing the skin or a mucous membrane
	Explanation	All CHANGE procedures are coded using the approach EXTERNAL
	Examples	Urinary catheter change, gastrostomy tube change
Control	Definition	Stopping, or attempting to stop, postprocedural bleeding
	Explanation	The site of the bleeding is coded as an anatomical region and not to a specific body part
	Examples	Control of post-prostatectomy hemorrhage, control of post-tonsillectomy hemorrhage
Creation	Definition	Making a new genital structure that does not take over the function of a body part
	Explanation	Used only for sex change operations
	Examples	Creation of vagina in a male, creation of penis in a female
Destruction	Definition	Physical eradication of all or a portion of a body part by the direct use of energy, force or a destructive agent
	Explanation	None of the body part is physically taken out
	Examples	Fulguration of rectal polyp, cautery of skin lesion
Detachment	Definition	Cutting off all or a portion of the upper or lower extremities
	Explanation	The body part value is the site of the detachment, with a qualifier if applicable to further specify the level where the extremity was detached
	Examples	Below knee amputation, disarticulation of shoulder
Dilation	Definition	Expanding an orifice or the lumen of a tubular body part
	Explanation	The orifice can be a natural orifice or an artificially created orifice. Accomplished by stretching a tubular body part using intraluminal pressure or by cutting part of the orifice or wall of the tubular body part
	Examples	Percutaneous transluminal angioplasty, pyloromyotomy
Division	Definition	Cutting into a body part without draining fluids and/or gases from the body part in order to separate or transect a body part
	Explanation	All or a portion of the body part is separated into two or more portions
	Examples	Spinal cordotomy, osteotomy

ROOT OPERATIONS		
Drainage	Definition	Taking or letting out fluids and/or gases from a body part
	Explanation	The qualifier DIAGNOSTIC is used to identify drainage procedures that are biopsies
	Examples	Thoracentesis, incision and drainage
Excision	Definition	Cutting out or off, without replacement, a portion of a body part
	Explanation	The qualifier DIAGNOSTIC is used to identify excision procedures that are biopsies
	Examples	Partial nephrectomy, liver biopsy
Extirpation	Definition	Taking or cutting out solid matter from a body part
	Explanation	The solid matter may be an abnormal byproduct of a biological function or a foreign body; it may be imbedded in a body part or in the lumen of a tubular body part. The solid matter may or may not have been previously broken into pieces
	Examples	Thrombectomy, choledocholithotomy
Extraction	Definition	Pulling or stripping out or off all or a portion of a body part by the use of force
	Explanation	The qualifier DIAGNOSTIC is used to identify extraction procedures that are biopsies
	Examples	Dilation and curettage, vein stripping
Fragmentation	Definition	Breaking solid matter in a body part into pieces
	Explanation	Physical force (e.g., manual, ultrasonic) applied directly or indirectly is used to break the solid matter into pieces. The solid matter may be an abnormal byproduct of a biological function or a foreign body. The pieces of solid matter are not taken out
	Examples	Extracorporeal shockwave lithotripsy, transurethral lithotripsy
Fusion	Definition	Joining together portions of an articular body part rendering the articular body part immobile
	Explanation	The body part is joined together by fixation device, bone graft, or other means
	Examples	Spinal fusion, ankle arthrodesis
Insertion	Definition	Putting in a nonbiological device that monitors, assists, performs or prevents a physiological function but does not physically take the place of a body part
	Explanation	N/A
	Examples	Insertion of radioactive implant, insertion of central venous catheter
Inspection	Definition	Visually and/or manually exploring a body part
	Explanation	Visual exploration may be performed with or without optical instrumentation. Manual exploration may be performed directly or through intervening body layers
	Examples	Diagnostic arthroscopy, exploratory laparotomy
Map	Definition	Locating the route of passage of electrical impulses and/or locating functional areas in a body part
	Explanation	Applicable only to the cardiac conduction mechanism and the central nervous system
	Examples	Cardiac mapping, cortical mapping
Occlusion	Definition	Completely closing an orifice or the lumen of a tubular body part
	Explanation	The orifice can be a natural orifice or an artificially created orifice
	Examples	Fallopian tube ligation, ligation of inferior vena cava

ROOT OPERATIONS		
Reattachment	Definition	Putting back in or on all or a portion of a separated body part to its normal location or other suitable location
	Explanation	Vascular circulation and nervous pathways may or may not be reestablished
	Examples	Reattachment of hand, reattachment of avulsed kidney
Release	Definition	Freeing a body part from an abnormal physical constraint by cutting or by use of force
	Explanation	Some of the restraining tissue may be taken out but none of the body part is taken out
	Examples	Adhesiolysis, carpal tunnel release
	Definition	Taking out or off a device from a body part
Removal	Explanation	If a device is taken out and a similar device put in without cutting or puncturing the skin or mucous membrane, the procedure is coded to the root operation CHANGE. Otherwise, the procedure for taking out a device is coded to the root operation REMOVAL
	Examples	Drainage tube removal, cardiac pacemaker removal
	Definition	Restoring, to the extent possible, a body part to its normal anatomic structure and function
Repair	Explanation	Used only when the method to accomplish the repair is not one of the other root operations
	Examples	Colostomy takedown, suture of laceration
	Definition	Putting in or on biological or synthetic material that physically takes the place and/or function of all or a portion of a body part
Replacement	Explanation	The body part may have been taken out or replaced, or may be taken out, physically eradicated, or rendered nonfunctional during the Replacement procedure. A Removal procedure is coded for taking out the device used in a previous replacement procedure
	Examples	Total hip replacement, bone graft, free skin graft
	Definition	Moving to its normal location, or other suitable location, all or a portion of a body part
Reposition	Explanation	The body part is moved to a new location from an abnormal location, or from a normal location where it is not functioning correctly. The body part may or may not be cut out or off to be moved to the new location
	Examples	Reposition of undescended testicle, fracture reduction
	Definition	Cutting out or off, without replacement, all of a body part
Resection	Explanation	N/A
	Examples	Total nephrectomy, total lobectomy of lung
	Definition	Partially closing an orifice or the lumen of a tubular body part
Restriction	Explanation	The orifice can be a natural orifice or an artificially created orifice
	Examples	Esophagogastric fundoplication, cervical cerclage
	Definition	Correcting, to the extent possible, a portion of a malfunctioning device or the position of a displaced device
Revision	Explanation	Revision can include correcting a malfunctioning or displaced device by taking out or putting in components of the device such as a screw or pin
	Examples	Adjustment of position of pacemaker lead, recementing of hip prosthesis
	Definition	Putting in or on biological or synthetic material that physically reinforces and/or augments the function of a portion of a body part
Supplement	Explanation	The biological material is non-living, or is living and from the same individual. The body part may have been previously replaced, and the Supplement procedure is performed to physically reinforce and/or augment the function of the replaced body part

ROOT OPERATIONS		
	Examples	Herniorrhaphy using mesh, free nerve graft, mitral valve ring annuloplasty, put a new acetabular liner in a previous hip replacement
	Definition	Moving, without taking out, all or a portion of a body part to another location to take over the function of all or a portion of a body part
Transfer	Explanation	The body part transferred remains connected to its vascular and nervous supply
	Examples	Tendon transfer, skin pedicle flap transfer
	Definition	Putting in or on all or a portion of a living body part taken from another individual or animal to physically take the place and/or function of all or a portion of a similar body part
Transplantation	Explanation	The native body part may or may not be taken out, and the transplanted body part may take over all or a portion of its function
	Examples	Kidney transplant, heart transplant

APPROACHES	
Open	Cutting through the skin or mucous membrane and any other body layers necessary to expose the site of the procedure
Percutaneous	Entry, by puncture or minor incision, of instrumentation through the skin or mucous membrane and any other body layers necessary to reach the site of the procedure
Percutaneous Endoscopic	Entry, by puncture or minor incision, of instrumentation through the skin or mucous membrane and any other body layers necessary to reach and visualize the site of the procedure
Via Natural or Artificial Opening	Entry of instrumentation through a natural or artificial external opening to reach the site of the procedure
Via Natural or Artificial Opening Endoscopic	Entry of instrumentation through a natural or artificial external opening to reach and visualize the site of the procedure
Via Natural or Artificial Opening With Percutaneous Endoscopic Assistance	Entry of instrumentation through a natural or artificial external opening and entry, by puncture or minor incision, of instrumentation through the skin or mucous membrane and any other body layers necessary to aid in the performance of the procedure
External	Procedures performed directly on the skin or mucous membrane and procedures performed indirectly by the application of external force through the skin or mucous membrane

ICD-10-PCS DEVICE AND SUBSTANCE CLASSIFICATION

This appendix discusses the distinguishing features of device, substance and equipment as classified in ICD-10-PCS, to provide further guidance for correct identification and coding. The appendix includes discussion of the ICD-10-PCS definitions and classification of device, substance and equipment, and is accompanied by specific coding instruction and examples.

ICD-10-PCS DEVICE CLASSIFICATION

In most ICD-10-PCS codes, the 6th character of the code is used to classify device. The 6th character device value "defines the material or appliance used to accomplish the objective of the procedure that remains in or on the procedure site at the end of the procedure." If the device is the means by which the procedural objective is accomplished, then a specific device value is coded in the 6th character. If no device is used to accomplish the objective of the procedure, the device value NO DEVICE is coded in the 6th character.

For example, an aortocoronary bypass that uses saphenous vein graft to accomplish the bypass is coded to the device value Autologous Venous Tissue in the 6th character of the ICD-10-PCS code. A coronary bypass that uses the patient's internal mammary artery directly to accomplish the bypass uses the device value NO DEVICE in the 6th character of the ICD-10-PCS code

DEVICE AND PROCEDURAL OBJECTIVE

Whether or not the material used in a procedure should be coded using a specific ICD-10-PCS device value can be determined primarily by asking the question

- Is this material central to achieving the objective of the procedure, or does it only support the performance of the procedure?

For example, radiological markers are put in the procedure site to guide the performance of a primary procedure such as excision of a tumor, whereas radioactive brachytherapy seeds are put in the procedure site as an end in themselves, to treat a malignant tumor. The radiological marker is not classified as a device in ICD-10-PCS, but the brachytherapy seeds are classified to the device value RADIOACTIVE ELEMENT in the root operation INSERTION.

The same device coded as a specific device value for one procedure may not be coded at all for another procedure where it is not central to the procedural objective. For example, a procedure performed specifically to place a drain in a body part for diagnostic or therapeutic purposes is coded to the root operation DRAINAGE with the specific device value DRAINAGE DEVICE in the 6th character of the code. However, a wound drain placed at an incision site at the conclusion of the procedure to promote healing is not central to the procedural objective and therefore not coded separately as a device in ICD-10-PCS. For this reason, materials such as wound dressings and operative site drains that support the performance of the procedure are not coded separately.

Sutures and suture alternatives (e.g., fibrin glue, Dermabond, specialized vessel closures) are not coded as devices in ICD-10-PCS, because in most cases using material to bring the edges of a procedure site together is not central to the procedural objective, but is used to support the performance of the procedure (to close the site). For procedures where the sole objective is to close a wound created by trauma or other incident, the procedure is coded to the root operation REPAIR with the device value NO DEVICE in the 6th character of the ICD-10-PCS code.

DEVICE AND LOCATION

Whether material or an appliance is coded as a device cannot be determined by the size, shape or complexity of the object or material being used. A device may be too small to be seen with the naked eye (microcoils used to occlude a vessel) or two feet long (external fixator for a long bone). A device may be of a predetermined shape (prosthetic heart valve) or no particular shape (morselized bone graft). A device may be a highly complex machine (cardiac synchronization pacemaker/defibrillator) or a simple piece of hardware (internal fixation bone screw).

However, material that is classified as a ICD-10-PCS device is distinguished from material classified as a ICD-10-PCS substance by the fact that it has a specific location. A device is intended to maintain a fixed location at the procedure site where it was put, whereas a substance is intended to disperse or be absorbed in the body. Indeed, a device that does not stay where it was put may need to be "revised" in a subsequent procedure, to move the device back to its intended location.

DEVICE AND REMOVABILITY

Material that is classified as a ICD-10-PCS device is also distinguishable by the fact that it is removable. Although it may not be *practical* to remove some types of devices once they become established at the site, it is *physically possible* to remove a device for some time after the procedure. A skin graft, once it "takes," may be nearly indistinguishable from the surrounding skin and so is no longer clearly identifiable as a device. Nevertheless, procedures that involve material coded as a device can for the most part be "reversed" by removing the device from the procedure site.

DEVICE DISTRIBUTION IN ICD-10-PCS

The general distribution and use of the 6th character when specified as a device is summarized in the table below. The sections and root operations that specify device in the 6th character are listed. Also included are examples of 6th character values and corresponding procedure examples.

PCS Section	Root Operation	Device Value Example	Procedure Example
Medical and Surgical	Alteration	Autologous Tissue Substitute	Nasal tip elevation using fat autograft
Medical and Surgical	Bypass	Synthetic Substitute	Femoral-popliteal bypass using synthetic graft
Medical and Surgical	Change	Drainage Device	Foley catheter exchange
Medical and Surgical	Creation	Nonautologous Tissue Substitute	Sex change operation using tissue bank graft material
Medical and Surgical	Dilation	Intraluminal Device	Percutaneous coronary angioplasty using stent
Medical and Surgical	Drainage	Drainage Device	Drainage of pleural effusion using chest tube
Medical and Surgical	Fusion	Interbody Fusion Device	Spinal interbody fusion
Medical and Surgical	Insertion	Infusion Pump	Insertion of infusion pump for pain control
Medical and Surgical	Occlusion	Extraluminal Device	Fallopian tube ligation using clips
Medical and Surgical	Removal	Spacer	Removal of joint spacer
Medical and Surgical	Replacement	Autologous Tissue Substitute	Skin graft using patient's own skin
Medical and Surgical	Reposition	Internal Fixation Device	Fracture reduction with plate and screw fixation
Medical and Surgical	Restriction	Extraluminal Device	Laparoscopic gastric banding, adjustable band
Medical and Surgical	Revision	Neurostimulator Lead	Reposition of spinal neurostimulator lead
Medical and Surgical	Supplement	Zooplastic Tissue	Pulmonary artery patch graft using bovine pericardium
Obstetrics	Insertion, Removal	Monitoring Electrode	Insertion of fetal monitoring electrode
Placement	Change	Cast	Forearm cast change
Placement	Compression	Pressure Dressing	Application of pressure dressing to lower leg
Placement	Dressing	Bandage	Application of bandage to chest wall

PCS Section	Root Operation	Device Value Example	Procedure Example
Placement	Immobilization	Splint	Splint placement to wrist
Placement	Packing	Packing Material	Nasal packing
Placement	Removal	Brace	Removal of back brace
Placement	Traction	Traction Apparatus	Skin traction of lower leg using traction device

ICD-10-PCS SUBSTANCE CLASSIFICATION

The 6th character substance value "defines the blood component or other liquid put in or on the body to accomplish the objective of the procedure." The 6th character is defined as substance in the ADMINISTRATION section. Administration is the only section where a substance is classified as a separate code, and not included as information in a more definitive procedure.

SUBSTANCE AND PROCEDURAL OBJECTIVE

Many different substances are typically put in or on the body in the course of an inpatient hospital stay, both during surgical procedures and at the bedside. Only those which meet UHDDS and facility coding guidelines are coded separately. Most material classified as a substance in the ADMINISTRATION section is in liquid form and intended to be immediately absorbed by the body or, in the case of blood and blood products, disseminated in the circulatory system. An exception is the substance value ADHESION BARRIER. It is a non-liquid substance classified in the Administration section, and coded separately for tracking purposes.

SUBSTANCE AND REMOVABILITY

Most substances cannot be removed once they are administered, because the whole point of administering them is for them to be dispersed and/or absorbed by the body. Imaging contrast is sometimes extracted from the bloodstream at the conclusion of a procedure to minimize the possibility of adverse effects.

SUBSTANCE DISTRIBUTION IN ADMINISTRATION SECTION

The general distribution and use of the 6th character specified as a substance in the ADMINISTRATION section is summarized in the table below. All root operations that specify substance in the 6th character are listed. Also included are examples of 6th character values and corresponding procedure examples.

Root Operation	Substance Value Example	Procedure Example
Introduction	Nutritional substance	Infusion of total parenteral nutrition
Irrigation	Irrigating Substance	Irrigation of eye
Transfusion	Frozen Plasma	Transfusion of frozen plasma

CLASSIFICATION OF SUBSTANCE IN ANCILLARY SECTIONS

Three ancillary sections record their own specific substance values as part of the ICD-10-PCS code, where a substance is used to support the objective of the procedure. They are the IMAGING, NUCLEAR MEDICINE and RADIATION ONCOLOGY sections, and they specify CONTRAST, RADIONUCLIDE and RADIOISOTOPE respectively. However, these substance values are unambiguously included as part of a more definitive procedure code, to be recorded when the substance is used to support the objective of the procedure. Substances in these three ancillary sections are therefore not likely to be confused with separately coded substances in the ADMINISTRATION section.

SUBSTANCE DISTRIBUTION IN ANCILLARY SECTIONS

The three ancillary sections that specify a type of substance used in the procedure are summarized in the table below. The sections and the type of substance classified are listed along with the ICD-10-PCS character where this information is recorded. Also included are examples of the values used and corresponding procedure examples.

PCS Section	Substance Classified	Substance Value Example	Procedure Example
Imaging	Contrast (5th character)	Low Osmolar Contrast	Left heart ventriculography using low osmolar contrast
Nuclear Medicine	Radionuclide (5th character)	Fluorine 18	PET scan of brain using Fluorine 18
Radiation oncology	Isotope (6th character)	Iodine 125	HDR brachytherapy of thyroid using Iodine 125

EQUIPMENT AND ICD-10-PCS CODING

For the most part, equipment used to assist in the performance of the procedure is not coded in ICD-10-PCS.

The only exception to this rule occurs in the REHABILITATION AND DIAGNOSTIC AUDIOLOGY section, where the 6th character is specified as *equipment*. The 6th character values in the REHABILITATION AND DIAGNOSTIC AUDIOLOGY section are used to capture information about the machine, physical aid, or other equipment used to assist in performing the procedure.

EQUIPMENT AND PROCEDURAL OBJECTIVE

For all other sections in ICD-10-PCS, equipment is distinguished from a codeable device by the fact that equipment is a method used to support the performance of a procedure. For example, the machine used to maintain cardiovascular circulation during an open heart bypass procedure is equipment that performs the circulatory functions for the heart so that the heart bypass can be performed. This support procedure is coded to the root operation PERFORMANCE in the EXTRACORPOREAL ASSISTANCE AND PERFORMANCE section, and the type of equipment used is not captured in the code. The primary procedure is coded to the root operation BYPASS in the MEDICAL AND SURGICAL section, and any graft material used is coded to the appropriate 6th character device value.

EQUIPMENT AND LOCATION

Equipment is also distinguished from a codeable device in ICD-10-PCS by the fact that equipment resides primarily outside the body during the procedure. Cardiopulmonary circulatory support is coded to the EXTRACORPOREAL ASSISTANCE AND PERFORMANCE section and the type of equipment used is not recorded in the ICD-10-PCS code. With cardiovascular support equipment, the machinery resides primarily outside the body. The outtake and return cannulae are the only portions of the machine directly connected to the patient.

On the other hand, insertion of intra-aortic balloon pump is coded as a separate INSERTION procedure in ICD-10-PCS, in addition to the ICD-10-PCS code in the EXTRACORPOREAL ASSISTANCE AND PERFOR-MANCE section specifying assistance with cardiac output. The intra-aortic balloon pump resides principally in the patient's body. The balloon mechanism that supports cardiac output is in the aorta itself.

Mechanical ventilation is also coded to the EXTRACORPOREAL ASSISTANCE AND PERFORMANCE section and the equipment used is not recorded in the ICD-10-PCS code. As with cardiovascular support equipment, the mechanical ventilation machine resides primarily outside the body. The endotracheal tube is the only portion of the machine directly connected to the patient. Insertion of the endotracheal tube as part of a mechanical ventilation procedure is not coded as a separate device insertion procedure, because it is merely the interface between the patient and the equipment used to perform the procedure, rather than an end in itself.

On the other hand, insertion of an endotracheal tube in order to maintain an airway in patients who are unconscious or unable to breathe on their own is the central objective of the procedure. Therefore, insertion of an endotracheal tube as an end in itself is coded to the root operation INSERTION and the device ENDOTRACHEAL AIRWAY.

EQUIPMENT AND REMOVABILITY

Equipment used solely to support the performance of a procedure and therefore not coded in ICD-10-PCS can be further distinguished by the fact that the equipment is used only for the duration of the procedure. Once the procedure is completed, any portions of the equipment attached to the patient are disconnected. For example, a patient no longer requiring mechanical ventilation is "extubated," or disconnected from the equipment that provides ventilation support.

SUMMARY

Three distinguishing features have been identified to enable correct identification and coding of device, substance and equipment: procedural objective, location, and removability. The procedural objective alone is sufficient in most cases to determine whether material or an appliance used in a procedure should be coded in ICD-10-PCS. Once it is determined that the information should be coded in ICD-10-PCS, location and removability are useful in determining whether the item is classified as a device or substance. The following table summarizes the distinguishing features of device, substance, and equipment in relation to each other, along with examples.

PCS 6th Character	Procedural Objective	Location	Removability	Procedure Example
Device	Material or appliance put in or on the body is central to accomplishing the procedural objective	Resides at the site of the procedure, not intended to change location	Capable of being removed from the procedure site	Neurostimulator lead insertion
Substance	Liquid or blood component is central to accomplishing the procedural objective	No fixed position, intended to be absorbed or dispersed	Not removable, once dispersed or absorbed	Antibiotic injection
Equipment	Machinery or other aid used to perform a procedure	Resides primarily outside the body	Temporary, used for the duration of the procedure only	Mechanical ventilation

ICD-10-PCS OFFICIAL GUIDELINES
FOR CODING AND REPORTING

The Centers for Medicare and Medicaid Services (CMS) and the National Center for Health Statistics (NCHS), two departments within the U.S. Federal Government's Department of Health and Human Services (DHHS) provide the following guidelines for coding and reporting using the International Classification of Diseases, 10th Revision, Procedure Coding System (ICD-10-PCS). These guidelines should be used as a companion document to the official version of the ICD-10-PCS as published on the CMS website. The ICD-10-PCS is a procedure classification published by the United States for classifying procedures performed in hospital inpatient health care settings.

These guidelines have been approved by the four organizations that make up the Cooperating Parties for the ICD-10-PCS: the American Hospital Association (AHA), the American Health Information Management Association (AHIMA), CMS, and NCHS.

These guidelines are a set of rules that have been developed to accompany and complement the official conventions and instructions provided within the ICD-10-PCS itself. The instructions and conventions of the classification take precedence over guidelines. These guidelines are based on the coding and sequencing instructions in the Tables, Index and Definitions of ICD-10-PCS, but provide additional instruction. Adherence to these guidelines when assigning ICD-10-PCS procedure codes is required under the Health Insurance Portability and Accountability Act (HIPAA). The procedure codes have been adopted under HIPAA for hospital inpatient healthcare settings. A joint effort between the healthcare provider and the coder is essential to achieve complete and accurate documentation, code assignment, and reporting of diagnoses and procedures. These guidelines have been developed to assist both the healthcare provider and the coder in identifying those procedures that are to be reported. The importance of consistent, complete documentation in the medical record cannot be overemphasized. Without such documentation accurate coding cannot be achieved.

CONVENTIONS

A1   ICD-10-PCS codes are composed of seven characters. Each character is an axis of classification that specifies information about the procedure performed. Within a defined code range, a character specifies the same type of information in that axis of classification.

Example: The fifth axis of classification specifies the approach in sections 0 through 4 and 7 through 9 of the system.

A2   One of 34 possible values can be assigned to each axis of classification in the seven-character code: they are the numbers 0 through 9 and the alphabet (except I and O because they are easily confused with the numbers 1 and 0). The number of unique values used in an axis of classification differs as needed.

Example: Where the fifth axis of classification specifies the approach, seven different approach values are currently used to specify the approach.

A3   The valid values for an axis of classification can be added to as needed.

Example: If a significantly distinct type of device is used in a new procedure, a new device value can be added to the system.

A4   As with words in their context, the meaning of any single value is a combination of its axis of classification and any preceding values on which it may be dependent.

Example: The meaning of a body part value in the Medical and Surgical section is always dependent on the body system value. The body part value 0 in the Central Nervous body system specifies Brain and the body part value 0 in the Peripheral Nervous body system specifies Cervical Plexus.

A5   As the system is expanded to become increasingly detailed, over time more values will depend on preceding values for their meaning.

Example: In the Lower Joints body system, the device value 3 in the root operation Insertion specifies Infusion Device and the device value 3 in the root operation Replacement specifies Ceramic Synthetic Substitute.

Example: In the Lower Joints body system, the device value 3 in the root operation Insertion specifies Infusion Device and the device value 3 in the root operation Replacement specifies Ceramic Synthetic Substitute.

A6   The purpose of the alphabetic index is to locate the appropriate table that contains all information necessary to construct a procedure code. The PCS Tables should always be consulted to find the most appropriate valid code.

A7   It is not required to consult the index first before proceeding to the tables to complete the code. A valid code may be chosen directly from the tables.

A8   All seven characters must be specified to be a valid code. If the documentation is incomplete for coding purposes, the physician should be queried for the necessary information.

A9   Within a PCS table, valid codes include all combinations of choices in characters 4 through 7 contained in the same row of the table. In the example below, 0JHT3VZ is a valid code, and 0JHW3VZ is *not* a valid code

Section:	0	Medical and Surgical		
Body System:	J	Subcutaneous Tissue and Fascia		
Operation:	H	Insertion: Putting in a nonbiological appliance that monitors, assists, performs, or prevents a physiological function but does not physically take the place of a body part		

Body Part	Approach	Device	Qualifier
S Subcutaneous Tissue and Fascia, Head and Neck V Subcutaneous Tissue and Fascia, Upper Extremity W Subcutaneous Tissue and Fascia, Lower Extremity	0 Open 3 Percutaneous	1 Radioactive Element 3 Infusion Device	Z No Qualifier
T Subcutaneous Tissue and Fascia, Trunk	0 Open 3 Percutaneous	1 Radioactive Element 3 Infusion Device V Infusion Pump	Z No Qualifier

A10   "And," when used in a code description, means "and/or."

Example: Lower Arm and Wrist Muscle means lower arm and/or wrist muscle.

A11   Many of the terms used to construct PCS codes are defined within the system. It is the coder's responsibility to determine what the documentation in the medical record equates to in the PCS definitions. The physician is not expected to use the terms used in PCS code descriptions, nor is the coder required to query the physician when the correlation between the documentation and the defined PCS terms is clear.

Example: When the physician documents "partial resection" the coder can independently correlate "partial resection" to the root operation Excision without querying the physician for clarification.

MEDICAL AND SURGICAL SECTION GUIDELINES (SECTION 0)

B2. Body System

General guidelines

B2.1a   The procedure codes in the general anatomical regions body systems can be used when the procedure is performed on an anatomical region rather than a specific body part (e.g., root operations Control and Detachment, Drainage of a body cavity) or on the rare occasion when no information is available to support assignment of a code to a specific body part.

Examples: Control of postoperative hemorrhage is coded to the root operation Control found in the general anatomical regions body systems.

Chest tube drainage of the pleural cavity is coded to the root operation Drainage found in the general anatomical regions body systems. Suture repair of the abdominal wall is coded to the root operation Repair in the general anatomical regions body system.

B2.1b Where the general body part values "upper" and "lower" are provided as an option in the Upper Arteries, Lower Arteries, Upper Veins, Lower Veins, Muscles and Tendons body systems, "upper" or "lower "specifies body parts located above or below the diaphragm respectively.

Example: Vein body parts above the diaphragm are found in the Upper Veins body system; vein body parts below the diaphragm are found in the Lower Veins body system.

B3. Root Operation

General guidelines

B3.1a In order to determine the appropriate root operation, the full definition of the root operation as contained in the PCS Tables must be applied.

B3.1b Components of a procedure specified in the root operation definition and explanation are not coded separately. Procedural steps necessary to reach the operative site and close the operative site, including anastomosis of a tubular body part, are also not coded separately.

Examples: Resection of a joint as part of a joint replacement procedure is included in the root operation definition of Replacement and is not coded separately.

Laparotomy performed to reach the site of an open liver biopsy is not coded separately. In a resection of sigmoid colon with anastomosis of descending colon to rectum, the anastomosis is not coded separately.

Multiple procedures

a. The same root operation is performed on different body parts as defined by distinct values of the body part character.

Examples: Diagnostic excision of liver and pancreas are coded separately. Excision of lesion in the ascending colon and excision of lesion in the transverse colon are coded separately.

b. The same root operation is repeated in multiple body parts, and those body parts are separate and distinct body parts classified to a single ICD-10-PCS body part value.

Examples: Excision of the sartorius muscle and excision of the gracilis muscle are both included in the upper leg muscle body part value, and multiple procedures are coded.

Extraction of multiple toenails are coded separately.

c. Multiple root operations with distinct objectives are performed on the same body part.

Example: Destruction of sigmoid lesion and bypass of sigmoid colon are coded separately.

d. The intended root operation is attempted using one approach, but is converted to a different approach.

Example: Laparoscopic cholecystectomy converted to an open cholecystectomy is coded as percutaneous endoscopic Inspection and open Resection.

Example: Laparoscopic cholecystectomy converted to an open cholecystectomy is coded as percutaneous endoscopic Inspection and open Resection.

Discontinued procedures

B3.3   If the intended procedure is discontinued, code the procedure to the root operation performed. If a procedure is discontinued before any other root operation is performed, code the root operation Inspection of the body part or anatomical region inspected.

Example: A planned aortic valve replacement procedure is discontinued after the initial thoracotomy and before any incision is made in the heart muscle, when the patient becomes hemodynamically unstable. This procedure is coded as an open Inspection of the mediastinum.

Biopsy procedures

B3.4a   Biopsy procedures are coded using the root operations Excision, Extraction, or Drainage and the qualifier Diagnostic.

Examples: Fine needle aspiration biopsy of fluid in the lung is coded to the root operation Drainage with the qualifier Diagnostic.

Biopsy of bone marrow is coded to the root operation Extraction with the qualifier Diagnostic. Lymph node sampling for biopsy is coded to the root operation Excision with the qualifier Diagnostic.

Biopsy followed by more definitive treatment

B3.4b   If a diagnostic Excision, Extraction, or Drainage procedure (biopsy) is followed by a more definitive procedure, such as Destruction, Excision or Resection at the same procedure site, both the biopsy and the more definitive treatment are coded.

Example: Biopsy of breast followed by partial mastectomy at the same procedure site, both the biopsy and the partial mastectomy procedure are coded.

Overlapping body layers

B3.5   If the root operations Excision, Repair or Inspection are performed on overlapping layers of the musculoskeletal system, the body part specifying the deepest layer is coded. *Example*: Excisional debridement that includes skin and subcutaneous tissue and muscle is coded to the muscle body part.

Bypass procedures

B3.6a   Bypass procedures are coded by identifying the body part bypassed "from" and the body part bypassed "to." The fourth character body part specifies the body part bypassed from, and the qualifier specifies the body part bypassed to.

Example: Bypass from stomach to jejunum, stomach is the body part and jejunum is the qualifier.

B3.6b   Coronary artery bypass procedures are coded differently than other bypass procedures as described in the previous guideline. Rather than identifying the body part bypassed from, the body part identifies the number of coronary artery sites bypassed to, and the qualifier specifies the vessel bypassed from.

Example: Aortocoronary artery bypass of the left anterior descending coronary artery and the obtuse marginal coronary artery is classified in the body part axis of classification as two coronary arteries, and the qualifier specifies the aorta as the body part bypassed from.

B3.6c   If multiple coronary arteries are bypassed, a separate procedure is coded for each coronary artery that uses a different device and/or qualifier.

Example: Aortocoronary artery bypass and internal mammary coronary artery bypass are coded separately.

Control vs. more definitive root operations

B3.7 The root operation Control is defined as, "Stopping, or attempting to stop, postprocedural or other acute bleeding." If an attempt to stop postprocedural or other acute bleeding is initially unsuccessful, and to stop the bleeding requires performing any of the definitive root operations Bypass, Detachment, Excision, Extraction, Reposition, Replacement, or Resection, then that root operation is coded instead of Control.

Example: Resection of spleen to stop bleeding is coded to Resection instead of Control.

Excision vs. Resection

B3.8 PCS contains specific body parts for anatomical subdivisions of a body part, such as lobes of the lungs or liver and regions of the intestine. Resection of the specific body part is coded whenever all of the body part is cut out or off, rather than coding Excision of a less specific body part.

Example: Left upper lung lobectomy is coded to Resection of Upper Lung Lobe, Left rather than Excision of Lung, Left.

Excision for graft

B3.9 If an autograft is obtained from a different procedure site in order to complete the objective of the procedure, a separate procedure is coded.

Example: Coronary bypass with excision of saphenous vein graft, excision of saphenous vein is coded separately.

Fusion procedures of the spine

B3.10a The body part coded for a spinal vertebral joint(s) rendered immobile by a spinal fusion procedure is classified by the level of the spine (e.g. thoracic). There are distinct body part values for a single vertebral joint and for multiple vertebral joints at each spinal level.

Example: Body part values specify Lumbar Vertebral Joint, Lumbar Vertebral Joints, 2 or More and Lumbosacral Vertebral Joint.

B3.10b If multiple vertebral joints are fused, a separate procedure is coded for each vertebral joint that uses a different device and/or qualifier.

Example: Fusion of lumbar vertebral joint, posterior approach, anterior column and fusion of lumbar vertebral joint, posterior approach, posterior column are coded separately.

B3.10c Combinations of devices and materials are often used on a vertebral joint to render the joint immobile. When combinations of devices are used on the same vertebral joint, the device value coded for the procedure is as follows:

- If an interbody fusion device is used to render the joint immobile (alone or containing other material like bone graft), the procedure is coded with the device value Interbody Fusion Device
- If bone graft is the *only* device used to render the joint immobile, the procedure is coded with the device value Nonautologous Tissue Substitute or Autologous Tissue Substitute
- If a mixture of autologous and nonautologous bone graft (with or without biological or synthetic extenders or binders) is used to render the joint immobile, code the procedure with the device value Autologous Tissue Substitute

Examples: Fusion of a vertebral joint using a cage style interbody fusion device containing morselized bone graft is coded to the device Interbody Fusion Device. Fusion of a vertebral joint using a bone dowel interbody fusion device made of cadaver bone and packed with a mixture of local morselized bone and demineralized bone matrix is coded to the device Interbody Fusion Device.

Fusion of a vertebral joint using both autologous bone graft and bone bank bone graft is coded to the device Autologous Tissue Substitute.

Inspection procedures

B3.11a   Inspection of a body part(s) performed in order to achieve the objective of a procedure is not coded separately.

Example: Fiberoptic bronchoscopy performed for irrigation of bronchus, only the irrigation procedure is coded.

B3.11b   If multiple tubular body parts are inspected, the most distal body part (the body part furthest from the starting point of the inspection) is coded. If multiple non-tubular body parts in a region are inspected, the body part that specifies the entire area inspected is coded.

Examples: Cystoureteroscopy with inspection of bladder and ureters is coded to the ureter body part value. Exploratory laparotomy with general inspection of abdominal contents is coded to the peritoneal cavity body part value.

B3.11c   When both an Inspection procedure and another procedure are performed on the same body part during the same episode, if the Inspection procedure is performed using a different approach than the other procedure, the Inspection procedure is coded separately.

Example: Endoscopic Inspection of the duodenum is coded separately when open Excision of the duodenum is performed during the same procedural episode.

Occlusion vs. Restriction for vessel embolization procedures

B3.12   If the objective of an embolization procedure is to completely close a vessel, the root operation Occlusion is coded. If the objective of an embolization procedure is to narrow the lumen of a vessel, the root operation Restriction is coded.

Examples: Tumor embolization is coded to the root operation Occlusion, because the objective of the procedure is to cut off the blood supply to the vessel.

Embolization of a cerebral aneurysm is coded to the root operation Restriction, because the objective of the procedure is not to close off the vessel entirely, but to narrow the lumen of the vessel at the site of the aneurysm where it is abnormally wide.

Release procedures

B3.13   In the root operation Release, the body part value coded is the body part being freed and not the tissue being manipulated or cut to free the body part.

Example: Lysis of intestinal adhesions is coded to the specific intestine body part value.

Release vs. Division

B3.14   If the sole objective of the procedure is freeing a body part without cutting the body part, the root operation is Release. If the sole objective of the procedure is separating or transecting a body part, the root operation is Division.

Examples: Freeing a nerve root from surrounding scar tissue to relieve pain is coded to the root operation Release. Severing a nerve root to relieve pain is coded to the root operation Division.

Reposition for fracture treatment

B3.15   Reduction of a displaced fracture is coded to the root operation Reposition and the application of a cast or splint in conjunction with the Reposition procedure is not coded separately. Treatment of a nondisplaced fracture is coded to the procedure performed.

Examples: Putting a pin in a nondisplaced fracture is coded to the root operation Insertion.

Casting of a nondisplaced fracture is coded to the root operation Immobilization in the Placement section.

Transplantation vs. Administration

B3.16   Putting in a mature and functioning living body part taken from another individual or animal is coded to the root operation Transplantation. Putting in autologous or nonautologous cells is coded to the Administration section.

Example: Putting in autologous or nonautologous bone marrow, pancreatic islet cells or stem cells is coded to the Administration section.

B4. Body Part

General guidelines

B4.1a   If a procedure is performed on a portion of a body part that does not have a separate body part value, code the body part value corresponding to the whole body part.

Example: A procedure performed on the alveolar process of the mandible is coded to the mandible body part.

B4.1b   If the prefix "peri" is combined with a body part to identify the site of the procedure, and the site of the procedure is not further specified, then the procedure is coded to the body part named. This guideline applies only when a more specific body part value is not available.

Examples: A procedure site identified as perirenal is coded to the kidney body part when the site of the procedure is not further specified.

A procedure site described in the documentation as peri-urethral, and the documentation also indicates that it is the vulvar tissue and not the urethral tissue that is the site of the procedure, then the procedure is coded to the vulva body part.

Branches of body parts

B4.2   Where a specific branch of a body part does not have its own body part value in PCS, the body part is typically coded to the closest proximal branch that has a specific body part value. In the cardiovascular body systems, if a general body part is available in the correct root operation table, and coding to a proximal branch would require assigning a code in a different body system, the procedure is coded using the general body part value.

Examples: A procedure performed on the mandibular branch of the trigeminal nerve is coded to the trigeminal nerve body part value.

Occlusion of the bronchial artery is coded to the body part value Upper Artery in the body system Upper Arteries, and not to the body part value Thoracic Aorta, Descending in the body system Heart and Great Vessels.

Bilateral body part values

B4.3   Bilateral body part values are available for a limited number of body parts. If the identical procedure is performed on contralateral body parts, and a bilateral body part value exists for that body part, a single procedure is coded using the bilateral body part value. If no bilateral body part value exists, each procedure is coded separately using the appropriate body part value.

Examples: The identical procedure performed on both fallopian tubes is coded once using the body part value Fallopian Tube, Bilateral.

The identical procedure performed on both knee joints is coded twice using the body part values Knee Joint, Right and Knee Joint, Left.

Coronary arteries

B4.4   The coronary arteries are classified as a single body part that is further specified by number of arteries treated. One procedure code specifying multiple arteries is used when the same procedure is performed, including the same device and qualifier values. Separate codes are used when the same procedure is performed on multiple sites in the coronary arteries.

Examples: Angioplasty of two distinct coronary arteries with placement of two stents is coded as Dilation of Coronary Arteries, Two Arteries, with Intraluminal Device.

Angioplasty of two distinct coronary arteries, one with stent placed and one without, is coded separately as Dilation of Coronary Artery, One Artery with Intraluminal Device, and Dilation of Coronary Artery, One Artery with no device.

Tendons, ligaments, bursae and fascia near a joint

B4.5   Procedures performed on tendons, ligaments, bursae and fascia supporting a joint are coded to the body part in the respective body system that is the focus of the procedure. Procedures performed on joint structures themselves are coded to the body part in the joint body systems.

Examples: Repair of the anterior cruciate ligament of the knee is coded to the knee bursa and ligament body part in the bursae and ligaments body system.

Knee arthroscopy with shaving of articular cartilage is coded to the knee joint body part in the Lower Joints body system.

Skin, subcutaneous tissue and fascia overlying a joint

B4.6   If a procedure is performed on the skin, subcutaneous tissue or fascia overlying a joint, the procedure is coded to the following body part:

- Shoulder is coded to Upper Arm
- Elbow is coded to Lower Arm
- Wrist is coded to Lower Arm
- Hip is coded to Upper Leg
- Knee is coded to Lower Leg
- Ankle is coded to Foot

Fingers and toes

B4.7   If a body system does not contain a separate body part value for fingers, procedures performed on the fingers are coded to the body part value for the hand. If a body system does not contain a separate body part value for toes, procedures performed on the toes are coded to the body part value for the foot.

Example: Excision of finger muscle is coded to one of the hand muscle body part values in the Muscles body system.

Upper and lower intestinal tract

B4.8   In the Gastrointestinal body system, the general body part values Upper Intestinal Tract and Lower Intestinal Tract are provided as an option for the root operations Change, Inspection, Removal and Revision. Upper Intestinal Tract includes the portion of the gastrointestinal tract from the esophagus down to and including the duodenum, and Lower Intestinal Tract includes the portion of the gastrointestinal tract from the jejunum down to and including the rectum and anus.

Example: In the root operation Change table, change of a device in the jejunum is coded using the body part Lower Intestinal Tract.

B5. Approach

Open approach with percutaneous endoscopic assistance

B5.2 Procedures performed using the open approach with percutaneous endoscopic assistance are coded to the approach Open.

Example: Laparoscopic-assisted sigmoidectomy is coded to the approach Open.

External approach

B5.3a Procedures performed within an orifice on structures that are visible without the aid of any instrumentation are coded to the approach External.

Example: Resection of tonsils is coded to the approach External.

B5.3b Procedures performed indirectly by the application of external force through the intervening body layers are coded to the approach External.

Example: Closed reduction of fracture is coded to the approach External.

Percutaneous procedure via device

B5.4 Procedures performed percutaneously via a device placed for the procedure are coded to the approach Percutaneous.

Example: Fragmentation of kidney stone performed via percutaneous nephrostomy is coded to the approach Percutaneous.

B6. Device

General guidelines

B6.1a A device is coded only if a device remains after the procedure is completed. If no device remains, the device value No Device is coded.

B6.1b Materials such as sutures, ligatures, radiological markers and temporary post-operative wound drains are considered integral to the performance of a procedure and are not coded as devices.

B6.1c Procedures performed on a device only and not on a body part are specified in the root operations Change, Irrigation, Removal and Revision, and are coded to the procedure performed.

Example: Irrigation of percutaneous nephrostomy tube is coded to the root operation Irrigation of indwelling device in the Administration section.

Drainage device

B6.2 A separate procedure to put in a drainage device is coded to the root operation Drainage with the device value Drainage Device.

Obstetric Section Guidelines (section 1)

C. Obstetrics Section

Products of conception

C1 Procedures performed on the products of conception are coded to the Obstetrics section. Procedures performed on the pregnant female other than the products of conception are coded to the appropriate root operation in the Medical and Surgical section.

Example: Amniocentesis is coded to the products of conception body part in the Obstetrics section. Repair of obstetric urethral laceration is coded to the urethra body part in the Medical and Surgical section.

Procedures following delivery or abortion

C2   Procedures performed following a delivery or abortion for curettage of the endometrium or evacuation of retained products of conception are all coded in the Obstetrics section, to the root operation Extraction and the body part Products of Conception, Retained. Diagnostic or therapeutic dilation and curettage performed during times other than the postpartum or post-abortion period are all coded in the Medical and Surgical section, to the root operation Extraction and the body part Endometrium.

New Technology Section Guidelines (section X)

D. New Technology Section

General guidelines

D1   Section X codes are standalone codes. They are not supplemental codes. Section X codes fully represent the specific procedure described in the code title, and do not require any additional codes from other sections of ICD-10-PCS. When section X contains a code title which describes a specific new technology procedure, only that X code is reported for the procedure. There is no need to report a broader, non-specific code in another section of ICD-10-PCS.

    Example: XW04321 Introduction of Ceftazidime-Avibactam Anti-infective into Central Vein, Percutaneous Approach, New Technology Group 1, can be coded to indicate that Ceftazidime-Avibactam Anti-infective was administered via a central vein. A separate code from table 3E0 in the Administration section of ICD-10-PCS is not coded in addition to this code.

Selection of Principal Procedure

The following instructions should be applied in the selection of principal procedure and clarification on the importance of the relation to the principal diagnosis when more than one procedure is performed:

1. Procedure performed for definitive treatment of both principal diagnosis and secondary diagnosis

    a. Sequence procedure performed for definitive treatment most related to principal diagnosis as principal procedure.

2. Procedure performed for definitive treatment and diagnostic procedures performed for both principal diagnosis and secondary diagnosis

    a. Sequence procedure performed for definitive treatment most related to principal diagnosis as principal procedure

3. A diagnostic procedure was performed for the principal diagnosis and a procedure is performed for definitive treatment of a secondary diagnosis.

    a. Sequence diagnostic procedure as principal procedure, since the procedure most related to the principal diagnosis takes precedence.

4. No procedures performed that are related to principal diagnosis; procedures performed for definitive treatment and diagnostic procedures were performed for secondary diagnosis

    a. Sequence procedure performed for definitive treatment of secondary diagnosis as principal procedure, since there are no procedures (definitive or nondefinitive treatment) related to principal diagnosis.

Anatomical Illustrations

A fundamental knowledge and understanding of basic human anatomy and physiology is a prerequisite for accurate diagnosis coding. While a comprehensive treatment of anatomy and physiology is beyond the scope of this text, the large scale, full color anatomical illustrations on the following pages are designed to facilitate the procedure coding process for both beginning and experienced coders.

The illustrations provide an anatomical perspective of procedure coding by providing a side-by-side view of the major systems of the human body and a corresponding list of the most common ICD-10-PCS categories used to report medical, surgical and diagnostic procedures performed on the illustrated system.

The ICD-10-PCS categories listed on the left facing page of each anatomical illustration are code ranges only and should not be used for coding. These categories are provided as "pointers" to the appropriate section of ICD-10-PCS, where the definitive code may be found.

PLATE 1. SKIN AND SUBCUTANEOUS TISSUE – MALE

Skin and Breast, Alteration	0H0
Skin and Breast, Change	0H2
Skin and Breast, Destruction	0H5
Skin and Breast, Division	0H8
Skin and Breast, Drainage	0H9
Skin and Breast, Excision	0HB
Skin and Breast, Extirpation	0HC
Skin and Breast, Extraction	0HD
Skin and Breast, Insertion	0HH
Skin and Breast, Inspection	0HJ
Skin and Breast, Reattachment	0HM
Skin and Breast, Release	0HN
Skin and Breast, Removal	0HP
Skin and Breast, Repair	0HQ
Skin and Breast, Replacement	0HR
Skin and Breast, Reposition	0HS
Skin and Breast, Resection	0HT
Skin and Breast, Supplement	0HU
Skin and Breast, Revision	0HW
Skin and Breast, Transfer	0HX
Subcutaneous Tissue and Fascia, Alteration	0J0
Subcutaneous Tissue and Fascia, Change	0J2
Subcutaneous Tissue and Fascia, Destruction	0J5
Subcutaneous Tissue and Fascia, Division	0J8
Subcutaneous Tissue and Fascia, Drainage	0J9
Subcutaneous Tissue and Fascia, Excision	0JB
Subcutaneous Tissue and Fascia, Extirpation	0JC
Subcutaneous Tissue and Fascia, Extraction	0JD
Subcutaneous Tissue and Fascia, Insertion	0JH
Subcutaneous Tissue and Fascia, Inspection	0JJ
Subcutaneous Tissue and Fascia, Release	0JN
Subcutaneous Tissue and Fascia, Removal	0JP
Subcutaneous Tissue and Fascia, Repair	0JQ
Subcutaneous Tissue and Fascia, Replacement	0JR
Subcutaneous Tissue and Fascia, Supplement	0JU
Subcutaneous Tissue and Fascia, Revision	0JW
Subcutaneous Tissue and Fascia, Transfer	0JX
Imaging, Skin, Subcutaneous Tissue and Breast, Plain Radiography	BH0
Imaging, Skin, Subcutaneous Tissue and Breast, Magnetic Resonance Imaging (MRI)	BH3
Imaging, Skin, Subcutaneous Tissue and Breast, Ultrasonography	BH4
Nuclear Medicine, Skin, Subcutaneous Tissue And Breast, Planar Nuclear Medicine Imaging	CH1
Nuclear Medicine, Skin, Subcutaneous Tissue and Breast, Tomographic (TOMO) Nuclear Medicine Imaging	CH2
Radiation Therapy, Skin, Beam Radiation	DH0
Radiation Therapy, Skin, Other Radiation	DHY

Male Figure
(Anterior View)

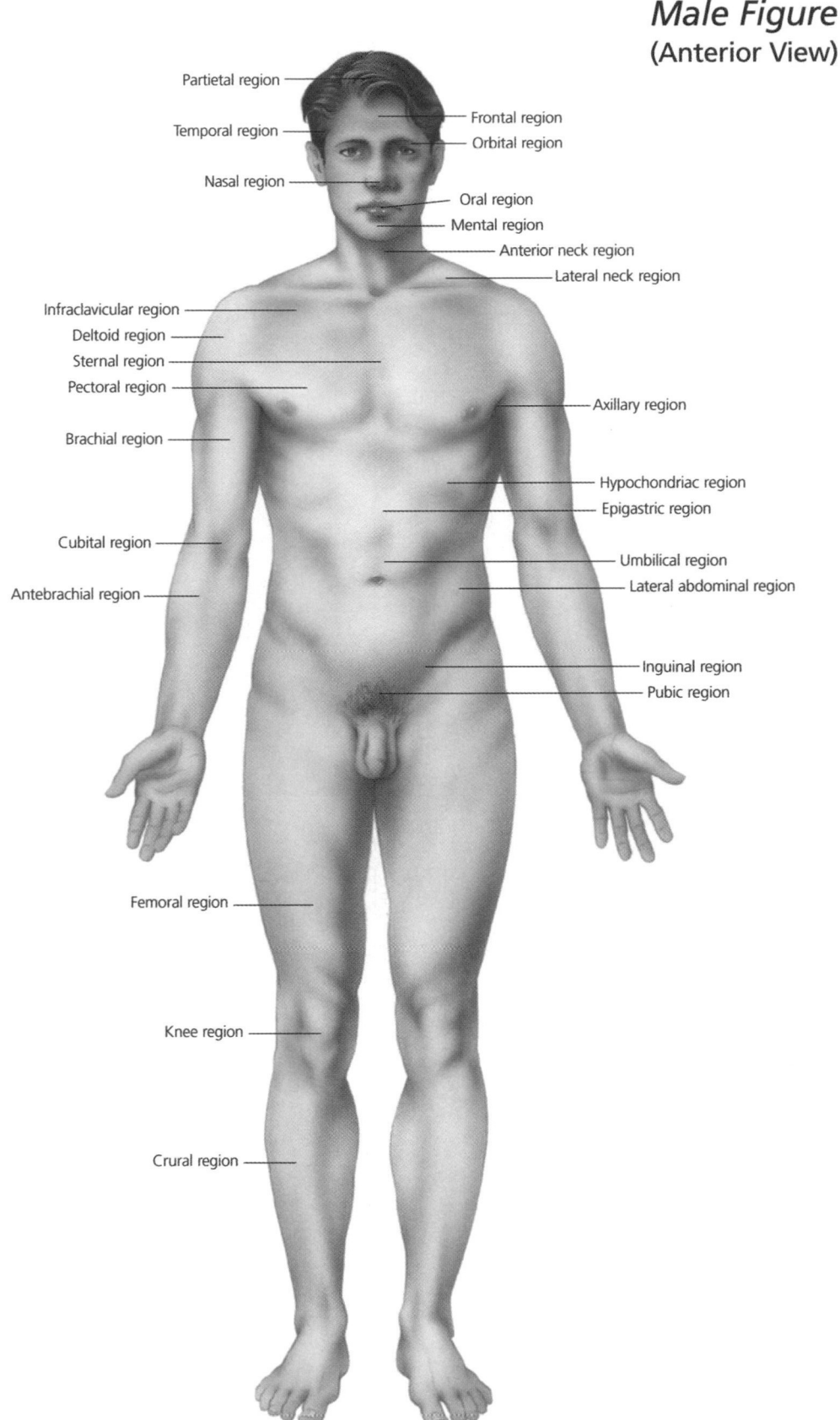

Partietal region

Temporal region

Nasal region

Frontal region

Orbital region

Oral region

Mental region

Anterior neck region

Lateral neck region

Infraclavicular region

Deltoid region

Sternal region

Pectoral region

Brachial region

Axillary region

Hypochondriac region

Epigastric region

Cubital region

Antebrachial region

Umbilical region

Lateral abdominal region

Inguinal region

Pubic region

Femoral region

Knee region

Crural region

PLATE 2. SKIN AND SUBCUTANEOUS TISSUE – FEMALE

Skin and Breast, Alteration	0H0
Skin and Breast, Change	0H2
Skin and Breast, Destruction	0H5
Skin and Breast, Division	0H8
Skin and Breast, Drainage	0H9
Skin and Breast, Excision	0HB
Skin and Breast, Extirpation	0HC
Skin and Breast, Extraction	0HD
Skin and Breast, Insertion	0HH
Skin and Breast, Inspection	0HJ
Skin and Breast, Reattachment	0HM
Skin and Breast, Release	0HN
Skin and Breast, Removal	0HP
Skin and Breast, Repair	0HQ
Skin and Breast, Replacement	0HR
Skin and Breast, Reposition	0HS
Skin and Breast, Resection	0HT
Skin and Breast, Supplement	0HU
Skin and Breast, Revision	0HW
Skin and Breast, Transfer	0HX
Subcutaneous Tissue and Fascia, Alteration	0J0
Subcutaneous Tissue and Fascia, Change	0J2
Subcutaneous Tissue and Fascia, Destruction	0J5
Subcutaneous Tissue and Fascia, Division	0J8
Subcutaneous Tissue and Fascia, Drainage	0J9
Subcutaneous Tissue and Fascia, Excision	0JB
Subcutaneous Tissue and Fascia, Extirpation	0JC
Subcutaneous Tissue and Fascia, Extraction	0JD
Subcutaneous Tissue and Fascia, Insertion	0JH
Subcutaneous Tissue and Fascia, Inspection	0JJ
Subcutaneous Tissue and Fascia, Release	0JN
Subcutaneous Tissue and Fascia, Removal	0JP
Subcutaneous Tissue and Fascia, Repair	0JQ
Subcutaneous Tissue and Fascia, Replacement	0JR
Subcutaneous Tissue and Fascia, Supplement	0JU
Subcutaneous Tissue and Fascia, Revision	0JW
Subcutaneous Tissue and Fascia, Transfer	0JX
Imaging, Skin, Subcutaneous Tissue and Breast, Plain Radiography	BH0
Imaging, Skin, Subcutaneous Tissue and Breast, Magnetic Resonance Imaging (MRI)	BH3
Imaging, Skin, Subcutaneous Tissue and Breast, Ultrasonography	BH4
Nuclear Medicine, Skin, Subcutaneous Tissue and Breast, Planar Nuclear Medicine Imaging	and CH1
Nuclear Medicine, Skin, Subcutaneous Tissue and Breast, Tomographic (TOMO) Nuclear Medicine Imaging	CH2
Radiation Therapy, Skin, Beam Radiation	DH0
Radiation Therapy, Skin, Other Radiation	DHY

Female Figure
(Anterior View)

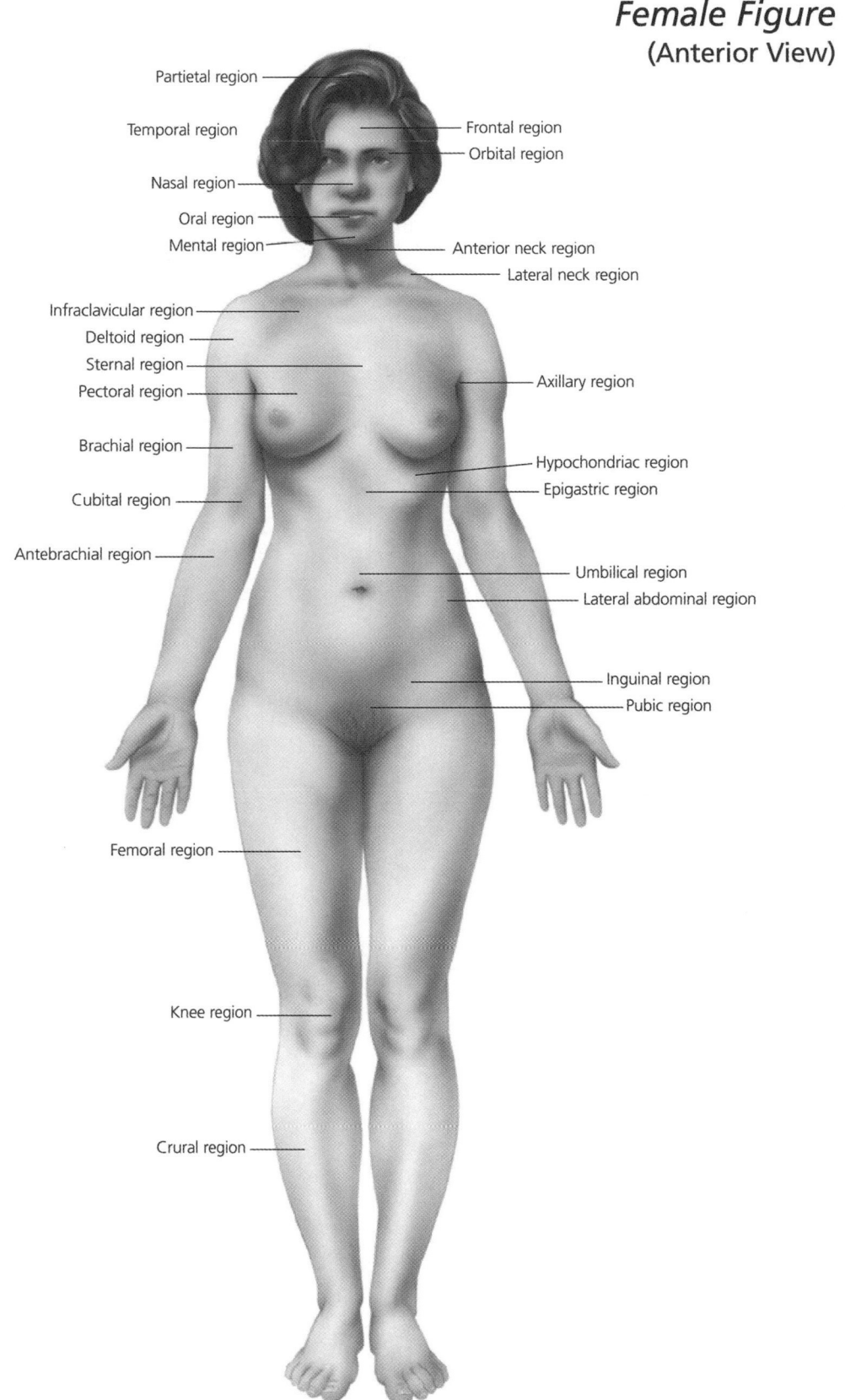

Partietal region

Temporal region

Nasal region

Oral region

Mental region

Frontal region

Orbital region

Anterior neck region

Lateral neck region

Infraclavicular region

Deltoid region

Sternal region

Pectoral region

Brachial region

Cubital region

Antebrachial region

Axillary region

Hypochondriac region

Epigastric region

Umbilical region

Lateral abdominal region

Inguinal region

Pubic region

Femoral region

Knee region

Crural region

PLATE 3. FEMALE BREAST

Skin and Breast, Alteration	0H0
Skin and Breast, Change	0H2
Skin and Breast, Destruction	0H5
Skin and Breast, Division	0H8
Skin and Breast, Drainage	0H9
Skin and Breast, Excision	0HB
Skin and Breast, Extirpation	0HC
Skin and Breast, Extraction	0HD
Skin and Breast, Insertion	0HH
Skin and Breast, Inspection	0HJ
Skin and Breast, Reattachment	0HM
Skin and Breast, Release	0HN
Skin and Breast, Removal	0HP
Skin and Breast, Repair	0HQ
Skin and Breast, Replacement	0HR
Skin and Breast, Reposition	0HS
Skin and Breast, Resection	0HT
Skin and Breast, Supplement	0HU
Skin and Breast, Revision	0HW
Skin and Breast, Transfer	0HX
Imaging, Skin, Subcutaneous Tissue and Breast, Plain Radiography	BH0
Imaging, Skin, Subcutaneous Tissue and Breast, Magnetic Resonance Imaging (MRI)	BH3
Imaging, Skin, Subcutaneous Tissue and Breast, Ultrasonography	BH4
Nuclear Medicine, Skin, Subcutaneous Tissue and Breast, Planar Nuclear Medicine Imaging	CH1
Nuclear Medicine, Skin, Subcutaneous Tissue and Breast, Tomographic (TOMO) Nuclear Medicine Imaging	CH2
Radiation Therapy, Breast, Beam Radiation	DM0
Radiation Therapy, Breast, Brachytherapy	DM1
Radiation Therapy, Breast, Stereotactic Radiosurgery	DM2
Radiation Therapy, Breast, Other Radiation	DMY

Female Breast

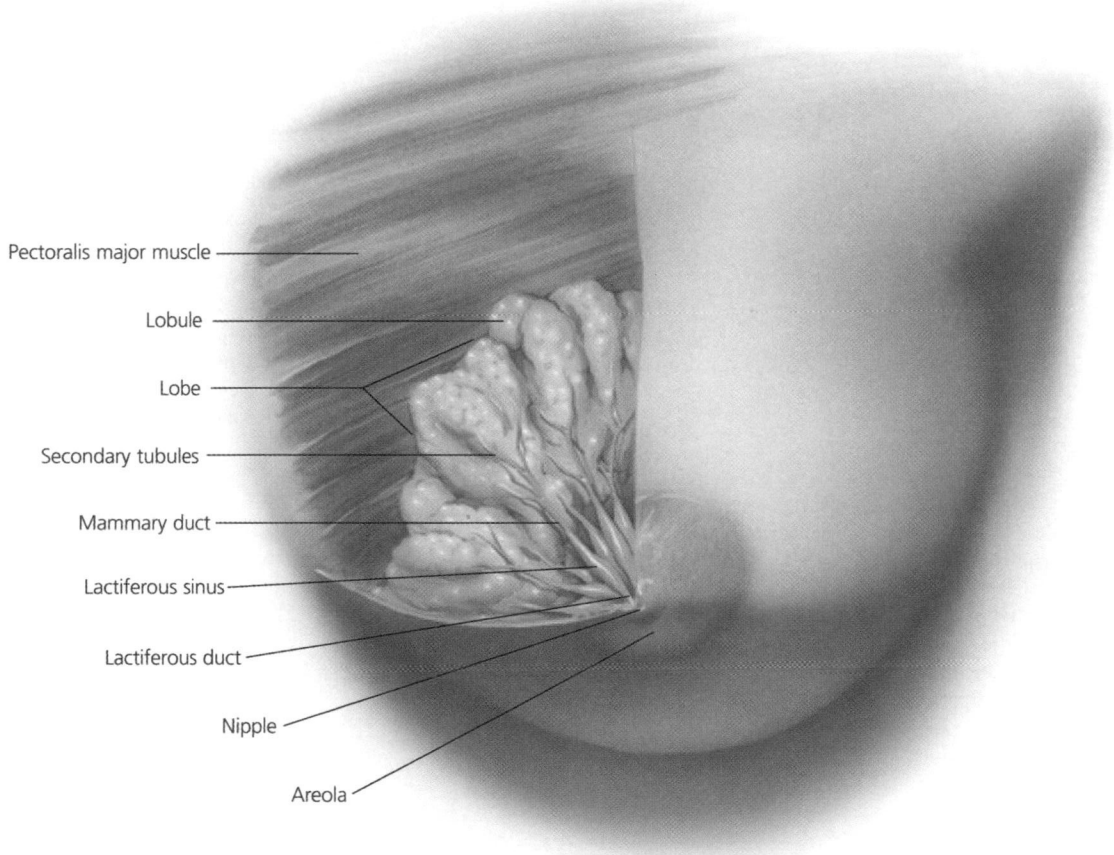

Pectoralis major muscle

Lobule

Lobe

Secondary tubules

Mammary duct

Lactiferous sinus

Lactiferous duct

Nipple

Areola

PLATE 4. MUSCULAR SYSTEM AND CONNECTIVE TISSUE – ANTERIOR VIEW

Muscles, Change	0K2
Muscles, Destruction	0K5
Muscles, Division	0K8
Muscles, Drainage	0K9
Muscles, Excision	0KB
Muscles, Extirpation	0KC
Muscles, Insertion	0KH
Muscles, Inspection	0KJ
Muscles, Reattachment	0KM
Muscles, Release	0KN
Muscles, Removal	0KP
Muscles, Repair	0KQ
Muscles, Reposition	0KS
Muscles, Resection	0KT
Muscles, Supplement	0KU
Muscles, Revision	0KW
Muscles, Transfer	0KX
Tendons, Change	0L2
Tendons, Destruction	0L5
Tendons, Division	0L8
Tendons, Drainage	0L9
Tendons, Excision	0LB
Tendons, Extirpation	0LC
Tendons, Inspection	0LJ
Tendons, Reattachment	0LM
Tendons, Release	0LN
Tendons, Removal	0LP
Tendons, Repair	0LQ
Tendons, Replacement	0LR
Tendons, Reposition	0LS
Tendons, Resection	0LT
Tendons, Supplement	0LU
Tendons, Revision	0LW
Tendons, Transfer	0LX
Bursae and Ligaments, Change	0M2
Bursae and Ligaments, Destruction	0M5
Bursae and Ligaments, Division	0M8
Bursae and Ligaments, Drainage	0M9
Bursae and Ligaments, Excision	0MB
Bursae and Ligaments, Extirpation	0MC
Bursae and Ligaments, Extraction	0MD
Bursae and Ligaments, Inspection	0MJ
Bursae and Ligaments, Reattachment	0MM
Bursae and Ligaments, Release	0MN
Bursae and Ligaments, Removal	0MP
Bursae and Ligaments, Repair	0MQ
Bursae and Ligaments, Reposition	0MS
Bursae and Ligaments, Resection	0MT
Bursae and Ligaments, Supplement	0MU
Bursae and Ligaments, Revision	0MW
Bursae and Ligaments, Transfer	0MX
Anatomical Regions, Upper Extremities, Alteration	0X0
Anatomical Regions, Upper Extremities, Change	0X2
Anatomical Regions, Upper Extremities, Control	0X3
Anatomical Regions, Upper Extremities, Detachment	0X6
Anatomical Regions, Upper Extremities, Drainage	0X9
Anatomical Regions, Upper Extremities, Excision	0XB
Anatomical Regions, Upper Extremities, Insertion	0XH
Anatomical Regions, Upper Extremities, Inspection	0XJ
Anatomical Regions, Upper Extremities, Reattachment	0XM

Anatomical Regions, Upper Extremities, Removal	0XP
Anatomical Regions, Upper Extremities, Repair	0XQ
Anatomical Regions, Upper Extremities, Replacement	0XR
Anatomical Regions, Upper Extremities, Supplement	0XU
Anatomical Regions, Upper Extremities, Revision	0XW
Anatomical Regions, Upper Extremities, Transfer	0XX
Anatomical Regions, Lower Extremities, Alteration	0Y0
Anatomical Regions, Lower Extremities, Change	0Y2
Anatomical Regions, Lower Extremities, Control	0Y3
Anatomical Regions, Lower Extremities, Detachment	0Y6
Anatomical Regions, Lower Extremities, Drainage	0Y9
Anatomical Regions, Lower Extremities, Excision	0YB
Anatomical Regions, Lower Extremities, Insertion	0YH
Anatomical Regions, Lower Extremities, Inspection	0YJ
Anatomical Regions, Lower Extremities, Reattachment	0YM
Anatomical Regions, Lower Extremities, Removal	0YP
Anatomical Regions, Lower Extremities, Repair	0YQ
Anatomical Regions, Lower Extremities, Supplement	0YU
Anatomical Regions, Lower Extremities, Revision	0YW
Nuclear Medicine, Musculoskeletal System, Planar Nuclear Medicine Imaging	CP1
Nuclear Medicine, Musculoskeletal System, Tomographic (TOMO) Nuclear Medicine Imaging	CP2
Nuclear Medicine, Musculoskeletal System, Nonimaging Nuclear Medicine Probe	CP5
Radiation Therapy, Musculoskeletal System, Beam Radiation	DP0
Radiation Therapy, Musculoskeletal System, Other Radiation	DPY

Muscular System
(Anterior View)

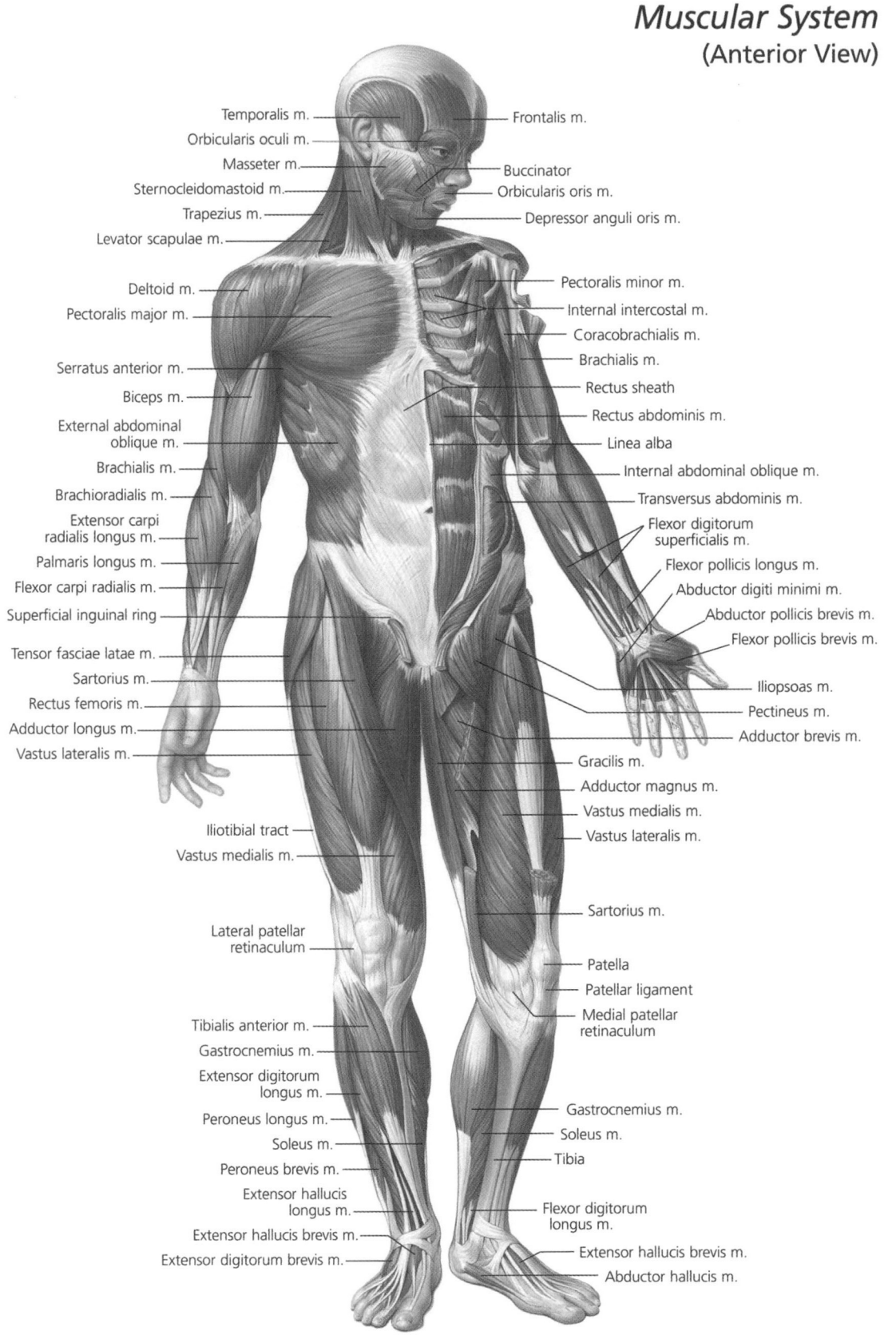

Temporalis m.
Orbicularis oculi m.
Masseter m.
Sternocleidomastoid m.
Trapezius m.
Levator scapulae m.

Frontalis m.
Buccinator
Orbicularis oris m.
Depressor anguli oris m.

Deltoid m.
Pectoralis major m.
Serratus anterior m.
Biceps m.
External abdominal oblique m.
Brachialis m.
Brachioradialis m.
Extensor carpi radialis longus m.
Palmaris longus m.
Flexor carpi radialis m.
Superficial inguinal ring
Tensor fasciae latae m.
Sartorius m.
Rectus femoris m.
Adductor longus m.
Vastus lateralis m.

Pectoralis minor m.
Internal intercostal m.
Coracobrachialis m.
Brachialis m.
Rectus sheath
Rectus abdominis m.
Linea alba
Internal abdominal oblique m.
Transversus abdominis m.
Flexor digitorum superficialis m.
Flexor pollicis longus m.
Abductor digiti minimi m.
Abductor pollicis brevis m.
Flexor pollicis brevis m.
Iliopsoas m.
Pectineus m.
Adductor brevis m.

Gracilis m.
Adductor magnus m.
Vastus medialis m.
Vastus lateralis m.

Iliotibial tract
Vastus medialis m.

Sartorius m.

Lateral patellar retinaculum

Patella
Patellar ligament
Medial patellar retinaculum

Tibialis anterior m.
Gastrocnemius m.
Extensor digitorum longus m.
Peroneus longus m.
Soleus m.
Peroneus brevis m.
Extensor hallucis longus m.
Extensor hallucis brevis m.
Extensor digitorum brevis m.

Gastrocnemius m.
Soleus m.
Tibia
Flexor digitorum longus m.
Extensor hallucis brevis m.
Abductor hallucis m.

PLATE 5. MUSCULAR SYSTEM AND CONNECTIVE TISSUE – POSTERIOR VIEW

Muscles, Change	0K2
Muscles, Destruction	0K5
Muscles, Division	0K8
Muscles, Drainage	0K9
Muscles, Excision	0KB
Muscles, Extirpation	0KC
Muscles, Insertion	0KH
Muscles, Inspection	0KJ
Muscles, Reattachment	0KM
Muscles, Release	0KN
Muscles, Removal	0KP
Muscles, Repair	0KQ
Muscles, Reposition	0KS
Muscles, Resection	0KT
Muscles, Supplement	0KU
Muscles, Revision	0KW
Muscles, Transfer	0KX
Tendons, Change	0L2
Tendons, Destruction	0L5
Tendons, Division	0L8
Tendons, Drainage	0L9
Tendons, Excision	0LB
Tendons, Extirpation	0LC
Tendons, Inspection	0LJ
Tendons, Reattachment	0LM
Tendons, Release	0LN
Tendons, Removal	0LP
Tendons, Repair	0LQ
Tendons, Replacement	0LR
Tendons, Reposition	0LS
Tendons, Resection	0LT
Tendons, Supplement	0LU
Tendons, Revision	0LW
Tendons, Transfer	0LX
Bursae and Ligaments, Change	0M2
Bursae and Ligaments, Destruction	0M5
Bursae and Ligaments, Division	0M8
Bursae and Ligaments, Drainage	0M9
Bursae and Ligaments, Excision	0MB
Bursae and Ligaments, Extirpation	0MC
Bursae and Ligaments, Extraction	0MD
Bursae and Ligaments, Inspection	0MJ
Bursae and Ligaments, Reattachment	0MM
Bursae and Ligaments, Release	0MN
Bursae and Ligaments, Removal	0MP
Bursae and Ligaments, Repair	0MQ
Bursae and Ligaments, Reposition	0MS
Bursae and Ligaments, Resection	0MT
Bursae and Ligaments, Supplement	0MU
Bursae and Ligaments, Revision	0MW
Bursae and Ligaments, Transfer	0MX
Anatomical Regions, Upper Extremities, Alteration	0X0
Anatomical Regions, Upper Extremities, Change	0X2
Anatomical Regions, Upper Extremities, Control	0X3
Anatomical Regions, Upper Extremities, Detachment	0X6
Anatomical Regions, Upper Extremities, Drainage	0X9
Anatomical Regions, Upper Extremities, Excision	0XB
Anatomical Regions, Upper Extremities, Insertion	0XH
Anatomical Regions, Upper Extremities, Inspection	0XJ
Anatomical Regions, Upper Extremities, Reattachment	0XM
Anatomical Regions, Upper Extremities, Removal	0XP
Anatomical Regions, Upper Extremities, Repair	0XQ
Anatomical Regions, Upper Extremities, Replacement	0XR
Anatomical Regions, Upper Extremities, Supplement	0XU
Anatomical Regions, Upper Extremities, Revision	0XW
Anatomical Regions, Upper Extremities, Transfer	0XX
Anatomical Regions, Lower Extremities, Alteration	0Y0
Anatomical Regions, Lower Extremities, Change	0Y2
Anatomical Regions, Lower Extremities, Control	0Y3
Anatomical Regions, Lower Extremities, Detachment	0Y6
Anatomical Regions, Lower Extremities, Drainage	0Y9
Anatomical Regions, Lower Extremities, Excision	0YB
Anatomical Regions, Lower Extremities, Insertion	0YH
Anatomical Regions, Lower Extremities, Inspection	0YJ
Anatomical Regions, Lower Extremities, Reattachment	0YM
Anatomical Regions, Lower Extremities, Removal	0YP
Anatomical Regions, Lower Extremities, Repair	0YQ
Anatomical Regions, Lower Extremities, Supplement	0YU
Anatomical Regions, Lower Extremities, Revision	0YW
Nuclear Medicine, Musculoskeletal System, Planar Nuclear Medicine Imaging	CP1
Nuclear Medicine, Musculoskeletal System, Tomographic (TOMO) Nuclear Medicine Imaging	CP2
Nuclear Medicine, Musculoskeletal System, Nonimaging Nuclear Medicine Probe	CP5
Radiation Therapy, Musculoskeletal System, Beam Radiation	DP0
Radiation Therapy, Musculoskeletal System, Other Radiation	DPY

Muscular System
(Posterior View)

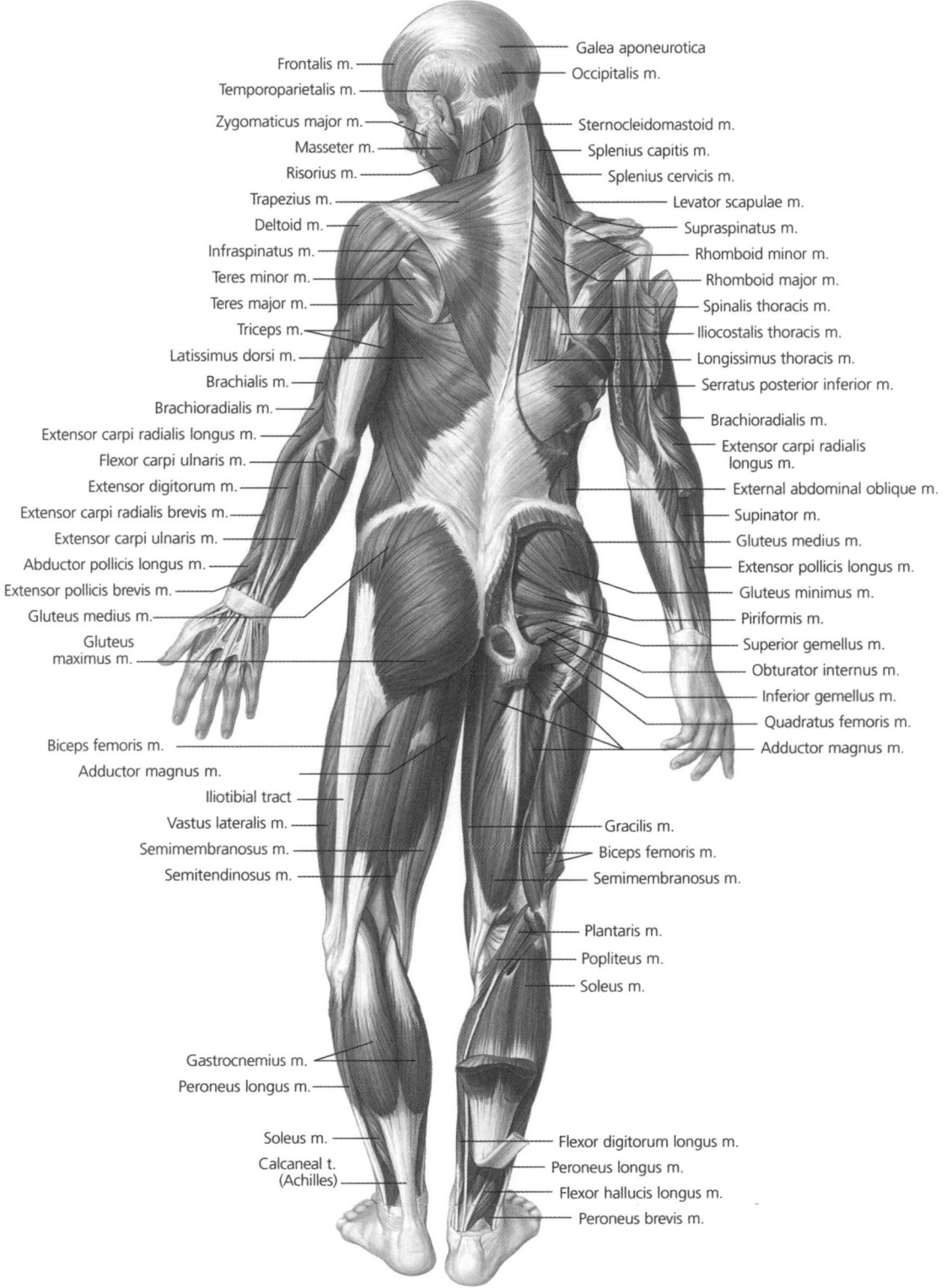

Frontalis m.
Temporoparietalis m.
Zygomaticus major m.
Masseter m.
Risorius m.
Trapezius m.
Deltoid m.
Infraspinatus m.
Teres minor m.
Teres major m.
Triceps m.
Latissimus dorsi m.
Brachialis m.
Brachioradialis m.
Extensor carpi radialis longus m.
Flexor carpi ulnaris m.
Extensor digitorum m.
Extensor carpi radialis brevis m.
Extensor carpi ulnaris m.
Abductor pollicis longus m.
Extensor pollicis brevis m.
Gluteus medius m.
Gluteus maximus m.
Biceps femoris m.
Adductor magnus m.
Iliotibial tract
Vastus lateralis m.
Semimembranosus m.
Semitendinosus m.
Gastrocnemius m.
Peroneus longus m.
Soleus m.
Calcaneal t. (Achilles)

Galea aponeurotica
Occipitalis m.
Sternocleidomastoid m.
Splenius capitis m.
Splenius cervicis m.
Levator scapulae m.
Supraspinatus m.
Rhomboid minor m.
Rhomboid major m.
Spinalis thoracis m.
Iliocostalis thoracis m.
Longissimus thoracis m.
Serratus posterior inferior m.
Brachioradialis m.
Extensor carpi radialis longus m.
External abdominal oblique m.
Supinator m.
Gluteus medius m.
Extensor pollicis longus m.
Gluteus minimus m.
Piriformis m.
Superior gemellus m.
Obturator internus m.
Inferior gemellus m.
Quadratus femoris m.
Adductor magnus m.
Gracilis m.
Biceps femoris m.
Semimembranosus m.
Plantaris m.
Popliteus m.
Soleus m.
Flexor digitorum longus m.
Peroneus longus m.
Flexor hallucis longus m.
Peroneus brevis m.

PLATE 6. MUSCULAR SYSTEM - SHOULDER AND ELBOW

Muscles, Change	0K2
Muscles, Destruction	0K5
Muscles, Division	0K8
Muscles, Drainage	0K9
Muscles, Excision	0KB
Muscles, Extirpation	0KC
Muscles, Insertion	0KH
Muscles, Inspection	0KJ
Muscles, Reattachment	0KM
Muscles, Release	0KN
Muscles, Removal	0KP
Muscles, Repair	0KQ
Muscles, Reposition	0KS
Muscles, Resection	0KT
Muscles, Supplement	0KU
Muscles, Revision	0KW
Muscles, Transfer	0KX
Tendons, Change	0L2
Tendons, Destruction	0L5
Tendons, Division	0L8
Tendons, Drainage	0L9
Tendons, Excision	0LB
Tendons, Extirpation	0LC
Tendons, Inspection	0LJ
Tendons, Reattachment	0LM
Tendons, Release	0LN
Tendons, Removal	0LP
Tendons, Repair	0LQ
Tendons, Replacement	0LR
Tendons, Reposition	0LS
Tendons, Resection	0LT
Tendons, Supplement	0LU
Tendons, Revision	0LW
Tendons, Transfer	0LX
Bursae and Ligaments, Change	0M2
Bursae and Ligaments, Destruction	0M5
Bursae and Ligaments, Division	0M8
Bursae and Ligaments, Drainage	0M9
Bursae and Ligaments, Excision	0MB
Bursae and Ligaments, Extirpation	0MC
Bursae and Ligaments, Extraction	0MD
Bursae and Ligaments, Inspection	0MJ
Bursae and Ligaments, Reattachment	0MM
Bursae and Ligaments, Release	0MN
Bursae and Ligaments, Removal	0MP
Bursae and Ligaments, Repair	0MQ
Bursae and Ligaments, Reposition	0MS
Bursae and Ligaments, Resection	0MT
Bursae and Ligaments, Supplement	0MU
Bursae and Ligaments, Revision	0MW
Bursae and Ligaments, Transfer	0MX
Anatomical Regions, Upper Extremities, Alteration	0X0
Anatomical Regions, Upper Extremities, Change	0X2
Anatomical Regions, Upper Extremities, Control	0X3
Anatomical Regions, Upper Extremities, Detachment	0X6
Anatomical Regions, Upper Extremities, Drainage	0X9
Anatomical Regions, Upper Extremities, Excision	0XB
Anatomical Regions, Upper Extremities, Insertion	0XH
Anatomical Regions, Upper Extremities, Inspection	0XJ
Anatomical Regions, Upper Extremities, Reattachment	0XM
Anatomical Regions, Upper Extremities, Removal	0XP

Anatomical Regions, Upper Extremities, Repair	0XQ
Anatomical Regions, Upper Extremities, Replacement	0XR
Anatomical Regions, Upper Extremities, Supplement	0XU
Anatomical Regions, Upper Extremities, Revision	0XW
Anatomical Regions, Upper Extremities, Transfer	0XX
Nuclear Medicine, Musculoskeletal System, Planar Nuclear Medicine Imaging	CP1
Nuclear Medicine, Musculoskeletal System, Tomographic (TOMO) Nuclear Medicine Imaging	CP2
Nuclear Medicine, Musculoskeletal System, Nonimaging Nuclear Medicine Probe	CP5
Radiation Therapy, Musculoskeletal System, Beam Radiation	DP0
Radiation Therapy, Musculoskeletal System, Other Radiation	DPY

Shoulder and Elbow
(Anterior View)

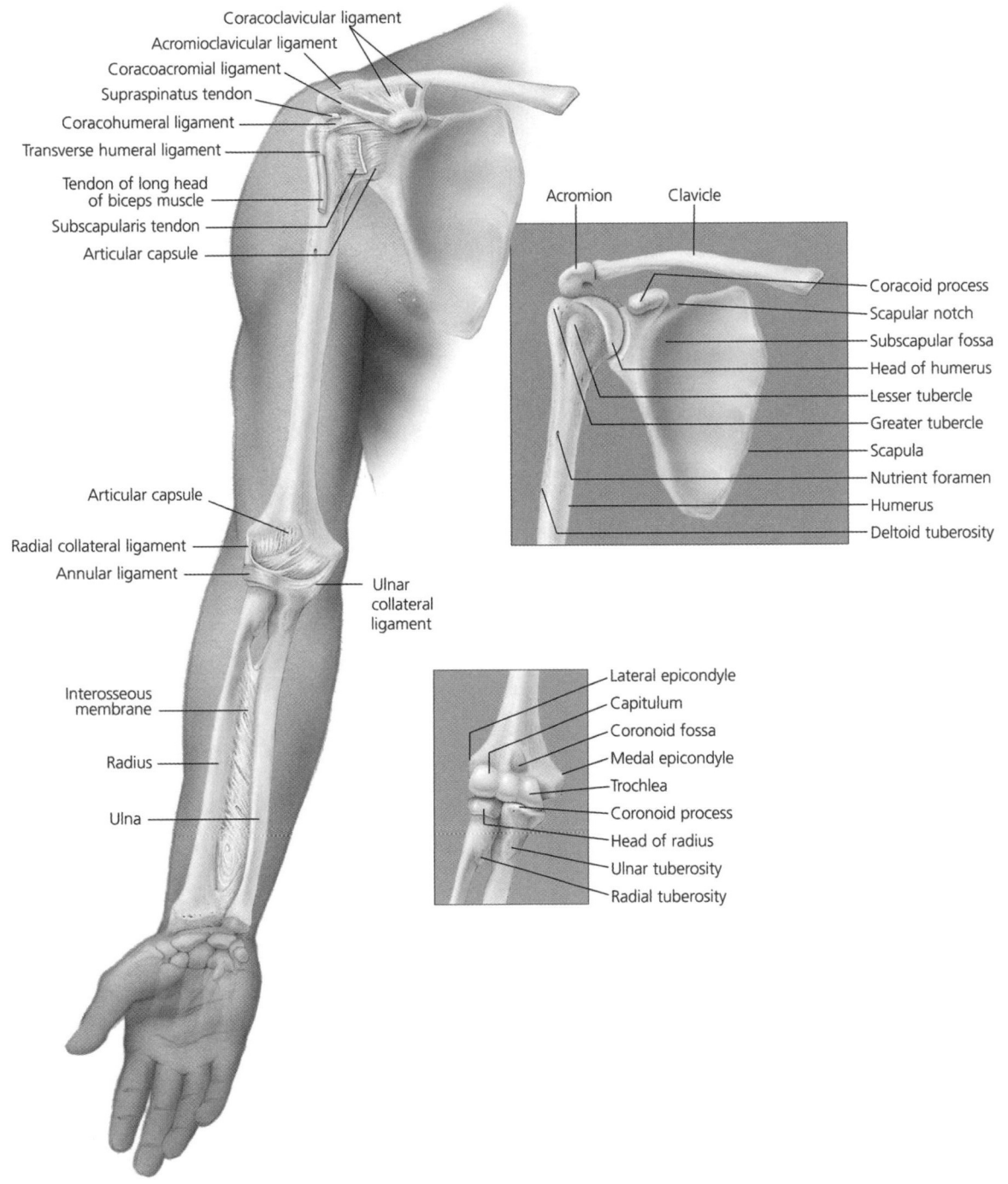

Coracoclavicular ligament

Acromioclavicular ligament

Coracoacromial ligament

Supraspinatus tendon

Coracohumeral ligament

Transverse humeral ligament

Tendon of long head of biceps muscle

Subscapularis tendon

Articular capsule

Articular capsule

Radial collateral ligament

Annular ligament

Ulnar collateral ligament

Interosseous membrane

Radius

Ulna

Acromion

Clavicle

Coracoid process

Scapular notch

Subscapular fossa

Head of humerus

Lesser tubercle

Greater tubercle

Scapula

Nutrient foramen

Humerus

Deltoid tuberosity

Lateral epicondyle

Capitulum

Coronoid fossa

Medal epicondyle

Trochlea

Coronoid process

Head of radius

Ulnar tuberosity

Radial tuberosity

PLATE 7. MUSCULAR SYSTEM - HAND AND WRIST

Muscles, Change	0K2
Muscles, Destruction	0K5
Muscles, Division	0K8
Muscles, Drainage	0K9
Muscles, Excision	0KB
Muscles, Extirpation	0KC
Muscles, Insertion	0KH
Muscles, Inspection	0KJ
Muscles, Reattachment	0KM
Muscles, Release	0KN
Muscles, Removal	0KP
Muscles, Repair	0KQ
Muscles, Reposition	0KS
Muscles, Resection	0KT
Muscles, Supplement	0KU
Muscles, Revision	0KW
Muscles, Transfer	0KX
Tendons, Change	0L2
Tendons, Destruction	0L5
Tendons, Division	0L8
Tendons, Drainage	0L9
Tendons, Excision	0LB
Tendons, Extirpation	0LC
Tendons, Inspection	0LJ
Tendons, Reattachment	0LM
Tendons, Release	0LN
Tendons, Removal	0LP
Tendons, Repair	0LQ
Tendons, Replacement	0LR
Tendons, Reposition	0LS
Tendons, Resection	0LT
Tendons, Supplement	0LU
Tendons, Revision	0LW
Tendons, Transfer	0LX
Bursae and Ligaments, Change	0M2
Bursae and Ligaments, Destruction	0M5
Bursae and Ligaments, Division	0M8
Bursae and Ligaments, Drainage	0M9
Bursae and Ligaments, Excision	0MB
Bursae and Ligaments, Extirpation	0MC
Bursae and Ligaments, Extraction	0MD
Bursae and Ligaments, Inspection	0MJ
Bursae and Ligaments, Reattachment	0MM
Bursae and Ligaments, Release	0MN
Bursae and Ligaments, Removal	0MP
Bursae and Ligaments, Repair	0MQ
Bursae and Ligaments, Reposition	0MS
Bursae and Ligaments, Resection	0MT
Bursae and Ligaments, Supplement	0MU
Bursae and Ligaments, Revision	0MW
Bursae and Ligaments, Transfer	0MX
Anatomical Regions, Upper Extremities, Alteration	0X0
Anatomical Regions, Upper Extremities, Change	0X2
Anatomical Regions, Upper Extremities, Control	0X3
Anatomical Regions, Upper Extremities, Detachment	0X6
Anatomical Regions, Upper Extremities, Drainage	0X9
Anatomical Regions, Upper Extremities, Excision	0XB
Anatomical Regions, Upper Extremities, Insertion	0XH
Anatomical Regions, Upper Extremities, Inspection	0XJ
Anatomical Regions, Upper Extremities, Reattachment	0XM
Anatomical Regions, Upper Extremities, Removal	0XP
Anatomical Regions, Upper Extremities, Repair	0XQ
Anatomical Regions, Upper Extremities, Replacement	0XR
Anatomical Regions, Upper Extremities, Supplement	0XU
Anatomical Regions, Upper Extremities, Revision	0XW
Anatomical Regions, Upper Extremities, Transfer	0XX
Nuclear Medicine, Musculoskeletal System, Planar Nuclear Medicine Imaging	CP1
Nuclear Medicine, Musculoskeletal System, Tomographic (TOMO) Nuclear Medicine Imaging	CP2
Nuclear Medicine, Musculoskeletal System, Nonimaging Nuclear Medicine Probe	CP5
Radiation Therapy, Musculoskeletal System, Beam Radiation	DP0
Radiation Therapy, Musculoskeletal System, Other Radiation	DPY

Hand and Wrist

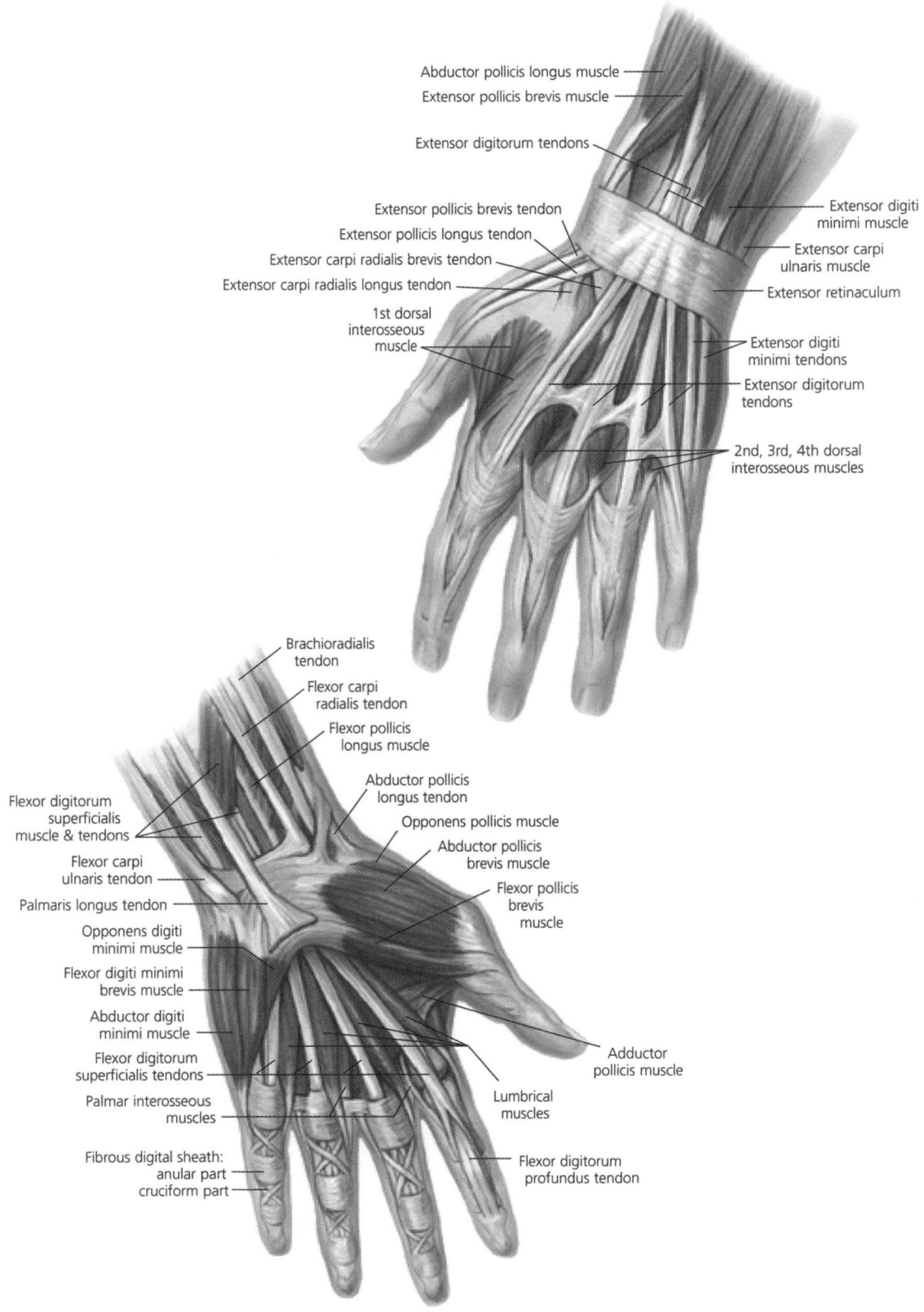

Abductor pollicis longus muscle

Extensor pollicis brevis muscle

Extensor digitorum tendons

Extensor pollicis brevis tendon

Extensor pollicis longus tendon

Extensor carpi radialis brevis tendon

Extensor carpi radialis longus tendon

1st dorsal interosseous muscle

Extensor digiti minimi muscle

Extensor carpi ulnaris muscle

Extensor retinaculum

Extensor digiti minimi tendons

Extensor digitorum tendons

2nd, 3rd, 4th dorsal interosseous muscles

Brachioradialis tendon

Flexor carpi radialis tendon

Flexor pollicis longus muscle

Abductor pollicis longus tendon

Flexor digitorum superficialis muscle & tendons

Opponens pollicis muscle

Abductor pollicis brevis muscle

Flexor carpi ulnaris tendon

Palmaris longus tendon

Flexor pollicis brevis muscle

Opponens digiti minimi muscle

Flexor digiti minimi brevis muscle

Abductor digiti minimi muscle

Adductor pollicis muscle

Flexor digitorum superficialis tendons

Lumbrical muscles

Palmar interosseous muscles

Fibrous digital sheath:
anular part
cruciform part

Flexor digitorum profundus tendon

PLATE 8. MUSCULOSKELETAL SYSTEM - HIP AND KNEE

Muscles, Change	0K2
Muscles, Destruction	0K5
Muscles, Division	0K8
Muscles, Drainage	0K9
Muscles, Excision	0KB
Muscles, Extirpation	0KC
Muscles, Insertion	0KH
Muscles, Inspection	0KJ
Muscles, Reattachment	0KM
Muscles, Release	0KN
Muscles, Removal	0KP
Muscles, Repair	0KQ
Muscles, Reposition	0KS
Muscles, Resection	0KT
Muscles, Supplement	0KU
Muscles, Revision	0KW
Muscles, Transfer	0KX
Tendons, Change	0L2
Tendons, Destruction	0L5
Tendons, Division	0L8
Tendons, Drainage	0L9
Tendons, Excision	0LB
Tendons, Extirpation	0LC
Tendons, Inspection	0LJ
Tendons, Reattachment	0LM
Tendons, Release	0LN
Tendons, Removal	0LP
Tendons, Repair	0LQ
Tendons, Replacement	0LR
Tendons, Reposition	0LS
Tendons, Resection	0LT
Tendons, Supplement	0LU
Tendons, Revision	0LW
Tendons, Transfer	0LX
Bursae and Ligaments, Change	0M2
Bursae and Ligaments, Destruction	0M5
Bursae and Ligaments, Division	0M8
Bursae and Ligaments, Drainage	0M9
Bursae and Ligaments, Excision	0MB
Bursae and Ligaments, Extirpation	0MC
Bursae and Ligaments, Extraction	0MD
Bursae and Ligaments, Inspection	0MJ
Bursae and Ligaments, Reattachment	0MM
Bursae and Ligaments, Release	0MN
Bursae and Ligaments, Removal	0MP
Bursae and Ligaments, Repair	0MQ
Bursae and Ligaments, Reposition	0MS
Bursae and Ligaments, Resection	0MT
Bursae and Ligaments, Supplement	0MU
Bursae and Ligaments, Revision	0MW
Bursae and Ligaments, Transfer	0MX
Anatomical Regions, Lower Extremities, Alteration	0Y0
Anatomical Regions, Lower Extremities, Change	0Y2
Anatomical Regions, Lower Extremities, Control	0Y3
Anatomical Regions, Lower Extremities, Detachment	0Y6
Anatomical Regions, Lower Extremities, Drainage	0Y9
Anatomical Regions, Lower Extremities, Excision	0YB
Anatomical Regions, Lower Extremities, Insertion	0YH
Anatomical Regions, Lower Extremities, Inspection	0YJ
Anatomical Regions, Lower Extremities, Reattachment	0YM

Anatomical Regions, Lower Extremities, Removal	0YP
Anatomical Regions, Lower Extremities, Repair	0YQ
Anatomical Regions, Lower Extremities, Supplement	0YU
Anatomical Regions, Lower Extremities, Revision	0YW
Nuclear Medicine, Musculoskeletal System, Planar Nuclear Medicine Imaging	CP1
Nuclear Medicine, Musculoskeletal System, Tomographic (TOMO) Nuclear Medicine Imaging	CP2
Nuclear Medicine, Musculoskeletal System, Nonimaging Nuclear Medicine Probe	CP5
Radiation Therapy, Musculoskeletal System, Beam Radiation	DP0
Radiation Therapy, Musculoskeletal System, Other Radiation	DPY

Hip and Knee
(Anterior View)

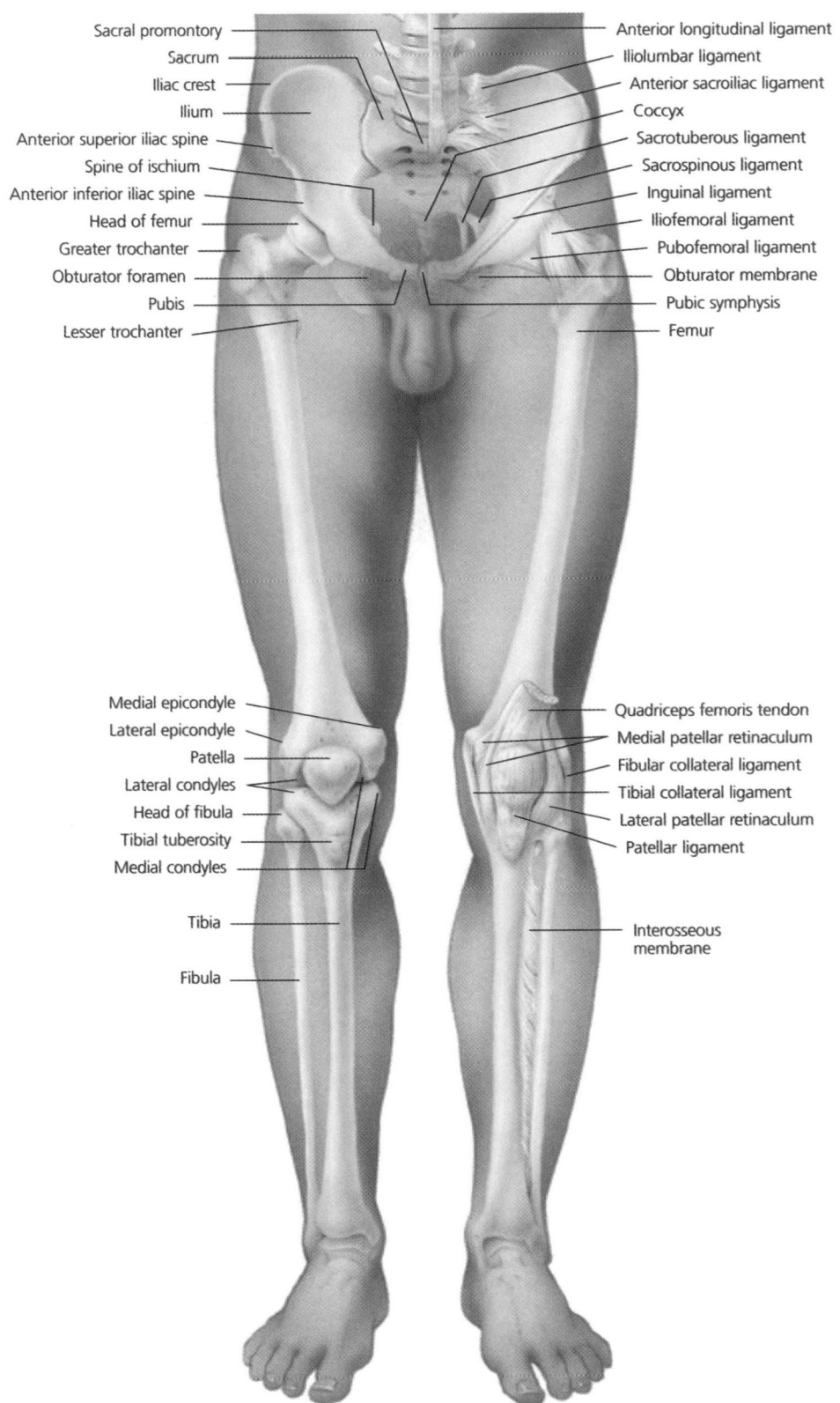

Sacral promontory

Sacrum

Iliac crest

Ilium

Anterior superior iliac spine

Spine of ischium

Anterior inferior iliac spine

Head of femur

Greater trochanter

Obturator foramen

Pubis

Lesser trochanter

Anterior longitudinal ligament

Iliolumbar ligament

Anterior sacroiliac ligament

Coccyx

Sacrotuberous ligament

Sacrospinous ligament

Inguinal ligament

Iliofemoral ligament

Pubofemoral ligament

Obturator membrane

Pubic symphysis

Femur

Medial epicondyle

Lateral epicondyle

Patella

Lateral condyles

Head of fibula

Tibial tuberosity

Medial condyles

Tibia

Fibula

Quadriceps femoris tendon

Medial patellar retinaculum

Fibular collateral ligament

Tibial collateral ligament

Lateral patellar retinaculum

Patellar ligament

Interosseous membrane

PLATE 9. MUSCULOSKELETAL SYSTEM – FOOT AND ANKLE

Muscles, Change	0K2
Muscles, Destruction	0K5
Muscles, Division	0K8
Muscles, Drainage	0K9
Muscles, Excision	0KB
Muscles, Extirpation	0KC
Muscles, Insertion	0KH
Muscles, Inspection	0KJ
Muscles, Reattachment	0KM
Muscles, Release	0KN
Muscles, Removal	0KP
Muscles, Repair	0KQ
Muscles, Reposition	0KS
Muscles, Resection	0KT
Muscles, Supplement	0KU
Muscles, Revision	0KW
Muscles, Transfer	0KX
Tendons, Change	0L2
Tendons, Destruction	0L5
Tendons, Division	0L8
Tendons, Drainage	0L9
Tendons, Excision	0LB
Tendons, Extirpation	0LC
Tendons, Inspection	0LJ
Tendons, Reattachment	0LM
Tendons, Release	0LN
Tendons, Removal	0LP
Tendons, Repair	0LQ
Tendons, Replacement	0LR
Tendons, Reposition	0LS
Tendons, Resection	0LT
Tendons, Supplement	0LU
Tendons, Revision	0LW
Tendons, Transfer	0LX
Bursae and Ligaments, Change	0M2
Bursae and Ligaments, Destruction	0M5
Bursae and Ligaments, Division	0M8
Bursae and Ligaments, Drainage	0M9
Bursae and Ligaments, Excision	0MB
Bursae and Ligaments, Extirpation	0MC
Bursae and Ligaments, Extraction	0MD
Bursae and Ligaments, Inspection	0MJ
Bursae and Ligaments, Reattachment	0MM
Bursae and Ligaments, Release	0MN
Bursae and Ligaments, Removal	0MP
Bursae and Ligaments, Repair	0MQ
Bursae and Ligaments, Reposition	0MS
Bursae and Ligaments, Resection	0MT
Bursae and Ligaments, Supplement	0MU
Bursae and Ligaments, Revision	0MW
Bursae and Ligaments, Transfer	0MX
Anatomical Regions, Lower Extremities, Alteration	0Y0
Anatomical Regions, Lower Extremities, Change	0Y2
Anatomical Regions, Lower Extremities, Control	0Y3
Anatomical Regions, Lower Extremities, Detachment	0Y6
Anatomical Regions, Lower Extremities, Drainage	0Y9
Anatomical Regions, Lower Extremities, Excision	0YB
Anatomical Regions, Lower Extremities, Insertion	0YH
Anatomical Regions, Lower Extremities, Inspection	0YJ
Anatomical Regions, Lower Extremities, Reattachment	0YM

Anatomical Regions, Lower Extremities, Removal	0YP
Anatomical Regions, Lower Extremities, Repair	0YQ
Anatomical Regions, Lower Extremities, Supplement	0YU
Anatomical Regions, Lower Extremities, Revision	0YW
Nuclear Medicine, Musculoskeletal System, Planar Nuclear Medicine Imaging	CP1
Nuclear Medicine, Musculoskeletal System, Tomographic (TOMO) Nuclear Medicine Imaging	CP2
Nuclear Medicine, Musculoskeletal System, Nonimaging Nuclear Medicine Probe	CP5
Radiation Therapy, Musculoskeletal System, Beam Radiation	DP0
Radiation Therapy, Musculoskeletal System, Other Radiation	DPY

Foot and Ankle

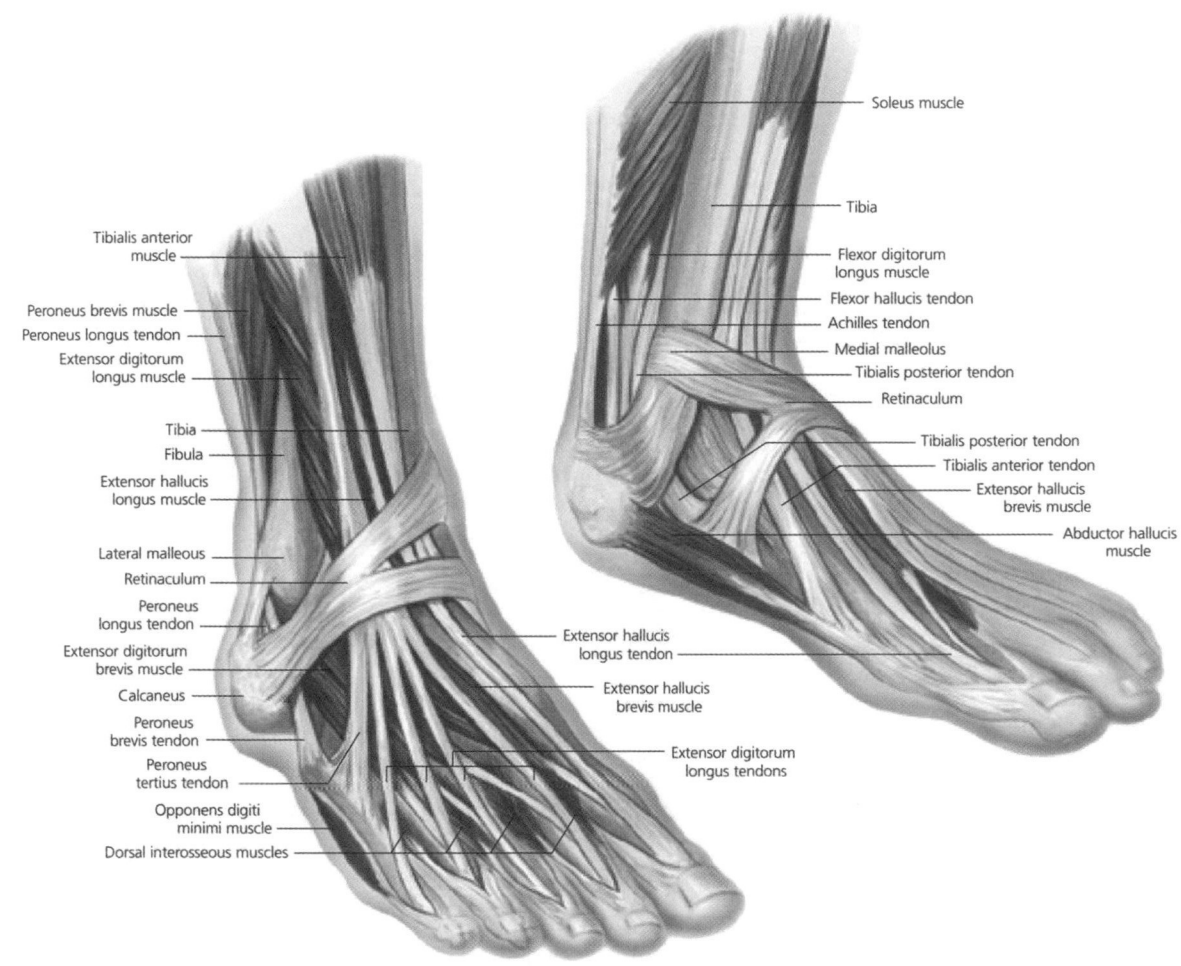

Soleus muscle

Tibia

Flexor digitorum longus muscle

Flexor hallucis tendon

Achilles tendon

Medial malleolus

Tibialis posterior tendon

Retinaculum

Tibialis posterior tendon

Tibialis anterior tendon

Extensor hallucis brevis muscle

Abductor hallucis muscle

Tibialis anterior muscle

Peroneus brevis muscle

Peroneus longus tendon

Extensor digitorum longus muscle

Tibia

Fibula

Extensor hallucis longus muscle

Lateral malleous

Retinaculum

Peroneus longus tendon

Extensor digitorum brevis muscle

Calcaneus

Peroneus brevis tendon

Peroneus tertius tendon

Opponens digiti minimi muscle

Dorsal interosseous muscles

Extensor hallucis longus tendon

Extensor hallucis brevis muscle

Extensor digitorum longus tendons

PLATE 10. SKELETAL SYSTEM - ANTERIOR VIEW

Head and Facial Bones, Change	0N2	Upper Joints, Reposition	0RS
Head and Facial Bones, Destruction	0N5	Upper Joints, Resection	0RT
Head and Facial Bones, Division	0N8	Upper Joints, Supplement	0RU
Head and Facial Bones, Drainage	0N9	Upper Joints, Revision	0RW
Head and Facial Bones, Excision	0NB	Lower Joints, Change	0S2
Head and Facial Bones, Extirpation	0NC	Lower Joints, Destruction	0S5
Head and Facial Bones, Insertion	0NH	Lower Joints, Drainage	0S9
Head and Facial Bones, Inspection	0NJ	Lower Joints, Excision	0SB
Head and Facial Bones, Release	0NN	Lower Joints, Extirpation	0SC
Head and Facial Bones, Removal	0NP	Lower Joints, Fusion	0SG
Head and Facial Bones, Repair	0NQ	Lower Joints, Insertion	0SH
Head and Facial Bones, Replacement	0NR	Lower Joints, Inspection	0SJ
Head and Facial Bones, Reposition	0NS	Lower Joints, Release	0SN
Head and Facial Bones, Resection	0NT	Lower Joints, Removal	0SP
Head and Facial Bones, Supplement	0NU	Lower Joints, Repair	0SQ
Head and Facial Bones, Revision	0NW	Lower Joints, Replacement	0SR
Upper Bones, Change	0P2	Lower Joints, Reposition	0SS
Upper Bones, Destruction	0P5	Lower Joints, Resection	0ST
Upper Bones, Division	0P8	Lower Joints, Supplement	0SU
Upper Bones, Drainage	0P9	Lower Joints, Revision	0SW
Upper Bones, Excision	0PB	Imaging, Skull and Facial Bones, Plain Radiography	BN0
Upper Bones, Extirpation	0PC	Imaging, Skull and Facial Bones, Fluoroscopy	BN1
Upper Bones, Insertion	0PH	Imaging, Skull and Facial Bones, Computerized Tomography (CT Scan)	BN2
Upper Bones, Inspection	0PJ		
Upper Bones, Release	0PN	Imaging, Skull and Facial Bones, Magnetic Resonance Imaging (MRI)	BN3
Upper Bones, Removal	0PP		
Upper Bones, Repair	0PQ	Imaging, Non-Axial Upper Bones, Plain Radiography	BP0
Upper Bones, Replacement	0PR	Imaging, Non-Axial Upper Bones, Fluoroscopy	BP1
Upper Bones, Reposition	0PS	Imaging, Non-Axial Upper Bones, Computerized Tomography (CT Scan)	BP2
Upper Bones, Resection	0PT		
Upper Bones, Supplement	0PU	Imaging, Non-Axial Upper Bones, Magnetic Resonance Imaging (MRI)	BP3
Upper Bones, Revision	0PW		
Lower Bones, Change	0Q2	Imaging, Non-Axial Upper Bones, Ultrasonography	BP4
Lower Bones, Destruction	0Q5	Imaging, Non-Axial Lower Bones, Plain Radiography	BQ0
Lower Bones, Division	0Q8	Imaging, Non-Axial Lower Bones, Fluoroscopy	BQ1
Lower Bones, Drainage	0Q9	Imaging, Non-Axial Lower Bones, Computerized Tomography (CT Scan)	BQ2
Lower Bones, Excision	0QB		
Lower Bones, Extirpation	0QC	Imaging, Non-Axial Lower Bones, Magnetic Resonance Imaging (MRI)	BQ3
Lower Bones, Insertion	0QH		
Lower Bones, Inspection	0QJ	Imaging, Non-Axial Lower Bones, Ultrasonography	BQ4
Lower Bones, Release	0QN	Imaging, Axial Skeleton, Except Skull and Facial Bones, Plain Radiography	BR0
Lower Bones, Removal	0QP		
Lower Bones, Repair	0QQ	Imaging, Axial Skeleton, Except Skull and Facial Bones, Fluoroscopy	BR1
Lower Bones, Replacement	0QR		
Lower Bones, Reposition	0QS	Imaging, Axial Skeleton, Except Skull and Facial Bones, Computerized Tomography (CT Scan)	BR2
Lower Bones, Resection	0QT		
Lower Bones, Supplement	0QU	Imaging, Axial Skeleton, Except Skull and Facial Bones, Magnetic Resonance Imaging (MRI)	BR3
Lower Bones, Revision	0QW		
Upper Joints, Change	0R2	Imaging, Axial Skeleton, Except Skull and Facial Bones, Ultrasonography	BR4
Upper Joints, Destruction	0R5		
Upper Joints, Drainage	0R9	Nuclear Medicine, Musculoskeletal System, Planar Nuclear Medicine Imaging	CP1
Upper Joints, Excision	0RB		
Upper Joints, Extirpation	0RC	Nuclear Medicine, Musculoskeletal System, Tomographic (TOMO) Nuclear Medicine Imaging	CP2
Upper Joints, Fusion	0RG		
Upper Joints, Insertion	0RH	Nuclear Medicine, Musculoskeletal System, Nonimaging Nuclear Medicine Probe	CP5
Upper Joints, Inspection	0RJ		
Upper Joints, Release	0RN	Radiation Therapy, Musculoskeletal System, Beam Radiation	DP0
Upper Joints, Removal	0RP	Radiation Therapy, Musculoskeletal System, Other Radiation	DPY
Upper Joints, Repair	0RQ	New Technology, Joints, Monitoring	XR2
Upper Joints, Replacement	0RR		

Skeletal System
(Anterior View)

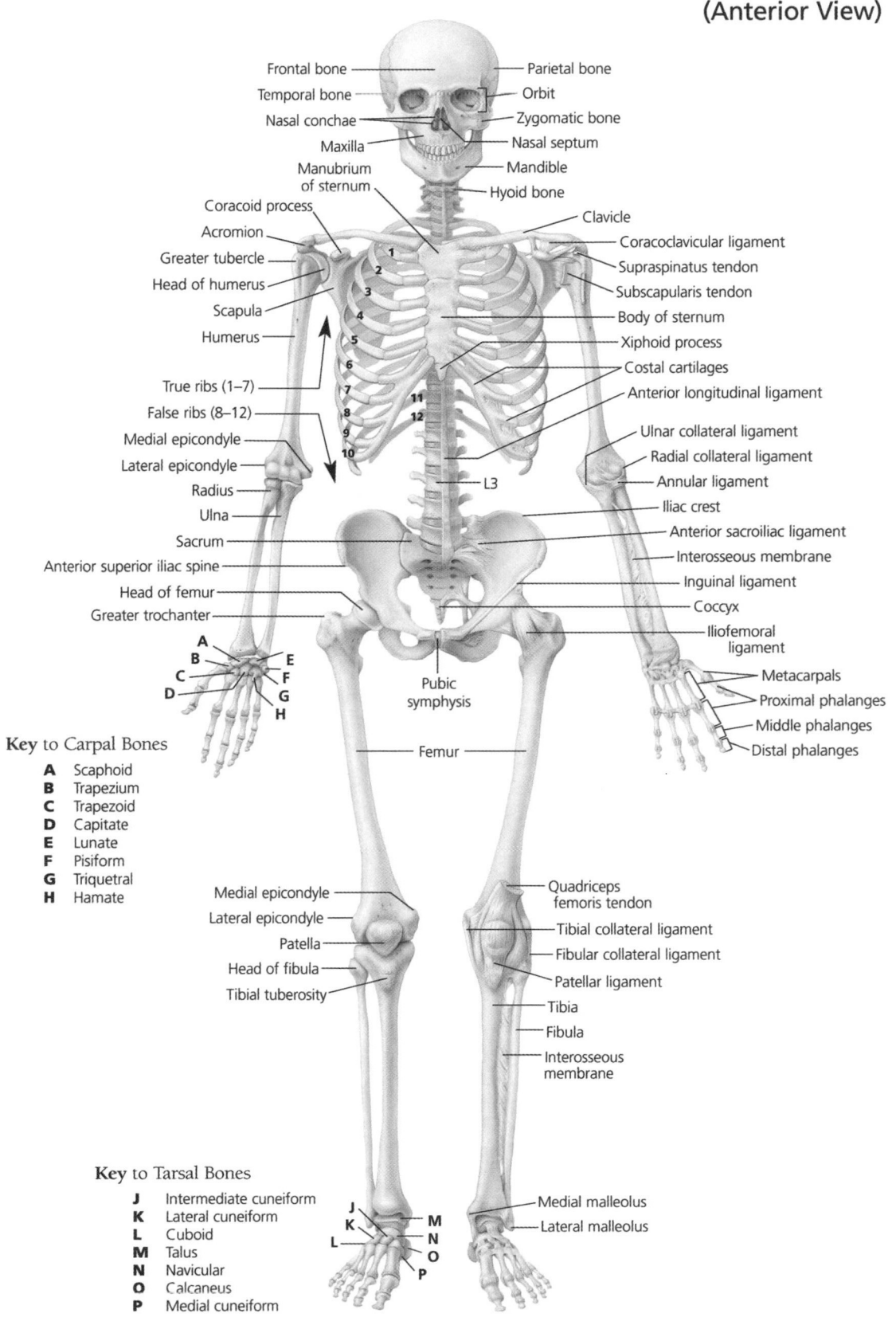

Frontal bone
Temporal bone
Nasal conchae
Maxilla
Manubrium of sternum
Coracoid process
Acromion
Greater tubercle
Head of humerus
Scapula
Humerus
True ribs (1–7)
False ribs (8–12)
Medial epicondyle
Lateral epicondyle
Radius
Ulna
Sacrum
Anterior superior iliac spine
Head of femur
Greater trochanter

Parietal bone
Orbit
Zygomatic bone
Nasal septum
Mandible
Hyoid bone
Clavicle
Coracoclavicular ligament
Supraspinatus tendon
Subscapularis tendon
Body of sternum
Xiphoid process
Costal cartilages
Anterior longitudinal ligament
Ulnar collateral ligament
Radial collateral ligament
Annular ligament
Iliac crest
Anterior sacroiliac ligament
Interosseous membrane
Inguinal ligament
Coccyx
Iliofemoral ligament
Metacarpals
Proximal phalanges
Middle phalanges
Distal phalanges

L3

Pubic symphysis
Femur

Key to Carpal Bones

A	Scaphoid
B	Trapezium
C	Trapezoid
D	Capitate
E	Lunate
F	Pisiform
G	Triquetral
H	Hamate

Medial epicondyle
Lateral epicondyle
Patella
Head of fibula
Tibial tuberosity

Quadriceps femoris tendon
Tibial collateral ligament
Fibular collateral ligament
Patellar ligament
Tibia
Fibula
Interosseous membrane

Key to Tarsal Bones

J	Intermediate cuneiform
K	Lateral cuneiform
L	Cuboid
M	Talus
N	Navicular
O	Calcaneus
P	Medial cuneiform

Medial malleolus
Lateral malleolus

PLATE 11. SKELETAL SYSTEM - POSTERIOR VIEW

Head and Facial Bones, Change	0N2	Upper Joints, Reposition	0RS
Head and Facial Bones, Destruction	0N5	Upper Joints, Resection	0RT
Head and Facial Bones, Division	0N8	Upper Joints, Supplement	0RU
Head and Facial Bones, Drainage	0N9	Upper Joints, Revision	0RW
Head and Facial Bones, Excision	0NB	Lower Joints, Change	0S2
Head and Facial Bones, Extirpation	0NC	Lower Joints, Destruction	0S5
Head and Facial Bones, Insertion	0NH	Lower Joints, Drainage	0S9
Head and Facial Bones, Inspection	0NJ	Lower Joints, Excision	0SB
Head and Facial Bones, Release	0NN	Lower Joints, Extirpation	0SC
Head and Facial Bones, Removal	0NP	Lower Joints, Fusion	0SG
Head and Facial Bones, Repair	0NQ	Lower Joints, Insertion	0SH
Head and Facial Bones, Replacement	0NR	Lower Joints, Inspection	0SJ
Head and Facial Bones, Reposition	0NS	Lower Joints, Release	0SN
Head and Facial Bones, Resection	0NT	Lower Joints, Removal	0SP
Head and Facial Bones, Supplement	0NU	Lower Joints, Repair	0SQ
Head and Facial Bones, Revision	0NW	Lower Joints, Replacement	0SR
Upper Bones, Change	0P2	Lower Joints, Reposition	0SS
Upper Bones, Destruction	0P5	Lower Joints, Resection	0ST
Upper Bones, Division	0P8	Lower Joints, Supplement	0SU
Upper Bones, Drainage	0P9	Lower Joints, Revision	0SW
Upper Bones, Excision	0PB	Imaging, Skull and Facial Bones, Plain Radiography	BN0
Upper Bones, Extirpation	0PC	Imaging, Skull and Facial Bones, Fluoroscopy	BN1
Upper Bones, Insertion	0PH	Imaging, Skull and Facial Bones, Computerized Tomography (CT Scan)	BN2
Upper Bones, Inspection	0PJ		
Upper Bones, Release	0PN	Imaging, Skull and Facial Bones, Magnetic Resonance Imaging (MRI)	BN3
Upper Bones, Removal	0PP		
Upper Bones, Repair	0PQ	Imaging, Non-Axial Upper Bones, Plain Radiography	BP0
Upper Bones, Replacement	0PR	Imaging, Non-Axial Upper Bones, Fluoroscopy	BP1
Upper Bones, Reposition	0PS	Imaging, Non-Axial Upper Bones, Computerized Tomography (CT Scan)	BP2
Upper Bones, Resection	0PT		
Upper Bones, Supplement	0PU	Imaging, Non-Axial Upper Bones, Magnetic Resonance Imaging (MRI)	BP3
Upper Bones, Revision	0PW		
Lower Bones, Change	0Q2	Imaging, Non-Axial Upper Bones, Ultrasonography	BP4
Lower Bones, Destruction	0Q5	Imaging, Non-Axial Lower Bones, Plain Radiography	BQ0
Lower Bones, Division	0Q8	Imaging, Non-Axial Lower Bones, Fluoroscopy	BQ1
Lower Bones, Drainage	0Q9	Imaging, Non-Axial Lower Bones, Computerized Tomography (CT Scan)	BQ2
Lower Bones, Excision	0QB		
Lower Bones, Extirpation	0QC	Imaging, Non-Axial Lower Bones, Magnetic Resonance Imaging (MRI)	BQ3
Lower Bones, Insertion	0QH		
Lower Bones, Inspection	0QJ	Imaging, Non-Axial Lower Bones, Ultrasonography	BQ4
Lower Bones, Release	0QN	Imaging, Axial Skeleton, Except Skull and Facial Bones, Plain Radiography	BR0
Lower Bones, Removal	0QP		
Lower Bones, Repair	0QQ	Imaging, Axial Skeleton, Except Skull and Facial Bones, Fluoroscopy	BR1
Lower Bones, Replacement	0QR		
Lower Bones, Reposition	0QS	Imaging, Axial Skeleton, Except Skull and Facial Bones, Computerized Tomography (CT Scan)	BR2
Lower Bones, Resection	0QT		
Lower Bones, Supplement	0QU	Imaging, Axial Skeleton, Except Skull and Facial Bones, Magnetic Resonance Imaging (MRI)	BR3
Lower Bones, Revision	0QW		
Upper Joints, Change	0R2	Imaging, Axial Skeleton, Except Skull and Facial Bones, Ultrasonography	BR4
Upper Joints, Destruction	0R5		
Upper Joints, Drainage	0R9	Nuclear Medicine, Musculoskeletal System, Planar Nuclear Medicine Imaging	CP1
Upper Joints, Excision	0RB		
Upper Joints, Extirpation	0RC	Nuclear Medicine, Musculoskeletal System, Tomographic (TOMO) Nuclear Medicine Imaging	CP2
Upper Joints, Fusion	0RG		
Upper Joints, Insertion	0RH	Nuclear Medicine, Musculoskeletal System, Nonimaging Nuclear Medicine Probe	CP5
Upper Joints, Inspection	0RJ		
Upper Joints, Release	0RN	Radiation Therapy, Musculoskeletal System, Beam Radiation	DP0
Upper Joints, Removal	0RP	Radiation Therapy, Musculoskeletal System, Other Radiation	DPY
Upper Joints, Repair	0RQ	New Technology, Joints, Monitoring	XR2
Upper Joints, Replacement	0RR		

Skeletal System
(Posterior View)

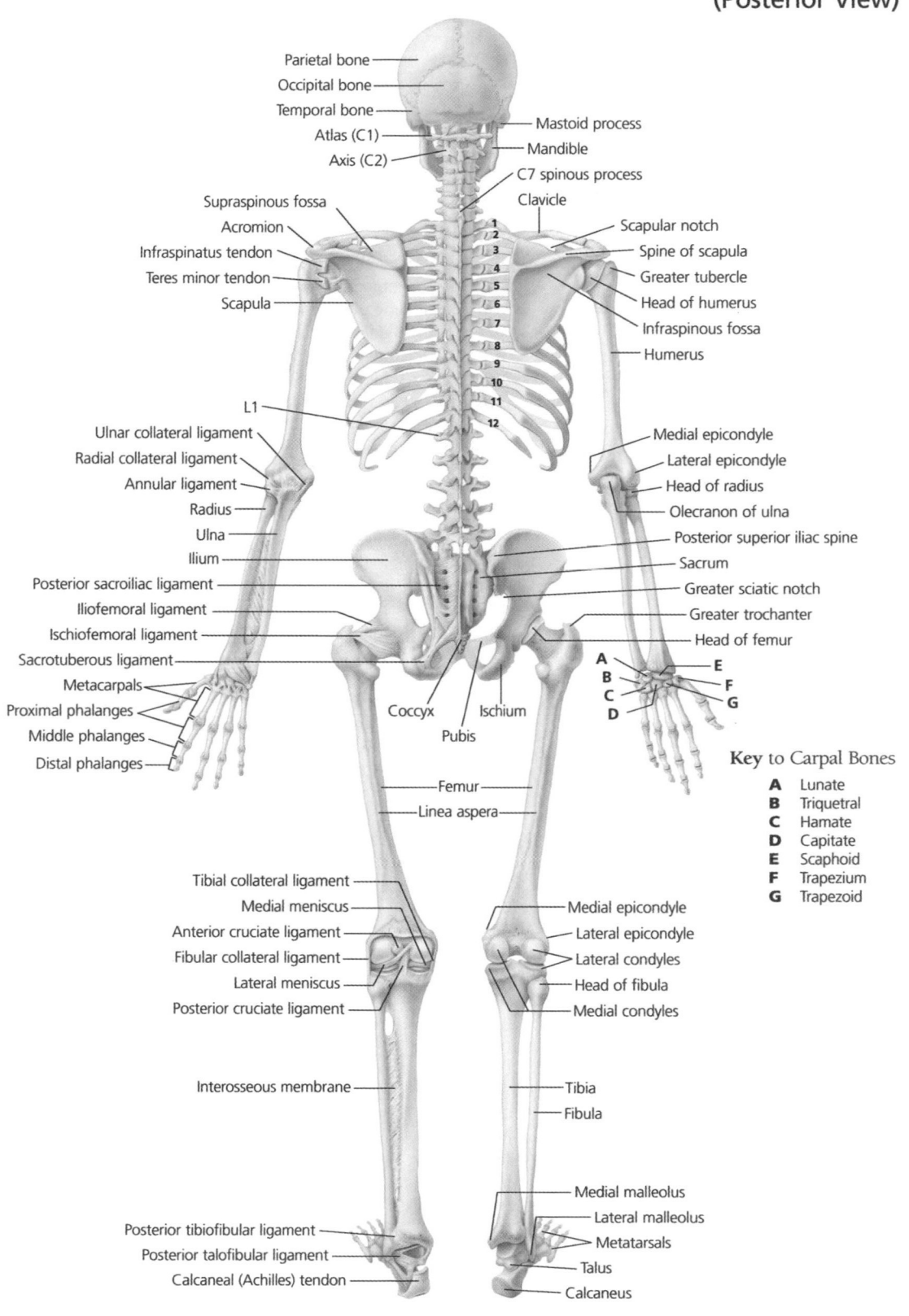

Parietal bone
Occipital bone
Temporal bone
Atlas (C1)
Axis (C2)
Supraspinous fossa
Acromion
Infraspinatus tendon
Teres minor tendon
Scapula
L1
Ulnar collateral ligament
Radial collateral ligament
Annular ligament
Radius
Ulna
Ilium
Posterior sacroiliac ligament
Iliofemoral ligament
Ischiofemoral ligament
Sacrotuberous ligament
Metacarpals
Proximal phalanges
Middle phalanges
Distal phalanges

Mastoid process
Mandible
C7 spinous process
Clavicle
Scapular notch
Spine of scapula
Greater tubercle
Head of humerus
Infraspinous fossa
Humerus
Medial epicondyle
Lateral epicondyle
Head of radius
Olecranon of ulna
Posterior superior iliac spine
Sacrum
Greater sciatic notch
Greater trochanter
Head of femur

Coccyx
Ischium
Pubis

A   E
B   F
C   G
D

Femur
Linea aspera

Key to Carpal Bones

A   Lunate
B   Triquetral
C   Hamate
D   Capitate
E   Scaphoid
F   Trapezium
G   Trapezoid

Tibial collateral ligament
Medial meniscus
Anterior cruciate ligament
Fibular collateral ligament
Lateral meniscus
Posterior cruciate ligament

Medial epicondyle
Lateral epicondyle
Lateral condyles
Head of fibula
Medial condyles

Interosseous membrane

Tibia
Fibula

Posterior tibiofibular ligament
Posterior talofibular ligament
Calcaneal (Achilles) tendon

Medial malleolus
Lateral malleolus
Metatarsals
Talus
Calcaneus

PLATE 12. SKELETAL SYSTEM - VERTEBRAL COLUMN

Upper Bones, Change	0P2	Lower Joints, Resection	0ST
Upper Bones, Destruction	0P5	Lower Joints, Supplement	0SU
Upper Bones, Division	0P8	Lower Joints, Revision	0SW
Upper Bones, Drainage	0P9	Imaging, Non-Axial Upper Bones, Plain Radiography	BP0
Upper Bones, Excision	0PB	Imaging, Non-Axial Upper Bones, Fluoroscopy	BP1
Upper Bones, Extirpation	0PC	Imaging, Non-Axial Upper Bones, Computerized	
Upper Bones, Insertion	0PH	Tomography (CT Scan)	BP2
Upper Bones, Inspection	0PJ	Imaging, Non-Axial Upper Bones, Magnetic Resonance	
Upper Bones, Release	0PN	Imaging (MRI)	BP3
Upper Bones, Removal	0PP	Imaging, Non-Axial Upper Bones, Ultrasonography	BP4
Upper Bones, Repair	0PQ	Imaging, Non-Axial Lower Bones, Plain Radiography	BQ0
Upper Bones, Replacement	0PR	Imaging, Non-Axial Lower Bones, Fluoroscopy	BQ1
Upper Bones, Reposition	0PS	Imaging, Non-Axial Lower Bones, Computerized	
Upper Bones, Resection	0PT	Tomography (CT Scan)	BQ2
Upper Bones, Supplement	0PU	Imaging, Non-Axial Lower Bones, Magnetic Resonance	
Upper Bones, Revision	0PW	Imaging (MRI)	BQ3
Lower Bones, Change	0Q2	Imaging, Non-Axial Lower Bones, Ultrasonography	BQ4
Lower Bones, Destruction	0Q5	Imaging, Axial Skeleton, Except Skull and Facial Bones,	
Lower Bones, Division	0Q8	Plain Radiography	BR0
Lower Bones, Drainage	0Q9	Imaging, Axial Skeleton, Except Skull and Facial Bones,	
Lower Bones, Excision	0QB	Fluoroscopy	BR1
Lower Bones, Extirpation	0QC	Imaging, Axial Skeleton, Except Skull and Facial Bones,	
Lower Bones, Insertion	0QH	Computerized Tomography (CT Scan)	BR2
Lower Bones, Inspection	0QJ	Imaging, Axial Skeleton, Except Skull and Facial Bones,	
Lower Bones, Release	0QN	Magnetic Resonance Imaging (MRI)	BR3
Lower Bones, Removal	0QP	Imaging, Axial Skeleton, Except Skull and Facial Bones,	
Lower Bones, Repair	0QQ	Ultrasonography	BR4
Lower Bones, Replacement	0QR	Nuclear Medicine, Musculoskeletal System, Planar Nuclear	
Lower Bones, Reposition	0QS	Medicine Imaging	CP1
Lower Bones, Resection	0QT	Nuclear Medicine, Musculoskeletal System, Tomographic	
Lower Bones, Supplement	0QU	(TOMO) Nuclear Medicine Imaging	CP2
Lower Bones, Revision	0QW	Nuclear Medicine, Musculoskeletal System, Nonimaging	
Upper Joints, Change	0R2	Nuclear Medicine Probe	CP5
Upper Joints, Destruction	0R5	Radiation Therapy, Musculoskeletal System, Beam Radiation	DP0
Upper Joints, Drainage	0R9	Radiation Therapy, Musculoskeletal System, Other Radiation	DPY
Upper Joints, Excision	0RB		
Upper Joints, Extirpation	0RC		
Upper Joints, Fusion	0RG		
Upper Joints, Insertion	0RH		
Upper Joints, Inspection	0RJ		
Upper Joints, Release	0RN		
Upper Joints, Removal	0RP		
Upper Joints, Repair	0RQ		
Upper Joints, Replacement	0RR		
Upper Joints, Reposition	0RS		
Upper Joints, Resection	0RT		
Upper Joints, Supplement	0RU		
Upper Joints, Revision	0RW		
Lower Joints, Change	0S2		
Lower Joints, Destruction	0S5		
Lower Joints, Drainage	0S9		
Lower Joints, Excision	0SB		
Lower Joints, Extirpation	0SC		
Lower Joints, Fusion	0SG		
Lower Joints, Insertion	0SH		
Lower Joints, Inspection	0SJ		
Lower Joints, Release	0SN		
Lower Joints, Removal	0SP		
Lower Joints, Repair	0SQ		
Lower Joints, Replacement	0SR		
Lower Joints, Reposition	0SS		

Vertebral Column
(Lateral View)

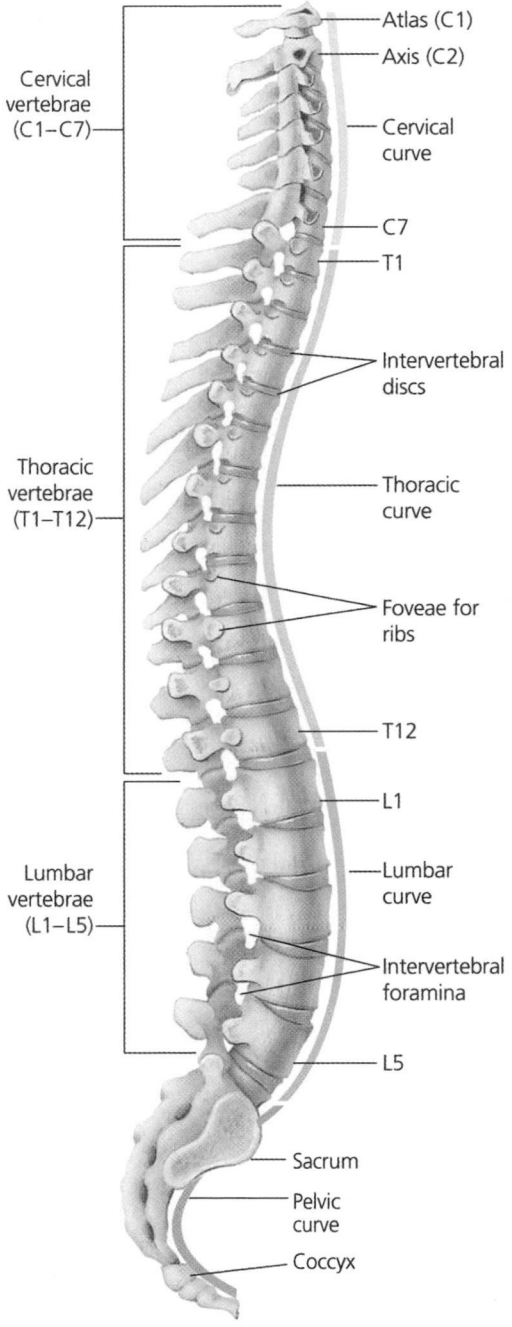

Cervical vertebrae (C1–C7)

Thoracic vertebrae (T1–T12)

Lumbar vertebrae (L1–L5)

Atlas (C1)

Axis (C2)

Cervical curve

C7

T1

Intervertebral discs

Thoracic curve

Foveae for ribs

T12

L1

Lumbar curve

Intervertebral foramina

L5

Sacrum

Pelvic curve

Coccyx

PLATE 13. RESPIRATORY SYSTEM

Respiratory System, Bypass	0B1
Respiratory System, Change	0B2
Respiratory System, Destruction	0B5
Respiratory System, Dilation	0B7
Respiratory System, Drainage	0B9
Respiratory System, Excision	0BB
Respiratory System, Extirpation	0BC
Respiratory System, Extraction	0BD
Respiratory System, Fragmentation	0BF
Respiratory System, Insertion	0BH
Respiratory System, Inspection	0BJ
Respiratory System, Occlusion	0BL
Respiratory System, Reattachment	0BM
Respiratory System, Release	0BN
Respiratory System, Removal	0BP
Respiratory System, Repair	0BQ
Respiratory System, Reposition	0BS
Respiratory System, Resection	0BT
Respiratory System, Supplement	0BU
Respiratory System, Restriction	0BV
Respiratory System, Revision	0BW
Respiratory System, Transplantation	0BY
Imaging, Respiratory System, Plain Radiography	BB0
Imaging, Respiratory System, Fluoroscopy	BB1
Imaging, Respiratory System, Computerized Tomography (CT Scan)	BB2
Imaging, Respiratory System, Magnetic Resonance Imaging (MRI)	BB3
Imaging, Respiratory System, Ultrasonography	BB4
Nuclear Medicine, Respiratory System, Planar Nuclear Medicine Imaging	CB1
Nuclear Medicine, Respiratory System, Tomographic (TOMO) Nuclear Medicine Imaging	CB2
Nuclear Medicine, Respiratory System, Positron Emission Tomographic (PET) Imaging	CB3
Radiation Therapy, Ear, Nose, Mouth and Throat, Beam Radiation	D90
Radiation Therapy, Ear, Nose, Mouth and Throat, Brachytherapy	D91
Radiation Therapy, Ear, Nose, Mouth and Throat, Stereotactic Radiosurgery	D92
Radiation Therapy, Ear, Nose, Mouth and Throat, Other Radiation	D9Y
Radiation Therapy, Respiratory System, Beam Radiation	DB0
Radiation Therapy, Respiratory System, Brachytherapy	DB1
Radiation Therapy, Respiratory System, Stereotactic Radiosurgery	DB2
Radiation Therapy, Respiratory System, Other Radiation	DBY

Respiratory System

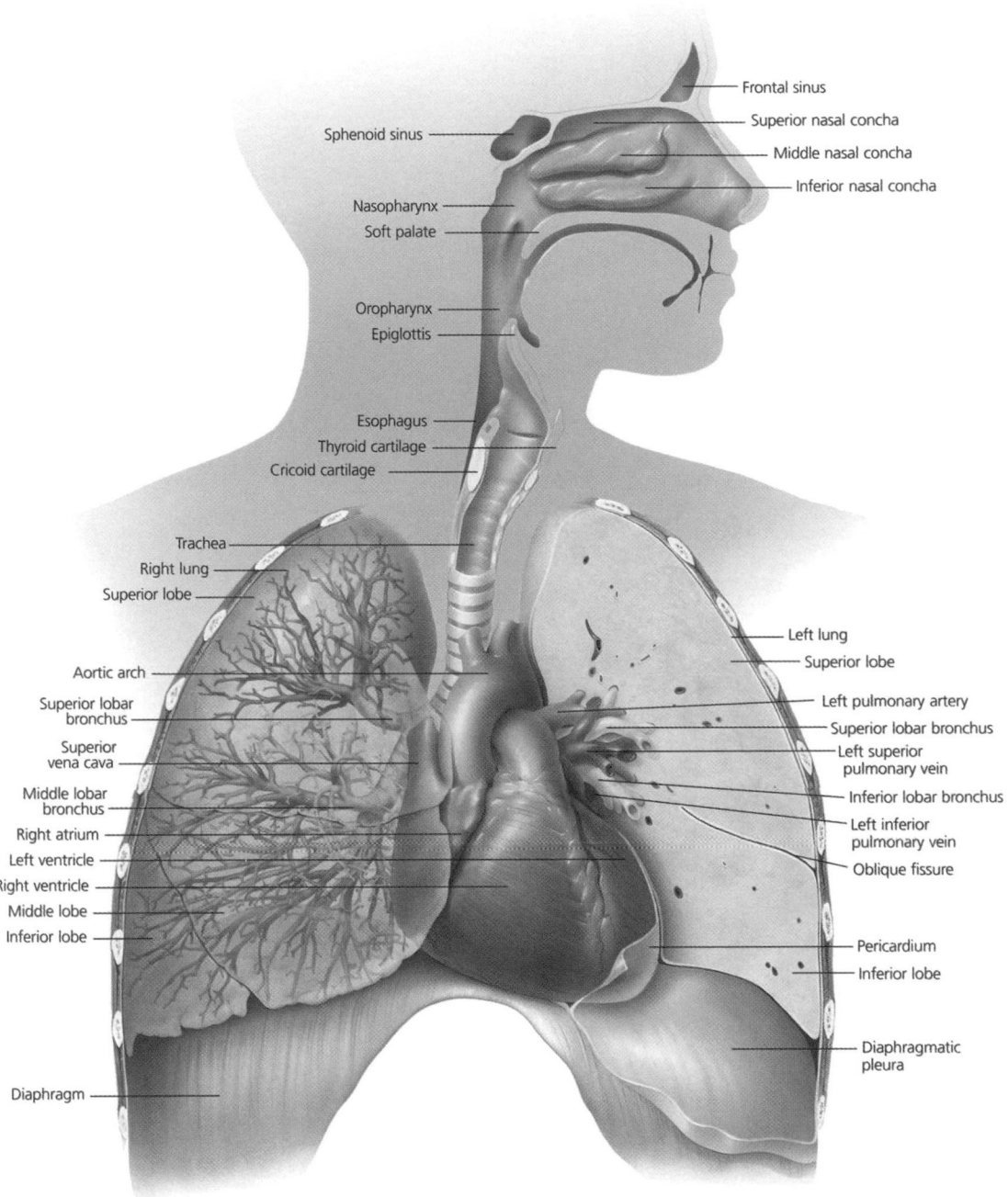

- Frontal sinus
- Sphenoid sinus
- Superior nasal concha
- Middle nasal concha
- Inferior nasal concha
- Nasopharynx
- Soft palate
- Oropharynx
- Epiglottis
- Esophagus
- Thyroid cartilage
- Cricoid cartilage
- Trachea
- Right lung
- Superior lobe
- Left lung
- Superior lobe
- Aortic arch
- Superior lobar bronchus
- Left pulmonary artery
- Superior lobar bronchus
- Left superior pulmonary vein
- Superior vena cava
- Middle lobar bronchus
- Inferior lobar bronchus
- Right atrium
- Left superior pulmonary vein
- Left inferior pulmonary vein
- Left ventricle
- Right ventricle
- Oblique fissure
- Middle lobe
- Inferior lobe
- Pericardium
- Inferior lobe
- Diaphragmatic pleura
- Diaphragm

PLATE 14. HEART AND PERICARDIUM

Heart and Great Vessels, Bypass	021
Heart and Great Vessels, Destruction	025
Heart and Great Vessels, Dilation	027
Heart and Great Vessels, Division	028
Heart and Great Vessels, Excision	02B
Heart and Great Vessels, Extirpation	02C
Heart and Great Vessels, Fragmentation	02F
Heart and Great Vessels, Insertion	02H
Heart and Great Vessels, Inspection	02J
Heart and Great Vessels, Map	02K
Heart and Great Vessels, Occlusion	02L
Heart and Great Vessels, Release	02N
Heart and Great Vessels, Removal	02P
Heart and Great Vessels, Repair	02Q
Heart and Great Vessels, Replacement	02R
Heart and Great Vessels, Reposition	02S
Heart and Great Vessels, Resection	02T
Heart and Great Vessels, Supplement	02U
Heart and Great Vessels, Restriction	02V
Heart and Great Vessels, Revision	02W
Heart and Great Vessels, Transplantation	02Y
Imaging, Heart, Plain Radiography	B20
Imaging, Heart, Fluoroscopy	B21
Imaging, Heart, Computerized Tomography (CT Scan)	B22
Imaging, Heart, Magnetic Resonance Imaging (MRI)	B23
Imaging, Heart, Ultrasonography	B24
Nuclear Medicine, Heart, Planar Nuclear Medicine Imaging	C21
Nuclear Medicine, Heart, Tomographic (TOMO) Nuclear Medicine Imaging	C22
Nuclear Medicine, Heart, Positron Emission Tomographic (PET) Imaging	C23
Nuclear Medicine, Heart, Nonimaging Nuclear Medicine Probe	C25
New Technology, Cardiovascular System, Extirpation	X2C

Heart
(External View)

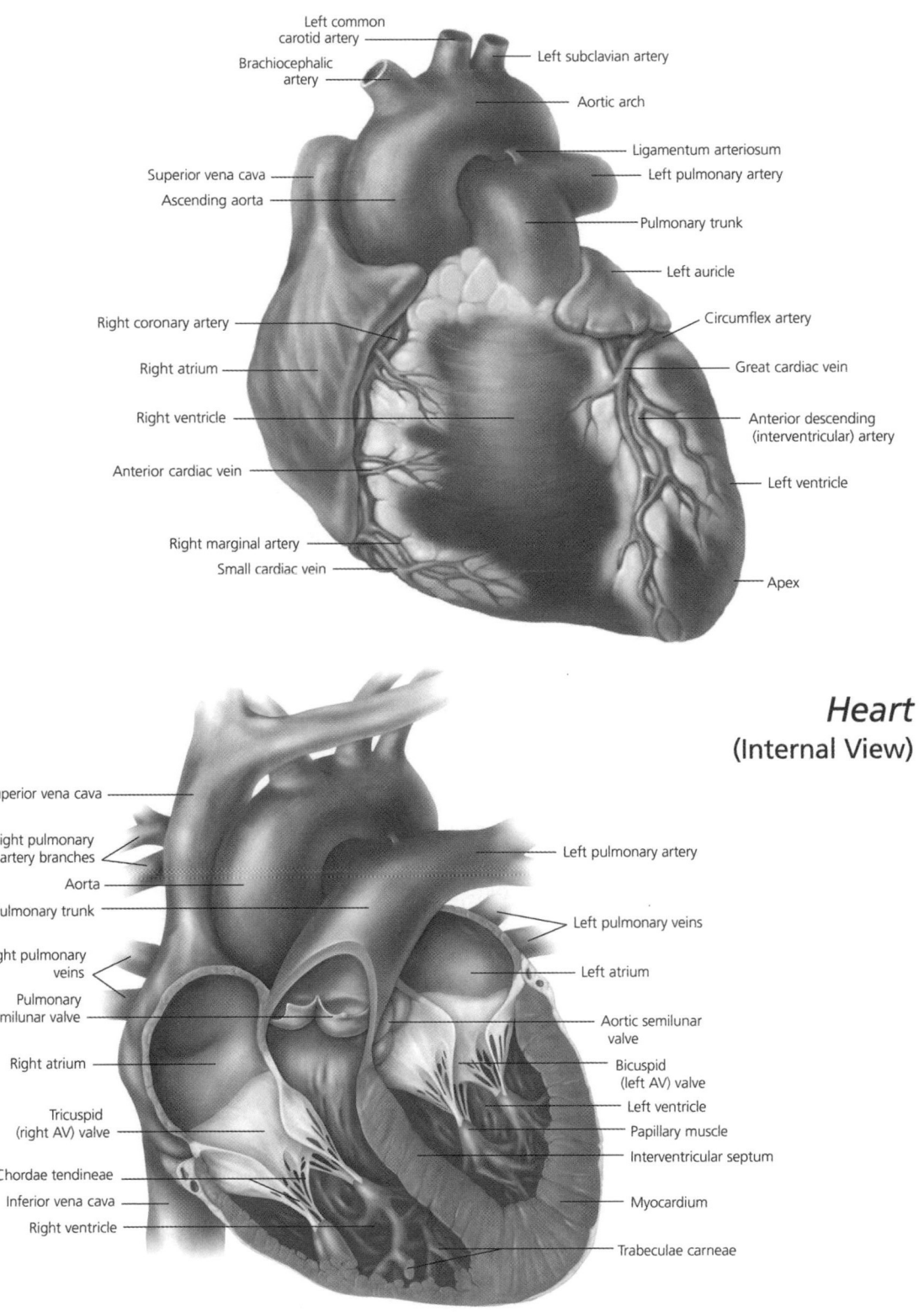

Left common
carotid artery

Brachiocephalic
artery

Left subclavian artery

Aortic arch

Ligamentum arteriosum

Superior vena cava

Left pulmonary artery

Ascending aorta

Pulmonary trunk

Left auricle

Right coronary artery

Circumflex artery

Right atrium

Great cardiac vein

Right ventricle

Anterior descending
(interventricular) artery

Anterior cardiac vein

Left ventricle

Right marginal artery

Small cardiac vein

Apex

Heart
(Internal View)

Superior vena cava

Right pulmonary
artery branches

Left pulmonary artery

Aorta

Pulmonary trunk

Left pulmonary veins

Right pulmonary
veins

Left atrium

Pulmonary
semilunar valve

Aortic semilunar
valve

Right atrium

Bicuspid
(left AV) valve

Tricuspid
(right AV) valve

Left ventricle

Papillary muscle

Chordae tendineae

Interventricular septum

Inferior vena cava

Myocardium

Right ventricle

Trabeculae carneae

PLATE 15. VASCULAR SYSTEM

Upper Arteries, Bypass	031	Lower Veins, Occlusion	06L
Upper Arteries, Destruction	035	Lower Veins, Release	06N
Upper Arteries, Dilation	037	Lower Veins, Removal	06P
Upper Arteries, Drainage	039	Lower Veins, Repair	06Q
Upper Arteries, Excision	03B	Lower Veins, Replacement	06R
Upper Arteries, Extirpation	03C	Lower Veins, Reposition	06S
Upper Arteries, Insertion	03H	Lower Veins, Supplement	06U
Upper Arteries, Inspection	03J	Lower Veins, Restriction	06V
Upper Arteries, Occlusion	03L	Lower Veins, Revision	06W
Upper Arteries, Release	03N	Imaging, Upper Arteries, Plain Radiography	B30
Upper Arteries, Removal	03P	Imaging, Upper Arteries, Fluoroscopy	B31
Upper Arteries, Repair	03Q	Imaging, Upper Arteries, Computerized Tomography	
Upper Arteries, Replacement	03R	(CT Scan)	B32
Upper Arteries, Reposition	03S	Imaging, Upper Arteries, Magnetic Resonance	
Upper Arteries, Supplement	03U	Imaging (MRI)	B33
Upper Arteries, Restriction	03V	Imaging, Upper Arteries, Ultrasonography	B34
Upper Arteries, Revision	03W	Imaging, Lower Arteries, Plain Radiography	B40
Lower Arteries, Bypass	041	Imaging, Lower Arteries, Fluoroscopy	B41
Lower Arteries, Destruction	045	Imaging, Lower Arteries, Computerized Tomography	
Lower Arteries, Dilation	047	(CT Scan)	B42
Lower Arteries, Drainage	049	Imaging, Lower Arteries, Magnetic Resonance	
Lower Arteries, Excision	04B	Imaging (MRI)	B43
Lower Arteries, Extirpation	04C	Imaging, Lower Arteries, Ultrasonography	B44
Lower Arteries, Insertion	04H	Imaging, Veins, Plain Radiography	B50
Lower Arteries, Inspection	04J	Imaging, Veins, Fluoroscopy	B51
Lower Arteries, Occlusion	04L	Imaging, Veins, Computerized Tomography (CT Scan)	B52
Lower Arteries, Release	04N	Imaging, Veins, Magnetic Resonance Imaging (MRI)	B53
Lower Arteries, Removal	04P	Imaging, Veins, Ultrasonography	B54
Lower Arteries, Repair	04Q	Nuclear Medicine, Veins, Planar Nuclear Medicine Imaging	C51
Lower Arteries, Replacement	04R		
Lower Arteries, Reposition	04S		
Lower Arteries, Supplement	04U		
Lower Arteries, Restriction	04V		
Lower Arteries, Revision	04W		
Upper Veins, Bypass	051		
Upper Veins, Destruction	055		
Upper Veins, Dilation	057		
Upper Veins, Drainage	059		
Upper Veins, Excision	05B		
Upper Veins, Extirpation	05C		
Upper Veins, Extraction	05D		
Upper Veins, Insertion	05H		
Upper Veins, Inspection	05J		
Upper Veins, Occlusion	05L		
Upper Veins, Release	05N		
Upper Veins, Removal	05P		
Upper Veins, Repair	05Q		
Upper Veins, Replacement	05R		
Upper Veins, Reposition	05S		
Upper Veins, Supplement	05U		
Upper Veins, Restriction	05V		
Upper Veins, Revision	05W		
Lower Veins, Bypass	061		
Lower Veins, Destruction	065		
Lower Veins, Dilation	067		
Lower Veins, Drainage	069		
Lower Veins, Excision	06B		
Lower Veins, Extirpation	06C		
Lower Veins, Extraction	06D		
Lower Veins, Insertion	06H		
Lower Veins, Inspection	06J		

Vascular System

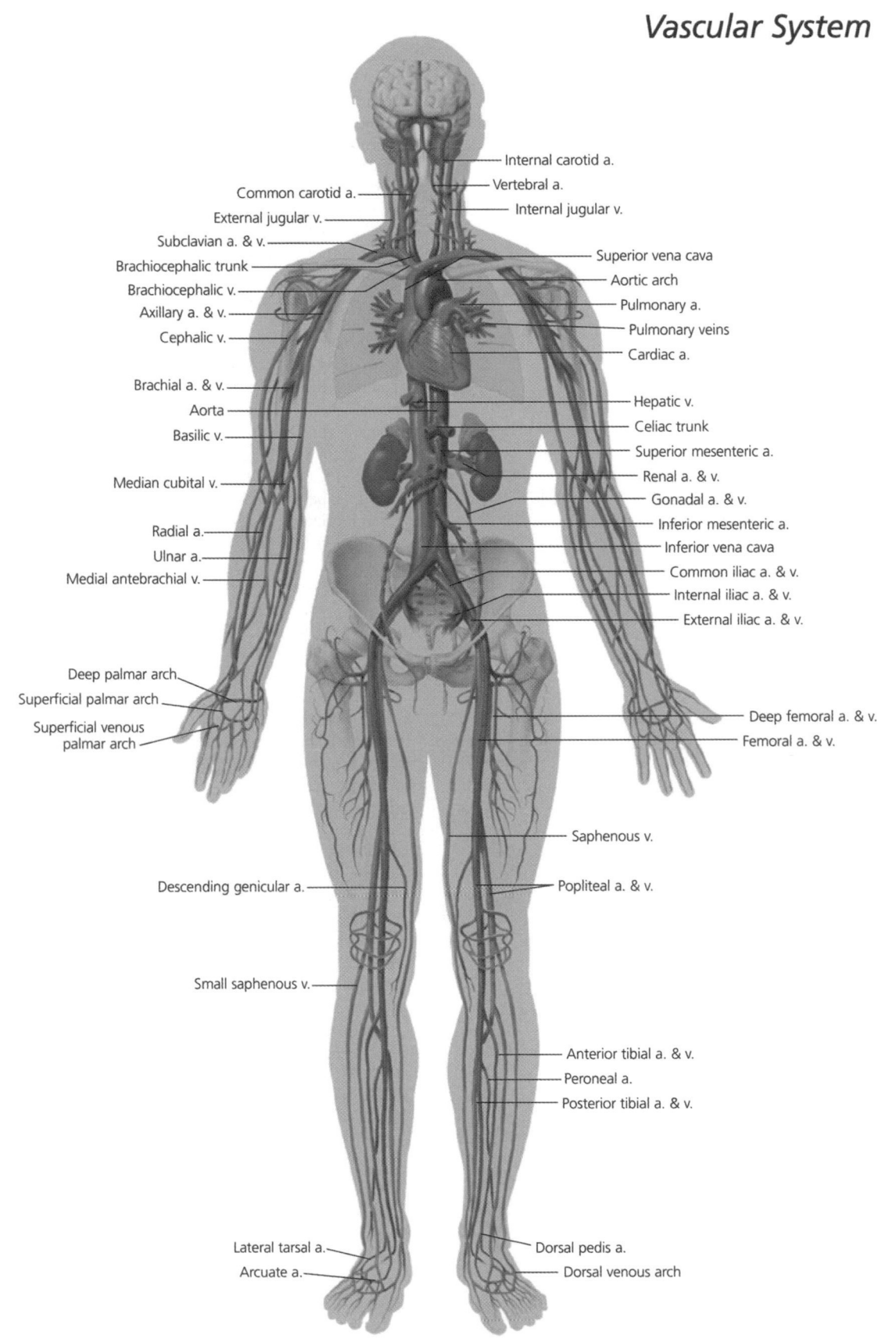

Internal carotid a.
Common carotid a.
Vertebral a.
External jugular v.
Internal jugular v.
Subclavian a. & v.
Brachiocephalic trunk
Superior vena cava
Brachiocephalic v.
Aortic arch
Axillary a. & v.
Pulmonary a.
Cephalic v.
Pulmonary veins
Cardiac a.
Brachial a. & v.
Hepatic v.
Aorta
Celiac trunk
Basilic v.
Superior mesenteric a.
Renal a. & v.
Median cubital v.
Gonadal a. & v.
Inferior mesenteric a.
Radial a.
Inferior vena cava
Ulnar a.
Common iliac a. & v.
Medial antebrachial v.
Internal iliac a. & v.
External iliac a. & v.
Deep palmar arch
Superficial palmar arch
Superficial venous palmar arch
Deep femoral a. & v.
Femoral a. & v.
Saphenous v.
Descending genicular a.
Popliteal a. & v.
Small saphenous v.
Anterior tibial a. & v.
Peroneal a.
Posterior tibial a. & v.
Lateral tarsal a.
Dorsal pedis a.
Arcuate a.
Dorsal venous arch

PLATE 16. DIGESTIVE SYSTEM

Mouth and Throat, Alteration	0C0
Mouth and Throat, Change	0C2
Mouth and Throat, Destruction	0C5
Mouth and Throat, Dilation	0C7
Mouth and Throat, Drainage	0C9
Mouth and Throat, Excision	0CB
Mouth and Throat, Extirpation	0CC
Mouth and Throat, Extraction	0CD
Mouth and Throat, Fragmentation	0CF
Mouth and Throat, Insertion	0CH
Mouth and Throat, Inspection	0CJ
Mouth and Throat, Occlusion	0CL
Mouth and Throat, Reattachment	0CM
Mouth and Throat, Release	0CN
Mouth and Throat, Removal	0CP
Mouth and Throat, Repair	0CQ
Mouth and Throat, Replacement	0CR
Mouth and Throat, Reposition	0CS
Mouth and Throat, Resection	0CT
Mouth and Throat, Supplement	0CU
Mouth and Throat, Restriction	0CV
Mouth and Throat, Revision	0CW
Mouth and Throat, Transfer	0CX
Gastrointestinal System, Bypass	0D1
Gastrointestinal System, Change	0D2
Gastrointestinal System, Destruction	0D5
Gastrointestinal System, Dilation	0D7
Gastrointestinal System, Division	0D8
Gastrointestinal System, Drainage	0D9
Gastrointestinal System, Excision	0DB
Gastrointestinal System, Extirpation	0DC
Gastrointestinal System, Fragmentation	0DF
Gastrointestinal System, Insertion	0DH
Gastrointestinal System, Inspection	0DJ
Gastrointestinal System, Occlusion	0DL
Gastrointestinal System, Reattachment	0DM
Gastrointestinal System, Release	0DN
Gastrointestinal System, Removal	0DP
Gastrointestinal System, Repair	0DQ
Gastrointestinal System, Replacement	0DR
Gastrointestinal System, Reposition	0DS
Gastrointestinal System, Resection	0DT
Gastrointestinal System, Supplement	0DU
Gastrointestinal System, Restriction	0DV
Gastrointestinal System, Revision	0DW
Gastrointestinal System, Transfer	0DX
Gastrointestinal System, Transplantation	0DY
Hepatobiliary System and Pancreas, Bypass	0F1
Hepatobiliary System and Pancreas, Change	0F2
Hepatobiliary System and Pancreas, Destruction	0F5
Hepatobiliary System and Pancreas, Dilation	0F7
Hepatobiliary System and Pancreas, Division	0F8
Hepatobiliary System and Pancreas, Drainage	0F9
Hepatobiliary System and Pancreas, Excision	0FB
Hepatobiliary System and Pancreas, Extirpation	0FC
Hepatobiliary System and Pancreas, Fragmentation	0FF
Hepatobiliary System and Pancreas, Insertion	0FH
Hepatobiliary System and Pancreas, Inspection	0FJ
Hepatobiliary System and Pancreas, Occlusion	0FL

Hepatobiliary System and Pancreas, Reattachment	0FM
Hepatobiliary System and Pancreas, Release	0FN
Hepatobiliary System and Pancreas, Removal	0FP
Hepatobiliary System and Pancreas, Repair	0FQ
Hepatobiliary System and Pancreas, Replacement	0FR
Hepatobiliary System and Pancreas, Reposition	0FS
Hepatobiliary System and Pancreas, Resection	0FT
Hepatobiliary System and Pancreas, Supplement	0FU
Hepatobiliary System and Pancreas, Restriction	0FV
Hepatobiliary System and Pancreas, Revision	0FW
Hepatobiliary System and Pancreas, Transplantation	0FY
Imaging, Gastrointestinal System, Fluoroscopy	BD1
Imaging, Gastrointestinal System, Computerized Tomography (CT Scan)	BD2
Imaging, Gastrointestinal System, Ultrasonography	BD4
Imaging, Hepatobiliary System and Pancreas, Plain Radiography	BF0
Imaging, Hepatobiliary System and Pancreas, Fluoroscopy	BF1
Imaging, Hepatobiliary System and Pancreas, Computerized Tomography (CT Scan)	BF2
Imaging, Hepatobiliary System and Pancreas, Magnetic Resonance Imaging (MRI)	BF3
Imaging, Hepatobiliary System and Pancreas, Ultrasonography	BF4
Nuclear Medicine, Gastrointestinal System, Planar Nuclear Medicine Imaging	CD1
Nuclear Medicine, Gastrointestinal System, Tomographic (TOMO) Nuclear Medicine Imaging	CD2
Nuclear Medicine, Hepatobiliary System and Pancreas, Planar Nuclear Medicine Imaging	CF1
Nuclear Medicine, Hepatobiliary System and Pancreas, Tomographic (TOMO) Nuclear Medicine Imaging	CF2
Radiation Therapy, Gastrointestinal System, Beam Radiation	DD0
Radiation Therapy, Gastrointestinal System, Brachytherapy	DD1
Radiation Therapy, Gastrointestinal System, Stereotactic Radiosurgery	DD2
Radiation Therapy, Gastrointestinal System, Other Radiation	DDY
Radiation Therapy, Hepatobiliary System and Pancreas, Beam Radiation	DF0
Radiation Therapy, Hepatobiliary System and Pancreas, Brachytherapy	DF1
Radiation Therapy, Hepatobiliary System and Pancreas, Stereotactic Radiosurgery	DF2
Radiation Therapy, Hepatobiliary System and Pancreas, Other Radiation	DFY

Digestive System

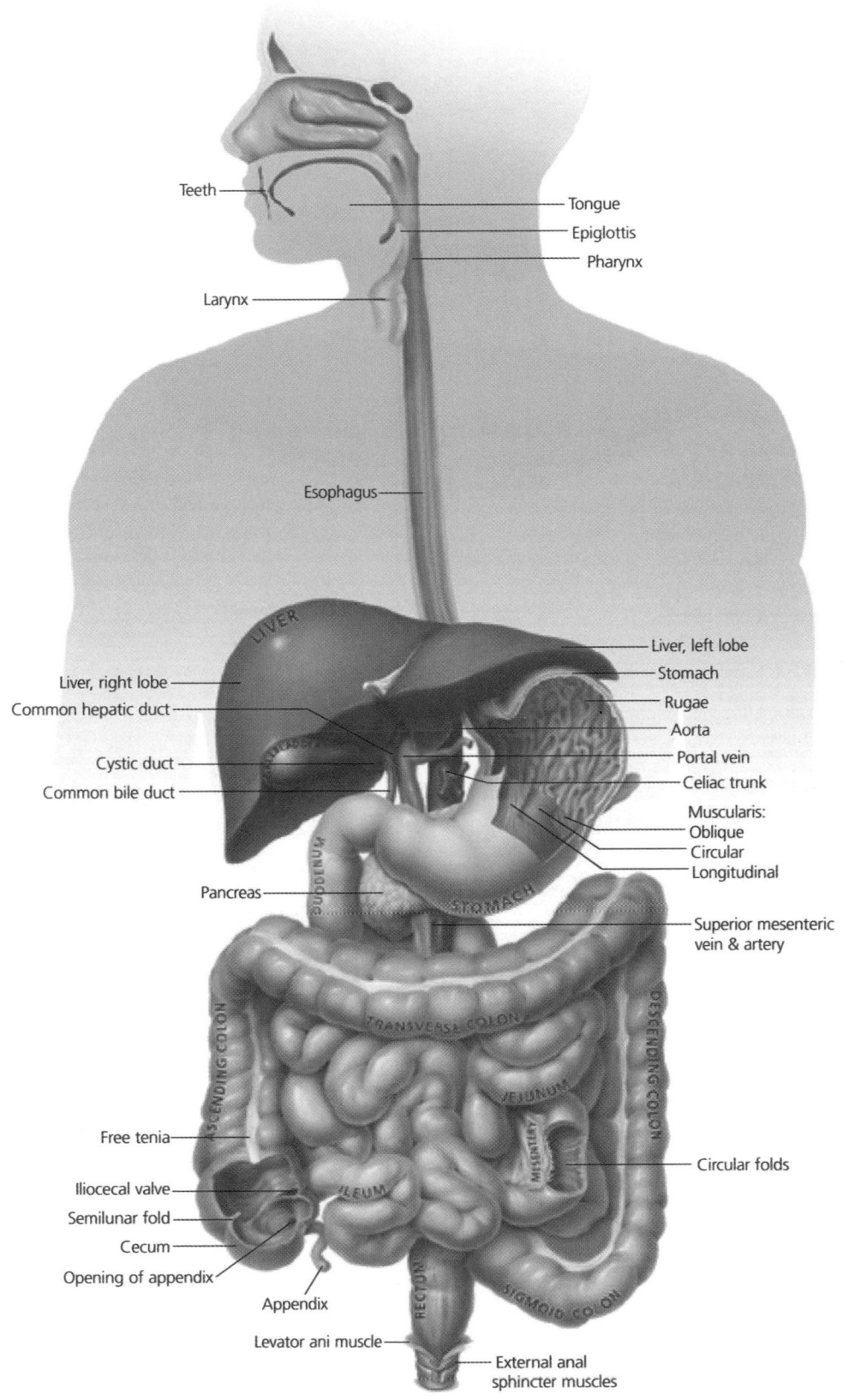

Teeth

Tongue

Epiglottis

Pharynx

Larynx

Esophagus

Liver, left lobe

Stomach

Liver, right lobe

Rugae

Common hepatic duct

Aorta

Portal vein

Cystic duct

Celiac trunk

Common bile duct

Muscularis:
Oblique
Circular
Longitudinal

Pancreas

Superior mesenteric
vein & artery

Free tenia

Circular folds

Iliocecal valve

Semilunar fold

Cecum

Opening of appendix

Appendix

Levator ani muscle

External anal
sphincter muscles

PLATE 17. GENITOURINARY SYSTEM

Urinary System, Bypass	0T1
Urinary System, Change	0T2
Urinary System, Destruction	0T5
Urinary System, Dilation	0T7
Urinary System, Division	0T8
Urinary System, Drainage	0T9
Urinary System, Excision	0TB
Urinary System, Extirpation	0TC
Urinary System, Extraction	0TD
Urinary System, Fragmentation	0TF
Urinary System, Insertion	0TH
Urinary System, Inspection	0TJ
Urinary System, Occlusion	0TL
Urinary System, Reattachment	0TM
Urinary System, Release	0TN
Urinary System, Removal	0TP
Urinary System, Repair	0TQ
Urinary System, Replacement	0TR
Urinary System, Reposition	0TS
Urinary System, Resection	0TT
Urinary System, Supplement	0TU
Urinary System, Restriction	0TV
Urinary System, Revision	0TW
Urinary System, Transplantation	0TY
Imaging, Urinary System, Plain Radiography	BT0
Imaging, Urinary System, Fluoroscopy	BT1
Imaging, Urinary System, Computerized Tomography (CT Scan)	BT2
Imaging, Urinary System, Magnetic Resonance Imaging (MRI)	BT3
Imaging, Urinary System, Ultrasonography	BT4
Nuclear Medicine, Urinary System, Planar Nuclear Medicine Imaging	CT1
Nuclear Medicine, Urinary System, Tomographic (TOMO) Nuclear Medicine Imaging	CT2
Nuclear Medicine, Urinary System, Nonimaging Nuclear Medicine Assay	CT6
Radiation Therapy, Urinary System, Beam Radiation	DT0
Radiation Therapy, Urinary System, Brachytherapy	DT1
Radiation Therapy, Urinary System, Stereotactic Radiosurgery	DT2
Radiation Therapy, Urinary System, Other Radiation	DTY

Urinary System

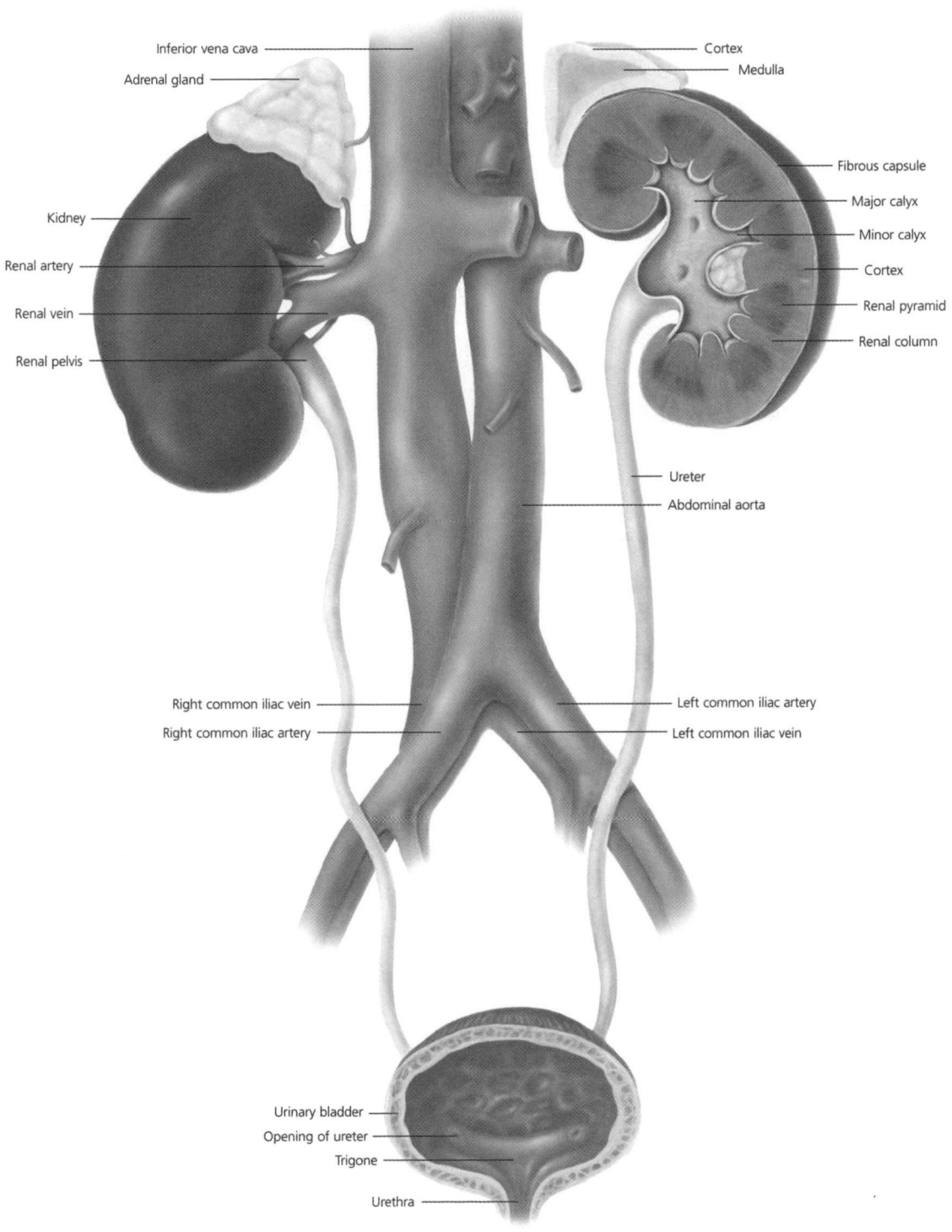

Inferior vena cava

Adrenal gland

Kidney

Renal artery

Renal vein

Renal pelvis

Cortex

Medulla

Fibrous capsule

Major calyx

Minor calyx

Cortex

Renal pyramid

Renal column

Ureter

Abdominal aorta

Right common iliac vein

Right common iliac artery

Left common iliac artery

Left common iliac vein

Urinary bladder

Opening of ureter

Trigone

Urethra

PLATE 18. MALE REPRODUCTIVE SYSTEM

Male Reproductive System, Bypass	0V1
Male Reproductive System, Change	0V2
Male Reproductive System, Destruction	0V5
Male Reproductive System, Dilation	0V7
Male Reproductive System, Drainage	0V9
Male Reproductive System, Excision	0VB
Male Reproductive System, Extirpation	0VC
Male Reproductive System, Insertion	0VH
Male Reproductive System, Inspection	0VJ
Male Reproductive System, Occlusion	0VL
Male Reproductive System, Reattachment	0VM
Male Reproductive System, Release	0VN
Male Reproductive System, Removal	0VP
Male Reproductive System, Repair	0VQ
Male Reproductive System, Replacement	0VR
Male Reproductive System, Reposition	0VS
Male Reproductive System, Resection	0VT
Male Reproductive System, Supplement	0VU
Male Reproductive System, Revision	0VW
Imaging, Male Reproductive System, Plain Radiography	BV0
Imaging, Male Reproductive System, Fluoroscopy	BV1
Imaging, Male Reproductive System, Computerized Tomography (CT Scan)	BV2
Imaging, Male Reproductive System, Magnetic Resonance Imaging (MRI)	BV3
Imaging, Male Reproductive System, Ultrasonography	BV4
Nuclear Medicine, Male Reproductive System, Planar Nuclear Medicine Imaging	CV1
Radiation Therapy, Male Reproductive System, Beam Radiation	DV0
Radiation Therapy, Male Reproductive System, Brachytherapy	DV1
Radiation Therapy, Male Reproductive System, Stereotactic Radiosurgery	DV2
Radiation Therapy, Male Reproductive System, Other Radiation	DVY

Male Reproductive System

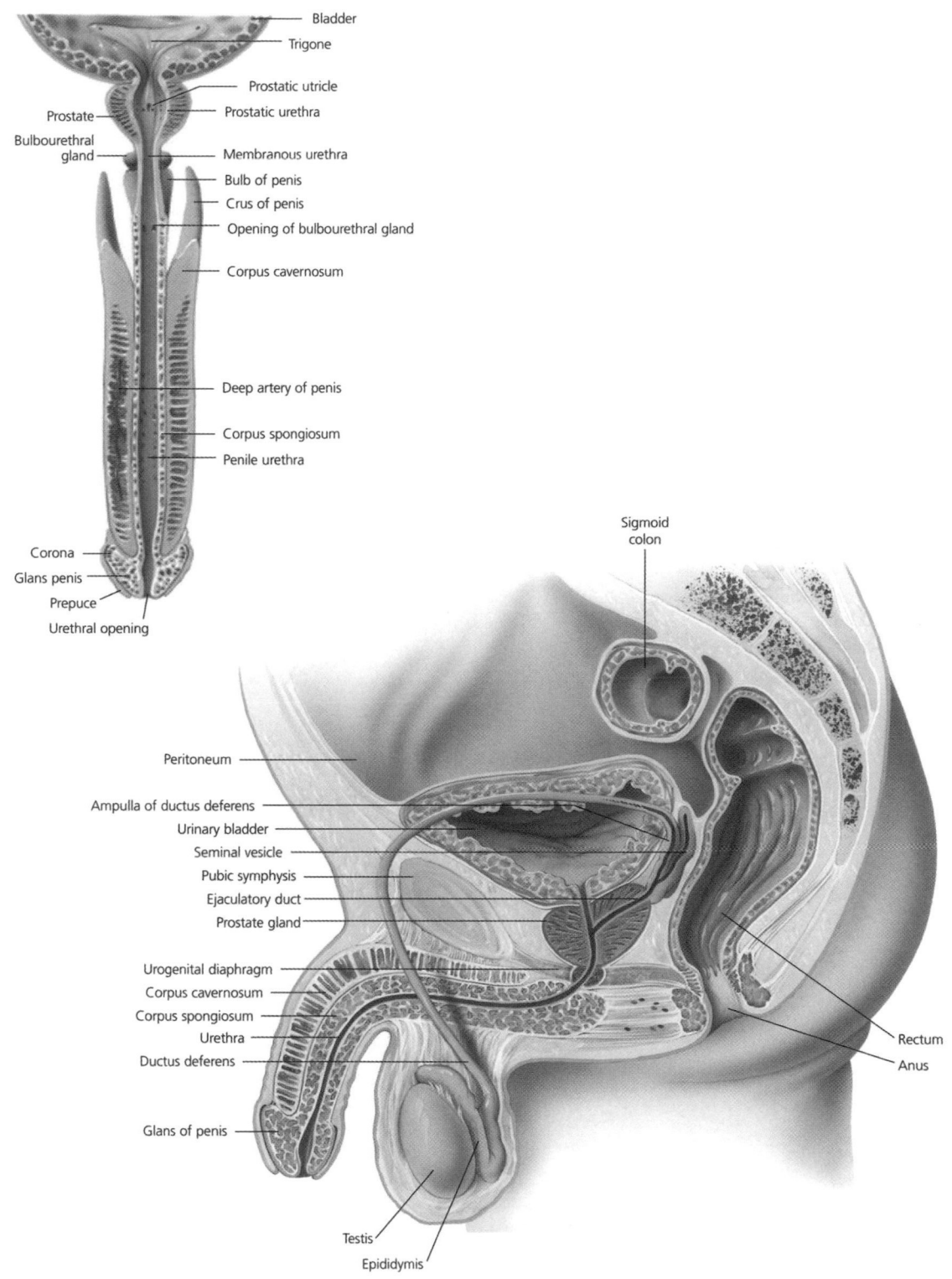

Bladder
Trigone
Prostatic utricle
Prostatic urethra
Prostate
Bulbourethral gland
Membranous urethra
Bulb of penis
Crus of penis
Opening of bulbourethral gland
Corpus cavernosum
Deep artery of penis
Corpus spongiosum
Penile urethra
Corona
Glans penis
Prepuce
Urethral opening

Sigmoid colon
Peritoneum
Ampulla of ductus deferens
Urinary bladder
Seminal vesicle
Pubic symphysis
Ejaculatory duct
Prostate gland
Urogenital diaphragm
Corpus cavernosum
Corpus spongiosum
Urethra
Ductus deferens
Glans of penis
Rectum
Anus
Testis
Epididymis

PLATE 19. FEMALE REPRODUCTIVE SYSTEM

Female Reproductive System, Bypass	0U1
Female Reproductive System, Change	0U2
Female Reproductive System, Destruction	0U5
Female Reproductive System, Dilation	0U7
Female Reproductive System, Division	0U8
Female Reproductive System, Drainage	0U9
Female Reproductive System, Excision	0UB
Female Reproductive System, Extirpation	0UC
Female Reproductive System, Extraction	0UD
Female Reproductive System, Fragmentation	0UF
Female Reproductive System, Insertion	0UH
Female Reproductive System, Inspection	0UJ
Female Reproductive System, Occlusion	0UL
Female Reproductive System, Reattachment	0UM
Female Reproductive System, Release	0UN
Female Reproductive System, Removal	0UP
Female Reproductive System, Repair	0UQ
Female Reproductive System, Reposition	0US
Female Reproductive System, Resection	0UT
Female Reproductive System, Supplement	0UU
Female Reproductive System, Restriction	0UV
Female Reproductive System, Revision	0UW
Female Reproductive System, Transplantation	0UY
Radiation Therapy, Female Reproductive System, Beam Radiation	DU0
Radiation Therapy, Female Reproductive System, Brachytherapy	DU1
Radiation Therapy, Female Reproductive System, Stereotactic Radiosurgery	DU2
Radiation Therapy, Female Reproductive System, Other Radiation	DUY

Female Reproductive System

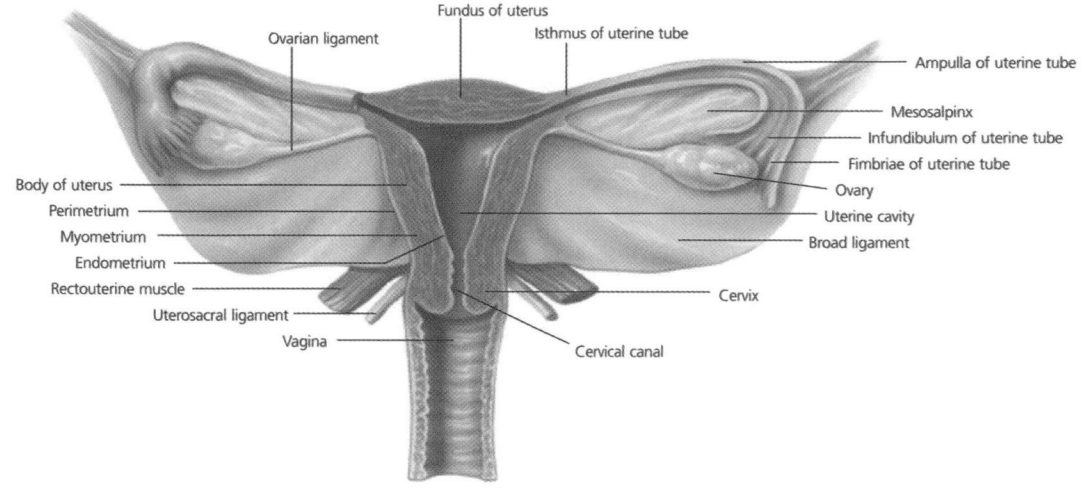

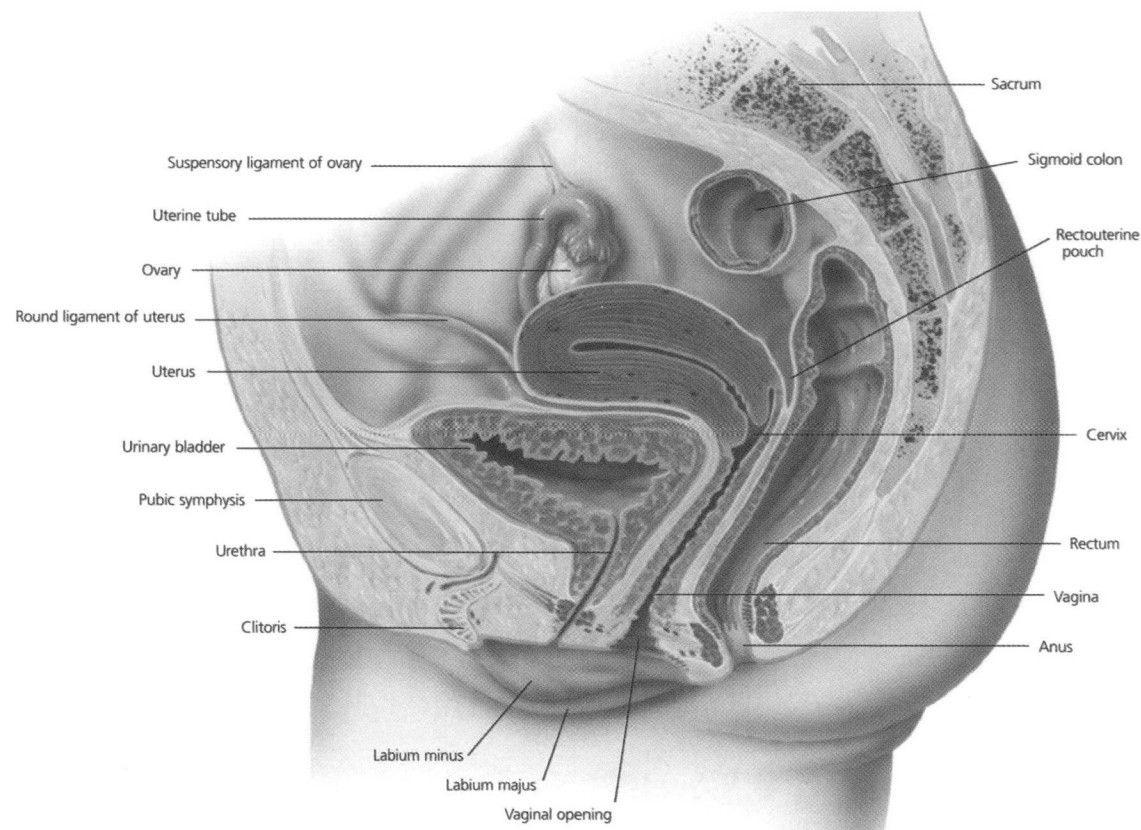

PLATE 20. PREGNANCY, CHILDBIRTH AND THE PUERPERIUM

Female Reproductive System: Pregnancy
(Lateral View)

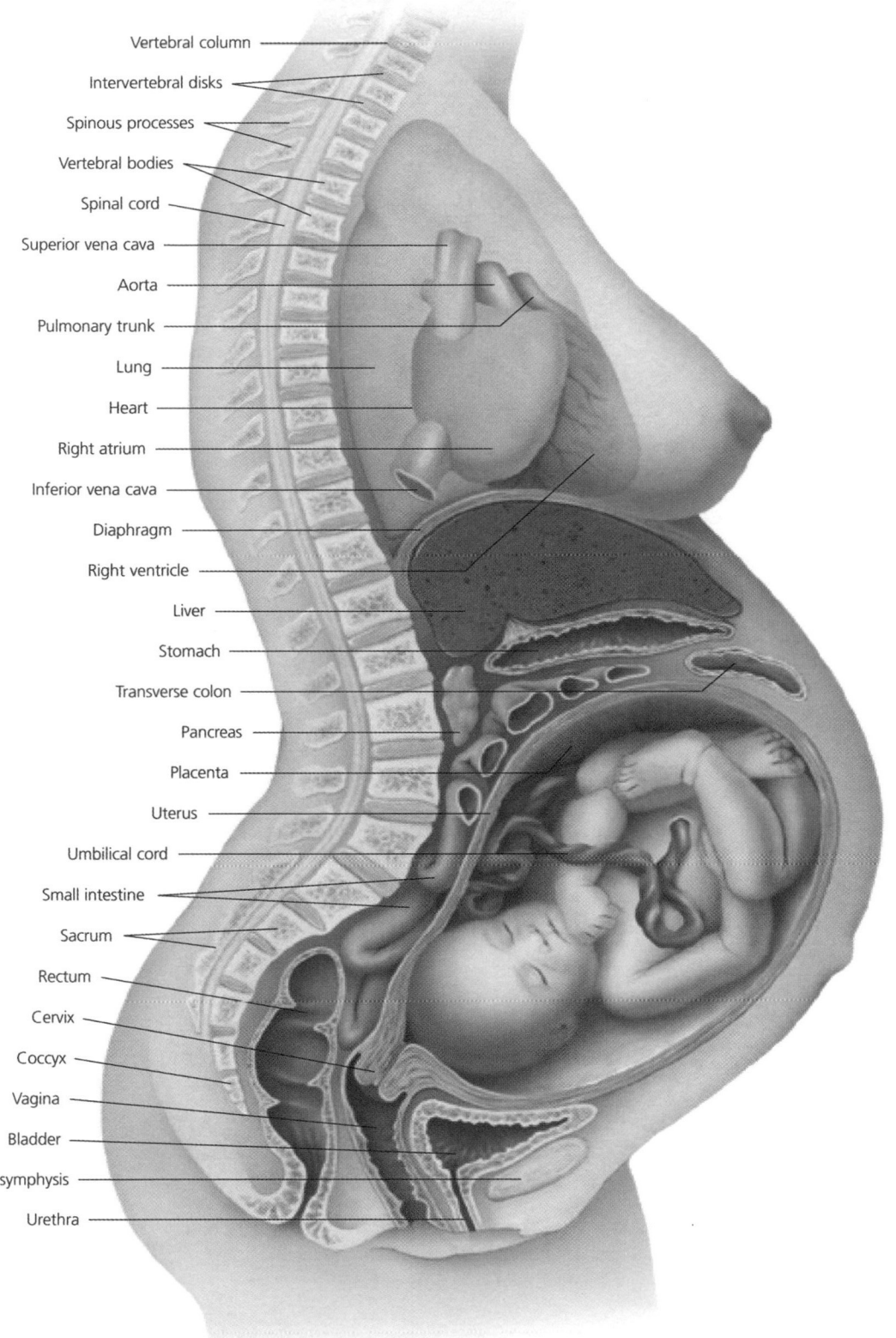

Vertebral column
Intervertebral disks
Spinous processes
Vertebral bodies
Spinal cord
Superior vena cava
Aorta
Pulmonary trunk
Lung
Heart
Right atrium
Inferior vena cava
Diaphragm
Right ventricle
Liver
Stomach
Transverse colon
Pancreas
Placenta
Uterus
Umbilical cord
Small intestine
Sacrum
Rectum
Cervix
Coccyx
Vagina
Bladder
Pubic symphysis
Urethra

PLATE 21. NERVOUS SYSTEM – BRAIN

Central Nervous System, Bypass	001
Central Nervous System, Change	002
Central Nervous System, Destruction	005
Central Nervous System, Division	008
Central Nervous System, Drainage	009
Central Nervous System, Excision	00B
Central Nervous System, Extirpation	00C
Central Nervous System, Extraction	00D
Central Nervous System, Fragmentation	00F
Central Nervous System, Insertion	00H
Central Nervous System, Inspection	00J
Central Nervous System, Map	00K
Central Nervous System, Release	00N
Central Nervous System, Removal	00P
Central Nervous System, Repair	00Q
Central Nervous System, Reposition	00S
Central Nervous System, Resection	00T
Central Nervous System, Supplement	00U
Central Nervous System, Revision	00W
Central Nervous System, Transfer	00X
Imaging, Central Nervous System, Plain Radiography	B00
Imaging, Central Nervous System, Fluoroscopy	B01
Imaging, Central Nervous System, Computerized Tomography (CT Scan)	B02
Imaging, Central Nervous System, Magnetic Resonance Imaging (MRI)	B03
Imaging, Central Nervous System, Ultrasonography	B04
Nuclear Medicine, Central Nervous System, Planar Nuclear Medicine Imaging	C01
Nuclear Medicine, Central Nervous System, Tomographic (TOMO) Nuclear Medicine Imaging	C02
Nuclear Medicine, Central Nervous System, Positron Emission Tomographic (PET) Imaging	C03
Nuclear Medicine, Central Nervous System, Nonimaging Nuclear Medicine Probe	C05
Radiation Therapy, Central and Peripheral Nervous System, Beam Radiation	D00
Radiation Therapy, Central and Peripheral Nervous System, Brachytherapy	D01
Radiation Therapy, Central and Peripheral Nervous System, Stereotactic Radiosurgery	D02
Radiation Therapy, Central and Peripheral Nervous System, Other Radiation	D0Y

Brain
(Base View)

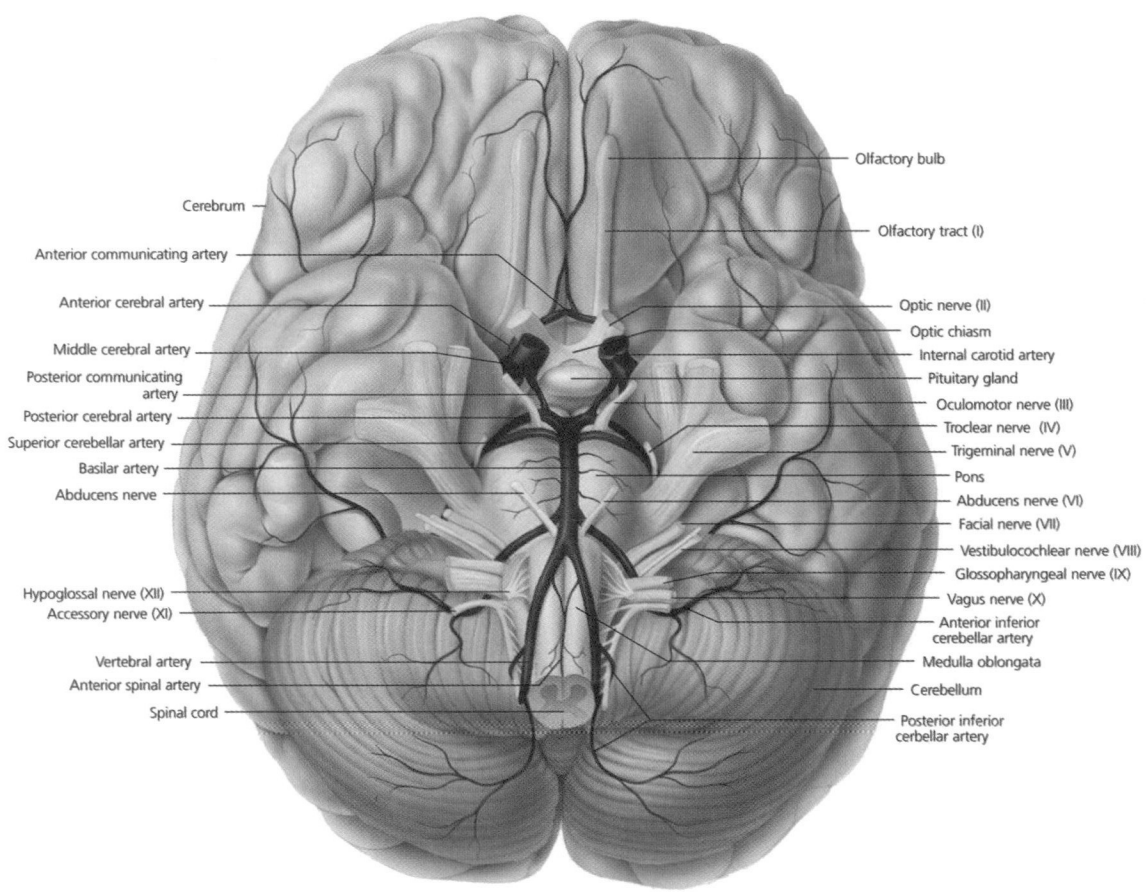

Cerebrum

Anterior communicating artery

Anterior cerebral artery

Middle cerebral artery

Posterior communicating artery

Posterior cerebral artery

Superior cerebellar artery

Basilar artery

Abducens nerve

Hypoglossal nerve (XII)

Accessory nerve (XI)

Vertebral artery

Anterior spinal artery

Spinal cord

Olfactory bulb

Olfactory tract (I)

Optic nerve (II)

Optic chiasm

Internal carotid artery

Pituitary gland

Oculomotor nerve (III)

Troclear nerve (IV)

Trigeminal nerve (V)

Pons

Abducens nerve (VI)

Facial nerve (VII)

Vestibulocochlear nerve (VIII)

Glossopharyngeal nerve (IX)

Vagus nerve (X)

Anterior inferior cerebellar artery

Medulla oblongata

Cerebellum

Posterior inferior cerbellar artery

PLATE 22. NERVOUS SYSTEM

Central Nervous System, Bypass	001
Central Nervous System, Change	002
Central Nervous System, Destruction	005
Central Nervous System, Division	008
Central Nervous System, Drainage	009
Central Nervous System, Excision	00B
Central Nervous System, Extirpation	00C
Central Nervous System, Extraction	00D
Central Nervous System, Fragmentation	00F
Central Nervous System, Insertion	00H
Central Nervous System, Inspection	00J
Central Nervous System, Map	00K
Central Nervous System, Release	00N
Central Nervous System, Removal	00P
Central Nervous System, Repair	00Q
Central Nervous System, Reposition	00S
Central Nervous System, Resection	00T
Central Nervous System, Supplement	00U
Central Nervous System, Revision	00W
Central Nervous System, Transfer	00X
Peripheral Nervous System, Change	012
Peripheral Nervous System, Destruction	015
Peripheral Nervous System, Division	018
Peripheral Nervous System, Drainage	019
Peripheral Nervous System, Excision	01B
Peripheral Nervous System, Extirpation	01C
Peripheral Nervous System, Extraction	01D
Peripheral Nervous System, Insertion	01H
Peripheral Nervous System, Inspection	01J
Peripheral Nervous System, Release	01N
Peripheral Nervous System, Removal	01P
Peripheral Nervous System, Repair	01Q
Peripheral Nervous System, Reposition	01S
Peripheral Nervous System, Supplement	01U
Peripheral Nervous System, Revision	01W
Peripheral Nervous System, Transfer	01X
Imaging, Central Nervous System, Plain Radiography	B00
Imaging, Central Nervous System, Fluoroscopy	B01
Imaging, Central Nervous System, Computerized Tomography (CT Scan)	B02
Imaging, Central Nervous System, Magnetic Resonance Imaging (MRI)	B03
Imaging, Central Nervous System, Ultrasonography	B04
Nuclear Medicine, Central Nervous System, Planar Nuclear Medicine Imaging	C01
Nuclear Medicine, Central Nervous System, Tomographic (TOMO) Nuclear Medicine Imaging	C02
Nuclear Medicine, Central Nervous System, Positron Emission Tomographic (PET) Imaging	C03
Nuclear Medicine, Central Nervous System, Nonimaging Nuclear Medicine Probe	C05
Radiation Therapy, Central and Peripheral Nervous System, Beam Radiation	D00
Radiation Therapy, Central and Peripheral Nervous System, Brachytherapy	D01
Radiation Therapy, Central and Peripheral Nervous System, Stereotactic Radiosurgery	D02
Radiation Therapy, Central and Peripheral Nervous System, Other Radiation	D0Y

Nervous System

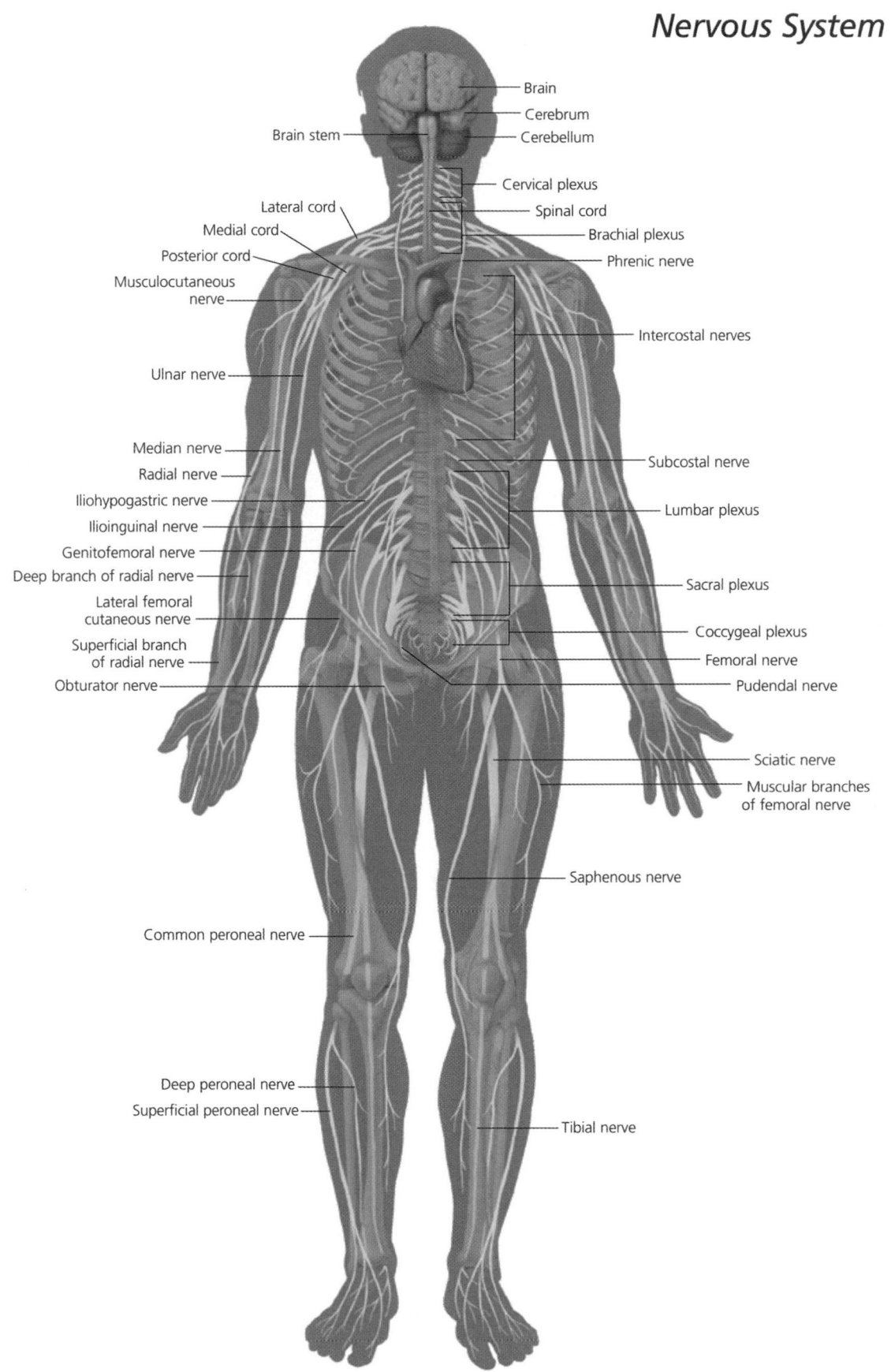

Brain
Cerebrum
Brain stem
Cerebellum
Cervical plexus
Lateral cord
Spinal cord
Medial cord
Brachial plexus
Posterior cord
Phrenic nerve
Musculocutaneous nerve
Intercostal nerves
Ulnar nerve
Median nerve
Radial nerve
Subcostal nerve
Iliohypogastric nerve
Ilioinguinal nerve
Lumbar plexus
Genitofemoral nerve
Deep branch of radial nerve
Sacral plexus
Lateral femoral cutaneous nerve
Coccygeal plexus
Superficial branch of radial nerve
Femoral nerve
Obturator nerve
Pudendal nerve
Sciatic nerve
Muscular branches of femoral nerve
Saphenous nerve
Common peroneal nerve
Deep peroneal nerve
Superficial peroneal nerve
Tibial nerve

PLATE 23. EYE AND OCULAR ADNEXA

Eye, Alteration	080
Eye, Bypass	081
Eye, Change	082
Eye, Destruction	085
Eye, Dilation	087
Eye, Drainage	089
Eye, Excision	08B
Eye, Extirpation	08C
Eye, Extraction	08D
Eye, Fragmentation	08F
Eye, Insertion	08H
Eye, Inspection	08J
Eye, Occlusion	08L
Eye, Reattachment	08M
Eye, Release	08N
Eye, Removal	08P
Eye, Repair	08Q
Eye, Replacement	08R
Eye, Reposition	08S
Eye, Resection	08T
Eye, Supplement	08U
Eye, Restriction	08V
Eye, Revision	08W
Eye, Transfer	08X
Imaging, Eye, Plain Radiography	B80
Imaging, Eye, Computerized Tomography (CT Scan)	B82
Imaging, Eye, Magnetic Resonance Imaging (MRI)	B83
Imaging, Eye, Ultrasonography	B84
Nuclear Medicine, Eye, Planar Nuclear Medicine Imaging	C81
Radiation Therapy, Eye, Beam Radiation	D80
Radiation Therapy, Eye, Brachytherapy	D81
Radiation Therapy, Eye, Stereotactic Radiosurgery	D82
Radiation Therapy, Eye, Other Radiation	D8Y

Right Eye
(Horizontal Section)

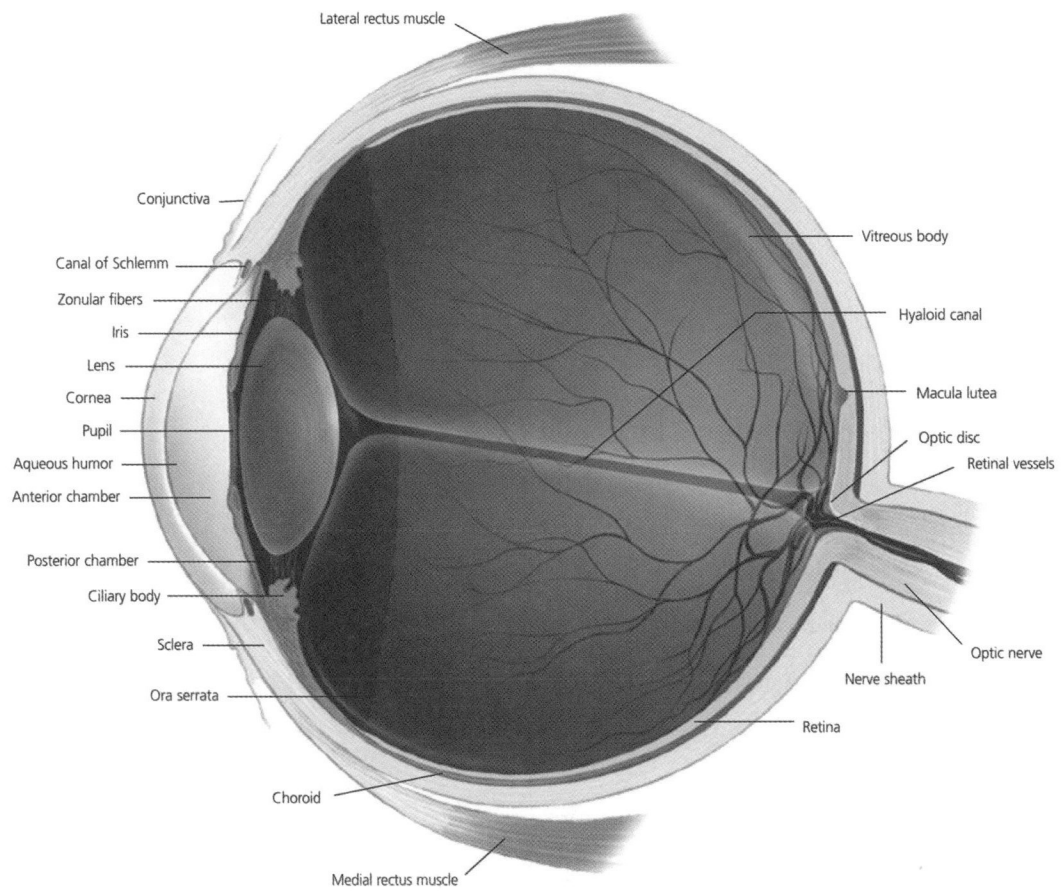

Lateral rectus muscle

Conjunctiva

Canal of Schlemm

Zonular fibers

Iris

Lens

Cornea

Pupil

Aqueous humor

Anterior chamber

Posterior chamber

Ciliary body

Sclera

Ora serrata

Choroid

Medial rectus muscle

Vitreous body

Hyaloid canal

Macula lutea

Optic disc

Retinal vessels

Optic nerve

Nerve sheath

Retina

PLATE 24. AUDITORY SYSTEM

Ear, Nose, Sinus, Alteration	090
Ear, Nose, Sinus, Bypass	091
Ear, Nose, Sinus, Change	092
Ear, Nose, Sinus, Destruction	095
Ear, Nose, Sinus, Dilation	097
Ear, Nose, Sinus, Division	098
Ear, Nose, Sinus, Drainage	099
Ear, Nose, Sinus, Excision	09B
Ear, Nose, Sinus, Extirpation	09C
Ear, Nose, Sinus, Extraction	09D
Ear, Nose, Sinus, Insertion	09H
Ear, Nose, Sinus, Inspection	09J
Ear, Nose, Sinus, Reattachment	09M
Ear, Nose, Sinus, Release	09N
Ear, Nose, Sinus, Removal	09P
Ear, Nose, Sinus, Repair	09Q
Ear, Nose, Sinus, Replacement	09R
Ear, Nose, Sinus, Reposition	09S
Ear, Nose, Sinus, Resection	09T
Ear, Nose, Sinus, Supplement	09U
Ear, Nose, Sinus, Revision	09W
Imaging, Ear, Nose, Mouth and Throat, Plain Radiography	B90
Imaging, Ear, Nose, Mouth and Throat, Fluoroscopy	B91
Imaging, Ear, Nose, Mouth and Throat, Computerized Tomography (CT Scan)	B92
Imaging, Ear, Nose, Mouth and Throat, Magnetic Resonance Imaging (MRI)	B93
Nuclear Medicine, Ear, Nose, Mouth and Throat, Planar Nuclear Medicine Imaging	C91
Radiation Therapy, Ear, Nose, Mouth and Throat, Beam Radiation	D90
Radiation Therapy, Ear, Nose, Mouth and Throat, Brachytherapy	D91
Radiation Therapy, Ear, Nose, Mouth and Throat, Stereotactic Radiosurgery	D92
Radiation Therapy, Ear, Nose, Mouth and Throat, Other Radiation	D9Y
Physical Rehabilitation and Diagnostic Audiology, Rehabilitation, Hearing Treatment	F09
Physical Rehabilitation and Diagnostic Audiology, Rehabilitation, Cochlear Implant Treatment	F0B
Physical Rehabilitation and Diagnostic Audiology, Rehabilitation, Vestibular Treatment	F0C
Physical Rehabilitation and Diagnostic Audiology, Rehabilitation, Device Fitting	F0D
Physical Rehabilitation and Diagnostic Audiology, Diagnostic Audiology, Hearing Assessment	F13
Physical Rehabilitation and Diagnostic Audiology, Diagnostic Audiology, Hearing Aid Assessment	F14
Physical Rehabilitation and Diagnostic Audiology, Diagnostic Audiology, Vestibular Assessment	F15

The Ear

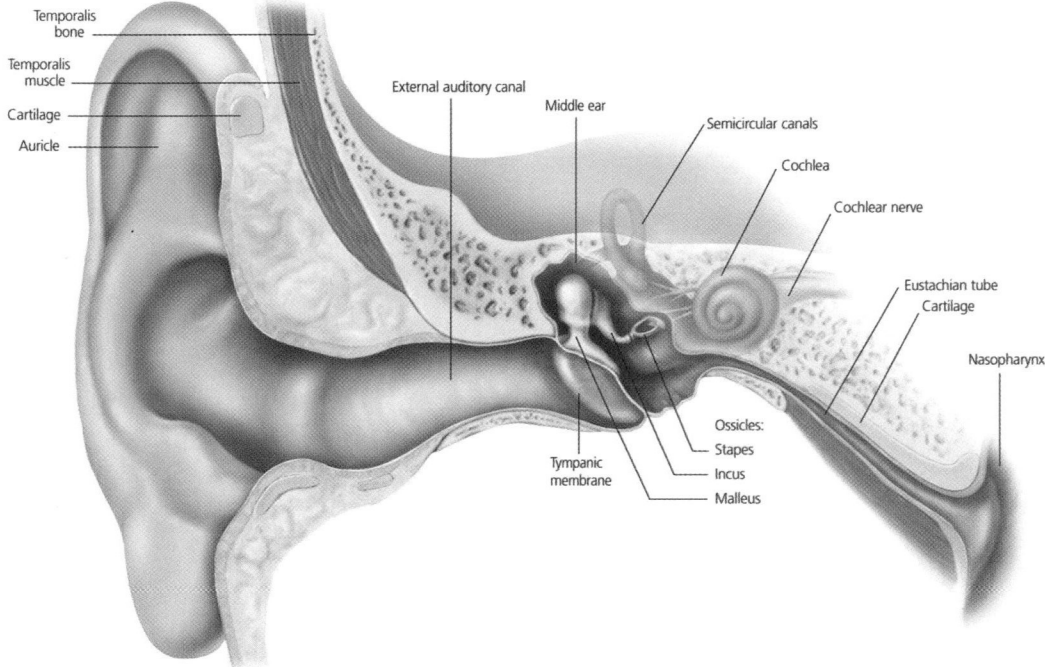

Temporalis bone

Temporalis muscle

Cartilage

Auricle

External auditory canal

Middle ear

Semicircular canals

Cochlea

Cochlear nerve

Eustachian tube

Cartilage

Nasopharynx

Ossicles:

Stapes

Incus

Malleus

Tympanic membrane

ICD-10-PCS TABLES

Section	0	Medical and Surgical		
Body System	0	Central Nervous System		
Operation	1	Bypass: Altering the route of passage of the contents of a tubular body part		

Body Part (Character 4)	Approach (Character 5)	Device (Character 6)	Qualifier (Character 7)
6 Cerebral Ventricle	0 Open 3 Percutaneous	7 Autologous Tissue Substitute J Synthetic Substitute K Nonautologous Tissue Substitute	0 Nasopharynx 1 Mastoid Sinus 2 Atrium 3 Blood Vessel 4 Pleural Cavity 5 Intestine 6 Peritoneal Cavity 7 Urinary Tract 8 Bone Marrow B Cerebral Cisterns
U Spinal Canal	0 Open 3 Percutaneous	7 Autologous Tissue Substitute J Synthetic Substitute K Nonautologous Tissue Substitute	4 Pleural Cavity 6 Peritoneal Cavity 7 Urinary Tract 9 Fallopian Tube

Section	0	Medical and Surgical		
Body System	0	Central Nervous System		
Operation	2	Change: Taking out or off a device from a body part and putting back an identical or similar device in or on the same body part without cutting or puncturing the skin or a mucous membrane		

Body Part (Character 4)	Approach (Character 5)	Device (Character 6)	Qualifier (Character 7)
0 Brain E Cranial Nerve U Spinal Canal	X External	0 Drainage Device Y Other Device	Z No Qualifier

Section	0	Medical and Surgical		
Body System	0	Central Nervous System		
Operation	5	Destruction: Physical eradication of all or a portion of a body part by the direct use of energy, force, or al destructive agent		

Body Part (Character 4)	Approach (Character 5)	Device (Character 6)	Qualifier (Character 7)
0 Brain 1 Cerebral Meninges 2 Dura Mater 6 Cerebral Ventricle 7 Cerebral Hemisphere 8 Basal Ganglia 9 Thalamus A Hypothalamus B Pons C Cerebellum D Medulla Oblongata F Olfactory Nerve G Optic Nerve H Oculomotor Nerve J Trochlear Nerve K Trigeminal Nerve L Abducens Nerve M Facial Nerve N Acoustic Nerve P Glossopharyngeal Nerve Q Vagus Nerve	0 Open 3 Percutaneous 4 Percutaneous Endoscopic	Z No Device	Z No Qualifier Continued on Next Page ▶

			Continued from ◀ Previous Page
R Accessory Nerve S Hypoglossal Nerve T Spinal Meninges W Cervical Spinal Cord X Thoracic Spinal Cord Y Lumbar Spinal Cord			

Section	0	Medical and Surgical		
Body System	0	Central Nervous System		
Operation	8	Division: Cutting into a body part, without draining fluids and/or gases from the body part, in order to separate or transect a body part		

Body Part (Character 4)	Approach (Character 5)	Device (Character 6)	Qualifier (Character 7)
0 Brain 7 Cerebral Hemisphere 8 Basal Ganglia F Olfactory Nerve G Optic Nerve H Oculomotor Nerve J Trochlear Nerve K Trigeminal Nerve L Abducens Nerve M Facial Nerve N Acoustic Nerve P Glossopharyngeal Nerve Q Vagus Nerve R Accessory Nerve S Hypoglossal Nerve W Cervical Spinal Cord X Thoracic Spinal Cord Y Lumbar Spinal Cord	0 Open 3 Percutaneous 4 Percutaneous Endoscopic	Z No Device	Z No Qualifier

Section	0	Medical and Surgical		
Body System	0	Central Nervous System		
Operation	9	Drainage: Taking or letting out fluids and/or gases from a body part		

Body Part (Character 4)	Approach (Character 5)	Device (Character 6)	Qualifier (Character 7)
0 Brain 1 Cerebral Meninges 2 Dura Mater 3 Epidural Space 4 Subdural Space 5 Subarachnoid Space 6 Cerebral Ventricle 7 Cerebral Hemisphere 8 Basal Ganglia 9 Thalamus A Hypothalamus B Pons C Cerebellum D Medulla Oblongata F Olfactory Nerve G Optic Nerve H Oculomotor Nerve J Trochlear Nerve K Trigeminal Nerve L Abducens Nerve M Facial Nerve	0 Open 3 Percutaneous 4 Percutaneous Endoscopic	0 Drainage Device	Z No Qualifier

Continued on Next Page ▶

			Continued from ◀ Previous Page
N Acoustic Nerve P Glossopharyngeal Nerve Q Vagus Nerve R Accessory Nerve S Hypoglossal Nerve T Spinal Meninges U Spinal Canal W Cervical Spinal Cord X Thoracic Spinal Cord Y Lumbar Spinal Cord			
0 Brain 1 Cerebral Meninges 2 Dura Mater 3 Epidural Space 4 Subdural Space 5 Subarachnoid Space 6 Cerebral Ventricle 7 Cerebral Hemisphere 8 Basal Ganglia 9 Thalamus A Hypothalamus B Pons C Cerebellum D Medulla Oblongata F Olfactory Nerve G Optic Nerve H Oculomotor Nerve J Trochlear Nerve K Trigeminal Nerve L Abducens Nerve M Facial Nerve N Acoustic Nerve P Glossopharyngeal Nerve Q Vagus Nerve R Accessory Nerve S Hypoglossal Nerve T Spinal Meninges U Spinal Canal W Cervical Spinal Cord X Thoracic Spinal Cord Y Lumbar Spinal Cord	0 Open 3 Percutaneous 4 Percutaneous Endoscopic	Z No Device	X Diagnostic Z No Qualifier

Section	0	Medical and Surgical	
Body System	0	Central Nervous System	
Operation	B	Excision: Cutting out or off, without replacement, a portion of a body part	

Body Part (Character 4)	Approach (Character 5)	Device (Character 6)	Qualifier (Character 7)
0 Brain 1 Cerebral Meninges 2 Dura Mater 6 Cerebral Ventricle 7 Cerebral Hemisphere 8 Basal Ganglia 9 Thalamus A Hypothalamus	0 Open 3 Percutaneous 4 Percutaneous Endoscopic	Z No Device	X Diagnostic Z No Qualifier

Continued on Next Page ▶ |

B Pons
C Cerebellum
D Medulla Oblongata
F Olfactory Nerve
G Optic Nerve
H Oculomotor Nerve
J Trochlear Nerve
K Trigeminal Nerve
L Abducens Nerve
M Facial Nerve
N Acoustic Nerve
P Glossopharyngeal Nerve
Q Vagus Nerve
R Accessory Nerve
S Hypoglossal Nerve
T Spinal Meninges
W Cervical Spinal Cord
X Thoracic Spinal Cord
Y Lumbar Spinal Cord

Continued from
◀ Previous Page

Section	0	Medical and Surgical
Body System	0	Central Nervous System
Operation	C	Extirpation: Taking or cutting out solid matter from a body part

Body Part (Character 4)	Approach (Character 5)	Device (Character 6)	Qualifier (Character 7)
0 Brain	**0** Open	**Z** No Device	**Z** No Qualifier
1 Cerebral Meninges	**3** Percutaneous		
2 Dura Mater	**4** Percutaneous Endoscopic		
3 Epidural Space			
4 Subdural Space			
5 Subarachnoid Space			
6 Cerebral Ventricle			
7 Cerebral Hemisphere			
8 Basal Ganglia			
9 Thalamus			
A Hypothalamus			
B Pons			
C Cerebellum			
D Medulla Oblongata			
F Olfactory Nerve			
G Optic Nerve			
H Oculomotor Nerve			
J Trochlear Nerve			
K Trigeminal Nerve			
L Abducens Nerve			
M Facial Nerve			
N Acoustic Nerve			
P Glossopharyngeal Nerve			
Q Vagus Nerve			
R Accessory Nerve			
S Hypoglossal Nerve			
T Spinal Meninges			
W Cervical Spinal Cord			
X Thoracic Spinal Cord			
Y Lumbar Spinal Cord			

Section	0	Medical and Surgical		
Body System	0	Central Nervous System		
Operation	D	Extraction: Pulling or stripping out or off all or a portion of a body part by the use of force		

Body Part (Character 4)	Approach (Character 5)	Device (Character 6)	Qualifier (Character 7)
1 Cerebral Meninges 2 Dura Mater F Olfactory Nerve G Optic Nerve H Oculomotor Nerve J Trochlear Nerve K Trigeminal Nerve L Abducens Nerve M Facial Nerve N Acoustic Nerve P Glossopharyngeal Nerve Q Vagus Nerve R Accessory Nerve S Hypoglossal Nerve T Spinal Meninges	0 Open 3 Percutaneous 4 Percutaneous Endoscopic	Z No Device	Z No Qualifier

Section	0	Medical and Surgical		
Body System	0	Central Nervous System		
Operation	F	Fragmentation: Breaking solid matter in a body part into pieces		

Body Part (Character 4)	Approach (Character 5)	Device (Character 6)	Qualifier (Character 7)
3 Epidural Space 4 Subdural Space 5 Subarachnoid Space 6 Cerebral Ventricle U Spinal Canal	0 Open 3 Percutaneous 4 Percutaneous Endoscopic X External	Z No Device	Z No Qualifier

Section	0	Medical and Surgical		
Body System	0	Central Nervous System		
Operation	H	Insertion: Putting in a nonbiological appliance that monitors, assists, performs, or prevents a physiological function but does not physically take the place of a body part		

Body Part (Character 4)	Approach (Character 5)	Device (Character 6)	Qualifier (Character 7)
0 Brain 6 Cerebral Ventricle E Cranial Nerve U Spinal Canal V Spinal Cord	0 Open 3 Percutaneous 4 Percutaneous Endoscopic	2 Monitoring Device 3 Infusion Device M Neurostimulator Lead	Z No Qualifier

Section	0	Medical and Surgical		
Body System	0	Central Nervous System		
Operation	J	Inspection: Visually and/or manually exploring a body part		

Body Part (Character 4)	Approach (Character 5)	Device (Character 6)	Qualifier (Character 7)
0 Brain E Cranial Nerve U Spinal Canal V Spinal Cord	0 Open 3 Percutaneous 4 Percutaneous Endoscopic	Z No Device	Z No Qualifier

Section	0	Medical and Surgical
Body System	0	Central Nervous System
Operation	K	Map: Locating the route of passage of electrical impulses and/or locating functional areas in a body part

Body Part (Character 4)	Approach (Character 5)	Device (Character 6)	Qualifier (Character 7)
0 Brain **7** Cerebral Hemisphere **8** Basal Ganglia **9** Thalamus **A** Hypothalamus **B** Pons **C** Cerebellum **D** Medulla Oblongata	**0** Open **3** Percutaneous **4** Percutaneous Endoscopic	**Z** No Device	**Z** No Qualifier

Section	0	Medical and Surgical
Body System	0	Central Nervous System
Operation	N	Release: Freeing a body part from an abnormal physical constraint by cutting or by the use of force

Body Part (Character 4)	Approach (Character 5)	Device (Character 6)	Qualifier (Character 7)
0 Brain **1** Cerebral Meninges **2** Dura Mater **6** Cerebral Ventricle **7** Cerebral Hemisphere **8** Basal Ganglia **9** Thalamus **A** Hypothalamus **B** Pons **C** Cerebellum **D** Medulla Oblongata **F** Olfactory Nerve **G** Optic Nerve **H** Oculomotor Nerve **J** Trochlear Nerve **K** Trigeminal Nerve **L** Abducens Nerve **M** Facial Nerve **N** Acoustic Nerve **P** Glossopharyngeal Nerve **Q** Vagus Nerve **R** Accessory Nerve **S** Hypoglossal Nerve **T** Spinal Meninges **W** Cervical Spinal Cord **X** Thoracic Spinal Cord **Y** Lumbar Spinal Cord	**0** Open **3** Percutaneous **4** Percutaneous Endoscopic	**Z** No Device	**Z** No Qualifier

Section	0	Medical and Surgical
Body System	0	Central Nervous System
Operation	P	Removal: Taking out or off a device from a body part

Body Part (Character 4)	Approach (Character 5)	Device (Character 6)	Qualifier (Character 7)
0 Brain **V** Spinal Cord	**0** Open **3** Percutaneous **4** Percutaneous Endoscopic	**0** Drainage Device **2** Monitoring Device **3** Infusion Device **7** Autologous Tissue Substitute **J** Synthetic Substitute **K** Nonautologous Tissue Substitute **M** Neurostimulator Lead	**Z** No Qualifier
0 Brain **V** Spinal Cord	**X** External	**0** Drainage Device **2** Monitoring Device **3** Infusion Device **M** Neurostimulator Lead	**Z** No Qualifier
6 Cerebral Ventricle **U** Spinal Canal	**0** Open **3** Percutaneous **4** Percutaneous Endoscopic	**0** Drainage Device **2** Monitoring Device **3** Infusion Device **J** Synthetic Substitute **M** Neurostimulator Lead	**Z** No Qualifier
6 Cerebral Ventricle **U** Spinal Canal	**X** External	**0** Drainage Device **2** Monitoring Device **3** Infusion Device **M** Neurostimulator Lead	**Z** No Qualifier
E Cranial Nerve	**0** Open **3** Percutaneous **4** Percutaneous Endoscopic	**0** Drainage Device **2** Monitoring Device **3** Infusion Device **7** Autologous Tissue Substitute **M** Neurostimulator Lead	**Z** No Qualifier
E Cranial Nerve	**X** External	**0** Drainage Device **2** Monitoring Device **3** Infusion Device **M** Neurostimulator Lead	**Z** No Qualifier

Section	0	Medical and Surgical
Body System	0	Central Nervous System
Operation	Q	Repair: Restoring, to the extent possible, a body part to its normal anatomic structure and function

Body Part (Character 4)	Approach (Character 5)	Device (Character 6)	Qualifier (Character 7)
0 Brain **1** Cerebral Meninges **2** Dura Mater **6** Cerebral Ventricle **7** Cerebral Hemisphere **8** Basal Ganglia **9** Thalamus **A** Hypothalamus **B** Pons **C** Cerebellum **D** Medulla Oblongata **F** Olfactory Nerve	**0** Open **3** Percutaneous **4** Percutaneous Endoscopic	**Z** No Device	**Z** No Qualifier

Continued on Next Page ▶

G Optic Nerve **H** Oculomotor Nerve **J** Trochlear Nerve **K** Trigeminal Nerve **L** Abducens Nerve **M** Facial Nerve **N** Acoustic Nerve **P** Glossopharyngeal Nerve **Q** Vagus Nerve **R** Accessory Nerve **S** Hypoglossal Nerve **T** Spinal Meninges **W** Cervical Spinal Cord **X** Thoracic Spinal Cord **Y** Lumbar Spinal Cord			Continued from ◀ Previous Page

Section	0	Medical and Surgical	
Body System	0	Central Nervous System	
Operation	S	Reposition: Moving to its normal location, or other suitable location, all or a portion of a body part	

Body Part (Character 4)	Approach (Character 5)	Device (Character 6)	Qualifier (Character 7)
F Olfactory Nerve **G** Optic Nerve **H** Oculomotor Nerve **J** Trochlear Nerve **K** Trigeminal Nerve **L** Abducens Nerve **M** Facial Nerve **N** Acoustic Nerve **P** Glossopharyngeal Nerve **Q** Vagus Nerve **R** Accessory Nerve **S** Hypoglossal Nerve **W** Cervical Spinal Cord **X** Thoracic Spinal Cord **Y** Lumbar Spinal Cord	**0** Open **3** Percutaneous **4** Percutaneous Endoscopic	**Z** No Device	**Z** No Qualifier

Section	0	Medical and Surgical	
Body System	0	Central Nervous System	
Operation	T	Resection: Cutting out or off, without replacement, all of a body part	

Body Part (Character 4)	Approach (Character 5)	Device (Character 6)	Qualifier (Character 7)
7 Cerebral Hemisphere	**0** Open **3** Percutaneous **4** Percutaneous Endoscopic	**Z** No Device	**Z** No Qualifier

Section	0	Medical and Surgical
Body System	0	Central Nervous System
Operation	U	Supplement: Putting in or on biological or synthetic material that physically reinforces and/or augments the function of a portion of a body part

Body Part (Character 4)	Approach (Character 5)	Device (Character 6)	Qualifier (Character 7)
1 Cerebral Meninges 2 Dura Mater T Spinal Meninges	0 Open 3 Percutaneous 4 Percutaneous Endoscopic	7 Autologous Tissue Substitute J Synthetic Substitute K Nonautologous Tissue Substitute	Z No Qualifier
F Olfactory Nerve G Optic Nerve H Oculomotor Nerve J Trochlear Nerve K Trigeminal Nerve L Abducens Nerve M Facial Nerve N Acoustic Nerve P Glossopharyngeal Nerve Q Vagus Nerve R Accessory Nerve S Hypoglossal Nerve	0 Open 3 Percutaneous 4 Percutaneous Endoscopic	7 Autologous Tissue Substitute	Z No Qualifier

Section	0	Medical and Surgical
Body System	0	Central Nervous System
Operation	W	Revision: Correcting, to the extent possible, a portion of a malfunctioning device or the position of a displaced device

Body Part (Character 4)	Approach (Character 5)	Device (Character 6)	Qualifier (Character 7)
0 Brain V Spinal Cord	0 Open 3 Percutaneous 4 Percutaneous Endoscopic X External	0 Drainage Device 2 Monitoring Device 3 Infusion Device 7 Autologous Tissue Substitute J Synthetic Substitute K Nonautologous Tissue Substitute M Neurostimulator Lead	Z No Qualifier
6 Cerebral Ventricle U Spinal Canal	0 Open 3 Percutaneous 4 Percutaneous Endoscopic X External	0 Drainage Device 2 Monitoring Device 3 Infusion Device J Synthetic Substitute M Neurostimulator Lead	Z No Qualifier
E Cranial Nerve	0 Open 3 Percutaneous 4 Percutaneous Endoscopic X External	0 Drainage Device 2 Monitoring Device 3 Infusion Device 7 Autologous Tissue Substitute M Neurostimulator Lead	Z No Qualifier

Section	0	Medical and Surgical				
Body System	0	Central Nervous System				
Operation	X	Transfer: Moving, without taking out, all or a portion of a body part to another location to take over the function of all or a portion of a body part				

Body Part (Character 4)	Approach (Character 5)	Device (Character 6)	Qualifier (Character 7)
F Olfactory Nerve	0 Open	Z No Device	F Olfactory Nerve
G Optic Nerve	4 Percutaneous Endoscopic		G Optic Nerve
H Oculomotor Nerve			H Oculomotor Nerve
J Trochlear Nerve			J Trochlear Nerve
K Trigeminal Nerve			K Trigeminal Nerve
L Abducens Nerve			L Abducens Nerve
M Facial Nerve			M Facial Nerve
N Acoustic Nerve			N Acoustic Nerve
P Glossopharyngeal Nerve			P Glossopharyngeal Nerve
Q Vagus Nerve			Q Vagus Nerve
R Accessory Nerve			R Accessory Nerve
S Hypoglossal Nerve			S Hypoglossal Nerve

Section	0	Medical and Surgical		
Body System	1	Peripheral Nervous System		
Operation	2	Change: Taking out or off a device from a body part and putting back an identical or similar device in or on the same body part without cutting or puncturing the skin or a mucous membrane		
Body Part (Character 4)		**Approach (Character 5)**	**Device (Character 6)**	**Qualifier (Character 7)**
Y Peripheral Nerve		X External	0 Drainage Device Y Other Device	Z No Qualifier

Section	0	Medical and Surgical		
Body System	1	Peripheral Nervous System		
Operation	5	Destruction: Physical eradication of all or a portion of a body part by the direct use of energy, force, or a destructive agent		
Body Part (Character 4)		**Approach (Character 5)**	**Device (Character 6)**	**Qualifier (Character 7)**
0 Cervical Plexus		0 Open	Z No Device	Z No Qualifier
1 Cervical Nerve		3 Percutaneous		
2 Phrenic Nerve		4 Percutaneous Endoscopic		
3 Brachial Plexus				
4 Ulnar Nerve				
5 Median Nerve				
6 Radial Nerve				
8 Thoracic Nerve				
9 Lumbar Plexus				
A Lumbosacral Plexus				
B Lumbar Nerve				
C Pudendal Nerve				
D Femoral Nerve				
F Sciatic Nerve				
G Tibial Nerve				
H Peroneal Nerve				
K Head and Neck Sympathetic Nerve				
L Thoracic Sympathetic Nerve				
M Abdominal Sympathetic Nerve				
N Lumbar Sympathetic Nerve				
P Sacral Sympathetic Nerve				
Q Sacral Plexus				
R Sacral Nerve				

Section	0	Medical and Surgical		
Body System	1	Peripheral Nervous System		
Operation	8	Division: Cutting into a body part, without draining fluids and/or gases from the body part, in order to separate or transect a body part		
Body Part (Character 4)		**Approach (Character 5)**	**Device (Character 6)**	**Qualifier (Character 7)**
0 Cervical Plexus		0 Open	Z No Device	Z No Qualifier
1 Cervical Nerve		3 Percutaneous		
2 Phrenic Nerve		4 Percutaneous Endoscopic		
3 Brachial Plexus				
4 Ulnar Nerve				
5 Median Nerve				
6 Radial Nerve				
8 Thoracic Nerve				**Continued on Next Page ▶**

			Continued from ◀ Previous Page
9 Lumbar Plexus			
A Lumbosacral Plexus			
B Lumbar Nerve			
C Pudendal Nerve			
D Femoral Nerve			
F Sciatic Nerve			
G Tibial Nerve			
H Peroneal Nerve			
K Head and Neck Sympathetic Nerve			
L Thoracic Sympathetic Nerve			
M Abdominal Sympathetic Nerve			
N Lumbar Sympathetic Nerve			
P Sacral Sympathetic Nerve			
Q Sacral Plexus			
R Sacral Nerve			

Section	0	Medical and Surgical	
Body System	1	Peripheral Nervous System	
Operation	9	Drainage: Taking or letting out fluids and/or gases from a body part	

Body Part (Character 4)	Approach (Character 5)	Device (Character 6)	Qualifier (Character 7)
0 Cervical Plexus	0 Open	0 Drainage Device	Z No Qualifier
1 Cervical Nerve	3 Percutaneous		
2 Phrenic Nerve	4 Percutaneous Endoscopic		
3 Brachial Plexus			
4 Ulnar Nerve			
5 Median Nerve			
6 Radial Nerve			
8 Thoracic Nerve			
9 Lumbar Plexus			
A Lumbosacral Plexus			
B Lumbar Nerve			
C Pudendal Nerve			
D Femoral Nerve			
F Sciatic Nerve			
G Tibial Nerve			
H Peroneal Nerve			
K Head and Neck Sympathetic Nerve			
L Thoracic Sympathetic Nerve			
M Abdominal Sympathetic Nerve			
N Lumbar Sympathetic Nerve			
P Sacral Sympathetic Nerve			
Q Sacral Plexus			
R Sacral Nerve			
0 Cervical Plexus	0 Open	Z No Device	X Diagnostic
1 Cervical Nerve	3 Percutaneous		Z No Qualifier
2 Phrenic Nerve	4 Percutaneous Endoscopic		
3 Brachial Plexus			

Continued on
Next Page ▶

4 Ulnar Nerve			Continued from ◀ Previous Page
5 Median Nerve			
6 Radial Nerve			
8 Thoracic Nerve			
9 Lumbar Plexus			
A Lumbosacral Plexus			
B Lumbar Nerve			
C Pudendal Nerve			
D Femoral Nerve			
F Sciatic Nerve			
G Tibial Nerve			
H Peroneal Nerve			
K Head and Neck Sympathetic Nerve			
L Thoracic Sympathetic Nerve			
M Abdominal Sympathetic Nerve			
N Lumbar Sympathetic Nerve			
P Sacral Sympathetic Nerve			
Q Sacral Plexus			
R Sacral Nerve			

Section	0	Medical and Surgical	
Body System	1	Peripheral Nervous System	
Operation	B	Excision: Cutting out or off, without replacement, a portion of a body part	

Body Part (Character 4)	Approach (Character 5)	Device (Character 6)	Qualifier (Character 7)
0 Cervical Plexus	0 Open	Z No Device	X Diagnostic
1 Cervical Nerve	3 Percutaneous		Z No Qualifier
2 Phrenic Nerve	4 Percutaneous Endoscopic		
3 Brachial Plexus			
4 Ulnar Nerve			
5 Median Nerve			
6 Radial Nerve			
8 Thoracic Nerve			
9 Lumbar Plexus			
A Lumbosacral Plexus			
B Lumbar Nerve			
C Pudendal Nerve			
D Femoral Nerve			
F Sciatic Nerve			
G Tibial Nerve			
H Peroneal Nerve			
K Head and Neck Sympathetic Nerve			
L Thoracic Sympathetic Nerve			
M Abdominal Sympathetic Nerve			
N Lumbar Sympathetic Nerve			
P Sacral Sympathetic Nerve			
Q Sacral Plexus			
R Sacral Nerve			

Section	0	Medical and Surgical		
Body System	1	Peripheral Nervous System		
Operation	C	Extirpation: Taking or cutting out solid matter from a body part		

Body Part (Character 4)	Approach (Character 5)	Device (Character 6)	Qualifier (Character 7)
0 Cervical Plexus	0 Open	Z No Device	Z No Device
1 Cervical Nerve	3 Percutaneous		
2 Phrenic Nerve	4 Percutaneous Endoscopic		
3 Brachial Plexus			
4 Ulnar Nerve			
5 Median Nerve			
6 Radial Nerve			
8 Thoracic Nerve			
9 Lumbar Plexus			
A Lumbosacral Plexus			
B Lumbar Nerve			
C Pudendal Nerve			
D Femoral Nerve			
F Sciatic Nerve			
G Tibial Nerve			
H Peroneal Nerve			
K Head and Neck Sympathetic Nerve			
L Thoracic Sympathetic Nerve			
M Abdominal Sympathetic Nerve			
N Lumbar Sympathetic Nerve			
P Sacral Sympathetic Nerve			
Q Sacral Plexus			
R Sacral Nerve			

Section	0	Medical and Surgical		
Body System	1	Peripheral Nervous System		
Operation	D	Extraction: Pulling or stripping out or off all or a portion of a body part by the use of force		

Body Part (Character 4)	Approach (Character 5)	Device (Character 6)	Qualifier (Character 7)
0 Cervical Plexus	0 Open	Z No Device	Z No Qualifier
1 Cervical Nerve	3 Percutaneous		
2 Phrenic Nerve	4 Percutaneous Endoscopic		
3 Brachial Plexus			
4 Ulnar Nerve			
5 Median Nerve			
6 Radial Nerve			
8 Thoracic Nerve			
9 Lumbar Plexus			
A Lumbosacral Plexus			
B Lumbar Nerve			
C Pudendal Nerve			
D Femoral Nerve			
F Sciatic Nerve			
G Tibial Nerve			
H Peroneal Nerve			
K Head and Neck Sympathetic Nerve			Continued on Next Page ▶

			Continued from ◄ Previous Page
L Thoracic Sympathetic Nerve			
M Abdominal Sympathetic Nerve			
N Lumbar Sympathetic Nerve			
P Sacral Sympathetic Nerve			
Q Sacral Plexus			
R Sacral Nerve			

Section	0	Medical and Surgical	
Body System	1	Peripheral Nervous System	
Operation	H	Insertion: Putting in a nonbiological appliance that monitors, assists, performs, or prevents a physiological function but does not physically take the place of a body part	

Body Part (Character 4)	Approach (Character 5)	Device (Character 6)	Qualifier (Character 7)
Y Peripheral Nerve	0 Open 3 Percutaneous 4 Percutaneous Endoscopic	2 Monitoring Device M Neurostimulator Lead	Z No Qualifier

Section	0	Medical and Surgical	
Body System	1	Peripheral Nervous System	
Operation	J	Inspection: Visually and/or manually exploring a body part	

Body Part (Character 4)	Approach (Character 5)	Device (Character 6)	Qualifier (Character 7)
Y Peripheral Nerve	0 Open 3 Percutaneous 4 Percutaneous Endoscopic	Z No Device	Z No Qualifier

Section	0	Medical and Surgical	
Body System	1	Peripheral Nervous System	
Operation	N	Release: Freeing a body part from an abnormal physical constraint by cutting or by the use of force	

Body Part (Character 4)	Approach (Character 5)	Device (Character 6)	Qualifier (Character 7)
0 Cervical Plexus 1 Cervical Nerve 2 Phrenic Nerve 3 Brachial Plexus 4 Ulnar Nerve 5 Median Nerve 6 Radial Nerve 8 Thoracic Nerve 9 Lumbar Plexus A Lumbosacral Plexus B Lumbar Nerve C Pudendal Nerve D Femoral Nerve F Sciatic Nerve G Tibial Nerve H Peroneal Nerve K Head and Neck Sympathetic Nerve L Thoracic Sympathetic Nerve M Abdominal Sympathetic Nerve	0 Open 3 Percutaneous 4 Percutaneous Endoscopic	Z No Device	Z No Qualifier

Continued on Next Page ▶

N Lumbar Sympathetic Nerve			Continued from ◀ Previous Page
P Sacral Sympathetic Nerve			
Q Sacral Plexus			
R Sacral Nerve			

Section	0	Medical and Surgical
Body System	1	Peripheral Nervous System
Operation	P	Removal: Taking out or off a device from a body part

Body Part (Character 4)	Approach (Character 5)	Device (Character 6)	Qualifier (Character 7)
Y Peripheral Nerve	**0** Open **3** Percutaneous **4** Percutaneous Endoscopic	**0** Drainage Device **2** Monitoring Device **7** Autologous Tissue Substitute **M** Neurostimulator Lead	**Z** No Qualifier
Y Peripheral Nerve	**X** External	**0** Drainage Device **2** Monitoring Device **M** Neurostimulator Lead	**Z** No Qualifier

Section	0	Medical and Surgical
Body System	1	Peripheral Nervous System
Operation	Q	Repair: Restoring, to the extent possible, a body part to its normal anatomic structure and function

Body Part (Character 4)	Approach (Character 5)	Device (Character 6)	Qualifier (Character 7)
0 Cervical Plexus **1** Cervical Nerve **2** Phrenic Nerve **3** Brachial Plexus **4** Ulnar Nerve **5** Median Nerve **6** Radial Nerve **8** Thoracic Nerve **9** Lumbar Plexus **A** Lumbosacral Plexus **B** Lumbar Nerve **C** Pudendal Nerve **D** Femoral Nerve **F** Sciatic Nerve **G** Tibial Nerve **H** Peroneal Nerve **K** Head and Neck Sympathetic Nerve **L** Thoracic Sympathetic Nerve **M** Abdominal Sympathetic Nerve **N** Lumbar Sympathetic Nerve **P** Sacral Sympathetic Nerve **Q** Sacral Plexus **R** Sacral Nerve	**0** Open **3** Percutaneous **4** Percutaneous Endoscopic	**Z** No Device	**Z** No Qualifier

Section	0	Medical and Surgical		
Body System	1	Peripheral Nervous System		
Operation	S	Reposition: Moving to its normal location, or other suitable location, all or a portion of a body part		

Body Part (Character 4)	Approach (Character 5)	Device (Character 6)	Qualifier (Character 7)
0 Cervical Plexus 1 Cervical Nerve 2 Phrenic Nerve 3 Brachial Plexus 4 Ulnar Nerve 5 Median Nerve 6 Radial Nerve 8 Thoracic Nerve 9 Lumbar Plexus A Lumbosacral Plexus B Lumbar Nerve C Pudendal Nerve D Femoral Nerve F Sciatic Nerve G Tibial Nerve H Peroneal Nerve Q Sacral Plexus R Sacral Nerve	0 Open 3 Percutaneous 4 Percutaneous Endoscopic	Z No Device	Z No Qualifier

Section	0	Medical and Surgical		
Body System	1	Peripheral Nervous System		
Operation	U	Supplement: Putting in or on biological or synthetic material that physically reinforces and/or augments the function of a portion of a body part		

Body Part (Character 4)	Approach (Character 5)	Device (Character 6)	Qualifier (Character 7)
1 Cervical Nerve 2 Phrenic Nerve 4 Ulnar Nerve 5 Median Nerve 6 Radial Nerve 8 Thoracic Nerve B Lumbar Nerve C Pudendal Nerve D Femoral Nerve F Sciatic Nerve G Tibial Nerve H Peroneal Nerve R Sacral Nerve	0 Open 3 Percutaneous 4 Percutaneous Endoscopic	7 Autologous Tissue Substitute	Z No Qualifier

Section	0	Medical and Surgical		
Body System	1	Peripheral Nervous System		
Operation	W	Revision: Correcting, to the extent possible, a portion of a malfunctioning device or the position of a displaced device		

Body Part (Character 4)	Approach (Character 5)	Device (Character 6)	Qualifier (Character 7)
Y Peripheral Nerve	0 Open 3 Percutaneous 4 Percutaneous Endoscopic X External	0 Drainage Device 2 Monitoring Device 7 Autologous Tissue Substitute M Neurostimulator Lead	Z No Qualifier

Section	0	Medical and Surgical		
Body System	1	Peripheral Nervous System		
Operation	X	Transfer: Moving, without taking out, all or a portion of a body part to another location to take over the function of all or a portion of a body part		

Body Part (Character 4)	Approach (Character 5)	Device (Character 6)	Qualifier (Character 7)
1 Cervical Nerve 2 Phrenic Nerve	0 Open 4 Percutaneous Endoscopic	Z No Device	1 Cervical Nerve 2 Phrenic Nerve
4 Ulnar Nerve 5 Median Nerve 6 Radial Nerve	0 Open 4 Percutaneous Endoscopic	Z No Device	4 Ulnar Nerve 5 Median Nerve 6 Radial Nerve
8 Thoracic Nerve	0 Open 4 Percutaneous Endoscopic	Z No Device	8 Thoracic Nerve
B Lumbar Nerve C Pudendal Nerve	0 Open 4 Percutaneous Endoscopic	Z No Device	B Lumbar Nerve C Perineal Nerve
D Femoral Nerve F Sciatic Nerve G Tibial Nerve H Peroneal Nerve	0 Open 4 Percutaneous Endoscopic	Z No Device	D Femoral Nerve F Sciatic Nerve G Tibial Nerve H Peroneal Nerve

Section	0	Medical and Surgical	
Body System	2	Heart and Great Vessels	
Operation	1	Bypass: Altering the route of passage of the contents of a tubular body part	

Body Part (Character 4)	Approach (Character 5)	Device (Character 6)	Qualifier (Character 7)
0 Coronary Artery, One Site **1** Coronary Artery, Two Sites **2** Coronary Artery, Three Sites **3** Coronary Artery, Four or More Sites	**0** Open	**8** Zooplastic Tissue **9** Autologous Venous Tissue **A** Autologous Arterial Tissue **J** Synthetic Substitute **K** Nonautologous Tissue Substitute	**3** Coronary Artery **8** Internal Mammary, Right **9** Internal Mammary, Left **C** Thoracic Artery **F** Abdominal Artery **W** Aorta
0 Coronary Artery, One Artery **1** Coronary Artery, Two Arteries **2** Coronary Artery, Three Arteries **3** Coronary Artery, Four or More Arteries	**0** Open	**Z** No Device	**3** Coronary Artery **8** Internal Mammary, Right **9** Internal Mammary, Left **C** Thoracic Artery **F** Abdominal Artery
0 Coronary Artery, One Artery **1** Coronary Artery, Two Arteries **2** Coronary Artery, Three Arteries **3** Coronary Artery, Four or More Arteries	**3** Percutaneous	**4** Intraluminal Device, Drug-eluting **D** Intraluminal Device	**4** Coronary Vein
0 Coronary Artery, One Artery **1** Coronary Artery, Two Arteries **2** Coronary Artery, Three Arteries **3** Coronary Artery, Four or More Arteries	**4** Percutaneous Endoscopic	**4** Intraluminal Device, Drug-eluting **D** Intraluminal Device	**4** Coronary Vein
0 Coronary Artery, One Site **1** Coronary Artery, Two Sites **2** Coronary Artery, Three Sites **3** Coronary Artery, Four or More Sites	**4** Percutaneous Endoscopic	**8** Zooplastic Tissue **9** Autologous Venous Tissue **A** Autologous Arterial Tissue **J** Synthetic Substitute **K** Nonautologous Tissue Substitute	**3** Coronary Artery **8** Internal Mammary, Right **9** Internal Mammary, Left **C** Thoracic Artery **F** Abdominal Artery **W** Aorta
0 Coronary Artery, One Artery **1** Coronary Artery, Two Arteries **2** Coronary Artery, Three Arteries **3** Coronary Artery, Four or More Arteries	**4** Percutaneous Endoscopic	**Z** No Device	**3** Coronary Artery **8** Internal Mammary, Right **9** Internal Mammary, Left **C** Thoracic Artery **F** Abdominal Artery
6 Atrium, Right	**0** Open **4** Percutaneous Endoscopic	**8** Zooplastic Tissue **9** Autologous Venous Tissue **A** Autologous Arterial Tissue **J** Synthetic Substitute **K** Nonautologous Tissue Substitute	**P** Pulmonary Trunk **Q** Pulmonary Artery, Right **R** Pulmonary Artery, Left

Section	0	Medical and Surgical		
Body System	2	Heart and Great Vessels		
Operation	1	Bypass: Altering the route of passage of the contents of a tubular body part		

Body Part (Character 4)	Approach (Character 5)	Device (Character 6)	Qualifier (Character 7)
6 Atrium, Right	0 Open 4 Percutaneous Endoscopic	Z No Device	7 Atrium, Left P Pulmonary Trunk Q Pulmonary Artery, Right R Pulmonary Artery, Left
7 Atrium, Left V Superior Vena Cava	0 Open 4 Percutaneous Endoscopic	8 Zooplastic Tissue 9 Autologous Venous Tissue A Autologous Arterial Tissue J Synthetic Substitute K Nonautologous Tissue Substitute Z No Device	P Pulmonary Trunk Q Pulmonary Artery, Right R Pulmonary Artery, Left S Pulmonary Vein, Right T Pulmonary Vein, Left U Pulmonary Vein, Confluence
K Ventricle, Right L Ventricle, Left	0 Open 4 Percutaneous Endoscopic	8 Zooplastic Tissue 9 Autologous Venous Tissue A Autologous Arterial Tissue J Synthetic Substitute K Nonautologous Tissue Substitute	P Pulmonary Trunk Q Pulmonary Artery, Right R Pulmonary Artery, Left
K Ventricle, Right L Ventricle, Left	0 Open 4 Percutaneous Endoscopic	Z No Device	5 Coronary Circulation 8 Internal Mammary, Right 9 Internal Mammary, Left C Thoracic Artery F Abdominal Artery P Pulmonary Trunk Q Pulmonary Artery, Right R Pulmonary Artery, Left W Aorta
P Pulmonary Trunk Q Pulmonary Artery, Right R Pulmonary Artery, Left	0 Open 4 Percutaneous Endoscopic	8 Zooplastic Tissue 9 Autologous Venous Tissue A Autologous Arterial Tissue J Synthetic Substitute K Nonautologous Tissue Substitute Z No Device	A Innominate Artery B Subclavian D Carotid
W Thoracic Aorta, Descending X Thoracic Aorta, Ascending/Arch	0 Open 4 Percutaneous Endoscopic	8 Zooplastic Tissue 9 Autologous Venous Tissue A Autologous Arterial Tissue J Synthetic Substitute K Nonautologous Tissue Substitute Z No Device	B Subclavian D Carotid P Pulmonary Trunk Q Pulmonary Artery, Right R Pulmonary Artery, Left

Section	0	Medical and Surgical		
Body System	2	Heart and Great Vessels		
Operation	4	Creation: Putting in or on biological or synthetic material to form a new body part that to the extent possible replicates the anatomic structure or function of an absent body part		

Body Part (Character 4)	Approach (Character 5)	Device (Character 6)	Qualifier (Character 7)

F Aortic Valve	0 Open	7 Autologous Tissue
		8 Substitute
		  Zooplastic Tissue
		J Synthetic Substitute
		K Nonautologous Tissue
		  Substitute
			J Truncal Valve

G Mitral Valve
J Tricuspid Valve
	0 Open	7 Autologous Tissue
		8 Substitute
		  Zooplastic Tissue
		J Synthetic Substitute
		K Nonautologous Tissue
		  Substitute
			2 Common Atrioventricular
			  Valve

Section	0	Medical and Surgical		
Body System	2	Heart and Great Vessels		
Operation	5	Destruction: Physical eradication of all or a portion of a body part by the direct use of energy, force, or a destructive agent		

Body Part (Character 4)	Approach (Character 5)	Device (Character 6)	Qualifier (Character 7)
4 Coronary Vein 5 Atrial Septum 6 Atrium, Right 8 Conduction Mechanism 9 Chordae Tendineae D Papillary Muscle F Aortic Valve G Mitral Valve H Pulmonary Valve J Tricuspid Valve K Ventricle, Right L Ventricle, Left M Ventricular Septum N Pericardium P Pulmonary Trunk Q Pulmonary Artery, Right R Pulmonary Artery, Left S Pulmonary Vein, Right T Pulmonary Vein, Left V Superior Vena Cava W Thoracic Aorta, Descending X Thoracic Aorta, Ascending/Arch	0 Open 3 Percutaneous 4 Percutaneous Endoscopic	Z No Device	Z No Qualifier
7 Atrium, Left	0 Open 3 Percutaneous 4 Percutaneous Endoscopic	Z No Device	K Left Atrial Appendage Z No Qualifier

Section	0	Medical and Surgical
Body System	2	Heart and Great Vessels
Operation	7	Dilation: Expanding an orifice or the lumen of a tubular body part

Body Part (Character 4)	Approach (Character 5)	Device (Character 6)	Qualifier (Character 7)
0 Coronary Artery, One Artery **1** Coronary Artery, Two Arteries **2** Coronary Artery, Three Arteries **3** Coronary Artery, Four Or More Arteries	**0** Open **3** Percutaneous **4** Percutaneous Endoscopic	**4** Intraluminal Device, Drug-eluting **D** Intraluminal Device **T** Intraluminal Device, Radioactive **Z** No Device	**6** Bifurcation **Z** No Qualifier
F Aortic Valve **G** Mitral Valve **H** Pulmonary Valve **J** Tricuspid Valve **K** Ventricle, Right **P** Pulmonary Trunk **Q** Pulmonary Artery, Right **S** Pulmonary Vein, Right **T** Pulmonary Vein, Left **V** Superior Vena Cava **W** Thoracic Aorta, Descending **X** Thoracic Aorta, Ascending/Arch	**0** Open **3** Percutaneous **4** Percutaneous Endoscopic	**4** Intraluminal Device, Drug-eluting **D** Intraluminal Device **Z** No Device	**Z** No Qualifier
R Pulmonary Artery, Left	**0** Open **3** Percutaneous **4** Percutaneous Endoscopic	**4** Intraluminal Device, Drug-eluting **D** Intraluminal Device **Z** No Device	**T** Ductus Arteriosus **Z** No Qualifier

Section	0	Medical and Surgical
Body System	2	Heart and Great Vessels
Operation	8	Division: Cutting into a body part, without draining fluids and/or gases from the body part, in order to separate or transect a body part

Body Part Character 4	Approach Character 5	Device Character 6	Qualifier Character 7
8 Conduction Mechanism **9** Chordae Tendineae **D** Papillary Muscle	**0** Open **3** Percutaneous **4** Percutaneous Endoscopic	**Z** No Device	**Z** No Qualifier

Section	0	Medical and Surgical
Body System	2	Heart and Great Vessels
Operation	B	Excision: Cutting out or off, without replacement, a portion of a body part

Body Part (Character 4)	Approach (Character 5)	Device (Character 6)	Qualifier (Character 7)
4 Coronary Vein **5** Atrial Septum **6** Atrium, Right **8** Conduction Mechanism **9** Chordae Tendineae **D** Papillary Muscle **F** Aortic Valve **G** Mitral Valve	**0** Open **3** Percutaneous **4** Percutaneous Endoscopic	**Z** No Device	**X** Diagnostic **Z** No Qualifier

Continued on Next Page ▶

H Pulmonary Valve J Tricuspid Valve K Ventricle, Right L Ventricle, Left M Ventricular Septum N Pericardium P Pulmonary Trunk Q Pulmonary Artery, Right R Pulmonary Artery, Left S Pulmonary Vein, Right T Pulmonary Vein, Left V Superior Vena Cava W Thoracic Aorta, Descending X Thoracic Aorta, Ascending/Arch			Continued from ◄ Previous Page
7 Atrium, Left	0 Open 3 Percutaneous 4 Percutaneous Endoscopic	Z No Device	K Left Atrial Appendage X Diagnostic Z No Qualifier

Section	0	Medical and Surgical
Body System	2	Heart and Great Vessels
Operation	C	Extirpation: Taking or cutting out solid matter from a body part

Body Part (Character 4)	Approach (Character 5)	Device (Character 6)	Qualifier (Character 7)
0 Coronary Artery, One Artery 1 Coronary Artery, Two Arteries 2 Coronary Artery, Three Arteries 3 Coronary Artery, Four or More Arteries	0 Open 3 Percutaneous 4 Percutaneous Endoscopic	Z No Device	6 Bifurcation Z No Qualifier
4 Coronary Vein 5 Atrial Septum 6 Atrium, Right 7 Atrium, Left 8 Conduction Mechanism 9 Chordae Tendineae D Papillary Muscle F Aortic Valve G Mitral Valve H Pulmonary Valve J Tricuspid Valve K Ventricle, Right L Ventricle, Left M Ventricular Septum N Pericardium P Pulmonary Trunk Q Pulmonary Artery, Right R Pulmonary Artery, Left S Pulmonary Vein, Right T Pulmonary Vein, Left V Superior Vena Cava	0 Open 3 Percutaneous 4 Percutaneous Endoscopic	Z No Device	Z No Qualifier Continued on Next Page ►

W Thoracic Aorta, Descending			**Continued from** ◄**Previous Page**
X Thoracic Aorta, Ascending/Arch			

Section	0	Medical and Surgical		
Body System	2	Heart and Great Vessels		
Operation	F	Fragmentation: Breaking solid matter in a body part into pieces		

Body Part (Character 4)	Approach (Character 5)	Device (Character 6)	Qualifier (Character 7)
N Pericardium	0 Open 3 Percutaneous 4 Percutaneous Endoscopic X External	Z No Device	Z No Qualifier

Section	0	Medical and Surgical		
Body System	2	Heart and Great Vessels		
Operation	H	Insertion: Putting in a nonbiological appliance that monitors, assists, performs, or prevents a physiological function but does not physically take the place of a body part		

Body Part (Character 4)	Approach (Character 5)	Device (Character 6)	Qualifier (Character 7)
4 Coronary Vein 6 Atrium, Right 7 Atrium, Left K Ventricle, Right L Ventricle, Left	0 Open 3 Percutaneous 4 Percutaneous Endoscopic	0 Monitoring Device, Pressure Sensor 2 Monitoring Device 3 Infusion Device D Intraluminal Device J Cardiac Lead, Pacemaker K Cardiac Lead, Defibrillator M Cardiac Lead N Intracardiac Pacemak	Z No Qualifier
A Heart	0 Open 3 Percutaneous 4 Percutaneous Endoscopic	Q Implantable Heart Assist System	Z No Qualifier
A Heart	0 Open 3 Percutaneous 4 Percutaneous Endoscopic	R External Heart Assist System	S Biventricular Z No Qualifier
N Pericardium	0 Open 3 Percutaneous 4 Percutaneous Endoscopic	0 Monitoring Device, Pressure Sensor 2 Monitoring Device J Cardiac Lead, Pacemaker K Cardiac Lead, Defibrillator M Cardiac Lead	Z No Qualifier
P Pulmonary Trunk Q Pulmonary Artery, Right R Pulmonary Artery, Left S Pulmonary Vein, Right T Pulmonary Vein, Left V Superior Vena Cava W Thoracic Aorta, Descending X Thoracic Aorta, Ascending/Arch	0 Open 3 Percutaneous 4 Percutaneous Endoscopic	0 Monitoring Device, Pressure Sensor 2 Monitoring Device 3 Infusion Device D Intraluminal Device	Z No Qualifier

Section	0	Medical and Surgical		
Body System	2	Heart and Great Vessels		
Operation	J	Inspection: Visually and/or manually exploring a body part		
Body Part (Character 4)		**Approach (Character 5)**	**Device (Character 6)**	**Qualifier (Character 7)**
A Heart Y Great Vessel		0 Open 3 Percutaneous 4 Percutaneous Endoscopic	Z No Device	Z No Qualifier

Section	0	Medical and Surgical		
Body System	2	Heart and Great Vessels		
Operation	K	Map: Locating the route of passage of electrical impulses and/or locating functional areas in a body part		
Body Part (Character 4)		**Approach (Character 5)**	**Device (Character 6)**	**Qualifier (Character 7)**
8 Conduction Mechanism		0 Open 3 Percutaneous 4 Percutaneous Endoscopic	Z No Device	Z No Qualifier

Section	0	Medical and Surgical		
Body System	2	Heart and Great Vessels		
Operation	L	Occlusion: Completely closing an orifice or the lumen of a tubular body part		
Body Part (Character 4)		**Approach (Character 5)**	**Device (Character 6)**	**Qualifier (Character 7)**
7 Atrium, Left		0 Open 3 Percutaneous 4 Percutaneous Endoscopic	C Extraluminal Device D Intraluminal Device Z No Device	K Left Atrial Appendage
H Pulmonary Valve S Pulmonary Vein, Right T Pulmonary Vein, Left V Superior Vena Cava		0 Open 3 Percutaneous 4 Percutaneous Endoscopic	C Extraluminal Device D Intraluminal Device Z No Device	Z No Qualifier
R Pulmonary Artery, Left		0 Open 3 Percutaneous 4 Percutaneous Endoscopic	C Extraluminal Device D Intraluminal Device Z No Device	T Ductus Arteriosus

Section	0	Medical and Surgical		
Body System	2	Heart and Great Vessels		
Operation	N	Release: Freeing a body part from an abnormal physical constraint by cutting or by the use of force		
Body Part (Character 4)		**Approach (Character 5)**	**Device (Character 6)**	**Qualifier (Character 7)**
4 Coronary Vein 5 Atrial Septum 6 Atrium, Right 7 Atrium, Left 8 Conduction Mechanism 9 Chordae Tendineae D Papillary Muscle F Aortic Valve G Mitral Valve H Pulmonary Valve J Tricuspid Valve K Ventricle, Right L Ventricle, Left M Ventricular Septum N Pericardium P Pulmonary Trunk Q Pulmonary Artery, Right		0 Open 3 Percutaneous 4 Percutaneous Endoscopic	Z No Device	Z No Qualifier **Continued on Next Page ▶**

R Pulmonary Artery, Left S Pulmonary Vein, Right T Pulmonary Vein, Left V Superior Vena Cava W Thoracic Aorta, Descending X Thoracic Aorta, Ascending/Arch			**Continued from ◄ Previous Page**

Section	0	Medical and Surgical
Body System	2	Heart and Great Vessels
Operation	P	Removal: Taking out or off a device from a body part

Body Part (Character 4)	Approach (Character 5)	Device (Character 6)	Qualifier (Character 7)
A Heart	0 Open 3 Percutaneous 4 Percutaneous Endoscopic	2 Monitoring Device 3 Infusion Device 7 Autologous Tissue Substitute 8 Zooplastic Tissue C Extraluminal Device D Intraluminal Device J Synthetic Substitute K Nonautologous Tissue Substitute M Cardiac Lead N Intracardiac Pacemaker Q Implantable Heart Assist System R External Heart Assist System	Z No Qualifier
A Heart	X External	2 Monitoring Device 3 Infusion Device D Intraluminal Device M Cardiac Lead	Z No Qualifier
Y Great Vessel	0 Open 3 Percutaneous 4 Percutaneous Endoscopic	2 Monitoring Device 3 Infusion Device 7 Autologous Tissue Substitute 8 Zooplastic Tissue C Extraluminal Device D Intraluminal Device J Synthetic Substitute K Nonautologous Tissue Substitute	Z No Qualifier
Y Great Vessel	X External	2 Monitoring Device 3 Infusion Device D Intraluminal Device	Z No Qualifier

Section	0	Medical and Surgical		
Body System	2	Heart and Great Vessels		
Operation	Q	Repair: Restoring, to the extent possible, a body part to its normal anatomic structure and function		

Body Part (Character 4)	Approach (Character 5)	Device (Character 6)	Qualifier (Character 7)
0 Coronary Artery, One Artery 1 Coronary Artery, Two Arteries 2 Coronary Artery, Three Arteries 3 Coronary Artery, Four or More Arteries 4 Coronary Vein 5 Atrial Septum 6 Atrium, Right 7 Atrium, Left 8 Conduction Mechanism 9 Chordae Tendineae A Heart B Heart, Right C Heart, Left D Papillary Muscle H Pulmonary Valve K Ventricle, Right L Ventricle, Left M Ventricular Septum N Pericardium P Pulmonary Trunk Q Pulmonary Artery, Right R Pulmonary Artery, Left S Pulmonary Vein, Right T Pulmonary Vein, Left V Superior Vena Cava W Thoracic Aorta, Descending X Thoracic Aorta, Ascending/Arch	0 Open 3 Percutaneous 4 Percutaneous Endoscopic	Z No Device	Z No Qualifier
F Aortic Valve	0 Open 3 Percutaneous 4 Percutaneous Endoscopic	Z No Device	J Truncal Valve Z No Qualifier
G Mitral Valve	0 Open 3 Percutaneous 4 Percutaneous Endoscopic	Z No Device	E Atrioventricular Valve, Left Z No Qualifier
J Tricuspid Valve	0 Open 3 Percutaneous 4 Percutaneous Endoscopic	Z No Device	G Atrioventricular Valve, Right Z No Qualifier

Section	0	Medical and Surgical		
Body System	2	Heart and Great Vessels		
Operation	R	Replacement: Putting in or on biological or synthetic material that physically takes the place and/or function of all or a portion of a body part		

Body Part (Character 4)	Approach (Character 5)	Device (Character 6)	Qualifier (Character 7)
5 Atrial Septum 6 Atrium, Right 7 Atrium, Left 9 Chordae Tendineae D Papillary Muscle J Tricuspid Valve K Ventricle, Right L Ventricle, Left M Ventricular Septum N Pericardium P Pulmonary Trunk Q Pulmonary Artery, Right R Pulmonary Artery, Left S Pulmonary Vein, Right T Pulmonary Vein, Left V Superior Vena Cava W Thoracic Aorta, Descending X Thoracic Aorta, Ascending/Arch	0 Open 4 Percutaneous Endoscopic	7 Autologous Tissue Substitute 8 Zooplastic Tissue J Synthetic Substitute K Nonautologous Tissue Substitute	Z No Qualifier
F Aortic Valve G Mitral Valve H Pulmonary Valve	0 Open 4 Percutaneous Endoscopic	7 Autologous Tissue Substitute 8 Zooplastic Tissue J Synthetic Substitute K Nonautologous Tissue Substitute	Z No Qualifier
F Aortic Valve G Mitral Valve H Pulmonary Valve	3 Percutaneous	7 Autologous Tissue Substitute 8 Zooplastic Tissue J Synthetic Substitute K Nonautologous Tissue Substitute	H Transapical Z No Qualifier

Section	0	Medical and Surgical		
Body System	2	Heart and Great Vessels		
Operation	S	Reposition: Moving to its normal location, or other suitable location, all or a portion of a body part		

Body Part (Character 4)	Approach (Character 5)	Device (Character 6)	Qualifier (Character 7)
0 Coronary Artery, One Artery 1 Coronary Artery, Two Arteries P Pulmonary Trunk Q Pulmonary Artery, Right R Pulmonary Artery, Left S Pulmonary Vein, Right T Pulmonary Vein, Left V Superior Vena Cava W Thoracic Aorta, Descending X Thoracic Aorta, Ascending/Arch	0 Open	Z No Device	Z No Qualifier

Section	0	Medical and Surgical			
Body System	2	Heart and Great Vessels			
Operation	T	Resection: Cutting out or off, without replacement, all of a body part			

Body Part (Character 4)	Approach (Character 5)	Device (Character 6)	Qualifier (Character 7)
5 Atrial Septum	0 Open	Z No Device	Z No Qualifier
8 Conduction Mechanism	3 Percutaneous		
9 Chordae Tendineae	4 Percutaneous Endoscopic		
D Papillary Muscle			
H Pulmonary Valve			
M Ventricular Septum			
N Pericardium			

Section	0	Medical and Surgical			
Body System	2	Heart and Great Vessels			
Operation	U	Supplement: Putting in or on biological or synthetic material that physically reinforces and/or augments the function of a portion of a body part			

Body Part (Character 4)	Approach (Character 5)	Device (Character 6)	Qualifier (Character 7)
5 Atrial Septum	0 Open	7 Autologous Tissue Substitute	Z No Qualifier
6 Atrium, Right	3 Percutaneous	8 Zooplastic Tissue	
7 Atrium, Left	4 Percutaneous Endoscopic	J Synthetic Substitute	
9 Chordae Tendineae		K Nonautologous Tissue Substitute	
A Heart			
D Papillary Muscle			
H Pulmonary Valve			
K Ventricle, Right			
L Ventricle, Left			
M Ventricular Septum			
N Pericardium			
P Pulmonary Trunk			
Q Pulmonary Artery, Right			
R Pulmonary Artery, Left			
S Pulmonary Vein, Right			
T Pulmonary Vein, Left			
V Superior Vena Cava			
W Thoracic Aorta, Descending			
X Thoracic Aorta, Ascending/Arch			

Section	0	Medical and Surgical		
Body System	2	Heart and Great Vessels		
Operation	V	Restriction: Partially closing an orifice or the lumen of a tubular body part		

Body Part (Character 4)	Approach (Character 5)	Device (Character 6)	Qualifier (Character 7)
A Heart	0 Open 3 Percutaneous 4 Percutaneous Endoscopic	C Extraluminal Device Z No Device	Z No Qualifier
P Pulmonary Trunk Q Pulmonary Artery, Right S Pulmonary Vein, Right T Pulmonary Vein, Left V Superior Vena Cava	0 Open 3 Percutaneous 4 Percutaneous Endoscopic	C Extraluminal Device D Intraluminal Device Z No Device	Z No Qualifier
R Pulmonary Artery, Left	0 Open 3 Percutaneous 4 Percutaneous Endoscopic	C Extraluminal Device D Intraluminal Device Z No Device	T Ductus Arteriosus Z No Qualifier
W Thoracic Aorta, Descending X Thoracic Aorta, Ascending/Arch	0 Open 3 Percutaneous 4 Percutaneous Endoscopic	C Extraluminal Device D Intraluminal Device E Intraluminal Device, Branched or Fenestrated, One or Two Arteries F Intraluminal Device, Branched or Fenestrated, Three or More Arteries Z No Device	Z No Qualifier

Section	0	Medical and Surgical		
Body System	2	Heart and Great Vessels		
Operation	W	Revision: Correcting, to the extent possible, a portion of a malfunctioning device or the position of a displaced device		

Body Part (Character 4)	Approach (Character 5)	Device (Character 6)	Qualifier (Character 7)
5 Atrial Septum M Ventricular Septum	0 Open 4 Percutaneous Endoscopic	J Synthetic Substitute	Z No Qualifier
A Heart	0 Open 3 Percutaneous 4 Percutaneous Endoscopic X External	2 Monitoring Device 3 Infusion Device 7 Autologous Tissue Substitute 8 Zooplastic Tissue C Extraluminal Device D Intraluminal Device J Synthetic Substitute K Nonautologous Tissue Substitute M Cardiac Lead N Intracardiac Pacemaker Q Implantable Heart Assist System R External Heart Assist System	Z No Qualifier
F Aortic Valve G Mitral Valve H Pulmonary Valve J Tricuspid Valve	0 Open 4 Percutaneous Endoscopic	7 Autologous Tissue Substitute 8 Zooplastic Tissue J Synthetic Substitute K Nonautologous Tissue Substitute	Z No Qualifier

Continued on Next Page ▶

			Continued from ◀ Previous Page
Y Great Vessel	**0** Open **3** Percutaneous **4** Percutaneous Endoscopic **X** External	**2** Monitoring Device **3** Infusion Device **7** Autologous Tissue Substitute **8** Zooplastic Tissue **C** Extraluminal Device **D** Intraluminal Device **J** Synthetic Substitute **K** Nonautologous Tissue Substitute	**Z** No Qualifier

Section	0	Medical and Surgical	
Body System	2	Heart and Great Vessels	
Operation	Y	Transplantation: Putting in or on all or a portion of a living body part taken from another individual or animal to physically take the place and/or function of all or a portion of a similar body part	

Body Part (Character 4)	Approach (Character 5)	Device (Character 6)	Qualifier (Character 7)
A Heart	**0** Open	**Z** No Device	**0** Allogeneic **1** Syngeneic **2** Zooplastic

Section	0	Medical and Surgical
Body System	3	Upper Arteries
Operation	1	Bypass: Altering the route of passage of the contents of a tubular body part

Body Part (Character 4)	Approach (Character 5)	Device (Character 6)	Qualifier (Character 7)
7 Brachial Artery, Right	0 Open	9 Autologous Venous Tissue A Autologous Arterial Tissue J Synthetic Substitute K Nonautologous Tissue Substitute Z No Device	0 Upper Arm Artery, Right 3 Lower Arm Artery, Right D Upper Arm Vein F Lower Arm Vein
8 Brachial Artery, Left	0 Open	9 Autologous Venous Tissue A Autologous Arterial Tissue J Synthetic Substitute K Nonautologous Tissue Substitute Z No Device	1 Upper Arm Artery, Left 4 Lower Arm Artery, Left D Upper Arm Vein F Lower Arm Vein
9 Ulnar Artery, Right B Radial Artery, Right	0 Open	9 Autologous Venous Tissue A Autologous Arterial Tissue J Synthetic Substitute K Nonautologous Tissue Substitute Z No Device	3 Lower Arm Artery, Right F Lower Arm Vein
A Ulnar Artery, Left C Radial Artery, Left	0 Open	9 Autologous Venous Tissue A Autologous Arterial Tissue J Synthetic Substitute K Nonautologous Tissue Substitute Z No Device	4 Lower Arm Artery, Left F Lower Arm Vein
G Intracranial Artery S Temporal Artery, Right T Temporal Artery, Left	0 Open	9 Autologous Venous Tissue A Autologous Arterial Tissue J Synthetic Substitute K Nonautologous Tissue Substitute Z No Device	G Intracranial Artery
H Common Carotid Artery, Right	0 Open	9 Autologous Venous Tissue A Autologous Arterial Tissue J Synthetic Substitute K Nonautologous Tissue Substitute Z No Device	G Intracranial Artery J Extracranial Artery, Right
J Common Carotid Artery, Left	0 Open	9 Autologous Venous Tissue A Autologous Arterial Tissue J Synthetic Substitute K Nonautologous Tissue Substitute Z No Device	G Intracranial Artery K Extracranial Artery, Left
K Internal Carotid Artery, Right M External Carotid Artery, Right	0 Open	9 Autologous Venous Tissue A Autologous Arterial Tissue J Synthetic Substitute K Nonautologous Tissue Substitute Z No Device	J Extracranial Artery, Right
L Internal Carotid Artery, Left N External Carotid Artery,	0 Open	9 Autologous Venous Tissue A Autologous Arterial Tissue J Synthetic Substitute	K Extracranial Artery, Left **Continued on Next Page ▶**

Left		K Nonautologous Tissue Substitute Z No Device	Continued from ◀ Previous Page

Section	0	Medical and Surgical	
Body System	3	Upper Arteries	
Operation	5	Destruction: Physical eradication of all or a portion of a body part by the direct use of energy, force, or a destructive agent	

Body Part (Character 4)	Approach (Character 5)	Device (Character 6)	Qualifier (Character 7)
0 Internal Mammary Artery, Right 1 Internal Mammary Artery, Left 2 Innominate Artery 3 Subclavian Artery, Right 4 Subclavian Artery, Left 5 Axillary Artery, Right 6 Axillary Artery, Left 7 Brachial Artery, Right 8 Brachial Artery, Left 9 Ulnar Artery, Right A Ulnar Artery, Left B Radial Artery, Right C Radial Artery, Left D Hand Artery, Right F Hand Artery, Left G Intracranial Artery H Common Carotid Artery, Right J Common Carotid Artery, Left K Internal Carotid Artery, Right L Internal Carotid Artery, Left M External Carotid Artery, Right N External Carotid Artery, Left P Vertebral Artery, Right Q Vertebral Artery, Left R Face Artery S Temporal Artery, Right T Temporal Artery, Left U Thyroid Artery, Right V Thyroid Artery, Left Y Upper Artery	0 Open 3 Percutaneous 4 Percutaneous Endoscopic	Z No Device	Z No Qualifier

Section	0	Medical and Surgical
Body System	3	Upper Arteries
Operation	7	Dilation: Expanding an orifice or the lumen of a tubular body part

Body Part (Character 4)	Approach (Character 5)	Device (Character 6)	Qualifier (Character 7)
0 Internal Mammary Artery, Right	0 Open	4 Intraluminal Device, Drugeluting	6 Bifurcation
1 Internal Mammary Artery, Left	3 Percutaneous	5 Intraluminal Device, Drugeluting, Two	Z No Qualifier
2 Innominate Artery	4 Percutaneous Endoscopic	6 Intraluminal Device, Drug eluting, Three	
3 Subclavian Artery, Right		7 Intraluminal Device, Drug eluting, Four or More	
4 Subclavian Artery, Left		D Intraluminal Device	
5 Axillary Artery, Right		E Intraluminal Device, Two	
6 Axillary Artery, Left		F Intraluminal Device, Three	
7 Brachial Artery, Right		G Intraluminal Device, Four or More Z No Device	
8 Brachial Artery, Left			
9 Ulnar Artery, Right			
A Ulnar Artery, Left			
B Radial Artery, Right			
C Radial Artery, Left			
D Hand Artery, Right			
F Hand Artery, Left			
G Intracranial Artery			
H Common Carotid Artery, Right			
J Common Carotid Artery, Left			
K Internal Carotid Artery, Right			
L Internal Carotid Artery, Left			
M External Carotid Artery, Right			
N External Carotid Artery, Left			
P Vertebral Artery, Right			
Q Vertebral Artery, Left			
R Face Artery			
S Temporal Artery, Right			
T Temporal Artery, Left			
U Thyroid Artery, Right			
V Thyroid Artery, Left			
Y Upper Artery			

Section	0	Medical and Surgical		
Body System	3	Upper Arteries		
Operation	9	Drainage: Taking or letting out fluids and/or gases from a body part		

Body Part (Character 4)	Approach (Character 5)	Device (Character 6)	Qualifier (Character 7)
0 Internal Mammary Artery, Right 1 Internal Mammary Artery, Left 2 Innominate Artery 3 Subclavian Artery, Right 4 Subclavian Artery, Left 5 Axillary Artery, Right 6 Axillary Artery, Left 7 Brachial Artery, Right 8 Brachial Artery, Left 9 Ulnar Artery, Right A Ulnar Artery, Left B Radial Artery, Right C Radial Artery, Left D Hand Artery, Right F Hand Artery, Left G Intracranial Artery H Common Carotid Artery, Right J Common Carotid Artery, Left K Internal Carotid Artery, Right L Internal Carotid Artery, Left M External Carotid Artery, Right N External Carotid Artery, Left P Vertebral Artery, Right Q Vertebral Artery, Left R Face Artery S Temporal Artery, Right T Temporal Artery, Left U Thyroid Artery, Right V Thyroid Artery, Left Y Upper Artery	0 Open 3 Percutaneous 4 Percutaneous Endoscopic	0 Drainage Device	Z No Qualifier
0 Internal Mammary Artery, Right 1 Internal Mammary Artery, Left 2 Innominate Artery 3 Subclavian Artery, Right 4 Subclavian Artery, Left 5 Axillary Artery, Right 6 Axillary Artery, Left 7 Brachial Artery, Right 8 Brachial Artery, Left 9 Ulnar Artery, Right A Ulnar Artery, Left	0 Open 3 Percutaneous 4 Percutaneous Endoscopic	Z No Device	X Diagnostic Z No Qualifier

Continued on Next Page ▶

B Radial Artery, Right C Radial Artery, Left D Hand Artery, Right F Hand Artery, Left G Intracranial Artery H Common Carotid Artery, Right J Common Carotid Artery, Left K Internal Carotid Artery, Right L Internal Carotid Artery, Left			Continued from ◀ Previous Page
M External Carotid Artery, Right N External Carotid Artery, Left P Vertebral Artery, Right Q Vertebral Artery, Left R Face Artery S Temporal Artery, Right T Temporal Artery, Left U Thyroid Artery, Right V Thyroid Artery, Left Y Upper Artery			

Section	0	Medical and Surgical	
Body System	3	Upper Arteries	
Operation	C	Extirpation: Taking or cutting out solid matter from a body part	

Body Part (Character 4)	Approach (Character 5)	Device (Character 6)	Qualifier (Character 7)
0 Internal Mammary Artery, Right 1 Internal Mammary Artery, Left 2 Innominate Artery 3 Subclavian Artery, Right 4 Subclavian Artery, Left 5 Axillary Artery, Right 6 Axillary Artery, Left 7 Brachial Artery, Right 8 Brachial Artery, Left 9 Ulnar Artery, Right A Ulnar Artery, Left B Radial Artery, Right C Radial Artery, Left D Hand Artery, Right F Hand Artery, Left G Intracranial Artery H Common Carotid Artery, Right J Common Carotid Artery, Left K Internal Carotid Artery, Right L Internal Carotid Artery, Left	0 Open 3 Percutaneous 4 Percutaneous Endoscopic	Z No Device	6 Bifurcation Z No Qualifier

Continued on
Next Page ▶

M External Carotid Artery, Right			Continued from ◄ Previous Page
N External Carotid Artery, Left			
P Vertebral Artery, Right			
Q Vertebral Artery, Left			
R Face Artery			
S Temporal Artery, Right			
T Temporal Artery, Left			
U Thyroid Artery, Right			
V Thyroid Artery, Left			
Y Upper Artery			

Section	0	Medical and Surgical
Body System	3	Upper Arteries
Operation	H	Insertion: Putting in a nonbiological appliance that monitors, assists, performs, or prevents a physiological function but does not physically take the place of a body part

Body Part (Character 4)	Approach (Character 5)	Device (Character 6)	Qualifier (Character 7)
0 Internal Mammary Artery, Right **1** Internal Mammary Artery, Left **2** Innominate Artery **3** Subclavian Artery, Right **4** Subclavian Artery, Left **5** Axillary Artery, Right **6** Axillary Artery, Left **7** Brachial Artery, Right **8** Brachial Artery, Left **9** Ulnar Artery, Right **A** Ulnar Artery, Left **B** Radial Artery, Right **C** Radial Artery, Left **D** Hand Artery, Right **F** Hand Artery, Left **G** Intracranial Artery **H** Common Carotid Artery, Right **J** Common Carotid Artery, Left **M** External Carotid Artery, Right **N** External Carotid Artery, Left **P** Vertebral Artery, Right **Q** Vertebral Artery, Left **R** Face Artery **S** Temporal Artery, Right **T** Temporal Artery, Left **U** Thyroid Artery, Right **V** Thyroid Artery, Left	**0** Open **3** Percutaneous **4** Percutaneous Endoscopic	**3** Infusion Device **D** Intraluminal Device	**Z** No Qualifier
K Internal Carotid Artery, Right **L** Internal Carotid Artery, Left	**0** Open **3** Percutaneous **4** Percutaneous Endoscopic	**3** Infusion Device **D** Intraluminal Device **M** Stimulator Lead	**Z** No Qualifier
Y Upper Artery	**0** Open **3** Percutaneous **4** Percutaneous Endoscopic	**2** Monitoring Device **3** Infusion Device **D** Intraluminal Device	**Z** No Qualifier

Section	0	Medical and Surgical		
Body System	3	Upper Arteries		
Operation	J	Inspection: Visually and/or manually exploring a body part		
Body Part (Character 4)		**Approach (Character 5)**	**Device (Character 6)**	**Qualifier (Character 7)**
Y Upper Artery		0 Open 3 Percutaneous 4 Percutaneous Endoscopic X External	Z No Device	Z No Qualifier

Section	0	Medical and Surgical		
Body System	3	Upper Arteries		
Operation	L	Occlusion: Completely closing an orifice or the lumen of a tubular body part		
Body Part (Character 4)		**Approach (Character 5)**	**Device (Character 6)**	**Qualifier (Character 7)**
0 Internal Mammary Artery, Right 1 Internal Mammary Artery, Left 2 Innominate Artery 3 Subclavian Artery, Right 4 Subclavian Artery, Left 5 Axillary Artery, Right 6 Axillary Artery, Left 7 Brachial Artery, Right 8 Brachial Artery, Left 9 Ulnar Artery, Right A Ulnar Artery, Left B Radial Artery, Right C Radial Artery, Left D Hand Artery, Right F Hand Artery, Left R Face Artery S Temporal Artery, Right T Temporal Artery, Left U Thyroid Artery, Right V Thyroid Artery, Left Y Upper Artery		0 Open 3 Percutaneous 4 Percutaneous Endoscopic	C Extraluminal Device D Intraluminal Device Z No Device	Z No Qualifier
G Intracranial Artery H Common Carotid Artery, Right J Common Carotid Artery, Left K Internal Carotid Artery, Right L Internal Carotid Artery, Left M External Carotid Artery, Right N External Carotid Artery, Left P Vertebral Artery, Right Q Vertebral Artery, Left		0 Open 3 Percutaneous 4 Percutaneous Endoscopic	B Intraluminal Device, Bioactive C Extraluminal Device D Intraluminal Device Z No Device	Z No Qualifier

Section	0	Medical and Surgical
Body System	3	Upper Arteries
Operation	N	Release: Freeing a body part from an abnormal physical constraint by cutting or by the use of force

Body Part (Character 4)	Approach (Character 5)	Device (Character 6)	Qualifier (Character 7)
0 Internal Mammary Artery, Right	0 Open	Z No Device	Z No Qualifier
1 Internal Mammary Artery, Left	3 Percutaneous		
2 Innominate Artery	4 Percutaneous Endoscopic		
3 Subclavian Artery, Right			
4 Subclavian Artery, Left			
5 Axillary Artery, Right			
6 Axillary Artery, Left			
7 Brachial Artery, Right			
8 Brachial Artery, Left			
9 Ulnar Artery, Right			
A Ulnar Artery, Left			
B Radial Artery, Right			
C Radial Artery, Left			
D Hand Artery, Right			
F Hand Artery, Left			
G Intracranial Artery			
H Common Carotid Artery, Right			
J Common Carotid Artery, Left			
K Internal Carotid Artery, Right			
L Internal Carotid Artery, Left			
M External Carotid Artery, Right			
N External Carotid Artery, Left			
P Vertebral Artery, Right			
Q Vertebral Artery, Left			
R Face Artery			
S Temporal Artery, Right			
T Temporal Artery, Left			
U Thyroid Artery, Right			
V Thyroid Artery, Left			
Y Upper Artery			

Section	0	Medical and Surgical		
Body System	3	Upper Arteries		
Operation	P	Removal: Taking out or off a device from a body part		

Body Part (Character 4)	Approach (Character 5)	Device (Character 6)	Qualifier (Character 7)
Y Upper Artery	**0** Open **3** Percutaneous **4** Percutaneous Endoscopic	**0** Drainage Device **2** Monitoring Device **3** Infusion Device **7** Autologous Tissue Substitute **C** Extraluminal Device **D** Intraluminal Device **J** Synthetic Substitute **K** Nonautologous Tissue Substitute **M** Stimulator Lead	**Z** No Qualifier
Y Upper Artery	**X** External	**0** Drainage Device **2** Monitoring Device **3** Infusion Device **D** Intraluminal Device **M** Stimulator Lead	**Z** No Qualifier

Section	0	Medical and Surgical		
Body System	3	Upper Arteries		
Operation	Q	Repair: Restoring, to the extent possible, a body part to its normal anatomic structure and function		

Body Part (Character 4)	Approach (Character 5)	Device (Character 6)	Qualifier (Character 7)
0 Internal Mammary Artery, Right **1** Internal Mammary Artery, Left **2** Innominate Artery **3** Subclavian Artery, Right **4** Subclavian Artery, Left **5** Axillary Artery, Right **6** Axillary Artery, Left **7** Brachial Artery, Right **8** Brachial Artery, Left **9** Ulnar Artery, Right **A** Ulnar Artery, Left **B** Radial Artery, Right **C** Radial Artery, Left **D** Hand Artery, Right **F** Hand Artery, Left **G** Intracranial Artery **H** Common Carotid Artery, Right **J** Common Carotid Artery, Left **K** Internal Carotid Artery, Right **L** Internal Carotid Artery, Left **M** External Carotid Artery, Right **N** External Carotid Artery, Left	**0** Open **3** Percutaneous **4** Percutaneous Endoscopic	**Z** No Device	**Z** No Qualifier

Continued on Next Page ▶

P Vertebral Artery, Right			Continued from ◀ Previous Page
Q Vertebral Artery, Left			
R Face Artery			
S Temporal Artery, Right			
T Temporal Artery, Left			
U Thyroid Artery, Right			
V Thyroid Artery, Left			
Y Upper Artery			

Section	0	Medical and Surgical	
Body System	3	Upper Arteries	
Operation	R	Replacement: Putting in or on biological or synthetic material that physically takes the place and/or function of all or a portion of a body part	

Body Part (Character 4)	Approach (Character 5)	Device (Character 6)	Qualifier (Character 7)
0 Internal Mammary Artery, Right	0 Open	7 Autologous Tissue Substitute	Z No Qualifier
1 Internal Mammary Artery, Left	4 Percutaneous Endoscopic	J Synthetic Substitute	
2 Innominate Artery		K Nonautologous Tissue Substitute	
3 Subclavian Artery, Right			
4 Subclavian Artery, Left			
5 Axillary Artery, Right			
6 Axillary Artery, Left			
7 Brachial Artery, Right			
8 Brachial Artery, Left			
9 Ulnar Artery, Right			
A Ulnar Artery, Left			
B Radial Artery, Right			
C Radial Artery, Left			
D Hand Artery, Right			
F Hand Artery, Left			
G Intracranial Artery			
H Common Carotid Artery, Right			
J Common Carotid Artery, Left			
K Internal Carotid Artery, Right			
L Internal Carotid Artery, Left			
M External Carotid Artery, Right			
N External Carotid Artery, Left			
P Vertebral Artery, Right			
Q Vertebral Artery, Left			
R Face Artery			
S Temporal Artery, Right			
T Temporal Artery, Left			
U Thyroid Artery, Right			
V Thyroid Artery, Left			
Y Upper Artery			

Section	0	Medical and Surgical	
Body System	3	Upper Arteries	
Operation	S	Reposition: Moving to its normal location, or other suitable location, all or a portion of a body part	

Body Part (Character 4)	Approach (Character 5)	Device (Character 6)	Qualifier (Character 7)
0 Internal Mammary Artery, Right	0 Open	Z No Device	Z No Qualifier
1 Internal Mammary Artery, Left	3 Percutaneous		
2 Innominate Artery	4 Percutaneous Endoscopic		
3 Subclavian Artery, Right			
4 Subclavian Artery, Left			
5 Axillary Artery, Right			
6 Axillary Artery, Left			
7 Brachial Artery, Right			
8 Brachial Artery, Left			
9 Ulnar Artery, Right			
A Ulnar Artery, Left			
B Radial Artery, Right			
C Radial Artery, Left			
D Hand Artery, Right			
F Hand Artery, Left			
G Intracranial Artery			
H Common Carotid Artery, Right			
J Common Carotid Artery, Left			
K Internal Carotid Artery, Right			
L Internal Carotid Artery, Left			
M External Carotid Artery, Right			
N External Carotid Artery, Left			
P Vertebral Artery, Right			
Q Vertebral Artery, Left			
R Face Artery			
S Temporal Artery, Right			
T Temporal Artery, Left			
U Thyroid Artery, Right			
V Thyroid Artery, Left			
Y Upper Artery			

Section	0	Medical and Surgical		
Body System	3	Upper Arteries		
Operation	U	Supplement: Putting in or on biological or synthetic material that physically reinforces and/or augments the function of a portion of a body part		

Body Part (Character 4)	Approach (Character 5)	Device (Character 6)	Qualifier (Character 7)
0 Internal Mammary Artery, Right	0 Open	7 Autologous Tissue Substitute	Z No Qualifier
1 Internal Mammary Artery, Left	3 Percutaneous	J Synthetic Substitute	
2 Innominate Artery	4 Percutaneous Endoscopic	K Nonautologous Tissue Substitute	
3 Subclavian Artery, Right			
4 Subclavian Artery, Left			
5 Axillary Artery, Right			
6 Axillary Artery, Left			
7 Brachial Artery, Right			
8 Brachial Artery, Left			
9 Ulnar Artery, Right			
A Ulnar Artery, Left			
B Radial Artery, Right			
C Radial Artery, Left			
D Hand Artery, Right			
F Hand Artery, Left			
G Intracranial Artery			
H Common Carotid Artery, Right			
J Common Carotid Artery, Left			
K Internal Carotid Artery, Right			
L Internal Carotid Artery, Left			
M External Carotid Artery, Right			
N External Carotid Artery, Left			
P Vertebral Artery, Right			
Q Vertebral Artery, Left			
R Face Artery			
S Temporal Artery, Right			
T Temporal Artery, Left			
U Thyroid Artery, Right			
V Thyroid Artery, Left			
Y Upper Artery			

Section	0	Medical and Surgical		
Body System	3	Upper Arteries		
Operation	V	Restriction: Partially closing an orifice or the lumen of a tubular body part		

Body Part (Character 4)	Approach (Character 5)	Device (Character 6)	Qualifier (Character 7)
0 Internal Mammary Artery, Right **1** Internal Mammary Artery, Left **2** Innominate Artery **3** Subclavian Artery, Right **4** Subclavian Artery, Left **5** Axillary Artery, Right **6** Axillary Artery, Left **7** Brachial Artery, Right **8** Brachial Artery, Left **9** Ulnar Artery, Right **A** Ulnar Artery, Left **B** Radial Artery, Right **C** Radial Artery, Left **D** Hand Artery, Right **F** Hand Artery, Left **R** Face Artery **S** Temporal Artery, Right **T** Temporal Artery, Left **U** Thyroid Artery, Right **V** Thyroid Artery, Left **Y** Upper Artery	**0** Open **3** Percutaneous **4** Percutaneous Endoscopic	**C** Extraluminal Device **D** Intraluminal Device **Z** No Device	**Z** No Qualifier
G Intracranial Artery **H** Common Carotid Artery, Right **J** Common Carotid Artery, Left **K** Internal Carotid Artery, Right **L** Internal Carotid Artery, Left **M** External Carotid Artery, Right **N** External Carotid Artery, Left **P** Vertebral Artery, Right **Q** Vertebral Artery, Left	**0** Open **3** Percutaneous **4** Percutaneous Endoscopic	**B** Intraluminal Device, Bioactive **C** Extraluminal Device **D** Intraluminal Device **Z** No Device	**Z** No Qualifier

Section	0	Medical and Surgical
Body System	3	Upper Arteries
Operation	W	Revision: Correcting, to the extent possible, a portion of a malfunctioning device or the position of a displaced device

Body Part (Character 4)	Approach (Character 5)	Device (Character 6)	Qualifier (Character 7)
Y Upper Artery	0 Open 3 Percutaneous 4 Percutaneous Endoscopic X External	0 Drainage Device 2 Monitoring Device 3 Infusion Device 7 Autologous Tissue Substitute C Extraluminal Device D Intraluminal Device J Synthetic Substitute K Nonautologous Tissue Substitute M Stimulator Lead	Z No Qualifier

Section	0	Medical and Surgical
Body System	4	Lower Arteries
Operation	1	Bypass: Altering the route of passage of the contents of a tubular body part

Body Part (Character 4)	Approach (Character 5)	Device (Character 6)	Qualifier (Character 7)
0 Abdominal Aorta **C** Common Iliac Artery, Right **D** Common Iliac Artery, Left	**0** Open **4** Percutaneous Endoscopic	**9** Autologous Venous Tissue **A** Autologous Arterial Tissue **J** Synthetic Substitute **K** Nonautologous Tissue Substitute **Z** No Device	**0** Abdominal Aorta **1** Celiac Artery **2** Mesenteric Artery **3** Renal Artery, Right **4** Renal Artery, Left **5** Renal Artery, Bilateral **6** Common Iliac Artery, Right **7** Common Iliac Artery, Left **8** Common Iliac Arteries, Bilateral **9** Internal Iliac Artery, Right **B** Internal Iliac Artery, Left **C** Internal Iliac Arteries, Bilateral **D** External Iliac Artery, Right **F** External Iliac Artery, Left **G** External Iliac Arteries, Bilateral **H** Femoral Artery, Right **J** Femoral Artery, Left **K** Femoral Arteries, Bilateral **Q** Lower Extremity Artery **R** Lower Artery
4 Splenic Artery	**0** Open **4** Percutaneous Endoscopic	**9** Autologous Venous Tissue **A** Autologous Arterial Tissue **J** Synthetic Substitute **K** Nonautologous Tissue Substitute **Z** No Device	**3** Renal Artery, Right **4** Renal Artery, Left **5** Renal Artery, Bilateral
E Internal Iliac Artery, Right **F** Internal Iliac Artery, Left **H** External Iliac Artery, Right **J** External Iliac Artery, Left	**0** Open **4** Percutaneous Endoscopic	**9** Autologous Venous Tissue **A** Autologous Arterial Tissue **J** Synthetic Substitute **K** Nonautologous Tissue Substitute **Z** No Device	**9** Internal Iliac Artery, Right **B** Internal Iliac Artery, Left **C** Internal Iliac Arteries, Bilateral **D** External Iliac Artery, Right **F** External Iliac Artery, Left **G** External Iliac Arteries, Bilateral **H** Femoral Artery, Right **J** Femoral Artery, Left **K** Femoral Arteries, Bilateral **P** Foot Artery **Q** Lower Extremity Artery

ICD-10-PCS 2017

Section	0	Medical and Surgical		
Body System	4	Lower Arteries		
Operation	1	Bypass: Altering the route of passage of the contents of a tubular body part		

Body Part (Character 4)	Approach (Character 5)	Device (Character 6)	Qualifier (Character 7)
K Femoral Artery, Right L Femoral Artery, Left	0 Open 4 Percutaneous Endoscopic	9 Autologous Venous Tissue A Autologous Arterial Tissue J Synthetic Substitute K Nonautologous Tissue Substitute Z No Device	H Femoral Artery, Right J Femoral Artery, Left K Femoral Arteries, Bilateral L Popliteal Artery M Peroneal Artery N Posterior Tibial Artery P Foot Artery Q Lower Extremity Artery S Lower Extremity Vein
M Popliteal Artery, Right N Popliteal Artery, Left	0 Open 4 Percutaneous Endoscopic	9 Autologous Venous Tissue A Autologous Arterial Tissue J Synthetic Substitute K Nonautologous Tissue Substitute Z No Device	L Popliteal Artery M Peroneal Artery P Foot Artery Q Lower Extremity Artery S Lower Extremity Vein

Section	0	Medical and Surgical		
Body System	4	Lower Arteries		
Operation	5	Destruction: Physical eradication of all or a portion of a body part by the direct use of energy, force, or a destructive agent		

Body Part (Character 4)	Approach (Character 5)	Device (Character 6)	Qualifier (Character 7)
0 Abdominal Aorta 1 Celiac Artery 2 Gastric Artery 3 Hepatic Artery 4 Splenic Artery 5 Superior Mesenteric Artery 6 Colic Artery, Right 7 Colic Artery, Left 8 Colic Artery, Middle 9 Renal Artery, Right A Renal Artery, Left B Inferior Mesenteric Artery C Common Iliac Artery, Right D Common Iliac Artery, Left E Internal Iliac Artery, Right F Internal Iliac Artery, Left H External Iliac Artery, Right J External Iliac Artery, Left K Femoral Artery, Right L Femoral Artery, Left M Popliteal Artery, Right N Popliteal Artery, Left P Anterior Tibial Artery, Right Q Anterior Tibial Artery, Left R Posterior Tibial Artery, Right S Posterior Tibial Artery, Left T Peroneal Artery, Right	0 Open 3 Percutaneous 4 Percutaneous Endoscopic	Z No Device	Z No Qualifier Continued on Next Page ▶

174

U Peroneal Artery, Left			Continued from ◄ Previous Page
V Foot Artery, Right			
W Foot Artery, Left			
Y Lower Artery			

Section	0	Medical and Surgical
Body System	4	Lower Arteries
Operation	7	Dilation: Expanding an orifice or the lumen of a tubular body part

Body Part (Character 4)	Approach (Character 5)	Device (Character 6)	Qualifier (Character 7)
0 Abdominal Aorta 1 Celiac Artery 2 Gastric Artery 3 Hepatic Artery 4 Splenic Artery 5 Superior Mesenteric Artery 6 Colic Artery, Right 7 Colic Artery, Left 8 Colic Artery, Middle 9 Renal Artery, Right A Renal Artery, Left B Inferior Mesenteric Artery C Common Iliac Artery, Right D Common Iliac Artery, Left E Internal Iliac Artery, Right F Internal Iliac Artery, Left H External Iliac Artery, Right J External Iliac Artery, Left P Anterior Tibial Artery, Right Q Anterior Tibial Artery, Left R Posterior Tibial Artery, Right S Posterior Tibial Artery, Left T Peroneal Artery, Right U Peroneal Artery, Left V Foot Artery, Right W Foot Artery, Left Y Lower Artery	0 Open 3 Percutaneous 4 Percutaneous Endoscopic	4 Intraluminal Device, Drug eluting 5 Intraluminal Device, Drug eluting, Two 6 Intraluminal Device, Drug eluting, Three 7 Intraluminal Device, Drug eluting, Four or More D Intraluminal Device E Intraluminal Device, Two F Intraluminal Device, Three G Intraluminal Device, Four or More Z No Device	6 Bifurcation Z No Qualifier
K Femoral Artery, Right L Femoral Artery, Left M Popliteal Artery, Right N Popliteal Artery, Left	0 Open 3 Percutaneous 4 Percutaneous Endoscopic	4 Intraluminal Device, Drug-eluting D Intraluminal Device Z No Device	1 Drug-Coated Balloon 6 Bifurcation Z No Qualifier
K Femoral Artery, Right L Femoral Artery, Left M Popliteal Artery, Right N Popliteal Artery, Left	0 Open 3 Percutaneous 4 Percutaneous Endoscopic	5 Intraluminal Device, Drug eluting, Two 6 Intraluminal Device, Drug eluting, Three 7 Drug eluting, Four or More E Intraluminal Device, Two F Intraluminal Device, Three G Intraluminal Device, Four or More	6 Bifurcation Z No Qualifier

Section	0	Medical and Surgical		
Body System	4	Lower Arteries		
Operation	9	Drainage: Taking or letting out fluids and/or gases from a body part		

Body Part (Character 4)	Approach (Character 5)	Device (Character 6)	Qualifier (Character 7)
0 Abdominal Aorta 1 Celiac Artery 2 Gastric Artery 3 Hepatic Artery 4 Splenic Artery 5 Superior Mesenteric Artery 6 Colic Artery, Right 7 Colic Artery, Left 8 Colic Artery, Middle 9 Renal Artery, Right A Renal Artery, Left B Inferior Mesenteric Artery C Common Iliac Artery, Right D Common Iliac Artery, Left E Internal Iliac Artery, Right F Internal Iliac Artery, Left H External Iliac Artery, Right J External Iliac Artery, Left K Femoral Artery, Right L Femoral Artery, Left M Popliteal Artery, Right N Popliteal Artery, Left P Anterior Tibial Artery, Right Q Anterior Tibial Artery, Left R Posterior Tibial Artery, Right S Posterior Tibial Artery, Left T Peroneal Artery, Right U Peroneal Artery, Left V Foot Artery, Right W Foot Artery, Left Y Lower Artery	0 Open 3 Percutaneous 4 Percutaneous Endoscopic	0 Drainage Device	Z No Qualifier
0 Abdominal Aorta 1 Celiac Artery 2 Gastric Artery 3 Hepatic Artery 4 Splenic Artery 5 Superior Mesenteric Artery 6 Colic Artery, Right 7 Colic Artery, Left 8 Colic Artery, Middle 9 Renal Artery, Right A Renal Artery, Left B Inferior Mesenteric Artery C Common Iliac Artery, Right D Common Iliac Artery, Left E Internal Iliac Artery, Right	0 Open 3 Percutaneous 4 Percutaneous Endoscopic	Z No Device	X Diagnostic Z No Qualifier

Continued on Next Page ▶

F Internal Iliac Artery, Left			Continued from ◀ Previous Page
H External Iliac Artery, Right			
J External Iliac Artery, Left			
K Femoral Artery, Right			
L Femoral Artery, Left			
M Popliteal Artery, Right			
N Popliteal Artery, Left			
P Anterior Tibial Artery, Right			
Q Anterior Tibial Artery, Left			
R Posterior Tibial Artery, Right			
S Posterior Tibial Artery, Left			
T Peroneal Artery, Right			
U Peroneal Artery, Left			
V Foot Artery, Right			
W Foot Artery, Left			
Y Lower Artery			

Section	0	Medical and Surgical	
Body System	4	Lower Arteries	
Operation	B	Excision: Cutting out or off, without replacement, a portion of a body part	

Body Part (Character 4)	Approach (Character 5)	Device (Character 6)	Qualifier (Character 7)
0 Abdominal Aorta	0 Open	Z No Device	X Diagnostic
1 Celiac Artery	3 Percutaneous		Z No Qualifier
2 Gastric Artery	4 Percutaneous Endoscopic		
3 Hepatic Artery			
4 Splenic Artery			
5 Superior Mesenteric Artery			
6 Colic Artery, Right			
7 Colic Artery, Left			
8 Colic Artery, Middle			
9 Renal Artery, Right			
A Renal Artery, Left			
B Inferior Mesenteric Artery			
C Common Iliac Artery, Right			
D Common Iliac Artery, Left			
E Internal Iliac Artery, Right			
F Internal Iliac Artery, Left			
H External Iliac Artery, Right			
J External Iliac Artery, Left			
K Femoral Artery, Right			
L Femoral Artery, Left			
M Popliteal Artery, Right			
N Popliteal Artery, Left			
P Anterior Tibial Artery, Right			
Q Anterior Tibial Artery, Left			
R Posterior Tibial Artery, Right			
S Posterior Tibial Artery, Left			Continued on Next Page ▶

T Peroneal Artery, Right			Continued from
U Peroneal Artery, Left			◄ Previous Page
V Foot Artery, Right			
W Foot Artery, Left			
Y Lower Artery			

Section	0	Medical and Surgical	
Body System	4	Lower Arteries	
Operation	C	Extirpation: Taking or cutting out solid matter from a body part	

Body Part (Character 4)	Approach (Character 5)	Device (Character 6)	Qualifier (Character 7)
0 Abdominal Aorta	0 Open	Z No Device	6 Bifurcation
1 Celiac Artery	3 Percutaneous		Z No Qualifier
2 Gastric Artery	4 Percutaneous Endoscopic		
3 Hepatic Artery			
4 Splenic Artery			
5 Superior Mesenteric Artery			
6 Colic Artery, Right			
7 Colic Artery, Left			
8 Colic Artery, Middle			
9 Renal Artery, Right			
A Renal Artery, Left			
B Inferior Mesenteric Artery			
C Common Iliac Artery, Right			
D Common Iliac Artery, Left			
E Internal Iliac Artery, Right			
F Internal Iliac Artery, Left			
H External Iliac Artery, Right			
J External Iliac Artery, Left			
K Femoral Artery, Right			
L Femoral Artery, Left			
M Popliteal Artery, Right			
N Popliteal Artery, Left			
P Anterior Tibial Artery, Right			
Q Anterior Tibial Artery, Left			
R Posterior Tibial Artery, Right			
S Posterior Tibial Artery, Left			
T Peroneal Artery, Right			
U Peroneal Artery, Left			
V Foot Artery, Right			
W Foot Artery, Left			
Y Lower Artery			

Section	0	Medical and Surgical		
Body System	4	Lower Arteries		
Operation	H	Insertion: Putting in a nonbiological appliance that monitors, assists, performs, or prevents a physiological function but does not physically take the place of a body part		

Body Part (Character 4)	Approach (Character 5)	Device (Character 6)	Qualifier (Character 7)
0 Abdominal Aorta **Y** Lower Artery	**0** Open **3** Percutaneous **4** Percutaneous Endoscopic	**2** Monitoring Device **3** Infusion Device **D** Intraluminal Device	**Z** No Qualifier
1 Celiac Artery **2** Gastric Artery **3** Hepatic Artery **4** Splenic Artery **5** Superior Mesenteric Artery **6** Colic Artery, Right **7** Colic Artery, Left **8** Colic Artery, Middle **9** Renal Artery, Right **A** Renal Artery, Left **B** Inferior Mesenteric Artery **C** Common Iliac Artery, Right **D** Common Iliac Artery, Left **E** Internal Iliac Artery, Right **F** Internal Iliac Artery, Left **H** External Iliac Artery, Right **J** External Iliac Artery, Left **K** Femoral Artery, Right **L** Femoral Artery, Left **M** Popliteal Artery, Right **N** Popliteal Artery, Left **P** Anterior Tibial Artery, Right **Q** Anterior Tibial Artery, Left **R** Posterior Tibial Artery, Right **S** Posterior Tibial Artery, Left **T** Peroneal Artery, Right **U** Peroneal Artery, Left **V** Foot Artery, Right **W** Foot Artery, Left	**0** Open **3** Percutaneous **4** Percutaneous Endoscopic	**3** Infusion Device **D** Intraluminal Device	**Z** No Qualifier

Section	0	Medical and Surgical		
Body System	4	Lower Arteries		
Operation	J	Inspection: Visually and/or manually exploring a body part		

Body Part (Character 4)	Approach (Character 5)	Device (Character 6)	Qualifier (Character 7)
Y Lower Artery	**0** Open **3** Percutaneous **4** Percutaneous Endoscopic **X** External	**Z** No Device	**Z** No Qualifier

Section	0	Medical and Surgical		
Body System	4	Lower Arteries		
Operation	L	Occlusion: Completely closing an orifice or the lumen of a tubular body part		

Body Part (Character 4)	Approach (Character 5)	Device (Character 6)	Qualifier (Character 7)
0 Abdominal Aorta 1 Celiac Artery 2 Gastric Artery 3 Hepatic Artery 4 Splenic Artery 5 Superior Mesenteric Artery 6 Colic Artery, Right 7 Colic Artery, Left 8 Colic Artery, Middle 9 Renal Artery, Right A Renal Artery, Left B Inferior Mesenteric Artery C Common Iliac Artery, Right D Common Iliac Artery, Left H External Iliac Artery, Right J External Iliac Artery, Left K Femoral Artery, Right L Femoral Artery, Left M Popliteal Artery, Right N Popliteal Artery, Left P Anterior Tibial Artery, Right Q Anterior Tibial Artery, Left R Posterior Tibial Artery, Right S Posterior Tibial Artery, Left T Peroneal Artery, Right U Peroneal Artery, Left V Foot Artery, Right W Foot Artery, Left Y Lower Artery	0 Open 3 Percutaneous 4 Percutaneous Endoscopic	C Extraluminal Device D Intraluminal Device Z No Device	Z No Qualifier
E Internal Iliac Artery, Right	0 Open 3 Percutaneous 4 Percutaneous Endoscopic	C Extraluminal Device D Intraluminal Device Z No Device	T Uterine Artery, Right Z No Qualifier
F Internal Iliac Artery, Left	0 Open 3 Percutaneous 4 Percutaneous Endoscopic	C Extraluminal Device D Intraluminal Device Z No Device	U Uterine Artery, Left Z No Qualifier

Section	0	Medical and Surgical
Body System	4	Lower Arteries
Operation	N	Release: Freeing a body part from an abnormal physical constraint by cutting or by the use of force

Body Part (Character 4)	Approach (Character 5)	Device (Character 6)	Qualifier (Character 7)
0 Abdominal Aorta	0 Open	Z No Device	Z No Qualifier
1 Celiac Artery	3 Percutaneous		
2 Gastric Artery	4 Percutaneous Endoscopic		
3 Hepatic Artery			
4 Splenic Artery			
5 Superior Mesenteric Artery			
6 Colic Artery, Right			
7 Colic Artery, Left			
8 Colic Artery, Middle			
9 Renal Artery, Right			
A Renal Artery, Left			
B Inferior Mesenteric Artery			
C Common Iliac Artery, Right			
D Common Iliac Artery, Left			
E Internal Iliac Artery, Right			
F Internal Iliac Artery, Left			
H External Iliac Artery, Right			
J External Iliac Artery, Left			
K Femoral Artery, Right			
L Femoral Artery, Left			
M Popliteal Artery, Right			
N Popliteal Artery, Left			
P Anterior Tibial Artery, Right			
Q Anterior Tibial Artery, Left			
R Posterior Tibial Artery, Right			
S Posterior Tibial Artery, Left			
T Peroneal Artery, Right			
U Peroneal Artery, Left			
V Foot Artery, Right			
W Foot Artery, Left			
Y Lower Artery			

Section	0	Medical and Surgical
Body System	4	Lower Arteries
Operation	P	Removal: Taking out or off a device from a body part

Body Part (Character 4)	Approach (Character 5)	Device (Character 6)	Qualifier (Character 7)
Y Lower Artery	0 Open 3 Percutaneous 4 Percutaneous Endoscopic	0 Drainage Device 2 Monitoring Device 3 Infusion Device 7 Autologous Tissue Substitute C Extraluminal Device D Intraluminal Device J Synthetic Substitute K Nonautologous Tissue Substitute	Z No Qualifier
Y Lower Artery	X External	0 Drainage Device 1 Radioactive Element 2 Monitoring Device 3 Infusion Device D Intraluminal Device	Z No Qualifier

Section	0	Medical and Surgical
Body System	4	Lower Arteries
Operation	Q	Repair: Restoring, to the extent possible, a body part to its normal anatomic structure and function

Body Part (Character 4)	Approach (Character 5)	Device (Character 6)	Qualifier (Character 7)
0 Abdominal Aorta 1 Celiac Artery 2 Gastric Artery 3 Hepatic Artery 4 Splenic Artery 5 Superior Mesenteric Artery 6 Colic Artery, Right 7 Colic Artery, Left 8 Colic Artery, Middle 9 Renal Artery, Right A Renal Artery, Left B Inferior Mesenteric Artery C Common Iliac Artery, Right D Common Iliac Artery, Left E Internal Iliac Artery, Right F Internal Iliac Artery, Left H External Iliac Artery, Right J External Iliac Artery, Left K Femoral Artery, Right L Femoral Artery, Left M Popliteal Artery, Right N Popliteal Artery, Left P Anterior Tibial Artery, Right Q Anterior Tibial Artery, Left R Posterior Tibial Artery, Right S Posterior Tibial Artery, Left T Peroneal Artery, Right	0 Open 3 Percutaneous 4 Percutaneous Endoscopic	Z No Device	Z No Qualifier

Continued on Next Page ▶

U Peroneal Artery, Left			Continued from ◄ Previous Page
V Foot Artery, Right			
W Foot Artery, Left			
Y Lower Artery			

Section	0	Medical and Surgical		
Body System	4	Lower Arteries		
Operation	R	Replacement: Putting in or on biological or synthetic material that physically takes the place and/or function of all or a portion of a body part		

Body Part (Character 4)	Approach (Character 5)	Device (Character 6)	Qualifier (Character 7)
0 Abdominal Aorta	0 Open	7 Autologous Tissue Substitute	Z No Qualifier
1 Celiac Artery	4 Percutaneous Endoscopic	J Synthetic Substitute	
2 Gastric Artery		K Nonautologous Tissue Substitute	
3 Hepatic Artery			
4 Splenic Artery			
5 Superior Mesenteric Artery			
6 Colic Artery, Right			
7 Colic Artery, Left			
8 Colic Artery, Middle			
9 Renal Artery, Right			
A Renal Artery, Left			
B Inferior Mesenteric Artery			
C Common Iliac Artery, Right			
D Common Iliac Artery, Left			
E Internal Iliac Artery, Right			
F Internal Iliac Artery, Left			
H External Iliac Artery, Right			
J External Iliac Artery, Left			
K Femoral Artery, Right			
L Femoral Artery, Left			
M Popliteal Artery, Right			
N Popliteal Artery, Left			
P Anterior Tibial Artery, Right			
Q Anterior Tibial Artery, Left			
R Posterior Tibial Artery, Right			
S Posterior Tibial Artery, Left			
T Peroneal Artery, Right			
U Peroneal Artery, Left			
V Foot Artery, Right			
W Foot Artery, Left			
Y Lower Artery			

Section	0	Medical and Surgical
Body System	4	Lower Arteries
Operation	S	Reposition: Moving to its normal location, or other suitable location, all or a portion of a body part

Body Part (Character 4)	Approach (Character 5)	Device (Character 6)	Qualifier (Character 7)
0 Abdominal Aorta	**0** Open	**Z** No Device	**Z** No Qualifier
1 Celiac Artery	**3** Percutaneous		
2 Gastric Artery	**4** Percutaneous Endoscopic		
3 Hepatic Artery			
4 Splenic Artery			
5 Superior Mesenteric Artery			
6 Colic Artery, Right			
7 Colic Artery, Left			
8 Colic Artery, Middle			
9 Renal Artery, Right			
A Renal Artery, Left			
B Inferior Mesenteric Artery			
C Common Iliac Artery, Right			
D Common Iliac Artery, Left			
E Internal Iliac Artery, Right			
F Internal Iliac Artery, Left			
H External Iliac Artery, Right			
J External Iliac Artery, Left			
K Femoral Artery, Right			
L Femoral Artery, Left			
M Popliteal Artery, Right			
N Popliteal Artery, Left			
P Anterior Tibial Artery, Right			
Q Anterior Tibial Artery, Left			
R Posterior Tibial Artery, Right			
S Posterior Tibial Artery, Left			
T Peroneal Artery, Right			
U Peroneal Artery, Left			
V Foot Artery, Right			
W Foot Artery, Left			
Y Lower Artery			

Section	0	Medical and Surgical
Body System	4	Lower Arteries
Operation	U	Supplement: Putting in or on biological or synthetic material that physically reinforces and/or augments the function of a portion of a body part

Body Part (Character 4)	Approach (Character 5)	Device (Character 6)	Qualifier (Character 7)
0 Abdominal Aorta	0 Open	7 Autologous Tissue Substitute	Z No Qualifier
1 Celiac Artery	3 Percutaneous	J Synthetic Substitute	
2 Gastric Artery	4 Percutaneous Endoscopic	K Nonautologous Tissue Substitute	
3 Hepatic Artery			
4 Splenic Artery			
5 Superior Mesenteric Artery			
6 Colic Artery, Right			
7 Colic Artery, Left			
8 Colic Artery, Middle			
9 Renal Artery, Right			
A Renal Artery, Left			
B Inferior Mesenteric Artery			
C Common Iliac Artery, Right			
D Common Iliac Artery, Left			
E Internal Iliac Artery, Right			
F Internal Iliac Artery, Left			
H External Iliac Artery, Right			
J External Iliac Artery, Left			
K Femoral Artery, Right			
L Femoral Artery, Left			
M Popliteal Artery, Right			
N Popliteal Artery, Left			
P Anterior Tibial Artery, Right			
Q Anterior Tibial Artery, Left			
R Posterior Tibial Artery, Right			
S Posterior Tibial Artery, Left			
T Peroneal Artery, Right			
U Peroneal Artery, Left			
V Foot Artery, Right			
W Foot Artery, Left			
Y Lower Artery			

Section	0	Medical and Surgical			
Body System	4	Lower Arteries			
Operation	V	Restriction: Partially closing an orifice or the lumen of a tubular body part			

Body Part (Character 4)	Approach (Character 5)	Device (Character 6)	Qualifier (Character 7)
0 Abdominal Aorta	**0** Open **3** Percutaneous **4** Percutaneous Endoscopic	**C** Extraluminal Device **E** Intraluminal Device, Branched or Fenestrated, One or Two Arteries **F** Intraluminal Device, Branched or Fenestrated, Three or More Arteries **Z** No Device	**6** Bifurcation **Z** No Qualifier
0 Abdominal Aorta	**0** Open **3** Percutaneous **4** Percutaneous Endoscopic	**D** Intraluminal Device	**6** Bifurcation **J** Temporary **Z** No Qualifier
1 Celiac Artery **2** Gastric Artery **3** Hepatic Artery **4** Splenic Artery **5** Superior Mesenteric Artery **6** Colic Artery, Right **7** Colic Artery, Left **8** Colic Artery, Middle **9** Renal Artery, Right **A** Renal Artery, Left **B** Inferior Mesenteric Artery **C** Common Iliac Artery, Right **D** Common Iliac Artery, Left **E** Internal Iliac Artery, Right **F** Internal Iliac Artery, Left **H** External Iliac Artery, Right **J** External Iliac Artery, Left **K** Femoral Artery, Right **L** Femoral Artery, Left **M** Popliteal Artery, Right **N** Popliteal Artery, Left **P** Anterior Tibial Artery, Right **Q** Anterior Tibial Artery, Left **R** Posterior Tibial Artery, Right **S** Posterior Tibial Artery, Left **T** Peroneal Artery, Right **U** Peroneal Artery, Left **V** Foot Artery, Right **W** Foot Artery, Left **Y** Lower Artery	**0** Open **3** Percutaneous **4** Percutaneous Endoscopic	**C** Extraluminal Device **D** Intraluminal Device **Z** No Device	**Z** No Qualifier
C Common Iliac Artery, Right **D** Common Iliac Artery, Left	**0** Open **3** Percutaneous **4** Percutaneous Endoscopic	**C** Extraluminal Device **D** Intraluminal Device **E** Intraluminal Device, Branched or Fenestrated, One or Two Arteries **F** Intraluminal Device, Branched or Fenestrated, Three or More Arteries **Z** No Device	**Z** No Qualifier

Section	0	Medical and Surgical		
Body System	4	Lower Arteries		
Operation	W	Revision: Correcting, to the extent possible, a portion of a malfunctioning device or the position of a displaced device		

Body Part (Character 4)	Approach (Character 5)	Device (Character 6)	Qualifier (Character 7)
Y Lower Artery	0 Open 3 Percutaneous 4 Percutaneous Endoscopic X External	0 Drainage Device 2 Monitoring Device 3 Infusion Device 7 Autologous Tissue Substitute C Extraluminal Device D Intraluminal Device J Synthetic Substitute K Nonautologous Tissue Substitute	Z No Qualifier

Section	0	Medical and Surgical		
Body System	5	Upper Veins		
Operation	1	Bypass: Altering the route of passage of the contents of a tubular body part		

Body Part (Character 4)	Approach (Character 5)	Device (Character 6)	Qualifier (Character 7)
0 Azygos Vein	0 Open	7 Autologous Tissue Substitute	Y Upper Vein
1 Hemiazygos Vein	4 Percutaneous Endoscopic	9 Autologous Venous Tissue	
3 Innominate Vein, Right		A Autologous Arterial Tissue	
4 Innominate Vein, Left		J Synthetic Substitute	
5 Subclavian Vein, Right		K Nonautologous Tissue Substitute	
6 Subclavian Vein, Left		Z No Device	
7 Axillary Vein, Right			
8 Axillary Vein, Left			
9 Brachial Vein, Right			
A Brachial Vein, Left			
B Basilic Vein, Right			
C Basilic Vein, Left			
D Cephalic Vein, Right			
F Cephalic Vein, Left			
G Hand Vein, Right			
H Hand Vein, Left			
L Intracranial Vein			
M Internal Jugular Vein, Right			
N Internal Jugular Vein, Left			
P External Jugular Vein, Right			
Q External Jugular Vein, Left			
R Vertebral Vein, Right			
S Vertebral Vein, Left			
T Face Vein, Right			
V Face Vein, Left			

Section	0	Medical and Surgical		
Body System	5	Upper Veins		
Operation	5	Destruction: Physical eradication of all or a portion of a body part by the direct use of energy, force, or a destructive agent		

Body Part (Character 4)	Approach (Character 5)	Device (Character 6)	Qualifier (Character 7)
0 Azygos Vein	0 Open	Z No Device	Z No Qualifier
1 Hemiazygos Vein	3 Percutaneous		
3 Innominate Vein, Right	4 Percutaneous Endoscopic		
4 Innominate Vein, Left			
5 Subclavian Vein, Right			
6 Subclavian Vein, Left			
7 Axillary Vein, Right			
8 Axillary Vein, Left			
9 Brachial Vein, Right			
A Brachial Vein, Left			
B Basilic Vein, Right			
C Basilic Vein, Left			
D Cephalic Vein, Right			
F Cephalic Vein, Left			
G Hand Vein, Right			
H Hand Vein, Left			
L Intracranial Vein			Continued on Next Page ▶

M Internal Jugular Vein, Right			**Continued from** ◀ **Previous Page**
N Internal Jugular Vein, Left			
P External Jugular Vein, Right			
Q External Jugular Vein, Left			
R Vertebral Vein, Right			
S Vertebral Vein, Left			
T Face Vein, Right			
V Face Vein, Left			
Y Upper Vein			

Section	0	Medical and Surgical		
Body System	**5**	**Upper Veins**		
Operation	**7**	**Dilation: Expanding an orifice or the lumen of a tubular body part**		

Body Part (Character 4)	Approach (Character 5)	Device (Character 6)	Qualifier (Character 7)
0 Azygos Vein	**0** Open	**D** Intraluminal Device	**Z** No Qualifier
1 Hemiazygos Vein	**3** Percutaneous	**Z** No Device	
3 Innominate Vein, Right	**4** Percutaneous Endoscopic		
4 Innominate Vein, Left			
5 Subclavian Vein, Right			
6 Subclavian Vein, Left			
7 Axillary Vein, Right			
8 Axillary Vein, Left			
9 Brachial Vein, Right			
A Brachial Vein, Left			
B Basilic Vein, Right			
C Basilic Vein, Left			
D Cephalic Vein, Right			
F Cephalic Vein, Left			
G Hand Vein, Right			
H Hand Vein, Left			
L Intracranial Vein			
M Internal Jugular Vein, Right			
N Internal Jugular Vein, Left			
P External Jugular Vein, Right			
Q External Jugular Vein, Left			
R Vertebral Vein, Right			
S Vertebral Vein, Left			
T Face Vein, Right			
V Face Vein, Left			
Y Upper Vein			

Section	0	Medical and Surgical		
Body System	5	Upper Veins		
Operation	9	Drainage: Taking or letting out fluids and/or gases from a body part		

Body Part (Character 4)	Approach (Character 5)	Device (Character 6)	Qualifier (Character 7)
0 Azygos Vein 1 Hemiazygos Vein 3 Innominate Vein, Right 4 Innominate Vein, Left 5 Subclavian Vein, Right 6 Subclavian Vein, Left 7 Axillary Vein, Right 8 Axillary Vein, Left 9 Brachial Vein, Right A Brachial Vein, Left B Basilic Vein, Right C Basilic Vein, Left D Cephalic Vein, Right F Cephalic Vein, Left G Hand Vein, Right H Hand Vein, Left L Intracranial Vein M Internal Jugular Vein, Right N Internal Jugular Vein, Left P External Jugular Vein, Right Q External Jugular Vein, Left R Vertebral Vein, Right S Vertebral Vein, Left T Face Vein, Right V Face Vein, Left Y Upper Vein	0 Open 3 Percutaneous 4 Percutaneous Endoscopic	0 Drainage Device	Z No Qualifier
0 Azygos Vein 1 Hemiazygos Vein 3 Innominate Vein, Right 4 Innominate Vein, Left 5 Subclavian Vein, Right 6 Subclavian Vein, Left 7 Axillary Vein, Right 8 Axillary Vein, Left 9 Brachial Vein, Right A Brachial Vein, Left B Basilic Vein, Right C Basilic Vein, Left D Cephalic Vein, Right F Cephalic Vein, Left G Hand Vein, Right H Hand Vein, Left L Intracranial Vein M Internal Jugular Vein, Right N Internal Jugular Vein, Left P External Jugular Vein, Right	0 Open 3 Percutaneous 4 Percutaneous Endoscopic	Z No Device	X Diagnostic Z No Qualifier

Continued on Next Page ▶

			Continued from ◀ Previous Page
Q External Jugular Vein, Left R Vertebral Vein, Right S Vertebral Vein, Left T Face Vein, Right V Face Vein, Left Y Upper Vein			

Section	0	Medical and Surgical
Body System	5	Upper Veins
Operation	B	Excision: Cutting out or off, without replacement, a portion of a body part

Body Part (Character 4)	Approach (Character 5)	Device (Character 6)	Qualifier (Character 7)
0 Azygos Vein 1 Hemiazygos Vein 3 Innominate Vein, Right 4 Innominate Vein, Left 5 Subclavian Vein, Right 6 Subclavian Vein, Left 7 Axillary Vein, Right 8 Axillary Vein, Left 9 Brachial Vein, Right A Brachial Vein, Left B Basilic Vein, Right C Basilic Vein, Left D Cephalic Vein, Right F Cephalic Vein, Left G Hand Vein, Right H Hand Vein, Left L Intracranial Vein M Internal Jugular Vein, Right N Internal Jugular Vein, Left P External Jugular Vein, Right Q External Jugular Vein, Left R Vertebral Vein, Right S Vertebral Vein, Left T Face Vein, Right V Face Vein, Left Y Upper Vein	0 Open 3 Percutaneous 4 Percutaneous Endoscopic	Z No Device	X Diagnostic Z No Qualifier

Section	0	Medical and Surgical		
Body System	5	Upper Veins		
Operation	C	Extirpation: Taking or cutting out solid matter from a body part		

Body Part (Character 4)	Approach (Character 5)	Device (Character 6)	Qualifier (Character 7)
0 Azygos Vein	0 Open	Z No Device	Z No Qualifier
1 Hemiazygos Vein	3 Percutaneous		
3 Innominate Vein, Right	4 Percutaneous Endoscopic		
4 Innominate Vein, Left			
5 Subclavian Vein, Right			
6 Subclavian Vein, Left			
7 Axillary Vein, Right			
8 Axillary Vein, Left			
9 Brachial Vein, Right			
A Brachial Vein, Left			
B Basilic Vein, Right			
C Basilic Vein, Left			
D Cephalic Vein, Right			
F Cephalic Vein, Left			
G Hand Vein, Right			
H Hand Vein, Left			
L Intracranial Vein			
M Internal Jugular Vein, Right			
N Internal Jugular Vein, Left			
P External Jugular Vein, Right			
Q External Jugular Vein, Left			
R Vertebral Vein, Right			
S Vertebral Vein, Left			
T Face Vein, Right			
V Face Vein, Left			
Y Upper Vein			

Section	0	Medical and Surgical		
Body System	5	Upper Veins		
Operation	D	Extraction: Pulling or stripping out or off all or a portion of a body part by the use of force		

Body Part (Character 4)	Approach (Character 5)	Device (Character 6)	Qualifier (Character 7)
9 Brachial Vein, Right	0 Open	Z No Device	Z No Qualifier
A Brachial Vein, Left	3 Percutaneous		
B Basilic Vein, Right			
C Basilic Vein, Left			
D Cephalic Vein, Right			
F Cephalic Vein, Left			
G Hand Vein, Right			
H Hand Vein, Left			
Y Upper Vein			

Section	0	Medical and Surgical
Body System	5	Upper Veins
Operation	H	Insertion: Putting in a nonbiological appliance that monitors, assists, performs, or prevents a physiological function but does not physically take the place of a body part

Body Part (Character 4)	Approach (Character 5)	Device (Character 6)	Qualifier (Character 7)
0 Azygos Vein	**0** Open **3** Percutaneous **4** Percutaneous Endoscopic	**2** Monitoring Device **3** Infusion Device **D** Intraluminal Device **M** Neurostimulator Lead	**Z** No Qualifier
1 Hemiazygos Vein **3** Innominate Vein, Right **4** Innominate Vein, Left **5** Subclavian Vein, Right **6** Subclavian Vein, Left **7** Axillary Vein, Right **8** Axillary Vein, Left **9** Brachial Vein, Right **A** Brachial Vein, Left **B** Basilic Vein, Right **C** Basilic Vein, Left **D** Cephalic Vein, Right **F** Cephalic Vein, Left **G** Hand Vein, Right **H** Hand Vein, Left **L** Intracranial Vein **M** Internal Jugular Vein, Right **N** Internal Jugular Vein, Left **P** External Jugular Vein, Right **Q** External Jugular Vein, Left **R** Vertebral Vein, Right **S** Vertebral Vein, Left **T** Face Vein, Right **V** Face Vein, Left	**0** Open **3** Percutaneous **4** Percutaneous Endoscopic	**3** Infusion Device **D** Intraluminal Device	**Z** No Qualifier
3 Innominate Vein, Right **4** Innominate Vein, Left	**0** Open **3** Percutaneous **4** Percutaneous Endoscopic	**3** Infusion Device **D** Intraluminal Device **M** Neurostimulator Lead	**Z** No Qualifier
Y Upper Vein	**0** Open **3** Percutaneous **4** Percutaneous Endoscopic	**2** Monitoring Device **3** Infusion Device **D** Intraluminal Device	**Z** No Qualifier

Section	0	Medical and Surgical
Body System	5	Upper Veins
Operation	J	Inspection: Visually and/or manually exploring a body part

Body Part (Character 4)	Approach (Character 5)	Device (Character 6)	Qualifier (Character 7)
Y Upper Vein	**0** Open **3** Percutaneous **4** Percutaneous Endoscopic **X** External	**Z** No Device	**Z** No Qualifier

Section	0	Medical and Surgical
Body System	5	Upper Veins
Operation	L	Occlusion: Completely closing an orifice or the lumen of a tubular body part

Body Part (Character 4)	Approach (Character 5)	Device (Character 6)	Qualifier (Character 7)
0 Azygos Vein	0 Open	C Extraluminal Device	Z No Qualifier
1 Hemiazygos Vein	3 Percutaneous	D Intraluminal Device	
3 Innominate Vein, Right	4 Percutaneous Endoscopic	Z No Device	
4 Innominate Vein, Left			
5 Subclavian Vein, Right			
6 Subclavian Vein, Left			
7 Axillary Vein, Right			
8 Axillary Vein, Left			
9 Brachial Vein, Right			
A Brachial Vein, Left			
B Basilic Vein, Right			
C Basilic Vein, Left			
D Cephalic Vein, Right			
F Cephalic Vein, Left			
G Hand Vein, Right			
H Hand Vein, Left			
L Intracranial Vein			
M Internal Jugular Vein, Right			
N Internal Jugular Vein, Left			
P External Jugular Vein, Right			
Q External Jugular Vein, Left			
R Vertebral Vein, Right			
S Vertebral Vein, Left			
T Face Vein, Right			
V Face Vein, Left			
Y Upper Vein			

Section	0	Medical and Surgical
Body System	5	Upper Veins
Operation	N	Release: Freeing a body part from an abnormal physical constraint by cutting or by the use of force

Body Part (Character 4)	Approach (Character 5)	Device (Character 6)	Qualifier (Character 7)
0 Azygos Vein	0 Open	Z No Device	Z No Qualifier
1 Hemiazygos Vein	3 Percutaneous		
3 Innominate Vein, Right	4 Percutaneous Endoscopic		
4 Innominate Vein, Left			
5 Subclavian Vein, Right			
6 Subclavian Vein, Left			
7 Axillary Vein, Right			
8 Axillary Vein, Left			
9 Brachial Vein, Right			
A Brachial Vein, Left			
B Basilic Vein, Right			
C Basilic Vein, Left			
D Cephalic Vein, Right			
F Cephalic Vein, Left			
G Hand Vein, Right			
H Hand Vein, Left			

Continued on Next Page ▶

L Intracranial Vein **M** Internal Jugular Vein, Right **N** Internal Jugular Vein, Left **P** External Jugular Vein, Right **Q** External Jugular Vein, Left **R** Vertebral Vein, Right **S** Vertebral Vein, Left **T** Face Vein, Right **V** Face Vein, Left **Y** Upper Vein			**Continued from** ◄ **Previous Page**

Section	0	Medical and Surgical
Body System	5	Upper Veins
Operation	P	Removal: Taking out or off a device from a body part

Body Part (Character 4)	Approach (Character 5)	Device (Character 6)	Qualifier (Character 7)
0 Azygos Vein	**0** Open **3** Percutaneous **4** Percutaneous Endoscopic **X** External	**2** Monitoring Device **M** Neurostimulator Lead	**Z** No Qualifier
3 Innominate Vein, Right **4** Innominate Vein, Left	**0** Open **3** Percutaneous **4** Percutaneous Endoscopic **X** External	**M** Neurostimulator Lead	**Z** No Qualifier
Y Upper Vein	**0** Open **3** Percutaneous **4** Percutaneous Endoscopic	**0** Drainage Device **2** Monitoring Device **3** Infusion Device **7** Autologous Tissue Substitute **C** Extraluminal Device **D** Intraluminal Device **J** Synthetic Substitute **K** Nonautologous Tissue Substitute	**Z** No Qualifier
Y Upper Vein	**X** External	**0** Drainage Device **2** Monitoring Device **3** Infusion Device **D** Intraluminal Device	**Z** No Qualifier

Section	0	Medical and Surgical
Body System	5	Upper Veins
Operation	Q	Repair: Restoring, to the extent possible, a body part to its normal anatomic structure and function

Body Part (Character 4)	Approach (Character 5)	Device (Character 6)	Qualifier (Character 7)
0 Azygos Vein **1** Hemiazygos Vein **3** Innominate Vein, Right **4** Innominate Vein, Left **5** Subclavian Vein, Right **6** Subclavian Vein, Left **7** Axillary Vein, Right **8** Axillary Vein, Left **9** Brachial Vein, Right	**0** Open **3** Percutaneous **4** Percutaneous Endoscopic	**Z** No Device	**Z** No Qualifier **Continued on** **Next Page ▶**

			Continued from ◄ Previous Page
A Brachial Vein, Left			
B Basilic Vein, Right			
C Basilic Vein, Left			
D Cephalic Vein, Right			
F Cephalic Vein, Left			
G Hand Vein, Right			
H Hand Vein, Left			
L Intracranial Vein			
M Internal Jugular Vein, Right			
N Internal Jugular Vein, Left			
P External Jugular Vein, Right			
Q External Jugular Vein, Left			
R Vertebral Vein, Right			
S Vertebral Vein, Left			
T Face Vein, Right			
V Face Vein, Left			
Y Upper Vein			

Section	0	Medical and Surgical
Body System	5	Upper Veins
Operation	R	Replacement: Putting in or on biological or synthetic material that physically takes the place and/or function of all or a portion of a body part

Body Part (Character 4)	Approach (Character 5)	Device (Character 6)	Qualifier (Character 7)
0 Azygos Vein	**0** Open	**7** Autologous Tissue Substitute	**Z** No Qualifier
1 Hemiazygos Vein	**4** Percutaneous Endoscopic	**J** Synthetic Substitute	
3 Innominate Vein, Right		**K** Nonautologous Tissue Substitute	
4 Innominate Vein, Left			
5 Subclavian Vein, Right			
6 Subclavian Vein, Left			
7 Axillary Vein, Right			
8 Axillary Vein, Left			
9 Brachial Vein, Right			
A Brachial Vein, Left			
B Basilic Vein, Right			
C Basilic Vein, Left			
D Cephalic Vein, Right			
F Cephalic Vein, Left			
G Hand Vein, Right			
H Hand Vein, Left			
L Intracranial Vein			
M Internal Jugular Vein, Right			
N Internal Jugular Vein, Left			
P External Jugular Vein, Right			
Q External Jugular Vein, Left			
R Vertebral Vein, Right			
S Vertebral Vein, Left			
T Face Vein, Right			
V Face Vein, Left			
Y Upper Vein			

Section	0	Medical and Surgical
Body System	5	Upper Veins
Operation	S	Reposition: Moving to its normal location, or other suitable location, all or a portion of a body part

Body Part (Character 4)	Approach (Character 5)	Device (Character 6)	Qualifier (Character 7)
0 Azygos Vein	**0** Open	**Z** No Device	**Z** No Qualifier
1 Hemiazygos Vein	**3** Percutaneous		
3 Innominate Vein, Right	**4** Percutaneous Endoscopic		
4 Innominate Vein, Left			
5 Subclavian Vein, Right			
6 Subclavian Vein, Left			
7 Axillary Vein, Right			
8 Axillary Vein, Left			
9 Brachial Vein, Right			
A Brachial Vein, Left			
B Basilic Vein, Right			
C Basilic Vein, Left			
D Cephalic Vein, Right			
F Cephalic Vein, Left			
G Hand Vein, Right			
H Hand Vein, Left			
L Intracranial Vein			
M Internal Jugular Vein, Right			
N Internal Jugular Vein, Left			
P External Jugular Vein, Right			
Q External Jugular Vein, Left			
R Vertebral Vein, Right			
S Vertebral Vein, Left			
T Face Vein, Right			
V Face Vein, Left			
Y Upper Vein			

Section	0	Medical and Surgical
Body System	5	Upper Veins
Operation	U	Supplement: Putting in or on biological or synthetic material that physically reinforces and/or augments the function of a portion of a body part

Body Part (Character 4)	Approach (Character 5)	Device (Character 6)	Qualifier (Character 7)
0 Azygos Vein	**0** Open	**7** Autologous Tissue Substitute	**Z** No Qualifier
1 Hemiazygos Vein	**3** Percutaneous	**J** Synthetic Substitute	
3 Innominate Vein, Right	**4** Percutaneous Endoscopic	**K** Nonautologous Tissue Substitute	
4 Innominate Vein, Left			
5 Subclavian Vein, Right			
6 Subclavian Vein, Left			
7 Axillary Vein, Right			
8 Axillary Vein, Left			
9 Brachial Vein, Right			
A Brachial Vein, Left			
B Basilic Vein, Right			
C Basilic Vein, Left			
D Cephalic Vein, Right			
F Cephalic Vein, Left			
G Hand Vein, Right			

Continued on Next Page ▶

			Continued from ◀ Previous Page
H Hand Vein, Left			
L Intracranial Vein			
M Internal Jugular Vein, Right			
N Internal Jugular Vein, Left			
P External Jugular Vein, Right			
Q External Jugular Vein, Left			
R Vertebral Vein, Right			
S Vertebral Vein, Left			
T Face Vein, Right			
V Face Vein, Left			
Y Upper Vein			

Section	0	Medical and Surgical
Body System	5	Upper Veins
Operation	V	Restriction: Partially closing an orifice or the lumen of a tubular body part

Body Part (Character 4)	Approach (Character 5)	Device (Character 6)	Qualifier (Character 7)
0 Azygos Vein	**0** Open	**C** Extraluminal Device	**Z** No Qualifier
1 Hemiazygos Vein	**3** Percutaneous	**D** Intraluminal Device	
3 Innominate Vein, Right	**4** Percutaneous Endoscopic	**Z** No Device	
4 Innominate Vein, Left			
5 Subclavian Vein, Right			
6 Subclavian Vein, Left			
7 Axillary Vein, Right			
8 Axillary Vein, Left			
9 Brachial Vein, Right			
A Brachial Vein, Left			
B Basilic Vein, Right			
C Basilic Vein, Left			
D Cephalic Vein, Right			
F Cephalic Vein, Left			
G Hand Vein, Right			
H Hand Vein, Left			
L Intracranial Vein			
M Internal Jugular Vein, Right			
N Internal Jugular Vein, Left			
P External Jugular Vein, Right			
Q External Jugular Vein, Left			
R Vertebral Vein, Right			
S Vertebral Vein, Left			
T Face Vein, Right			
V Face Vein, Left			
Y Upper Vein			

Section	0	Medical and Surgical		
Body System	5	Upper Veins		
Operation	W	Revision: Correcting, to the extent possible, a portion of a malfunctioning device or the position of a displaced device		

Body Part (Character 4)	Approach (Character 5)	Device (Character 6)	Qualifier (Character 7)
0 Azygos Vein	**0** Open **3** Percutaneous **4** Percutaneous Endoscopic **X** External	**2** Monitoring Device **M** Neurostimulator Lead	**Z** No Qualifier
3 Innominate Vein, Right **4** Innominate Vein, Left	**0** Open **3** Percutaneous **4** Percutaneous Endoscopic **X** External	**M** Neurostimulator Lead	**Z** No Qualifier
Y Upper Vein	**0** Open **3** Percutaneous **4** Percutaneous Endoscopic **X** External	**0** Drainage Device **2** Monitoring Device **3** Infusion Device **7** Autologous Tissue Substitute **C** Extraluminal Device **D** Intraluminal Device **J** Synthetic Substitute **K** Nonautologous Tissue Substitute	**Z** No Qualifier

Section	0	Medical and Surgical	
Body System	6	Lower Veins	
Operation	1	Bypass: Altering the route of passage of the contents of a tubular body part	

Body Part (Character 4)	Approach (Character 5)	Device (Character 6)	Qualifier (Character 7)
0 Inferior Vena Cava	0 Open 4 Percutaneous Endoscopic	7 Autologous Tissue Substitute 9 Autologous Venous Tissue A Autologous Arterial Tissue J Synthetic Substitute K Nonautologous Tissue Substitute Z No Device	5 Superior Mesenteric Vein 6 Inferior Mesenteric Vein Y Lower Vein
1 Splenic Vein	0 Open 4 Percutaneous Endoscopic	7 Autologous Tissue Substitute 9 Autologous Venous Tissue A Autologous Arterial Tissue J Synthetic Substitute K Nonautologous Tissue Substitute Z No Device	9 Renal Vein, Right B Renal Vein, Left Y Lower Vein
2 Gastric Vein 3 Esophageal Vein 4 Hepatic Vein 5 Superior Mesenteric Vein 6 Inferior Mesenteric Vein 7 Colic Vein 9 Renal Vein, Right B Renal Vein, Left C Common Iliac Vein, Right D Common Iliac Vein, Left F External Iliac Vein, Right G External Iliac Vein, Left H Hypogastric Vein, Right J Hypogastric Vein, Left M Femoral Vein, Right N Femoral Vein, Left P Greater Saphenous Vein, Right Q Greater Saphenous Vein, Left R Lesser Saphenous Vein, Right S Lesser Saphenous Vein, Left T Foot Vein, Right V Foot Vein, Left	0 Open 4 Percutaneous Endoscopic	7 Autologous Tissue Substitute 9 Autologous Venous Tissue A Autologous Arterial Tissue J Synthetic Substitute K Nonautologous Tissue Substitute Z No Device	Y Lower Vein
8 Portal Vein	0 Open	7 Autologous Tissue Substitute 9 Autologous Venous Tissue A Autologous Arterial Tissue J Synthetic Substitute K Nonautologous Tissue Substitute Z No Device	9 Renal Vein, Right B Renal Vein, Left Y Lower Vein

Continued on Next Page ▶

			Continued from ◀ Previous Page
8 Portal Vein	3 Percutaneous	D Intraluminal Device	Y Lower Vein
8 Portal Vein	4 Percutaneous Endoscopic	7 Autologous Tissue Substitute 9 Autologous Venous Tissue A Autologous Arterial Tissue J Synthetic Substitute K Nonautologous Tissue Substitute Z No Device	9 Renal Vein, Right B Renal Vein, Left Y Lower Vein
8 Portal Vein	4 Percutaneous Endoscopic	D Intraluminal Device	Y Lower Vein

Section	0	Medical and Surgical
Body System	6	Lower Veins
Operation	5	Destruction: Physical eradication of all or a portion of a body part by the direct use of energy, force, or a destructive agent

Body Part (Character 4)	Approach (Character 5)	Device (Character 6)	Qualifier (Character 7)
0 Inferior Vena Cava 1 Splenic Vein 2 Gastric Vein 3 Esophageal Vein 4 Hepatic Vein 5 Superior Mesenteric Vein 6 Inferior Mesenteric Vein 7 Colic Vein 8 Portal Vein 9 Renal Vein, Right B Renal Vein, Left C Common Iliac Vein, Right D Common Iliac Vein, Left F External Iliac Vein, Right G External Iliac Vein, Left H Hypogastric Vein, Right J Hypogastric Vein, Left M Femoral Vein, Right N Femoral Vein, Left P Greater Saphenous Vein, Right Q Greater Saphenous Vein, Left R Lesser Saphenous Vein, Right S Lesser Saphenous Vein, Left T Foot Vein, Right V Foot Vein, Left	0 Open 3 Percutaneous 4 Percutaneous Endoscopic	Z No Device	Z No Qualifier
Y Lower Vein	0 Open 3 Percutaneous 4 Percutaneous Endoscopic	Z No Device	C Hemorrhoidal Plexus Z No Qualifier

Section	0	Medical and Surgical		
Body System	6	Lower Veins		
Operation	7	Dilation: Expanding an orifice or the lumen of a tubular body part		

Body Part (Character 4)	Approach (Character 5)	Device (Character 6)	Qualifier (Character 7)
0 Inferior Vena Cava	0 Open	D Intraluminal Device	Z No Qualifier
1 Splenic Vein	3 Percutaneous	Z No Device	
2 Gastric Vein	4 Percutaneous Endoscopic		
3 Esophageal Vein			
4 Hepatic Vein			
5 Superior Mesenteric Vein			
6 Inferior Mesenteric Vein			
7 Colic Vein			
8 Portal Vein			
9 Renal Vein, Right			
B Renal Vein, Left			
C Common Iliac Vein, Right			
D Common Iliac Vein, Left			
F External Iliac Vein, Right			
G External Iliac Vein, Left			
H Hypogastric Vein, Right			
J Hypogastric Vein, Left			
M Femoral Vein, Right			
N Femoral Vein, Left			
P Greater Saphenous Vein, Right			
Q Greater Saphenous Vein, Left			
R Lesser Saphenous Vein, Right			
S Lesser Saphenous Vein, Left			
T Foot Vein, Right			
V Foot Vein, Left			
Y Lower Vein			

Section	0	Medical and Surgical		
Body System	6	Lower Veins		
Operation	9	Drainage: Taking or letting out fluids and/or gases from a body part		

Body Part (Character 4)	Approach (Character 5)	Device (Character 6)	Qualifier (Character 7)
0 Inferior Vena Cava	0 Open	0 Drainage Device	Z No Qualifier
1 Splenic Vein	3 Percutaneous		
2 Gastric Vein	4 Percutaneous Endoscopic		
3 Esophageal Vein			
4 Hepatic Vein			
5 Superior Mesenteric Vein			
6 Inferior Mesenteric Vein			
7 Colic Vein			
8 Portal Vein			
9 Renal Vein, Right			
B Renal Vein, Left			
C Common Iliac Vein, Right			
D Common Iliac Vein, Left			
F External Iliac Vein, Right			
G External Iliac Vein, Left			Continued on Next Page ▶

			Continued from ◀ Previous Page
H Hypogastric Vein, Right **J** Hypogastric Vein, Left **M** Femoral Vein, Right **N** Femoral Vein, Left **P** Greater Saphenous Vein, Right **Q** Greater Saphenous Vein, Left **R** Lesser Saphenous Vein, Right **S** Lesser Saphenous Vein, Left **T** Foot Vein, Right **V** Foot Vein, Left **Y** Lower Vein			
0 Inferior Vena Cava **1** Splenic Vein **2** Gastric Vein **3** Esophageal Vein **4** Hepatic Vein **5** Superior Mesenteric Vein **6** Inferior Mesenteric Vein **7** Colic Vein **8** Portal Vein **9** Renal Vein, Right **B** Renal Vein, Left **C** Common Iliac Vein, Right **D** Common Iliac Vein, Left **F** External Iliac Vein, Right **G** External Iliac Vein, Left **H** Hypogastric Vein, Right **J** Hypogastric Vein, Left **M** Femoral Vein, Right **N** Femoral Vein, Left **P** Greater Saphenous Vein, Right **Q** Greater Saphenous Vein, Left **R** Lesser Saphenous Vein, Right **S** Lesser Saphenous Vein, Left **T** Foot Vein, Right **V** Foot Vein, Left **Y** Lower Vein	**0** Open **3** Percutaneous **4** Percutaneous Endoscopic	**Z** No Device	**X** Diagnostic **Z** No Qualifier

Section	0	Medical and Surgical		
Body System	6	Lower Veins		
Operation	B	Excision: Cutting out or off, without replacement, a portion of a body part		

Body Part (Character 4)	Approach (Character 5)	Device (Character 6)	Qualifier (Character 7)
0 Inferior Vena Cava	0 Open	Z No Device	X Diagnostic
1 Splenic Vein	3 Percutaneous		Z No Qualifier
2 Gastric Vein	4 Percutaneous Endoscopic		
3 Esophageal Vein			
4 Hepatic Vein			
5 Superior Mesenteric Vein			
6 Inferior Mesenteric Vein			
7 Colic Vein			
8 Portal Vein			
9 Renal Vein, Right			
B Renal Vein, Left			
C Common Iliac Vein, Right			
D Common Iliac Vein, Left			
F External Iliac Vein, Right			
G External Iliac Vein, Left			
H Hypogastric Vein, Right			
J Hypogastric Vein, Left			
M Femoral Vein, Right			
N Femoral Vein, Left			
P Greater Saphenous Vein, Right			
Q Greater Saphenous Vein, Left			
R Lesser Saphenous Vein, Right			
S Lesser Saphenous Vein, Left			
T Foot Vein, Right			
V Foot Vein, Left			
Y Lower Vein	0 Open	Z No Device	C Hemorrhoidal Plexus
	3 Percutaneous		X Diagnostic
	4 Percutaneous Endoscopic		Z No Qualifier

Section	0	Medical and Surgical		
Body System	6	Lower Veins		
Operation	C	Extirpation: Taking or cutting out solid matter from a body part		

Body Part (Character 4)	Approach (Character 5)	Device (Character 6)	Qualifier (Character 7)
0 Inferior Vena Cava	0 Open	Z No Device	Z No Qualifier
1 Splenic Vein	3 Percutaneous		
2 Gastric Vein	4 Percutaneous Endoscopic		
3 Esophageal Vein			
4 Hepatic Vein			
5 Superior Mesenteric Vein			
6 Inferior Mesenteric Vein			
7 Colic Vein			
8 Portal Vein			
9 Renal Vein, Right			
B Renal Vein, Left			
C Common Iliac Vein, Right			
D Common Iliac Vein, Left			

Continued on Next Page ▶

			Continued from ◀ Previous Page
F External Iliac Vein, Right **G** External Iliac Vein, Left **H** Hypogastric Vein, Right **J** Hypogastric Vein, Left **M** Femoral Vein, Right **N** Femoral Vein, Left **P** Greater Saphenous Vein, Right **Q** Greater Saphenous Vein, Left **R** Lesser Saphenous Vein, Right **S** Lesser Saphenous Vein, Left **T** Foot Vein, Right **V** Foot Vein, Left **Y** Lower Vein			

Section	0	Medical and Surgical
Body System	6	Lower Veins
Operation	D	Extraction: Pulling or stripping out or off all or a portion of a body part by the use of force

Body Part (Character 4)	Approach (Character 5)	Device (Character 6)	Qualifier (Character 7)
M Femoral Vein, Right **N** Femoral Vein, Left **P** Greater Saphenous Vein, Right **Q** Greater Saphenous Vein, Left **R** Lesser Saphenous Vein, Right **S** Lesser Saphenous Vein, Left **T** Foot Vein, Right **V** Foot Vein, Left **Y** Lower Vein	**0** Open **3** Percutaneous **4** Percutaneous Endoscopic	**Z** No Device	**Z** No Qualifier

Section	0	Medical and Surgical
Body System	6	Lower Veins
Operation	H	Insertion: Putting in a nonbiological appliance that monitors, assists, performs, or prevents a physiological function but does not physically take the place of a body part

Body Part (Character 4)	Approach (Character 5)	Device (Character 6)	Qualifier (Character 7)
0 Inferior Vena Cava	**0** Open **3** Percutaneous	**3** Infusion Device	**T** Via Umbilical Vein **Z** No Qualifier
0 Inferior Vena Cava	**0** Open **3** Percutaneous	**D** Intraluminal Device	**Z** No Qualifier
0 Inferior Vena Cava	**4** Percutaneous Endoscopic	**3** Infusion Device **D** Intraluminal Device	**Z** No Qualifier
1 Splenic Vein **2** Gastric Vein **3** Esophageal Vein **4** Hepatic Vein **5** Superior Mesenteric Vein **6** Inferior Mesenteric Vein **7** Colic Vein **8** Portal Vein	**0** Open **3** Percutaneous **4** Percutaneous Endoscopic	**3** Infusion Device **D** Intraluminal Device	**Z** No Qualifier

Continued on Next Page ▶

			Continued from ◀ Previous Page
9 Renal Vein, Right			
B Renal Vein, Left			
C Common Iliac Vein, Right			
D Common Iliac Vein, Left			
F External Iliac Vein, Right			
G External Iliac Vein, Left			
H Hypogastric Vein, Right			
J Hypogastric Vein, Left			
M Femoral Vein, Right			
N Femoral Vein, Left			
P Greater Saphenous Vein, Right			
Q Greater Saphenous Vein, Left			
R Lesser Saphenous Vein, Right			
S Lesser Saphenous Vein, Left			
T Foot Vein, Right			
V Foot Vein, Left			
Y Lower Vein	0 Open 3 Percutaneous 4 Percutaneous Endoscopic	2 Monitoring Device 3 Infusion Device D Intraluminal Device	Z No Qualifier

Section	0	Medical and Surgical	
Body System	6	Lower Veins	
Operation	J	Inspection: Visually and/or manually exploring a body part	
Body Part (Character 4)	**Approach (Character 5)**	**Device (Character 6)**	**Qualifier (Character 7)**
Y Lower Vein	0 Open 3 Percutaneous 4 Percutaneous Endoscopic X External	Z No Device	Z No Qualifier

Section	0	Medical and Surgical	
Body System	6	Lower Veins	
Operation	L	Occlusion: Completely closing an orifice or the lumen of a tubular body part	
Body Part (Character 4)	**Approach (Character 5)**	**Device (Character 6)**	**Qualifier (Character 7)**
0 Inferior Vena Cava 1 Splenic Vein 2 Gastric Vein 3 Esophageal Vein 4 Hepatic Vein 5 Superior Mesenteric Vein 6 Inferior Mesenteric Vein 7 Colic Vein 8 Portal Vein 9 Renal Vein, Right B Renal Vein, Left C Common Iliac Vein, Right D Common Iliac Vein, Left F External Iliac Vein, Right G External Iliac Vein, Left H Hypogastric Vein, Right J Hypogastric Vein, Left	0 Open 3 Percutaneous 4 Percutaneous Endoscopic	C Extraluminal Device D Intraluminal Device Z No Device	Z No Qualifier

Continued on Next Page ▶

			Continued from ◀ Previous Page
M Femoral Vein, Right **N** Femoral Vein, Left **P** Greater Saphenous Vein, Right **Q** Greater Saphenous Vein, Left **R** Lesser Saphenous Vein, Right **S** Lesser Saphenous Vein, Left **T** Foot Vein, Right **V** Foot Vein, Left			
Y Lower Vein	**0** Open **3** Percutaneous **4** Percutaneous Endoscopic	**C** Extraluminal Device **D** Intraluminal Device **Z** No Device	**C** Hemorrhoidal Plexus **Z** No Qualifier

Section	0	Medical and Surgical
Body System	6	Lower Veins
Operation	N	Release: Freeing a body part from an abnormal physical constraint by cutting or by the use of force

Body Part (Character 4)	Approach (Character 5)	Device (Character 6)	Qualifier (Character 7)
0 Inferior Vena Cava **1** Splenic Vein **2** Gastric Vein **3** Esophageal Vein **4** Hepatic Vein **5** Superior Mesenteric Vein **6** Inferior Mesenteric Vein **7** Colic Vein **8** Portal Vein **9** Renal Vein, Right **B** Renal Vein, Left **C** Common Iliac Vein, Right **D** Common Iliac Vein, Left **F** External Iliac Vein, Right **G** External Iliac Vein, Left **H** Hypogastric Vein, Right **J** Hypogastric Vein, Left **M** Femoral Vein, Right **N** Femoral Vein, Left **P** Greater Saphenous Vein, Right **Q** Greater Saphenous Vein, Left **R** Lesser Saphenous Vein, Right **S** Lesser Saphenous Vein, Left **T** Foot Vein, Right **V** Foot Vein, Left **Y** Lower Vein	**0** Open **3** Percutaneous **4** Percutaneous Endoscopic	**Z** No Device	**Z** No Qualifier

Section	0	Medical and Surgical		
Body System	6	Lower Veins		
Operation	P	Removal: Taking out or off a device from a body part		

Body Part (Character 4)	Approach (Character 5)	Device (Character 6)	Qualifier (Character 7)
Y Lower Vein	0 Open 3 Percutaneous 4 Percutaneous Endoscopic	0 Drainage Device 2 Monitoring Device 3 Infusion Device 7 Autologous Tissue Substitute C Extraluminal Device D Intraluminal Device J Synthetic Substitute K Nonautologous Tissue Substitute	Z No Qualifier
Y Lower Vein	X External	0 Drainage Device 2 Monitoring Device 3 Infusion Device D Intraluminal Device	Z No Qualifier

Section	0	Medical and Surgical		
Body System	6	Lower Veins		
Operation	Q	Repair: Restoring, to the extent possible, a body part to its normal anatomic structure and function		

Body Part (Character 4)	Approach (Character 5)	Device (Character 6)	Qualifier (Character 7)
0 Inferior Vena Cava 1 Splenic Vein 2 Gastric Vein 3 Esophageal Vein 4 Hepatic Vein 5 Superior Mesenteric Vein 6 Inferior Mesenteric Vein 7 Colic Vein 8 Portal Vein 9 Renal Vein, Right B Renal Vein, Left C Common Iliac Vein, Right D Common Iliac Vein, Left F External Iliac Vein, Right G External Iliac Vein, Left H Hypogastric Vein, Right J Hypogastric Vein, Left M Femoral Vein, Right N Femoral Vein, Left P Greater Saphenous Vein, Right Q Greater Saphenous Vein, Left R Lesser Saphenous Vein, Right S Lesser Saphenous Vein, Left T Foot Vein, Right V Foot Vein, Left Y Lower Vein	0 Open 3 Percutaneous 4 Percutaneous Endoscopic	Z No Device	Z No Qualifier

Section	0	Medical and Surgical		
Body System	6	Lower Veins		
Operation	R	Replacement: Putting in or on biological or synthetic material that physically takes the place and/or function of all or a portion of a body part		

Body Part (Character 4)	Approach (Character 5)	Device (Character 6)	Qualifier (Character 7)
0 Inferior Vena Cava 1 Splenic Vein 2 Gastric Vein 3 Esophageal Vein 4 Hepatic Vein 5 Superior Mesenteric Vein 6 Inferior Mesenteric Vein 7 Colic Vein 8 Portal Vein 9 Renal Vein, Right B Renal Vein, Left C Common Iliac Vein, Right D Common Iliac Vein, Left F External Iliac Vein, Right G External Iliac Vein, Left H Hypogastric Vein, Right J Hypogastric Vein, Left M Femoral Vein, Right N Femoral Vein, Left P Greater Saphenous Vein, Right Q Greater Saphenous Vein, Left R Lesser Saphenous Vein, Right S Lesser Saphenous Vein, Left T Foot Vein, Right V Foot Vein, Left Y Lower Vein	0 Open 4 Percutaneous Endoscopic	7 Autologous Tissue Substitute J Synthetic Substitute K Nonautologous Tissue Substitute	Z No Qualifier

Section	0	Medical and Surgical		
Body System	6	Lower Veins		
Operation	S	Reposition: Moving to its normal location, or other suitable location, all or a portion of a body part		

Body Part (Character 4)	Approach (Character 5)	Device (Character 6)	Qualifier (Character 7)
0 Inferior Vena Cava 1 Splenic Vein 2 Gastric Vein 3 Esophageal Vein 4 Hepatic Vein 5 Superior Mesenteric Vein 6 Inferior Mesenteric Vein 7 Colic Vein 8 Portal Vein 9 Renal Vein, Right B Renal Vein, Left C Common Iliac Vein, Right D Common Iliac Vein, Left F External Iliac Vein, Right	0 Open 3 Percutaneous 4 Percutaneous Endoscopic	Z No Device	Z No Qualifier

Continued on Next Page ▶

G External Iliac Vein, Left			Continued from ◀ Previous Page
H Hypogastric Vein, Right			
J Hypogastric Vein, Left			
M Femoral Vein, Right			
N Femoral Vein, Left			
P Greater Saphenous Vein, Right			
Q Greater Saphenous Vein, Left			
R Lesser Saphenous Vein, Right			
S Lesser Saphenous Vein, Left			
T Foot Vein, Right			
V Foot Vein, Left			
Y Lower Vein			

Section	0	Medical and Surgical
Body System	6	Lower Veins
Operation	U	Supplement: Putting in or on biological or synthetic material that physically reinforces and/or augments the function of a portion of a body part

Body Part (Character 4)	Approach (Character 5)	Device (Character 6)	Qualifier (Character 7)
0 Inferior Vena Cava	**0** Open	**7** Autologous Tissue Substitute	**Z** No Qualifier
1 Splenic Vein	**3** Percutaneous	**J** Synthetic Substitute	
2 Gastric Vein	**4** Percutaneous Endoscopic	**K** Nonautologous Tissue Substitute	
3 Esophageal Vein			
4 Hepatic Vein			
5 Superior Mesenteric Vein			
6 Inferior Mesenteric Vein			
7 Colic Vein			
8 Portal Vein			
9 Renal Vein, Right			
B Renal Vein, Left			
C Common Iliac Vein, Right			
D Common Iliac Vein, Left			
F External Iliac Vein, Right			
G External Iliac Vein, Left			
H Hypogastric Vein, Right			
J Hypogastric Vein, Left			
M Femoral Vein, Right			
N Femoral Vein, Left			
P Greater Saphenous Vein, Right			
Q Greater Saphenous Vein, Left			
R Lesser Saphenous Vein, Right			
S Lesser Saphenous Vein, Left			
T Foot Vein, Right			
V Foot Vein, Left			
Y Lower Vein			

Section	0	Medical and Surgical		
Body System	6	Lower Veins		
Operation	V	Restriction: Partially closing an orifice or the lumen of a tubular body part		

Body Part (Character 4)	Approach (Character 5)	Device (Character 6)	Qualifier (Character 7)
0 Inferior Vena Cava	0 Open	C Extraluminal Device	Z No Qualifier
1 Splenic Vein	3 Percutaneous	D Intraluminal Device	
2 Gastric Vein	4 Percutaneous Endoscopic	Z No Device	
3 Esophageal Vein			
4 Hepatic Vein			
5 Superior Mesenteric Vein			
6 Inferior Mesenteric Vein			
7 Colic Vein			
8 Portal Vein			
9 Renal Vein, Right			
B Renal Vein, Left			
C Common Iliac Vein, Right			
D Common Iliac Vein, Left			
F External Iliac Vein, Right			
G External Iliac Vein, Left			
H Hypogastric Vein, Right			
J Hypogastric Vein, Left			
M Femoral Vein, Right			
N Femoral Vein, Left			
P Greater Saphenous Vein, Right			
Q Greater Saphenous Vein, Left			
R Lesser Saphenous Vein, Right			
S Lesser Saphenous Vein, Left			
T Foot Vein, Right			
V Foot Vein, Left			
Y Lower Vein			

Section	0	Medical and Surgical		
Body System	6	Lower Veins		
Operation	W	Revision: Correcting, to the extent possible, a portion of a malfunctioning device or the position of a displaced device		

Body Part (Character 4)	Approach (Character 5)	Device (Character 6)	Qualifier (Character 7)
Y Lower Vein	0 Open	0 Drainage Device	Z No Qualifier
	3 Percutaneous	2 Monitoring Device	
	4 Percutaneous Endoscopic	3 Infusion Device	
	X External	7 Autologous Tissue Substitute	
		C Extraluminal Device	
		D Intraluminal Device	
		J Synthetic Substitute	
		K Nonautologous Tissue Substitute	

Section	0	Medical and Surgical
Body System	7	Lymphatic and Hemic Systems
Operation	2	Change: Taking out or off a device from a body part and putting back an identical or similar device in or on the same body part without cutting or puncturing the skin or a mucous membrane

Body Part (Character 4)	Approach (Character 5)	Device (Character 6)	Qualifier (Character 7)
K Thoracic Duct L Cisterna Chyli M Thymus N Lymphatic P Spleen T Bone Marrow	X External	0 Drainage Device Y Other Device	Z No Qualifier

Section	0	Medical and Surgical
Body System	7	Lymphatic and Hemic Systems
Operation	5	Destruction: Physical eradication of all or a portion of a body part by the direct use of energy, force, or a destructive agent

Body Part (Character 4)	Approach (Character 5)	Device (Character 6)	Qualifier (Character 7)
0 Lymphatic, Head 1 Lymphatic, Right Neck 2 Lymphatic, Left Neck 3 Lymphatic, Right Upper Extremity 4 Lymphatic, Left Upper Extremity 5 Lymphatic, Right Axillary 6 Lymphatic, Left Axillary 7 Lymphatic, Thorax 8 Lymphatic, Internal Mammary, Right 9 Lymphatic, Internal Mammary, Left B Lymphatic, Mesenteric C Lymphatic, Pelvis D Lymphatic, Aortic F Lymphatic, Right Lower Extremity G Lymphatic, Left Lower Extremity H Lymphatic, Right Inguinal J Lymphatic, Left Inguinal K Thoracic Duct L Cisterna Chyli M Thymus P Spleen	0 Open 3 Percutaneous 4 Percutaneous Endoscopic	Z No Device	Z No Qualifier

Section	0	Medical and Surgical
Body System	7	Lymphatic and Hemic Systems
Operation	9	Drainage: Taking or letting out fluids and/or gases from a body part

Body Part (Character 4)	Approach (Character 5)	Device (Character 6)	Qualifier (Character 7)
0 Lymphatic, Head 1 Lymphatic, Right Neck 2 Lymphatic, Left Neck 3 Lymphatic, Right Upper Extremity 4 Lymphatic, Left Upper Extremity 5 Lymphatic, Right Axillary 6 Lymphatic, Left Axillary 7 Lymphatic, Thorax 8 Lymphatic, Internal Mammary, Right 9 Lymphatic, Internal Mammary, Left B Lymphatic, Mesenteric C Lymphatic, Pelvis D Lymphatic, Aortic F Lymphatic, Right Lower Extremity G Lymphatic, Left Lower Extremity H Lymphatic, Right Inguinal J Lymphatic, Left Inguinal K Thoracic Duct L Cisterna Chyli M Thymus P Spleen T Bone Marrow	0 Open 3 Percutaneous 4 Percutaneous Endoscopic	0 Drainage Device	Z No Qualifier
0 Lymphatic, Head 1 Lymphatic, Right Neck 2 Lymphatic, Left Neck 3 Lymphatic, Right Upper Extremity 4 Lymphatic, Left Upper Extremity 5 Lymphatic, Right Axillary 6 Lymphatic, Left Axillary 7 Lymphatic, Thorax 8 Lymphatic, Internal Mammary, Right 9 Lymphatic, Internal Mammary, Left B Lymphatic, Mesenteric C Lymphatic, Pelvis D Lymphatic, Aortic F Lymphatic, Right Lower Extremity G Lymphatic, Left Lower Extremity H Lymphatic, Right Inguinal J Lymphatic, Left Inguinal K Thoracic Duct L Cisterna Chyli M Thymus P Spleen T Bone Marrow	0 Open 3 Percutaneous 4 Percutaneous Endoscopic	Z No Device	X Diagnostic Z No Qualifier

Section	0	Medical and Surgical		
Body System	7	Lymphatic and Hemic Systems		
Operation	B	Excision: Cutting out or off, without replacement, a portion of a body part		
Body Part (Character 4)		Approach (Character 5)	Device (Character 6)	Qualifier (Character 7)
0 Lymphatic, Head		0 Open	Z No Device	X Diagnostic
1 Lymphatic, Right Neck		3 Percutaneous		Z No Qualifier
2 Lymphatic, Left Neck		4 Percutaneous Endoscopic		
3 Lymphatic, Right Upper Extremity				
4 Lymphatic, Left Upper Extremity				
5 Lymphatic, Right Axillary				
6 Lymphatic, Left Axillary				
7 Lymphatic, Thorax				
8 Lymphatic, Internal Mammary, Right				
9 Lymphatic, Internal Mammary, Left				
B Lymphatic, Mesenteric				
C Lymphatic, Pelvis				
D Lymphatic, Aortic				
F Lymphatic, Right Lower Extremity				
G Lymphatic, Left Lower Extremity				
H Lymphatic, Right Inguinal				
J Lymphatic, Left Inguinal				
K Thoracic Duct				
L Cisterna Chyli				
M Thymus				
P Spleen				

Section	0	Medical and Surgical		
Body System	7	Lymphatic and Hemic Systems		
Operation	C	Extirpation: Taking or cutting out solid matter from a body part		
Body Part (Character 4)		Approach (Character 5)	Device (Character 6)	Qualifier (Character 7)
0 Lymphatic, Head		0 Open	Z No Device	Z No Qualifier
1 Lymphatic, Right Neck		3 Percutaneous		
2 Lymphatic, Left Neck		4 Percutaneous Endoscopic		
3 Lymphatic, Right Upper Extremity				
4 Lymphatic, Left Upper Extremity				
5 Lymphatic, Right Axillary				
6 Lymphatic, Left Axillary				
7 Lymphatic, Thorax				
8 Lymphatic, Internal Mammary, Right				
9 Lymphatic, Internal Mammary, Left				
B Lymphatic, Mesenteric				
C Lymphatic, Pelvis				
D Lymphatic, Aortic				
F Lymphatic, Right Lower Extremity				
G Lymphatic, Left Lower				

Continued on Next Page ▶

Extremity			Continued from ◀ Previous Page
H Lymphatic, Right Inguinal			
J Lymphatic, Left Inguinal			
K Thoracic Duct			
L Cisterna Chyli			
M Thymus			
P Spleen			

Section	0	Medical and Surgical		
Body System	7	Lymphatic and Hemic Systems		
Operation	D	Extraction: Pulling or stripping out or off all or a portion of a body part by the use of force		
Body Part (Character 4)	**Approach (Character 5)**		**Device (Character 6)**	**Qualifier (Character 7)**
Q Bone Marrow, Sternum	0 Open		Z No Device	X Diagnostic
R Bone Marrow, Iliac	3 Percutaneous			Z No Qualifier
S Bone Marrow, Vertebral				

Section	0	Medical and Surgical		
Body System	7	Lymphatic and Hemic Systems		
Operation	H	Insertion: Putting in a nonbiological appliance that monitors, assists, performs, or prevents a physiological function but does not physically take the place of a body part		
Body Part (Character 4)	**Approach (Character 5)**		**Device (Character 6)**	**Qualifier (Character 7)**
K Thoracic Duct	0 Open		3 Infusion Device	Z No Qualifier
L Cisterna Chyli	3 Percutaneous			
M Thymus	4 Percutaneous Endoscopic			
N Lymphatic				
P Spleen				

Section	0	Medical and Surgical		
Body System	7	Lymphatic and Hemic Systems		
Operation	J	Inspection: Visually and/or manually exploring a body part		
Body Part (Character 4)	**Approach (Character 5)**		**Device (Character 6)**	**Qualifier (Character 7)**
K Thoracic Duct	0 Open		Z No Device	Z No Qualifier
L Cisterna Chyli	3 Percutaneous			
M Thymus	4 Percutaneous Endoscopic			
T Bone Marrow				
N Lymphatic	0 Open		Z No Device	Z No Qualifier
P Spleen	3 Percutaneous			
	4 Percutaneous Endoscopic			
	X External			

Section	0	Medical and Surgical		
Body System	7	Lymphatic and Hemic Systems		
Operation	L	Occlusion: Completely closing an orifice or the lumen of a tubular body part		
Body Part (Character 4)	**Approach (Character 5)**		**Device (Character 6)**	**Qualifier (Character 7)**
0 Lymphatic, Head	0 Open		C Extraluminal Device	Z No Qualifier
1 Lymphatic, Right Neck	3 Percutaneous		D Intraluminal Device	
2 Lymphatic, Left Neck	4 Percutaneous Endoscopic		Z No Device	
3 Lymphatic, Right Upper Extremity				
4 Lymphatic, Left Upper Extremity				
5 Lymphatic, Right Axillary				
6 Lymphatic, Left Axillary				Continued on Next Page ▶
7 Lymphatic, Thorax				

			Continued from ◄ Previous Page
8 Lymphatic, Internal Mammary, Right			
9 Lymphatic, Internal Mammary, Left			
B Lymphatic, Mesenteric			
C Lymphatic, Pelvis			
D Lymphatic, Aortic			
F Lymphatic, Right Lower Extremity			
G Lymphatic, Left Lower Extremity			
H Lymphatic, Right Inguinal			
J Lymphatic, Left Inguinal			
K Thoracic Duct			
L Cisterna Chyli			

Section	0	Medical and Surgical	
Body System	7	Lymphatic and Hemic Systems	
Operation	N	Release: Freeing a body part from an abnormal physical constraint by cutting or by the use of force	

Body Part (Character 4)	Approach (Character 5)	Device (Character 6)	Qualifier (Character 7)
0 Lymphatic, Head	0 Open	Z No Device	Z No Qualifier
1 Lymphatic, Right Neck	3 Percutaneous		
2 Lymphatic, Left Neck	4 Percutaneous Endoscopic		
3 Lymphatic, Right Upper Extremity			
4 Lymphatic, Left Upper Extremity			
5 Lymphatic, Right Axillary			
6 Lymphatic, Left Axillary			
7 Lymphatic, Thorax			
8 Lymphatic, Internal Mammary, Right			
9 Lymphatic, Internal Mammary, Left			
B Lymphatic, Mesenteric			
C Lymphatic, Pelvis			
D Lymphatic, Aortic			
F Lymphatic, Right Lower Extremity			
G Lymphatic, Left Lower Extremity			
H Lymphatic, Right Inguinal			
J Lymphatic, Left Inguinal			
K Thoracic Duct			
L Cisterna Chyli			
M Thymus			
P Spleen			

Section	0	Medical and Surgical		
Body System	7	Lymphatic and Hemic Systems		
Operation	P	Removal: Taking out or off a device from a body part		

Body Part (Character 4)	Approach (Character 5)	Device (Character 6)	Qualifier (Character 7)
K Thoracic Duct L Cisterna Chyli N Lymphatic	0 Open 3 Percutaneous 4 Percutaneous Endoscopic	0 Drainage Device 3 Infusion Device 7 Autologous Tissue Substitute C Extraluminal Device D Intraluminal Device J Synthetic Substitute K Nonautologous Tissue Substitute	Z No Qualifier
K Thoracic Duct L Cisterna Chyli N Lymphatic	X External	0 Drainage Device 3 Infusion Device D Intraluminal Device	Z No Qualifier
M Thymus P Spleen	0 Open 3 Percutaneous 4 Percutaneous Endoscopic X External	0 Drainage Device 3 Infusion Device	Z No Qualifier
T Bone Marrow	0 Open 3 Percutaneous 4 Percutaneous Endoscopic X External	0 Drainage Device	Z No Qualifier

Section	0	Medical and Surgical		
Body System	7	Lymphatic and Hemic Systems		
Operation	Q	Repair: Restoring, to the extent possible, a body part to its normal anatomic structure and function		

Body Part (Character 4)	Approach (Character 5)	Device (Character 6)	Qualifier (Character 7)
0 Lymphatic, Head 1 Lymphatic, Right Neck 2 Lymphatic, Left Neck 3 Lymphatic, Right Upper Extremity 4 Lymphatic, Left Upper Extremity 5 Lymphatic, Right Axillary 6 Lymphatic, Left Axillary 7 Lymphatic, Thorax 8 Lymphatic, Internal Mammary, Right 9 Lymphatic, Internal Mammary, Left B Lymphatic, Mesenteric C Lymphatic, Pelvis D Lymphatic, Aortic F Lymphatic, Right Lower Extremity G Lymphatic, Left Lower Extremity H Lymphatic, Right Inguinal J Lymphatic, Left Inguinal K Thoracic Duct L Cisterna Chyli M Thymus P Spleen	0 Open 3 Percutaneous 4 Percutaneous Endoscopic	Z No Device	Z No Qualifier

Section	0	Medical and Surgical		
Body System	7	Lymphatic and Hemic Systems		
Operation	S	Reposition: Moving to its normal location, or other suitable location, all or a portion of a body part		

Body Part (Character 4)	Approach (Character 5)	Device (Character 6)	Qualifier (Character 7)
M Thymus P Spleen	0 Open	Z No Device	Z No Qualifier

Section	0	Medical and Surgical		
Body System	7	Lymphatic and Hemic Systems		
Operation	T	Resection: Cutting out or off, without replacement, all of a body part		

Body Part (Character 4)	Approach (Character 5)	Device (Character 6)	Qualifier (Character 7)
0 Lymphatic, Head 1 Lymphatic, Right Neck 2 Lymphatic, Left Neck 3 Lymphatic, Right Upper Extremity 4 Lymphatic, Left Upper Extremity 5 Lymphatic, Right Axillary 6 Lymphatic, Left Axillary 7 Lymphatic, Thorax 8 Lymphatic, Internal Mammary, Right 9 Lymphatic, Internal Mammary, Left B Lymphatic, Mesenteric C Lymphatic, Pelvis D Lymphatic, Aortic F Lymphatic, Right Lower Extremity G Lymphatic, Left Lower Extremity H Lymphatic, Right Inguinal J Lymphatic, Left Inguinal K Thoracic Duct L Cisterna Chyli M Thymus P Spleen	0 Open 4 Percutaneous Endoscopic	Z No Device	Z No Qualifier

Section	0	Medical and Surgical		
Body System	7	Lymphatic and Hemic Systems		
Operation	U	Supplement: Putting in or on biological or synthetic material that physically reinforces and/or augments the function of a portion of a body part		

Body Part (Character 4)	Approach (Character 5)	Device (Character 6)	Qualifier (Character 7)
0 Lymphatic, Head 1 Lymphatic, Right Neck 2 Lymphatic, Left Neck 3 Lymphatic, Right Upper Extremity 4 Lymphatic, Left Upper Extremity 5 Lymphatic, Right Axillary 6 Lymphatic, Left Axillary 7 Lymphatic, Thorax	0 Open 4 Percutaneous Endoscopic	7 Autologous Tissue Substitute J Synthetic Substitute K Nonautologous Tissue Substitute	Z No Qualifier

Continued on Next Page ▶

8 Lymphatic, Internal Mammary, Right			Continued from ◀ Previous Page
9 Lymphatic, Internal Mammary, Left			
B Lymphatic, Mesenteric			
C Lymphatic, Pelvis			
D Lymphatic, Aortic			
F Lymphatic, Right Lower Extremity			
G Lymphatic, Left Lower Extremity			
H Lymphatic, Right Inguinal			
J Lymphatic, Left Inguinal			
K Thoracic Duct			
L Cisterna Chyli			

Section	0	Medical and Surgical	
Body System	7	Lymphatic and Hemic Systems	
Operation	V	Restriction: Partially closing an orifice or the lumen of a tubular body part	

Body Part (Character 4)	Approach (Character 5)	Device (Character 6)	Qualifier (Character 7)
0 Lymphatic, Head	0 Open	C Extraluminal Device	Z No Qualifier
1 Lymphatic, Right Neck	3 Percutaneous	D Intraluminal Device	
2 Lymphatic, Left Neck	4 Percutaneous Endoscopic	Z No Device	
3 Lymphatic, Right Upper Extremity			
4 Lymphatic, Left Upper Extremity			
5 Lymphatic, Right Axillary			
6 Lymphatic, Left Axillary			
7 Lymphatic, Thorax			
8 Lymphatic, Internal Mammary, Right			
9 Lymphatic, Internal Mammary, Left			
B Lymphatic, Mesenteric			
C Lymphatic, Pelvis			
D Lymphatic, Aortic			
F Lymphatic, Right Lower Extremity			
G Lymphatic, Left Lower Extremity			
H Lymphatic, Right Inguinal			
J Lymphatic, Left Inguinal			
K Thoracic Duct			
L Cisterna Chyli			

Section	0	Medical and Surgical		
Body System	7	Lymphatic and Hemic Systems		
Operation	W	Revision: Correcting, to the extent possible, a portion of a malfunctioning device or the position of a displaced device		

Body Part (Character 4)	Approach (Character 5)	Device (Character 6)	Qualifier (Character 7)
K Thoracic Duct L Cisterna Chyli N Lymphatic	0 Open 3 Percutaneous 4 Percutaneous Endoscopic X External	0 Drainage Device 3 Infusion Device 7 Autologous Tissue Substitute C Extraluminal Device D Intraluminal Device J Synthetic Substitute K Nonautologous Tissue Substitute	Z No Qualifier
M Thymus P Spleen	0 Open 3 Percutaneous 4 Percutaneous Endoscopic X External	0 Drainage Device 3 Infusion Device	Z No Qualifier
T Bone Marrow	0 Open 3 Percutaneous 4 Percutaneous Endoscopic X External	0 Drainage Device	Z No Qualifier

Section	0	Medical and Surgical		
Body System	7	Lymphatic and Hemic Systems		
Operation	Y	Transplantation: Putting in or on all or a portion of a living body part taken from another individual or animal to physically take the place and/or function of all or a portion of a similar body part		

Body Part (Character 4)	Approach (Character 5)	Device (Character 6)	Qualifier (Character 7)
M Thymus P Spleen	0 Open	Z No Device	0 Allogeneic 1 Syngeneic 2 Zooplastic

Section	0	Medical and Surgical
Body System	8	Eye
Operation	0	Alteration: Modifying the anatomic structure of a body part without affecting the function of the body part

Body Part (Character 4)	Approach (Character 5)	Device (Character 6)	Qualifier (Character 7)
N Upper Eyelid, Right P Upper Eyelid, Left Q Lower Eyelid, Right R Lower Eyelid, Left	0 Open 3 Percutaneous X External	7 Autologous Tissue Substitute J Synthetic Substitute K Nonautologous Tissue Substitute Z No Device	Z No Qualifier

Section	0	Medical and Surgical
Body System	8	Eye
Operation	1	Bypass: Altering the route of passage of the contents of a tubular body part

Body Part (Character 4)	Approach (Character 5)	Device (Character 6)	Qualifier (Character 7)
2 Anterior Chamber, Right 3 Anterior Chamber, Left	3 Percutaneous	J Synthetic Substitute K Nonautologous Tissue Substitute Z No Device	4 Sclera
X Lacrimal Duct, Right Y Lacrimal Duct, Left	0 Open 3 Percutaneous	J Synthetic Substitute K Nonautologous Tissue Substitute Z No Device	3 Nasal Cavity

Section	0	Medical and Surgical
Body System	8	Eye
Operation	2	Change: Taking out or off a device from a body part and putting back an identical or similar device in or on the same body part without cutting or puncturing the skin or a mucous membrane

Body Part (Character 4)	Approach (Character 5)	Device (Character 6)	Qualifier (Character 7)
0 Eye, Right 1 Eye, Left	X External	0 Drainage Device Y Other Device	Z No Qualifier

Section	0	Medical and Surgical
Body System	8	Eye
Operation	5	Destruction: Physical eradication of all or a portion of a body part by the direct use of energy, force, or a destructive agent

Body Part (Character 4)	Approach (Character 5)	Device (Character 6)	Qualifier (Character 7)
0 Eye, Right 1 Eye, Left 6 Sclera, Right 7 Sclera, Left 8 Cornea, Right 9 Cornea, Left S Conjunctiva, Right T Conjunctiva, Left	X External	Z No Device	Z No Qualifier
2 Anterior Chamber, Right 3 Anterior Chamber, Left 4 Vitreous, Right 5 Vitreous, Left C Iris, Right D Iris, Left E Retina, Right F Retina, Left	3 Percutaneous	Z No Device	Z No Qualifier Continued on Next Page ▶

G Retinal Vessel, Right H Retinal Vessel, Left J Lens, Right K Lens, Left			Continued from ◄ Previous Page
A Choroid, Right B Choroid, Left L Extraocular Muscle, Right M Extraocular Muscle, Left V Lacrimal Gland, Right W Lacrimal Gland, Left	0 Open 3 Percutaneous	Z No Device	Z No Qualifier
N Upper Eyelid, Right P Upper Eyelid, Left Q Lower Eyelid, Right R Lower Eyelid, Left	0 Open 3 Percutaneous X External	Z No Device	Z No Qualifier
X Lacrimal Duct, Right Y Lacrimal Duct, Left	0 Open 3 Percutaneous 7 Via Natural or Artificial Opening 8 Via Natural or Artificial Opening Endoscopic	Z No Device	Z No Qualifier

Section	0	Medical and Surgical
Body System	8	Eye
Operation	7	Dilation: Expanding an orifice or the lumen of a tubular body part

Body Part (Character 4)	Approach (Character 5)	Device (Character 6)	Qualifier (Character 7)
X Lacrimal Duct, Right Y Lacrimal Duct, Left	0 Open 3 Percutaneous 7 Via Natural or Artificial Opening 8 Via Natural or Artificial Opening Endoscopic	D Intraluminal Device Z No Device	Z No Qualifier

Section	0	Medical and Surgical
Body System	8	Eye
Operation	9	Drainage: Taking or letting out fluids and/or gases from a body part

Body Part (Character 4)	Approach (Character 5)	Device (Character 6)	Qualifier (Character 7)
0 Eye, Right 1 Eye, Left 6 Sclera, Right 7 Sclera, Left 8 Cornea, Right 9 Cornea, Left S Conjunctiva, Right T Conjunctiva, Left	X External	0 Drainage Device	Z No Qualifier
0 Eye, Right 1 Eye, Left 6 Sclera, Right 7 Sclera, Left 8 Cornea, Right 9 Cornea, Left S Conjunctiva, Right T Conjunctiva, Left	X External	Z No Device	X Diagnostic Z No Qualifier
2 Anterior Chamber, Right 3 Anterior Chamber, Left	3 Percutaneous	0 Drainage Device	Z No Qualifier Continued on Next Page ►

			Continued from ◀ Previous Page
4 Vitreous, Right **5** Vitreous, Left **C** Iris, Right **D** Iris, Left **E** Retina, Right **F** Retina, Left **G** Retinal Vessel, Right **H** Retinal Vessel, Left **J** Lens, Right **K** Lens, Left			
2 Anterior Chamber, Right **3** Anterior Chamber, Left **4** Vitreous, Right **5** Vitreous, Left **C** Iris, Right **D** Iris, Left **E** Retina, Right **F** Retina, Left **G** Retinal Vessel, Right **H** Retinal Vessel, Left **J** Lens, Right **K** Lens, Left	**3** Percutaneous	**Z** No Device	**X** Diagnostic **Z** No Qualifier
A Choroid, Right **B** Choroid, Left **L** Extraocular Muscle, Right **M** Extraocular Muscle, Left **V** Lacrimal Gland, Right **W** Lacrimal Gland, Left	**0** Open **3** Percutaneous	**0** Drainage Device	**Z** No Qualifier
A Choroid, Right **B** Choroid, Left **L** Extraocular Muscle, Right **M** Extraocular Muscle, Left **V** Lacrimal Gland, Right **W** Lacrimal Gland, Left	**0** Open **3** Percutaneous	**Z** No Device	**X** Diagnostic **Z** No Qualifier
N Upper Eyelid, Right **P** Upper Eyelid, Left **Q** Lower Eyelid, Right **R** Lower Eyelid, Left	**0** Open **3** Percutaneous **X** External	**0** Drainage Device	**Z** No Qualifier
N Upper Eyelid, Right **P** Upper Eyelid, Left **Q** Lower Eyelid, Right **R** Lower Eyelid, Left	**0** Open **3** Percutaneous **X** External	**Z** No Device	**X** Diagnostic **Z** No Qualifier
X Lacrimal Duct, Right **Y** Lacrimal Duct, Left	**0** Open **3** Percutaneous **7** Via Natural or Artificial Opening **8** Via Natural or Artificial Opening Endoscopic	**0** Drainage Device	**Z** No Qualifier
X Lacrimal Duct, Right **Y** Lacrimal Duct, Left	**0** Open **3** Percutaneous **7** Via Natural or Artificial Opening **8** Via Natural or Artificial Opening Endoscopic	**Z** No Device	**X** Diagnostic **Z** No Qualifier

Section	0	Medical and Surgical
Body System	8	Eye
Operation	B	Excision: Cutting out or off, without replacement, a portion of a body part

Body Part (Character 4)	Approach (Character 5)	Device (Character 6)	Qualifier (Character 7)
0 Eye, Right 1 Eye, Left N Upper Eyelid, Right P Upper Eyelid, Left Q Lower Eyelid, Right R Lower Eyelid, Left	0 Open 3 Percutaneous X External	Z No Device	X Diagnostic Z No Qualifier
4 Vitreous, Right 5 Vitreous, Left C Iris, Right D Iris, Left E Retina, Right F Retina, Left J Lens, Right K Lens, Left	3 Percutaneous	Z No Device	X Diagnostic Z No Qualifier
6 Sclera, Right 7 Sclera, Left 8 Cornea, Right 9 Cornea, Left S Conjunctiva, Right T Conjunctiva, Left	X External	Z No Device	X Diagnostic Z No Qualifier
A Choroid, Right B Choroid, Left L Extraocular Muscle, Right M Extraocular Muscle, Left V Lacrimal Gland, Right W Lacrimal Gland, Left	0 Open 3 Percutaneous	Z No Device	X Diagnostic Z No Qualifier
X Lacrimal Duct, Right Y Lacrimal Duct, Left	0 Open 3 Percutaneous 7 Via Natural or Artificial Opening 8 Via Natural or Artificial Opening Endoscopic	Z No Device	X Diagnostic Z No Qualifier

Section	0	Medical and Surgical
Body System	8	Eye
Operation	C	Extirpation: Taking or cutting out solid matter from a body part

Body Part (Character 4)	Approach (Character 5)	Device (Character 6)	Qualifier (Character 7)
0 Eye, Right 1 Eye, Left 6 Sclera, Right 7 Sclera, Left 8 Cornea, Right 9 Cornea, Left S Conjunctiva, Right T Conjunctiva, Left	X External	Z No Device	Z No Qualifier
2 Anterior Chamber, Right 3 Anterior Chamber, Left 4 Vitreous, Right 5 Vitreous, Left C Iris, Right	3 Percutaneous X External	Z No Device	Z No Qualifier

Continued on Next Page ▶

			Continued from ◄ Previous Page
D Iris, Left **E** Retina, Right **F** Retina, Left **G** Retinal Vessel, Right **H** Retinal Vessel, Left **J** Lens, Right **K** Lens, Left			
A Choroid, Right **B** Choroid, Left **L** Extraocular Muscle, Right **M** Extraocular Muscle, Left **N** Upper Eyelid, Right **P** Upper Eyelid, Left **Q** Lower Eyelid, Right **R** Lower Eyelid, Left **V** Lacrimal Gland, Right **W** Lacrimal Gland, Left	**0** Open **3** Percutaneous **X** External	**Z** No Device	**Z** No Qualifier
X Lacrimal Duct, Right **Y** Lacrimal Duct, Left	**0** Open **3** Percutaneous **7** Via Natural or Artificial Opening **8** Via Natural or Artificial Opening Endoscopic	**Z** No Device	**Z** No Qualifier

Section	0	Medical and Surgical		
Body System	**8**	**Eye**		
Operation	**D**	**Extraction: Pulling or stripping out or off all or a portion of a body part by the use of force**		

Body Part (Character 4)	Approach (Character 5)	Device (Character 6)	Qualifier (Character 7)
8 Cornea, Right **9** Cornea, Left	**X** External	**Z** No Device	**X** Diagnostic **Z** No Qualifier
J Lens, Right **K** Lens, Left	**3** Percutaneous	**Z** No Device	**Z** No Qualifier

Section	0	Medical and Surgical		
Body System	**8**	**Eye**		
Operation	**F**	**Fragmentation: Breaking solid matter in a body part into pieces**		

Body Part (Character 4)	Approach (Character 5)	Device (Character 6)	Qualifier (Character 7)
4 Vitreous, Right **5** Vitreous, Left	**3** Percutaneous **X** External	**Z** No Device	**Z** No Qualifier

Section	0	Medical and Surgical		
Body System	**8**	**Eye**		
Operation	**H**	**Insertion: Putting in a nonbiological appliance that monitors, assists, performs, or prevents a physiological function but does not physically take the place of a body part**		

Body Part (Character 4)	Approach (Character 5)	Device (Character 6)	Qualifier (Character 7)
0 Eye, Right **1** Eye, Left	**0** Open	**3** Epiretinal Visual Prosthesis	**Z** No Qualifier
0 Eye, Right **1** Eye, Left	**3** Percutaneous **X** External	**1** Radioactive Element **3** Infusion Device	**Z** No Qualifier

Section	0	Medical and Surgical		
Body System	8	Eye		
Operation	J	Inspection: Visually and/or manually exploring a body part		
Body Part (Character 4)	**Approach (Character 5)**		**Device (Character 6)**	**Qualifier (Character 7)**
0 Eye, Right 1 Eye, Left J Lens, Right K Lens, Left	X External		Z No Device	Z No Qualifier
L Extraocular Muscle, Right M Extraocular Muscle, Left	0 Open X External		Z No Device	Z No Qualifier

Section	0	Medical and Surgical		
Body System	8	Eye		
Operation	L	Occlusion: Completely closing an orifice or the lumen of a tubular body part		
Body Part (Character 4)	**Approach (Character 5)**		**Device (Character 6)**	**Qualifier (Character 7)**
X Lacrimal Duct, Right Y Lacrimal Duct, Left	0 Open 3 Percutaneous		C Extraluminal Device D Intraluminal Device Z No Device	Z No Qualifier
X Lacrimal Duct, Right Y Lacrimal Duct, Left	7 Via Natural or Artificial Opening 8 Via Natural or Artificial Opening Endoscopic		D Intraluminal Device Z No Device	Z No Qualifier

Section	0	Medical and Surgical		
Body System	8	Eye		
Operation	M	Reattachment Putting back in or on all or a portion of a separated body part to its normal location or other suitable location		
Body Part (Character 4)	**Approach (Character 5)**		**Device (Character 6)**	**Qualifier (Character 7)**
N Upper Eyelid, Right P Upper Eyelid, Left Q Lower Eyelid, Right R Lower Eyelid, Left	X External		Z No Device	Z No Qualifier

Section	0	Medical and Surgical		
Body System	8	Eye		
Operation	N	Release: Freeing a body part from an abnormal physical constraint by cutting or by the use of force		
Body Part (Character 4)	**Approach (Character 5)**		**Device (Character 6)**	**Qualifier (Character 7)**
0 Eye, Right 1 Eye, Left 6 Sclera, Right 7 Sclera, Left 8 Cornea, Right 9 Cornea, Left S Conjunctiva, Right T Conjunctiva, Left	X External		Z No Device	Z No Qualifier
2 Anterior Chamber, Right 3 Anterior Chamber, Left 4 Vitreous, Right 5 Vitreous, Left C Iris, Right D Iris, Left E Retina, Right F Retina, Left	3 Percutaneous		Z No Device	Z No Qualifier

Continued on Next Page ▶

G Retinal Vessel, Right **H** Retinal Vessel, Left **J** Lens, Right **K** Lens, Left			Continued from ◀ Previous Page
A Choroid, Right **B** Choroid, Left **L** Extraocular Muscle, Right **M** Extraocular Muscle, Left **V** Lacrimal Gland, Right **W** Lacrimal Gland, Left	**0** Open **3** Percutaneous	**Z** No Device	**Z** No Qualifier
N Upper Eyelid, Right **P** Upper Eyelid, Left **Q** Lower Eyelid, Right **R** Lower Eyelid, Left	**0** Open **3** Percutaneous **X** External	**Z** No Device	**Z** No Qualifier
X Lacrimal Duct, Right **Y** Lacrimal Duct, Left	**0** Open **3** Percutaneous **7** Via Natural or Artificial Opening **8** Via Natural or Artificial Opening Endoscopic	**Z** No Device	**Z** No Qualifier

Section	0	Medical and Surgical	
Body System	8	Eye	
Operation	P	Removal: Taking out or off a device from a body part	

Body Part (Character 4)	Approach (Character 5)	Device (Character 6)	Qualifier (Character 7)
0 Eye, Right **1** Eye, Left	**0** Open **3** Percutaneous **7** Via Natural or Artificial Opening **8** Via Natural or Artificial Opening Endoscopic **X** External	**0** Drainage Device **1** Radioactive Element **3** Infusion Device **7** Autologous Tissue Substitute **C** Extraluminal Device **D** Intraluminal Device **J** Synthetic Substitute **K** Nonautologous Tissue Substitute	**Z** No Qualifier
J Lens, Right **K** Lens, Left	**3** Percutaneous	**J** Synthetic Substitute	**Z** No Qualifier
L Extraocular Muscle, Right **M** Extraocular Muscle, Left	**0** Open **3** Percutaneous	**0** Drainage Device **7** Autologous Tissue Substitute **J** Synthetic Substitute **K** Nonautologous Tissue Substitute	**Z** No Qualifier

Section	0	Medical and Surgical			
Body System	8	Eye			
Operation	Q	Repair: Restoring, to the extent possible, a body part to its normal anatomic structure and function			

Body Part (Character 4)	Approach (Character 5)	Device (Character 6)	Qualifier (Character 7)
0 Eye, Right 1 Eye, Left 6 Sclera, Right 7 Sclera, Left 8 Cornea, Right 9 Cornea, Left S Conjunctiva, Right T Conjunctiva, Left	X External	Z No Device	Z No Qualifier
2 Anterior Chamber, Right 3 Anterior Chamber, Left 4 Vitreous, Right 5 Vitreous, Left C Iris, Right D Iris, Left E Retina, Right F Retina, Left G Retinal Vessel, Right H Retinal Vessel, Left J Lens, Right K Lens, Left	3 Percutaneous	Z No Device	Z No Qualifier
A Choroid, Right B Choroid, Left L Extraocular Muscle, Right M Extraocular Muscle, Left V Lacrimal Gland, Right W Lacrimal Gland, Left	0 Open 3 Percutaneous	Z No Device	Z No Qualifier
N Upper Eyelid, Right P Upper Eyelid, Left Q Lower Eyelid, Right R Lower Eyelid, Left	0 Open 3 Percutaneous X External	Z No Device	Z No Qualifier
X Lacrimal Duct, Right Y Lacrimal Duct, Left	0 Open 3 Percutaneous 7 Via Natural or Artificial Opening 8 Via Natural or Artificial Opening Endoscopic	Z No Device	Z No Qualifier

Section	0	Medical and Surgical
Body System	8	Eye
Operation	R	Replacement: Putting in or on biological or synthetic material that physically takes the place and/or function of all or a portion of a body part

Body Part (Character 4)	Approach (Character 5)	Device (Character 6)	Qualifier (Character 7)
0 Eye, Right 1 Eye, Left A Choroid, Right B Choroid, Left	0 Open 3 Percutaneous	7 Autologous Tissue Substitute J Synthetic Substitute K Nonautologous Tissue Substitute	Z No Qualifier
4 Vitreous, Right 5 Vitreous, Left C Iris, Right D Iris, Left G Retinal Vessel, Right H Retinal Vessel, Left	3 Percutaneous	7 Autologous Tissue Substitute J Synthetic Substitute K Nonautologous Tissue Substitute	Z No Qualifier
6 Sclera, Right 7 Sclera, Left S Conjunctiva, Right T Conjunctiva, Left	X External	7 Autologous Tissue Substitute J Synthetic Substitute K Nonautologous Tissue Substitute	Z No Qualifier
8 Cornea, Right 9 Cornea, Left	3 Percutaneous X External	7 Autologous Tissue Substitute J Synthetic Substitute K Nonautologous Tissue Substitute	Z No Qualifier
J Lens, Right K Lens, Left	3 Percutaneous	0 Synthetic Substitute, Intraocular Telescope 7 Autologous Tissue Substitute J Synthetic Substitute K Nonautologous Tissue Substitute	Z No Qualifier
N Upper Eyelid, Right P Upper Eyelid, Left Q Lower Eyelid, Right R Lower Eyelid, Left	0 Open 3 Percutaneous X External	7 Autologous Tissue Substitute J Synthetic Substitute K Nonautologous Tissue Substitute	Z No Qualifier
X Lacrimal Duct, Right Y Lacrimal Duct, Left	0 Open 3 Percutaneous 7 Via Natural or Artificial Opening 8 Via Natural or Artificial Opening Endoscopic	7 Autologous Tissue Substitute J Synthetic Substitute K Nonautologous Tissue Substitute	Z No Qualifier

Section	0	Medical and Surgical		
Body System	8	Eye		
Operation	S	Reposition: Moving to its normal location, or other suitable location, all or a portion of a body part		

Body Part (Character 4)	Approach (Character 5)	Device (Character 6)	Qualifier (Character 7)
C Iris, Right **D** Iris, Left **G** Retinal Vessel, Right **H** Retinal Vessel, Left **J** Lens, Right **K** Lens, Left	**3** Percutaneous	**Z** No Device	**Z** No Qualifier
L Extraocular Muscle, Right **M** Extraocular Muscle, Left **V** Lacrimal Gland, Right **W** Lacrimal Gland, Left	**0** Open **3** Percutaneous	**Z** No Device	**Z** No Qualifier
N Upper Eyelid, Right **P** Upper Eyelid, Left **Q** Lower Eyelid, Right **R** Lower Eyelid, Left	**0** Open **3** Percutaneous **X** External	**Z** No Device	**Z** No Qualifier
X Lacrimal Duct, Right **Y** Lacrimal Duct, Left	**0** Open **3** Percutaneous **7** Via Natural or Artificial Opening **8** Via Natural or Artificial Opening Endoscopic	**Z** No Device	**Z** No Qualifier

Section	0	Medical and Surgical		
Body System	8	Eye		
Operation	T	Resection: Cutting out or off, without replacement, all of a body part		

Body Part (Character 4)	Approach (Character 5)	Device (Character 6)	Qualifier (Character 7)
0 Eye, Right **1** Eye, Left **8** Cornea, Right **9** Cornea, Left	**X** External	**Z** No Device	**Z** No Qualifier
4 Vitreous, Right **5** Vitreous, Left **C** Iris, Right **D** Iris, Left **J** Lens, Right **K** Lens, Left	**3** Percutaneous	**Z** No Device	**Z** No Qualifier
L Extraocular Muscle, Right **M** Extraocular Muscle, Left **V** Lacrimal Gland, Right **W** Lacrimal Gland, Left	**0** Open **3** Percutaneous	**Z** No Device	**Z** No Qualifier
N Upper Eyelid, Right **P** Upper Eyelid, Left **Q** Lower Eyelid, Right **R** Lower Eyelid, Left	**0** Open **X** External	**Z** No Device	**Z** No Qualifier
X Lacrimal Duct, Right **Y** Lacrimal Duct, Left	**0** Open **3** Percutaneous **7** Via Natural or Artificial Opening **8** Via Natural or Artificial Opening Endoscopic	**Z** No Device	**Z** No Qualifier

Section	0	Medical and Surgical
Body System	8	Eye
Operation	U	Supplement: Putting in or on biological or synthetic material that physically reinforces and/or augments the function of a portion of a body part

Body Part (Character 4)	Approach (Character 5)	Device (Character 6)	Qualifier (Character 7)
0 Eye, Right 1 Eye, Left C Iris, Right D Iris, Left E Retina, Right F Retina, Left G Retinal Vessel, Right H Retinal Vessel, Left L Extraocular Muscle, Right M Extraocular Muscle, Left	0 Open 3 Percutaneous	7 Autologous Tissue Substitute J Synthetic Substitute K Nonautologous Tissue Substitute	Z No Qualifier
8 Cornea, Right 9 Cornea, Left N Upper Eyelid, Right P Upper Eyelid, Left Q Lower Eyelid, Right R Lower Eyelid, Left	0 Open 3 Percutaneous X External	7 Autologous Tissue Substitute J Synthetic Substitute K Nonautologous Tissue Substitute	Z No Qualifier
X Lacrimal Duct, Right Y Lacrimal Duct, Left	0 Open 3 Percutaneous 7 Via Natural or Artificial Opening 8 Via Natural or Artificial Opening Endoscopic	7 Autologous Tissue Substitute J Synthetic Substitute K Nonautologous Tissue Substitute	Z No Qualifier

Section	0	Medical and Surgical
Body System	8	Eye
Operation	V	Restriction: Partially closing an orifice or the lumen of a tubular body part

Body Part (Character 4)	Approach (Character 5)	Device (Character 6)	Qualifier (Character 7)
X Lacrimal Duct, Right Y Lacrimal Duct, Left	0 Open 3 Percutaneous	C Extraluminal Device D Intraluminal Device Z No Device	Z No Qualifier
X Lacrimal Duct, Right Y Lacrimal Duct, Left	7 Via Natural or Artificial Opening 8 Via Natural or Artificial Opening Endoscopic	D Intraluminal Device Z No Device	Z No Qualifier

Section	0	Medical and Surgical		
Body System	8	Eye		
Operation	W	Revision: Correcting, to the extent possible, a portion of a malfunctioning device or the position of a displaced device		

Body Part (Character 4)	Approach (Character 5)	Device (Character 6)	Qualifier (Character 7)
0 Eye, Right **1** Eye, Left	**0** Open **3** Percutaneous **7** Via Natural or Artificial Opening **8** Via Natural or Artificial Opening Endoscopic **X** External	**0** Drainage Device **3** Infusion Device **7** Autologous Tissue Substitute **C** Extraluminal Device **D** Intraluminal Device **J** Synthetic Substitute **K** Nonautologous Tissue Substitute	**Z** No Qualifier
J Lens, Right **K** Lens, Left	**3** Percutaneous **X** External	**J** Synthetic Substitute	**Z** No Qualifier
L Extraocular Muscle, Right **M** Extraocular Muscle, Left	**0** Open **3** Percutaneous	**0** Drainage Device **7** Autologous Tissue Substitute **J** Synthetic Substitute **K** Nonautologous Tissue Substitute	**Z** No Qualifier

Section	0	Medical and Surgical		
Body System	8	Eye		
Operation	X	Transfer: Moving, without taking out, all or a portion of a body part to another location to take over the function of all or a portion of a body part		

Body Part (Character 4)	Approach (Character 5)	Device (Character 6)	Qualifier (Character 7)
L Extraocular Muscle, Right	**0** Open	**Z** No Device	**Z** No Qualifier
M Extraocular Muscle, Left	**3** Percutaneous		

Section	0	Medical and Surgical		
Body System	9	Ear, Nose, Sinus		
Operation	0	Alteration: Modifying the anatomic structure of a body part without affecting the function of the body part		

Body Part (Character 4)	Approach (Character 5)	Device (Character 6)	Qualifier (Character 7)
0 External Ear, Right 1 External Ear, Left 2 External Ear, Bilateral K Nose	0 Open 3 Percutaneous 4 Percutaneous Endoscopic X External	7 Autologous Tissue Substitute J Synthetic Substitute K Nonautologous Tissue Substitute Z No Device	Z No Qualifier

Section	0	Medical and Surgical		
Body System	9	Ear, Nose, Sinus		
Operation	1	Bypass: Altering the route of passage of the contents of a tubular body part		

Body Part Character 4	Approach Character 5	Device Character 6	Qualifier
D Inner Ear, Right E Inner Ear, Left	0 Open	7 Autologous Tissue Substitute J Synthetic Substitute K Nonautologous Tissue Substitute Z No Device	0 Endolymphatic

Section	0	Medical and Surgical		
Body System	9	Ear, Nose, Sinus		
Operation	2	Change: Taking out or off a device from a body part and putting back an identical or similar device in or on the same body part without cutting or puncturing the skin or a mucous membrane		

Body Part (Character 4)	Approach (Character 5)	Device (Character 6)	Qualifier (Character 7)
H Ear, Right J Ear, Left K Nose Y Sinus	X External	0 Drainage Device Y Other Device	Z No Qualifier

Section	0	Medical and Surgical		
Body System	9	Ear, Nose, Sinus		
Operation	5	Destruction: Physical eradication of all or a portion of a body part by the direct use of energy, force, or a destructive agent		

Body Part (Character 4)	Approach (Character 5)	Device (Character 6)	Qualifier (Character 7)
0 External Ear, Right 1 External Ear, Left K Nose	0 Open 3 Percutaneous 4 Percutaneous Endoscopic X External	Z No Device	Z No Qualifier
3 External Auditory Canal, Right 4 External Auditory Canal, Left	0 Open 3 Percutaneous 4 Percutaneous Endoscopic 7 Via Natural or Artificial Opening 8 Via Natural or Artificial Opening Endoscopic X External	Z No Device	Z No Qualifier
5 Middle Ear, Right 6 Middle Ear, Left 9 Auditory Ossicle, Right	0 Open	Z No Device	Z No Qualifier

Continued on Next Page ▶

A Auditory Ossicle, Left D Inner Ear, Right E Inner Ear, Left			Continued from ◀ Previous Page
7 Tympanic Membrane, Right 8 Tympanic Membrane, Left F Eustachian Tube, Right G Eustachian Tube, Left L Nasal Turbinate N Nasopharynx	0 Open 3 Percutaneous 4 Percutaneous Endoscopic 7 Via Natural or Artificial Opening 8 Via Natural or Artificial Opening Endoscopic	Z No Device	Z No Qualifier
B Mastoid Sinus, Right C Mastoid Sinus, Left M Nasal Septum P Accessory Sinus Q Maxillary Sinus, Right R Maxillary Sinus, Left S Frontal Sinus, Right T Frontal Sinus, Left U Ethmoid Sinus, Right V Ethmoid Sinus, Left W Sphenoid Sinus, Right X Sphenoid Sinus, Left	0 Open 3 Percutaneous 4 Percutaneous Endoscopic	Z No Device	Z No Qualifier

Section	0	Medical and Surgical
Body System	9	Ear, Nose, Sinus
Operation	7	Dilation: Expanding an orifice or the lumen of a tubular body part

Body Part (Character 4)	Approach (Character 5)	Device (Character 6)	Qualifier (Character 7)
F Eustachian Tube, Right G Eustachian Tube, Left	0 Open 7 Via Natural or Artificial Opening 8 Via Natural or Artificial Opening Endoscopic	D Intraluminal Device Z No Device	Z No Qualifier
F Eustachian Tube, Right G Eustachian Tube, Left	3 Percutaneous 4 Percutaneous Endoscopic	Z No Device	Z No Qualifier

Section	0	Medical and Surgical
Body System	9	Ear, Nose, Sinus
Operation	8	Division: Cutting into a body part, without draining fluids and/or gases from the body part, in order to separate or transect a body part

Body Part (Character 4)	Approach (Character 5)	Device (Character 6)	Qualifier (Character 7)
L Nasal Turbinate	0 Open 3 Percutaneous 4 Percutaneous Endoscopic 7 Via Natural or Artificial Opening 8 Via Natural or Artificial Opening Endoscopic	Z No Device	Z No Qualifier

Section	0	Medical and Surgical		
Body System	9	Ear, Nose, Sinus		
Operation	9	Drainage: Taking or letting out fluids and/or gases from a body part		

Body Part (Character 4)	Approach (Character 5)	Device (Character 6)	Qualifier (Character 7)
0 External Ear, Right 1 External Ear, Left K Nose	0 Open 3 Percutaneous 4 Percutaneous Endoscopic X External	0 Drainage Device	Z No Qualifier
0 External Ear, Right 1 External Ear, Left K Nose	0 Open 3 Percutaneous 4 Percutaneous Endoscopic X External	Z No Device	X Diagnostic Z No Qualifier
3 External Auditory Canal, Right 4 External Auditory Canal, Left	0 Open 3 Percutaneous 4 Percutaneous Endoscopic 7 Via Natural or Artificial Opening 8 Via Natural or Artificial Opening Endoscopic X External	0 Drainage Device	Z No Qualifier
3 External Auditory Canal, Right 4 External Auditory Canal, Left	0 Open 3 Percutaneous 4 Percutaneous Endoscopic 7 Via Natural or Artificial Opening 8 Via Natural or Artificial Opening Endoscopic X External	Z No Device	X Diagnostic Z No Qualifier
5 Middle Ear, Right 6 Middle Ear, Left 9 Auditory Ossicle, Right A Auditory Ossicle, Left D Inner Ear, Right E Inner Ear, Left	0 Open	0 Drainage Device	Z No Qualifier
5 Middle Ear, Right 6 Middle Ear, Left 9 Auditory Ossicle, Right A Auditory Ossicle, Left D Inner Ear, Right E Inner Ear, Left	0 Open	Z No Device	X Diagnostic Z No Qualifier
7 Tympanic Membrane, Right 8 Tympanic Membrane, Left F Eustachian Tube, Right G Eustachian Tube, Left L Nasal Turbinate N Nasopharynx	0 Open 3 Percutaneous 4 Percutaneous Endoscopic 7 Via Natural or Artificial Opening 8 Via Natural or Artificial Opening Endoscopic	0 Drainage Device	Z No Qualifier
7 Tympanic Membrane, Right 8 Tympanic Membrane, Left F Eustachian Tube, Right G Eustachian Tube, Left L Nasal Turbinate N Nasopharynx	0 Open 3 Percutaneous 4 Percutaneous Endoscopic 7 Via Natural or Artificial Opening 8 Via Natural or Artificial Opening Endoscopic	Z No Device	X Diagnostic Z No Qualifier

Continued on Next Page ▶

			Continued from ◀ Previous Page
7 Tympanic Membrane, Right 8 Tympanic Membrane, Left F Eustachian Tube, Right G Eustachian Tube, Left L Nasal Turbinate N Nasopharynx	0 Open 3 Percutaneous 4 Percutaneous Endoscopic 7 Via Natural or Artificial Opening 8 Via Natural or Artificial Opening Endoscopic	Z No Device	X Diagnostic Z No Qualifier
B Mastoid Sinus, Right C Mastoid Sinus, Left M Nasal Septum P Accessory Sinus Q Maxillary Sinus, Right R Maxillary Sinus, Left S Frontal Sinus, Right T Frontal Sinus, Left U Ethmoid Sinus, Right V Ethmoid Sinus, Left W Sphenoid Sinus, Right X Sphenoid Sinus, Left	0 Open 3 Percutaneous 4 Percutaneous Endoscopic	0 Drainage Device	Z No Qualifier
B Mastoid Sinus, Right C Mastoid Sinus, Left M Nasal Septum P Accessory Sinus Q Maxillary Sinus, Right R Maxillary Sinus, Left S Frontal Sinus, Right T Frontal Sinus, Left U Ethmoid Sinus, Right V Ethmoid Sinus, Left W Sphenoid Sinus, Right X Sphenoid Sinus, Left	0 Open 3 Percutaneous 4 Percutaneous Endoscopic	Z No Device	X Diagnostic Z No Qualifier

Section	0	Medical and Surgical
Body System	9	Ear, Nose, Sinus
Operation	B	Excision: Cutting out or off, without replacement, a portion of a body part

Body Part (Character 4)	Approach (Character 5)	Device (Character 6)	Qualifier (Character 7)
0 External Ear, Right 1 External Ear, Left K Nose	0 Open 3 Percutaneous 4 Percutaneous Endoscopic X External	Z No Device	X Diagnostic Z No Qualifier
3 External Auditory Canal, Right 4 External Auditory Canal, Left	0 Open 3 Percutaneous 4 Percutaneous Endoscopic 7 Via Natural or Artificial Opening 8 Via Natural or Artificial Opening Endoscopic X External	Z No Device	X Diagnostic Z No Qualifier
5 Middle Ear, Right 6 Middle Ear, Left 9 Auditory Ossicle, Right A Auditory Ossicle, Left	0 Open	Z No Device	X Diagnostic Z No Qualifier

Continued on Next Page ▶

			Continued from ◀ Previous Page
D Inner Ear, Right E Inner Ear, Left			
7 Tympanic Membrane, Right 8 Tympanic Membrane, Left F Eustachian Tube, Right G Eustachian Tube, Left L Nasal Turbinate N Nasopharynx	0 Open 3 Percutaneous 4 Percutaneous Endoscopic 7 Via Natural or Artificial Opening 8 Via Natural or Artificial Opening Endoscopic	Z No Device	X Diagnostic Z No Qualifier
B Mastoid Sinus, Right C Mastoid Sinus, Left M Nasal Septum P Accessory Sinus Q Maxillary Sinus, Right R Maxillary Sinus, Left S Frontal Sinus, Right T Frontal Sinus, Left U Ethmoid Sinus, Right V Ethmoid Sinus, Left W Sphenoid Sinus, Right X Sphenoid Sinus, Left	0 Open 3 Percutaneous 4 Percutaneous Endoscopic	Z No Device	X Diagnostic Z No Qualifier

Section	0	Medical and Surgical
Body System	9	Ear, Nose, Sinus
Operation	C	Extirpation: Taking or cutting out solid matter from a body part

Body Part (Character 4)	Approach (Character 5)	Device (Character 6)	Qualifier (Character 7)
0 External Ear, Right 1 External Ear, Left K Nose	0 Open 3 Percutaneous 4 Percutaneous Endoscopic X External	Z No Device	Z No Qualifier
3 External Auditory Canal, Right 4 External Auditory Canal, Left	0 Open 3 Percutaneous 4 Percutaneous Endoscopic 7 Via Natural or Artificial Opening 8 Via Natural or Artificial Opening Endoscopic X External	Z No Device	Z No Qualifier
5 Middle Ear, Right 6 Middle Ear, Left 9 Auditory Ossicle, Right A Auditory Ossicle, Left D Inner Ear, Right E Inner Ear, Left	0 Open	Z No Device	Z No Qualifier
7 Tympanic Membrane, Right 8 Tympanic Membrane, Left F Eustachian Tube, Right G Eustachian Tube, Left L Nasal Turbinate N Nasopharynx	0 Open 3 Percutaneous 4 Percutaneous Endoscopic 7 Via Natural or Artificial Opening 8 Via Natural or Artificial Opening Endoscopic	Z No Device	Z No Qualifier
B Mastoid Sinus, Right C Mastoid Sinus, Left M Nasal Septum	0 Open 3 Percutaneous 4 Percutaneous Endoscopic	Z No Device	Z No Qualifier Continued on Next Page ▶

			Continued from ◀ Previous Page
P Accessory Sinus **Q** Maxillary Sinus, Right **R** Maxillary Sinus, Left **S** Frontal Sinus, Right **T** Frontal Sinus, Left **U** Ethmoid Sinus, Right **V** Ethmoid Sinus, Left **W** Sphenoid Sinus, Right **X** Sphenoid Sinus, Left			

Section	0	Medical and Surgical
Body System	9	Ear, Nose, Sinus
Operation	D	Extraction: Pulling or stripping out or off all or a portion of a body part by the use of force

Body Part (Character 4)	Approach (Character 5)	Device (Character 6)	Qualifier (Character 7)
7 Tympanic Membrane, Right **8** Tympanic Membrane, Left **L** Nasal Turbinate	**0** Open **3** Percutaneous **4** Percutaneous Endoscopic **7** Via Natural or Artificial Opening **8** Via Natural or Artificial Opening Endoscopic	**Z** No Device	**Z** No Qualifier
9 Auditory Ossicle, Right **A** Auditory Ossicle, Left	**0** Open	**Z** No Device	**Z** No Qualifier
B Mastoid Sinus, Right **C** Mastoid Sinus, Left **M** Nasal Septum **P** Accessory Sinus **Q** Maxillary Sinus, Right **R** Maxillary Sinus, Left **S** Frontal Sinus, Right **T** Frontal Sinus, Left **U** Ethmoid Sinus, Right **V** Ethmoid Sinus, Left **W** Sphenoid Sinus, Right **X** Sphenoid Sinus, Left	**0** Open **3** Percutaneous **4** Percutaneous Endoscopic	**Z** No Device	**Z** No Qualifier

Section	0	Medical and Surgical
Body System	9	Ear, Nose, Sinus
Operation	H	Insertion: Putting in a nonbiological appliance that monitors, assists, performs, or prevents a physiological function but does not physically take the place of a body part

Body Part (Character 4)	Approach (Character 5)	Device (Character 6)	Qualifier (Character 7)
D Inner Ear, Right **E** Inner Ear, Left	**0** Open **3** Percutaneous **4** Percutaneous Endoscopic	**4** Hearing Device, Bone Conduction **5** Hearing Device, Single Channel Cochlear Prosthesis **6** Hearing Device, Multiple Channel Cochlear Prosthesis **S** Hearing Device	**Z** No Qualifier
N Nasopharynx	**7** Via Natural or Artificial Opening **8** Via Natural or Artificial Opening Endoscopic	**B** Intraluminal Device, Airway	**Z** No Qualifier

Section	0	Medical and Surgical
Body System	9	Ear, Nose, Sinus
Operation	J	Inspection: Visually and/or manually exploring a body part

Body Part (Character 4)	Approach (Character 5)	Device (Character 6)	Qualifier (Character 7)
7 Tympanic Membrane, Right 8 Tympanic Membrane, Left H Ear, Right J Ear, Left	0 Open 3 Percutaneous 4 Percutaneous Endoscopic 7 Via Natural or Artificial Opening 8 Via Natural or Artificial Opening Endoscopic X External	Z No Device	Z No Qualifier
D Inner Ear, Right E Inner Ear, Left K Nose Y Sinus	0 Open 3 Percutaneous 4 Percutaneous Endoscopic X External	Z No Device	Z No Qualifier

Section	0	Medical and Surgical
Body System	9	Ear, Nose, Sinus
Operation	M	Reattachment Putting back in or on all or a portion of a separated body part to its normal location or other suitable location

Body Part (Character 4)	Approach (Character 5)	Device (Character 6)	Qualifier (Character 7)
0 External Ear, Right 1 External Ear, Left K Nose	X External	Z No Device	Z No Qualifier

Section	0	Medical and Surgical
Body System	9	Ear, Nose, Sinus
Operation	N	Release: Freeing a body part from an abnormal physical constraint by cutting or by the use of force

Body Part (Character 4)	Approach (Character 5)	Device (Character 6)	Qualifier (Character 7)
0 External Ear, Right 1 External Ear, Left K Nose	0 Open 3 Percutaneous 4 Percutaneous Endoscopic X External	Z No Device	Z No Qualifier
3 External Auditory Canal, Right 4 External Auditory Canal, Left	0 Open 3 Percutaneous 4 Percutaneous Endoscopic 7 Via Natural or Artificial Opening 8 Via Natural or Artificial Opening Endoscopic X External	Z No Device	Z No Qualifier
5 Middle Ear, Right 6 Middle Ear, Left 9 Auditory Ossicle, Right A Auditory Ossicle, Left D Inner Ear, Right E Inner Ear, Left	0 Open	Z No Device	Z No Qualifier
7 Tympanic Membrane, Right 8 Tympanic Membrane, Left F Eustachian Tube, Right G Eustachian Tube, Left L Nasal Turbinate	0 Open 3 Percutaneous 4 Percutaneous Endoscopic 7 Via Natural or Artificial Opening 8 Via Natural or Artificial	Z No Device	Z No Qualifier **Continued on Next Page ▶**

N Nasopharynx	Opening Endoscopic		**Continued from** ◄ **Previous Page**
B Mastoid Sinus, Right C Mastoid Sinus, Left M Nasal Septum P Accessory Sinus Q Maxillary Sinus, Right R Maxillary Sinus, Left S Frontal Sinus, Right T Frontal Sinus, Left U Ethmoid Sinus, Right V Ethmoid Sinus, Left W Sphenoid Sinus, Right X Sphenoid Sinus, Left	0 Open 3 Percutaneous 4 Percutaneous Endoscopic	Z No Device	Z No Qualifier

Section	0	Medical and Surgical	
Body System	9	Ear, Nose, Sinus	
Operation	P	Removal: Taking out or off a device from a body part	

Body Part (Character 4)	Approach (Character 5)	Device (Character 6)	Qualifier (Character 7)
7 Tympanic Membrane, Right 8 Tympanic Membrane, Left	0 Open 7 Via Natural or Artificial Opening 8 Via Natural or Artificial Opening Endoscopic X External	0 Drainage Device	Z No Qualifier
D Inner Ear, Right E Inner Ear, Left	0 Open 7 Via Natural or Artificial Opening 8 Via Natural or Artificial Opening Endoscopic	S Hearing Device	Z No Qualifier
H Ear, Right J Ear, Left K Nose	0 Open 3 Percutaneous 4 Percutaneous Endoscopic 7 Via Natural or Artificial Opening 8 Via Natural or Artificial Opening Endoscopic X External	0 Drainage Device 7 Autologous Tissue Substitute D Intraluminal Device J Synthetic Substitute K Nonautologous Tissue Substitute	Z No Qualifier
Y Sinus	0 Open 3 Percutaneous 4 Percutaneous Endoscopic X External	0 Drainage Device	Z No Qualifier

Section	0	Medical and Surgical		
Body System	9	Ear, Nose, Sinus		
Operation	Q	Repair: Restoring, to the extent possible, a body part to its normal anatomic structure and function		

Body Part (Character 4)	Approach (Character 5)	Device (Character 6)	Qualifier (Character 7)
0 External Ear, Right **1** External Ear, Left **2** External Ear, Bilateral **K** Nose	**0** Open **3** Percutaneous **4** Percutaneous Endoscopic **X** External	**Z** No Device	**Z** No Qualifier
3 External Auditory Canal, Right **4** External Auditory Canal, Left **F** Eustachian Tube, Right **G** Eustachian Tube, Left	**0** Open **3** Percutaneous **4** Percutaneous Endoscopic **7** Via Natural or Artificial Opening **8** Via Natural or Artificial Opening Endoscopic **X** External	**Z** No Device	**Z** No Qualifier
5 Middle Ear, Right **6** Middle Ear, Left **9** Auditory Ossicle, Right **A** Auditory Ossicle, Left **D** Inner Ear, Right **E** Inner Ear, Left	**0** Open	**Z** No Device	**Z** No Qualifier
7 Tympanic Membrane, Right **8** Tympanic Membrane, Left **L** Nasal Turbinate **N** Nasopharynx	**0** Open **3** Percutaneous **4** Percutaneous Endoscopic **7** Via Natural or Artificial Opening **8** Via Natural or Artificial Opening Endoscopic	**Z** No Device	**Z** No Qualifier
B Mastoid Sinus, Right **C** Mastoid Sinus, Left **M** Nasal Septum **P** Accessory Sinus **Q** Maxillary Sinus, Right **R** Maxillary Sinus, Left **S** Frontal Sinus, Right **T** Frontal Sinus, Left **U** Ethmoid Sinus, Right **V** Ethmoid Sinus, Left **W** Sphenoid Sinus, Right **X** Sphenoid Sinus, Left	**0** Open **3** Percutaneous **4** Percutaneous Endoscopic	**Z** No Device	**Z** No Qualifier

Section	0	Medical and Surgical		
Body System	9	Ear, Nose, Sinus		
Operation	R	Replacement: Putting in or on biological or synthetic material that physically takes the place and/or function of all or a portion of a body part		

Body Part (Character 4)	Approach (Character 5)	Device (Character 6)	Qualifier (Character 7)
0 External Ear, Right 1 External Ear, Left 2 External Ear, Bilateral K Nose	0 Open X External	7 Autologous Tissue Substitute J Synthetic Substitute K Nonautologous Tissue Substitute	Z No Qualifier
5 Middle Ear, Right 6 Middle Ear, Left 9 Auditory Ossicle, Right A Auditory Ossicle, Left D Inner Ear, Right E Inner Ear, Left	0 Open	7 Autologous Tissue Substitute J Synthetic Substitute K Nonautologous Tissue Substitute	Z No Qualifier
7 Tympanic Membrane, Right 8 Tympanic Membrane, Left N Nasopharynx	0 Open 7 Via Natural or Artificial Opening 8 Via Natural or Artificial Opening Endoscopic	7 Autologous Tissue Substitute J Synthetic Substitute K Nonautologous Tissue Substitute	Z No Qualifier
L Nasal Turbinate	0 Open 3 Percutaneous 4 Percutaneous Endoscopic 7 Via Natural or Artificial Opening 8 Via Natural or Artificial Opening Endoscopic	7 Autologous Tissue Substitute J Synthetic Substitute K Nonautologous Tissue Substitute	Z No Qualifier
M Nasal Septum	0 Open 3 Percutaneous 4 Percutaneous Endoscopic	7 Autologous Tissue Substitute J Synthetic Substitute K Nonautologous Tissue Substitute	Z No Qualifier

Section	0	Medical and Surgical		
Body System	9	Ear, Nose, Sinus		
Operation	S	Reposition: Moving to its normal location, or other suitable location, all or a portion of a body part		

Body Part (Character 4)	Approach (Character 5)	Device (Character 6)	Qualifier (Character 7)
0 External Ear, Right 1 External Ear, Left 2 External Ear, Bilateral K Nose	0 Open 4 Percutaneous Endoscopic X External	Z No Device	Z No Qualifier
7 Tympanic Membrane, Right 8 Tympanic Membrane, Left F Eustachian Tube, Right G Eustachian Tube, Left L Nasal Turbinate	0 Open 4 Percutaneous Endoscopic 7 Via Natural or Artificial Opening 8 Via Natural or Artificial Opening Endoscopic	Z No Device	Z No Qualifier
9 Auditory Ossicle, Right A Auditory Ossicle, Left M Nasal Septum	0 Open 4 Percutaneous Endoscopic	Z No Device	Z No Qualifier

Section	0	Medical and Surgical		
Body System	9	Ear, Nose, Sinus		
Operation	T	Resection: Cutting out or off, without replacement, all of a body part		

Body Part (Character 4)	Approach (Character 5)	Device (Character 6)	Qualifier (Character 7)
0 External Ear, Right 1 External Ear, Left K Nose	0 Open 4 Percutaneous Endoscopic X External	Z No Device	Z No Qualifier
5 Middle Ear, Right 6 Middle Ear, Left 9 Auditory Ossicle, Right A Auditory Ossicle, Left D Inner Ear, Right E Inner Ear, Left	0 Open	Z No Device	Z No Qualifier
7 Tympanic Membrane, Right 8 Tympanic Membrane, Left F Eustachian Tube, Right G Eustachian Tube, Left L Nasal Turbinate N Nasopharynx	0 Open 4 Percutaneous Endoscopic 7 Via Natural or Artificial Opening 8 Via Natural or Artificial Opening Endoscopic	Z No Device	Z No Qualifier
B Mastoid Sinus, Right C Mastoid Sinus, Left M Nasal Septum P Accessory Sinus Q Maxillary Sinus, Right R Maxillary Sinus, Left S Frontal Sinus, Right T Frontal Sinus, Left U Ethmoid Sinus, Right V Ethmoid Sinus, Left W Sphenoid Sinus, Right X Sphenoid Sinus, Left	0 Open 4 Percutaneous Endoscopic	Z No Device	Z No Qualifier

Section	0	Medical and Surgical		
Body System	9	Ear, Nose, Sinus		
Operation	U	Supplement: Putting in or on biological or synthetic material that physically reinforces and/or augments the function of a portion of a body part		

Body Part (Character 4)	Approach (Character 5)	Device (Character 6)	Qualifier (Character 7)
0 External Ear, Right 1 External Ear, Left 2 External Ear, Bilateral K Nose	0 Open X External	7 Autologous Tissue Substitute J Synthetic Substitute K Nonautologous Tissue Substitute	Z No Qualifier
5 Middle Ear, Right 6 Middle Ear, Left 9 Auditory Ossicle, Right A Auditory Ossicle, Left D Inner Ear, Right E Inner Ear, Left	0 Open	7 Autologous Tissue Substitute J Synthetic Substitute K Nonautologous Tissue Substitute	Z No Qualifier
7 Tympanic Membrane, Right 8 Tympanic Membrane, Left N Nasopharynx	0 Open 7 Via Natural or Artificial Opening 8 Via Natural or Artificial Opening Endoscopic	7 Autologous Tissue Substitute J Synthetic Substitute K Nonautologous Tissue Substitute	Z No Qualifier

Continued on Next Page ▶

			Continued from ◀ Previous Page
L Nasal Turbinate	**0** Open **3** Percutaneous **4** Percutaneous Endoscopic **7** Via Natural or Artificial Opening **8** Via Natural or Artificial Opening Endoscopic	**7** Autologous Tissue Substitute **J** Synthetic Substitute **K** Nonautologous Tissue Substitute	**Z** No Qualifier
M Nasal Septum	**0** Open **3** Percutaneous **4** Percutaneous Endoscopic	**7** Autologous Tissue Substitute **J** Synthetic Substitute **K** Nonautologous Tissue Substitute	**Z** No Qualifier

Section	0	Medical and Surgical	
Body System	9	Ear, Nose, Sinus	
Operation	W	Revision: Correcting, to the extent possible, a portion of a malfunctioning device or the position of a displaced device	

Body Part (Character 4)	Approach (Character 5)	Device (Character 6)	Qualifier (Character 7)
7 Tympanic Membrane, Right **8** Tympanic Membrane, Left **9** Auditory Ossicle, Right **A** Auditory Ossicle, Left	**0** Open **7** Via Natural or Artificial Opening **8** Via Natural or Artificial Opening Endoscopic	**7** Autologous Tissue Substitute **J** Synthetic Substitute **K** Nonautologous Tissue Substitute	**Z** No Qualifier
D Inner Ear, Right **E** Inner Ear, Left	**0** Open **7** Via Natural or Artificial Opening **8** Via Natural or Artificial Opening Endoscopic	**S** Hearing Device	**Z** No Qualifier
H Ear, Right **J** Ear, Left **K** Nose	**0** Open **3** Percutaneous **4** Percutaneous Endoscopic **7** Via Natural or Artificial Opening **8** Via Natural or Artificial Opening Endoscopic **X** External	**0** Drainage Device **7** Autologous Tissue Substitute **D** Intraluminal Device **J** Synthetic Substitute **K** Nonautologous Tissue Substitute	**Z** No Qualifier
Y Sinus	**0** Open **3** Percutaneous **4** Percutaneous Endoscopic **X** External	**0** Drainage Device	**Z** No Qualifier

Section	0	Medical and Surgical
Body System	B	Respiratory System
Operation	1	Bypass: Altering the route of passage of the contents of a tubular body part

Body Part (Character 4)	Approach (Character 5)	Device (Character 6)	Qualifier (Character 7)
1 Trachea	0 Open	D Intraluminal Device	6 Esophagus
1 Trachea	0 Open	F Tracheostomy Device Z No Device	4 Cutaneous
1 Trachea	3 Percutaneous 4 Percutaneous Endoscopic	F Tracheostomy Device Z No Device	4 Cutaneous

Section	0	Medical and Surgical
Body System	B	Respiratory System
Operation	2	Change: Taking out or off a device from a body part and putting back an identical or similar device in or on the same body part without cutting or puncturing the skin or a mucous membrane

Body Part (Character 4)	Approach (Character 5)	Device (Character 6)	Qualifier (Character 7)
0 Tracheobronchial Tree K Lung, Right L Lung, Left Q Pleura T Diaphragm	X External	0 Drainage Device Y Other Device	Z No Qualifier
1 Trachea	X External	0 Drainage Device E Intraluminal Device, Endotracheal Airway F Tracheostomy Device Y Other Device	Z No Qualifier

Section	0	Medical and Surgical
Body System	B	Respiratory System
Operation	5	Destruction: Physical eradication of all or a portion of a body part by the direct use of energy, force, or a destructive agent

Body Part (Character 4)	Approach (Character 5)	Device (Character 6)	Qualifier (Character 7)
1 Trachea 2 Carina 3 Main Bronchus, Right 4 Upper Lobe Bronchus, Right 5 Middle Lobe Bronchus, Right 6 Lower Lobe Bronchus, Right 7 Main Bronchus, Left 8 Upper Lobe Bronchus, Left 9 Lingula Bronchus B Lower Lobe Bronchus, Left C Upper Lung Lobe, Right D Middle Lung Lobe, Right F Lower Lung Lobe, Right G Upper Lung Lobe, Left H Lung Lingula J Lower Lung Lobe, Left K Lung, Right L Lung, Left M Lungs, Bilateral	0 Open 3 Percutaneous 4 Percutaneous Endoscopic 7 Via Natural or Artificial Opening 8 Via Natural or Artificial Opening Endoscopic	Z No Device	Z No Qualifier

Continued on Next Page ▶

			Continued from ◀ Previous Page
N Pleura, Right P Pleura, Left R Diaphragm, Right S Diaphragm, Left	0 Open 3 Percutaneous 4 Percutaneous Endoscopic	Z No Device	Z No Qualifier

Section	0	Medical and Surgical	
Body System	B	Respiratory System	
Operation	7	Dilation: Expanding an orifice or the lumen of a tubular body part	

Body Part (Character 4)	Approach (Character 5)	Device (Character 6)	Qualifier (Character 7)
1 Trachea 2 Carina 3 Main Bronchus, Right 4 Upper Lobe Bronchus, Right 5 Middle Lobe Bronchus, Right 6 Lower Lobe Bronchus, Right 7 Main Bronchus, Left 8 Upper Lobe Bronchus, Left 9 Lingula Bronchus B Lower Lobe Bronchus, Left	0 Open 3 Percutaneous 4 Percutaneous Endoscopic 7 Via Natural or Artificial Opening 8 Via Natural or Artificial Opening Endoscopic	D Intraluminal Device Z No Device	Z No Qualifier

Section	0	Medical and Surgical	
Body System	B	Respiratory System	
Operation	9	Drainage: Taking or letting out fluids and/or gases from a body part	

Body Part (Character 4)	Approach (Character 5)	Device (Character 6)	Qualifier (Character 7)
1 Trachea 2 Carina 3 Main Bronchus, Right 4 Upper Lobe Bronchus, Right 5 Middle Lobe Bronchus, Right 6 Lower Lobe Bronchus, Right 7 Main Bronchus, Left 8 Upper Lobe Bronchus, Left 9 Lingula Bronchus B Lower Lobe Bronchus, Left C Upper Lung Lobe, Right D Middle Lung Lobe, Right F Lower Lung Lobe, Right G Upper Lung Lobe, Left H Lung Lingula J Lower Lung Lobe, Left K Lung, Right L Lung, Left M Lungs, Bilateral	0 Open 3 Percutaneous 4 Percutaneous Endoscopic 7 Via Natural or Artificial Opening 8 Via Natural or Artificial Opening Endoscopic	0 Drainage Device	Z No Qualifier

Continued on Next Page ▶

Continued from
◀ Previous Page

1 Trachea 2 Carina 3 Main Bronchus, Right 4 Upper Lobe Bronchus, Right 5 Middle Lobe Bronchus, Right 6 Lower Lobe Bronchus, Right 7 Main Bronchus, Left 8 Upper Lobe Bronchus, Left 9 Lingula Bronchus B Lower Lobe Bronchus, Left C Upper Lung Lobe, Right D Middle Lung Lobe, Right F Lower Lung Lobe, Right G Upper Lung Lobe, Left H Lung Lingula J Lower Lung Lobe, Left K Lung, Right L Lung, Left M Lungs, Bilateral	0 Open 3 Percutaneous 4 Percutaneous Endoscopic 7 Via Natural or Artificial Opening 8 Via Natural or Artificial Opening Endoscopic	Z No Device	X Diagnostic Z No Qualifier
N Pleura, Right P Pleura, Left R Diaphragm, Right S Diaphragm, Left	0 Open 3 Percutaneous 4 Percutaneous Endoscopic	0 Drainage Device	Z No Qualifier
N Pleura, Right P Pleura, Left R Diaphragm, Right S Diaphragm, Left	0 Open 3 Percutaneous 4 Percutaneous Endoscopic	Z No Device	X Diagnostic Z No Qualifier

Section	0	Medical and Surgical	
Body System	B	Respiratory System	
Operation	B	Excision: Cutting out or off, without replacement, a portion of a body part	

Body Part (Character 4)	Approach (Character 5)	Device (Character 6)	Qualifier (Character 7)
1 Trachea 2 Carina 3 Main Bronchus, Right 4 Upper Lobe Bronchus, Right 5 Middle Lobe Bronchus, Right 6 Lower Lobe Bronchus, Right 7 Main Bronchus, Left 8 Upper Lobe Bronchus, Left 9 Lingula Bronchus B Lower Lobe Bronchus, Left C Upper Lung Lobe, Right D Middle Lung Lobe, Right F Lower Lung Lobe, Right	0 Open 3 Percutaneous 4 Percutaneous Endoscopic 7 Via Natural or Artificial Opening 8 Via Natural or Artificial Opening Endoscopic	Z No Device	X Diagnostic Z No Qualifier

Continued on
Next Page ▶

			Continued from ◀ Previous Page
G Upper Lung Lobe, Left **H** Lung Lingula **J** Lower Lung Lobe, Left **K** Lung, Right **L** Lung, Left **M** Lungs, Bilateral			
N Pleura, Right **P** Pleura, Left **R** Diaphragm, Right **S** Diaphragm, Left	**0** Open **3** Percutaneous **4** Percutaneous Endoscopic	**Z** No Device	**X** Diagnostic **Z** No Qualifier

Section	0	Medical and Surgical
Body System	B	Respiratory System
Operation	C	Extirpation: Taking or cutting out solid matter from a body part

Body Part (Character 4)	Approach (Character 5)	Device (Character 6)	Qualifier (Character 7)
1 Trachea **2** Carina **3** Main Bronchus, Right **4** Upper Lobe Bronchus, Right **5** Middle Lobe Bronchus, Right **6** Lower Lobe Bronchus, Right **7** Main Bronchus, Left **8** Upper Lobe Bronchus, Left **9** Lingula Bronchus **B** Lower Lobe Bronchus, Left **C** Upper Lung Lobe, Right **D** Middle Lung Lobe, Right **F** Lower Lung Lobe, Right **G** Upper Lung Lobe, Left **H** Lung Lingula **J** Lower Lung Lobe, Left **K** Lung, Right **L** Lung, Left **M** Lungs, Bilateral	**0** Open **3** Percutaneous **4** Percutaneous Endoscopic **7** Via Natural or Artificial Opening **8** Via Natural or Artificial Opening Endoscopic	**Z** No Device	**Z** No Qualifier
N Pleura, Right **P** Pleura, Left **R** Diaphragm, Right **S** Diaphragm, Left	**0** Open **3** Percutaneous **4** Percutaneous Endoscopic	**Z** No Device	**Z** No Qualifier

Section	0	Medical and Surgical
Body System	B	Respiratory System
Operation	D	Extraction: Pulling or stripping out or off all or a portion of a body part by the use of force

Body Part (Character 4)	Approach (Character 5)	Device (Character 6)	Qualifier (Character 7)
N Pleura, Right **P** Pleura, Left	**0** Open **3** Percutaneous **4** Percutaneous Endoscopic	**Z** No Device	**X** Diagnostic **Z** No Qualifier

Section	0	Medical and Surgical			
Body System	B	Respiratory System			
Operation	F	Fragmentation: Breaking solid matter in a body part into pieces			

Body Part (Character 4)	Approach (Character 5)	Device (Character 6)	Qualifier (Character 7)
1 Trachea 2 Carina 3 Main Bronchus, Right 4 Upper Lobe Bronchus, Right 5 Middle Lobe Bronchus, Right 6 Lower Lobe Bronchus, Right 7 Main Bronchus, Left 8 Upper Lobe Bronchus, Left 9 Lingula Bronchus B Lower Lobe Bronchus, Left	0 Open 3 Percutaneous 4 Percutaneous Endoscopic 7 Via Natural or Artificial Opening 8 Via Natural or Artificial Opening Endoscopic X External	Z No Device	Z No Qualifier

Section	0	Medical and Surgical			
Body System	B	Respiratory System			
Operation	H	Insertion: Putting in a nonbiological appliance that monitors, assists, performs, or prevents a physiological function but does not physically take the place of a body part			

Body Part (Character 4)	Approach (Character 5)	Device (Character 6)	Qualifier (Character 7)
0 Tracheobronchial Tree	0 Open 3 Percutaneous 4 Percutaneous Endoscopic 7 Via Natural or Artificial Opening 8 Via Natural or Artificial Opening Endoscopic	1 Radioactive Element 2 Monitoring Device 3 Infusion Device D Intraluminal Device	Z No Qualifier
1 Trachea	0 Open	2 Monitoring Device D Intraluminal Device	Z No Qualifier
1 Trachea	3 Percutaneous	D Intraluminal Device E Intraluminal Device, Endotracheal Airway	Z No Qualifier
1 Trachea	4 Percutaneous Endoscopic	D Intraluminal Device	Z No Qualifier
1 Trachea	7 Via Natural or Artificial Opening 8 Via Natural or Artificial Opening Endoscopic	2 Monitoring Device D Intraluminal Device E Intraluminal Device, Endotracheal Airway	Z No Qualifier
3 Main Bronchus, Right 4 Upper Lobe Bronchus, Right 5 Middle Lobe Bronchus, Right 6 Lower Lobe Bronchus, Right 7 Main Bronchus, Left 8 Upper Lobe Bronchus, Left 9 Lingula Bronchus B Lower Lobe Bronchus, Left	0 Open 3 Percutaneous 4 Percutaneous Endoscopic 7 Via Natural or Artificial Opening 8 Via Natural or Artificial Opening Endoscopic	G Intraluminal Device, Endobronchial Valve	Z No Qualifier
K Lung, Right L Lung, Left	0 Open 3 Percutaneous 4 Percutaneous Endoscopic	1 Radioactive Element 2 Monitoring Device 3 Infusion Device	Z No Qualifier **Continued on Next Page ▶**

	7 Via Natural or Artificial Opening 8 Via Natural or Artificial Opening Endoscopic		Continued from ◀ Previous Page
R Diaphragm, Right S Diaphragm, Left	0 Open 3 Percutaneous 4 Percutaneous Endoscopic	2 Monitoring Device M Diaphragmatic Pacemaker Lead	Z No Qualifier

Section	0	Medical and Surgical
Body System	B	Respiratory System
Operation	J	Inspection: Visually and/or manually exploring a body part

Body Part (Character 4)	Approach (Character 5)	Device (Character 6)	Qualifier (Character 7)
0 Tracheobronchial Tree 1 Trachea K Lung, Right L Lung, Left Q Pleura T Diaphragm	0 Open 3 Percutaneous 4 Percutaneous Endoscopic 7 Via Natural or Artificial Opening 8 Via Natural or Artificial Opening Endoscopic X External	Z No Device	Z No Qualifier

Section	0	Medical and Surgical
Body System	B	Respiratory System
Operation	L	Occlusion: Completely closing an orifice or the lumen of a tubular body part

Body Part (Character 4)	Approach (Character 5)	Device (Character 6)	Qualifier (Character 7)
1 Trachea 2 Carina 3 Main Bronchus, Right 4 Upper Lobe Bronchus, Right 5 Middle Lobe Bronchus, Right 6 Lower Lobe Bronchus, Right 7 Main Bronchus, Left 8 Upper Lobe Bronchus, Left 9 Lingula Bronchus B Lower Lobe Bronchus, Left	0 Open 3 Percutaneous 4 Percutaneous Endoscopic	C Extraluminal Device D Intraluminal Device Z No Device	Z No Qualifier
1 Trachea 2 Carina 3 Main Bronchus, Right 4 Upper Lobe Bronchus, Right 5 Middle Lobe Bronchus, Right 6 Lower Lobe Bronchus, Right 7 Main Bronchus, Left 8 Upper Lobe Bronchus, Left 9 Lingula Bronchus B Lower Lobe Bronchus, Left	7 Via Natural or Artificial Opening 8 Via Natural or Artificial Opening Endoscopic	D Intraluminal Device Z No Device	Z No Qualifier

Section	0	Medical and Surgical		
Body System	B	Respiratory System		
Operation	M	Reattachment Putting back in or on all or a portion of a separated body part to its normal location or other suitable location		

Body Part (Character 4)	Approach (Character 5)	Device (Character 6)	Qualifier (Character 7)
1 Trachea	0 Open	Z No Device	Z No Qualifier
2 Carina			
3 Main Bronchus, Right			
4 Upper Lobe Bronchus, Right			
5 Middle Lobe Bronchus, Right			
6 Lower Lobe Bronchus, Right			
7 Main Bronchus, Left			
8 Upper Lobe Bronchus, Left			
9 Lingula Bronchus			
B Lower Lobe Bronchus, Left			
C Upper Lung Lobe, Right			
D Middle Lung Lobe, Right			
F Lower Lung Lobe, Right			
G Upper Lung Lobe, Left			
H Lung Lingula			
J Lower Lung Lobe, Left			
K Lung, Right			
L Lung, Left			
R Diaphragm, Right			
S Diaphragm, Left			

Section	0	Medical and Surgical		
Body System	B	Respiratory System		
Operation	N	Release: Freeing a body part from an abnormal physical constraint by cutting or by the use of force		

Body Part (Character 4)	Approach (Character 5)	Device (Character 6)	Qualifier (Character 7)
1 Trachea	0 Open	Z No Device	Z No Qualifier
2 Carina	3 Percutaneous		
3 Main Bronchus, Right	4 Percutaneous Endoscopic		
4 Upper Lobe Bronchus, Right	7 Via Natural or Artificial Opening		
5 Middle Lobe Bronchus, Right	8 Via Natural or Artificial Opening Endoscopic		
6 Lower Lobe Bronchus, Right			
7 Main Bronchus, Left			
8 Upper Lobe Bronchus, Left			
9 Lingula Bronchus			
B Lower Lobe Bronchus, Left			
C Upper Lung Lobe, Right			
D Middle Lung Lobe, Right			
F Lower Lung Lobe, Right			
G Upper Lung Lobe, Left			
H Lung Lingula			
J Lower Lung Lobe, Left			Continued on Next Page ▶

K Lung, Right L Lung, Left M Lungs, Bilateral			Continued from ◀ Previous Page
N Pleura, Right P Pleura, Left R Diaphragm, Right S Diaphragm, Left	0 Open 3 Percutaneous 4 Percutaneous Endoscopic	Z No Device	Z No Qualifier

Section	0	Medical and Surgical
Body System	B	Respiratory System
Operation	P	Removal: Taking out or off a device from a body part

Body Part (Character 4)	Approach (Character 5)	Device (Character 6)	Qualifier (Character 7)
0 Tracheobronchial Tree	0 Open 3 Percutaneous 4 Percutaneous Endoscopic 7 Via Natural or Artificial Opening 8 Via Natural or Artificial Opening Endoscopic	0 Drainage Device 1 Radioactive Element 2 Monitoring Device 3 Infusion Device 7 Autologous Tissue Substitute C Extraluminal Device D Intraluminal Device J Synthetic Substitute K Nonautologous Tissue Substitute	Z No Qualifier
0 Tracheobronchial Tree	X External	0 Drainage Device 1 Radioactive Element 2 Monitoring Device 3 Infusion Device D Intraluminal Device	Z No Qualifier
1 Trachea	0 Open 3 Percutaneous 4 Percutaneous Endoscopic 7 Via Natural or Artificial Opening 8 Via Natural or Artificial Opening Endoscopic	0 Drainage Device 2 Monitoring Device 7 Autologous Tissue Substitute C Extraluminal Device D Intraluminal Device F Tracheostomy Device J Synthetic Substitute K Nonautologous Tissue Substitute	Z No Qualifier
1 Trachea	X External	0 Drainage Device 2 Monitoring Device D Intraluminal Device F Tracheostomy Device	Z No Qualifier
K Lung, Right L Lung, Left	0 Open 3 Percutaneous 4 Percutaneous Endoscopic 7 Via Natural or Artificial Opening 8 Via Natural or Artificial Opening Endoscopic X External	0 Drainage Device 1 Radioactive Element 2 Monitoring Device 3 Infusion Device	Z No Qualifier
Q Pleura	0 Open 3 Percutaneous 4 Percutaneous Endoscopic 7 Via Natural or Artificial Opening	0 Drainage Device 1 Radioactive Element 2 Monitoring Device	Z No Qualifier

Continued on Next Page ▶

	8 Via Natural or Artificial Opening Endoscopic X External		Continued from ◀ Previous Page
T Diaphragm	0 Open 3 Percutaneous 4 Percutaneous Endoscopic 7 Via Natural or Artificial Opening 8 Via Natural or Artificial Opening Endoscopic	0 Drainage Device 2 Monitoring Device 7 Autologous Tissue Substitute J Synthetic Substitute K Nonautologous Tissue Substitute M Diaphragmatic Pacemaker Lead	Z No Qualifier
T Diaphragm	X External	0 Drainage Device 2 Monitoring Device M Diaphragmatic Pacemaker Lead	Z No Qualifier

Section	0	Medical and Surgical
Body System	B	Respiratory System
Operation	Q	Repair: Restoring, to the extent possible, a body part to its normal anatomic structure and function

Body Part (Character 4)	Approach (Character 5)	Device (Character 6)	Qualifier (Character 7)
1 Trachea 2 Carina 3 Main Bronchus, Right 4 Upper Lobe Bronchus, Right 5 Middle Lobe Bronchus, Right 6 Lower Lobe Bronchus, Right 7 Main Bronchus, Left 8 Upper Lobe Bronchus, Left 9 Lingula Bronchus B Lower Lobe Bronchus, Left C Upper Lung Lobe, Right D Middle Lung Lobe, Right F Lower Lung Lobe, Right G Upper Lung Lobe, Left H Lung Lingula J Lower Lung Lobe, Left K Lung, Right L Lung, Left M Lungs, Bilateral	0 Open 3 Percutaneous 4 Percutaneous Endoscopic 7 Via Natural or Artificial Opening 8 Via Natural or Artificial Opening Endoscopic	Z No Device	Z No Qualifier
N Pleura, Right P Pleura, Left R Diaphragm, Right S Diaphragm, Left	0 Open 3 Percutaneous 4 Percutaneous Endoscopic	Z No Device	Z No Qualifier

Section	0	Medical and Surgical		
Body System	B	Respiratory System		
Operation	S	Reposition: Moving to its normal location, or other suitable location, all or a portion of a body part		

Body Part (Character 4)	Approach (Character 5)	Device (Character 6)	Qualifier (Character 7)
1 Trachea	0 Open	Z No Device	Z No Qualifier
2 Carina			
3 Main Bronchus, Right			
4 Upper Lobe Bronchus, Right			
5 Middle Lobe Bronchus, Right			
6 Lower Lobe Bronchus, Right			
7 Main Bronchus, Left			
8 Upper Lobe Bronchus, Left			
9 Lingula Bronchus			
B Lower Lobe Bronchus, Left			
C Upper Lung Lobe, Right			
D Middle Lung Lobe, Right			
F Lower Lung Lobe, Right			
G Upper Lung Lobe, Left			
H Lung Lingula			
J Lower Lung Lobe, Left			
K Lung, Right			
L Lung, Left			
R Diaphragm, Right			
S Diaphragm, Left			

Section	0	Medical and Surgical		
Body System	B	Respiratory System		
Operation	T	Resection: Cutting out or off, without replacement, all of a body part		

Body Part (Character 4)	Approach (Character 5)	Device (Character 6)	Qualifier (Character 7)
1 Trachea	0 Open	Z No Device	Z No Qualifier
2 Carina	4 Percutaneous Endoscopic		
3 Main Bronchus, Right			
4 Upper Lobe Bronchus, Right			
5 Middle Lobe Bronchus, Right			
6 Lower Lobe Bronchus, Right			
7 Main Bronchus, Left			
8 Upper Lobe Bronchus, Left			
9 Lingula Bronchus			
B Lower Lobe Bronchus, Left			
C Upper Lung Lobe, Right			
D Middle Lung Lobe, Right			
F Lower Lung Lobe, Right			
G Upper Lung Lobe, Left			
H Lung Lingula			
J Lower Lung Lobe, Left			
K Lung, Right			Continued on Next Page ▶

L Lung, Left			Continued from
M Lungs, Bilateral			◀ Previous Page
R Diaphragm, Right			
S Diaphragm, Left			

Section	0	Medical and Surgical	
Body System	B	Respiratory System	
Operation	U	Supplement: Putting in or on biological or synthetic material that physically reinforces and/or augments the function of a portion of a body part	

Body Part (Character 4)	Approach (Character 5)	Device (Character 6)	Qualifier (Character 7)
1 Trachea 2 Carina 3 Main Bronchus, Right 4 Upper Lobe Bronchus, Right 5 Middle Lobe Bronchus, Right 6 Lower Lobe Bronchus, Right 7 Main Bronchus, Left 8 Upper Lobe Bronchus, Left 9 Lingula Bronchus B Lower Lobe Bronchus, Left R Diaphragm, Right S Diaphragm, Left	0 Open 4 Percutaneous Endoscopic	7 Autologous Tissue Substitute J Synthetic Substitute K Nonautologous Tissue Substitute	Z No Qualifier

Section	0	Medical and Surgical	
Body System	B	Respiratory System	
Operation	V	Restriction: Partially closing an orifice or the lumen of a tubular body part	

Body Part (Character 4)	Approach (Character 5)	Device (Character 6)	Qualifier (Character 7)
1 Trachea 2 Carina 3 Main Bronchus, Right 4 Upper Lobe Bronchus, Right 5 Middle Lobe Bronchus, Right 6 Lower Lobe Bronchus, Right 7 Main Bronchus, Left 8 Upper Lobe Bronchus, Left 9 Lingula Bronchus B Lower Lobe Bronchus, Left	0 Open 3 Percutaneous 4 Percutaneous Endoscopic	C Extraluminal Device D Intraluminal Device Z No Device	Z No Qualifier
1 Trachea 2 Carina 3 Main Bronchus, Right 4 Upper Lobe Bronchus, Right 5 Middle Lobe Bronchus, Right 6 Lower Lobe Bronchus, Right 7 Main Bronchus, Left 8 Upper Lobe Bronchus, Left 9 Lingula Bronchus B Lower Lobe Bronchus, Left	7 Via Natural or Artificial Opening 8 Via Natural or Artificial Opening Endoscopic	D Intraluminal Device Z No Device	Z No Qualifier

Section	0	Medical and Surgical	
Body System	B	Respiratory System	
Operation	W	Revision: Correcting, to the extent possible, a portion of a malfunctioning device or the position of a displaced device	

Body Part (Character 4)	Approach (Character 5)	Device (Character 6)	Qualifier (Character 7)
0 Tracheobronchial Tree	0 Open 3 Percutaneous 4 Percutaneous Endoscopic 7 Via Natural or Artificial Opening 8 Via Natural or Artificial Opening Endoscopic X External	0 Drainage Device 2 Monitoring Device 3 Infusion Device 7 Autologous Tissue Substitute C Extraluminal Device D Intraluminal Device J Synthetic Substitute K Nonautologous Tissue Substitute	Z No Qualifier
1 Trachea	0 Open 3 Percutaneous 4 Percutaneous Endoscopic 7 Via Natural or Artificial Opening 8 Via Natural or Artificial Opening Endoscopic X External	0 Drainage Device 2 Monitoring Device 7 Autologous Tissue Substitute C Extraluminal Device D Intraluminal Device F Tracheostomy Device J Synthetic Substitute K Nonautologous Tissue Substitute	Z No Qualifier
K Lung, Right L Lung, Left	0 Open 3 Percutaneous 4 Percutaneous Endoscopic 7 Via Natural or Artificial Opening 8 Via Natural or Artificial Opening Endoscopic X External	0 Drainage Device 2 Monitoring Device 3 Infusion Device	Z No Qualifier
Q Pleura	0 Open 3 Percutaneous 4 Percutaneous Endoscopic 7 Via Natural or Artificial Opening 8 Via Natural or Artificial Opening Endoscopic X External	0 Drainage Device 2 Monitoring Device	Z No Qualifier
T Diaphragm	0 Open 3 Percutaneous 4 Percutaneous Endoscopic 7 Via Natural or Artificial Opening 8 Via Natural or Artificial Opening Endoscopic X External	0 Drainage Device 2 Monitoring Device 7 Autologous Tissue Substitute J Synthetic Substitute K Nonautologous Tissue Substitute M Diaphragmatic Pacemaker Lead	Z No Qualifier

Section	0	Medical and Surgical
Body System	B	Respiratory System
Operation	Y	Transplantation: Putting in or on all or a portion of a living body part taken from another individual or animal to physically take the place and/or function of all or a portion of a similar body part

Body Part (Character 4)	Approach (Character 5)	Device (Character 6)	Qualifier (Character 7)
C Upper Lung Lobe, Right	0 Open	Z No Device	0 Allogeneic
D Middle Lung Lobe, Right			1 Syngeneic
F Lower Lung Lobe, Right			2 Zooplastic
G Upper Lung Lobe, Left			
H Lung Lingula			
J Lower Lung Lobe, Left			
K Lung, Right			
L Lung, Left			
M Lungs, Bilateral			

Section	0	Medical and Surgical
Body System	C	Mouth and Throat
Operation	0	Alteration: Modifying the anatomic structure of a body part without affecting the function of the body part

Body Part (Character 4)	Approach (Character 5)	Device (Character 6)	Qualifier (Character 7)
0 Upper Lip 1 Lower Lip	X External	7 Autologous Tissue Substitute J Synthetic Substitute K Nonautologous Tissue Substitute Z No Device	Z No Qualifier

Section	0	Medical and Surgical
Body System	C	Mouth and Throat
Operation	2	Change: Taking out or off a device from a body part and putting back an identical or similar device in or on the same body part without cutting or puncturing the skin or a mucous membrane

Body Part (Character 4)	Approach (Character 5)	Device (Character 6)	Qualifier (Character 7)
A Salivary Gland S Larynx Y Mouth and Throat	X External	0 Drainage Device Y Other Device	Z No Qualifier

Section	0	Medical and Surgical
Body System	C	Mouth and Throat
Operation	5	Destruction: Physical eradication of all or a portion of a body part by the direct use of energy, force, or a destructive agent

Body Part (Character 4)	Approach (Character 5)	Device (Character 6)	Qualifier (Character 7)
0 Upper Lip 1 Lower Lip 2 Hard Palate 3 Soft Palate 4 Buccal Mucosa 5 Upper Gingiva 6 Lower Gingiva 7 Tongue N Uvula P Tonsils Q Adenoids	0 Open 3 Percutaneous X External	Z No Device	Z No Qualifier
8 Parotid Gland, Right 9 Parotid Gland, Left B Parotid Duct, Right C Parotid Duct, Left D Sublingual Gland, Right F Sublingual Gland, Left G Submaxillary Gland, Right H Submaxillary Gland, Left J Minor Salivary Gland	0 Open 3 Percutaneous	Z No Device	Z No Qualifier
M Pharynx R Epiglottis S Larynx T Vocal Cord, Right V Vocal Cord, Left	0 Open 3 Percutaneous 4 Percutaneous Endoscopic 7 Via Natural or Artificial Opening 8 Via Natural or Artificial Opening Endoscopic	Z No Device	Z No Qualifier

Continued on Next Page ▶

			Continued from ◀ Previous Page
W Upper Tooth **X** Lower Tooth	**0** Open **X** External	**Z** No Device	**0** Single **1** Multiple **2** All

Section	0	Medical and Surgical	
Body System	C	Mouth and Throat	
Operation	7	Dilation: Expanding an orifice or the lumen of a tubular body part	

Body Part (Character 4)	Approach (Character 5)	Device (Character 6)	Qualifier (Character 7)
B Parotid Duct, Right **C** Parotid Duct, Left	**0** Open **3** Percutaneous **7** Via Natural or Artificial Opening	**D** Intraluminal Device **Z** No Device	**Z** No Qualifier
M Pharynx	**7** Via Natural or Artificial Opening **8** Via Natural or Artificial Opening Endoscopic	**D** Intraluminal Device **Z** No Device	**Z** No Qualifier
S Larynx	**0** Open **3** Percutaneous **4** Percutaneous Endoscopic **7** Via Natural or Artificial Opening **8** Via Natural or Artificial Opening Endoscopic	**D** Intraluminal Device **Z** No Device	**Z** No Qualifier

Section	0	Medical and Surgical	
Body System	C	Mouth and Throat	
Operation	9	Drainage: Taking or letting out fluids and/or gases from a body part	

Body Part (Character 4)	Approach (Character 5)	Device (Character 6)	Qualifier (Character 7)
0 Upper Lip **1** Lower Lip **2** Hard Palate **3** Soft Palate **4** Buccal Mucosa **5** Upper Gingiva **6** Lower Gingiva **7** Tongue **N** Uvula **P** Tonsils **Q** Adenoids	**0** Open **3** Percutaneous **X** External	**0** Drainage Device	**Z** No Qualifier
0 Upper Lip **1** Lower Lip **2** Hard Palate **3** Soft Palate **4** Buccal Mucosa **5** Upper Gingiva **6** Lower Gingiva **7** Tongue **N** Uvula **P** Tonsils **Q** Adenoids	**0** Open **3** Percutaneous **X** External	**Z** No Device	**X** Diagnostic **Z** No Qualifier
8 Parotid Gland, Right **9** Parotid Gland, Left	**0** Open **3** Percutaneous	**0** Drainage Device	**Z** No Qualifier

Continued on Next Page ▶

			Continued from ◀ Previous Page
B Parotid Duct, Right **C** Parotid Duct, Left **D** Sublingual Gland, Right **F** Sublingual Gland, Left **G** Submaxillary Gland, Right **H** Submaxillary Gland, Left **J** Minor Salivary Gland			
8 Parotid Gland, Right **9** Parotid Gland, Left **B** Parotid Duct, Right **C** Parotid Duct, Left **D** Sublingual Gland, Right **F** Sublingual Gland, Left **G** Submaxillary Gland, Right **H** Submaxillary Gland, Left **J** Minor Salivary Gland	**0** Open **3** Percutaneous	**Z** No Device	**X** Diagnostic **Z** No Qualifier
M Pharynx **R** Epiglottis **S** Larynx **T** Vocal Cord, Right **V** Vocal Cord, Left	**0** Open **3** Percutaneous **4** Percutaneous Endoscopic **7** Via Natural or Artificial Opening **8** Via Natural or Artificial Opening Endoscopic	**0** Drainage Device	**Z** No Qualifier
M Pharynx **R** Epiglottis **S** Larynx **T** Vocal Cord, Right **V** Vocal Cord, Left	**0** Open **3** Percutaneous **4** Percutaneous Endoscopic **7** Via Natural or Artificial Opening **8** Via Natural or Artificial Opening Endoscopic	**Z** No Device	**X** Diagnostic **Z** No Qualifier
W Upper Tooth **X** Lower Tooth	**0** Open **X** External	**0** Drainage Device **Z** No Device	**0** Single **1** Multiple **2** All

Section	0	Medical and Surgical	
Body System	C	Mouth and Throat	
Operation	B	Excision: Cutting out or off, without replacement, a portion of a body part	
Body Part (Character 4)	**Approach (Character 5)**	**Device (Character 6)**	**Qualifier (Character 7)**
0 Upper Lip **1** Lower Lip **2** Hard Palate **3** Soft Palate **4** Buccal Mucosa **5** Upper Gingiva **6** Lower Gingiva **7** Tongue **N** Uvula **P** Tonsils **Q** Adenoids	**0** Open **3** Percutaneous **X** External	**Z** No Device	**X** Diagnostic **Z** No Qualifier
8 Parotid Gland, Right **9** Parotid Gland, Left **B** Parotid Duct, Right **C** Parotid Duct, Left **D** Sublingual Gland, Right	**0** Open **3** Percutaneous	**Z** No Device	**X** Diagnostic **Z** No Qualifier Continued on Next Page ▶

F Sublingual Gland, Left			Continued from
G Submaxillary Gland, Right			◄ Previous Page
H Submaxillary Gland, Left			
J Minor Salivary Gland			
M Pharynx	0 Open	Z No Device	X Diagnostic
R Epiglottis	3 Percutaneous		Z No Qualifier
S Larynx	4 Percutaneous Endoscopic		
T Vocal Cord, Right	7 Via Natural or Artificial Opening		
V Vocal Cord, Left	8 Via Natural or Artificial Opening Endoscopic		
W Upper Tooth	0 Open	Z No Device	0 Single
X Lower Tooth	X External		1 Multiple
			2 All

Section	0	Medical and Surgical	
Body System	C	Mouth and Throat	
Operation	C	Extirpation: Taking or cutting out solid matter from a body part	

Body Part (Character 4)	Approach (Character 5)	Device (Character 6)	Qualifier (Character 7)
0 Upper Lip	0 Open	Z No Device	Z No Qualifier
1 Lower Lip	3 Percutaneous		
2 Hard Palate	X External		
3 Soft Palate			
4 Buccal Mucosa			
5 Upper Gingiva			
6 Lower Gingiva			
7 Tongue			
N Uvula			
P Tonsils			
Q Adenoids			
8 Parotid Gland, Right	0 Open	Z No Device	Z No Qualifier
9 Parotid Gland, Left	3 Percutaneous		
B Parotid Duct, Right			
C Parotid Duct, Left			
D Sublingual Gland, Right			
F Sublingual Gland, Left			
G Submaxillary Gland, Right			
H Submaxillary Gland, Left			
J Minor Salivary Gland			
M Pharynx	0 Open	Z No Device	Z No Qualifier
R Epiglottis	3 Percutaneous		
S Larynx	4 Percutaneous Endoscopic		
T Vocal Cord, Right	7 Via Natural or Artificial Opening		
V Vocal Cord, Left	8 Via Natural or Artificial Opening Endoscopic		
W Upper Tooth	0 Open	Z No Device	0 Single
X Lower Tooth	X External		1 Multiple
			2 All

Section	0	Medical and Surgical		
Body System	C	Mouth and Throat		
Operation	D	Extraction: Pulling or stripping out or off all or a portion of a body part by the use of force		
Body Part (Character 4)	Approach (Character 5)		Device (Character 6)	Qualifier (Character 7)
T Vocal Cord, Right V Vocal Cord, Left	0 Open 3 Percutaneous 4 Percutaneous Endoscopic 7 Via Natural or Artificial Opening 8 Via Natural or Artificial Opening Endoscopic		Z No Device	Z No Qualifier
W Upper Tooth X Lower Tooth	X External		Z No Device	0 Single 1 Multiple 2 All

Section	0	Medical and Surgical		
Body System	C	Mouth and Throat		
Operation	F	Fragmentation: Breaking solid matter in a body part into pieces		
Body Part (Character 4)	Approach (Character 5)		Device (Character 6)	Qualifier (Character 7)
B Parotid Duct, Right C Parotid Duct, Left	0 Open 3 Percutaneous 7 Via Natural or Artificial Opening X External		Z No Device	Z No Qualifier

Section	0	Medical and Surgical		
Body System	C	Mouth and Throat		
Operation	H	Insertion: Putting in a nonbiological appliance that monitors, assists, performs, or prevents a physiological function but does not physically take the place of a body part		
Body Part (Character 4)	Approach (Character 5)		Device (Character 6)	Qualifier (Character 7)
7 Tongue	0 Open 3 Percutaneous X External		1 Radioactive Element	Z No Qualifier
Y Mouth and Throat	7 Via Natural or Artificial Opening 8 Via Natural or Artificial Opening Endoscopic		B Intraluminal Device, Airway	Z No Qualifier

Section	0	Medical and Surgical		
Body System	C	Mouth and Throat		
Operation	J	Inspection: Visually and/or manually exploring a body part		
Body Part (Character 4)	Approach (Character 5)		Device (Character 6)	Qualifier (Character 7)
A Salivary Gland	0 Open 3 Percutaneous X External		Z No Device	Z No Qualifier
S Larynx Y Mouth and Throat	0 Open 3 Percutaneous 4 Percutaneous Endoscopic 7 Via Natural or Artificial Opening 8 Via Natural or Artificial Opening Endoscopic X External		Z No Device	Z No Qualifier

Section	0	Medical and Surgical		
Body System	C	Mouth and Throat		
Operation	L	Occlusion: Completely closing an orifice or the lumen of a tubular body part		

Body Part (Character 4)	Approach (Character 5)	Device (Character 6)	Qualifier (Character 7)
B Parotid Duct, Right C Parotid Duct, Left	0 Open 3 Percutaneous 4 Percutaneous Endoscopic	C Extraluminal Device D Intraluminal Device Z No Device	Z No Qualifier
B Parotid Duct, Right C Parotid Duct, Left	7 Via Natural or Artificial Opening 8 Via Natural or Artificial Opening Endoscopic	D Intraluminal Device Z No Device	Z No Qualifier

Section	0	Medical and Surgical		
Body System	C	Mouth and Throat		
Operation	M	Reattachment Putting back in or on all or a portion of a separated body part to its normal location or other suitable location		

Body Part (Character 4)	Approach (Character 5)	Device (Character 6)	Qualifier (Character 7)
0 Upper Lip 1 Lower Lip 3 Soft Palate 7 Tongue N Uvula	0 Open	Z No Device	Z No Qualifier
W Upper Tooth X Lower Tooth	0 Open X External	Z No Device	0 Single 1 Multiple 2 All

Section	0	Medical and Surgical		
Body System	C	Mouth and Throat		
Operation	N	Release: Freeing a body part from an abnormal physical constraint by cutting or by the use of force		

Body Part (Character 4)	Approach (Character 5)	Device (Character 6)	Qualifier (Character 7)
0 Upper Lip 1 Lower Lip 2 Hard Palate 3 Soft Palate 4 Buccal Mucosa 5 Upper Gingiva 6 Lower Gingiva 7 Tongue N Uvula P Tonsils Q Adenoids	0 Open 3 Percutaneous X External	Z No Device	Z No Qualifier
8 Parotid Gland, Right 9 Parotid Gland, Left B Parotid Duct, Right C Parotid Duct, Left D Sublingual Gland, Right F Sublingual Gland, Left G Submaxillary Gland, Right H Submaxillary Gland, Left J Minor Salivary Gland	0 Open 3 Percutaneous	Z No Device	Z No Qualifier
M Pharynx R Epiglottis S Larynx	0 Open 3 Percutaneous 4 Percutaneous Endoscopic	Z No Device	Z No Qualifier

Continued on Next Page ▶

T Vocal Cord, Right V Vocal Cord, Left	7 Via Natural or Artificial Opening 8 Via Natural or Artificial Opening Endoscopic		Continued from ◀ Previous Page
W Upper Tooth X Lower Tooth	0 Open X External	Z No Device	0 Single 1 Multiple 2 All

Section	0	Medical and Surgical	
Body System	C	Mouth and Throat	
Operation	P	Removal: Taking out or off a device from a body part	

Body Part (Character 4)	Approach (Character 5)	Device (Character 6)	Qualifier (Character 7)
A Salivary Gland	0 Open 3 Percutaneous	0 Drainage Device C Extraluminal Device	Z No Qualifier
S Larynx	0 Open 3 Percutaneous 7 Via Natural or Artificial Opening 8 Via Natural or Artificial Opening Endoscopic X External	0 Drainage Device 7 Autologous Tissue Substitute D Intraluminal Device J Synthetic Substitute K Nonautologous Tissue Substitute	Z No Qualifier
Y Mouth and Throat	0 Open 3 Percutaneous 7 Via Natural or Artificial Opening 8 Via Natural or Artificial Opening Endoscopic X External	0 Drainage Device 1 Radioactive Element 7 Autologous Tissue Substitute D Intraluminal Device J Synthetic Substitute K Nonautologous Tissue Substitute	Z No Qualifier

Section	0	Medical and Surgical	
Body System	C	Mouth and Throat	
Operation	Q	Repair: Restoring, to the extent possible, a body part to its normal anatomic structure and function	

Body Part (Character 4)	Approach (Character 5)	Device (Character 6)	Qualifier (Character 7)
0 Upper Lip 1 Lower Lip 2 Hard Palate 3 Soft Palate 4 Buccal Mucosa 5 Upper Gingiva 6 Lower Gingiva 7 Tongue N Uvula P Tonsils Q Adenoids	0 Open 3 Percutaneous X External	Z No Device	Z No Qualifier
8 Parotid Gland, Right 9 Parotid Gland, Left B Parotid Duct, Right C Parotid Duct, Left D Sublingual Gland, Right F Sublingual Gland, Left G Submaxillary Gland, Right H Submaxillary Gland, Left J Minor Salivary Gland	0 Open 3 Percutaneous	Z No Device	Z No Qualifier Continued on Next Page ▶

			Continued from ◀ Previous Page
M Pharynx R Epiglottis S Larynx T Vocal Cord, Right V Vocal Cord, Left	0 Open 3 Percutaneous 4 Percutaneous Endoscopic 7 Via Natural or Artificial Opening 8 Via Natural or Artificial Opening Endoscopic	Z No Device	Z No Qualifier
W Upper Tooth X Lower Tooth	0 Open X External	Z No Device	0 Single 1 Multiple 2 All

Section	0	Medical and Surgical
Body System	C	Mouth and Throat
Operation	R	Replacement: Putting in or on biological or synthetic material that physically takes the place and/or function of all or a portion of a body part

Body Part (Character 4)	Approach (Character 5)	Device (Character 6)	Qualifier (Character 7)
0 Upper Lip 1 Lower Lip 2 Hard Palate 3 Soft Palate 4 Buccal Mucosa 5 Upper Gingiva 6 Lower Gingiva 7 Tongue N Uvula	0 Open 3 Percutaneous X External	7 Autologous Tissue Substitute J Synthetic Substitute K Nonautologous Tissue Substitute	Z No Qualifier
B Parotid Duct, Right C Parotid Duct, Left	0 Open 3 Percutaneous	7 Autologous Tissue Substitute J Synthetic Substitute K Nonautologous Tissue Substitute	Z No Qualifier
M Pharynx R Epiglottis S Larynx T Vocal Cord, Right V Vocal Cord, Left	0 Open 7 Via Natural or Artificial Opening 8 Via Natural or Artificial Opening Endoscopic	7 Autologous Tissue Substitute J Synthetic Substitute K Nonautologous Tissue Substitute	Z No Qualifier
W Upper Tooth X Lower Tooth	0 Open X External	7 Autologous Tissue Substitute J Synthetic Substitute K Nonautologous Tissue Substitute	0 Single 1 Multiple 2 All

Section	0	Medical and Surgical		
Body System	C	Mouth and Throat		
Operation	S	Reposition: Moving to its normal location, or other suitable location, all or a portion of a body part		

Body Part (Character 4)	Approach (Character 5)	Device (Character 6)	Qualifier (Character 7)
0 Upper Lip 1 Lower Lip 2 Hard Palate 3 Soft Palate 7 Tongue N Uvula	0 Open X External	Z No Device	Z No Qualifier
B Parotid Duct, Right C Parotid Duct, Left	0 Open 3 Percutaneous	Z No Device	Z No Qualifier
R Epiglottis T Vocal Cord, Right V Vocal Cord, Left	0 Open 7 Via Natural or Artificial Opening 8 Via Natural or Artificial Opening Endoscopic	Z No Device	Z No Qualifier
W Upper Tooth X Lower Tooth	0 Open X External	5 External Fixation Device Z No Device	0 Single 1 Multiple 2 All

Section	0	Medical and Surgical		
Body System	C	Mouth and Throat		
Operation	T	Resection: Cutting out or off, without replacement, all of a body part		

Body Part (Character 4)	Approach (Character 5)	Device (Character 6)	Qualifier (Character 7)
0 Upper Lip 1 Lower Lip 2 Hard Palate 3 Soft Palate 7 Tongue N Uvula P Tonsils Q Adenoids	0 Open X External	Z No Device	Z No Qualifier
8 Parotid Gland, Right 9 Parotid Gland, Left B Parotid Duct, Right C Parotid Duct, Left D Sublingual Gland, Right F Sublingual Gland, Left G Submaxillary Gland, Right H Submaxillary Gland, Left J Minor Salivary Gland	0 Open	Z No Device	Z No Qualifier
M Pharynx R Epiglottis S Larynx T Vocal Cord, Right V Vocal Cord, Left	0 Open 4 Percutaneous Endoscopic 7 Via Natural or Artificial Opening 8 Via Natural or Artificial Opening Endoscopic	Z No Device	Z No Qualifier
W Upper Tooth X Lower Tooth	0 Open	Z No Device	0 Single 1 Multiple 2 All

Section	0	Medical and Surgical		
Body System	C	Mouth and Throat		
Operation	U	Supplement: Putting in or on biological or synthetic material that physically reinforces and/or augments the function of a portion of a body part		

Body Part (Character 4)	Approach (Character 5)	Device (Character 6)	Qualifier (Character 7)
0 Upper Lip 1 Lower Lip 2 Hard Palate 3 Soft Palate 4 Buccal Mucosa 5 Upper Gingiva 6 Lower Gingiva 7 Tongue N Uvula	0 Open 3 Percutaneous X External	7 Autologous Tissue Substitute J Synthetic Substitute K Nonautologous Tissue Substitute	Z No Qualifier
M Pharynx R Epiglottis S Larynx T Vocal Cord, Right V Vocal Cord, Left	0 Open 7 Via Natural or Artificial Opening 8 Via Natural or Artificial Opening Endoscopic	7 Autologous Tissue Substitute J Synthetic Substitute K Nonautologous Tissue Substitute	Z No Qualifier

Section	0	Medical and Surgical		
Body System	C	Mouth and Throat		
Operation	V	Restriction: Partially closing an orifice or the lumen of a tubular body part		

Body Part (Character 4)	Approach (Character 5)	Device (Character 6)	Qualifier (Character 7)
B Parotid Duct, Right C Parotid Duct, Left	0 Open 3 Percutaneous	C Extraluminal Device D Intraluminal Device Z No Device	Z No Qualifier
B Parotid Duct, Right C Parotid Duct, Left	7 Via Natural or Artificial Opening 8 Via Natural or Artificial Opening Endoscopic	D Intraluminal Device Z No Device	Z No Qualifier

Section	0	Medical and Surgical		
Body System	C	Mouth and Throat		
Operation	W	Revision: Correcting, to the extent possible, a portion of a malfunctioning device or the position of a displaced device		

Body Part (Character 4)	Approach (Character 5)	Device (Character 6)	Qualifier (Character 7)
A Salivary Gland	0 Open 3 Percutaneous X External	0 Drainage Device C Extraluminal Device	Z No Qualifier
S Larynx	0 Open 3 Percutaneous 7 Via Natural or Artificial Opening 8 Via Natural or Artificial Opening Endoscopic X External	0 Drainage Device 7 Autologous Tissue Substitute D Intraluminal Device J Synthetic Substitute K Nonautologous Tissue Substitute	Z No Qualifier
Y Mouth and Throat	0 Open 3 Percutaneous 7 Via Natural or Artificial Opening 8 Via Natural or Artificial Opening Endoscopic X External	0 Drainage Device 1 Radioactive Element 7 Autologous Tissue Substitute D Intraluminal Device J Synthetic Substitute K Nonautologous Tissue Substitute	Z No Qualifier

Section	0	Medical and Surgical		
Body System	C	Mouth and Throat		
Operation	X	Transfer: Moving, without taking out, all or a portion of a body part to another location to take over the function of all or a portion of a body part		

Body Part (Character 4)	Approach (Character 5)	Device (Character 6)	Qualifier (Character 7)
0 Upper Lip 1 Lower Lip 3 Soft Palate 4 Buccal Mucosa 5 Upper Gingiva 6 Lower Gingiva 7 Tongue	0 Open X External	Z No Device	Z No Qualifier

Section	0	Medical and Surgical	
Body System	D	Gastrointestinal System	
Operation	1	Bypass: Altering the route of passage of the contents of a tubular body part	

Body Part (Character 4)	Approach (Character 5)	Device (Character 6)	Qualifier (Character 7)
1 Esophagus, Upper 2 Esophagus, Middle 3 Esophagus, Lower 5 Esophagus	0 Open 4 Percutaneous Endoscopic 8 Via Natural or Artificial Opening Endoscopic	7 Autologous Tissue Substitute J Synthetic Substitute K Nonautologous Tissue Substitute Z No Device	4 Cutaneous 6 Stomach 9 Duodenum A Jejunum B Ileum
1 Esophagus, Upper 2 Esophagus, Middle 3 Esophagus, Lower 5 Esophagus	3 Percutaneous	J Synthetic Substitute	4 Cutaneous
6 Stomach 9 Duodenum	0 Open 4 Percutaneous Endoscopic 8 Via Natural or Artificial Opening Endoscopic	7 Autologous Tissue Substitute J Synthetic Substitute K Nonautologous Tissue Substitute Z No Device	4 Cutaneous 9 Duodenum A Jejunum B Ileum L Transverse Colon
6 Stomach 9 Duodenum	3 Percutaneous	J Synthetic Substitute	4 Cutaneous
A Jejunum	0 Open 4 Percutaneous Endoscopic 8 Via Natural or Artificial Opening Endoscopic	7 Autologous Tissue Substitute J Synthetic Substitute K Nonautologous Tissue Substitute Z No Device	4 Cutaneous A Jejunum B Ileum H Cecum K Ascending Colon L Transverse Colon M Descending Colon N Sigmoid Colon P Rectum Q Anus
A Jejunum	3 Percutaneous	J Synthetic Substitute	4 Cutaneous
B Ileum	0 Open 4 Percutaneous Endoscopic 8 Via Natural or Artificial Opening Endoscopic	7 Autologous Tissue Substitute J Synthetic Substitute K Nonautologous Tissue Substitute Z No Device	4 Cutaneous B Ileum H Cecum K Ascending Colon L Transverse Colon M Descending Colon N Sigmoid Colon P Rectum Q Anus
B Ileum	3 Percutaneous	J Synthetic Substitute	4 Cutaneous
H Cecum	0 Open 4 Percutaneous Endoscopic 8 Via Natural or Artificial Opening Endoscopic	7 Autologous Tissue Substitute J Synthetic Substitute K Nonautologous Tissue Substitute Z No Device	4 Cutaneous H Cecum K Ascending Colon L Transverse Colon M Descending Colon N Sigmoid Colon P Rectum
H Cecum	3 Percutaneous	J Synthetic Substitute	4 Cutaneous
K Ascending Colon	0 Open 4 Percutaneous Endoscopic 8 Via Natural or Artificial	7 Autologous Tissue Substitute J Synthetic Substitute	4 Cutancous K Ascending Colon

Continued on Next Page ▶

	Opening Endoscopic	K Nonautologous Tissue Substitute Z No Device	Continued from ◀ Previous Page L Transverse Colon M Descending Colon N Sigmoid Colon P Rectum
K Ascending Colon	3 Percutaneous	J Synthetic Substitute	4 Cutaneous
L Transverse Colon	0 Open 4 Percutaneous Endoscopic 8 Via Natural or Artificial Opening Endoscopic	7 Autologous Tissue Substitute J Synthetic Substitute K Nonautologous Tissue Substitute Z No Device	4 Cutaneous L Transverse Colon M Descending Colon N Sigmoid Colon P Rectum
L Transverse Colon	3 Percutaneous	J Synthetic Substitute	4 Cutaneous
M Descending Colon	0 Open 4 Percutaneous Endoscopic 8 Via Natural or Artificial Opening Endoscopic	7 Autologous Tissue Substitute J Synthetic Substitute K Nonautologous Tissue Substitute Z No Device	4 Cutaneous M Descending Colon N Sigmoid Colon P Rectum
M Descending Colon	3 Percutaneous	J Synthetic Substitute	4 Cutaneous
N Sigmoid Colon	0 Open 4 Percutaneous Endoscopic 8 Via Natural or Artificial Opening Endoscopic	7 Autologous Tissue Substitute J Synthetic Substitute K Nonautologous Tissue Substitute Z No Device	4 Cutaneous N Sigmoid Colon P Rectum
N Sigmoid Colon	3 Percutaneous	J Synthetic Substitute	4 Cutaneous

Section	0	Medical and Surgical
Body System	D	Gastrointestinal System
Operation	2	Change: Taking out or off a device from a body part and putting back an identical or similar device in or on the same body part without cutting or puncturing the skin or a mucous membrane

Body Part (Character 4)	Approach (Character 5)	Device (Character 6)	Qualifier (Character 7)
0 Upper Intestinal Tract D Lower Intestinal Tract	X External	0 Drainage Device U Feeding Device Y Other Device	Z No Qualifier
U Omentum V Mesentery W Peritoneum	X External	0 Drainage Device Y Other Device	Z No Qualifier

Section	0	Medical and Surgical
Body System	D	Gastrointestinal System
Operation	5	Destruction: Physical eradication of all or a portion of a body part by the direct use of energy, force, or a destructive agent

Body Part (Character 4)	Approach (Character 5)	Device (Character 6)	Qualifier (Character 7)
1 Esophagus, Upper 2 Esophagus, Middle 3 Esophagus, Lower 4 Esophagogastric Junction 5 Esophagus 6 Stomach 7 Stomach, Pylorus 8 Small Intestine	0 Open 3 Percutaneous 4 Percutaneous Endoscopic 7 Via Natural or Artificial Opening 8 Via Natural or Artificial Opening Endoscopic	Z No Device	Z No Qualifier Continued on Next Page ▶

			Continued from ◀ Previous Page
9 Duodenum A Jejunum B Ileum C Ileocecal Valve E Large Intestine F Large Intestine, Right G Large Intestine, Left H Cecum J Appendix K Ascending Colon L Transverse Colon M Descending Colon N Sigmoid Colon P Rectum			
Q Anus	0 Open 3 Percutaneous 4 Percutaneous Endoscopic 7 Via Natural or Artificial Opening 8 Via Natural or Artificial Opening Endoscopic X External	Z No Device	Z No Qualifier
R Anal Sphincter S Greater Omentum T Lesser Omentum V Mesentery W Peritoneum	0 Open 3 Percutaneous 4 Percutaneous Endoscopic	Z No Device	Z No Qualifier

Section	0	Medical and Surgical
Body System	D	Gastrointestinal System
Operation	7	Dilation: Expanding an orifice or the lumen of a tubular body part

Body Part (Character 4)	Approach (Character 5)	Device (Character 6)	Qualifier (Character 7)
1 Esophagus, Upper 2 Esophagus, Middle 3 Esophagus, Lower 4 Esophagogastric Junction 5 Esophagus 6 Stomach 7 Stomach, Pylorus 8 Small Intestine 9 Duodenum A Jejunum B Ileum C Ileocecal Valve E Large Intestine F Large Intestine, Right G Large Intestine, Left H Cecum K Ascending Colon L Transverse Colon M Descending Colon N Sigmoid Colon P Rectum Q Anus	0 Open 3 Percutaneous 4 Percutaneous Endoscopic 7 Via Natural or Artificial Opening 8 Via Natural or Artificial Opening Endoscopic	D Intraluminal Device Z No Device	Z No Qualifier

Section	0	Medical and Surgical		
Body System	D	Gastrointestinal System		
Operation	8	Division: Cutting into a body part, without draining fluids and/or gases from the body part, in order to separate or transect a body part		

Body Part (Character 4)	Approach (Character 5)	Device (Character 6)	Qualifier (Character 7)
4 Esophagogastric Junction 7 Stomach, Pylorus	0 Open 3 Percutaneous 4 Percutaneous Endoscopic 7 Via Natural or Artificial Opening 8 Via Natural or Artificial Opening Endoscopic	Z No Device	Z No Qualifier
R Anal Sphincter	0 Open 3 Percutaneous	Z No Device	Z No Qualifier

Section	0	Medical and Surgical		
Body System	D	Gastrointestinal System		
Operation	9	Drainage: Taking or letting out fluids and/or gases from a body part		

Body Part (Character 4)	Approach (Character 5)	Device (Character 6)	Qualifier (Character 7)
1 Esophagus, Upper 2 Esophagus, Middle 3 Esophagus, Lower 4 Esophagogastric Junction 5 Esophagus 6 Stomach 7 Stomach, Pylorus 8 Small Intestine 9 Duodenum A Jejunum B Ileum C Ileocecal Valve E Large Intestine F Large Intestine, Right G Large Intestine, Left H Cecum J Appendix K Ascending Colon L Transverse Colon M Descending Colon N Sigmoid Colon P Rectum	0 Open 3 Percutaneous 4 Percutaneous Endoscopic 7 Via Natural or Artificial Opening 8 Via Natural or Artificial Opening Endoscopic	0 Drainage Device	Z No Qualifier
1 Esophagus, Upper 2 Esophagus, Middle 3 Esophagus, Lower 4 Esophagogastric Junction 5 Esophagus 6 Stomach 7 Stomach, Pylorus 8 Small Intestine 9 Duodenum A Jejunum B Ileum C Ileocecal Valve E Large Intestine	0 Open 3 Percutaneous 4 Percutaneous Endoscopic 7 Via Natural or Artificial Opening 8 Via Natural or Artificial Opening Endoscopic	Z No Device	X Diagnostic Z No Qualifier

Continued on Next Page ▶

			Continued from ◀ Previous Page
F Large Intestine, Right **G** Large Intestine, Left **H** Cecum **J** Appendix **K** Ascending Colon **L** Transverse Colon **M** Descending Colon **N** Sigmoid Colon **P** Rectum			
Q Anus	**0** Open **3** Percutaneous **4** Percutaneous Endoscopic **7** Via Natural or Artificial Opening **8** Via Natural or Artificial Opening Endoscopic **X** External	**0** Drainage Device	**Z** No Qualifier
Q Anus	**0** Open **3** Percutaneous **4** Percutaneous Endoscopic **7** Via Natural or Artificial Opening **8** Via Natural or Artificial Opening Endoscopic **X** External	**Z** No Device	**X** Diagnostic **Z** No Qualifier
R Anal Sphincter **S** Greater Omentum **T** Lesser Omentum **V** Mesentery **W** Peritoneum	**0** Open **3** Percutaneous **4** Percutaneous Endoscopic	**0** Drainage Device	**Z** No Qualifier
R Anal Sphincter **S** Greater Omentum **T** Lesser Omentum **V** Mesentery **W** Peritoneum	**0** Open **3** Percutaneous **4** Percutaneous Endoscopic	**Z** No Device	**X** Diagnostic **Z** No Qualifier

Section	0	Medical and Surgical
Body System	**D**	**Gastrointestinal System**
Operation	**B**	**Excision: Cutting out or off, without replacement, a portion of a body part**

Body Part (Character 4)	Approach (Character 5)	Device (Character 6)	Qualifier (Character 7)
1 Esophagus, Upper **2** Esophagus, Middle **3** Esophagus, Lower **4** Esophagogastric Junction **5** Esophagus **7** Stomach, Pylorus **8** Small Intestine **9** Duodenum **A** Jejunum **B** Ileum **C** Ileocecal Valve **E** Large Intestine **F** Large Intestine, Right **G** Large Intestine, Left	**0** Open **3** Percutaneous **4** Percutaneous Endoscopic **7** Via Natural or Artificial Opening **8** Via Natural or Artificial Opening Endoscopic	**Z** No Device	**X** Diagnostic **Z** No Qualifier
			Continued on Next Page ▶

			Continued from ◀ Previous Page
H Cecum J Appendix K Ascending Colon L Transverse Colon M Descending Colon N Sigmoid Colon P Rectum			
6 Stomach	0 Open 3 Percutaneous 4 Percutaneous Endoscopic 7 Via Natural or Artificial Opening 8 Via Natural or Artificial Opening Endoscopic	Z No Device	3 Vertical X Diagnostic Z No Qualifier
Q Anus	0 Open 3 Percutaneous 4 Percutaneous Endoscopic 7 Via Natural or Artificial Opening 8 Via Natural or Artificial Opening Endoscopic X External	Z No Device	X Diagnostic Z No Qualifier
R Anal Sphincter S Greater Omentum T Lesser Omentum V Mesentery W Peritoneum	0 Open 3 Percutaneous 4 Percutaneous Endoscopic	Z No Device	X Diagnostic Z No Qualifier

Section	0	Medical and Surgical
Body System	D	Gastrointestinal System
Operation	C	Extirpation: Taking or cutting out solid matter from a body part

Body Part (Character 4)	Approach (Character 5)	Device (Character 6)	Qualifier (Character 7)
1 Esophagus, Upper 2 Esophagus, Middle 3 Esophagus, Lower 4 Esophagogastric Junction 5 Esophagus 6 Stomach 7 Stomach, Pylorus 8 Small Intestine 9 Duodenum A Jejunum B Ileum C Ileocecal Valve E Large Intestine F Large Intestine, Right G Large Intestine, Left H Cecum J Appendix K Ascending Colon L Transverse Colon M Descending Colon N Sigmoid Colon P Rectum	0 Open 3 Percutaneous 4 Percutaneous Endoscopic 7 Via Natural or Artificial Opening 8 Via Natural or Artificial Opening Endoscopic	Z No Device	Z No Qualifier

Continued on Next Page ▶

			Continued from ◀ Previous Page
Q Anus	**0** Open **3** Percutaneous **4** Percutaneous Endoscopic **7** Via Natural or Artificial Opening **8** Via Natural or Artificial Opening Endoscopic **X** External	**Z** No Device	**Z** No Qualifier
R Anal Sphincter **S** Greater Omentum **T** Lesser Omentum **V** Mesentery **W** Peritoneum	**0** Open **3** Percutaneous **4** Percutaneous Endoscopic	**Z** No Device	**Z** No Qualifier

Section	0	Medical and Surgical	
Body System	D	Gastrointestinal System	
Operation	F	Fragmentation: Breaking solid matter in a body part into pieces	

Body Part (Character 4)	Approach (Character 5)	Device (Character 6)	Qualifier (Character 7)
5 Esophagus **6** Stomach **8** Small Intestine **9** Duodenum **A** Jejunum **B** Ileum **E** Large Intestine **F** Large Intestine, Right **G** Large Intestine, Left **H** Cecum **J** Appendix **K** Ascending Colon **L** Transverse Colon **M** Descending Colon **N** Sigmoid Colon **P** Rectum **Q** Anus	**0** Open **3** Percutaneous **4** Percutaneous Endoscopic **7** Via Natural or Artificial Opening **8** Via Natural or Artificial Opening Endoscopic **X** External	**Z** No Device	**Z** No Qualifier

Section	0	Medical and Surgical	
Body System	D	Gastrointestinal System	
Operation	H	Insertion: Putting in a nonbiological appliance that monitors, assists, performs, or prevents a physiological function but does not physically take the place of a body part	

Body Part (Character 4)	Approach (Character 5)	Device (Character 6)	Qualifier (Character 7)
5 Esophagus	**0** Open **3** Percutaneous **4** Percutaneous Endoscopic	**1** Radioactive Element **2** Monitoring Device **3** Infusion Device **D** Intraluminal Device **U** Feeding Device	**Z** No Qualifier
5 Esophagus	**7** Via Natural or Artificial Opening **8** Via Natural or Artificial Opening Endoscopic	**1** Radioactive Element **2** Monitoring Device **3** Infusion Device **B** Intraluminal Device, Airway **D** Intraluminal Device **U** Feeding Device	**Z** No Qualifier **Continued on Next Page ▶**

			Continued from ◀ Previous Page
6 Stomach	**0** Open **3** Percutaneous **4** Percutaneous Endoscopic	**2** Monitoring Device **3** Infusion Device **D** Intraluminal Device **M** Stimulator Lead **U** Feeding Device	**Z** No Qualifier
6 Stomach	**7** Via Natural or Artificial Opening **8** Via Natural or Artificial Opening Endoscopic	**2** Monitoring Device **3** Infusion Device **D** Intraluminal Device **U** Feeding Device	**Z** No Qualifier
8 Small Intestine **9** Duodenum **A** Jejunum **B** Ileum	**0** Open **3** Percutaneous **4** Percutaneous Endoscopic **7** Via Natural or Artificial Opening **8** Via Natural or Artificial Opening Endoscopic	**2** Monitoring Device **3** Infusion Device **D** Intraluminal Device **U** Feeding Device	**Z** No Qualifier
E Large Intestine	**0** Open **3** Percutaneous **4** Percutaneous Endoscopic **7** Via Natural or Artificial Opening **8** Via Natural or Artificial Opening Endoscopic	**D** Intraluminal Device	**Z** No Qualifier
P Rectum	**0** Open **3** Percutaneous **4** Percutaneous Endoscopic **7** Via Natural or Artificial Opening **8** Via Natural or Artificial Opening Endoscopic	**1** Radioactive Element **D** Intraluminal Device	**Z** No Qualifier
Q Anus	**0** Open **3** Percutaneous **4** Percutaneous Endoscopic	**D** Intraluminal Device **L** Artificial Sphincter	**Z** No Qualifier
Q Anus	**7** Via Natural or Artificial Opening **8** Via Natural or Artificial Opening Endoscopic	**D** Intraluminal Device	**Z** No Qualifier
R Anal Sphincter	**0** Open **3** Percutaneous **4** Percutaneous Endoscopic	**M** Stimulator Lead	**Z** No Qualifier

Section	0	Medical and Surgical		
Body System	D	Gastrointestinal System		
Operation	J	Inspection: Visually and/or manually exploring a body part		

Body Part (Character 4)	Approach (Character 5)	Device (Character 6)	Qualifier (Character 7)
0 Upper Intestinal Tract **6** Stomach **D** Lower Intestinal Tract	**0** Open **3** Percutaneous **4** Percutaneous Endoscopic **7** Via Natural or Artificial Opening **8** Via Natural or Artificial Opening Endoscopic **X** External	**Z** No Device	**Z** No Qualifier
U Omentum **V** Mesentery **W** Peritoneum	**0** Open **3** Percutaneous **4** Percutaneous Endoscopic **X** External	**Z** No Device	**Z** No Qualifier

Section	0	Medical and Surgical		
Body System	D	Gastrointestinal System		
Operation	L	Occlusion: Completely closing an orifice or the lumen of a tubular body part		

Body Part (Character 4)	Approach (Character 5)	Device (Character 6)	Qualifier (Character 7)
1 Esophagus, Upper **2** Esophagus, Middle **3** Esophagus, Lower **4** Esophagogastric Junction **5** Esophagus **6** Stomach **7** Stomach, Pylorus **8** Small Intestine **9** Duodenum **A** Jejunum **B** Ileum **C** Ileocecal Valve **E** Large Intestine **F** Large Intestine, Right **G** Large Intestine, Left **H** Cecum **K** Ascending Colon **L** Transverse Colon **M** Descending Colon **N** Sigmoid Colon **P** Rectum	**0** Open **3** Percutaneous **4** Percutaneous Endoscopic	**C** Extraluminal Device **D** Intraluminal Device **Z** No Device	**Z** No Qualifier
1 Esophagus, Upper **2** Esophagus, Middle **3** Esophagus, Lower **4** Esophagogastric Junction **5** Esophagus **6** Stomach **7** Stomach, Pylorus **8** Small Intestine **9** Duodenum **A** Jejunum **B** Ileum **C** Ileocecal Valve	**7** Via Natural or Artificial Opening **8** Via Natural or Artificial Opening Endoscopic	**D** Intraluminal Device **Z** No Device	**Z** No Qualifier

Continued on Next Page ▶

E Large Intestine			Continued from
F Large Intestine, Right			◀ Previous Page
G Large Intestine, Left			
H Cecum			
K Ascending Colon			
L Transverse Colon			
M Descending Colon			
N Sigmoid Colon			
P Rectum			
Q Anus	0 Open	C Extraluminal Device	Z No Qualifier
	3 Percutaneous	D Intraluminal Device	
	4 Percutaneous Endoscopic	Z No Device	
	X External		
Q Anus	7 Via Natural or Artificial Opening	D Intraluminal Device	Z No Qualifier
	8 Via Natural or Artificial Opening Endoscopic	Z No Device	

Section	0	Medical and Surgical
Body System	D	Gastrointestinal System
Operation	M	Reattachment Putting back in or on all or a portion of a separated body part to its normal location or other suitable location

Body Part (Character 4)	Approach (Character 5)	Device (Character 6)	Qualifier (Character 7)
5 Esophagus	0 Open	Z No Device	Z No Qualifier
6 Stomach	4 Percutaneous Endoscopic		
8 Small Intestine			
9 Duodenum			
A Jejunum			
B Ileum			
E Large Intestine			
F Large Intestine, Right			
G Large Intestine, Left			
H Cecum			
K Ascending Colon			
L Transverse Colon			
M Descending Colon			
N Sigmoid Colon			
P Rectum			

Section	0	Medical and Surgical
Body System	D	Gastrointestinal System
Operation	N	Release: Freeing a body part from an abnormal physical constraint by cutting or by the use of force

Body Part (Character 4)	Approach (Character 5)	Device (Character 6)	Qualifier (Character 7)
1 Esophagus, Upper	0 Open	Z No Device	Z No Qualifier
2 Esophagus, Middle	3 Percutaneous		
3 Esophagus, Lower	4 Percutaneous Endoscopic		
4 Esophagogastric Junction	7 Via Natural or Artificial Opening		
5 Esophagus	8 Via Natural or Artificial Opening Endoscopic		
6 Stomach			
7 Stomach, Pylorus			
8 Small Intestine			
9 Duodenum			
A Jejunum			Continued on Next Page ▶

			Continued from ◀ Previous Page
B Ileum **C** Ileocecal Valve **E** Large Intestine **F** Large Intestine, Right **G** Large Intestine, Left **H** Cecum **J** Appendix **K** Ascending Colon **L** Transverse Colon **M** Descending Colon **N** Sigmoid Colon **P** Rectum			
Q Anus	**0** Open **3** Percutaneous **4** Percutaneous Endoscopic **7** Via Natural or Artificial Opening **8** Via Natural or Artificial Opening Endoscopic **X** External	**Z** No Device	**Z** No Qualifier
R Anal Sphincter **S** Greater Omentum **T** Lesser Omentum **V** Mesentery **W** Peritoneum	**0** Open **3** Percutaneous **4** Percutaneous Endoscopic	**Z** No Device	**Z** No Qualifier

Section	0	Medical and Surgical	
Body System	**D**	**Gastrointestinal System**	
Operation	**P**	**Removal: Taking out or off a device from a body part**	

Body Part (Character 4)	Approach (Character 5)	Device (Character 6)	Qualifier (Character 7)
0 Upper Intestinal Tract **D** Lower Intestinal Tract	**0** Open **3** Percutaneous **4** Percutaneous Endoscopic **7** Via Natural or Artificial Opening **8** Via Natural or Artificial Opening Endoscopic	**0** Drainage Device **2** Monitoring Device **3** Infusion Device **7** Autologous Tissue Substitute **C** Extraluminal Device **D** Intraluminal Device **J** Synthetic Substitute **K** Nonautologous Tissue Substitute **U** Feeding Device	**Z** No Qualifier
0 Upper Intestinal Tract **D** Lower Intestinal Tract	**X** External	**0** Drainage Device **2** Monitoring Device **3** Infusion Device **D** Intraluminal Device **U** Feeding Device	**Z** No Qualifier
5 Esophagus	**0** Open **3** Percutaneous **4** Percutaneous Endoscopic	**1** Radioactive Element **2** Monitoring Device **3** Infusion Device **U** Feeding Device	**Z** No Qualifier
5 Esophagus	**7** Via Natural or Artificial Opening **8** Via Natural or Artificial Opening Endoscopic	**1** Radioactive Element **D** Intraluminal Device	**Z** No Qualifier

Continued on Next Page ▶

			Continued from ◀ Previous Page
5 Esophagus	**X** External	**1** Radioactive Element **2** Monitoring Device **3** Infusion Device **D** Intraluminal Device **U** Feeding Device	**Z** No Qualifier
6 Stomach	**0** Open **3** Percutaneous **4** Percutaneous Endoscopic	**0** Drainage Device **2** Monitoring Device **3** Infusion Device **7** Autologous Tissue Substitute **C** Extraluminal Device **D** Intraluminal Device **J** Synthetic Substitute **K** Nonautologous Tissue Substitute **M** Stimulator Lead **U** Feeding Device	**Z** No Qualifier
6 Stomach	**7** Via Natural or Artificial Opening **8** Via Natural or Artificial Opening Endoscopic	**0** Drainage Device **2** Monitoring Device **3** Infusion Device **7** Autologous Tissue Substitute **C** Extraluminal Device **D** Intraluminal Device **J** Synthetic Substitute **K** Nonautologous Tissue Substitute **U** Feeding Device	**Z** No Qualifier
6 Stomach	**X** External	**0** Drainage Device **2** Monitoring Device **3** Infusion Device **D** Intraluminal Device **U** Feeding Device	**Z** No Qualifier
P Rectum	**0** Open **3** Percutaneous **4** Percutaneous Endoscopic **7** Via Natural or Artificial Opening **8** Via Natural or Artificial Opening Endoscopic **X** External	**1** Radioactive Element	**Z** No Qualifier
Q Anus	**0** Open **3** Percutaneous **4** Percutaneous Endoscopic **7** Via Natural or Artificial Opening **8** Via Natural or Artificial Opening Endoscopic	**L** Artificial Sphincter	**Z** No Qualifier
R Anal Sphincter	**0** Open **3** Percutaneous **4** Percutaneous Endoscopic	**M** Stimulator Lead	**Z** No Qualifier

Continued on Next Page ▶

			Continued from ◀ Previous Page
U Omentum V Mesentery W Peritoneum	0 Open 3 Percutaneous 4 Percutaneous Endoscopic	0 Drainage Device 1 Radioactive Element 7 Autologous Tissue Substitute J Synthetic Substitute K Nonautologous Tissue Substitute	Z No Qualifier

Section	0	Medical and Surgical
Body System	D	Gastrointestinal System
Operation	Q	Repair: Restoring, to the extent possible, a body part to its normal anatomic structure and function

Body Part (Character 4)	Approach (Character 5)	Device (Character 6)	Qualifier (Character 7)
1 Esophagus, Upper 2 Esophagus, Middle 3 Esophagus, Lower 4 Esophagogastric Junction 5 Esophagus 6 Stomach 7 Stomach, Pylorus 8 Small Intestine 9 Duodenum A Jejunum B Ileum C Ileocecal Valve E Large Intestine F Large Intestine, Right G Large Intestine, Left H Cecum J Appendix K Ascending Colon L Transverse Colon M Descending Colon N Sigmoid Colon P Rectum	0 Open 3 Percutaneous 4 Percutaneous Endoscopic 7 Via Natural or Artificial Opening 8 Via Natural or Artificial Opening Endoscopic	Z No Device	Z No Qualifier
Q Anus	0 Open 3 Percutaneous 4 Percutaneous Endoscopic 7 Via Natural or Artificial Opening 8 Via Natural or Artificial Opening Endoscopic X External	Z No Device	Z No Qualifier
R Anal Sphincter S Greater Omentum T Lesser Omentum V Mesentery W Peritoneum	0 Open 3 Percutaneous 4 Percutaneous Endoscopic	Z No Device	Z No Qualifier

Section	0	Medical and Surgical		
Body System	D	Gastrointestinal System		
Operation	R	Replacement: Putting in or on biological or synthetic material that physically takes the place and/or function of all or a portion of a body part		

Body Part (Character 4)	Approach (Character 5)	Device (Character 6)	Qualifier (Character 7)
5 Esophagus	0 Open 4 Percutaneous Endoscopic 7 Via Natural or Artificial Opening 8 Via Natural or Artificial Opening Endoscopic	7 Autologous Tissue Substitute J Synthetic Substitute K Nonautologous Tissue Substitute	Z No Qualifier
R Anal Sphincter S Greater Omentum T Lesser Omentum V Mesentery W Peritoneum	0 Open 4 Percutaneous Endoscopic	7 Autologous Tissue Substitute J Synthetic Substitute K Nonautologous Tissue Substitute	Z No Qualifier

Section	0	Medical and Surgical		
Body System	D	Gastrointestinal System		
Operation	S	Reposition: Moving to its normal location, or other suitable location, all or a portion of a body part		

Body Part (Character 4)	Approach (Character 5)	Device (Character 6)	Qualifier (Character 7)
5 Esophagus 6 Stomach 9 Duodenum A Jejunum B Ileum H Cecum K Ascending Colon L Transverse Colon M Descending Colon N Sigmoid Colon P Rectum Q Anus	0 Open 4 Percutaneous Endoscopic 7 Via Natural or Artificial Opening 8 Via Natural or Artificial Opening Endoscopic X External	Z No Device	Z No Qualifier

Section	0	Medical and Surgical		
Body System	D	Gastrointestinal System		
Operation	T	Resection: Cutting out or off, without replacement, all of a body part		

Body Part (Character 4)	Approach (Character 5)	Device (Character 6)	Qualifier (Character 7)
1 Esophagus, Upper 2 Esophagus, Middle 3 Esophagus, Lower 4 Esophagogastric Junction 5 Esophagus 6 Stomach 7 Stomach, Pylorus 8 Small Intestine 9 Duodenum A Jejunum B Ileum C Ileocecal Valve E Large Intestine F Large Intestine, Right G Large Intestine, Left	0 Open 4 Percutaneous Endoscopic 7 Via Natural or Artificial Opening 8 Via Natural or Artificial Opening Endoscopic	Z No Device	Z No Qualifier

Continued on Next Page ▶

			Continued from ◀ Previous Page
H Cecum **J** Appendix **K** Ascending Colon **L** Transverse Colon **M** Descending Colon **N** Sigmoid Colon **P** Rectum **Q** Anus			
R Anal Sphincter **S** Greater Omentum **T** Lesser Omentum	**0** Open **4** Percutaneous Endoscopic	**Z** No Device	**Z** No Qualifier

Section	0	Medical and Surgical
Body System	D	Gastrointestinal System
Operation	U	Supplement: Putting in or on biological or synthetic material that physically reinforces and/or augments the function of a portion of a body part

Body Part (Character 4)	Approach (Character 5)	Device (Character 6)	Qualifier (Character 7)
1 Esophagus, Upper **2** Esophagus, Middle **3** Esophagus, Lower **4** Esophagogastric Junction **5** Esophagus **6** Stomach **7** Stomach, Pylorus **8** Small Intestine **9** Duodenum **A** Jejunum **B** Ileum **C** Ileocecal Valve **E** Large Intestine **F** Large Intestine, Right **G** Large Intestine, Left **H** Cecum **K** Ascending Colon **L** Transverse Colon **M** Descending Colon **N** Sigmoid Colon **P** Rectum	**0** Open **4** Percutaneous Endoscopic **7** Via Natural or Artificial Opening **8** Via Natural or Artificial Opening Endoscopic	**7** Autologous Tissue Substitute **J** Synthetic Substitute **K** Nonautologous Tissue Substitute	**Z** No Qualifier
Q Anus	**0** Open **4** Percutaneous Endoscopic **7** Via Natural or Artificial Opening **8** Via Natural or Artificial Opening Endoscopic **X** External	**7** Autologous Tissue Substitute **J** Synthetic Substitute **K** Nonautologous Tissue Substitute	**Z** No Qualifier
R Anal Sphincter **S** Greater Omentum **T** Lesser Omentum **V** Mesentery **W** Peritoneum	**0** Open **4** Percutaneous Endoscopic	**7** Autologous Tissue Substitute **J** Synthetic Substitute **K** Nonautologous Tissue Substitute	**Z** No Qualifier

Section	0	Medical and Surgical		
Body System	D	Gastrointestinal System		
Operation	V	Restriction: Partially closing an orifice or the lumen of a tubular body part		

Body Part (Character 4)	Approach (Character 5)	Device (Character 6)	Qualifier (Character 7)
1 Esophagus, Upper 2 Esophagus, Middle 3 Esophagus, Lower 4 Esophagogastric Junction 5 Esophagus 6 Stomach 7 Stomach, Pylorus 8 Small Intestine 9 Duodenum A Jejunum B Ileum C Ileocecal Valve E Large Intestine F Large Intestine, Right G Large Intestine, Left H Cecum K Ascending Colon L Transverse Colon M Descending Colon N Sigmoid Colon P Rectum	0 Open 3 Percutaneous 4 Percutaneous Endoscopic	C Extraluminal Device D Intraluminal Device Z No Device	Z No Qualifier
1 Esophagus, Upper 2 Esophagus, Middle 3 Esophagus, Lower 4 Esophagogastric Junction 5 Esophagus 6 Stomach 7 Stomach, Pylorus 8 Small Intestine 9 Duodenum A Jejunum B Ileum C Ileocecal Valve E Large Intestine F Large Intestine, Right G Large Intestine, Left H Cecum K Ascending Colon L Transverse Colon M Descending Colon N Sigmoid Colon P Rectum	7 Via Natural or Artificial Opening 8 Via Natural or Artificial Opening Endoscopic	D Intraluminal Device Z No Device	Z No Qualifier
Q Anus	0 Open 3 Percutaneous 4 Percutaneous Endoscopic X External	C Extraluminal Device D Intraluminal Device Z No Device	Z No Qualifier
Q Anus	7 Via Natural or Artificial Opening 8 Via Natural or Artificial Opening Endoscopic	D Intraluminal Device Z No Device	Z No Qualifier

Section	0	Medical and Surgical
Body System	D	Gastrointestinal System
Operation	W	Revision: Correcting, to the extent possible, a portion of a malfunctioning device or the position of a displaced device

Body Part (Character 4)	Approach (Character 5)	Device (Character 6)	Qualifier (Character 7)
0 Upper Intestinal Tract **D** Lower Intestinal Tract	**0** Open **3** Percutaneous **4** Percutaneous Endoscopic **7** Via Natural or Artificial Opening **8** Via Natural or Artificial Opening Endoscopic **X** External	**0** Drainage Device **2** Monitoring Device **3** Infusion Device **7** Autologous Tissue Substitute **C** Extraluminal Device **D** Intraluminal Device **J** Synthetic Substitute **K** Nonautologous Tissue Substitute **U** Feeding Device	**Z** No Qualifier
5 Esophagus	**7** Via Natural or Artificial Opening **8** Via Natural or Artificial Opening Endoscopic **X** External	**D** Intraluminal Device	**Z** No Qualifier
6 Stomach	**0** Open **3** Percutaneous **4** Percutaneous Endoscopic	**0** Drainage Device **2** Monitoring Device **3** Infusion Device **7** Autologous Tissue Substitute **C** Extraluminal Device **D** Intraluminal Device **J** Synthetic Substitute **K** Nonautologous Tissue Substitute **M** Stimulator Lead **U** Feeding Device	**Z** No Qualifier
6 Stomach	**7** Via Natural or Artificial Opening **8** Via Natural or Artificial Opening Endoscopic **X** External	**0** Drainage Device **2** Monitoring Device **3** Infusion Device **7** Autologous Tissue Substitute **C** Extraluminal Device **D** Intraluminal Device **J** Synthetic Substitute **K** Nonautologous Tissue Substitute **U** Feeding Device	**Z** No Qualifier
8 Small Intestine **E** Large Intestine	**0** Open **4** Percutaneous Endoscopic **7** Via Natural or Artificial Opening **8** Via Natural or Artificial Opening Endoscopic	**7** Autologous Tissue Substitute **J** Synthetic Substitute **K** Nonautologous Tissue Substitute	**Z** No Qualifier
Q Anus	**0** Open **3** Percutaneous **4** Percutaneous Endoscopic **7** Via Natural or Artificial Opening	**L** Artificial Sphincter	**Z** No Qualifier

Continued on Next Page ▶

	8 Via Natural or Artificial Opening Endoscopic		Continued from ◀ Previous Page
R Anal Sphincter	**0** Open **3** Percutaneous **4** Percutaneous Endoscopic	**M** Stimulator Lead	**Z** No Qualifier
U Omentum **V** Mesentery **W** Peritoneum	**0** Open **3** Percutaneous **4** Percutaneous Endoscopic	**0** Drainage Device **7** Autologous Tissue Substitute **J** Synthetic Substitute **K** Nonautologous Tissue Substitute	**Z** No Qualifier

Section	0	Medical and Surgical
Body System	D	Gastrointestinal System
Operation	X	Transfer: Moving, without taking out, all or a portion of a body part to another location to take over the function of all or a portion of a body part

Body Part (Character 4)	Approach (Character 5)	Device (Character 6)	Qualifier (Character 7)
6 Stomach **8** Small Intestine **E** Large Intestine	**0** Open **4** Percutaneous Endoscopic	**Z** No Device	**5** Esophagus

Section	0	Medical and Surgical
Body System	D	Gastrointestinal System
Operation	Y	Transplantation: Putting in or on all or a portion of a living body part taken from another individual or animal to physically take the place and/or function of all or a portion of a similar body part

Body Part (Character 4)	Approach (Character 5)	Device (Character 6)	Qualifier (Character 7)
5 Esophagus **6** Stomach **8** Small Intestine **E** Large Intestine	**0** Open	**Z** No Device	**0** Allogeneic **1** Syngeneic **2** Zooplastic

Section	0	Medical and Surgical
Body System	F	Hepatobiliary System and Pancreas
Operation	1	Bypass: Altering the route of passage of the contents of a tubular body part

Body Part (Character 4)	Approach (Character 5)	Device (Character 6)	Qualifier (Character 7)
4 Gallbladder 5 Hepatic Duct, Right 6 Hepatic Duct, Left 8 Cystic Duct 9 Common Bile Duct	0 Open 4 Percutaneous Endoscopic	D Intraluminal Device Z No Device	3 Duodenum 4 Stomach 5 Hepatic Duct, Right 6 Hepatic Duct, Left 7 Hepatic Duct, Caudate 8 Cystic Duct 9 Common Bile Duct B Small Intestine
D Pancreatic Duct F Pancreatic Duct, Accessory G Pancreas	0 Open 4 Percutaneous Endoscopic	D Intraluminal Device Z No Device	3 Duodenum B Small Intestine C Large Intestine

Section	0	Medical and Surgical
Body System	F	Hepatobiliary System and Pancreas
Operation	2	Change: Taking out or off a device from a body part and putting back an identical or similar device in or on the same body part without cutting or puncturing the skin or a mucous membrane

Body Part (Character 4)	Approach (Character 5)	Device (Character 6)	Qualifier (Character 7)
0 Liver 4 Gallbladder B Hepatobiliary Duct D Pancreatic Duct G Pancreas	X External	0 Drainage Device Y Other Device	Z No Qualifier

Section	0	Medical and Surgical
Body System	F	Hepatobiliary System and Pancreas
Operation	5	Destruction: Physical eradication of all or a portion of a body part by the direct use of energy, force, or a destructive agent

Body Part (Character 4)	Approach (Character 5)	Device (Character 6)	Qualifier (Character 7)
0 Liver 1 Liver, Right Lobe 2 Liver, Left Lobe 4 Gallbladder G Pancreas	0 Open 3 Percutaneous 4 Percutaneous Endoscopic	Z No Device	Z No Qualifier
5 Hepatic Duct, Right 6 Hepatic Duct, Left 8 Cystic Duct 9 Common Bile Duct C Ampulla of Vater D Pancreatic Duct F Pancreatic Duct, Accessory	0 Open 3 Percutaneous 4 Percutaneous Endoscopic 7 Via Natural or Artificial Opening 8 Via Natural or Artificial Opening Endoscopic	Z No Device	Z No Qualifier

Section	0	Medical and Surgical		
Body System	F	Hepatobiliary System and Pancreas		
Operation	7	Dilation: Expanding an orifice or the lumen of a tubular body part		

Body Part (Character 4)	Approach (Character 5)	Device (Character 6)	Qualifier (Character 7)
5 Hepatic Duct, Right 6 Hepatic Duct, Left 8 Cystic Duct 9 Common Bile Duct C Ampulla of Vater D Pancreatic Duct F Pancreatic Duct, Accessory	0 Open 3 Percutaneous 4 Percutaneous Endoscopic 7 Via Natural or Artificial Opening 8 Via Natural or Artificial Opening Endoscopic	D Intraluminal Device Z No Device	Z No Qualifier

Section	0	Medical and Surgical		
Body System	F	Hepatobiliary System and Pancreas		
Operation	8	Division: Cutting into a body part, without draining fluids and/or gases from the body part, in order to separate or transect a body part		

Body Part (Character 4)	Approach (Character 5)	Device (Character 6)	Qualifier (Character 7)
G Pancreas	0 Open 3 Percutaneous 4 Percutaneous Endoscopic	Z No Device	Z No Qualifier

Section	0	Medical and Surgical		
Body System	F	Hepatobiliary System and Pancreas		
Operation	9	Drainage: Taking or letting out fluids and/or gases from a body part		

Body Part (Character 4)	Approach (Character 5)	Device (Character 6)	Qualifier (Character 7)
0 Liver 1 Liver, Right Lobe 2 Liver, Left Lobe 4 Gallbladder G Pancreas	0 Open 3 Percutaneous 4 Percutaneous Endoscopic	0 Drainage Device	Z No Qualifier
0 Liver 1 Liver, Right Lobe 2 Liver, Left Lobe 4 Gallbladder G Pancreas	0 Open 3 Percutaneous 4 Percutaneous Endoscopic	Z No Device	X Diagnostic Z No Qualifier
5 Hepatic Duct, Right 6 Hepatic Duct, Left 8 Cystic Duct 9 Common Bile Duct C Ampulla of Vater D Pancreatic Duct F Pancreatic Duct, Accessory	0 Open 3 Percutaneous 4 Percutaneous Endoscopic 7 Via Natural or Artificial Opening 8 Via Natural or Artificial Opening Endoscopic	0 Drainage Device	Z No Qualifier
5 Hepatic Duct, Right 6 Hepatic Duct, Left 8 Cystic Duct 9 Common Bile Duct C Ampulla of Vater D Pancreatic Duct F Pancreatic Duct, Accessory	0 Open 3 Percutaneous 4 Percutaneous Endoscopic 7 Via Natural or Artificial Opening 8 Via Natural or Artificial Opening Endoscopic	Z No Device	X Diagnostic Z No Qualifier

Section	0	Medical and Surgical		
Body System	F	Hepatobiliary System and Pancreas		
Operation	B	Excision: Cutting out or off, without replacement, a portion of a body part		

Body Part (Character 4)	Approach (Character 5)	Device (Character 6)	Qualifier (Character 7)
0 Liver **1** Liver, Right Lobe **2** Liver, Left Lobe **4** Gallbladder **G** Pancreas	**0** Open **3** Percutaneous **4** Percutaneous Endoscopic	**Z** No Device	**X** Diagnostic **Z** No Qualifier
5 Hepatic Duct, Right **6** Hepatic Duct, Left **8** Cystic Duct **9** Common Bile Duct **C** Ampulla of Vater **D** Pancreatic Duct **F** Pancreatic Duct, Accessory	**0** Open **3** Percutaneous **4** Percutaneous Endoscopic **7** Via Natural or Artificial Opening **8** Via Natural or Artificial Opening Endoscopic	**Z** No Device	**X** Diagnostic **Z** No Qualifier

Section	0	Medical and Surgical		
Body System	F	Hepatobiliary System and Pancreas		
Operation	C	Extirpation: Taking or cutting out solid matter from a body part		

Body Part (Character 4)	Approach (Character 5)	Device (Character 6)	Qualifier (Character 7)
0 Liver **1** Liver, Right Lobe **2** Liver, Left Lobe **4** Gallbladder **G** Pancreas	**0** Open **3** Percutaneous **4** Percutaneous Endoscopic	**Z** No Device	**Z** No Qualifier
5 Hepatic Duct, Right **6** Hepatic Duct, Left **8** Cystic Duct **9** Common Bile Duct **C** Ampulla of Vater **D** Pancreatic Duct **F** Pancreatic Duct, Accessory	**0** Open **3** Percutaneous **4** Percutaneous Endoscopic **7** Via Natural or Artificial Opening **8** Via Natural or Artificial Opening Endoscopic	**Z** No Device	**Z** No Qualifier

Section	0	Medical and Surgical		
Body System	F	Hepatobiliary System and Pancreas		
Operation	F	Fragmentation: Breaking solid matter in a body part into pieces		

Body Part (Character 4)	Approach (Character 5)	Device (Character 6)	Qualifier (Character 7)
4 Gallbladder **5** Hepatic Duct, Right **6** Hepatic Duct, Left **8** Cystic Duct **9** Common Bile Duct **C** Ampulla of Vater **D** Pancreatic Duct **F** Pancreatic Duct, Accessory	**0** Open **3** Percutaneous **4** Percutaneous Endoscopic **7** Via Natural or Artificial Opening **8** Via Natural or Artificial Opening Endoscopic **X** External	**Z** No Device	**Z** No Qualifier

Section	0	Medical and Surgical		
Body System	F	Hepatobiliary System and Pancreas		
Operation	H	Insertion: Putting in a nonbiological appliance that monitors, assists, performs, or prevents a physiological function but does not physically take the place of a body part		

Body Part (Character 4)	Approach (Character 5)	Device (Character 6)	Qualifier (Character 7)
0 Liver 1 Liver, Right Lobe 2 Liver, Left Lobe 4 Gallbladder G Pancreas	0 Open 3 Percutaneous 4 Percutaneous Endoscopic	2 Monitoring Device 3 Infusion Device	Z No Qualifier
B Hepatobiliary Duct D Pancreatic Duct	0 Open 3 Percutaneous 4 Percutaneous Endoscopic 7 Via Natural or Artificial Opening 8 Via Natural or Artificial Opening Endoscopic	1 Radioactive Element 2 Monitoring Device 3 Infusion Device D Intraluminal Device	Z No Qualifier

Section	0	Medical and Surgical		
Body System	F	Hepatobiliary System and Pancreas		
Operation	J	Inspection: Visually and/or manually exploring a body part		

Body Part (Character 4)	Approach (Character 5)	Device (Character 6)	Qualifier (Character 7)
0 Liver 4 Gallbladder G Pancreas	0 Open 3 Percutaneous 4 Percutaneous Endoscopic X External	Z No Device	Z No Qualifier
B Hepatobiliary Duct D Pancreatic Duct	0 Open 3 Percutaneous 4 Percutaneous Endoscopic 7 Via Natural or Artificial Opening 8 Via Natural or Artificial Opening Endoscopic	Z No Device	Z No Qualifier

Section	0	Medical and Surgical		
Body System	F	Hepatobiliary System and Pancreas		
Operation	L	Occlusion: Completely closing an orifice or the lumen of a tubular body part		

Body Part (Character 4)	Approach (Character 5)	Device (Character 6)	Qualifier (Character 7)
5 Hepatic Duct, Right 6 Hepatic Duct, Left 8 Cystic Duct 9 Common Bile Duct C Ampulla of Vater D Pancreatic Duct F Pancreatic Duct, Accessory	0 Open 3 Percutaneous 4 Percutaneous Endoscopic	C Extraluminal Device D Intraluminal Device Z No Device	Z No Qualifier
5 Hepatic Duct, Right 6 Hepatic Duct, Left 8 Cystic Duct 9 Common Bile Duct C Ampulla of Vater D Pancreatic Duct F Pancreatic Duct, Accessory	7 Via Natural or Artificial Opening 8 Via Natural or Artificial Opening Endoscopic	D Intraluminal Device Z No Device	Z No Qualifier

Section	0	Medical and Surgical
Body System	F	Hepatobiliary System and Pancreas
Operation	M	Reattachment Putting back in or on all or a portion of a separated body part to its normal location or other suitable location

Body Part (Character 4)	Approach (Character 5)	Device (Character 6)	Qualifier (Character 7)
0 Liver 1 Liver, Right Lobe 2 Liver, Left Lobe 4 Gallbladder 5 Hepatic Duct, Right 6 Hepatic Duct, Left 8 Cystic Duct 9 Common Bile Duct C Ampulla of Vater D Pancreatic Duct F Pancreatic Duct, Accessory G Pancreas	0 Open 4 Percutaneous Endoscopic	Z No Device	Z No Qualifier

Section	0	Medical and Surgical
Body System	F	Hepatobiliary System and Pancreas
Operation	N	Release: Freeing a body part from an abnormal physical constraint by cutting or by the use of force

Body Part (Character 4)	Approach (Character 5)	Device (Character 6)	Qualifier (Character 7)
0 Liver 1 Liver, Right Lobe 2 Liver, Left Lobe 4 Gallbladder G Pancreas	0 Open 3 Percutaneous 4 Percutaneous Endoscopic	Z No Device	Z No Qualifier
5 Hepatic Duct, Right 6 Hepatic Duct, Left 8 Cystic Duct 9 Common Bile Duct C Ampulla of Vater D Pancreatic Duct F Pancreatic Duct, Accessory	0 Open 3 Percutaneous 4 Percutaneous Endoscopic 7 Via Natural or Artificial Opening 8 Via Natural or Artificial Opening Endoscopic	Z No Device	Z No Qualifier

Section	0	Medical and Surgical
Body System	F	Hepatobiliary System and Pancreas
Operation	P	Removal: Taking out or off a device from a body part

Body Part (Character 4)	Approach (Character 5)	Device (Character 6)	Qualifier (Character 7)
0 Liver	0 Open 3 Percutaneous 4 Percutaneous Endoscopic X External	0 Drainage Device 2 Monitoring Device 3 Infusion Device	Z No Qualifier
4 Gallbladder G Pancreas	0 Open 3 Percutaneous 4 Percutaneous Endoscopic X External	0 Drainage Device 2 Monitoring Device 3 Infusion Device D Intraluminal Device	Z No Qualifier
B Hepatobiliary Duct D Pancreatic Duct	0 Open 3 Percutaneous 4 Percutaneous Endoscopic 7 Via Natural or Artificial	0 Drainage Device 1 Radioactive Element 2 Monitoring Device 3 Infusion Device	Z No Qualifier **Continued on Next Page ▶**

	Opening **8** Via Natural or Artificial Opening Endoscopic	**7** Autologous Tissue Substitute **C** Extraluminal Device **D** Intraluminal Device **J** Synthetic Substitute **K** Nonautologous Tissue Substitute	Continued from ◀ Previous Page
B Hepatobiliary Duct **D** Pancreatic Duct	**X** External	**0** Drainage Device **1** Radioactive Element **2** Monitoring Device **3** Infusion Device **D** Intraluminal Device	**Z** No Qualifier

Section	0	Medical and Surgical
Body System	F	Hepatobiliary System and Pancreas
Operation	Q	Repair: Restoring, to the extent possible, a body part to its normal anatomic structure and function

Body Part (Character 4)	Approach (Character 5)	Device (Character 6)	Qualifier (Character 7)
0 Liver **1** Liver, Right Lobe **2** Liver, Left Lobe **4** Gallbladder **G** Pancreas	**0** Open **3** Percutaneous **4** Percutaneous Endoscopic	**Z** No Device	**Z** No Qualifier
5 Hepatic Duct, Right **6** Hepatic Duct, Left **8** Cystic Duct **9** Common Bile Duct **C** Ampulla of Vater **D** Pancreatic Duct **F** Pancreatic Duct, Accessory	**0** Open **3** Percutaneous **4** Percutaneous Endoscopic **7** Via Natural or Artificial Opening **8** Via Natural or Artificial Opening Endoscopic	**Z** No Device	**Z** No Qualifier

Section	0	Medical and Surgical
Body System	F	Hepatobiliary System and Pancreas
Operation	R	Replacement: Putting in or on biological or synthetic material that physically takes the place and/or function of all or a portion of a body part

Body Part (Character 4)	Approach (Character 5)	Device (Character 6)	Qualifier (Character 7)
5 Hepatic Duct, Right **6** Hepatic Duct, Left **8** Cystic Duct **9** Common Bile Duct **C** Ampulla of Vater **D** Pancreatic Duct **F** Pancreatic Duct, Accessory	**0** Open **4** Percutaneous Endoscopic	**7** Autologous Tissue Substitute **J** Synthetic Substitute **K** Nonautologous Tissue Substitute	**Z** No Qualifier

Section	0	Medical and Surgical
Body System	F	Hepatobiliary System and Pancreas
Operation	S	Reposition: Moving to its normal location, or other suitable location, all or a portion of a body part

Body Part (Character 4)	Approach (Character 5)	Device (Character 6)	Qualifier (Character 7)
0 Liver 4 Gallbladder 5 Hepatic Duct, Right 6 Hepatic Duct, Left 8 Cystic Duct 9 Common Bile Duct C Ampulla of Vater D Pancreatic Duct F Pancreatic Duct, Accessory G Pancreas	0 Open 4 Percutaneous Endoscopic	Z No Device	Z No Qualifier

Section	0	Medical and Surgical
Body System	F	Hepatobiliary System and Pancreas
Operation	T	Resection: Cutting out or off, without replacement, all of a body part

Body Part (Character 4)	Approach (Character 5)	Device (Character 6)	Qualifier (Character 7)
0 Liver 1 Liver, Right Lobe 2 Liver, Left Lobe 4 Gallbladder G Pancreas	0 Open 4 Percutaneous Endoscopic	Z No Device	Z No Qualifier
5 Hepatic Duct, Right 6 Hepatic Duct, Left 8 Cystic Duct 9 Common Bile Duct C Ampulla of Vater D Pancreatic Duct F Pancreatic Duct, Accessory	0 Open 4 Percutaneous Endoscopic 7 Via Natural or Artificial Opening 8 Via Natural or Artificial Opening Endoscopic	Z No Device	Z No Qualifier

Section	0	Medical and Surgical
Body System	F	Hepatobiliary System and Pancreas
Operation	U	Supplement: Putting in or on biological or synthetic material that physically reinforces and/or augments the function of a portion of a body part

Body Part (Character 4)	Approach (Character 5)	Device (Character 6)	Qualifier (Character 7)
5 Hepatic Duct, Right 6 Hepatic Duct, Left 8 Cystic Duct 9 Common Bile Duct C Ampulla of Vater D Pancreatic Duct F Pancreatic Duct, Accessory	0 Open 3 Percutaneous 4 Percutaneous Endoscopic	7 Autologous Tissue Substitute J Synthetic Substitute K Nonautologous Tissue Substitute	Z No Qualifier

Section	0	Medical and Surgical		
Body System	F	Hepatobiliary System and Pancreas		
Operation	V	Restriction: Partially closing an orifice or the lumen of a tubular body part		

Body Part (Character 4)	Approach (Character 5)	Device (Character 6)	Qualifier (Character 7)
5 Hepatic Duct, Right 6 Hepatic Duct, Left 8 Cystic Duct 9 Common Bile Duct C Ampulla of Vater D Pancreatic Duct F Pancreatic Duct, Accessory	0 Open 3 Percutaneous 4 Percutaneous Endoscopic	C Extraluminal Device D Intraluminal Device Z No Device	Z No Qualifier
5 Hepatic Duct, Right 6 Hepatic Duct, Left 8 Cystic Duct 9 Common Bile Duct C Ampulla of Vater D Pancreatic Duct F Pancreatic Duct, Accessory	7 Via Natural or Artificial Opening 8 Via Natural or Artificial Opening Endoscopic	D Intraluminal Device Z No Device	Z No Qualifier

Section	0	Medical and Surgical		
Body System	F	Hepatobiliary System and Pancreas		
Operation	W	Revision: Correcting, to the extent possible, a portion of a malfunctioning device or the position of a displaced device		

Body Part (Character 4)	Approach (Character 5)	Device (Character 6)	Qualifier (Character 7)
0 Liver	0 Open 3 Percutaneous 4 Percutaneous Endoscopic X External	0 Drainage Device 2 Monitoring Device 3 Infusion Device	Z No Qualifier
4 Gallbladder G Pancreas	0 Open 3 Percutaneous 4 Percutaneous Endoscopic X External	0 Drainage Device 2 Monitoring Device 3 Infusion Device D Intraluminal Device	Z No Qualifier
B Hepatobiliary Duct D Pancreatic Duct	0 Open 3 Percutaneous 4 Percutaneous Endoscopic 7 Via Natural or Artificial Opening 8 Via Natural or Artificial Opening Endoscopic X External	0 Drainage Device 2 Monitoring Device 3 Infusion Device 7 Autologous Tissue Substitute C Extraluminal Device D Intraluminal Device J Synthetic Substitute K Nonautologous Tissue Substitute	Z No Qualifier

Section	0	Medical and Surgical		
Body System	F	Hepatobiliary System and Pancreas		
Operation	Y	Transplantation: Putting in or on all or a portion of a living body part taken from another individual or animal to physically take the place and/or function of all or a portion of a similar body part		

Body Part (Character 4)	Approach (Character 5)	Device (Character 6)	Qualifier (Character 7)
0 Liver G Pancreas	0 Open	Z No Device	0 Allogeneic 1 Syngeneic 2 Zooplastic

Section	0	Medical and Surgical		
Body System	G	Endocrine System		
Operation	2	Change: Taking out or off a device from a body part and putting back an identical or similar device in or on the same body part without cutting or puncturing the skin or a mucous membrane		

Body Part (Character 4)	Approach (Character 5)	Device (Character 6)	Qualifier (Character 7)
0 Pituitary Gland 1 Pineal Body 5 Adrenal Gland K Thyroid Gland R Parathyroid Gland S Endocrine Gland	X External	0 Drainage Device Y Other Device	Z No Qualifier

Section	0	Medical and Surgical		
Body System	G	Endocrine System		
Operation	5	Destruction: Physical eradication of all or a portion of a body part by the direct use of energy, force, or a destructive agent		

Body Part (Character 4)	Approach (Character 5)	Device (Character 6)	Qualifier (Character 7)
0 Pituitary Gland 1 Pineal Body 2 Adrenal Gland, Left 3 Adrenal Gland, Right 4 Adrenal Glands, Bilateral 6 Carotid Body, Left 7 Carotid Body, Right 8 Carotid Bodies, Bilateral 9 Para-aortic Body B Coccygeal Glomus C Glomus Jugulare D Aortic Body F Paraganglion Extremity G Thyroid Gland Lobe, Left H Thyroid Gland Lobe, Right K Thyroid Gland L Superior Parathyroid Gland, Right M Superior Parathyroid Gland, Left N Inferior Parathyroid Gland, Right P Inferior Parathyroid Gland, Left Q Parathyroid Glands, Multiple R Parathyroid Gland	0 Open 3 Percutaneous 4 Percutaneous Endoscopic	Z No Device	Z No Qualifier

Section	0	Medical and Surgical		
Body System	G	Endocrine System		
Operation	8	Division: Cutting into a body part, without draining fluids and/or gases from the body part, in order to separate or transect a body part		

Body Part (Character 4)	Approach (Character 5)	Device (Character 6)	Qualifier (Character 7)
0 Pituitary Gland J Thyroid Gland Isthmus	0 Open 3 Percutaneous 4 Percutaneous Endoscopic	Z No Device	Z No Qualifier

Section	0	Medical and Surgical		
Body System	G	Endocrine System		
Operation	9	Drainage: Taking or letting out fluids and/or gases from a body part		

Body Part (Character 4)	Approach (Character 5)	Device (Character 6)	Qualifier (Character 7)
0 Pituitary Gland 1 Pineal Body 2 Adrenal Gland, Left 3 Adrenal Gland, Right 4 Adrenal Glands, Bilateral 6 Carotid Body, Left 7 Carotid Body, Right 8 Carotid Bodies, Bilateral 9 Para-aortic Body B Coccygeal Glomus C Glomus Jugulare D Aortic Body F Paraganglion Extremity G Thyroid Gland Lobe, Left H Thyroid Gland Lobe, Right K Thyroid Gland L Superior Parathyroid Gland, Right M Superior Parathyroid Gland, Left N Inferior Parathyroid Gland, Right P Inferior Parathyroid Gland, Left Q Parathyroid Glands, Multiple R Parathyroid Gland	0 Open 3 Percutaneous 4 Percutaneous Endoscopic	0 Drainage Device	Z No Qualifier
0 Pituitary Gland 1 Pineal Body 2 Adrenal Gland, Left 3 Adrenal Gland, Right 4 Adrenal Glands, Bilateral 6 Carotid Body, Left 7 Carotid Body, Right 8 Carotid Bodies, Bilateral 9 Para-aortic Body B Coccygeal Glomus C Glomus Jugulare D Aortic Body F Paraganglion Extremity G Thyroid Gland Lobe, Left H Thyroid Gland Lobe, Right K Thyroid Gland L Superior Parathyroid Gland, Right M Superior Parathyroid Gland, Left N Inferior Parathyroid Gland, Right P Inferior Parathyroid Gland, Left Q Parathyroid Glands, Multiple R Parathyroid Gland	0 Open 3 Percutaneous 4 Percutaneous Endoscopic	Z No Device	X Diagnostic Z No Qualifier

Section	0	Medical and Surgical		
Body System	G	Endocrine System		
Operation	B	Excision: Cutting out or off, without replacement, a portion of a body part		

Body Part (Character 4)	Approach (Character 5)	Device (Character 6)	Qualifier (Character 7)
0 Pituitary Gland	0 Open	Z No Device	X Diagnostic
1 Pineal Body	3 Percutaneous		Z No Qualifier
2 Adrenal Gland, Left	4 Percutaneous Endoscopic		
3 Adrenal Gland, Right			
4 Adrenal Glands, Bilateral			
6 Carotid Body, Left			
7 Carotid Body, Right			
8 Carotid Bodies, Bilateral			
9 Para-aortic Body			
B Coccygeal Glomus			
C Glomus Jugulare			
D Aortic Body			
F Paraganglion Extremity			
G Thyroid Gland Lobe, Left			
H Thyroid Gland Lobe, Right			
L Superior Parathyroid Gland, Right			
M Superior Parathyroid Gland, Left			
N Inferior Parathyroid Gland, Right			
P Inferior Parathyroid Gland, Left			
Q Parathyroid Glands, Multiple			
R Parathyroid Gland			

Section	0	Medical and Surgical		
Body System	G	Endocrine System		
Operation	C	Extirpation: Taking or cutting out solid matter from a body part		

Body Part (Character 4)	Approach (Character 5)	Device (Character 6)	Qualifier (Character 7)
0 Pituitary Gland	0 Open	Z No Device	Z No Qualifier
1 Pineal Body	3 Percutaneous		
2 Adrenal Gland, Left	4 Percutaneous Endoscopic		
3 Adrenal Gland, Right			
4 Adrenal Glands, Bilateral			
6 Carotid Body, Left			
7 Carotid Body, Right			
8 Carotid Bodies, Bilateral			
9 Para-aortic Body			
B Coccygeal Glomus			
C Glomus Jugulare			
D Aortic Body			
F Paraganglion Extremity			
G Thyroid Gland Lobe, Left			
H Thyroid Gland Lobe, Right			
K Thyroid Gland			
L Superior Parathyroid Gland, Right			
M Superior Parathyroid Gland, Left			Continued on Next Page ▶

			Continued from ◄ Previous Page
N Inferior Parathyroid Gland, Right P Inferior Parathyroid Gland, Left Q Parathyroid Glands, Multiple R Parathyroid Gland			

Section	0	Medical and Surgical
Body System	G	Endocrine System
Operation	H	Insertion: Putting in a nonbiological appliance that monitors, assists, performs, or prevents a physiological function but does not physically take the place of a body part

Body Part (Character 4)	Approach (Character 5)	Device (Character 6)	Qualifier (Character 7)
S Endocrine Gland	0 Open 3 Percutaneous 4 Percutaneous Endoscopic	2 Monitoring Device 3 Infusion Device	Z No Qualifier

Section	0	Medical and Surgical
Body System	G	Endocrine System
Operation	J	Inspection: Visually and/or manually exploring a body part

Body Part (Character 4)	Approach (Character 5)	Device (Character 6)	Qualifier (Character 7)
0 Pituitary Gland 1 Pineal Body 5 Adrenal Gland K Thyroid Gland R Parathyroid Gland S Endocrine Gland	0 Open 3 Percutaneous 4 Percutaneous Endoscopic	Z No Device	Z No Qualifier

Section	0	Medical and Surgical
Body System	G	Endocrine System
Operation	M	Reattachment Putting back in or on all or a portion of a separated body part to its normal location or other suitable location

Body Part (Character 4)	Approach (Character 5)	Device (Character 6)	Qualifier (Character 7)
2 Adrenal Gland, Left 3 Adrenal Gland, Right G Thyroid Gland Lobe, Left H Thyroid Gland Lobe, Right L Superior Parathyroid Gland, Right M Superior Parathyroid Gland, Left N Inferior Parathyroid Gland, Right P Inferior Parathyroid Gland, Left Q Parathyroid Glands, Multiple R Parathyroid Gland	0 Open 4 Percutaneous Endoscopic	Z No Device	Z No Qualifier

Section	0	Medical and Surgical	
Body System	G	Endocrine System	
Operation	N	Release: Freeing a body part from an abnormal physical constraint by cutting or by the use of force	

Body Part (Character 4)	Approach (Character 5)	Device (Character 6)	Qualifier (Character 7)
0 Pituitary Gland	0 Open	Z No Device	Z No Qualifier
1 Pineal Body	3 Percutaneous		
2 Adrenal Gland, Left	4 Percutaneous Endoscopic		
3 Adrenal Gland, Right			
4 Adrenal Glands, Bilateral			
6 Carotid Body, Left			
7 Carotid Body, Right			
8 Carotid Bodies, Bilateral			
9 Para-aortic Body			
B Coccygeal Glomus			
C Glomus Jugulare			
D Aortic Body			
F Paraganglion Extremity			
G Thyroid Gland Lobe, Left			
H Thyroid Gland Lobe, Right			
K Thyroid Gland			
L Superior Parathyroid Gland, Right			
M Superior Parathyroid Gland, Left			
N Inferior Parathyroid Gland, Right			
P Inferior Parathyroid Gland, Left			
Q Parathyroid Glands, Multiple			
R Parathyroid Gland			

Section	0	Medical and Surgical	
Body System	G	Endocrine System	
Operation	P	Removal: Taking out or off a device from a body part	

Body Part (Character 4)	Approach (Character 5)	Device (Character 6)	Qualifier (Character 7)
0 Pituitary Gland	0 Open	0 Drainage Device	Z No Qualifier
1 Pineal Body	3 Percutaneous		
5 Adrenal Gland	4 Percutaneous Endoscopic		
K Thyroid Gland	X External		
R Parathyroid Gland			
S Endocrine Gland	0 Open	0 Drainage Device	Z No Qualifier
	3 Percutaneous	2 Monitoring Device	
	4 Percutaneous Endoscopic	3 Infusion Device	
	X External		

Section	0	Medical and Surgical		
Body System	G	Endocrine System		
Operation	Q	Repair: Restoring, to the extent possible, a body part to its normal anatomic structure and function		

Body Part (Character 4)	Approach (Character 5)	Device (Character 6)	Qualifier (Character 7)
0 Pituitary Gland	0 Open	Z No Device	Z No Qualifier
1 Pineal Body	3 Percutaneous		
2 Adrenal Gland, Left	4 Percutaneous Endoscopic		
3 Adrenal Gland, Right			
4 Adrenal Glands, Bilateral			
6 Carotid Body, Left			
7 Carotid Body, Right			
8 Carotid Bodies, Bilateral			
9 Para-aortic Body			
B Coccygeal Glomus			
C Glomus Jugulare			
D Aortic Body			
F Paraganglion Extremity			
G Thyroid Gland Lobe, Left			
H Thyroid Gland Lobe, Right			
J Thyroid Gland Isthmus			
K Thyroid Gland			
L Superior Parathyroid Gland, Right			
M Superior Parathyroid Gland, Left			
N Inferior Parathyroid Gland, Right			
P Inferior Parathyroid Gland, Left			
Q Parathyroid Glands, Multiple			
R Parathyroid Gland			

Section	0	Medical and Surgical		
Body System	G	Endocrine System		
Operation	S	Reposition: Moving to its normal location, or other suitable location, all or a portion of a body part		

Body Part (Character 4)	Approach (Character 5)	Device (Character 6)	Qualifier (Character 7)
2 Adrenal Gland, Left	0 Open	Z No Device	Z No Qualifier
3 Adrenal Gland, Right	4 Percutaneous Endoscopic		
G Thyroid Gland Lobe, Left			
H Thyroid Gland Lobe, Right			
L Superior Parathyroid Gland, Right			
M Superior Parathyroid Gland, Left			
N Inferior Parathyroid Gland, Right			
P Inferior Parathyroid Gland, Left			
Q Parathyroid Glands, Multiple			
R Parathyroid Gland			

Section	0	Medical and Surgical		
Body System	G	Endocrine System		
Operation	T	Resection: Cutting out or off, without replacement, all of a body part		

Body Part (Character 4)	Approach (Character 5)	Device (Character 6)	Qualifier (Character 7)
0 Pituitary Gland	0 Open	Z No Device	Z No Qualifier
1 Pineal Body	4 Percutaneous Endoscopic		
2 Adrenal Gland, Left			
3 Adrenal Gland, Right			
4 Adrenal Glands, Bilateral			
6 Carotid Body, Left			
7 Carotid Body, Right			
8 Carotid Bodies, Bilateral			
9 Para-aortic Body			
B Coccygeal Glomus			
C Glomus Jugulare			
D Aortic Body			
F Paraganglion Extremity			
G Thyroid Gland Lobe, Left			
H Thyroid Gland Lobe, Right			
K Thyroid Gland			
L Superior Parathyroid Gland, Right			
M Superior Parathyroid Gland, Left			
N Inferior Parathyroid Gland, Right			
P Inferior Parathyroid Gland, Left			
Q Parathyroid Glands, Multiple			
R Parathyroid Gland			

Section	0	Medical and Surgical		
Body System	G	Endocrine System		
Operation	W	Revision: Correcting, to the extent possible, a portion of a malfunctioning device or the position of a displaced device		

Body Part (Character 4)	Approach (Character 5)	Device (Character 6)	Qualifier (Character 7)
0 Pituitary Gland	0 Open	0 Drainage Device	Z No Qualifier
1 Pineal Body	3 Percutaneous		
5 Adrenal Gland	4 Percutaneous Endoscopic		
K Thyroid Gland	X External		
R Parathyroid Gland			
S Endocrine Gland	0 Open	0 Drainage Device	Z No Qualifier
	3 Percutaneous	2 Monitoring Device	
	4 Percutaneous Endoscopic	3 Infusion Device	
	X External		

Section	0	Medical and Surgical		
Body System	H	Skin and Breast		
Operation	0	Alteration: Modifying the anatomic structure of a body part without affecting the function of the body part		

Body Part (Character 4)	Approach (Character 5)	Device (Character 6)	Qualifier (Character 7)
T Breast, Right U Breast, Left V Breast, Bilateral	0 Open 3 Percutaneous X External	7 Autologous Tissue Substitute J Synthetic Substitute K Nonautologous Tissue Substitute Z No Device	Z No Qualifier

Section	0	Medical and Surgical		
Body System	H	Skin and Breast		
Operation	2	Change: Taking out or off a device from a body part and putting back an identical or similar device in or on the same body part without cutting or puncturing the skin or a mucous membrane		

Body Part (Character 4)	Approach (Character 5)	Device (Character 6)	Qualifier (Character 7)
P Skin T Breast, Right U Breast, Left	X External	0 Drainage Device Y Other Device	Z No Qualifier

Section	0	Medical and Surgical		
Body System	H	Skin and Breast		
Operation	5	Destruction: Physical eradication of all or a portion of a body part by the direct use of energy, force, or a destructive agent		

Body Part (Character 4)	Approach (Character 5)	Device (Character 6)	Qualifier (Character 7)
0 Skin, Scalp 1 Skin, Face 2 Skin, Right Ear 3 Skin, Left Ear 4 Skin, Neck 5 Skin, Chest 6 Skin, Back 7 Skin, Abdomen 8 Skin, Buttock 9 Skin, Perineum A Skin, Genitalia B Skin, Right Upper Arm C Skin, Left Upper Arm D Skin, Right Lower Arm E Skin, Left Lower Arm F Skin, Right Hand G Skin, Left Hand H Skin, Right Upper Leg J Skin, Left Upper Leg K Skin, Right Lower Leg L Skin, Left Lower Leg M Skin, Right Foot N Skin, Left Foot	X External	Z No Device	D Multiple Z No Qualifier
Q Finger Nail R Toe Nail	X External	Z No Device	Z No Qualifier

Continued on Next Page ▶

			Continued from ◀ Previous Page
T Breast, Right U Breast, Left V Breast, Bilateral W Nipple, Right X Nipple, Left	0 Open 3 Percutaneous 7 Via Natural or Artificial Opening 8 Via Natural or Artificial Opening Endoscopic X External	Z No Device	Z No Qualifier

Section	0	Medical and Surgical	
Body System	H	Skin and Breast	
Operation	8	Division: Cutting into a body part, without draining fluids and/or gases from the body part, in order to separate or transect a body part	

Body Part (Character 4)	Approach (Character 5)	Device (Character 6)	Qualifier (Character 7)
0 Skin, Scalp 1 Skin, Face 2 Skin, Right Ear 3 Skin, Left Ear 4 Skin, Neck 5 Skin, Chest 6 Skin, Back 7 Skin, Abdomen 8 Skin, Buttock 9 Skin, Perineum A Skin, Genitalia B Skin, Right Upper Arm C Skin, Left Upper Arm D Skin, Right Lower Arm E Skin, Left Lower Arm F Skin, Right Hand G Skin, Left Hand H Skin, Right Upper Leg J Skin, Left Upper Leg K Skin, Right Lower Leg L Skin, Left Lower Leg M Skin, Right Foot N Skin, Left Foot	X External	Z No Device	Z No Qualifier

Section	0	Medical and Surgical	
Body System	H	Skin and Breast	
Operation	9	Drainage: Taking or letting out fluids and/or gases from a body part	

Body Part (Character 4)	Approach (Character 5)	Device (Character 6)	Qualifier (Character 7)
0 Skin, Scalp 1 Skin, Face 2 Skin, Right Ear 3 Skin, Left Ear 4 Skin, Neck 5 Skin, Chest 6 Skin, Back 7 Skin, Abdomen 8 Skin, Buttock 9 Skin, Perineum A Skin, Genitalia	X External	0 Drainage Device	Z No Qualifier Continued on Next Page ▶

			Continued from ◀ Previous Page
B Skin, Right Upper Arm **C** Skin, Left Upper Arm **D** Skin, Right Lower Arm **E** Skin, Left Lower Arm **F** Skin, Right Hand **G** Skin, Left Hand **H** Skin, Right Upper Leg **J** Skin, Left Upper Leg **K** Skin, Right Lower Leg **L** Skin, Left Lower Leg **M** Skin, Right Foot **N** Skin, Left Foot **Q** Finger Nail **R** Toe Nail			
0 Skin, Scalp **1** Skin, Face **2** Skin, Right Ear **3** Skin, Left Ear **4** Skin, Neck **5** Skin, Chest **6** Skin, Back **7** Skin, Abdomen **8** Skin, Buttock **9** Skin, Perineum **A** Skin, Genitalia **B** Skin, Right Upper Arm **C** Skin, Left Upper Arm **D** Skin, Right Lower Arm **E** Skin, Left Lower Arm **F** Skin, Right Hand **G** Skin, Left Hand **H** Skin, Right Upper Leg **J** Skin, Left Upper Leg **K** Skin, Right Lower Leg **L** Skin, Left Lower Leg **M** Skin, Right Foot **N** Skin, Left Foot **Q** Finger Nail **R** Toe Nail	**X** External	**Z** No Device	**X** Diagnostic **Z** No Qualifier
T Breast, Right **U** Breast, Left **V** Breast, Bilateral **W** Nipple, Right **X** Nipple, Left	**0** Open **3** Percutaneous **7** Via Natural or Artificial Opening **8** Via Natural or Artificial Opening Endoscopic **X** External	**0** Drainage Device	**Z** No Qualifier
T Breast, Right **U** Breast, Left **V** Breast, Bilateral **W** Nipple, Right **X** Nipple, Left	**0** Open **3** Percutaneous **7** Via Natural or Artificial Opening **8** Via Natural or Artificial Opening Endoscopic **X** External	**Z** No Device	**X** Diagnostic **Z** No Qualifier

Section	0	Medical and Surgical		
Body System	H	Skin and Breast		
Operation	B	Excision: Cutting out or off, without replacement, a portion of a body part		

Body Part (Character 4)	Approach (Character 5)	Device (Character 6)	Qualifier (Character 7)
0 Skin, Scalp 1 Skin, Face 2 Skin, Right Ear 3 Skin, Left Ear 4 Skin, Neck 5 Skin, Chest 6 Skin, Back 7 Skin, Abdomen 8 Skin, Buttock 9 Skin, Perineum A Skin, Genitalia B Skin, Right Upper Arm C Skin, Left Upper Arm D Skin, Right Lower Arm E Skin, Left Lower Arm F Skin, Right Hand G Skin, Left Hand H Skin, Right Upper Leg J Skin, Left Upper Leg K Skin, Right Lower Leg L Skin, Left Lower Leg M Skin, Right Foot N Skin, Left Foot Q Finger Nail R Toe Nail	X External	Z No Device	X Diagnostic Z No Qualifier
T Breast, Right U Breast, Left V Breast, Bilateral W Nipple, Right X Nipple, Left Y Supernumerary Breast	0 Open 3 Percutaneous 7 Via Natural or Artificial Opening 8 Via Natural or Artificial Opening Endoscopic X External	Z No Device	X Diagnostic Z No Qualifier

Section	0	Medical and Surgical		
Body System	H	Skin and Breast		
Operation	C	Extirpation: Taking or cutting out solid matter from a body part		

Body Part (Character 4)	Approach (Character 5)	Device (Character 6)	Qualifier (Character 7)
0 Skin, Scalp 1 Skin, Face 2 Skin, Right Ear 3 Skin, Left Ear 4 Skin, Neck 5 Skin, Chest 6 Skin, Back 7 Skin, Abdomen 8 Skin, Buttock 9 Skin, Perineum A Skin, Genitalia B Skin, Right Upper Arm C Skin, Left Upper Arm	X External	Z No Device	Z No Qualifier Continued on Next Page ▶

D Skin, Right Lower Arm E Skin, Left Lower Arm F Skin, Right Hand G Skin, Left Hand H Skin, Right Upper Leg J Skin, Left Upper Leg K Skin, Right Lower Leg L Skin, Left Lower Leg M Skin, Right Foot N Skin, Left Foot Q Finger Nail R Toe Nail			Continued from ◀ Previous Page

T Breast, Right
U Breast, Left
V Breast, Bilateral
W Nipple, Right
X Nipple, Left
	0 Open
	3 Percutaneous
	7 Via Natural or Artificial
	   Opening
	8 Via Natural or Artificial
	   Opening Endoscopic
	X External
		Z No Device	Z No Qualifier

Section	0	Medical and Surgical	
Body System	H	Skin and Breast	
Operation	D	Extraction: Pulling or stripping out or off all or a portion of a body part by the use of force	

Body Part (Character 4)	Approach (Character 5)	Device (Character 6)	Qualifier (Character 7)
0 Skin, Scalp 1 Skin, Face 2 Skin, Right Ear 3 Skin, Left Ear 4 Skin, Neck 5 Skin, Chest 6 Skin, Back 7 Skin, Abdomen 8 Skin, Buttock 9 Skin, Perineum A Skin, Genitalia B Skin, Right Upper Arm C Skin, Left Upper Arm D Skin, Right Lower Arm E Skin, Left Lower Arm F Skin, Right Hand G Skin, Left Hand H Skin, Right Upper Leg J Skin, Left Upper Leg K Skin, Right Lower Leg L Skin, Left Lower Leg M Skin, Right Foot N Skin, Left Foot Q Finger Nail R Toe Nail S Hair	X External	Z No Device	Z No Qualifier

Section	0	Medical and Surgical
Body System	H	Skin and Breast
Operation	H	Insertion: Putting in a nonbiological appliance that monitors, assists, performs, or prevents a physiological function but does not physically take the place of a body part

Body Part (Character 4)	Approach (Character 5)	Device (Character 6)	Qualifier (Character 7)
T Breast, Right U Breast, Left V Breast, Bilateral W Nipple, Right X Nipple, Left	0 Open 3 Percutaneous 7 Via Natural or Artificial Opening 8 Via Natural or Artificial Opening Endoscopic	1 Radioactive Element N Tissue Expander	Z No Qualifier
T Breast, Right U Breast, Left V Breast, Bilateral W Nipple, Right X Nipple, Left	X External	1 Radioactive Element	Z No Qualifier

Section	0	Medical and Surgical
Body System	H	Skin and Breast
Operation	J	Inspection: Visually and/or manually exploring a body part

Body Part (Character 4)	Approach (Character 5)	Device (Character 6)	Qualifier (Character 7)
P Skin Q Finger Nail R Toe Nail	X External	Z No Device	Z No Qualifier
T Breast, Right U Breast, Left	0 Open 3 Percutaneous 7 Via Natural or Artificial Opening 8 Via Natural or Artificial Opening Endoscopic X External	Z No Device	Z No Qualifier

Section	0	Medical and Surgical
Body System	H	Skin and Breast
Operation	M	Reattachment Putting back in or on all or a portion of a separated body part to its normal location or other suitable location

Body Part (Character 4)	Approach (Character 5)	Device (Character 6)	Qualifier (Character 7)
0 Skin, Scalp 1 Skin, Face 2 Skin, Right Ear 3 Skin, Left Ear 4 Skin, Neck 5 Skin, Chest 6 Skin, Back 7 Skin, Abdomen 8 Skin, Buttock 9 Skin, Perineum A Skin, Genitalia B Skin, Right Upper Arm C Skin, Left Upper Arm D Skin, Right Lower Arm E Skin, Left Lower Arm F Skin, Right Hand G Skin, Left Hand H Skin, Right Upper Leg	X External	Z No Device	Z No Qualifier

Continued on Next Page ▶

J Skin, Left Upper Leg			**Continued from** ◄ **Previous Page**
K Skin, Right Lower Leg			
L Skin, Left Lower Leg			
M Skin, Right Foot			
N Skin, Left Foot			
T Breast, Right			
U Breast, Left			
V Breast, Bilateral			
W Nipple, Right			
X Nipple, Left			

Section	0	Medical and Surgical
Body System	H	Skin and Breast
Operation	N	Release: Freeing a body part from an abnormal physical constraint by cutting or by the use of force

Body Part (Character 4)	Approach (Character 5)	Device (Character 6)	Qualifier (Character 7)
0 Skin, Scalp	X External	Z No Device	Z No Qualifier
1 Skin, Face			
2 Skin, Right Ear			
3 Skin, Left Ear			
4 Skin, Neck			
5 Skin, Chest			
6 Skin, Back			
7 Skin, Abdomen			
8 Skin, Buttock			
9 Skin, Perineum			
A Skin, Genitalia			
B Skin, Right Upper Arm			
C Skin, Left Upper Arm			
D Skin, Right Lower Arm			
E Skin, Left Lower Arm			
F Skin, Right Hand			
G Skin, Left Hand			
H Skin, Right Upper Leg			
J Skin, Left Upper Leg			
K Skin, Right Lower Leg			
L Skin, Left Lower Leg			
M Skin, Right Foot			
N Skin, Left Foot			
Q Finger Nail			
R Toe Nail			
T Breast, Right	0 Open	Z No Device	Z No Qualifier
U Breast, Left	3 Percutaneous		
V Breast, Bilateral	7 Via Natural or Artificial Opening		
W Nipple, Right	8 Via Natural or Artificial Opening Endoscopic		
X Nipple, Left	X External		

Section	0	Medical and Surgical		
Body System	H	Skin and Breast		
Operation	P	Removal: Taking out or off a device from a body part		

Body Part (Character 4)	Approach (Character 5)	Device (Character 6)	Qualifier (Character 7)
P Skin Q Finger Nail R Toe Nail	X External	0 Drainage Device 7 Autologous Tissue Substitute J Synthetic Substitute K Nonautologous Tissue Substitute	Z No Qualifier
S Hair	X External	7 Autologous Tissue Substitute J Synthetic Substitute K Nonautologous Tissue Substitute	Z No Qualifier
T Breast, Right U Breast, Left	0 Open 3 Percutaneous 7 Via Natural or Artificial Opening 8 Via Natural or Artificial Opening Endoscopic	0 Drainage Device 1 Radioactive Element 7 Autologous Tissue Substitute J Synthetic Substitute K Nonautologous Tissue Substitute N Tissue Expander	Z No Qualifier
T Breast, Right U Breast, Left	X External	0 Drainage Device 1 Radioactive Element 7 Autologous Tissue Substitute J Synthetic Substitute K Nonautologous Tissue Substitute	Z No Qualifier

Section	0	Medical and Surgical		
Body System	H	Skin and Breast		
Operation	Q	Repair: Restoring, to the extent possible, a body part to its normal anatomic structure and function		

Body Part (Character 4)	Approach (Character 5)	Device (Character 6)	Qualifier (Character 7)
0 Skin, Scalp 1 Skin, Face 2 Skin, Right Ear 3 Skin, Left Ear 4 Skin, Neck 5 Skin, Chest 6 Skin, Back 7 Skin, Abdomen 8 Skin, Buttock 9 Skin, Perineum A Skin, Genitalia B Skin, Right Upper Arm C Skin, Left Upper Arm D Skin, Right Lower Arm E Skin, Left Lower Arm F Skin, Right Hand G Skin, Left Hand H Skin, Right Upper Leg J Skin, Left Upper Leg	X External	Z No Device	Z No Qualifier

Continued on Next Page ▶

			Continued from ◀ Previous Page
K Skin, Right Lower Leg L Skin, Left Lower Leg M Skin, Right Foot N Skin, Left Foot Q Finger Nail R Toe Nail			
T Breast, Right U Breast, Left V Breast, Bilateral W Nipple, Right X Nipple, Left Y Supernumerary Breast	0 Open 3 Percutaneous 7 Via Natural or Artificial Opening 8 Via Natural or Artificial Opening Endoscopic X External	Z No Device	Z No Qualifier

Section	0	Medical and Surgical
Body System	H	Skin and Breast
Operation	R	Replacement: Putting in or on biological or synthetic material that physically takes the place and/or function of all or a portion of a body part

Body Part (Character 4)	Approach (Character 5)	Device (Character 6)	Qualifier (Character 7)
0 Skin, Scalp 1 Skin, Face 2 Skin, Right Ear 3 Skin, Left Ear 4 Skin, Neck 5 Skin, Chest 6 Skin, Back 7 Skin, Abdomen 8 Skin, Buttock 9 Skin, Perineum A Skin, Genitalia B Skin, Right Upper Arm C Skin, Left Upper Arm D Skin, Right Lower Arm E Skin, Left Lower Arm F Skin, Right Hand G Skin, Left Hand H Skin, Right Upper Leg J Skin, Left Upper Leg K Skin, Right Lower Leg L Skin, Left Lower Leg M Skin, Right Foot N Skin, Left Foot	X External	7 Autologous Tissue Substitute K Nonautologous Tissue Substitute	3 Full Thickness 4 Partial Thickness
0 Skin, Scalp 1 Skin, Face 2 Skin, Right Ear 3 Skin, Left Ear 4 Skin, Neck 5 Skin, Chest 6 Skin, Back 7 Skin, Abdomen 8 Skin, Buttock 9 Skin, Perineum A Skin, Genitalia B Skin, Right Upper Arm	X External	J Synthetic Substitute	3 Full Thickness 4 Partial Thickness Z No Qualifier Continued on Next Page ▶

			Continued from ◀ Previous Page
C Skin, Left Upper Arm **D** Skin, Right Lower Arm **E** Skin, Left Lower Arm **F** Skin, Right Hand **G** Skin, Left Hand **H** Skin, Right Upper Leg **J** Skin, Left Upper Leg **K** Skin, Right Lower Leg **L** Skin, Left Lower Leg **M** Skin, Right Foot **N** Skin, Left Foot			
Q Finger Nail **R** Toe Nail **S** Hair	**X** External	**7** Autologous Tissue Substitute **J** Synthetic Substitute **K** Nonautologous Tissue Substitute	**Z** No Qualifier
T Breast, Right **U** Breast, Left **V** Breast, Bilateral	**0** Open	**7** Autologous Tissue Substitute	**5** Latissimus Dorsi Myocutaneous Flap **6** Transverse Rectus Abdominis Myocutaneous Flap **7** Deep Inferior Epigastric Artery Perforator Flap **8** Superficial Inferior Epigastric Artery Flap **9** Gluteal Artery Perforator Flap **Z** No Qualifier
T Breast, Right **U** Breast, Left **V** Breast, Bilateral	**0** Open	**J** Synthetic Substitute **K** Nonautologous Tissue Substitute	**Z** No Qualifier
T Breast, Right **U** Breast, Left **V** Breast, Bilateral	**3** Percutaneous **X** External	**7** Autologous Tissue Substitute **J** Synthetic Substitute **K** Nonautologous Tissue Substitute	**Z** No Qualifier
W Nipple, Right **X** Nipple, Left	**0** Open **3** Percutaneous **X** External	**7** Autologous Tissue Substitute **J** Synthetic Substitute **K** Nonautologous Tissue Substitute	**Z** No Qualifier

Section	0	Medical and Surgical	
Body System	H	Skin and Breast	
Operation	S	Reposition: Moving to its normal location, or other suitable location, all or a portion of a body part	

Body Part (Character 4)	Approach (Character 5)	Device (Character 6)	Qualifier (Character 7)
S Hair **W** Nipple, Right **X** Nipple, Left	**X** External	**Z** No Device	**Z** No Qualifier
T Breast, Right **U** Breast, Left **V** Breast, Bilateral	**0** Open	**Z** No Device	**Z** No Qualifier

Section	0	Medical and Surgical		
Body System	H	Skin and Breast		
Operation	T	Resection: Cutting out or off, without replacement, all of a body part		

Body Part (Character 4)	Approach (Character 5)	Device (Character 6)	Qualifier (Character 7)
Q Finger Nail R Toe Nail W Nipple, Right X Nipple, Left	X External	Z No Device	Z No Qualifier
T Breast, Right U Breast, Left V Breast, Bilateral Y Supernumerary Breast	0 Open	Z No Device	Z No Qualifier

Section	0	Medical and Surgical		
Body System	H	Skin and Breast		
Operation	U	Supplement: Putting in or on biological or synthetic material that physically reinforces and/or augments the function of a portion of a body part		

Body Part (Character 4)	Approach (Character 5)	Device (Character 6)	Qualifier (Character 7)
T Breast, Right U Breast, Left V Breast, Bilateral W Nipple, Right X Nipple, Left	0 Open 3 Percutaneous 7 Via Natural or Artificial Opening 8 Via Natural or Artificial Opening Endoscopic X External	7 Autologous Tissue Substitute J Synthetic Substitute K Nonautologous Tissue Substitute	Z No Qualifier

Section	0	Medical and Surgical		
Body System	H	Skin and Breast		
Operation	W	Revision: Correcting, to the extent possible, a portion of a malfunctioning device or the position of a displaced device		

Body Part (Character 4)	Approach (Character 5)	Device (Character 6)	Qualifier (Character 7)
P Skin Q Finger Nail R Toe Nail	X External	0 Drainage Device 7 Autologous Tissue Substitute J Synthetic Substitute K Nonautologous Tissue Substitute	Z No Qualifier
S Hair	X External	7 Autologous Tissue Substitute J Synthetic Substitute K Nonautologous Tissue Substitute	Z No Qualifier
T Breast, Right U Breast, Left	0 Open 3 Percutaneous 7 Via Natural or Artificial Opening 8 Via Natural or Artificial Opening Endoscopic	0 Drainage Device 7 Autologous Tissue Substitute J Synthetic Substitute K Nonautologous Tissue Substitute N Tissue Expander	Z No Qualifier
T Breast, Right U Breast, Left	X External	0 Drainage Device 7 Autologous Tissue Substitute J Synthetic Substitute K Nonautologous Tissue Substitute	Z No Qualifier

Section	0	Medical and Surgical		
Body System	H	Skin and Breast		
Operation	X	Transfer: Moving, without taking out, all or a portion of a body part to another location to take over the function of all or a portion of a body part		

Body Part (Character 4)	Approach (Character 5)	Device (Character 6)	Qualifier (Character 7)
0 Skin, Scalp	X External	Z No Device	Z No Qualifier
1 Skin, Face			
2 Skin, Right Ear			
3 Skin, Left Ear			
4 Skin, Neck			
5 Skin, Chest			
6 Skin, Back			
7 Skin, Abdomen			
8 Skin, Buttock			
9 Skin, Perineum			
A Skin, Genitalia			
B Skin, Right Upper Arm			
C Skin, Left Upper Arm			
D Skin, Right Lower Arm			
E Skin, Left Lower Arm			
F Skin, Right Hand			
G Skin, Left Hand			
H Skin, Right Upper Leg			
J Skin, Left Upper Leg			
K Skin, Right Lower Leg			
L Skin, Left Lower Leg			
M Skin, Right Foot			
N Skin, Left Foot			

Section	0	Medical and Surgical	
Body System	J	Subcutaneous Tissue and Fascia	
Operation	0	Alteration: Modifying the anatomic structure of a body part without affecting the function of the body part	

Body Part (Character 4)	Approach (Character 5)	Device (Character 6)	Qualifier (Character 7)
1 Subcutaneous Tissue and Fascia, Face	0 Open	Z No Device	Z No Qualifier
4 Subcutaneous Tissue and Fascia, Anterior Neck	3 Percutaneous		
5 Subcutaneous Tissue and Fascia, Posterior Neck			
6 Subcutaneous Tissue and Fascia, Chest			
7 Subcutaneous Tissue and Fascia, Back			
8 Subcutaneous Tissue and Fascia, Abdomen			
9 Subcutaneous Tissue and Fascia, Buttock			
D Subcutaneous Tissue and Fascia, Right Upper Arm			
F Subcutaneous Tissue and Fascia, Left Upper Arm			
G Subcutaneous Tissue and Fascia, Right Lower Arm			
H Subcutaneous Tissue and Fascia, Left Lower Arm			
L Subcutaneous Tissue and Fascia, Right Upper Leg			
M Subcutaneous Tissue and Fascia, Left Upper Leg			
N Subcutaneous Tissue and Fascia, Right Lower Leg			
P Subcutaneous Tissue and Fascia, Left Lower Leg			

Section	0	Medical and Surgical	
Body System	J	Subcutaneous Tissue and Fascia	
Operation	2	Change: Taking out or off a device from a body part and putting back an identical or similar device in or on the same body part without cutting or puncturing the skin or a mucous membrane	

Body Part (Character 4)	Approach (Character 5)	Device (Character 6)	Qualifier (Character 7)
S Subcutaneous Tissue and Fascia, Head and Neck	X External	0 Drainage Device	Z No Qualifier
T Subcutaneous Tissue and Fascia, Trunk		Y Other Device	
V Subcutaneous Tissue and Fascia, Upper Extremity			
W Subcutaneous Tissue and Fascia, Lower Extremity			

Section	0	Medical and Surgical		
Body System	J	Subcutaneous Tissue and Fascia		
Operation	5	Destruction: Physical eradication of all or a portion of a body part by the direct use of energy, force, or a destructive agent		

Body Part (Character 4)	Approach (Character 5)	Device (Character 6)	Qualifier (Character 7)
0 Subcutaneous Tissue and Fascia, Scalp	0 Open	Z No Device	Z No Qualifier
1 Subcutaneous Tissue and Fascia, Face	3 Percutaneous		
4 Subcutaneous Tissue and Fascia, Anterior Neck			
5 Subcutaneous Tissue and Fascia, Posterior Neck			
6 Subcutaneous Tissue and Fascia, Chest			
7 Subcutaneous Tissue and Fascia, Back			
8 Subcutaneous Tissue and Fascia, Abdomen			
9 Subcutaneous Tissue and Fascia, Buttock			
B Subcutaneous Tissue and Fascia, Perineum			
C Subcutaneous Tissue and Fascia, Pelvic Region			
D Subcutaneous Tissue and Fascia, Right Upper Arm			
F Subcutaneous Tissue and Fascia, Left Upper Arm			
G Subcutaneous Tissue and Fascia, Right Lower Arm			
H Subcutaneous Tissue and Fascia, Left Lower Arm			
J Subcutaneous Tissue and Fascia, Right Hand			
K Subcutaneous Tissue and Fascia, Left Hand			
L Subcutaneous Tissue and Fascia, Right Upper Leg			
M Subcutaneous Tissue and Fascia, Left Upper Leg			
N Subcutaneous Tissue and Fascia, Right Lower Leg			
P Subcutaneous Tissue and Fascia, Left Lower Leg			
Q Subcutaneous Tissue and Fascia, Right Foot			
R Subcutaneous Tissue and Fascia, Left Foot			

Section	0	Medical and Surgical		
Body System	J	Subcutaneous Tissue and Fascia		
Operation	8	Division: Cutting into a body part, without draining fluids and/or gases from the body part, in order to separate or transect a body part		

Body Part (Character 4)	Approach (Character 5)	Device (Character 6)	Qualifier (Character 7)
0 Subcutaneous Tissue and Fascia, Scalp	**0** Open	**Z** No Device	**Z** No Qualifier
1 Subcutaneous Tissue and Fascia, Face	**3** Percutaneous		
4 Subcutaneous Tissue and Fascia, Anterior Neck			
5 Subcutaneous Tissue and Fascia, Posterior Neck			
6 Subcutaneous Tissue and Fascia, Chest			
7 Subcutaneous Tissue and Fascia, Back			
8 Subcutaneous Tissue and Fascia, Abdomen			
9 Subcutaneous Tissue and Fascia, Buttock			
B Subcutaneous Tissue and Fascia, Perineum			
C Subcutaneous Tissue and Fascia, Pelvic Region			
D Subcutaneous Tissue and Fascia, Right Upper Arm			
F Subcutaneous Tissue and Fascia, Left Upper Arm			
G Subcutaneous Tissue and Fascia, Right Lower Arm			
H Subcutaneous Tissue and Fascia, Left Lower Arm			
J Subcutaneous Tissue and Fascia, Right Hand			
K Subcutaneous Tissue and Fascia, Left Hand			
L Subcutaneous Tissue and Fascia, Right Upper Leg			
M Subcutaneous Tissue and Fascia, Left Upper Leg			
N Subcutaneous Tissue and Fascia, Right Lower Leg			
P Subcutaneous Tissue and Fascia, Left Lower Leg			
Q Subcutaneous Tissue and Fascia, Right Foot			
R Subcutaneous Tissue and Fascia, Left Foot			
S Subcutaneous Tissue and Fascia, Head and Neck			
T Subcutaneous Tissue and Fascia, Trunk			
V Subcutaneous Tissue and Fascia, Upper Extremity			
W Subcutaneous Tissue and Fascia, Lower Extremity			

Section	0	Medical and Surgical			
Body System	J	Subcutaneous Tissue and Fascia			
Operation	9	Drainage: Taking or letting out fluids and/or gases from a body part			

Body Part (Character 4)	Approach (Character 5)	Device (Character 6)	Qualifier (Character 7)
0 Subcutaneous Tissue and Fascia, Scalp	**0** Open	**Z** No Device	**X** Diagnostic
1 Subcutaneous Tissue and Fascia, Face	**3** Percutaneous		**Z** No Qualifier
4 Subcutaneous Tissue and Fascia, Anterior Neck			
5 Subcutaneous Tissue and Fascia, Posterior Neck			
6 Subcutaneous Tissue and Fascia, Chest			
7 Subcutaneous Tissue and Fascia, Back			
8 Subcutaneous Tissue and Fascia, Abdomen			
9 Subcutaneous Tissue and Fascia, Buttock			
B Subcutaneous Tissue and Fascia, Perineum			
C Subcutaneous Tissue and Fascia, Pelvic Region			
D Subcutaneous Tissue and Fascia, Right Upper Arm			
F Subcutaneous Tissue and Fascia, Left Upper Arm			
G Subcutaneous Tissue and Fascia, Right Lower Arm			
H Subcutaneous Tissue and Fascia, Left Lower Arm			
J Subcutaneous Tissue and Fascia, Right Hand			
K Subcutaneous Tissue and Fascia, Left Hand			
L Subcutaneous Tissue and Fascia, Right Upper Leg			
M Subcutaneous Tissue and Fascia, Left Upper Leg			
N Subcutaneous Tissue and Fascia, Right Lower Leg			
P Subcutaneous Tissue and Fascia, Left Lower Leg			
Q Subcutaneous Tissue and Fascia, Right Foot			
R Subcutaneous Tissue and Fascia, Left Foot			

Section	0	Medical and Surgical		
Body System	J	Subcutaneous Tissue and Fascia		
Operation	B	Excision: Cutting out or off, without replacement, a portion of a body part		

Body Part (Character 4)	Approach (Character 5)	Device (Character 6)	Qualifier (Character 7)
0 Subcutaneous Tissue and Fascia, Scalp **1** Subcutaneous Tissue and Fascia, Face **4** Subcutaneous Tissue and Fascia, Anterior Neck **5** Subcutaneous Tissue and Fascia, Posterior Neck **6** Subcutaneous Tissue and Fascia, Chest **7** Subcutaneous Tissue and Fascia, Back **8** Subcutaneous Tissue and Fascia, Abdomen **9** Subcutaneous Tissue and Fascia, Buttock **B** Subcutaneous Tissue and Fascia, Perineum **C** Subcutaneous Tissue and Fascia, Pelvic Region **D** Subcutaneous Tissue and Fascia, Right Upper Arm **F** Subcutaneous Tissue and Fascia, Left Upper Arm **G** Subcutaneous Tissue and Fascia, Right Lower Arm **H** Subcutaneous Tissue and Fascia, Left Lower Arm **J** Subcutaneous Tissue and Fascia, Right Hand **K** Subcutaneous Tissue and Fascia, Left Hand **L** Subcutaneous Tissue and Fascia, Right Upper Leg **M** Subcutaneous Tissue and Fascia, Left Upper Leg **N** Subcutaneous Tissue and Fascia, Right Lower Leg **P** Subcutaneous Tissue and Fascia, Left Lower Leg **Q** Subcutaneous Tissue and Fascia, Right Foot **R** Subcutaneous Tissue and Fascia, Left Foot	**0** Open **3** Percutaneous	**Z** No Device	**X** Diagnostic **Z** No Qualifier

Section	0	Medical and Surgical		
Body System	J	Subcutaneous Tissue and Fascia		
Operation	C	Extirpation: Taking or cutting out solid matter from a body part		

Body Part (Character 4)	Approach (Character 5)	Device (Character 6)	Qualifier (Character 7)
0 Subcutaneous Tissue and Fascia, Scalp **1** Subcutaneous Tissue and Fascia, Face **4** Subcutaneous Tissue and Fascia, Anterior Neck **5** Subcutaneous Tissue and Fascia, Posterior Neck **6** Subcutaneous Tissue and Fascia, Chest **7** Subcutaneous Tissue and Fascia, Back **8** Subcutaneous Tissue and Fascia, Abdomen **9** Subcutaneous Tissue and Fascia, Buttock **B** Subcutaneous Tissue and Fascia, Perineum **C** Subcutaneous Tissue and Fascia, Pelvic Region **D** Subcutaneous Tissue and Fascia, Right Upper Arm **F** Subcutaneous Tissue and Fascia, Left Upper Arm **G** Subcutaneous Tissue and Fascia, Right Lower Arm **H** Subcutaneous Tissue and Fascia, Left Lower Arm **J** Subcutaneous Tissue and Fascia, Right Hand **K** Subcutaneous Tissue and Fascia, Left Hand **L** Subcutaneous Tissue and Fascia, Right Upper Leg **M** Subcutaneous Tissue and Fascia, Left Upper Leg **N** Subcutaneous Tissue and Fascia, Right Lower Leg **P** Subcutaneous Tissue and Fascia, Left Lower Leg **Q** Subcutaneous Tissue and Fascia, Right Foot **R** Subcutaneous Tissue and Fascia, Left Foot	**0** Open **3** Percutaneous	**Z** No Device	**Z** No Qualifier

Section	0	Medical and Surgical			
Body System	J	Subcutaneous Tissue and Fascia			
Operation	D	Extraction: Pulling or stripping out or off all or a portion of a body part by the use of force			

Body Part (Character 4)	Approach (Character 5)	Device (Character 6)	Qualifier (Character 7)
0 Subcutaneous Tissue and Fascia, Scalp	0 Open	Z No Device	Z No Qualifier
1 Subcutaneous Tissue and Fascia, Face	3 Percutaneous		
4 Subcutaneous Tissue and Fascia, Anterior Neck			
5 Subcutaneous Tissue and Fascia, Posterior Neck			
6 Subcutaneous Tissue and Fascia, Chest			
7 Subcutaneous Tissue and Fascia, Back			
8 Subcutaneous Tissue and Fascia, Abdomen			
9 Subcutaneous Tissue and Fascia, Buttock			
B Subcutaneous Tissue and Fascia, Perineum			
C Subcutaneous Tissue and Fascia, Pelvic Region			
D Subcutaneous Tissue and Fascia, Right Upper Arm			
F Subcutaneous Tissue and Fascia, Left Upper Arm			
G Subcutaneous Tissue and Fascia, Right Lower Arm			
H Subcutaneous Tissue and Fascia, Left Lower Arm			
J Subcutaneous Tissue and Fascia, Right Hand			
K Subcutaneous Tissue and Fascia, Left Hand			
L Subcutaneous Tissue and Fascia, Right Upper Leg			
M Subcutaneous Tissue and Fascia, Left Upper Leg			
N Subcutaneous Tissue and Fascia, Right Lower Leg			
P Subcutaneous Tissue and Fascia, Left Lower Leg			
Q Subcutaneous Tissue and Fascia, Right Foot			
R Subcutaneous Tissue and Fascia, Left Foot			

Section	0	Medical and Surgical
Body System	J	Subcutaneous Tissue and Fascia
Operation	H	Insertion: Putting in a nonbiological appliance that monitors, assists, performs, or prevents a physiological function but does not physically take the place of a body part

Body Part (Character 4)	Approach (Character 5)	Device (Character 6)	Qualifier (Character 7)
0 Subcutaneous Tissue and Fascia, Scalp **1** Subcutaneous Tissue and Fascia, Face **4** Subcutaneous Tissue and Fascia, Anterior Neck **5** Subcutaneous Tissue and Fascia, Posterior Neck **9** Subcutaneous Tissue and Fascia, Buttock **B** Subcutaneous Tissue and Fascia, Perineum **C** Subcutaneous Tissue and Fascia, Pelvic Region **J** Subcutaneous Tissue and Fascia, Right Hand **K** Subcutaneous Tissue and Fascia, Left Hand **Q** Subcutaneous Tissue and Fascia, Right Foot **R** Subcutaneous Tissue and Fascia, Left Foot	**0** Open **3** Percutaneous	**N** Tissue Expander **0** Monitoring Device,	**Z** No Qualifier
6 Subcutaneous Tissue and Fascia, Chest **8** Subcutaneous Tissue and Fascia, Abdomen	**0** Open **3** Percutaneous	**0** Monitoring Device, Hemodynamic **2** Monitoring Device **4** Pacemaker, Single Chamber **5** Pacemaker, Single Chamber Rate Responsive **6** Pacemaker, Dual Chamber **7** Cardiac Resynchronization Pacemaker Pulse Generator **8** Defibrillator Generator **9** Cardiac Resynchronization Defibrillator Pulse Generator **A** Contractility Modulation Device **B** Stimulator Generator, Single Array **C** Stimulator Generator, Single Array Rechargeable **D** Stimulator Generator, Multiple Array **E** Stimulator Generator, Multiple Array Rechargeable **H** Contraceptive Device	**Z** No Qualifier

Continued on Next Page ▶

		M Stimulator Generator	Continued from ◀ Previous Page
		N Tissue Expander	
		P Cardiac Rhythm Related Device	
		V Infusion Device, Pump	
		W Vascular Access Device, Reservoir	
		X Vascular Access Device	
7 Subcutaneous Tissue and Fascia, Back	**0** Open **3** Percutaneous	**B** Stimulator Generator, Single Array **C** Stimulator Generator, Single Array Rechargeable **D** Stimulator Generator, Multiple Array **E** Stimulator Generator, Multiple Array Rechargeable **M** Stimulator Generator **N** Tissue Expander **V** Infusion Device, Pump	**Z** No Qualifier
D Subcutaneous Tissue and Fascia, Right Upper Arm **F** Subcutaneous Tissue and Fascia, Left Upper Arm **G** Subcutaneous Tissue and Fascia, Right Lower Arm **H** Subcutaneous Tissue and Fascia, Left Lower Arm **L** Subcutaneous Tissue and Fascia, Right Upper Leg **M** Subcutaneous Tissue and Fascia, Left Upper Leg **N** Subcutaneous Tissue and Fascia, Right Lower Leg **P** Subcutaneous Tissue and Fascia, Left Lower Leg	**0** Open **3** Percutaneous	**H** Contraceptive Device **N** Tissue Expander **V** Infusion Device, Pump **W** Vascular Access Device, Reservoir **X** Vascular Access Device	**Z** No Qualifier
S Subcutaneous Tissue and Fascia, Head and Neck **V** Subcutaneous Tissue and Fascia, Upper Extremity **W** Subcutaneous Tissue and Fascia, Lower Extremity	**0** Open **3** Percutaneous	**1** Radioactive Element **3** Infusion Device	**Z** No Qualifier
T Subcutaneous Tissue and Fascia, Trunk	**0** Open **3** Percutaneous	**1** Radioactive Element **3** Infusion Device **V** Infusion Device, Pump	**Z** No Qualifier

Section	0	Medical and Surgical		
Body System	J	Subcutaneous Tissue and Fascia		
Operation	J	Inspection: Visually and/or manually exploring a body part		

Body Part (Character 4)	Approach (Character 5)	Device (Character 6)	Qualifier (Character 7)
S Subcutaneous Tissue and Fascia, Head and Neck T Subcutaneous Tissue and Fascia, Trunk V Subcutaneous Tissue and Fascia, Upper Extremity W Subcutaneous Tissue and Fascia, Lower Extremity	0 Open 3 Percutaneous X External	Z No Device	Z No Qualifier

Section	0	Medical and Surgical		
Body System	J	Subcutaneous Tissue and Fascia		
Operation	N	Release: Freeing a body part from an abnormal physical constraint by cutting or by the use of force		

Body Part (Character 4)	Approach (Character 5)	Device (Character 6)	Qualifier (Character 7)
0 Subcutaneous Tissue and Fascia, Scalp 1 Subcutaneous Tissue and Fascia, Face 4 Subcutaneous Tissue and Fascia, Anterior Neck 5 Subcutaneous Tissue and Fascia, Posterior Neck 6 Subcutaneous Tissue and Fascia, Chest 7 Subcutaneous Tissue and Fascia, Back 8 Subcutaneous Tissue and Fascia, Abdomen 9 Subcutaneous Tissue and Fascia, Buttock B Subcutaneous Tissue and Fascia, Perineum C Subcutaneous Tissue and Fascia, Pelvic Region D Subcutaneous Tissue and Fascia, Right Upper Arm F Subcutaneous Tissue and Fascia, Left Upper Arm G Subcutaneous Tissue and Fascia, Right Lower Arm H Subcutaneous Tissue and Fascia, Left Lower Arm J Subcutaneous Tissue and Fascia, Right Hand K Subcutaneous Tissue and Fascia, Left Hand L Subcutaneous Tissue and Fascia, Right Upper Leg M Subcutaneous Tissue and Fascia, Left Upper Leg N Subcutaneous Tissue and Fascia, Right Lower Leg P Subcutaneous Tissue and Fascia, Left Lower Leg	0 Open 3 Percutaneous X External	Z No Device	Z No Qualifier

Continued on Next Page ▶

| Q Subcutaneous Tissue and Fascia, Right Foot
R Subcutaneous Tissue and Fascia, Left Foot | | | **Continued from**
◀ **Previous Page** |

Section	0	Medical and Surgical
Body System	J	Subcutaneous Tissue and Fascia
Operation	P	Removal: Taking out or off a device from a body part

Body Part (Character 4)	Approach (Character 5)	Device (Character 6)	Qualifier (Character 7)
S Subcutaneous Tissue and Fascia, Head and Neck	0 Open 3 Percutaneous	0 Drainage Device 1 Radioactive Element 3 Infusion Device 7 Autologous Tissue Substitute J Synthetic Substitute K Nonautologous Tissue Substitute N Tissue Expander	Z No Qualifier
S Subcutaneous Tissue and Fascia, Head and Neck	X External	0 Drainage Device 1 Radioactive Element 3 Infusion Device	Z No Qualifier
T Subcutaneous Tissue and Fascia, Trunk	0 Open 3 Percutaneous	0 Drainage Device 1 Radioactive Element 2 Monitoring Device 3 Infusion Device 7 Autologous Tissue Substitute H Contraceptive Device J Synthetic Substitute K Nonautologous Tissue Substitute M Stimulator Generator N Tissue Expander P Cardiac Rhythm Related Device V Infusion Device, Pump W Vascular Access Device, Reservoir X Vascular Access Device	Z No Qualifier
T Subcutaneous Tissue and Fascia, Trunk	X External	0 Drainage Device 1 Radioactive Element 2 Monitoring Device 3 Infusion Device H Contraceptive Device V Infusion Device, Pump X Vascular Access Device	Z No Qualifier
V Subcutaneous Tissue and Fascia, Upper Extremity W Subcutaneous Tissue and Fascia, Lower Extremity	0 Open 3 Percutaneous	0 Drainage Device 1 Radioactive Element 3 Infusion Device 7 Autologous Tissue Substitute H Contraceptive Device J Synthetic Substitute K Nonautologous Tissue Substitute N Tissue Expander	Z No Qualifier

Continued on Next Page ▶

		V Infusion Device, Pump W Vascular Access Device, Reservoir X Vascular Access Device	Continued from ◀ Previous Page
V Subcutaneous Tissue and Fascia, Upper Extremity W Subcutaneous Tissue and Fascia, Lower Extremity	X External	0 Drainage Device 1 Radioactive Element 3 Infusion Device H Contraceptive Device V Infusion Device, Pump X Vascular Access Device	Z No Qualifier

Section	0	Medical and Surgical	
Body System	J	Subcutaneous Tissue and Fascia	
Operation	Q	Repair: Restoring, to the extent possible, a body part to its normal anatomic structure and function	

Body Part (Character 4)	Approach (Character 5)	Device (Character 6)	Qualifier (Character 7)
0 Subcutaneous Tissue and Fascia, Scalp 1 Subcutaneous Tissue and Fascia, Face 4 Subcutaneous Tissue and Fascia, Anterior Neck 5 Subcutaneous Tissue and Fascia, Posterior Neck 6 Subcutaneous Tissue and Fascia, Chest 7 Subcutaneous Tissue and Fascia, Back 8 Subcutaneous Tissue and Fascia, Abdomen 9 Subcutaneous Tissue and Fascia, Buttock B Subcutaneous Tissue and Fascia, Perineum C Subcutaneous Tissue and Fascia, Pelvic Region D Subcutaneous Tissue and Fascia, Right Upper Arm F Subcutaneous Tissue and Fascia, Left Upper Arm G Subcutaneous Tissue and Fascia, Right Lower Arm H Subcutaneous Tissue and Fascia, Left Lower Arm J Subcutaneous Tissue and Fascia, Right Hand K Subcutaneous Tissue and Fascia, Left Hand L Subcutaneous Tissue and Fascia, Right Upper Leg M Subcutaneous Tissue and Fascia, Left Upper Leg N Subcutaneous Tissue and Fascia, Right Lower Leg P Subcutaneous Tissue and Fascia, Left Lower Leg Q Subcutaneous Tissue and Fascia, Right Foot R Subcutaneous Tissue and Fascia, Left Foot	0 Open 3 Percutaneous	Z No Device	Z No Qualifier

Section	0	Medical and Surgical		
Body System	J	Subcutaneous Tissue and Fascia		
Operation	W	Revision: Correcting, to the extent possible, a portion of a malfunctioning device or the position of a displaced device		

Body Part (Character 4)	Approach (Character 5)	Device (Character 6)	Qualifier (Character 7)
S Subcutaneous Tissue and Fascia, Head and Neck	0 Open 3 Percutaneous X External	0 Drainage Device 3 Infusion Device 7 Autologous Tissue Substitute J Synthetic Substitute K Nonautologous Tissue Substitute N Tissue Expander	Z No Qualifier
T Subcutaneous Tissue and Fascia, Trunk	0 Open 3 Percutaneous X External	0 Drainage Device 2 Monitoring Device 3 Infusion Device 7 Autologous Tissue Substitute H Contraceptive Device J Synthetic Substitute K Nonautologous Tissue Substitute M Stimulator Generator N Tissue Expander P Cardiac Rhythm Related Device V Infusion Device, Pump W Vascular Access Device, Reservoir X Vascular Access Device	Z No Qualifier
V Subcutaneous Tissue and Fascia, Upper Extremity W Subcutaneous Tissue and Fascia, Lower Extremity	0 Open 3 Percutaneous X External	0 Drainage Device 3 Infusion Device 7 Autologous Tissue Substitute H Contraceptive Device J Synthetic Substitute K Nonautologous Tissue Substitute N Tissue Expander V Infusion Device, Pump W Vascular Access Device, Reservoir X Vascular Access Device	Z No Qualifier

Section	0	Medical and Surgical		
Body System	J	Subcutaneous Tissue and Fascia		
Operation	X	Transfer: Moving, without taking out, all or a portion of a body part to another location to take over the function of all or a portion of a body part		

Body Part (Character 4)	Approach (Character 5)	Device (Character 6)	Qualifier (Character 7)
0 Subcutaneous Tissue and Fascia, Scalp 1 Subcutaneous Tissue and Fascia, Face 4 Subcutaneous Tissue and Fascia, Anterior Neck 5 Subcutaneous Tissue and Fascia, Posterior Neck 6 Subcutaneous Tissue and Fascia, Chest 7 Subcutaneous Tissue and Fascia, Back 8 Subcutaneous Tissue and Fascia, Abdomen 9 Subcutaneous Tissue and Fascia, Buttock B Subcutaneous Tissue and Fascia, Perineum C Subcutaneous Tissue and Fascia, Pelvic Region D Subcutaneous Tissue and Fascia, Right Upper Arm F Subcutaneous Tissue and Fascia, Left Upper Arm G Subcutaneous Tissue and Fascia, Right Lower Arm H Subcutaneous Tissue and Fascia, Left Lower Arm J Subcutaneous Tissue and Fascia, Right Hand K Subcutaneous Tissue and Fascia, Left Hand L Subcutaneous Tissue and Fascia, Right Upper Leg M Subcutaneous Tissue and Fascia, Left Upper Leg N Subcutaneous Tissue and Fascia, Right Lower Leg P Subcutaneous Tissue and Fascia, Left Lower Leg Q Subcutaneous Tissue and Fascia, Right Foot R Subcutaneous Tissue and Fascia, Left Foot	0 Open 3 Percutaneous	Z No Device	B Skin and Subcutaneous Tissue C Skin, Subcutaneous Tissue and Fascia Z No Qualifier

Section	0	Medical and Surgical			
Body System	K	Muscles			
Operation	2	Change: Taking out or off a device from a body part and putting back an identical or similar device in or on the same body part without cutting or puncturing the skin or a mucous membrane			

Body Part (Character 4)	Approach (Character 5)	Device (Character 6)	Qualifier (Character 7)
X Upper Muscle	X External	0 Drainage Device	Z No Qualifier
Y Lower Muscle		Y Other Device	

Section	0	Medical and Surgical			
Body System	K	Muscles			
Operation	5	Destruction: Physical eradication of all or a portion of a body part by the direct use of energy, force, or a destructive agent			

Body Part (Character 4)	Approach (Character 5)	Device (Character 6)	Qualifier (Character 7)
0 Head Muscle	0 Open	Z No Device	Z No Qualifier
1 Facial Muscle	3 Percutaneous		
2 Neck Muscle, Right	4 Percutaneous Endoscopic		
3 Neck Muscle, Left			
4 Tongue, Palate, Pharynx Muscle			
5 Shoulder Muscle, Right			
6 Shoulder Muscle, Left			
7 Upper Arm Muscle, Right			
8 Upper Arm Muscle, Left			
9 Lower Arm and Wrist Muscle, Right			
B Lower Arm and Wrist Muscle, Left			
C Hand Muscle, Right			
D Hand Muscle, Left			
F Trunk Muscle, Right			
G Trunk Muscle, Left			
H Thorax Muscle, Right			
J Thorax Muscle, Left			
K Abdomen Muscle, Right			
L Abdomen Muscle, Left			
M Perineum Muscle			
N Hip Muscle, Right			
P Hip Muscle, Left			
Q Upper Leg Muscle, Right			
R Upper Leg Muscle, Left			
S Lower Leg Muscle, Right			
T Lower Leg Muscle, Left			
V Foot Muscle, Right			
W Foot Muscle, Left			

Section	0	Medical and Surgical		
Body System	K	Muscles		
Operation	8	Division: Cutting into a body part, without draining fluids and/or gases from the body part, in order to separate or transect a body part		

Body Part (Character 4)	Approach (Character 5)	Device (Character 6)	Qualifier (Character 7)
0 Head Muscle	**0** Open	**Z** No Device	**Z** No Qualifier
1 Facial Muscle	**3** Percutaneous		
2 Neck Muscle, Right	**4** Percutaneous Endoscopic		
3 Neck Muscle, Left			
4 Tongue, Palate, Pharynx Muscle			
5 Shoulder Muscle, Right			
6 Shoulder Muscle, Left			
7 Upper Arm Muscle, Right			
8 Upper Arm Muscle, Left			
9 Lower Arm and Wrist Muscle, Right			
B Lower Arm and Wrist Muscle, Left			
C Hand Muscle, Right			
D Hand Muscle, Left			
F Trunk Muscle, Right			
G Trunk Muscle, Left			
H Thorax Muscle, Right			
J Thorax Muscle, Left			
K Abdomen Muscle, Right			
L Abdomen Muscle, Left			
M Perineum Muscle			
N Hip Muscle, Right			
P Hip Muscle, Left			
Q Upper Leg Muscle, Right			
R Upper Leg Muscle, Left			
S Lower Leg Muscle, Right			
T Lower Leg Muscle, Left			
V Foot Muscle, Right			
W Foot Muscle, Left			

Section	0	Medical and Surgical		
Body System	K	Muscles		
Operation	9	Drainage: Taking or letting out fluids and/or gases from a body part		

Body Part (Character 4)	Approach (Character 5)	Device (Character 6)	Qualifier (Character 7)
0 Head Muscle	**0** Open	**0** Drainage Device	**Z** No Qualifier
1 Facial Muscle	**3** Percutaneous		
2 Neck Muscle, Right	**4** Percutaneous Endoscopic		
3 Neck Muscle, Left			
4 Tongue, Palate, Pharynx Muscle			
5 Shoulder Muscle, Right			
6 Shoulder Muscle, Left			
7 Upper Arm Muscle, Right			
8 Upper Arm Muscle, Left			
9 Lower Arm and Wrist Muscle, Right			
B Lower Arm and Wrist Muscle, Left			**Continued on Next Page ▶**

Continued on Next Page ▶

			Continued from ◀ Previous Page
C Hand Muscle, Right			
D Hand Muscle, Left			
F Trunk Muscle, Right			
G Trunk Muscle, Left			
H Thorax Muscle, Right			
J Thorax Muscle, Left			
K Abdomen Muscle, Right			
L Abdomen Muscle, Left			
M Perineum Muscle			
N Hip Muscle, Right			
P Hip Muscle, Left			
Q Upper Leg Muscle, Right			
R Upper Leg Muscle, Left			
S Lower Leg Muscle, Right			
T Lower Leg Muscle, Left			
V Foot Muscle, Right			
W Foot Muscle, Left			
0 Head Muscle	0 Open	Z No Device	X Diagnostic
1 Facial Muscle	3 Percutaneous		Z No Qualifier
2 Neck Muscle, Right	4 Percutaneous Endoscopic		
3 Neck Muscle, Left			
4 Tongue, Palate, Pharynx Muscle			
5 Shoulder Muscle, Right			
6 Shoulder Muscle, Left			
7 Upper Arm Muscle, Right			
8 Upper Arm Muscle, Left			
9 Lower Arm and Wrist Muscle, Right			
B Lower Arm and Wrist Muscle, Left			
C Hand Muscle, Right			
D Hand Muscle, Left			
F Trunk Muscle, Right			
G Trunk Muscle, Left			
H Thorax Muscle, Right			
J Thorax Muscle, Left			
K Abdomen Muscle, Right			
L Abdomen Muscle, Left			
M Perineum Muscle			
N Hip Muscle, Right			
P Hip Muscle, Left			
Q Upper Leg Muscle, Right			
R Upper Leg Muscle, Left			
S Lower Leg Muscle, Right			
T Lower Leg Muscle, Left			
V Foot Muscle, Right			
W Foot Muscle, Left			

Section	0	Medical and Surgical		
Body System	K	Muscles		
Operation	B	Excision: Cutting out or off, without replacement, a portion of a body part		

Body Part (Character 4)	Approach (Character 5)	Device (Character 6)	Qualifier (Character 7)
0 Head Muscle	**0** Open	**Z** No Device	**X** Diagnostic
1 Facial Muscle	**3** Percutaneous		**Z** No Qualifier
2 Neck Muscle, Right	**4** Percutaneous Endoscopic		
3 Neck Muscle, Left			
4 Tongue, Palate, Pharynx Muscle			
5 Shoulder Muscle, Right			
6 Shoulder Muscle, Left			
7 Upper Arm Muscle, Right			
8 Upper Arm Muscle, Left			
9 Lower Arm and Wrist Muscle, Right			
B Lower Arm and Wrist Muscle, Left			
C Hand Muscle, Right			
D Hand Muscle, Left			
F Trunk Muscle, Right			
G Trunk Muscle, Left			
H Thorax Muscle, Right			
J Thorax Muscle, Left			
K Abdomen Muscle, Right			
L Abdomen Muscle, Left			
M Perineum Muscle			
N Hip Muscle, Right			
P Hip Muscle, Left			
Q Upper Leg Muscle, Right			
R Upper Leg Muscle, Left			
S Lower Leg Muscle, Right			
T Lower Leg Muscle, Left			
V Foot Muscle, Right			
W Foot Muscle, Left			

Section	0	Medical and Surgical		
Body System	K	Muscles		
Operation	C	Extirpation: Taking or cutting out solid matter from a body part		

Body Part (Character 4)	Approach (Character 5)	Device (Character 6)	Qualifier (Character 7)
0 Head Muscle	**0** Open	**Z** No Device	**Z** No Qualifier
1 Facial Muscle	**3** Percutaneous		
2 Neck Muscle, Right	**4** Percutaneous Endoscopic		
3 Neck Muscle, Left			
4 Tongue, Palate, Pharynx Muscle			
5 Shoulder Muscle, Right			
6 Shoulder Muscle, Left			
7 Upper Arm Muscle, Right			
8 Upper Arm Muscle, Left			
9 Lower Arm and Wrist Muscle, Right			
B Lower Arm and Wrist Muscle, Left			
C Hand Muscle, Right			Continued on Next Page ▶

D Hand Muscle, Left			Continued from ◀ Previous Page
F Trunk Muscle, Right			
G Trunk Muscle, Left			
H Thorax Muscle, Right			
J Thorax Muscle, Left			
K Abdomen Muscle, Right			
L Abdomen Muscle, Left			
M Perineum Muscle			
N Hip Muscle, Right			
P Hip Muscle, Left			
Q Upper Leg Muscle, Right			
R Upper Leg Muscle, Left			
S Lower Leg Muscle, Right			
T Lower Leg Muscle, Left			
V Foot Muscle, Right			
W Foot Muscle, Left			

Section	0	Medical and Surgical		
Body System	K	Muscles		
Operation	H	Insertion: Putting in a nonbiological appliance that monitors, assists, performs, or prevents a physiological function but does not physically take the place of a body part		

Body Part (Character 4)	Approach (Character 5)	Device (Character 6)	Qualifier (Character 7)
X Upper Muscle	**0** Open	**M** Stimulator Lead	**Z** No Qualifier
Y Lower Muscle	**3** Percutaneous		
	4 Percutaneous Endoscopic		

Section	0	Medical and Surgical		
Body System	K	Muscles		
Operation	J	Inspection: Visually and/or manually exploring a body part		

Body Part (Character 4)	Approach (Character 5)	Device (Character 6)	Qualifier (Character 7)
X Upper Muscle	**0** Open	**Z** No Device	**Z** No Qualifier
Y Lower Muscle	**3** Percutaneous		
	4 Percutaneous Endoscopic		
	X External		

Section	0	Medical and Surgical		
Body System	K	Muscles		
Operation	M	Reattachment Putting back in or on all or a portion of a separated body part to its normal location or other suitable location		

Body Part (Character 4)	Approach (Character 5)	Device (Character 6)	Qualifier (Character 7)
0 Head Muscle	**0** Open	**Z** No Device	**Z** No Qualifier
1 Facial Muscle	**4** Percutaneous Endoscopic		
2 Neck Muscle, Right			
3 Neck Muscle, Left			
4 Tongue, Palate, Pharynx Muscle			
5 Shoulder Muscle, Right			
6 Shoulder Muscle, Left			
7 Upper Arm Muscle, Right			
8 Upper Arm Muscle, Left			
9 Lower Arm and Wrist Muscle, Right			
B Lower Arm and Wrist Muscle, Left			Continued on Next Page ▶

			Continued from ◀ Previous Page
C Hand Muscle, Right			
D Hand Muscle, Left			
F Trunk Muscle, Right			
G Trunk Muscle, Left			
H Thorax Muscle, Right			
J Thorax Muscle, Left			
K Abdomen Muscle, Right			
L Abdomen Muscle, Left			
M Perineum Muscle			
N Hip Muscle, Right			
P Hip Muscle, Left			
Q Upper Leg Muscle, Right			
R Upper Leg Muscle, Left			
S Lower Leg Muscle, Right			
T Lower Leg Muscle, Left			
V Foot Muscle, Right			
W Foot Muscle, Left			

Section	0	Medical and Surgical
Body System	K	Muscles
Operation	N	Release: Freeing a body part from an abnormal physical constraint by cutting or by the use of force

Body Part (Character 4)	Approach (Character 5)	Device (Character 6)	Qualifier (Character 7)
0 Head Muscle	0 Open	Z No Device	Z No Qualifier
1 Facial Muscle	3 Percutaneous		
2 Neck Muscle, Right	4 Percutaneous Endoscopic		
3 Neck Muscle, Left	X External		
4 Tongue, Palate, Pharynx Muscle			
5 Shoulder Muscle, Right			
6 Shoulder Muscle, Left			
7 Upper Arm Muscle, Right			
8 Upper Arm Muscle, Left			
9 Lower Arm and Wrist Muscle, Right			
B Lower Arm and Wrist Muscle, Left			
C Hand Muscle, Right			
D Hand Muscle, Left			
F Trunk Muscle, Right			
G Trunk Muscle, Left			
H Thorax Muscle, Right			
J Thorax Muscle, Left			
K Abdomen Muscle, Right			
L Abdomen Muscle, Left			
M Perineum Muscle			
N Hip Muscle, Right			
P Hip Muscle, Left			
Q Upper Leg Muscle, Right			
R Upper Leg Muscle, Left			
S Lower Leg Muscle, Right			
T Lower Leg Muscle, Left			
V Foot Muscle, Right			
W Foot Muscle, Left			

Section	0	Medical and Surgical
Body System	K	Muscles
Operation	P	Removal: Taking out or off a device from a body part

Body Part (Character 4)	Approach (Character 5)	Device (Character 6)	Qualifier (Character 7)
X Upper Muscle Y Lower Muscle	0 Open 3 Percutaneous 4 Percutaneous Endoscopic	0 Drainage Device 7 Autologous Tissue Substitute J Synthetic Substitute K Nonautologous Tissue Substitute M Stimulator Lead	Z No Qualifier
X Upper Muscle Y Lower Muscle	X External	0 Drainage Device M Stimulator Lead	Z No Qualifier

Section	0	Medical and Surgical
Body System	K	Muscles
Operation	Q	Repair: Restoring, to the extent possible, a body part to its normal anatomic structure and function

Body Part (Character 4)	Approach (Character 5)	Device (Character 6)	Qualifier (Character 7)
0 Head Muscle 1 Facial Muscle 2 Neck Muscle, Right 3 Neck Muscle, Left 4 Tongue, Palate, Pharynx Muscle 5 Shoulder Muscle, Right 6 Shoulder Muscle, Left 7 Upper Arm Muscle, Right 8 Upper Arm Muscle, Left 9 Lower Arm and Wrist Muscle, Right B Lower Arm and Wrist Muscle, Left C Hand Muscle, Right D Hand Muscle, Left F Trunk Muscle, Right G Trunk Muscle, Left H Thorax Muscle, Right J Thorax Muscle, Left K Abdomen Muscle, Right L Abdomen Muscle, Left M Perineum Muscle N Hip Muscle, Right P Hip Muscle, Left Q Upper Leg Muscle, Right R Upper Leg Muscle, Left S Lower Leg Muscle, Right T Lower Leg Muscle, Left V Foot Muscle, Right W Foot Muscle, Left	0 Open 3 Percutaneous 4 Percutaneous Endoscopic	Z No Device	Z No Qualifier

Section	0	Medical and Surgical		
Body System	K	Muscles		
Operation	S	Reposition: Moving to its normal location, or other suitable location, all or a portion of a body part		

Body Part (Character 4)	Approach (Character 5)	Device (Character 6)	Qualifier (Character 7)
0 Head Muscle	**0** Open	**Z** No Device	**Z** No Qualifier
1 Facial Muscle	**4** Percutaneous Endoscopic		
2 Neck Muscle, Right			
3 Neck Muscle, Left			
4 Tongue, Palate, Pharynx Muscle			
5 Shoulder Muscle, Right			
6 Shoulder Muscle, Left			
7 Upper Arm Muscle, Right			
8 Upper Arm Muscle, Left			
9 Lower Arm and Wrist Muscle, Right			
B Lower Arm and Wrist Muscle, Left			
C Hand Muscle, Right			
D Hand Muscle, Left			
F Trunk Muscle, Right			
G Trunk Muscle, Left			
H Thorax Muscle, Right			
J Thorax Muscle, Left			
K Abdomen Muscle, Right			
L Abdomen Muscle, Left			
M Perineum Muscle			
N Hip Muscle, Right			
P Hip Muscle, Left			
Q Upper Leg Muscle, Right			
R Upper Leg Muscle, Left			
S Lower Leg Muscle, Right			
T Lower Leg Muscle, Left			
V Foot Muscle, Right			
W Foot Muscle, Left			

Section	0	Medical and Surgical		
Body System	K	Muscles		
Operation	T	Resection: Cutting out or off, without replacement, all of a body part		

Body Part (Character 4)	Approach (Character 5)	Device (Character 6)	Qualifier (Character 7)
0 Head Muscle	**0** Open	**Z** No Device	**Z** No Qualifier
1 Facial Muscle	**4** Percutaneous Endoscopic		
2 Neck Muscle, Right			
3 Neck Muscle, Left			
4 Tongue, Palate, Pharynx Muscle			
5 Shoulder Muscle, Right			
6 Shoulder Muscle, Left			
7 Upper Arm Muscle, Right			
8 Upper Arm Muscle, Left			
9 Lower Arm and Wrist Muscle, Right			
B Lower Arm and Wrist Muscle, Left			

Continued on Next Page ▶

			Continued from ◀ Previous Page
C Hand Muscle, Right			
D Hand Muscle, Left			
F Trunk Muscle, Right			
G Trunk Muscle, Left			
H Thorax Muscle, Right			
J Thorax Muscle, Left			
K Abdomen Muscle, Right			
L Abdomen Muscle, Left			
M Perineum Muscle			
N Hip Muscle, Right			
P Hip Muscle, Left			
Q Upper Leg Muscle, Right			
R Upper Leg Muscle, Left			
S Lower Leg Muscle, Right			
T Lower Leg Muscle, Left			
V Foot Muscle, Right			
W Foot Muscle, Left			

Section	0	Medical and Surgical
Body System	K	Muscles
Operation	U	Supplement: Putting in or on biological or synthetic material that physically reinforces and/or augments the function of a portion of a body part

Body Part (Character 4)	Approach (Character 5)	Device (Character 6)	Qualifier (Character 7)
0 Head Muscle	**0** Open	**7** Autologous Tissue Substitute	**Z** No Qualifier
1 Facial Muscle	**4** Percutaneous Endoscopic	**J** Synthetic Substitute	
2 Neck Muscle, Right		**K** Nonautologous Tissue Substitute	
3 Neck Muscle, Left			
4 Tongue, Palate, Pharynx Muscle			
5 Shoulder Muscle, Right			
6 Shoulder Muscle, Left			
7 Upper Arm Muscle, Right			
8 Upper Arm Muscle, Left			
9 Lower Arm and Wrist Muscle, Right			
B Lower Arm and Wrist Muscle, Left			
C Hand Muscle, Right			
D Hand Muscle, Left			
F Trunk Muscle, Right			
G Trunk Muscle, Left			
H Thorax Muscle, Right			
J Thorax Muscle, Left			
K Abdomen Muscle, Right			
L Abdomen Muscle, Left			
M Perineum Muscle			
N Hip Muscle, Right			
P Hip Muscle, Left			
Q Upper Leg Muscle, Right			
R Upper Leg Muscle, Left			
S Lower Leg Muscle, Right			
T Lower Leg Muscle, Left			
V Foot Muscle, Right			
W Foot Muscle, Left			

Section	0	Medical and Surgical		
Body System	K	Muscles		
Operation	W	Revision: Correcting, to the extent possible, a portion of a malfunctioning device or the position of a displaced device		

Body Part (Character 4)	Approach (Character 5)	Device (Character 6)	Qualifier (Character 7)
X Upper Muscle Y Lower Muscle	0 Open 3 Percutaneous 4 Percutaneous Endoscopic X External	0 Drainage Device 7 Autologous Tissue Substitute J Synthetic Substitute K Nonautologous Tissue Substitute M Stimulator Lead	Z No Qualifier

Section	0	Medical and Surgical		
Body System	K	Muscles		
Operation	X	Transfer: Moving, without taking out, all or a portion of a body part to another location to take over the function of all or a portion of a body part		

Body Part (Character 4)	Approach (Character 5)	Device (Character 6)	Qualifier (Character 7)
0 Head Muscle 1 Facial Muscle 2 Neck Muscle, Right 3 Neck Muscle, Left 4 Tongue, Palate, Pharynx Muscle 5 Shoulder Muscle, Right 6 Shoulder Muscle, Left 7 Upper Arm Muscle, Right 8 Upper Arm Muscle, Left 9 Lower Arm and Wrist Muscle, Right B Lower Arm and Wrist Muscle, Left C Hand Muscle, Right D Hand Muscle, Left F Trunk Muscle, Right G Trunk Muscle, Left H Thorax Muscle, Right J Thorax Muscle, Left M Perineum Muscle N Hip Muscle, Right P Hip Muscle, Left Q Upper Leg Muscle, Right R Upper Leg Muscle, Left S Lower Leg Muscle, Right T Lower Leg Muscle, Left V Foot Muscle, Right W Foot Muscle, Left	0 Open 4 Percutaneous Endoscopic	Z No Device	0 Skin 1 Subcutaneous Tissue 2 Skin and Subcutaneous Tissue Z No Qualifier
K Abdomen Muscle, Right L Abdomen Muscle, Left	0 Open 4 Percutaneous Endoscopic	Z No Device	0 Skin 1 Subcutaneous Tissue 2 Skin and Subcutaneous Tissue 6 Transverse Rectus Abdominis Myocutaneous Flap Z No Qualifier

Section	0	Medical and Surgical		
Body System	L	Tendons		
Operation	2	Change: Taking out or off a device from a body part and putting back an identical or similar device in or on the same body part without cutting or puncturing the skin or a mucous membrane		

Body Part (Character 4)	Approach (Character 5)	Device (Character 6)	Qualifier (Character 7)
X Upper Tendon	X External	0 Drainage Device	Z No Qualifier
Y Lower Tendon		Y Other Device	

Section	0	Medical and Surgical		
Body System	L	Tendons		
Operation	5	Destruction: Physical eradication of all or a portion of a body part by the direct use of energy, force, or a destructive agent		

Body Part (Character 4)	Approach (Character 5)	Device (Character 6)	Qualifier (Character 7)
0 Head and Neck Tendon	0 Open	Z No Device	Z No Qualifier
1 Shoulder Tendon, Right	3 Percutaneous		
2 Shoulder Tendon, Left	4 Percutaneous Endoscopic		
3 Upper Arm Tendon, Right			
4 Upper Arm Tendon, Left			
5 Lower Arm and Wrist Tendon, Right			
6 Lower Arm and Wrist Tendon, Left			
7 Hand Tendon, Right			
8 Hand Tendon, Left			
9 Trunk Tendon, Right			
B Trunk Tendon, Left			
C Thorax Tendon, Right			
D Thorax Tendon, Left			
F Abdomen Tendon, Right			
G Abdomen Tendon, Left			
H Perineum Tendon			
J Hip Tendon, Right			
K Hip Tendon, Left			
L Upper Leg Tendon, Right			
M Upper Leg Tendon, Left			
N Lower Leg Tendon, Right			
P Lower Leg Tendon, Left			
Q Knee Tendon, Right			
R Knee Tendon, Left			
S Ankle Tendon, Right			
T Ankle Tendon, Left			
V Foot Tendon, Right			
W Foot Tendon, Left			

Section	0	Medical and Surgical		
Body System	L	Tendons		
Operation	8	Division: Cutting into a body part, without draining fluids and/or gases from the body part, in order to separate or transect a body part		
Body Part (Character 4)	Approach (Character 5)	Device (Character 6)	Qualifier (Character 7)
0 Head and Neck Tendon	0 Open	Z No Device	Z No Qualifier
1 Shoulder Tendon, Right	3 Percutaneous		
2 Shoulder Tendon, Left	4 Percutaneous Endoscopic		
3 Upper Arm Tendon, Right			
4 Upper Arm Tendon, Left			
5 Lower Arm and Wrist Tendon, Right			
6 Lower Arm and Wrist Tendon, Left			
7 Hand Tendon, Right			
8 Hand Tendon, Left			
9 Trunk Tendon, Right			
B Trunk Tendon, Left			
C Thorax Tendon, Right			
D Thorax Tendon, Left			
F Abdomen Tendon, Right			
G Abdomen Tendon, Left			
H Perineum Tendon			
J Hip Tendon, Right			
K Hip Tendon, Left			
L Upper Leg Tendon, Right			
M Upper Leg Tendon, Left			
N Lower Leg Tendon, Right			
P Lower Leg Tendon, Left			
Q Knee Tendon, Right			
R Knee Tendon, Left			
S Ankle Tendon, Right			
T Ankle Tendon, Left			
V Foot Tendon, Right			
W Foot Tendon, Left			

Section	0	Medical and Surgical		
Body System	L	Tendons		
Operation	9	Drainage: Taking or letting out fluids and/or gases from a body part		
Body Part (Character 4)	Approach (Character 5)	Device (Character 6)	Qualifier (Character 7)
0 Head and Neck Tendon	0 Open	0 Drainage Device	Z No Qualifier
1 Shoulder Tendon, Right	3 Percutaneous		
2 Shoulder Tendon, Left	4 Percutaneous Endoscopic		
3 Upper Arm Tendon, Right			
4 Upper Arm Tendon, Left			
5 Lower Arm and Wrist Tendon, Right			
6 Lower Arm and Wrist Tendon, Left			
7 Hand Tendon, Right			
8 Hand Tendon, Left			
9 Trunk Tendon, Right			
B Trunk Tendon, Left			
C Thorax Tendon, Right			
D Thorax Tendon, Left			Continued on Next Page ▶

F Abdomen Tendon, Right			**Continued from ◀ Previous Page**
G Abdomen Tendon, Left			
H Perineum Tendon			
J Hip Tendon, Right			
K Hip Tendon, Left			
L Upper Leg Tendon, Right			
M Upper Leg Tendon, Left			
N Lower Leg Tendon, Right			
P Lower Leg Tendon, Left			
Q Knee Tendon, Right			
R Knee Tendon, Left			
S Ankle Tendon, Right			
T Ankle Tendon, Left			
V Foot Tendon, Right			
W Foot Tendon, Left			
0 Head and Neck Tendon	**0** Open	**Z** No Device	**X** Diagnostic
1 Shoulder Tendon, Right	**3** Percutaneous		**Z** No Qualifier
2 Shoulder Tendon, Left	**4** Percutaneous Endoscopic		
3 Upper Arm Tendon, Right			
4 Upper Arm Tendon, Left			
5 Lower Arm and Wrist Tendon, Right			
6 Lower Arm and Wrist Tendon, Left			
7 Hand Tendon, Right			
8 Hand Tendon, Left			
9 Trunk Tendon, Right			
B Trunk Tendon, Left			
C Thorax Tendon, Right			
D Thorax Tendon, Left			
F Abdomen Tendon, Right			
G Abdomen Tendon, Left			
H Perineum Tendon			
J Hip Tendon, Right			
K Hip Tendon, Left			
L Upper Leg Tendon, Right			
M Upper Leg Tendon, Left			
N Lower Leg Tendon, Right			
P Lower Leg Tendon, Left			
Q Knee Tendon, Right			
R Knee Tendon, Left			
S Ankle Tendon, Right			
T Ankle Tendon, Left			
V Foot Tendon, Right			
W Foot Tendon, Left			

Section	0	Medical and Surgical		
Body System	L	Tendons		
Operation	B	Excision: Cutting out or off, without replacement, a portion of a body part		

Body Part (Character 4)	Approach (Character 5)	Device (Character 6)	Qualifier (Character 7)
0 Head and Neck Tendon	0 Open	Z No Device	X Diagnostic
1 Shoulder Tendon, Right	3 Percutaneous		Z No Qualifier
2 Shoulder Tendon, Left	4 Percutaneous Endoscopic		
3 Upper Arm Tendon, Right			
4 Upper Arm Tendon, Left			
5 Lower Arm and Wrist Tendon, Right			
6 Lower Arm and Wrist Tendon, Left			
7 Hand Tendon, Right			
8 Hand Tendon, Left			
9 Trunk Tendon, Right			
B Trunk Tendon, Left			
C Thorax Tendon, Right			
D Thorax Tendon, Left			
F Abdomen Tendon, Right			
G Abdomen Tendon, Left			
H Perineum Tendon			
J Hip Tendon, Right			
K Hip Tendon, Left			
L Upper Leg Tendon, Right			
M Upper Leg Tendon, Left			
N Lower Leg Tendon, Right			
P Lower Leg Tendon, Left			
Q Knee Tendon, Right			
R Knee Tendon, Left			
S Ankle Tendon, Right			
T Ankle Tendon, Left			
V Foot Tendon, Right			
W Foot Tendon, Left			

Section	0	Medical and Surgical		
Body System	L	Tendons		
Operation	C	Extirpation: Taking or cutting out solid matter from a body part		

Body Part (Character 4)	Approach (Character 5)	Device (Character 6)	Qualifier (Character 7)
0 Head and Neck Tendon	0 Open	Z No Device	Z No Qualifier
1 Shoulder Tendon, Right	3 Percutaneous		
2 Shoulder Tendon, Left	4 Percutaneous Endoscopic		
3 Upper Arm Tendon, Right			
4 Upper Arm Tendon, Left			
5 Lower Arm and Wrist Tendon, Right			
6 Lower Arm and Wrist Tendon, Left			
7 Hand Tendon, Right			
8 Hand Tendon, Left			
9 Trunk Tendon, Right			
B Trunk Tendon, Left			
C Thorax Tendon, Right			
D Thorax Tendon, Left			

Continued on Next Page ▶

			Continued from ◀ Previous Page
F Abdomen Tendon, Right			
G Abdomen Tendon, Left			
H Perineum Tendon			
J Hip Tendon, Right			
K Hip Tendon, Left			
L Upper Leg Tendon, Right			
M Upper Leg Tendon, Left			
N Lower Leg Tendon, Right			
P Lower Leg Tendon, Left			
Q Knee Tendon, Right			
R Knee Tendon, Left			
S Ankle Tendon, Right			
T Ankle Tendon, Left			
V Foot Tendon, Right			
W Foot Tendon, Left			

Section	0	Medical and Surgical	
Body System	L	Tendons	
Operation	J	Inspection: Visually and/or manually exploring a body part	

Body Part (Character 4)	Approach (Character 5)	Device (Character 6)	Qualifier (Character 7)
X Upper Tendon	**0** Open	**Z** No Device	**Z** No Qualifier
Y Lower Tendon	**3** Percutaneous		
	4 Percutaneous Endoscopic		
	X External		

Section	0	Medical and Surgical	
Body System	L	Tendons	
Operation	M	Reattachment Putting back in or on all or a portion of a separated body part to its normal location or other suitable location	

Body Part (Character 4)	Approach (Character 5)	Device (Character 6)	Qualifier (Character 7)
0 Head and Neck Tendon	**0** Open	**Z** No Device	**Z** No Qualifier
1 Shoulder Tendon, Right	**4** Percutaneous Endoscopic		
2 Shoulder Tendon, Left			
3 Upper Arm Tendon, Right			
4 Upper Arm Tendon, Left			
5 Lower Arm and Wrist Tendon, Right			
6 Lower Arm and Wrist Tendon, Left			
7 Hand Tendon, Right			
8 Hand Tendon, Left			
9 Trunk Tendon, Right			
B Trunk Tendon, Left			
C Thorax Tendon, Right			
D Thorax Tendon, Left			
F Abdomen Tendon, Right			
G Abdomen Tendon, Left			
H Perineum Tendon			
J Hip Tendon, Right			
K Hip Tendon, Left			
L Upper Leg Tendon, Right			
M Upper Leg Tendon, Left			
N Lower Leg Tendon, Right			Continued on Next Page ▶
P Lower Leg Tendon, Left			

Q Knee Tendon, Right **R** Knee Tendon, Left **S** Ankle Tendon, Right **T** Ankle Tendon, Left **V** Foot Tendon, Right **W** Foot Tendon, Left			Continued from ◄ Previous Page

Section	0	Medical and Surgical
Body System	L	Tendons
Operation	N	Release: Freeing a body part from an abnormal physical constraint by cutting or by the use of force

Body Part (Character 4)	Approach (Character 5)	Device (Character 6)	Qualifier (Character 7)
0 Head and Neck Tendon **1** Shoulder Tendon, Right **2** Shoulder Tendon, Left **3** Upper Arm Tendon, Right **4** Upper Arm Tendon, Left **5** Lower Arm and Wrist Tendon, Right **6** Lower Arm and Wrist Tendon, Left **7** Hand Tendon, Right **8** Hand Tendon, Left **9** Trunk Tendon, Right **B** Trunk Tendon, Left **C** Thorax Tendon, Right **D** Thorax Tendon, Left **F** Abdomen Tendon, Right **G** Abdomen Tendon, Left **H** Perineum Tendon **J** Hip Tendon, Right **K** Hip Tendon, Left **L** Upper Leg Tendon, Right **M** Upper Leg Tendon, Left **N** Lower Leg Tendon, Right **P** Lower Leg Tendon, Left **Q** Knee Tendon, Right **R** Knee Tendon, Left **S** Ankle Tendon, Right **T** Ankle Tendon, Left **V** Foot Tendon, Right **W** Foot Tendon, Left	**0** Open **3** Percutaneous **4** Percutaneous Endoscopic **X** External	**Z** No Device	**Z** No Qualifier

Section	0	Medical and Surgical
Body System	L	Tendons
Operation	P	Removal: Taking out or off a device from a body part

Body Part (Character 4)	Approach (Character 5)	Device (Character 6)	Qualifier (Character 7)
X Upper Tendon **Y** Lower Tendon	**0** Open **3** Percutaneous **4** Percutaneous Endoscopic	**0** Drainage Device **7** Autologous Tissue Substitute **J** Synthetic Substitute **K** Nonautologous Tissue Substitute	**Z** No Qualifier
X Upper Tendon **Y** Lower Tendon	**X** External	**0** Drainage Device	**Z** No Qualifier

Section	0	Medical and Surgical		
Body System	L	Tendons		
Operation	Q	Repair: Restoring, to the extent possible, a body part to its normal anatomic structure and function		

Body Part (Character 4)	Approach (Character 5)	Device (Character 6)	Qualifier (Character 7)
0 Head and Neck Tendon	0 Open	Z No Device	Z No Qualifier
1 Shoulder Tendon, Right	3 Percutaneous		
2 Shoulder Tendon, Left	4 Percutaneous Endoscopic		
3 Upper Arm Tendon, Right			
4 Upper Arm Tendon, Left			
5 Lower Arm and Wrist Tendon, Right			
6 Lower Arm and Wrist Tendon, Left			
7 Hand Tendon, Right			
8 Hand Tendon, Left			
9 Trunk Tendon, Right			
B Trunk Tendon, Left			
C Thorax Tendon, Right			
D Thorax Tendon, Left			
F Abdomen Tendon, Right			
G Abdomen Tendon, Left			
H Perineum Tendon			
J Hip Tendon, Right			
K Hip Tendon, Left			
L Upper Leg Tendon, Right			
M Upper Leg Tendon, Left			
N Lower Leg Tendon, Right			
P Lower Leg Tendon, Left			
Q Knee Tendon, Right			
R Knee Tendon, Left			
S Ankle Tendon, Right			
T Ankle Tendon, Left			
V Foot Tendon, Right			
W Foot Tendon, Left			

Section	0	Medical and Surgical		
Body System	L	Tendons		
Operation	R	Replacement: Putting in or on biological or synthetic material that physically takes the place and/or function of all or a portion of a body part		

Body Part (Character 4)	Approach (Character 5)	Device (Character 6)	Qualifier (Character 7)
0 Head and Neck Tendon	0 Open	7 Autologous Tissue Substitute	Z No Qualifier
1 Shoulder Tendon, Right	4 Percutaneous Endoscopic	J Synthetic Substitute	
2 Shoulder Tendon, Left		K Nonautologous Tissue Substitute	
3 Upper Arm Tendon, Right			
4 Upper Arm Tendon, Left			
5 Lower Arm and Wrist Tendon, Right			
6 Lower Arm and Wrist Tendon, Left			
7 Hand Tendon, Right			
8 Hand Tendon, Left			
9 Trunk Tendon, Right			
B Trunk Tendon, Left			
C Thorax Tendon, Right			

Continued on Next Page ▶

D Thorax Tendon, Left			**Continued from** ◀ **Previous Page**
F Abdomen Tendon, Right			
G Abdomen Tendon, Left			
H Perineum Tendon			
J Hip Tendon, Right			
K Hip Tendon, Left			
L Upper Leg Tendon, Right			
M Upper Leg Tendon, Left			
N Lower Leg Tendon, Right			
P Lower Leg Tendon, Left			
Q Knee Tendon, Right			
R Knee Tendon, Left			
S Ankle Tendon, Right			
T Ankle Tendon, Left			
V Foot Tendon, Right			
W Foot Tendon, Left			

Section	0	Medical and Surgical
Body System	L	Tendons
Operation	S	Reposition: Moving to its normal location, or other suitable location, all or a portion of a body part

Body Part (Character 4)	Approach (Character 5)	Device (Character 6)	Qualifier (Character 7)
0 Head and Neck Tendon	0 Open	Z No Device	Z No Qualifier
1 Shoulder Tendon, Right	4 Percutaneous Endoscopic		
2 Shoulder Tendon, Left			
3 Upper Arm Tendon, Right			
4 Upper Arm Tendon, Left			
5 Lower Arm and Wrist Tendon, Right			
6 Lower Arm and Wrist Tendon, Left			
7 Hand Tendon, Right			
8 Hand Tendon, Left			
9 Trunk Tendon, Right			
B Trunk Tendon, Left			
C Thorax Tendon, Right			
D Thorax Tendon, Left			
F Abdomen Tendon, Right			
G Abdomen Tendon, Left			
H Perineum Tendon			
J Hip Tendon, Right			
K Hip Tendon, Left			
L Upper Leg Tendon, Right			
M Upper Leg Tendon, Left			
N Lower Leg Tendon, Right			
P Lower Leg Tendon, Left			
Q Knee Tendon, Right			
R Knee Tendon, Left			
S Ankle Tendon, Right			
T Ankle Tendon, Left			
V Foot Tendon, Right			
W Foot Tendon, Left			

Section	0	Medical and Surgical				
Body System	L	Tendons				
Operation	T	Resection: Cutting out or off, without replacement, all of a body part				

Body Part (Character 4)	Approach (Character 5)	Device (Character 6)	Qualifier (Character 7)
0 Head and Neck Tendon	**0** Open	**Z** No Device	**Z** No Qualifier
1 Shoulder Tendon, Right	**4** Percutaneous Endoscopic		
2 Shoulder Tendon, Left			
3 Upper Arm Tendon, Right			
4 Upper Arm Tendon, Left			
5 Lower Arm and Wrist Tendon, Right			
6 Lower Arm and Wrist Tendon, Left			
7 Hand Tendon, Right			
8 Hand Tendon, Left			
9 Trunk Tendon, Right			
B Trunk Tendon, Left			
C Thorax Tendon, Right			
D Thorax Tendon, Left			
F Abdomen Tendon, Right			
G Abdomen Tendon, Left			
H Perineum Tendon			
J Hip Tendon, Right			
K Hip Tendon, Left			
L Upper Leg Tendon, Right			
M Upper Leg Tendon, Left			
N Lower Leg Tendon, Right			
P Lower Leg Tendon, Left			
Q Knee Tendon, Right			
R Knee Tendon, Left			
S Ankle Tendon, Right			
T Ankle Tendon, Left			
V Foot Tendon, Right			
W Foot Tendon, Left			

Section	0	Medical and Surgical				
Body System	L	Tendons				
Operation	U	Supplement: Putting in or on biological or synthetic material that physically reinforces and/or augments the function of a portion of a body part				

Body Part (Character 4)	Approach (Character 5)	Device (Character 6)	Qualifier (Character 7)
0 Head and Neck Tendon	**0** Open	**7** Autologous Tissue Substitute	**Z** No Qualifier
1 Shoulder Tendon, Right	**4** Percutaneous Endoscopic	**J** Synthetic Substitute	
2 Shoulder Tendon, Left		**K** Nonautologous Tissue Substitute	
3 Upper Arm Tendon, Right			
4 Upper Arm Tendon, Left			
5 Lower Arm and Wrist Tendon, Right			
6 Lower Arm and Wrist Tendon, Left			
7 Hand Tendon, Right			
8 Hand Tendon, Left			
9 Trunk Tendon, Right			
B Trunk Tendon, Left			
C Thorax Tendon, Right			
D Thorax Tendon, Left			Continued on Next Page ▶

F Abdomen Tendon, Right			Continued from ◀ Previous Page
G Abdomen Tendon, Left			
H Perineum Tendon			
J Hip Tendon, Right			
K Hip Tendon, Left			
L Upper Leg Tendon, Right			
M Upper Leg Tendon, Left			
N Lower Leg Tendon, Right			
P Lower Leg Tendon, Left			
Q Knee Tendon, Right			
R Knee Tendon, Left			
S Ankle Tendon, Right			
T Ankle Tendon, Left			
V Foot Tendon, Right			
W Foot Tendon, Left			

Section	0	Medical and Surgical
Body System	L	Tendons
Operation	W	Revision: Correcting, to the extent possible, a portion of a malfunctioning device or the position of a displaced device

Body Part (Character 4)	Approach (Character 5)	Device (Character 6)	Qualifier (Character 7)
X Upper Tendon	0 Open	0 Drainage Device	Z No Qualifier
Y Lower Tendon	3 Percutaneous	7 Autologous Tissue Substitute	
	4 Percutaneous Endoscopic	J Synthetic Substitute	
	X External	K Nonautologous Tissue Substitute	

Section	0	Medical and Surgical
Body System	L	Tendons
Operation	X	Transfer: Moving, without taking out, all or a portion of a body part to another location to take over the function of all or a portion of a body part

Body Part (Character 4)	Approach (Character 5)	Device (Character 6)	Qualifier (Character 7)
0 Head and Neck Tendon	0 Open	Z No Device	Z No Qualifier
1 Shoulder Tendon, Right	4 Percutaneous Endoscopic		
2 Shoulder Tendon, Left			
3 Upper Arm Tendon, Right			
4 Upper Arm Tendon, Left			
5 Lower Arm and Wrist Tendon, Right			
6 Lower Arm and Wrist Tendon, Left			
7 Hand Tendon, Right			
8 Hand Tendon, Left			
9 Trunk Tendon, Right			
B Trunk Tendon, Left			
C Thorax Tendon, Right			
D Thorax Tendon, Left			
F Abdomen Tendon, Right			
G Abdomen Tendon, Left			
H Perineum Tendon			
J Hip Tendon, Right			
K Hip Tendon, Left			
L Upper Leg Tendon, Right			Continued on Next Page ▶
M Upper Leg Tendon, Left			

N Lower Leg Tendon, Right **P** Lower Leg Tendon, Left **Q** Knee Tendon, Right **R** Knee Tendon, Left **S** Ankle Tendon, Right **T** Ankle Tendon, Left **V** Foot Tendon, Right **W** Foot Tendon, Left		**Continued from** ◄ **Previous Page**

Section	0	Medical and Surgical			
Body System	M	Bursae and Ligaments			
Operation	2	Change: Taking out or off a device from a body part and putting back an identical or similar device in or on the same body part without cutting or puncturing the skin or a mucous membrane			

Body Part (Character 4)	Approach (Character 5)	Device (Character 6)	Qualifier (Character 7)
X Upper Bursa and Ligament	X External	0 Drainage Device	Z No Qualifier
Y Lower Bursa and Ligament		Y Other Device	

Section	0	Medical and Surgical			
Body System	M	Bursae and Ligaments			
Operation	5	Destruction: Physical eradication of all or a portion of a body part by the direct use of energy, force, or a destructive agent			

Body Part (Character 4)	Approach (Character 5)	Device (Character 6)	Qualifier (Character 7)
0 Head and Neck Bursa and Ligament	0 Open	Z No Device	Z No Qualifier
1 Shoulder Bursa and Ligament, Right	3 Percutaneous		
2 Shoulder Bursa and Ligament, Left	4 Percutaneous Endoscopic		
3 Elbow Bursa and Ligament, Right			
4 Elbow Bursa and Ligament, Left			
5 Wrist Bursa and Ligament, Right			
6 Wrist Bursa and Ligament, Left			
7 Hand Bursa and Ligament, Right			
8 Hand Bursa and Ligament, Left			
9 Upper Extremity Bursa and Ligament, Right			
B Upper Extremity Bursa and Ligament, Left			
C Trunk Bursa and Ligament, Right			
D Trunk Bursa and Ligament, Left			
F Thorax Bursa and Ligament, Right			
G Thorax Bursa and Ligament, Left			
H Abdomen Bursa and Ligament, Right			
J Abdomen Bursa and Ligament, Left			
K Perineum Bursa and Ligament			
L Hip Bursa and Ligament, Right			
M Hip Bursa and Ligament, Left			
N Knee Bursa and Ligament, Right			
P Knee Bursa and Ligament, Left			Continued on Next Page ▶

			Continued from ◀ Previous Page
Q Ankle Bursa and Ligament, Right			
R Ankle Bursa and Ligament, Left			
S Foot Bursa and Ligament, Right			
T Foot Bursa and Ligament, Left			
V Lower Extremity Bursa and Ligament, Right			
W Lower Extremity Bursa and Ligament, Left			

Section	0	Medical and Surgical
Body System	M	Bursae and Ligaments
Operation	8	Division: Cutting into a body part, without draining fluids and/or gases from the body part, in order to separate or transect a body part

Body Part (Character 4)	Approach (Character 5)	Device (Character 6)	Qualifier (Character 7)
0 Head and Neck Bursa and Ligament	**0** Open	**Z** No Device	**Z** No Qualifier
1 Shoulder Bursa and Ligament, Right	**3** Percutaneous		
2 Shoulder Bursa and Ligament, Left	**4** Percutaneous Endoscopic		
3 Elbow Bursa and Ligament, Right			
4 Elbow Bursa and Ligament, Left			
5 Wrist Bursa and Ligament, Right			
6 Wrist Bursa and Ligament, Left			
7 Hand Bursa and Ligament, Right			
8 Hand Bursa and Ligament, Left			
9 Upper Extremity Bursa and Ligament, Right			
B Upper Extremity Bursa and Ligament, Left			
C Trunk Bursa and Ligament, Right			
D Trunk Bursa and Ligament, Left			
F Thorax Bursa and Ligament, Right			
G Thorax Bursa and Ligament, Left			
H Abdomen Bursa and Ligament, Right			
J Abdomen Bursa and Ligament, Left			
K Perineum Bursa and Ligament			
L Hip Bursa and Ligament, Right			
M Hip Bursa and Ligament, Left			Continued on Next Page ▶

N Knee Bursa and Ligament, Right			**Continued from** ◀ **Previous Page**
P Knee Bursa and Ligament, Left			
Q Ankle Bursa and Ligament, Right			
R Ankle Bursa and Ligament, Left			
S Foot Bursa and Ligament, Right			
T Foot Bursa and Ligament, Left			
V Lower Extremity Bursa and Ligament, Right			
W Lower Extremity Bursa and Ligament, Left			

Section	0	Medical and Surgical
Body System	M	Bursae and Ligaments
Operation	9	Drainage: Taking or letting out fluids and/or gases from a body part

Body Part (Character 4)	Approach (Character 5)	Device (Character 6)	Qualifier (Character 7)
0 Head and Neck Bursa and Ligament **1** Shoulder Bursa and Ligament, Right **2** Shoulder Bursa and Ligament, Left **3** Elbow Bursa and Ligament, Right **4** Elbow Bursa and Ligament, Left **5** Wrist Bursa and Ligament, Right **6** Wrist Bursa and Ligament, Left **7** Hand Bursa and Ligament, Right **8** Hand Bursa and Ligament, Left **9** Upper Extremity Bursa and Ligament, Right **B** Upper Extremity Bursa and Ligament, Left **C** Trunk Bursa and Ligament, Right **D** Trunk Bursa and Ligament, Left **F** Thorax Bursa and Ligament, Right **G** Thorax Bursa and Ligament, Left **H** Abdomen Bursa and Ligament, Right **J** Abdomen Bursa and Ligament, Left **K** Perineum Bursa and Ligament	**0** Open **3** Percutaneous **4** Percutaneous Endoscopic	**0** Drainage Device	**Z** No Qualifier

Continued on
Next Page ▶

L Hip Bursa and Ligament, Right			Continued from ◀ Previous Page
M Hip Bursa and Ligament, Left			
N Knee Bursa and Ligament, Right			
P Knee Bursa and Ligament, Left			
Q Ankle Bursa and Ligament, Right			
R Ankle Bursa and Ligament, Left			
S Foot Bursa and Ligament, Right			
T Foot Bursa and Ligament, Left			
V Lower Extremity Bursa and Ligament, Right			
W Lower Extremity Bursa and Ligament, Left			
0 Head and Neck Bursa and Ligament	**0** Open	**Z** No Device	**X** Diagnostic
1 Shoulder Bursa and Ligament, Right	**3** Percutaneous		**Z** No Qualifier
2 Shoulder Bursa and Ligament, Left	**4** Percutaneous Endoscopic		
3 Elbow Bursa and Ligament, Right			
4 Elbow Bursa and Ligament, Left			
5 Wrist Bursa and Ligament, Right			
6 Wrist Bursa and Ligament, Left			
7 Hand Bursa and Ligament, Right			
8 Hand Bursa and Ligament, Left			
9 Upper Extremity Bursa and Ligament, Right			
B Upper Extremity Bursa and Ligament, Left			
C Trunk Bursa and Ligament, Right			
D Trunk Bursa and Ligament, Left			
F Thorax Bursa and Ligament, Right			
G Thorax Bursa and Ligament, Left			
H Abdomen Bursa and Ligament, Right			
J Abdomen Bursa and Ligament, Left			
K Perineum Bursa and Ligament			
L Hip Bursa and Ligament, Right			Continued on Next Page ▶

M Hip Bursa and Ligament, Left			Continued from ◄ Previous Page
N Knee Bursa and Ligament, Right			
P Knee Bursa and Ligament, Left			
Q Ankle Bursa and Ligament, Right			
R Ankle Bursa and Ligament, Left			
S Foot Bursa and Ligament, Right			
T Foot Bursa and Ligament, Left			
V Lower Extremity Bursa and Ligament, Right			
W Lower Extremity Bursa and Ligament, Left			

Section	0	Medical and Surgical		
Body System	M	Bursae and Ligaments		
Operation	B	Excision: Cutting out or off, without replacement, a portion of a body part		

Body Part (Character 4)	Approach (Character 5)	Device (Character 6)	Qualifier (Character 7)
0 Head and Neck Bursa and Ligament	**0** Open	**Z** No Device	**X** Diagnostic
1 Shoulder Bursa and Ligament, Right	**3** Percutaneous		**Z** No Qualifier
2 Shoulder Bursa and Ligament, Left	**4** Percutaneous Endoscopic		
3 Elbow Bursa and Ligament, Right			
4 Elbow Bursa and Ligament, Left			
5 Wrist Bursa and Ligament, Right			
6 Wrist Bursa and Ligament, Left			
7 Hand Bursa and Ligament, Right			
8 Hand Bursa and Ligament, Left			
9 Upper Extremity Bursa and Ligament, Right			
B Upper Extremity Bursa and Ligament, Left			
C Trunk Bursa and Ligament, Right			
D Trunk Bursa and Ligament, Left			
F Thorax Bursa and Ligament, Right			
G Thorax Bursa and Ligament, Left			
H Abdomen Bursa and Ligament, Right			
J Abdomen Bursa and Ligament, Left			Continued on Next Page ▶

			Continued from ◀ Previous Page
K Perineum Bursa and Ligament			
L Hip Bursa and Ligament, Right			
M Hip Bursa and Ligament, Left			
N Knee Bursa and Ligament, Right			
P Knee Bursa and Ligament, Left			
Q Ankle Bursa and Ligament, Right			
R Ankle Bursa and Ligament, Left			
S Foot Bursa and Ligament, Right			
T Foot Bursa and Ligament, Left			
V Lower Extremity Bursa and Ligament, Right			
W Lower Extremity Bursa and Ligament, Left			

Section	0	Medical and Surgical
Body System	M	Bursae and Ligaments
Operation	C	Extirpation: Taking or cutting out solid matter from a body part

Body Part (Character 4)	Approach (Character 5)	Device (Character 6)	Qualifier (Character 7)
0 Head and Neck Bursa and Ligament	**0** Open	**Z** No Device	**Z** No Qualifier
1 Shoulder Bursa and Ligament, Right	**3** Percutaneous		
2 Shoulder Bursa and Ligament, Left	**4** Percutaneous Endoscopic		
3 Elbow Bursa and Ligament, Right			
4 Elbow Bursa and Ligament, Left			
5 Wrist Bursa and Ligament, Right			
6 Wrist Bursa and Ligament, Left			
7 Hand Bursa and Ligament, Right			
8 Hand Bursa and Ligament, Left			
9 Upper Extremity Bursa and Ligament, Right			
B Upper Extremity Bursa and Ligament, Left			
C Trunk Bursa and Ligament, Right			
D Trunk Bursa and Ligament, Left			
F Thorax Bursa and Ligament, Right			
G Thorax Bursa and Ligament, Left			

Continued on Next Page ▶

H Abdomen Bursa and Ligament, Right			Continued from ◀ Previous Page
J Abdomen Bursa and Ligament, Left			
K Perineum Bursa and Ligament			
L Hip Bursa and Ligament, Right			
M Hip Bursa and Ligament, Left			
N Knee Bursa and Ligament, Right			
P Knee Bursa and Ligament, Left			
Q Ankle Bursa and Ligament, Right			
R Ankle Bursa and Ligament, Left			
S Foot Bursa and Ligament, Right			
T Foot Bursa and Ligament, Left			
V Lower Extremity Bursa and Ligament, Right			
W Lower Extremity Bursa and Ligament, Left			

Section	0	Medical and Surgical		
Body System	M	Bursae and Ligaments		
Operation	D	Extraction: Pulling or stripping out or off all or a portion of a body part by the use of force		

Body Part (Character 4)	Approach (Character 5)	Device (Character 6)	Qualifier (Character 7)
0 Head and Neck Bursa and Ligament	0 Open	Z No Device	Z No Qualifier
1 Shoulder Bursa and Ligament, Right	3 Percutaneous		
2 Shoulder Bursa and Ligament, Left	4 Percutaneous Endoscopic		
3 Elbow Bursa and Ligament, Right			
4 Elbow Bursa and Ligament, Left			
5 Wrist Bursa and Ligament, Right			
6 Wrist Bursa and Ligament, Left			
7 Hand Bursa and Ligament, Right			
8 Hand Bursa and Ligament, Left			
9 Upper Extremity Bursa and Ligament, Right			
B Upper Extremity Bursa and Ligament, Left			
C Trunk Bursa and Ligament, Right			
D Trunk Bursa and Ligament, Left			Continued on Next Page ▶

F Thorax Bursa and Ligament, Right **G** Thorax Bursa and Ligament, Left **H** Abdomen Bursa and Ligament, Right **J** Abdomen Bursa and Ligament, Left **K** Perineum Bursa and Ligament **L** Hip Bursa and Ligament, Right **M** Hip Bursa and Ligament, Left **N** Knee Bursa and Ligament, Right **P** Knee Bursa and Ligament, Left **Q** Ankle Bursa and Ligament, Right **R** Ankle Bursa and Ligament, Left **S** Foot Bursa and Ligament, Right **T** Foot Bursa and Ligament, Left **V** Lower Extremity Bursa and Ligament, Right **W** Lower Extremity Bursa and Ligament, Left			**Continued from** ◀ **Previous Page**

Section	0	Medical and Surgical
Body System	M	Bursae and Ligaments
Operation	J	Inspection: Visually and/or manually exploring a body part

Body Part (Character 4)	Approach (Character 5)	Device (Character 6)	Qualifier (Character 7)
X Upper Bursa and Ligament **Y** Lower Bursa and Ligament	**0** Open **3** Percutaneous **4** Percutaneous Endoscopic **X** External	**Z** No Device	**Z** No Qualifier

Section	0	Medical and Surgical
Body System	M	Bursae and Ligaments
Operation	M	Reattachment Putting back in or on all or a portion of a separated body part to its normal location or other suitable location

Body Part (Character 4)	Approach (Character 5)	Device (Character 6)	Qualifier (Character 7)
0 Head and Neck Bursa and Ligament **1** Shoulder Bursa and Ligament, Right **2** Shoulder Bursa and Ligament, Left **3** Elbow Bursa and Ligament, Right **4** Elbow Bursa and Ligament, Left **5** Wrist Bursa and Ligament, Right	**0** Open **4** Percutaneous Endoscopic	**Z** No Device	**Z** No Qualifier *Continued on Next Page ▶*

6 Wrist Bursa and Ligament, Left			Continued from ◀ Previous Page
7 Hand Bursa and Ligament, Right			
8 Hand Bursa and Ligament, Left			
9 Upper Extremity Bursa and Ligament, Right			
B Upper Extremity Bursa and Ligament, Left			
C Trunk Bursa and Ligament, Right			
D Trunk Bursa and Ligament, Left			
F Thorax Bursa and Ligament, Right			
G Thorax Bursa and Ligament, Left			
H Abdomen Bursa and Ligament, Right			
J Abdomen Bursa and Ligament, Left			
K Perineum Bursa and Ligament			
L Hip Bursa and Ligament, Right			
M Hip Bursa and Ligament, Left			
N Knee Bursa and Ligament, Right			
P Knee Bursa and Ligament, Left			
Q Ankle Bursa and Ligament, Right			
R Ankle Bursa and Ligament, Left			
S Foot Bursa and Ligament, Right			
T Foot Bursa and Ligament, Left			
V Lower Extremity Bursa and Ligament, Right			
W Lower Extremity Bursa and Ligament, Left			

Section	0	Medical and Surgical
Body System	M	Bursae and Ligaments
Operation	N	Release: Freeing a body part from an abnormal physical constraint by cutting or by the use of force

Body Part (Character 4)	Approach (Character 5)	Device (Character 6)	Qualifier (Character 7)
0 Head and Neck Bursa and Ligament	**0** Open	**Z** No Device	**Z** No Qualifier
1 Shoulder Bursa and Ligament, Right	**3** Percutaneous		
2 Shoulder Bursa and Ligament, Left	**4** Percutaneous Endoscopic		
3 Elbow Bursa and Ligament, Right	**X** External		Continued on Next Page ▶

Continued from
◀ **Previous Page**

4 Elbow Bursa and Ligament, Left

5 Wrist Bursa and Ligament, Right

6 Wrist Bursa and Ligament, Left

7 Hand Bursa and Ligament, Right

8 Hand Bursa and Ligament, Left

9 Upper Extremity Bursa and Ligament, Right

B Upper Extremity Bursa and Ligament, Left

C Trunk Bursa and Ligament, Right

D Trunk Bursa and Ligament, Left

F Thorax Bursa and Ligament, Right

G Thorax Bursa and Ligament, Left

H Abdomen Bursa and Ligament, Right

J Abdomen Bursa and Ligament, Left

K Perineum Bursa and Ligament

L Hip Bursa and Ligament, Right

M Hip Bursa and Ligament, Left

N Knee Bursa and Ligament, Right

P Knee Bursa and Ligament, Left

Q Ankle Bursa and Ligament, Right

R Ankle Bursa and Ligament, Left

S Foot Bursa and Ligament, Right

T Foot Bursa and Ligament, Left

V Lower Extremity Bursa and Ligament, Right

W Lower Extremity Bursa and Ligament, Left

Section	0	Medical and Surgical
Body System	M	Bursae and Ligaments
Operation	P	Removal: Taking out or off a device from a body part

Body Part (Character 4)	Approach (Character 5)	Device (Character 6)	Qualifier (Character 7)
X Upper Bursa and Ligament Y Lower Bursa and Ligament	0 Open 3 Percutaneous 4 Percutaneous Endoscopic	0 Drainage Device 7 Autologous Tissue Substitute J Synthetic Substitute K Nonautologous Tissue Substitute	Z No Qualifier
X Upper Bursa and Ligament Y Lower Bursa and Ligament	X External	0 Drainage Device	Z No Qualifier

Section	0	Medical and Surgical
Body System	M	Bursae and Ligaments
Operation	Q	Repair: Restoring, to the extent possible, a body part to its normal anatomic structure and function

Body Part (Character 4)	Approach (Character 5)	Device (Character 6)	Qualifier (Character 7)
0 Head and Neck Bursa and Ligament 1 Shoulder Bursa and Ligament, Right 2 Shoulder Bursa and Ligament, Left 3 Elbow Bursa and Ligament, Right 4 Elbow Bursa and Ligament, Left 5 Wrist Bursa and Ligament, Right 6 Wrist Bursa and Ligament, Left 7 Hand Bursa and Ligament, Right 8 Hand Bursa and Ligament, Left 9 Upper Extremity Bursa and Ligament, Right B Upper Extremity Bursa and Ligament, Left C Trunk Bursa and Ligament, Right D Trunk Bursa and Ligament, Left F Thorax Bursa and Ligament, Right G Thorax Bursa and Ligament, Left H Abdomen Bursa and Ligament, Right J Abdomen Bursa and Ligament, Left K Perineum Bursa and Ligament L Hip Bursa and Ligament, Right M Hip Bursa and Ligament,	0 Open 3 Percutaneous 4 Percutaneous Endoscopic	Z No Device	Z No Qualifier

Continued on Next Page ▶

Left

N Knee Bursa and Ligament, Right

P Knee Bursa and Ligament, Left

Q Ankle Bursa and Ligament, Right

R Ankle Bursa and Ligament, Left

S Foot Bursa and Ligament, Right

T Foot Bursa and Ligament, Left

V Lower Extremity Bursa and Ligament, Right

W Lower Extremity Bursa and Ligament, Left

Continued from
◄ Previous Page

Section	0	Medical and Surgical	
Body System	M	Bursae and Ligaments	
Operation	S	Reposition: Moving to its normal location, or other suitable location, all or a portion of a body part	

Body Part (Character 4)	Approach (Character 5)	Device (Character 6)	Qualifier (Character 7)
0 Head and Neck Bursa and Ligament	0 Open	Z No Device	Z No Qualifier
1 Shoulder Bursa and Ligament, Right	4 Percutaneous Endoscopic		
2 Shoulder Bursa and Ligament, Left			
3 Elbow Bursa and Ligament, Right			
4 Elbow Bursa and Ligament, Left			
5 Wrist Bursa and Ligament, Right			
6 Wrist Bursa and Ligament, Left			
7 Hand Bursa and Ligament, Right			
8 Hand Bursa and Ligament, Left			
9 Upper Extremity Bursa and Ligament, Right			
B Upper Extremity Bursa and Ligament, Left			
C Trunk Bursa and Ligament, Right			
D Trunk Bursa and Ligament, Left			
F Thorax Bursa and Ligament, Right			
G Thorax Bursa and Ligament, Left			
H Abdomen Bursa and Ligament, Right			
J Abdomen Bursa and Ligament, Left			

Continued on
Next Page ►

K Perineum Bursa and Ligament			Continued from ◀ Previous Page
L Hip Bursa and Ligament, Right			
M Hip Bursa and Ligament, Left			
N Knee Bursa and Ligament, Right			
P Knee Bursa and Ligament, Left			
Q Ankle Bursa and Ligament, Right			
R Ankle Bursa and Ligament, Left			
S Foot Bursa and Ligament, Right			
T Foot Bursa and Ligament, Left			
V Lower Extremity Bursa and Ligament, Right			
W Lower Extremity Bursa and Ligament, Left			

Section	0	Medical and Surgical
Body System	M	Bursae and Ligaments
Operation	T	Resection: Cutting out or off, without replacement, all of a body part

Body Part (Character 4)	Approach (Character 5)	Device (Character 6)	Qualifier (Character 7)
0 Head and Neck Bursa and Ligament	**0** Open	**Z** No Device	**Z** No Qualifier
1 Shoulder Bursa and Ligament, Right	**4** Percutaneous Endoscopic		
2 Shoulder Bursa and Ligament, Left			
3 Elbow Bursa and Ligament, Right			
4 Elbow Bursa and Ligament, Left			
5 Wrist Bursa and Ligament, Right			
6 Wrist Bursa and Ligament, Left			
7 Hand Bursa and Ligament, Right			
8 Hand Bursa and Ligament, Left			
9 Upper Extremity Bursa and Ligament, Right			
B Upper Extremity Bursa and Ligament, Left			
C Trunk Bursa and Ligament, Right			
D Trunk Bursa and Ligament, Left			
F Thorax Bursa and Ligament, Right			
G Thorax Bursa and Ligament, Left			Continued on Next Page ▶

			Continued from ◀ Previous Page
H Abdomen Bursa and Ligament, Right			
J Abdomen Bursa and Ligament, Left			
K Perineum Bursa and Ligament			
L Hip Bursa and Ligament, Right			
M Hip Bursa and Ligament, Left			
N Knee Bursa and Ligament, Right			
P Knee Bursa and Ligament, Left			
Q Ankle Bursa and Ligament, Right			
R Ankle Bursa and Ligament, Left			
S Foot Bursa and Ligament, Right			
T Foot Bursa and Ligament, Left			
V Lower Extremity Bursa and Ligament, Right			
W Lower Extremity Bursa and Ligament, Left			

Section	0	Medical and Surgical
Body System	M	Bursae and Ligaments
Operation	U	Supplement: Putting in or on biological or synthetic material that physically reinforces and/or augments the function of a portion of a body part

Body Part (Character 4)	Approach (Character 5)	Device (Character 6)	Qualifier (Character 7)
0 Head and Neck Bursa and Ligament 1 Shoulder Bursa and Ligament, Right 2 Shoulder Bursa and Ligament, Left 3 Elbow Bursa and Ligament, Right 4 Elbow Bursa and Ligament, Left 5 Wrist Bursa and Ligament, Right 6 Wrist Bursa and Ligament, Left 7 Hand Bursa and Ligament, Right 8 Hand Bursa and Ligament, Left 9 Upper Extremity Bursa and Ligament, Right B Upper Extremity Bursa and Ligament, Left C Trunk Bursa and Ligament, Right D Trunk Bursa and Ligament, Left	0 Open 4 Percutaneous Endoscopic	7 Autologous Tissue Substitute J Synthetic Substitute K Nonautologous Tissue Substitute	Z No Qualifier

Continued on Next Page ▶

F Thorax Bursa and Ligament, Right			**Continued from** ◀ **Previous Page**
G Thorax Bursa and Ligament, Left			
H Abdomen Bursa and Ligament, Right			
J Abdomen Bursa and Ligament, Left			
K Perineum Bursa and Ligament			
L Hip Bursa and Ligament, Right			
M Hip Bursa and Ligament, Left			
N Knee Bursa and Ligament, Right			
P Knee Bursa and Ligament, Left			
Q Ankle Bursa and Ligament, Right			
R Ankle Bursa and Ligament, Left			
S Foot Bursa and Ligament, Right			
T Foot Bursa and Ligament, Left			
V Lower Extremity Bursa and Ligament, Right			
W Lower Extremity Bursa and Ligament, Left			

Section	0	Medical and Surgical
Body System	M	Bursae and Ligaments
Operation	W	Revision: Correcting, to the extent possible, a portion of a malfunctioning device or the position of a displaced device

Body Part (Character 4)	Approach (Character 5)	Device (Character 6)	Qualifier (Character 7)
X Upper Bursa and Ligament	**0** Open	**0** Drainage Device	**Z** No Qualifier
Y Lower Bursa and Ligament	**3** Percutaneous	**7** Autologous Tissue Substitute	
	4 Percutaneous Endoscopic	**J** Synthetic Substitute	
	X External	**K** Nonautologous Tissue Substitute	

Section	0	Medical and Surgical
Body System	M	Bursae and Ligaments
Operation	X	Transfer: Moving, without taking out, all or a portion of a body part to another location to take over the function of all or a portion of a body part

Body Part (Character 4)	Approach (Character 5)	Device (Character 6)	Qualifier (Character 7)
0 Head and Neck Bursa and Ligament	**0** Open	**Z** No Device	**Z** No Qualifier
1 Shoulder Bursa and Ligament, Right	**4** Percutaneous Endoscopic		
2 Shoulder Bursa and Ligament, Left			
3 Elbow Bursa and Ligament, Right			
4 Elbow Bursa and Ligament, Left			**Continued on Next Page** ▶

Continued from
◄ Previous Page

5 Wrist Bursa and Ligament, Right

6 Wrist Bursa and Ligament, Left

7 Hand Bursa and Ligament, Right

8 Hand Bursa and Ligament, Left

9 Upper Extremity Bursa and Ligament, Right

B Upper Extremity Bursa and Ligament, Left

C Trunk Bursa and Ligament, Right

D Trunk Bursa and Ligament, Left

F Thorax Bursa and Ligament, Right

G Thorax Bursa and Ligament, Left

H Abdomen Bursa and Ligament, Right

J Abdomen Bursa and Ligament, Left

K Perineum Bursa and Ligament

L Hip Bursa and Ligament, Right

M Hip Bursa and Ligament, Left

N Knee Bursa and Ligament, Right

P Knee Bursa and Ligament, Left

Q Ankle Bursa and Ligament, Right

R Ankle Bursa and Ligament, Left

S Foot Bursa and Ligament, Right

T Foot Bursa and Ligament, Left

V Lower Extremity Bursa and Ligament, Right

W Lower Extremity Bursa and Ligament, Left

Section	0	Medical and Surgical		
Body System	N	Head and Facial Bones		
Operation	2	Change: Taking out or off a device from a body part and putting back an identical or similar device in or on the same body part without cutting or puncturing the skin or a mucous membrane		

Body Part (Character 4)	Approach (Character 5)	Device (Character 6)	Qualifier (Character 7)
0 Skull **B** Nasal Bone **W** Facial Bone	**X** External	**0** Drainage Device **Y** Other Device	**Z** No Qualifier

Section	0	Medical and Surgical		
Body System	N	Head and Facial Bones		
Operation	5	Destruction: Physical eradication of all or a portion of a body part by the direct use of energy, force, or a destructive agent		

Body Part (Character 4)	Approach (Character 5)	Device (Character 6)	Qualifier (Character 7)
0 Skull **1** Frontal Bone, Right **2** Frontal Bone, Left **3** Parietal Bone, Right **4** Parietal Bone, Left **5** Temporal Bone, Right **6** Temporal Bone, Left **7** Occipital Bone, Right **8** Occipital Bone, Left **B** Nasal Bone **C** Sphenoid Bone, Right **D** Sphenoid Bone, Left **F** Ethmoid Bone, Right **G** Ethmoid Bone, Left **H** Lacrimal Bone, Right **J** Lacrimal Bone, Left **K** Palatine Bone, Right **L** Palatine Bone, Left **M** Zygomatic Bone, Right **N** Zygomatic Bone, Left **P** Orbit, Right **Q** Orbit, Left **R** Maxilla, Right **S** Maxilla, Left **T** Mandible, Right **V** Mandible, Left **X** Hyoid Bone	**0** Open **3** Percutaneous **4** Percutaneous Endoscopic	**Z** No Device	**Z** No Qualifier

Section	0	Medical and Surgical		
Body System	N	Head and Facial Bones		
Operation	8	Division: Cutting into a body part, without draining fluids and/or gases from the body part, in order to separate or transect a body part		

Body Part (Character 4)	Approach (Character 5)	Device (Character 6)	Qualifier (Character 7)
0 Skull **1** Frontal Bone, Right **2** Frontal Bone, Left **3** Parietal Bone, Right **4** Parietal Bone, Left **5** Temporal Bone, Right	**0** Open **3** Percutaneous **4** Percutaneous Endoscopic	**Z** No Device	**Z** No Qualifier

Continued on Next Page ▶

6 Temporal Bone, Left			Continued from
7 Occipital Bone, Right			◄ Previous Page
8 Occipital Bone, Left			
B Nasal Bone			
C Sphenoid Bone, Right			
D Sphenoid Bone, Left			
F Ethmoid Bone, Right			
G Ethmoid Bone, Left			
H Lacrimal Bone, Right			
J Lacrimal Bone, Left			
K Palatine Bone, Right			
L Palatine Bone, Left			
M Zygomatic Bone, Right			
N Zygomatic Bone, Left			
P Orbit, Right			
Q Orbit, Left			
R Maxilla, Right			
S Maxilla, Left			
T Mandible, Right			
V Mandible, Left			
X Hyoid Bone			

Section	0	Medical and Surgical
Body System	N	Head and Facial Bones
Operation	9	Drainage: Taking or letting out fluids and/or gases from a body part

Body Part (Character 4)	Approach (Character 5)	Device (Character 6)	Qualifier (Character 7)
0 Skull	**0** Open	**0** Drainage Device	**Z** No Qualifier
1 Frontal Bone, Right	**3** Percutaneous		
2 Frontal Bone, Left	**4** Percutaneous Endoscopic		
3 Parietal Bone, Right			
4 Parietal Bone, Left			
5 Temporal Bone, Right			
6 Temporal Bone, Left			
7 Occipital Bone, Right			
8 Occipital Bone, Left			
B Nasal Bone			
C Sphenoid Bone, Right			
D Sphenoid Bone, Left			
F Ethmoid Bone, Right			
G Ethmoid Bone, Left			
H Lacrimal Bone, Right			
J Lacrimal Bone, Left			
K Palatine Bone, Right			
L Palatine Bone, Left			
M Zygomatic Bone, Right			
N Zygomatic Bone, Left			
P Orbit, Right			
Q Orbit, Left			
R Maxilla, Right			
S Maxilla, Left			
T Mandible, Right			
V Mandible, Left			
X Hyoid Bone			Continued on Next Page ►

			Continued from ◀ Previous Page
0 Skull	0 Open	Z No Device	X Diagnostic
1 Frontal Bone, Right	3 Percutaneous		Z No Qualifier
2 Frontal Bone, Left	4 Percutaneous Endoscopic		
3 Parietal Bone, Right			
4 Parietal Bone, Left			
5 Temporal Bone, Right			
6 Temporal Bone, Left			
7 Occipital Bone, Right			
8 Occipital Bone, Left			
B Nasal Bone			
C Sphenoid Bone, Right			
D Sphenoid Bone, Left			
F Ethmoid Bone, Right			
G Ethmoid Bone, Left			
H Lacrimal Bone, Right			
J Lacrimal Bone, Left			
K Palatine Bone, Right			
L Palatine Bone, Left			
M Zygomatic Bone, Right			
N Zygomatic Bone, Left			
P Orbit, Right			
Q Orbit, Left			
R Maxilla, Right			
S Maxilla, Left			
T Mandible, Right			
V Mandible, Left			
X Hyoid Bone			

Section	0	Medical and Surgical		
Body System	N	Head and Facial Bones		
Operation	B	Excision: Cutting out or off, without replacement, a portion of a body part		

Body Part (Character 4)	Approach (Character 5)	Device (Character 6)	Qualifier (Character 7)
0 Skull	0 Open	Z No Device	X Diagnostic
1 Frontal Bone, Right	3 Percutaneous		Z No Qualifier
2 Frontal Bone, Left	4 Percutaneous Endoscopic		
3 Parietal Bone, Right			
4 Parietal Bone, Left			
5 Temporal Bone, Right			
6 Temporal Bone, Left			
7 Occipital Bone, Right			
8 Occipital Bone, Left			
B Nasal Bone			
C Sphenoid Bone, Right			
D Sphenoid Bone, Left			
F Ethmoid Bone, Right			
G Ethmoid Bone, Left			
H Lacrimal Bone, Right			
J Lacrimal Bone, Left			
K Palatine Bone, Right			
L Palatine Bone, Left			
M Zygomatic Bone, Right			
N Zygomatic Bone, Left			Continued on Next Page ▶

P Orbit, Right **Q** Orbit, Left **R** Maxilla, Right **S** Maxilla, Left **T** Mandible, Right **V** Mandible, Left **X** Hyoid Bone			Continued from ◀ Previous Page

Section	0	Medical and Surgical
Body System	N	Head and Facial Bones
Operation	C	Extirpation: Taking or cutting out solid matter from a body part

Body Part (Character 4)	Approach (Character 5)	Device (Character 6)	Qualifier (Character 7)
1 Frontal Bone, Right **2** Frontal Bone, Left **3** Parietal Bone, Right **4** Parietal Bone, Left **5** Temporal Bone, Right **6** Temporal Bone, Left **7** Occipital Bone, Right **8** Occipital Bone, Left **B** Nasal Bone **C** Sphenoid Bone, Right **D** Sphenoid Bone, Left **F** Ethmoid Bone, Right **G** Ethmoid Bone, Left **H** Lacrimal Bone, Right **J** Lacrimal Bone, Left **K** Palatine Bone, Right **L** Palatine Bone, Left **M** Zygomatic Bone, Right **N** Zygomatic Bone, Left **P** Orbit, Right **Q** Orbit, Left **R** Maxilla, Right **S** Maxilla, Left **T** Mandible, Right **V** Mandible, Left **X** Hyoid Bone	**0** Open **3** Percutaneous **4** Percutaneous Endoscopic	**Z** No Device	**Z** No Qualifier

Section	0	Medical and Surgical
Body System	N	Head and Facial Bones
Operation	H	Insertion: Putting in a nonbiological appliance that monitors, assists, performs, or prevents a physiological function but does not physically take the place of a body part

Body Part (Character 4)	Approach (Character 5)	Device (Character 6)	Qualifier (Character 7)
0 Skull	**0** Open	**4** Internal Fixation Device **5** External Fixation Device **M** Bone Growth Stimulator **N** Neurostimulator Generator	**Z** No Qualifier
0 Skull	**3** Percutaneous **4** Percutaneous Endoscopic	**4** Internal Fixation Device **5** External Fixation Device **M** Bone Growth Stimulator	**Z** No Qualifier

Continued on
Next Page ▶

Continued from
◀ Previous Page

1 Frontal Bone, Right 2 Frontal Bone, Left 3 Parietal Bone, Right 4 Parietal Bone, Left 7 Occipital Bone, Right 8 Occipital Bone, Left C Sphenoid Bone, Right D Sphenoid Bone, Left F Ethmoid Bone, Right G Ethmoid Bone, Left H Lacrimal Bone, Right J Lacrimal Bone, Left K Palatine Bone, Right L Palatine Bone, Left M Zygomatic Bone, Right N Zygomatic Bone, Left P Orbit, Right Q Orbit, Left X Hyoid Bone	0 Open 3 Percutaneous 4 Percutaneous Endoscopic	4 Internal Fixation Device	Z No Qualifier
5 Temporal Bone, Right 6 Temporal Bone, Left	0 Open 3 Percutaneous 4 Percutaneous Endoscopic	4 Internal Fixation Device 5 Hearing Device	Z No Qualifier
B Nasal Bone	0 Open 3 Percutaneous 4 Percutaneous Endoscopic	4 Internal Fixation Device M Bone Growth Stimulator	Z No Qualifier
R Maxilla, Right S Maxilla, Left T Mandible, Right V Mandible, Left	0 Open 3 Percutaneous 4 Percutaneous Endoscopic	4 Internal Fixation Device 5 External Fixation Device	Z No Qualifier
W Facial Bone	0 Open 3 Percutaneous 4 Percutaneous Endoscopic	M Bone Growth Stimulator	Z No Qualifier

Section	0	Medical and Surgical	
Body System	N	Head and Facial Bones	
Operation	J	Inspection: Visually and/or manually exploring a body part	
Body Part (Character 4)	**Approach (Character 5)**	**Device (Character 6)**	**Qualifier (Character 7)**
0 Skull B Nasal Bone W Facial Bone	0 Open 3 Percutaneous 4 Percutaneous Endoscopic X External	Z No Device	Z No Qualifier

Section	0	Medical and Surgical	
Body System	N	Head and Facial Bones	
Operation	N	Release: Freeing a body part from an abnormal physical constraint by cutting or by the use of force	
Body Part (Character 4)	**Approach (Character 5)**	**Device (Character 6)**	**Qualifier (Character 7)**
1 Frontal Bone, Right 2 Frontal Bone, Left 3 Parietal Bone, Right 4 Parietal Bone, Left 5 Temporal Bone, Right	0 Open 3 Percutaneous 4 Percutaneous Endoscopic	Z No Device	Z No Qualifier

**Continued on
Next Page ▶**

			Continued from ◀ Previous Page
6 Temporal Bone, Left			
7 Occipital Bone, Right			
8 Occipital Bone, Left			
B Nasal Bone			
C Sphenoid Bone, Right			
D Sphenoid Bone, Left			
F Ethmoid Bone, Right			
G Ethmoid Bone, Left			
H Lacrimal Bone, Right			
J Lacrimal Bone, Left			
K Palatine Bone, Right			
L Palatine Bone, Left			
M Zygomatic Bone, Right			
N Zygomatic Bone, Left			
P Orbit, Right			
Q Orbit, Left			
R Maxilla, Right			
S Maxilla, Left			
T Mandible, Right			
V Mandible, Left			
X Hyoid Bone			

Section	0	Medical and Surgical
Body System	N	Head and Facial Bones
Operation	P	Removal: Taking out or off a device from a body part

Body Part (Character 4)	Approach (Character 5)	Device (Character 6)	Qualifier (Character 7)
0 Skull	**0** Open	**0** Drainage Device **4** Internal Fixation Device **5** External Fixation Device **7** Autologous Tissue Substitute **J** Synthetic Substitute **K** Nonautologous Tissue Substitute **M** Bone Growth Stimulator **N** Neurostimulator Generator **S** Hearing Device	**Z** No Qualifier
0 Skull	**3** Percutaneous **4** Percutaneous Endoscopic	**0** Drainage Device **4** Internal Fixation Device **5** External Fixation Device **7** Autologous Tissue Substitute **J** Synthetic Substitute **K** Nonautologous Tissue Substitute **M** Bone Growth Stimulator **S** Hearing Device	**Z** No Qualifier
0 Skull	**X** External	**0** Drainage Device **4** Internal Fixation Device **5** External Fixation Device **M** Bone Growth Stimulator **S** Hearing Device	**Z** No Qualifier

Continued on Next Page ▶

			Continued from ◀ **Previous Page**
B Nasal Bone **W** Facial Bone	**0** Open **3** Percutaneous **4** Percutaneous Endoscopic	**0** Drainage Device **4** Internal Fixation Device **7** Autologous Tissue Substitute **J** Synthetic Substitute **K** Nonautologous Tissue Substitute **M** Bone Growth Stimulator	**Z** No Qualifier
B Nasal Bone **W** Facial Bone	**X** External	**0** Drainage Device **4** Internal Fixation Device **M** Bone Growth Stimulator	**Z** No Qualifier

Section	0	Medical and Surgical
Body System	N	Head and Facial Bones
Operation	Q	Repair: Restoring, to the extent possible, a body part to its normal anatomic structure and function

Body Part (Character 4)	Approach (Character 5)	Device (Character 6)	Qualifier (Character 7)
0 Skull **1** Frontal Bone, Right **2** Frontal Bone, Left **3** Parietal Bone, Right **4** Parietal Bone, Left **5** Temporal Bone, Right **6** Temporal Bone, Left **7** Occipital Bone, Right **8** Occipital Bone, Left **B** Nasal Bone **C** Sphenoid Bone, Right **D** Sphenoid Bone, Left **F** Ethmoid Bone, Right **G** Ethmoid Bone, Left **H** Lacrimal Bone, Right **J** Lacrimal Bone, Left **K** Palatine Bone, Right **L** Palatine Bone, Left **M** Zygomatic Bone, Right **N** Zygomatic Bone, Left **P** Orbit, Right **Q** Orbit, Left **R** Maxilla, Right **S** Maxilla, Left **T** Mandible, Right **V** Mandible, Left **X** Hyoid Bone	**0** Open **3** Percutaneous **4** Percutaneous Endoscopic **X** External	**Z** No Device	**Z** No Qualifier

Section	0	Medical and Surgical		
Body System	N	Head and Facial Bones		
Operation	R	Replacement: Putting in or on biological or synthetic material that physically takes the place and/or function of all or a portion of a body part		

Body Part (Character 4)	Approach (Character 5)	Device (Character 6)	Qualifier (Character 7)
0 Skull 1 Frontal Bone, Right 2 Frontal Bone, Left 3 Parietal Bone, Right 4 Parietal Bone, Left 5 Temporal Bone, Right 6 Temporal Bone, Left 7 Occipital Bone, Right 8 Occipital Bone, Left B Nasal Bone C Sphenoid Bone, Right D Sphenoid Bone, Left F Ethmoid Bone, Right G Ethmoid Bone, Left H Lacrimal Bone, Right J Lacrimal Bone, Left K Palatine Bone, Right L Palatine Bone, Left M Zygomatic Bone, Right N Zygomatic Bone, Left P Orbit, Right Q Orbit, Left R Maxilla, Right S Maxilla, Left T Mandible, Right V Mandible, Left X Hyoid Bone	0 Open 3 Percutaneous 4 Percutaneous Endoscopic	7 Autologous Tissue Substitute J Synthetic Substitute K Nonautologous Tissue Substitute	Z No Qualifier

Section	0	Medical and Surgical		
Body System	N	Head and Facial Bones		
Operation	S	Reposition: Moving to its normal location, or other suitable location, all or a portion of a body part		

Body Part (Character 4)	Approach (Character 5)	Device (Character 6)	Qualifier (Character 7)
0 Skull R Maxilla, Right S Maxilla, Left T Mandible, Right V Mandible, Left	0 Open 3 Percutaneous 4 Percutaneous Endoscopic	4 Internal Fixation Device 5 External Fixation Device Z No Device	Z No Qualifier
0 Skull R Maxilla, Right S Maxilla, Left T Mandible, Right V Mandible, Left	X External	Z No Device	Z No Qualifier
1 Frontal Bone, Right 2 Frontal Bone, Left 3 Parietal Bone, Right 4 Parietal Bone, Left 5 Temporal Bone, Right 6 Temporal Bone, Left	0 Open 3 Percutaneous 4 Percutaneous Endoscopic	4 Internal Fixation Device Z No Device	Z No Qualifier

Continued on Next Page ▶

			Continued from ◀ Previous Page
7 Occipital Bone, Right 8 Occipital Bone, Left B Nasal Bone C Sphenoid Bone, Right D Sphenoid Bone, Left F Ethmoid Bone, Right G Ethmoid Bone, Left H Lacrimal Bone, Right J Lacrimal Bone, Left K Palatine Bone, Right L Palatine Bone, Left M Zygomatic Bone, Right N Zygomatic Bone, Left P Orbit, Right Q Orbit, Left X Hyoid Bone			
1 Frontal Bone, Right 2 Frontal Bone, Left 3 Parietal Bone, Right 4 Parietal Bone, Left 5 Temporal Bone, Right 6 Temporal Bone, Left 7 Occipital Bone, Right 8 Occipital Bone, Left B Nasal Bone C Sphenoid Bone, Right D Sphenoid Bone, Left F Ethmoid Bone, Right G Ethmoid Bone, Left H Lacrimal Bone, Right J Lacrimal Bone, Left K Palatine Bone, Right L Palatine Bone, Left M Zygomatic Bone, Right N Zygomatic Bone, Left P Orbit, Right Q Orbit, Left X Hyoid Bone	X External	Z No Device	Z No Qualifier

Section	0	Medical and Surgical
Body System	N	Head and Facial Bones
Operation	T	Resection: Cutting out or off, without replacement, all of a body part

Body Part (Character 4)	Approach (Character 5)	Device (Character 6)	Qualifier (Character 7)
1 Frontal Bone, Right 2 Frontal Bone, Left 3 Parietal Bone, Right 4 Parietal Bone, Left 5 Temporal Bone, Right 6 Temporal Bone, Left 7 Occipital Bone, Right 8 Occipital Bone, Left B Nasal Bone C Sphenoid Bone, Right D Sphenoid Bone, Left	0 Open	Z No Device	Z No Qualifier Continued on Next Page ▶

			Continued from ◄ Previous Page
F Ethmoid Bone, Right			
G Ethmoid Bone, Left			
H Lacrimal Bone, Right			
J Lacrimal Bone, Left			
K Palatine Bone, Right			
L Palatine Bone, Left			
M Zygomatic Bone, Right			
N Zygomatic Bone, Left			
P Orbit, Right			
Q Orbit, Left			
R Maxilla, Right			
S Maxilla, Left			
T Mandible, Right			
V Mandible, Left			
X Hyoid Bone			

Section	0	Medical and Surgical
Body System	N	Head and Facial Bones
Operation	U	Supplement: Putting in or on biological or synthetic material that physically reinforces and/or augments the function of a portion of a body part

Body Part (Character 4)	Approach (Character 5)	Device (Character 6)	Qualifier (Character 7)
0 Skull	0 Open	7 Autologous Tissue Substitute	Z No Qualifier
1 Frontal Bone, Right	3 Percutaneous	J Synthetic Substitute	
2 Frontal Bone, Left	4 Percutaneous Endoscopic	K Nonautologous Tissue Substitute	
3 Parietal Bone, Right			
4 Parietal Bone, Left			
5 Temporal Bone, Right			
6 Temporal Bone, Left			
7 Occipital Bone, Right			
8 Occipital Bone, Left			
B Nasal Bone			
C Sphenoid Bone, Right			
D Sphenoid Bone, Left			
F Ethmoid Bone, Right			
G Ethmoid Bone, Left			
H Lacrimal Bone, Right			
J Lacrimal Bone, Left			
K Palatine Bone, Right			
L Palatine Bone, Left			
M Zygomatic Bone, Right			
N Zygomatic Bone, Left			
P Orbit, Right			
Q Orbit, Left			
R Maxilla, Right			
S Maxilla, Left			
T Mandible, Right			
V Mandible, Left			
X Hyoid Bone			

Section	0	Medical and Surgical
Body System	N	Head and Facial Bones
Operation	W	Revision: Correcting, to the extent possible, a portion of a malfunctioning device or the position of a displaced device

Body Part (Character 4)	Approach (Character 5)	Device (Character 6)	Qualifier (Character 7)
0 Skull	**0** Open	**0** Drainage Device **4** Internal Fixation Device **5** External Fixation Device **7** Autologous Tissue Substitute **J** Synthetic Substitute **K** Nonautologous Tissue Substitute **M** Bone Growth Stimulator **N** Neurostimulator Generator **S** Hearing Device	**Z** No Qualifier
0 Skull	**3** Percutaneous **4** Percutaneous Endoscopic **X** External	**0** Drainage Device **4** Internal Fixation Device **5** External Fixation Device **7** Autologous Tissue Substitute **J** Synthetic Substitute **K** Nonautologous Tissue Substitute **M** Bone Growth Stimulator **S** Hearing Device	**Z** No Qualifier
B Nasal Bone **W** Facial Bone	**0** Open **3** Percutaneous **4** Percutaneous Endoscopic **X** External	**0** Drainage Device **4** Internal Fixation Device **7** Autologous Tissue Substitute **J** Synthetic Substitute **K** Nonautologous Tissue Substitute **M** Bone Growth Stimulator	**Z** No Qualifier

Section	0	Medical and Surgical		
Body System	P	Upper Bones		
Operation	2	Change: Taking out or off a device from a body part and putting back an identical or similar device in or on the same body part without cutting or puncturing the skin or a mucous membrane		

Body Part (Character 4)	Approach (Character 5)	Device (Character 6)	Qualifier (Character 7)
Y Upper Bone	X External	0 Drainage Device Y Other Device	Z No Qualifier

Section	0	Medical and Surgical		
Body System	P	Upper Bones		
Operation	5	Destruction: Physical eradication of all or a portion of a body part by the direct use of energy, force, or a destructive agent		

Body Part (Character 4)	Approach (Character 5)	Device (Character 6)	Qualifier (Character 7)
0 Sternum	0 Open	Z No Device	Z No Qualifier
1 Rib, Right	3 Percutaneous		
2 Rib, Left	4 Percutaneous Endoscopic		
3 Cervical Vertebra			
4 Thoracic Vertebra			
5 Scapula, Right			
6 Scapula, Left			
7 Glenoid Cavity, Right			
8 Glenoid Cavity, Left			
9 Clavicle, Right			
B Clavicle, Left			
C Humeral Head, Right			
D Humeral Head, Left			
F Humeral Shaft, Right			
G Humeral Shaft, Left			
H Radius, Right			
J Radius, Left			
K Ulna, Right			
L Ulna, Left			
M Carpal, Right			
N Carpal, Left			
P Metacarpal, Right			
Q Metacarpal, Left			
R Thumb Phalanx, Right			
S Thumb Phalanx, Left			
T Finger Phalanx, Right			
V Finger Phalanx, Left			

Section	0	Medical and Surgical		
Body System	P	Upper Bones		
Operation	8	Division: Cutting into a body part, without draining fluids and/or gases from the body part, in order to separate or transect a body part		

Body Part (Character 4)	Approach (Character 5)	Device (Character 6)	Qualifier (Character 7)
0 Sternum	0 Open	Z No Device	Z No Qualifier
1 Rib, Right	3 Percutaneous		
2 Rib, Left	4 Percutaneous Endoscopic		
3 Cervical Vertebra			
4 Thoracic Vertebra			
5 Scapula, Right			
6 Scapula, Left			Continued on Next Page ▶

7 Glenoid Cavity, Right			Continued from ◀ Previous Page
8 Glenoid Cavity, Left			
9 Clavicle, Right			
B Clavicle, Left			
C Humeral Head, Right			
D Humeral Head, Left			
F Humeral Shaft, Right			
G Humeral Shaft, Left			
H Radius, Right			
J Radius, Left			
K Ulna, Right			
L Ulna, Left			
M Carpal, Right			
N Carpal, Left			
P Metacarpal, Right			
Q Metacarpal, Left			
R Thumb Phalanx, Right			
S Thumb Phalanx, Left			
T Finger Phalanx, Right			
V Finger Phalanx, Left			

Section	0	Medical and Surgical	
Body System	P	Upper Bones	
Operation	9	Drainage: Taking or letting out fluids and/or gases from a body part	

Body Part (Character 4)	Approach (Character 5)	Device (Character 6)	Qualifier (Character 7)
0 Sternum	0 Open	0 Drainage Device	Z No Qualifier
1 Rib, Right	3 Percutaneous		
2 Rib, Left	4 Percutaneous Endoscopic		
3 Cervical Vertebra			
4 Thoracic Vertebra			
5 Scapula, Right			
6 Scapula, Left			
7 Glenoid Cavity, Right			
8 Glenoid Cavity, Left			
9 Clavicle, Right			
B Clavicle, Left			
C Humeral Head, Right			
D Humeral Head, Left			
F Humeral Shaft, Right			
G Humeral Shaft, Left			
H Radius, Right			
J Radius, Left			
K Ulna, Right			
L Ulna, Left			
M Carpal, Right			
N Carpal, Left			
P Metacarpal, Right			
Q Metacarpal, Left			
R Thumb Phalanx, Right			
S Thumb Phalanx, Left			
T Finger Phalanx, Right			
V Finger Phalanx, Left			
			Continued on Next Page ▶

			Continued from ◀ Previous Page
0 Sternum 1 Rib, Right 2 Rib, Left 3 Cervical Vertebra 4 Thoracic Vertebra 5 Scapula, Right 6 Scapula, Left 7 Glenoid Cavity, Right 8 Glenoid Cavity, Left 9 Clavicle, Right B Clavicle, Left C Humeral Head, Right D Humeral Head, Left F Humeral Shaft, Right G Humeral Shaft, Left H Radius, Right J Radius, Left K Ulna, Right L Ulna, Left M Carpal, Right N Carpal, Left P Metacarpal, Right Q Metacarpal, Left R Thumb Phalanx, Right S Thumb Phalanx, Left T Finger Phalanx, Right V Finger Phalanx, Left	0 Open 3 Percutaneous 4 Percutaneous Endoscopic	Z No Device	X Diagnostic Z No Qualifier

Section	0	Medical and Surgical	
Body System	P	Upper Bones	
Operation	B	Excision: Cutting out or off, without replacement, a portion of a body part	

Body Part (Character 4)	Approach (Character 5)	Device (Character 6)	Qualifier (Character 7)
0 Sternum 1 Rib, Right 2 Rib, Left 3 Cervical Vertebra 4 Thoracic Vertebra 5 Scapula, Right 6 Scapula, Left 7 Glenoid Cavity, Right 8 Glenoid Cavity, Left 9 Clavicle, Right B Clavicle, Left C Humeral Head, Right D Humeral Head, Left F Humeral Shaft, Right G Humeral Shaft, Left H Radius, Right J Radius, Left K Ulna, Right L Ulna, Left M Carpal, Right	0 Open 3 Percutaneous 4 Percutaneous Endoscopic	Z No Device	X Diagnostic Z No Qualifier Continued on Next Page ▶

			Continued from ◀ Previous Page
N Carpal, Left			
P Metacarpal, Right			
Q Metacarpal, Left			
R Thumb Phalanx, Right			
S Thumb Phalanx, Left			
T Finger Phalanx, Right			
V Finger Phalanx, Left			

Section	0	Medical and Surgical
Body System	P	Upper Bones
Operation	C	Extirpation: Taking or cutting out solid matter from a body part

Body Part (Character 4)	Approach (Character 5)	Device (Character 6)	Qualifier (Character 7)
0 Sternum	0 Open	Z No Device	Z No Qualifier
1 Rib, Right	3 Percutaneous		
2 Rib, Left	4 Percutaneous Endoscopic		
3 Cervical Vertebra			
4 Thoracic Vertebra			
5 Scapula, Right			
6 Scapula, Left			
7 Glenoid Cavity, Right			
8 Glenoid Cavity, Left			
9 Clavicle, Right			
B Clavicle, Left			
C Humeral Head, Right			
D Humeral Head, Left			
F Humeral Shaft, Right			
G Humeral Shaft, Left			
H Radius, Right			
J Radius, Left			
K Ulna, Right			
L Ulna, Left			
M Carpal, Right			
N Carpal, Left			
P Metacarpal, Right			
Q Metacarpal, Left			
R Thumb Phalanx, Right			
S Thumb Phalanx, Left			
T Finger Phalanx, Right			
V Finger Phalanx, Left			

Section	0	Medical and Surgical
Body System	P	Upper Bones
Operation	H	Insertion: Putting in a nonbiological appliance that monitors, assists, performs, or prevents a physiological function but does not physically take the place of a body part

Body Part (Character 4)	Approach (Character 5)	Device (Character 6)	Qualifier (Character 7)
0 Sternum	0 Open 3 Percutaneous 4 Percutaneous Endoscopic	0 Internal Fixation Device, Rigid Plate 4 Internal Fixation Device	Z No Qualifier
1 Rib, Right 2 Rib, Left 3 Cervical Vertebra 4 Thoracic Vertebra 5 Scapula, Right 6 Scapula, Left	0 Open 3 Percutaneous 4 Percutaneous Endoscopic	4 Internal Fixation Device	Z No Qualifier

Continued on Next Page ▶

			Continued from ◀ Previous Page
7 Glenoid Cavity, Right **8** Glenoid Cavity, Left **9** Clavicle, Right **B** Clavicle, Left			
C Humeral Head, Right **D** Humeral Head, Left **F** Humeral Shaft, Right **G** Humeral Shaft, Left **H** Radius, Right **J** Radius, Left **K** Ulna, Right **L** Ulna, Left	**0** Open **3** Percutaneous **4** Percutaneous Endoscopic	**4** Internal Fixation Device **5** External Fixation Device **6** Internal Fixation Device, Intramedullary **8** External Fixation Device, Limb Lengthening **B** External Fixation Device, Monoplanar **C** External Fixation Device, Ring **D** External Fixation Device, Hybrid	**Z** No Qualifier
M Carpal, Right **N** Carpal, Left **P** Metacarpal, Right **Q** Metacarpal, Left **R** Thumb Phalanx, Right **S** Thumb Phalanx, Left **T** Finger Phalanx, Right **V** Finger Phalanx, Left	**0** Open **3** Percutaneous **4** Percutaneous Endoscopic	**4** Internal Fixation Device **5** External Fixation Device	**Z** No Qualifier
Y Upper Bone	**0** Open **3** Percutaneous **4** Percutaneous Endoscopic	**M** Bone Growth Stimulator	**Z** No Qualifier

Section	0	Medical and Surgical
Body System	P	Upper Bones
Operation	J	Inspection: Visually and/or manually exploring a body part

Body Part (Character 4)	Approach (Character 5)	Device (Character 6)	Qualifier (Character 7)
Y Upper Bone	**0** Open **3** Percutaneous **4** Percutaneous Endoscopic **X** External	**Z** No Device	**Z** No Qualifier

Section	0	Medical and Surgical
Body System	P	Upper Bones
Operation	N	Release: Freeing a body part from an abnormal physical constraint by cutting or by the use of force

Body Part (Character 4)	Approach (Character 5)	Device (Character 6)	Qualifier (Character 7)
0 Sternum 1 Rib, Right 2 Rib, Left 3 Cervical Vertebra 4 Thoracic Vertebra 5 Scapula, Right 6 Scapula, Left 7 Glenoid Cavity, Right 8 Glenoid Cavity, Left 9 Clavicle, Right B Clavicle, Left C Humeral Head, Right D Humeral Head, Left	**0** Open **3** Percutaneous **4** Percutaneous Endoscopic	**Z** No Device	**Z** No Qualifier Continued on Next Page ▶

F Humeral Shaft, Right			Continued from ◄ Previous Page
G Humeral Shaft, Left			
H Radius, Right			
J Radius, Left			
K Ulna, Right			
L Ulna, Left			
M Carpal, Right			
N Carpal, Left			
P Metacarpal, Right			
Q Metacarpal, Left			
R Thumb Phalanx, Right			
S Thumb Phalanx, Left			
T Finger Phalanx, Right			
V Finger Phalanx, Left			

Section	0	Medical and Surgical
Body System	P	Upper Bones
Operation	P	Removal: Taking out or off a device from a body part

Body Part (Character 4)	Approach (Character 5)	Device (Character 6)	Qualifier (Character 7)
0 Sternum 1 Rib, Right 2 Rib, Left 3 Cervical Vertebra 4 Thoracic Vertebra 5 Scapula, Right 6 Scapula, Left 7 Glenoid Cavity, Right 8 Glenoid Cavity, Left 9 Clavicle, Right B Clavicle, Left	0 Open 3 Percutaneous 4 Percutaneous Endoscopic	4 Internal Fixation Device 7 Autologous Tissue Substitute J Synthetic Substitute K Nonautologous Tissue Substitute	Z No Qualifier
0 Sternum 1 Rib, Right 2 Rib, Left 3 Cervical Vertebra 4 Thoracic Vertebra 5 Scapula, Right 6 Scapula, Left 7 Glenoid Cavity, Right 8 Glenoid Cavity, Left 9 Clavicle, Right B Clavicle, Left	X External	4 Internal Fixation Device	Z No Qualifier
C Humeral Head, Right D Humeral Head, Left F Humeral Shaft, Right G Humeral Shaft, Left H Radius, Right J Radius, Left K Ulna, Right L Ulna, Left M Carpal, Right N Carpal, Left P Metacarpal, Right Q Metacarpal, Left R Thumb Phalanx, Right	0 Open 3 Percutaneous 4 Percutaneous Endoscopic	4 Internal Fixation Device 5 External Fixation Device 7 Autologous Tissue Substitute J Synthetic Substitute K Nonautologous Tissue Substitute	Z No Qualifier

Continued on Next Page ►

			Continued from ◀ Previous Page
S Thumb Phalanx, Left T Finger Phalanx, Right V Finger Phalanx, Left			
C Humeral Head, Right D Humeral Head, Left F Humeral Shaft, Right G Humeral Shaft, Left H Radius, Right J Radius, Left K Ulna, Right L Ulna, Left M Carpal, Right N Carpal, Left P Metacarpal, Right Q Metacarpal, Left R Thumb Phalanx, Right S Thumb Phalanx, Left T Finger Phalanx, Right V Finger Phalanx, Left	X External	4 Internal Fixation Device 5 External Fixation Device	Z No Qualifier
Y Upper Bone	0 Open 3 Percutaneous 4 Percutaneous Endoscopic X External	0 Drainage Device M Bone Growth Stimulator	Z No Qualifier

Section	0	Medical and Surgical
Body System	P	Upper Bones
Operation	Q	Repair: Restoring, to the extent possible, a body part to its normal anatomic structure and function

Body Part (Character 4)	Approach (Character 5)	Device (Character 6)	Qualifier (Character 7)
0 Sternum 1 Rib, Right 2 Rib, Left 3 Cervical Vertebra 4 Thoracic Vertebra 5 Scapula, Right 6 Scapula, Left 7 Glenoid Cavity, Right 8 Glenoid Cavity, Left 9 Clavicle, Right B Clavicle, Left C Humeral Head, Right D Humeral Head, Left F Humeral Shaft, Right G Humeral Shaft, Left H Radius, Right J Radius, Left K Ulna, Right L Ulna, Left M Carpal, Right N Carpal, Left P Metacarpal, Right Q Metacarpal, Left R Thumb Phalanx, Right S Thumb Phalanx, Left T Finger Phalanx, Right V Finger Phalanx, Left	0 Open 3 Percutaneous 4 Percutaneous Endoscopic X External	Z No Device	Z No Qualifier

Section	0	Medical and Surgical		
Body System	P	Upper Bones		
Operation	R	Replacement: Putting in or on biological or synthetic material that physically takes the place and/or function of all or a portion of a body part		

Body Part (Character 4)	Approach (Character 5)	Device (Character 6)	Qualifier (Character 7)
0 Sternum 1 Rib, Right 2 Rib, Left 3 Cervical Vertebra 4 Thoracic Vertebra 5 Scapula, Right 6 Scapula, Left 7 Glenoid Cavity, Right 8 Glenoid Cavity, Left 9 Clavicle, Right B Clavicle, Left C Humeral Head, Right D Humeral Head, Left F Humeral Shaft, Right G Humeral Shaft, Left H Radius, Right J Radius, Left K Ulna, Right L Ulna, Left M Carpal, Right N Carpal, Left P Metacarpal, Right Q Metacarpal, Left R Thumb Phalanx, Right S Thumb Phalanx, Left T Finger Phalanx, Right V Finger Phalanx, Left	0 Open 3 Percutaneous 4 Percutaneous Endoscopic	7 Autologous Tissue Substitute J Synthetic Substitute K Nonautologous Tissue Substitute	Z No Qualifier

Section	0	Medical and Surgical		
Body System	P	Upper Bones		
Operation	S	Reposition: Moving to its normal location, or other suitable location, all or a portion of a body part		

Body Part (Character 4)	Approach (Character 5)	Device (Character 6)	Qualifier (Character 7)
0 Sternum	0 Open 3 Percutaneous 4 Percutaneous Endoscopic	0 Internal Fixation Device, Rigid Plate 4 Internal Fixation Device Z No Device	Z No Qualifier
0 Sternum	X External	Z No Device	Z No Qualifier
1 Rib, Right 2 Rib, Left 3 Cervical Vertebra 4 Thoracic Vertebra 5 Scapula, Right 6 Scapula, Left 7 Glenoid Cavity, Right 8 Glenoid Cavity, Left 9 Clavicle, Right B Clavicle, Left	0 Open 3 Percutaneous 4 Percutaneous Endoscopic	4 Internal Fixation Device Z No Device	Z No Qualifier

Continued on Next Page ▶

			Continued from ◀ Previous Page
1 Rib, Right 2 Rib, Left 3 Cervical Vertebra 4 Thoracic Vertebra 5 Scapula, Right 6 Scapula, Left 7 Glenoid Cavity, Right 8 Glenoid Cavity, Left 9 Clavicle, Right B Clavicle, Left	X External	Z No Device	Z No Qualifier
C Humeral Head, Right D Humeral Head, Left F Humeral Shaft, Right G Humeral Shaft, Left H Radius, Right J Radius, Left K Ulna, Right L Ulna, Left	0 Open 3 Percutaneous 4 Percutaneous Endoscopic	4 Internal Fixation Device 5 External Fixation Device 6 Internal Fixation Device, Intramedullary B External Fixation Device, Monoplanar C External Fixation Device, Ring D External Fixation Device, Hybrid Z No Device	Z No Qualifier
C Humeral Head, Right D Humeral Head, Left F Humeral Shaft, Right G Humeral Shaft, Left H Radius, Right J Radius, Left K Ulna, Right L Ulna, Left	X External	Z No Device	Z No Qualifier
M Carpal, Right N Carpal, Left P Metacarpal, Right Q Metacarpal, Left R Thumb Phalanx, Right S Thumb Phalanx, Left T Finger Phalanx, Right V Finger Phalanx, Left	0 Open 3 Percutaneous 4 Percutaneous Endoscopic	4 Internal Fixation Device 5 External Fixation Device Z No Device	Z No Qualifier
M Carpal, Right N Carpal, Left P Metacarpal, Right Q Metacarpal, Left R Thumb Phalanx, Right S Thumb Phalanx, Left T Finger Phalanx, Right V Finger Phalanx, Left	X External	Z No Device	Z No Qualifier

Section	0	Medical and Surgical		
Body System	P	Upper Bones		
Operation	T	Resection: Cutting out or off, without replacement, all of a body part		

Body Part (Character 4)	Approach (Character 5)	Device (Character 6)	Qualifier (Character 7)
0 Sternum 1 Rib, Right 2 Rib, Left 5 Scapula, Right 6 Scapula, Left 7 Glenoid Cavity, Right 8 Glenoid Cavity, Left 9 Clavicle, Right B Clavicle, Left C Humeral Head, Right D Humeral Head, Left F Humeral Shaft, Right G Humeral Shaft, Left H Radius, Right J Radius, Left K Ulna, Right L Ulna, Left M Carpal, Right N Carpal, Left P Metacarpal, Right Q Metacarpal, Left R Thumb Phalanx, Right S Thumb Phalanx, Left T Finger Phalanx, Right V Finger Phalanx, Left	0 Open	Z No Device	Z No Qualifier

Section	0	Medical and Surgical		
Body System	P	Upper Bones		
Operation	U	Supplement: Putting in or on biological or synthetic material that physically reinforces and/or augments the function of a portion of a body part		

Body Part (Character 4)	Approach (Character 5)	Device (Character 6)	Qualifier (Character 7)
0 Sternum 1 Rib, Right 2 Rib, Left 3 Cervical Vertebra 4 Thoracic Vertebra 5 Scapula, Right 6 Scapula, Left 7 Glenoid Cavity, Right 8 Glenoid Cavity, Left 9 Clavicle, Right B Clavicle, Left C Humeral Head, Right D Humeral Head, Left F Humeral Shaft, Right G Humeral Shaft, Left H Radius, Right J Radius, Left K Ulna, Right L Ulna, Left	0 Open 3 Percutaneous 4 Percutaneous Endoscopic	7 Autologous Tissue Substitute J Synthetic Substitute K Nonautologous Tissue Substitute	Z No Qualifier

Continued on Next Page ▶

			Continued from ◀ Previous Page
M Carpal, Right N Carpal, Left P Metacarpal, Right Q Metacarpal, Left R Thumb Phalanx, Right S Thumb Phalanx, Left T Finger Phalanx, Right V Finger Phalanx, Left			

Section	0	Medical and Surgical
Body System	P	Upper Bones
Operation	W	Revision: Correcting, to the extent possible, a portion of a malfunctioning device or the position of a displaced device

Body Part (Character 4)	Approach (Character 5)	Device (Character 6)	Qualifier (Character 7)
0 Sternum 1 Rib, Right 2 Rib, Left 3 Cervical Vertebra 4 Thoracic Vertebra 5 Scapula, Right 6 Scapula, Left 7 Glenoid Cavity, Right 8 Glenoid Cavity, Left 9 Clavicle, Right B Clavicle, Left	0 Open 3 Percutaneous 4 Percutaneous Endoscopic X External	4 Internal Fixation Device 7 Autologous Tissue Substitute J Synthetic Substitute K Nonautologous Tissue Substitute	Z No Qualifier
C Humeral Head, Right D Humeral Head, Left F Humeral Shaft, Right G Humeral Shaft, Left H Radius, Right J Radius, Left K Ulna, Right L Ulna, Left M Carpal, Right N Carpal, Left P Metacarpal, Right Q Metacarpal, Left R Thumb Phalanx, Right S Thumb Phalanx, Left T Finger Phalanx, Right V Finger Phalanx, Left	0 Open 3 Percutaneous 4 Percutaneous Endoscopic X External	4 Internal Fixation Device 5 External Fixation Device 7 Autologous Tissue Substitute J Synthetic Substitute K Nonautologous Tissue Substitute	Z No Qualifier
Y Upper Bone	0 Open 3 Percutaneous 4 Percutaneous Endoscopic X External	0 Drainage Device M Bone Growth Stimulator	Z No Qualifier

Section	0	Medical and Surgical		
Body System	Q	Lower Bones		
Operation	2	Change: Taking out or off a device from a body part and putting back an identical or similar device in or on the same body part without cutting or puncturing the skin or a mucous membrane		

Body Part (Character 4)	Approach (Character 5)	Device (Character 6)	Qualifier (Character 7)
Y Lower Bone	X External	0 Drainage Device Y Other Device	Z No Qualifier

Section	0	Medical and Surgical		
Body System	Q	Lower Bones		
Operation	5	Destruction: Physical eradication of all or a portion of a body part by the direct use of energy, force, or a destructive agent		

Body Part (Character 4)	Approach (Character 5)	Device (Character 6)	Qualifier (Character 7)
0 Lumbar Vertebra	0 Open	Z No Device	Z No Qualifier
1 Sacrum	3 Percutaneous		
2 Pelvic Bone, Right	4 Percutaneous Endoscopic		
3 Pelvic Bone, Left			
4 Acetabulum, Right			
5 Acetabulum, Left			
6 Upper Femur, Right			
7 Upper Femur, Left			
8 Femoral Shaft, Right			
9 Femoral Shaft, Left			
B Lower Femur, Right			
C Lower Femur, Left			
D Patella, Right			
F Patella, Left			
G Tibia, Right			
H Tibia, Left			
J Fibula, Right			
K Fibula, Left			
L Tarsal, Right			
M Tarsal, Left			
N Metatarsal, Right			
P Metatarsal, Left			
Q Toe Phalanx, Right			
R Toe Phalanx, Left			
S Coccyx			

Section	0	Medical and Surgical		
Body System	Q	Lower Bones		
Operation	8	Division: Cutting into a body part, without draining fluids and/or gases from the body part, in order to separate or transect a body part		

Body Part (Character 4)	Approach (Character 5)	Device (Character 6)	Qualifier (Character 7)
0 Lumbar Vertebra	0 Open	Z No Device	Z No Qualifier
1 Sacrum	3 Percutaneous		
2 Pelvic Bone, Right	4 Percutaneous Endoscopic		
3 Pelvic Bone, Left			
4 Acetabulum, Right			
5 Acetabulum, Left			
6 Upper Femur, Right			
7 Upper Femur, Left			
8 Femoral Shaft, Right			**Continued on Next Page ▶**

			Continued from ◀ Previous Page
9 Femoral Shaft, Left			
B Lower Femur, Right			
C Lower Femur, Left			
D Patella, Right			
F Patella, Left			
G Tibia, Right			
H Tibia, Left			
J Fibula, Right			
K Fibula, Left			
L Tarsal, Right			
M Tarsal, Left			
N Metatarsal, Right			
P Metatarsal, Left			
Q Toe Phalanx, Right			
R Toe Phalanx, Left			
S Coccyx			

Section	0	Medical and Surgical	
Body System	Q	Lower Bones	
Operation	9	Drainage: Taking or letting out fluids and/or gases from a body part	

Body Part (Character 4)	Approach (Character 5)	Device (Character 6)	Qualifier (Character 7)
0 Lumbar Vertebra	**0** Open	**0** Drainage Device	**Z** No Qualifier
1 Sacrum	**3** Percutaneous		
2 Pelvic Bone, Right	**4** Percutaneous Endoscopic		
3 Pelvic Bone, Left			
4 Acetabulum, Right			
5 Acetabulum, Left			
6 Upper Femur, Right			
7 Upper Femur, Left			
8 Femoral Shaft, Right			
9 Femoral Shaft, Left			
B Lower Femur, Right			
C Lower Femur, Left			
D Patella, Right			
F Patella, Left			
G Tibia, Right			
H Tibia, Left			
J Fibula, Right			
K Fibula, Left			
L Tarsal, Right			
M Tarsal, Left			
N Metatarsal, Right			
P Metatarsal, Left			
Q Toe Phalanx, Right			
R Toe Phalanx, Left			
S Coccyx			
0 Lumbar Vertebra	**0** Open	**Z** No Device	**X** Diagnostic
1 Sacrum	**3** Percutaneous		**Z** No Qualifier
2 Pelvic Bone, Right	**4** Percutaneous Endoscopic		
3 Pelvic Bone, Left			
4 Acetabulum, Right			
5 Acetabulum, Left			
6 Upper Femur, Right			
7 Upper Femur, Left			

Continued on Next Page ▶

8 Femoral Shaft, Right			Continued from ◀ Previous Page
9 Femoral Shaft, Left			
B Lower Femur, Right			
C Lower Femur, Left			
D Patella, Right			
F Patella, Left			
G Tibia, Right			
H Tibia, Left			
J Fibula, Right			
K Fibula, Left			
L Tarsal, Right			
M Tarsal, Left			
N Metatarsal, Right			
P Metatarsal, Left			
Q Toe Phalanx, Right			
R Toe Phalanx, Left			
S Coccyx			

Section	0	Medical and Surgical	
Body System	Q	Lower Bones	
Operation	B	Excision: Cutting out or off, without replacement, a portion of a body part	

Body Part (Character 4)	Approach (Character 5)	Device (Character 6)	Qualifier (Character 7)
0 Lumbar Vertebra	0 Open	Z No Device	X Diagnostic
1 Sacrum	3 Percutaneous		Z No Qualifier
2 Pelvic Bone, Right	4 Percutaneous Endoscopic		
3 Pelvic Bone, Left			
4 Acetabulum, Right			
5 Acetabulum, Left			
6 Upper Femur, Right			
7 Upper Femur, Left			
8 Femoral Shaft, Right			
9 Femoral Shaft, Left			
B Lower Femur, Right			
C Lower Femur, Left			
D Patella, Right			
F Patella, Left			
G Tibia, Right			
H Tibia, Left			
J Fibula, Right			
K Fibula, Left			
L Tarsal, Right			
M Tarsal, Left			
N Metatarsal, Right			
P Metatarsal, Left			
Q Toe Phalanx, Right			
R Toe Phalanx, Left			
S Coccyx			

Section	0	Medical and Surgical		
Body System	Q	Lower Bones		
Operation	C	Extirpation: Taking or cutting out solid matter from a body part		

Body Part (Character 4)	Approach (Character 5)	Device (Character 6)	Qualifier (Character 7)
0 Lumbar Vertebra 1 Sacrum 2 Pelvic Bone, Right 3 Pelvic Bone, Left 4 Acetabulum, Right 5 Acetabulum, Left 6 Upper Femur, Right 7 Upper Femur, Left 8 Femoral Shaft, Right 9 Femoral Shaft, Left B Lower Femur, Right C Lower Femur, Left D Patella, Right F Patella, Left G Tibia, Right H Tibia, Left J Fibula, Right K Fibula, Left L Tarsal, Right M Tarsal, Left N Metatarsal, Right P Metatarsal, Left Q Toe Phalanx, Right R Toe Phalanx, Left S Coccyx	0 Open 3 Percutaneous 4 Percutaneous Endoscopic	Z No Device	Z No Qualifier

Section	0	Medical and Surgical		
Body System	Q	Lower Bones		
Operation	H	Insertion: Putting in a nonbiological appliance that monitors, assists, performs, or prevents a physiological function but does not physically take the place of a body part		

Body Part (Character 4)	Approach (Character 5)	Device (Character 6)	Qualifier (Character 7)
0 Lumbar Vertebra 1 Sacrum 2 Pelvic Bone, Right 3 Pelvic Bone, Left 4 Acetabulum, Right 5 Acetabulum, Left D Patella, Right F Patella, Left L Tarsal, Right M Tarsal, Left N Metatarsal, Right P Metatarsal, Left Q Toe Phalanx, Right R Toe Phalanx, Left S Coccyx	0 Open 3 Percutaneous 4 Percutaneous Endoscopic	4 Internal Fixation Device 5 External Fixation Device	Z No Qualifier
6 Upper Femur, Right 7 Upper Femur, Left 8 Femoral Shaft, Right 9 Femoral Shaft, Left	0 Open 3 Percutaneous 4 Percutaneous Endoscopic	4 Internal Fixation Device 5 External Fixation Device 6 Internal Fixation Device, Intramedullary	Z No Qualifier **Continued on Next Page ▶**

| B Lower Femur, Right
C Lower Femur, Left
G Tibia, Right
H Tibia, Left
J Fibula, Right
K Fibula, Left | | 8 External Fixation Device, Limb Lengthening
B External Fixation Device, Monoplanar
C External Fixation Device, Ring
D External Fixation Device, Hybrid | Continued from
◀ Previous Page |
| Y Lower Bone | 0 Open
3 Percutaneous
4 Percutaneous Endoscopic | M Bone Growth Stimulator | Z No Qualifier |

Section	0	Medical and Surgical		
Body System	Q	Lower Bones		
Operation	J	Inspection: Visually and/or manually exploring a body part		
Body Part (Character 4)		Approach (Character 5)	Device (Character 6)	Qualifier (Character 7)
Y Lower Bone		0 Open 3 Percutaneous 4 Percutaneous Endoscopic X External	Z No Device	Z No Qualifier

Section	0	Medical and Surgical		
Body System	Q	Lower Bones		
Operation	N	Release: Freeing a body part from an abnormal physical constraint by cutting or by the use of force		
Body Part (Character 4)		Approach (Character 5)	Device (Character 6)	Qualifier (Character 7)
0 Lumbar Vertebra 1 Sacrum 2 Pelvic Bone, Right 3 Pelvic Bone, Left 4 Acetabulum, Right 5 Acetabulum, Left 6 Upper Femur, Right 7 Upper Femur, Left 8 Femoral Shaft, Right 9 Femoral Shaft, Left B Lower Femur, Right C Lower Femur, Left D Patella, Right F Patella, Left G Tibia, Right H Tibia, Left J Fibula, Right K Fibula, Left L Tarsal, Right M Tarsal, Left N Metatarsal, Right P Metatarsal, Left Q Toe Phalanx, Right R Toe Phalanx, Left S Coccyx		0 Open 3 Percutaneous 4 Percutaneous Endoscopic	Z No Device	Z No Qualifier

Section	0	Medical and Surgical	
Body System	Q	Lower Bones	
Operation	P	Removal: Taking out or off a device from a body part	

Body Part (Character 4)	Approach (Character 5)	Device (Character 6)	Qualifier (Character 7)
0 Lumbar Vertebra **1** Sacrum **4** Acetabulum, Right **5** Acetabulum, Left **S** Coccyx	**0** Open **3** Percutaneous **4** Percutaneous Endoscopic	**4** Internal Fixation Device **7** Autologous Tissue Substitute **J** Synthetic Substitute **K** Nonautologous Tissue Substitute	**Z** No Qualifier
0 Lumbar Vertebra **1** Sacrum **4** Acetabulum, Right **5** Acetabulum, Left **S** Coccyx	**X** External	**4** Internal Fixation Device	**Z** No Qualifier
2 Pelvic Bone, Right **3** Pelvic Bone, Left **6** Upper Femur, Right **7** Upper Femur, Left **8** Femoral Shaft, Right **9** Femoral Shaft, Left **B** Lower Femur, Right **C** Lower Femur, Left **D** Patella, Right **F** Patella, Left **G** Tibia, Right **H** Tibia, Left **J** Fibula, Right **K** Fibula, Left **L** Tarsal, Right **M** Tarsal, Left **N** Metatarsal, Right **P** Metatarsal, Left **Q** Toe Phalanx, Right **R** Toe Phalanx, Left	**0** Open **3** Percutaneous **4** Percutaneous Endoscopic	**4** Internal Fixation Device **5** External Fixation Device **7** Autologous Tissue Substitute **J** Synthetic Substitute **K** Nonautologous Tissue Substitute	**Z** No Qualifier
2 Pelvic Bone, Right **3** Pelvic Bone, Left **6** Upper Femur, Right **7** Upper Femur, Left **8** Femoral Shaft, Right **9** Femoral Shaft, Left **B** Lower Femur, Right **C** Lower Femur, Left **D** Patella, Right **F** Patella, Left **G** Tibia, Right **H** Tibia, Left **J** Fibula, Right **K** Fibula, Left **L** Tarsal, Right **M** Tarsal, Left **N** Metatarsal, Right **P** Metatarsal, Left **Q** Toe Phalanx, Right	**X** External	**4** Internal Fixation Device **5** External Fixation Device	**Z** No Qualifier

Continued on Next Page ▶

			Continued from ◀ Previous Page
R Toe Phalanx, Left			
Y Lower Bone	**0** Open **3** Percutaneous **4** Percutaneous Endoscopic **X** External	**0** Drainage Device **M** Bone Growth Stimulator	**Z** No Qualifier

Section	0	Medical and Surgical
Body System	Q	Lower Bones
Operation	Q	Repair: Restoring, to the extent possible, a body part to its normal anatomic structure and function

Body Part (Character 4)	Approach (Character 5)	Device (Character 6)	Qualifier (Character 7)
0 Lumbar Vertebra **1** Sacrum **2** Pelvic Bone, Right **3** Pelvic Bone, Left **4** Acetabulum, Right **5** Acetabulum, Left **6** Upper Femur, Right **7** Upper Femur, Left **8** Femoral Shaft, Right **9** Femoral Shaft, Left **B** Lower Femur, Right **C** Lower Femur, Left **D** Patella, Right **F** Patella, Left **G** Tibia, Right **H** Tibia, Left **J** Fibula, Right **K** Fibula, Left **L** Tarsal, Right **M** Tarsal, Left **N** Metatarsal, Right **P** Metatarsal, Left **Q** Toe Phalanx, Right **R** Toe Phalanx, Left **S** Coccyx	**0** Open **3** Percutaneous **4** Percutaneous Endoscopic **X** External	**Z** No Device	**Z** No Qualifier

Section	0	Medical and Surgical
Body System	Q	Lower Bones
Operation	R	Replacement: Putting in or on biological or synthetic material that physically takes the place and/or function of all or a portion of a body part

Body Part (Character 4)	Approach (Character 5)	Device (Character 6)	Qualifier (Character 7)
0 Lumbar Vertebra **1** Sacrum **2** Pelvic Bone, Right **3** Pelvic Bone, Left **4** Acetabulum, Right **5** Acetabulum, Left **6** Upper Femur, Right **7** Upper Femur, Left **8** Femoral Shaft, Right **9** Femoral Shaft, Left	**0** Open **3** Percutaneous **4** Percutaneous Endoscopic	**7** Autologous Tissue Substitute **J** Synthetic Substitute **K** Nonautologous Tissue Substitute	**Z** No Qualifier

Continued on Next Page ▶

			Continued from ◀ Previous Page
B Lower Femur, Right			
C Lower Femur, Left			
D Patella, Right			
F Patella, Left			
G Tibia, Right			
H Tibia, Left			
J Fibula, Right			
K Fibula, Left			
L Tarsal, Right			
M Tarsal, Left			
N Metatarsal, Right			
P Metatarsal, Left			
Q Toe Phalanx, Right			
R Toe Phalanx, Left			
S Coccyx			

Section	0	Medical and Surgical	
Body System	Q	Lower Bones	
Operation	S	Reposition: Moving to its normal location, or other suitable location, all or a portion of a body part	

Body Part (Character 4)	Approach (Character 5)	Device (Character 6)	Qualifier (Character 7)
0 Lumbar Vertebra **1** Sacrum **4** Acetabulum, Right **5** Acetabulum, Left **S** Coccyx	**0** Open **3** Percutaneous **4** Percutaneous Endoscopic	**4** Internal Fixation Device **Z** No Device	**Z** No Qualifier
0 Lumbar Vertebra **1** Sacrum **4** Acetabulum, Right **5** Acetabulum, Left **S** Coccyx	**X** External	**Z** No Device	**Z** No Qualifier
2 Pelvic Bone, Right **3** Pelvic Bone, Left **D** Patella, Right **F** Patella, Left **L** Tarsal, Right **M** Tarsal, Left **N** Metatarsal, Right **P** Metatarsal, Left **Q** Toe Phalanx, Right **R** Toe Phalanx, Left	**0** Open **3** Percutaneous **4** Percutaneous Endoscopic	**4** Internal Fixation Device **5** External Fixation Device **Z** No Device	**Z** No Qualifier
2 Pelvic Bone, Right **3** Pelvic Bone, Left **D** Patella, Right **F** Patella, Left **L** Tarsal, Right **M** Tarsal, Left **N** Metatarsal, Right **P** Metatarsal, Left **Q** Toe Phalanx, Right **R** Toe Phalanx, Left	**X** External	**Z** No Device	**Z** No Qualifier
6 Upper Femur, Right **7** Upper Femur, Left **8** Femoral Shaft, Right	**0** Open **3** Percutaneous **4** Percutaneous Endoscopic	**4** Internal Fixation Device **5** External Fixation Device	**Z** No Qualifier **Continued on Next Page ▶**

		6 Internal Fixation Device, Intramedullary	Continued from ◀ Previous Page
9 Femoral Shaft, Left			
B Lower Femur, Right		B External Fixation Device, Monoplanar	
C Lower Femur, Left		C External Fixation Device, Ring	
G Tibia, Right			
H Tibia, Left		D External Fixation Device, Hybrid	
J Fibula, Right			
K Fibula, Left		Z No Device	
6 Upper Femur, Right	X External	Z No Device	Z No Qualifier
7 Upper Femur, Left			
8 Femoral Shaft, Right			
9 Femoral Shaft, Left			
B Lower Femur, Right			
C Lower Femur, Left			
G Tibia, Right			
H Tibia, Left			
J Fibula, Right			
K Fibula, Left			

Section	0	Medical and Surgical	
Body System	Q	Lower Bones	
Operation	T	Resection: Cutting out or off, without replacement, all of a body part	

Body Part (Character 4)	Approach (Character 5)	Device (Character 6)	Qualifier (Character 7)
2 Pelvic Bone, Right	0 Open	Z No Device	Z No Qualifier
3 Pelvic Bone, Left			
4 Acetabulum, Right			
5 Acetabulum, Left			
6 Upper Femur, Right			
7 Upper Femur, Left			
8 Femoral Shaft, Right			
9 Femoral Shaft, Left			
B Lower Femur, Right			
C Lower Femur, Left			
D Patella, Right			
F Patella, Left			
G Tibia, Right			
H Tibia, Left			
J Fibula, Right			
K Fibula, Left			
L Tarsal, Right			
M Tarsal, Left			
N Metatarsal, Right			
P Metatarsal, Left			
Q Toe Phalanx, Right			
R Toe Phalanx, Left			
S Coccyx			

Section	0	Medical and Surgical		
Body System	Q	Lower Bones		
Operation	U	Supplement: Putting in or on biological or synthetic material that physically reinforces and/or augments the function of a portion of a body part		

Body Part (Character 4)	Approach (Character 5)	Device (Character 6)	Qualifier (Character 7)
0 Lumbar Vertebra 1 Sacrum 2 Pelvic Bone, Right 3 Pelvic Bone, Left 4 Acetabulum, Right 5 Acetabulum, Left 6 Upper Femur, Right 7 Upper Femur, Left 8 Femoral Shaft, Right 9 Femoral Shaft, Left B Lower Femur, Right C Lower Femur, Left D Patella, Right F Patella, Left G Tibia, Right H Tibia, Left J Fibula, Right K Fibula, Left L Tarsal, Right M Tarsal, Left N Metatarsal, Right P Metatarsal, Left Q Toe Phalanx, Right R Toe Phalanx, Left S Coccyx	0 Open 3 Percutaneous 4 Percutaneous Endoscopic	7 Autologous Tissue Substitute J Synthetic Substitute K Nonautologous Tissue Substitute	Z No Qualifier

Section	0	Medical and Surgical		
Body System	Q	Lower Bones		
Operation	W	Revision: Correcting, to the extent possible, a portion of a malfunctioning device or the position of a displaced device		

Body Part (Character 4)	Approach (Character 5)	Device (Character 6)	Qualifier (Character 7)
0 Lumbar Vertebra 1 Sacrum 4 Acetabulum, Right 5 Acetabulum, Left S Coccyx	0 Open 3 Percutaneous 4 Percutaneous Endoscopic X External	4 Internal Fixation Device 7 Autologous Tissue Substitute J Synthetic Substitute K Nonautologous Tissue Substitute	Z No Qualifier
2 Pelvic Bone, Right 3 Pelvic Bone, Left 6 Upper Femur, Right 7 Upper Femur, Left 8 Femoral Shaft, Right 9 Femoral Shaft, Left B Lower Femur, Right C Lower Femur, Left D Patella, Right F Patella, Left G Tibia, Right H Tibia, Left	0 Open 3 Percutaneous 4 Percutaneous Endoscopic X External	4 Internal Fixation Device 5 External Fixation Device 7 Autologous Tissue Substitute J Synthetic Substitute K Nonautologous Tissue Substitute	Z No Qualifier

Continued on Next Page ▶

J Fibula, Right **K** Fibula, Left **L** Tarsal, Right **M** Tarsal, Left **N** Metatarsal, Right **P** Metatarsal, Left **Q** Toe Phalanx, Right **R** Toe Phalanx, Left			Continued from ◀ Previous Page
Y Lower Bone	**0** Open **3** Percutaneous **4** Percutaneous Endoscopic **X** External	**0** Drainage Device **M** Bone Growth Stimulator	**Z** No Qualifier

Section	0	Medical and Surgical			
Body System	R	Upper Joints			
Operation	2	Change: Taking out or off a device from a body part and putting back an identical or similar device in or on the same body part without cutting or puncturing the skin or a mucous membrane			

Body Part (Character 4)	Approach (Character 5)	Device (Character 6)	Qualifier (Character 7)
Y Upper Joint	X External	0 Drainage Device Y Other Device	Z No Qualifier

Section	0	Medical and Surgical			
Body System	R	Upper Joints			
Operation	5	Destruction: Physical eradication of all or a portion of a body part by the direct use of energy, force, or a destructive agent			

Body Part (Character 4)	Approach (Character 5)	Device (Character 6)	Qualifier (Character 7)
0 Occipital-cervical Joint	0 Open	Z No Device	Z No Qualifier
1 Cervical Vertebral Joint	3 Percutaneous		
3 Cervical Vertebral Disc	4 Percutaneous Endoscopic		
4 Cervicothoracic Vertebral Joint			
5 Cervicothoracic Vertebral Disc			
6 Thoracic Vertebral Joint			
9 Thoracic Vertebral Disc			
A Thoracolumbar Vertebral Joint			
B Thoracolumbar Vertebral Disc			
C Temporomandibular Joint, Right			
D Temporomandibular Joint, Left			
E Sternoclavicular Joint, Right			
F Sternoclavicular Joint, Left			
G Acromioclavicular Joint, Right			
H Acromioclavicular Joint, Left			
J Shoulder Joint, Right			
K Shoulder Joint, Left			
L Elbow Joint, Right			
M Elbow Joint, Left			
N Wrist Joint, Right			
P Wrist Joint, Left			
Q Carpal Joint, Right			
R Carpal Joint, Left			
S Metacarpocarpal Joint, Right			
T Metacarpocarpal Joint, Left			
U Metacarpophalangeal Joint, Right			
V Metacarpophalangeal Joint, Left			
W Finger Phalangeal Joint, Right			
X Finger Phalangeal Joint, Left			

Section	0	Medical and Surgical
Body System	R	Upper Joints
Operation	9	Drainage: Taking or letting out fluids and/or gases from a body part

Body Part (Character 4)	Approach (Character 5)	Device (Character 6)	Qualifier (Character 7)
0 Occipital-cervical Joint	0 Open	0 Drainage Device	Z No Qualifier
1 Cervical Vertebral Joint	3 Percutaneous		
3 Cervical Vertebral Disc	4 Percutaneous Endoscopic		
4 Cervicothoracic Vertebral Joint			
5 Cervicothoracic Vertebral Disc			
6 Thoracic Vertebral Joint			
9 Thoracic Vertebral Disc			
A Thoracolumbar Vertebral Joint			
B Thoracolumbar Vertebral Disc			
C Temporomandibular Joint, Right			
D Temporomandibular Joint, Left			
E Sternoclavicular Joint, Right			
F Sternoclavicular Joint, Left			
G Acromioclavicular Joint, Right			
H Acromioclavicular Joint, Left			
J Shoulder Joint, Right			
K Shoulder Joint, Left			
L Elbow Joint, Right			
M Elbow Joint, Left			
N Wrist Joint, Right			
P Wrist Joint, Left			
Q Carpal Joint, Right			
R Carpal Joint, Left			
S Metacarpocarpal Joint, Right			
T Metacarpocarpal Joint, Left			
U Metacarpophalangeal Joint, Right			
V Metacarpophalangeal Joint, Left			
W Finger Phalangeal Joint, Right			
X Finger Phalangeal Joint, Left			
0 Occipital-cervical Joint	0 Open	Z No Device	X Diagnostic
1 Cervical Vertebral Joint	3 Percutaneous		Z No Qualifier
3 Cervical Vertebral Disc	4 Percutaneous Endoscopic		
4 Cervicothoracic Vertebral Joint			
5 Cervicothoracic Vertebral Disc			
6 Thoracic Vertebral Joint			
9 Thoracic Vertebral Disc			
A Thoracolumbar Vertebral Joint			
B Thoracolumbar Vertebral Disc			Continued on Next Page ▶

C Temporomandibular Joint, Right			Continued from ◀ Previous Page
D Temporomandibular Joint, Left			
E Sternoclavicular Joint, Right			
F Sternoclavicular Joint, Left			
G Acromioclavicular Joint, Right			
H Acromioclavicular Joint, Left			
J Shoulder Joint, Right			
K Shoulder Joint, Left			
L Elbow Joint, Right			
M Elbow Joint, Left			
N Wrist Joint, Right			
P Wrist Joint, Left			
Q Carpal Joint, Right			
R Carpal Joint, Left			
S Metacarpocarpal Joint, Right			
T Metacarpocarpal Joint, Left			
U Metacarpophalangeal Joint, Right			
V Metacarpophalangeal Joint, Left			
W Finger Phalangeal Joint, Right			
X Finger Phalangeal Joint, Left			

Section	0	Medical and Surgical	
Body System	R	Upper Joints	
Operation	B	Excision: Cutting out or off, without replacement, a portion of a body part	

Body Part (Character 4)	Approach (Character 5)	Device (Character 6)	Qualifier (Character 7)
0 Occipital-cervical Joint	**0** Open	**Z** No Device	**X** Diagnostic
1 Cervical Vertebral Joint	**3** Percutaneous		**Z** No Qualifier
3 Cervical Vertebral Disc	**4** Percutaneous Endoscopic		
4 Cervicothoracic Vertebral Joint			
5 Cervicothoracic Vertebral Disc			
6 Thoracic Vertebral Joint			
9 Thoracic Vertebral Disc			
A Thoracolumbar Vertebral Joint			
B Thoracolumbar Vertebral Disc			
C Temporomandibular Joint, Right			
D Temporomandibular Joint, Left			
E Sternoclavicular Joint, Right			
F Sternoclavicular Joint, Left			
G Acromioclavicular Joint, Right			
H Acromioclavicular Joint, Left			
J Shoulder Joint, Right			
K Shoulder Joint, Left			Continued on Next Page ▶
L Elbow Joint, Right			

			Continued from ◀ Previous Page
M Elbow Joint, Left			
N Wrist Joint, Right			
P Wrist Joint, Left			
Q Carpal Joint, Right			
R Carpal Joint, Left			
S Metacarpocarpal Joint, Right			
T Metacarpocarpal Joint, Left			
U Metacarpophalangeal Joint, Right			
V Metacarpophalangeal Joint, Left			
W Finger Phalangeal Joint, Right			
X Finger Phalangeal Joint, Left			

Section	0	Medical and Surgical
Body System	R	Upper Joints
Operation	C	Extirpation: Taking or cutting out solid matter from a body part

Body Part (Character 4)	Approach (Character 5)	Device (Character 6)	Qualifier (Character 7)
0 Occipital-cervical Joint	0 Open	Z No Device	Z No Qualifier
1 Cervical Vertebral Joint	3 Percutaneous		
3 Cervical Vertebral Disc	4 Percutaneous Endoscopic		
4 Cervicothoracic Vertebral Joint			
5 Cervicothoracic Vertebral Disc			
6 Thoracic Vertebral Joint			
9 Thoracic Vertebral Disc			
A Thoracolumbar Vertebral Joint			
B Thoracolumbar Vertebral Disc			
C Temporomandibular Joint, Right			
D Temporomandibular Joint, Left			
E Sternoclavicular Joint, Right			
F Sternoclavicular Joint, Left			
G Acromioclavicular Joint, Right			
H Acromioclavicular Joint, Left			
J Shoulder Joint, Right			
K Shoulder Joint, Left			
L Elbow Joint, Right			
M Elbow Joint, Left			
N Wrist Joint, Right			
P Wrist Joint, Left			
Q Carpal Joint, Right			
R Carpal Joint, Left			
S Metacarpocarpal Joint, Right			
T Metacarpocarpal Joint, Left			
U Metacarpophalangeal Joint, Right			
V Metacarpophalangeal Joint, Left			
W Finger Phalangeal Joint, Right			
X Finger Phalangeal Joint, Left			

Section	0	Medical and Surgical
Body System	R	Upper Joints
Operation	G	Fusion: Joining together portions of an articular body part rendering the articular body part immobile

Body Part (Character 4)	Approach (Character 5)	Device (Character 6)	Qualifier (Character 7)
0 Occipital-cervical Joint 1 Cervical Vertebral Joint 2 Cervical Vertebral Joints, 2 or more 4 Cervicothoracic Vertebral Joint 6 Thoracic Vertebral Joint 7 Thoracic Vertebral Joints, 2-7 8 Thoracic Vertebral Joints, 8 or more A Thoracolumbar Vertebral Joint	0 Open 3 Percutaneous 4 Percutaneous Endoscopic	7 Autologous Tissue Substitute A Interbody Fusion Device J Synthetic Substitute K Nonautologous Tissue Substitute Z No Device	0 Anterior Approach, Anterior Column 1 Posterior Approach, Posterior Column J Posterior Approach, Anterior Column
C Temporomandibular Joint, Right D Temporomandibular Joint, Left E Sternoclavicular Joint, Right F Sternoclavicular Joint, Left G Acromioclavicular Joint, Right H Acromioclavicular Joint, Left J Shoulder Joint, Right K Shoulder Joint, Left	0 Open 3 Percutaneous 4 Percutaneous Endoscopic	4 Internal Fixation Device 7 Autologous Tissue Substitute J Synthetic Substitute K Nonautologous Tissue Substitute Z No Device	Z No Qualifier
L Elbow Joint, Right M Elbow Joint, Left N Wrist Joint, Right P Wrist Joint, Left Q Carpal Joint, Right R Carpal Joint, Left S Metacarpocarpal Joint, Right T Metacarpocarpal Joint, Left U Metacarpophalangeal Joint, Right V Metacarpophalangeal Joint, Left W Finger Phalangeal Joint, Right X Finger Phalangeal Joint, Left	0 Open 3 Percutaneous 4 Percutaneous Endoscopic	4 Internal Fixation Device 5 External Fixation Device 7 Autologous Tissue Substitute J Synthetic Substitute K Nonautologous Tissue Substitute Z No Device	Z No Qualifier

Section	0	Medical and Surgical
Body System	R	Upper Joints
Operation	H	Insertion: Putting in a nonbiological appliance that monitors, assists, performs, or prevents a physiological function but does not physically take the place of a body part

Body Part (Character 4)	Approach (Character 5)	Device (Character 6)	Qualifier (Character 7)
0 Occipital-cervical Joint 1 Cervical Vertebral Joint 4 Cervicothoracic Vertebral Joint 6 Thoracic Vertebral Joint A Thoracolumbar Vertebral Joint	0 Open 3 Percutaneous 4 Percutaneous Endoscopic	3 Infusion Device 4 Internal Fixation Device 8 Spacer B Spinal Stabilization Device, Interspinous Process C Spinal Stabilization Device, Pedicle-Based D Spinal Stabilization Device, Facet Replacement	Z No Qualifier
3 Cervical Vertebral Disc 5 Cervicothoracic Vertebral Disc 9 Thoracic Vertebral Disc B Thoracolumbar Vertebral Disc	0 Open 3 Percutaneous 4 Percutaneous Endoscopic	3 Infusion Device	Z No Qualifier
C Temporomandibular Joint, Right D Temporomandibular Joint, Left E Sternoclavicular Joint, Right F Sternoclavicular Joint, Left G Acromioclavicular Joint, Right H Acromioclavicular Joint, Left J Shoulder Joint, Right K Shoulder Joint, Left	0 Open 3 Percutaneous 4 Percutaneous Endoscopic	3 Infusion Device 4 Internal Fixation Device 8 Spacer	Z No Qualifier
L Elbow Joint, Right M Elbow Joint, Left N Wrist Joint, Right P Wrist Joint, Left Q Carpal Joint, Right R Carpal Joint, Left S Metacarpocarpal Joint, Right T Metacarpocarpal Joint, Left U Metacarpophalangeal Joint, Right V Metacarpophalangeal Joint, Left W Finger Phalangeal Joint, Right X Finger Phalangeal Joint, Left	0 Open 3 Percutaneous 4 Percutaneous Endoscopic	3 Infusion Device 4 Internal Fixation Device 5 External Fixation Device 8 Spacer	Z No Qualifier

Section	0	Medical and Surgical		
Body System	R	Upper Joints		
Operation	J	Inspection: Visually and/or manually exploring a body part		

Body Part (Character 4)	Approach (Character 5)	Device (Character 6)	Qualifier (Character 7)
0 Occipital-cervical Joint	0 Open	Z No Device	Z No Qualifier
1 Cervical Vertebral Joint	3 Percutaneous		
3 Cervical Vertebral Disc	4 Percutaneous Endoscopic		
4 Cervicothoracic Vertebral Joint	X External		
5 Cervicothoracic Vertebral Disc			
6 Thoracic Vertebral Joint			
9 Thoracic Vertebral Disc			
A Thoracolumbar Vertebral Joint			
B Thoracolumbar Vertebral Disc			
C Temporomandibular Joint, Right			
D Temporomandibular Joint, Left			
E Sternoclavicular Joint, Right			
F Sternoclavicular Joint, Left			
G Acromioclavicular Joint, Right			
H Acromioclavicular Joint, Left			
J Shoulder Joint, Right			
K Shoulder Joint, Left			
L Elbow Joint, Right			
M Elbow Joint, Left			
N Wrist Joint, Right			
P Wrist Joint, Left			
Q Carpal Joint, Right			
R Carpal Joint, Left			
S Metacarpocarpal Joint, Right			
T Metacarpocarpal Joint, Left			
U Metacarpophalangeal Joint, Right			
V Metacarpophalangeal Joint, Left			
W Finger Phalangeal Joint, Right			
X Finger Phalangeal Joint, Left			

Section	0	Medical and Surgical
Body System	R	Upper Joints
Operation	N	Release: Freeing a body part from an abnormal physical constraint by cutting or by the use of force

Body Part (Character 4)	Approach (Character 5)	Device (Character 6)	Qualifier (Character 7)
0 Occipital-cervical Joint	0 Open	Z No Device	Z No Qualifier
1 Cervical Vertebral Joint	3 Percutaneous		
3 Cervical Vertebral Disc	4 Percutaneous Endoscopic		
4 Cervicothoracic Vertebral Joint	X External		
5 Cervicothoracic Vertebral Disc			
6 Thoracic Vertebral Joint			
9 Thoracic Vertebral Disc			
A Thoracolumbar Vertebral Joint			
B Thoracolumbar Vertebral Disc			
C Temporomandibular Joint, Right			
D Temporomandibular Joint, Left			
E Sternoclavicular Joint, Right			
F Sternoclavicular Joint, Left			
G Acromioclavicular Joint, Right			
H Acromioclavicular Joint, Left			
J Shoulder Joint, Right			
K Shoulder Joint, Left			
L Elbow Joint, Right			
M Elbow Joint, Left			
N Wrist Joint, Right			
P Wrist Joint, Left			
Q Carpal Joint, Right			
R Carpal Joint, Left			
S Metacarpocarpal Joint, Right			
T Metacarpocarpal Joint, Left			
U Metacarpophalangeal Joint, Right			
V Metacarpophalangeal Joint, Left			
W Finger Phalangeal Joint, Right			
X Finger Phalangeal Joint, Left			

Section	0	Medical and Surgical
Body System	R	Upper Joints
Operation	P	Removal: Taking out or off a device from a body part

Body Part (Character 4)	Approach (Character 5)	Device (Character 6)	Qualifier (Character 7)
0 Occipital-cervical Joint 1 Cervical Vertebral Joint 4 Cervicothoracic Vertebral Joint 6 Thoracic Vertebral Joint A Thoracolumbar Vertebral Joint	0 Open 3 Percutaneous 4 Percutaneous Endoscopic	0 Drainage Device 3 Infusion Device 4 Internal Fixation Device 7 Autologous Tissue Substitute 8 Spacer A Interbody Fusion Device J Synthetic Substitute K Nonautologous Tissue Substitute	Z No Qualifier
0 Occipital-cervical Joint 1 Cervical Vertebral Joint 4 Cervicothoracic Vertebral Joint 6 Thoracic Vertebral Joint A Thoracolumbar Vertebral Joint	X External	0 Drainage Device 3 Infusion Device 4 Internal Fixation Device	Z No Qualifier
3 Cervical Vertebral Disc 5 Cervicothoracic Vertebral Disc 9 Thoracic Vertebral Disc B Thoracolumbar Vertebral Disc	0 Open 3 Percutaneous 4 Percutaneous Endoscopic	0 Drainage Device 3 Infusion Device 7 Autologous Tissue Substitute J Synthetic Substitute K Nonautologous Tissue Substitute	Z No Qualifier
3 Cervical Vertebral Disc 5 Cervicothoracic Vertebral Disc 9 Thoracic Vertebral Disc B Thoracolumbar Vertebral Disc	X External	0 Drainage Device 3 Infusion Device	Z No Qualifier
C Temporomandibular Joint, Right D Temporomandibular Joint, Left E Sternoclavicular Joint, Right F Sternoclavicular Joint, Left G Acromioclavicular Joint, Right H Acromioclavicular Joint, Left J Shoulder Joint, Right K Shoulder Joint, Left	0 Open 3 Percutaneous 4 Percutaneous Endoscopic	0 Drainage Device 3 Infusion Device 4 Internal Fixation Device 7 Autologous Tissue Substitute 8 Spacer J Synthetic Substitute K Nonautologous Tissue Substitute	Z No Qualifier
C Temporomandibular Joint, Right D Temporomandibular Joint, Left E Sternoclavicular Joint, Right F Sternoclavicular Joint, Left G Acromioclavicular Joint, Right H Acromioclavicular Joint, Left J Shoulder Joint, Right K Shoulder Joint, Left	X External	0 Drainage Device 3 Infusion Device 4 Internal Fixation Device	Z No Qualifier

Continued on Next Page ▶

			Continued from ◀ Previous Page
L Elbow Joint, Right **M** Elbow Joint, Left **N** Wrist Joint, Right **P** Wrist Joint, Left **Q** Carpal Joint, Right **R** Carpal Joint, Left **S** Metacarpocarpal Joint, Right **T** Metacarpocarpal Joint, Left **U** Metacarpophalangeal Joint, Right **V** Metacarpophalangeal Joint, Left **W** Finger Phalangeal Joint, Right **X** Finger Phalangeal Joint, Left	**0** Open **3** Percutaneous **4** Percutaneous Endoscopic	**0** Drainage Device **3** Infusion Device **4** Internal Fixation Device **5** External Fixation Device **7** Autologous Tissue Substitute **8** Spacer **J** Synthetic Substitute **K** Nonautologous Tissue Substitute	**Z** No Qualifier
L Elbow Joint, Right **M** Elbow Joint, Left **N** Wrist Joint, Right **P** Wrist Joint, Left **Q** Carpal Joint, Right **R** Carpal Joint, Left **S** Metacarpocarpal Joint, Right **T** Metacarpocarpal Joint, Left **U** Metacarpophalangeal Joint, Right **V** Metacarpophalangeal Joint, Left **W** Finger Phalangeal Joint, Right **X** Finger Phalangeal Joint, Left	**X** External	**0** Drainage Device **3** Infusion Device **4** Internal Fixation Device **5** External Fixation Device	**Z** No Qualifier

Section	0	Medical and Surgical	
Body System	R	Upper Joints	
Operation	Q	Repair: Restoring, to the extent possible, a body part to its normal anatomic structure and function	

Body Part (Character 4)	Approach (Character 5)	Device (Character 6)	Qualifier (Character 7)
0 Occipital-cervical Joint **1** Cervical Vertebral Joint **3** Cervical Vertebral Disc **4** Cervicothoracic Vertebral Joint **5** Cervicothoracic Vertebral Disc **6** Thoracic Vertebral Joint **9** Thoracic Vertebral Disc **A** Thoracolumbar Vertebral Joint **B** Thoracolumbar Vertebral Disc **C** Temporomandibular Joint, Right **D** Temporomandibular Joint, Left **E** Sternoclavicular Joint, Right	**0** Open **3** Percutaneous **4** Percutaneous Endoscopic **X** External	**Z** No Device	**Z** No Qualifier

Continued on Next Page ▶

			Continued from ◀ Previous Page
F Sternoclavicular Joint, Left			
G Acromioclavicular Joint, Right			
H Acromioclavicular Joint, Left			
J Shoulder Joint, Right			
K Shoulder Joint, Left			
L Elbow Joint, Right			
M Elbow Joint, Left			
N Wrist Joint, Right			
P Wrist Joint, Left			
Q Carpal Joint, Right			
R Carpal Joint, Left			
S Metacarpocarpal Joint, Right			
T Metacarpocarpal Joint, Left			
U Metacarpophalangeal Joint, Right			
V Metacarpophalangeal Joint, Left			
W Finger Phalangeal Joint, Right			
X Finger Phalangeal Joint, Left			

Section	0	Medical and Surgical
Body System	R	Upper Joints
Operation	R	Replacement: Putting in or on biological or synthetic material that physically takes the place and/or function of all or a portion of a body part

Body Part (Character 4)	Approach (Character 5)	Device (Character 6)	Qualifier (Character 7)
0 Occipital-cervical Joint	**0** Open	**7** Autologous Tissue Substitute	**Z** No Qualifier
1 Cervical Vertebral Joint		**J** Synthetic Substitute	
3 Cervical Vertebral Disc		**K** Nonautologous Tissue Substitute	
4 Cervicothoracic Vertebral Joint			
5 Cervicothoracic Vertebral Disc			
6 Thoracic Vertebral Joint			
9 Thoracic Vertebral Disc			
A Thoracolumbar Vertebral Joint			
B Thoracolumbar Vertebral Disc			
C Temporomandibular Joint, Right			
D Temporomandibular Joint, Left			
E Sternoclavicular Joint, Right			
F Sternoclavicular Joint, Left			
G Acromioclavicular Joint, Right			
H Acromioclavicular Joint, Left			
L Elbow Joint, Right			
M Elbow Joint, Left			
N Wrist Joint, Right			
P Wrist Joint, Left			
Q Carpal Joint, Right			
R Carpal Joint, Left			Continued on Next Page ▶
S Metacarpocarpal Joint, Right			

			Continued from ◀ Previous Page
T Metacarpocarpal Joint, Left U Metacarpophalangeal Joint, Right V Metacarpophalangeal Joint, Left W Finger Phalangeal Joint, Right X Finger Phalangeal Joint, Left			
J Shoulder Joint, Right K Shoulder Joint, Left	0 Open	0 Synthetic Substitute, Reverse Ball and Socket 7 Autologous Tissue Substitute K Nonautologous Tissue Substitute	Z No Qualifier
J Shoulder Joint, Right K Shoulder Joint, Left	0 Open	J Synthetic Substitute	6 Humeral Surface 7 Glenoid Surface Z No Qualifier

Section	0	Medical and Surgical
Body System	R	Upper Joints
Operation	S	Reposition: Moving to its normal location, or other suitable location, all or a portion of a body part

Body Part (Character 4)	Approach (Character 5)	Device (Character 6)	Qualifier (Character 7)
0 Occipital-cervical Joint 1 Cervical Vertebral Joint 4 Cervicothoracic Vertebral Joint 6 Thoracic Vertebral Joint A Thoracolumbar Vertebral Joint C Temporomandibular Joint, Right D Temporomandibular Joint, Left E Sternoclavicular Joint, Right F Sternoclavicular Joint, Left G Acromioclavicular Joint, Right H Acromioclavicular Joint, Left J Shoulder Joint, Right K Shoulder Joint, Left	0 Open 3 Percutaneous 4 Percutaneous Endoscopic X External	4 Internal Fixation Device Z No Device	Z No Qualifier
L Elbow Joint, Right M Elbow Joint, Left N Wrist Joint, Right P Wrist Joint, Left Q Carpal Joint, Right R Carpal Joint, Left S Metacarpocarpal Joint, Right T Metacarpocarpal Joint, Left U Metacarpophalangeal Joint, Right V Metacarpophalangeal Joint, Left W Finger Phalangeal Joint, Right X Finger Phalangeal Joint, Left	0 Open 3 Percutaneous 4 Percutaneous Endoscopic X External	4 Internal Fixation Device 5 External Fixation Device Z No Device	Z No Qualifier

Section	0	Medical and Surgical		
Body System	R	Upper Joints		
Operation	T	Resection: Cutting out or off, without replacement, all of a body part		

Body Part (Character 4)	Approach (Character 5)	Device (Character 6)	Qualifier (Character 7)
3 Cervical Vertebral Disc	0 Open	Z No Device	Z No Qualifier
4 Cervicothoracic Vertebral Joint			
5 Cervicothoracic Vertebral Disc			
9 Thoracic Vertebral Disc			
B Thoracolumbar Vertebral Disc			
C Temporomandibular Joint, Right			
D Temporomandibular Joint, Left			
E Sternoclavicular Joint, Right			
F Sternoclavicular Joint, Left			
G Acromioclavicular Joint, Right			
H Acromioclavicular Joint, Left			
J Shoulder Joint, Right			
K Shoulder Joint, Left			
L Elbow Joint, Right			
M Elbow Joint, Left			
N Wrist Joint, Right			
P Wrist Joint, Left			
Q Carpal Joint, Right			
R Carpal Joint, Left			
S Metacarpocarpal Joint, Right			
T Metacarpocarpal Joint, Left			
U Metacarpophalangeal Joint, Right			
V Metacarpophalangeal Joint, Left			
W Finger Phalangeal Joint, Right			
X Finger Phalangeal Joint, Left			

Section	0	Medical and Surgical		
Body System	R	Upper Joints		
Operation	U	Supplement: Putting in or on biological or synthetic material that physically reinforces and/or augments the function of a portion of a body part		

Body Part (Character 4)	Approach (Character 5)	Device (Character 6)	Qualifier (Character 7)
0 Occipital-cervical Joint	0 Open	7 Autologous Tissue Substitute	Z No Qualifier
1 Cervical Vertebral Joint	3 Percutaneous	J Synthetic Substitute	
3 Cervical Vertebral Disc	4 Percutaneous Endoscopic	K Nonautologous Tissue Substitute	
4 Cervicothoracic Vertebral Joint			
5 Cervicothoracic Vertebral Disc			
6 Thoracic Vertebral Joint			
9 Thoracic Vertebral Disc			
A Thoracolumbar Vertebral Joint			

Continued on Next Page ▶

B Thoracolumbar Vertebral Disc			**Continued from** ◀ **Previous Page**
C Temporomandibular Joint, Right			
D Temporomandibular Joint, Left			
E Sternoclavicular Joint, Right			
F Sternoclavicular Joint, Left			
G Acromioclavicular Joint, Right			
H Acromioclavicular Joint, Left			
J Shoulder Joint, Right			
K Shoulder Joint, Left			
L Elbow Joint, Right			
M Elbow Joint, Left			
N Wrist Joint, Right			
P Wrist Joint, Left			
Q Carpal Joint, Right			
R Carpal Joint, Left			
S Metacarpocarpal Joint, Right			
T Metacarpocarpal Joint, Left			
U Metacarpophalangeal Joint, Right			
V Metacarpophalangeal Joint, Left			
W Finger Phalangeal Joint, Right			
X Finger Phalangeal Joint, Left			

Section	0	Medical and Surgical
Body System	R	Upper Joints
Operation	W	Revision: Correcting, to the extent possible, a portion of a malfunctioning device or the position of a displaced device

Body Part (Character 4)	Approach (Character 5)	Device (Character 6)	Qualifier (Character 7)
0 Occipital-cervical Joint **1** Cervical Vertebral Joint **4** Cervicothoracic Vertebral Joint **6** Thoracic Vertebral Joint **A** Thoracolumbar Vertebral Joint	**0** Open **3** Percutaneous **4** Percutaneous Endoscopic **X** External	**0** Drainage Device **3** Infusion Device **4** Internal Fixation Device **7** Autologous Tissue Substitute **8** Spacer **A** Interbody Fusion Device **J** Synthetic Substitute **K** Nonautologous Tissue Substitute	**Z** No Qualifier
3 Cervical Vertebral Disc **5** Cervicothoracic Vertebral Disc **9** Thoracic Vertebral Disc **B** Thoracolumbar Vertebral Disc	**0** Open **3** Percutaneous **4** Percutaneous Endoscopic **X** External	**0** Drainage Device **3** Infusion Device **7** Autologous Tissue Substitute **J** Synthetic Substitute **K** Nonautologous Tissue Substitute	**Z** No Qualifier
C Temporomandibular Joint, Right **D** Temporomandibular Joint, Left **E** Sternoclavicular Joint, Right	**0** Open **3** Percutaneous **4** Percutaneous Endoscopic **X** External	**0** Drainage Device **3** Infusion Device **4** Internal Fixation Device **7** Autologous Tissue Substitute	**Z** No Qualifier **Continued on Next Page ▶**

F Sternoclavicular Joint, Left **G** Acromioclavicular Joint, Right **H** Acromioclavicular Joint, Left **J** Shoulder Joint, Right **K** Shoulder Joint, Left		**8** Spacer **J** Synthetic Substitute **K** Nonautologous Tissue Substitute	**Continued from** ◀ **Previous Page**
L Elbow Joint, Right **M** Elbow Joint, Left **N** Wrist Joint, Right **P** Wrist Joint, Left **Q** Carpal Joint, Right **R** Carpal Joint, Left **S** Metacarpocarpal Joint, Right **T** Metacarpocarpal Joint, Left **U** Metacarpophalangeal Joint, Right **V** Metacarpophalangeal Joint, Left **W** Finger Phalangeal Joint, Right **X** Finger Phalangeal Joint, Left	**0** Open **3** Percutaneous **4** Percutaneous Endoscopic **X** External	**0** Drainage Device **3** Infusion Device **4** Internal Fixation Device **5** External Fixation Device **7** Autologous Tissue Substitute **8** Spacer **J** Synthetic Substitute **K** Nonautologous Tissue Substitute	**Z** No Qualifier

Section	0	Medical and Surgical		
Body System	S	Lower Joints		
Operation	2	Change: Taking out or off a device from a body part and putting back an identical or similar device in or on the same body part without cutting or puncturing the skin or a mucous membrane		

Body Part (Character 4)	Approach (Character 5)	Device (Character 6)	Qualifier (Character 7)
Y Lower Joint	X External	0 Drainage Device Y Other Device	Z No Qualifier

Section	0	Medical and Surgical		
Body System	S	Lower Joints		
Operation	5	Destruction: Physical eradication of all or a portion of a body part by the direct use of energy, force, or a destructive agent		

Body Part (Character 4)	Approach (Character 5)	Device (Character 6)	Qualifier (Character 7)
0 Lumbar Vertebral Joint	0 Open	Z No Device	Z No Qualifier
2 Lumbar Vertebral Disc	3 Percutaneous		
3 Lumbosacral Joint	4 Percutaneous Endoscopic		
4 Lumbosacral Disc			
5 Sacrococcygeal Joint			
6 Coccygeal Joint			
7 Sacroiliac Joint, Right			
8 Sacroiliac Joint, Left			
9 Hip Joint, Right			
B Hip Joint, Left			
C Knee Joint, Right			
D Knee Joint, Left			
F Ankle Joint, Right			
G Ankle Joint, Left			
H Tarsal Joint, Right			
J Tarsal Joint, Left			
K Metatarsal-Tarsal Joint, Right			
L Metatarsal-Tarsal Joint, Left			
M Metatarsal-Phalangeal Joint, Right			
N Metatarsal-Phalangeal Joint, Left			
P Toe Phalangeal Joint, Right			
Q Toe Phalangeal Joint, Left			

Section	0	Medical and Surgical		
Body System	S	Lower Joints		
Operation	9	Drainage: Taking or letting out fluids and/or gases from a body part		

Body Part (Character 4)	Approach (Character 5)	Device (Character 6)	Qualifier (Character 7)
0 Lumbar Vertebral Joint	0 Open	0 Drainage Device	Z No Qualifier
2 Lumbar Vertebral Disc	3 Percutaneous		
3 Lumbosacral Joint	4 Percutaneous Endoscopic		
4 Lumbosacral Disc			
5 Sacrococcygeal Joint			
6 Coccygeal Joint			
7 Sacroiliac Joint, Right			
8 Sacroiliac Joint, Left			
9 Hip Joint, Right			
B Hip Joint, Left			Continued on Next Page ▶
C Knee Joint, Right			

Continued from
◀ Previous Page

D Knee Joint, Left
F Ankle Joint, Right
G Ankle Joint, Left
H Tarsal Joint, Right
J Tarsal Joint, Left
K Metatarsal-Tarsal Joint, Right
L Metatarsal-Tarsal Joint, Left
M Metatarsal-Phalangeal Joint, Right
N Metatarsal-Phalangeal Joint, Left
P Toe Phalangeal Joint, Right
Q Toe Phalangeal Joint, Left

Body Part (Character 4)	Approach (Character 5)	Device (Character 6)	Qualifier (Character 7)
0 Lumbar Vertebral Joint **2** Lumbar Vertebral Disc **3** Lumbosacral Joint **4** Lumbosacral Disc **5** Sacrococcygeal Joint **6** Coccygeal Joint **7** Sacroiliac Joint, Right **8** Sacroiliac Joint, Left **9** Hip Joint, Right **B** Hip Joint, Left **C** Knee Joint, Right **D** Knee Joint, Left **F** Ankle Joint, Right **G** Ankle Joint, Left **H** Tarsal Joint, Right **J** Tarsal Joint, Left **K** Metatarsal-Tarsal Joint, Right **L** Metatarsal-Tarsal Joint, Left **M** Metatarsal-Phalangeal Joint, Right **N** Metatarsal-Phalangeal Joint, Left **P** Toe Phalangeal Joint, Right **Q** Toe Phalangeal Joint, Left	**0** Open **3** Percutaneous **4** Percutaneous Endoscopic	**Z** No Device	**X** Diagnostic **Z** No Qualifier

Section	0	Medical and Surgical
Body System	S	Lower Joints
Operation	B	Excision: Cutting out or off, without replacement, a portion of a body part

Body Part (Character 4)	Approach (Character 5)	Device (Character 6)	Qualifier (Character 7)
0 Lumbar Vertebral Joint **2** Lumbar Vertebral Disc **3** Lumbosacral Joint **4** Lumbosacral Disc **5** Sacrococcygeal Joint **6** Coccygeal Joint **7** Sacroiliac Joint, Right **8** Sacroiliac Joint, Left **9** Hip Joint, Right **B** Hip Joint, Left **C** Knee Joint, Right	**0** Open **3** Percutaneous **4** Percutaneous Endoscopic	**Z** No Device	**X** Diagnostic **Z** No Qualifier Continued on Next Page ▶

D Knee Joint, Left			Continued from ◄ Previous Page
F Ankle Joint, Right			
G Ankle Joint, Left			
H Tarsal Joint, Right			
J Tarsal Joint, Left			
K Metatarsal-Tarsal Joint, Right			
L Metatarsal-Tarsal Joint, Left			
M Metatarsal-Phalangeal Joint, Right			
N Metatarsal-Phalangeal Joint, Left			
P Toe Phalangeal Joint, Right			
Q Toe Phalangeal Joint, Left			

Section	0	Medical and Surgical	
Body System	S	Lower Joints	
Operation	C	Extirpation: Taking or cutting out solid matter from a body part	

Body Part (Character 4)	Approach (Character 5)	Device (Character 6)	Qualifier (Character 7)
0 Lumbar Vertebral Joint	0 Open	Z No Device	Z No Qualifier
2 Lumbar Vertebral Disc	3 Percutaneous		
3 Lumbosacral Joint	4 Percutaneous Endoscopic		
4 Lumbosacral Disc			
5 Sacrococcygeal Joint			
6 Coccygeal Joint			
7 Sacroiliac Joint, Right			
8 Sacroiliac Joint, Left			
9 Hip Joint, Right			
B Hip Joint, Left			
C Knee Joint, Right			
D Knee Joint, Left			
F Ankle Joint, Right			
G Ankle Joint, Left			
H Tarsal Joint, Right			
J Tarsal Joint, Left			
K Metatarsal-Tarsal Joint, Right			
L Metatarsal-Tarsal Joint, Left			
M Metatarsal-Phalangeal Joint, Right			
N Metatarsal-Phalangeal Joint, Left			
P Toe Phalangeal Joint, Right			
Q Toe Phalangeal Joint, Left			

Section	0	Medical and Surgical		
Body System	S	Lower Joints		
Operation	G	Fusion: Joining together portions of an articular body part rendering the articular body part immobile		

Body Part (Character 4)	Approach (Character 5)	Device (Character 6)	Qualifier (Character 7)
0 Lumbar Vertebral Joint 1 Lumbar Vertebral Joints, 2 or more 3 Lumbosacral Joint	0 Open 3 Percutaneous 4 Percutaneous Endoscopic	7 Autologous Tissue Substitute A Interbody Fusion Device J Synthetic Substitute K Nonautologous Tissue Substitute Z No Device	0 Anterior Approach, Anterior Column 1 Posterior Approach, Posterior Column J Posterior Approach, Anterior Column
5 Sacrococcygeal Joint 6 Coccygeal Joint 7 Sacroiliac Joint, Right 8 Sacroiliac Joint, Left	0 Open 3 Percutaneous 4 Percutaneous Endoscopic	4 Internal Fixation Device 7 Autologous Tissue Substitute J Synthetic Substitute K Nonautologous Tissue Substitute Z No Device	Z No Qualifier
9 Hip Joint, Right B Hip Joint, Left C Knee Joint, Right D Knee Joint, Left F Ankle Joint, Right G Ankle Joint, Left H Tarsal Joint, Right J Tarsal Joint, Left K Metatarsal-Tarsal Joint, Right L Metatarsal-Tarsal Joint, Left M Metatarsal-Phalangeal Joint, Right N Metatarsal-Phalangeal Joint, Left P Toe Phalangeal Joint, Right Q Toe Phalangeal Joint, Left	0 Open 3 Percutaneous 4 Percutaneous Endoscopic	4 Internal Fixation Device 5 External Fixation Device 7 Autologous Tissue Substitute J Synthetic Substitute K Nonautologous Tissue Substitute Z No Device	Z No Qualifier

Section	0	Medical and Surgical		
Body System	S	Lower Joints		
Operation	H	Insertion: Putting in a nonbiological appliance that monitors, assists, performs, or prevents a physiological function but does not physically take the place of a body part		

Body Part (Character 4)	Approach (Character 5)	Device (Character 6)	Qualifier (Character 7)
0 Lumbar Vertebral Joint 3 Lumbosacral Joint	0 Open 3 Percutaneous 4 Percutaneous Endoscopic	3 Infusion Device 4 Internal Fixation Device 8 Spacer B Spinal Stabilization Device, Interspinous Process C Spinal Stabilization Device, Pedicle-Based D Spinal Stabilization Device, Facet Replacement	Z No Qualifier
2 Lumbar Vertebral Disc 4 Lumbosacral Disc	0 Open 3 Percutaneous 4 Percutaneous Endoscopic	3 Infusion Device 8 Spacer	Z No Qualifier **Continued on Next Page ▶**

			Continued from ◀ Previous Page
5 Sacrococcygeal Joint **6** Coccygeal Joint **7** Sacroiliac Joint, Right **8** Sacroiliac Joint, Left	**0** Open **3** Percutaneous **4** Percutaneous Endoscopic	**3** Infusion Device **4** Internal Fixation Device **8** Spacer	**Z** No Qualifier
9 Hip Joint, Right **B** Hip Joint, Left **C** Knee Joint, Right **D** Knee Joint, Left **F** Ankle Joint, Right **G** Ankle Joint, Left **H** Tarsal Joint, Right **J** Tarsal Joint, Left **K** Metatarsal-Tarsal Joint, Right **L** Metatarsal-Tarsal Joint, Left **M** Metatarsal-Phalangeal Joint, Right **N** Metatarsal-Phalangeal Joint, Left **P** Toe Phalangeal Joint, Right **Q** Toe Phalangeal Joint, Left	**0** Open **3** Percutaneous **4** Percutaneous Endoscopic	**3** Infusion Device **4** Internal Fixation Device **5** External Fixation Device **8** Spacer	**Z** No Qualifier

Section	0	Medical and Surgical	
Body System	**S**	**Lower Joints**	
Operation	**J**	**Inspection: Visually and/or manually exploring a body part**	
Body Part (Character 4)	**Approach (Character 5)**	**Device (Character 6)**	**Qualifier (Character 7)**
0 Lumbar Vertebral Joint **2** Lumbar Vertebral Disc **3** Lumbosacral Joint **4** Lumbosacral Disc **5** Sacrococcygeal Joint **6** Coccygeal Joint **7** Sacroiliac Joint, Right **8** Sacroiliac Joint, Left **9** Hip Joint, Right **B** Hip Joint, Left **C** Knee Joint, Right **D** Knee Joint, Left **F** Ankle Joint, Right **G** Ankle Joint, Left **H** Tarsal Joint, Right **J** Tarsal Joint, Left **K** Metatarsal-Tarsal Joint, Right **L** Metatarsal-Tarsal Joint, Left **M** Metatarsal-Phalangeal Joint, Right **N** Metatarsal-Phalangeal Joint, Left **P** Toe Phalangeal Joint, Right **Q** Toe Phalangeal Joint, Left	**0** Open **3** Percutaneous **4** Percutaneous Endoscopic **X** External	**Z** No Device	**Z** No Qualifier

Section	0	Medical and Surgical		
Body System	S	**Lower Joints**		
Operation	N	Release: Freeing a body part from an abnormal physical constraint by cutting or by the use of force		

Body Part (Character 4)	Approach (Character 5)	Device (Character 6)	Qualifier (Character 7)
0 Lumbar Vertebral Joint	**0** Open	**Z** No Device	**Z** No Qualifier
2 Lumbar Vertebral Disc	**3** Percutaneous		
3 Lumbosacral Joint	**4** Percutaneous Endoscopic		
4 Lumbosacral Disc	**X** External		
5 Sacrococcygeal Joint			
6 Coccygeal Joint			
7 Sacroiliac Joint, Right			
8 Sacroiliac Joint, Left			
9 Hip Joint, Right			
B Hip Joint, Left			
C Knee Joint, Right			
D Knee Joint, Left			
F Ankle Joint, Right			
G Ankle Joint, Left			
H Tarsal Joint, Right			
J Tarsal Joint, Left			
K Metatarsal-Tarsal Joint, Right			
L Metatarsal-Tarsal Joint, Left			
M Metatarsal-Phalangeal Joint, Right			
N Metatarsal-Phalangeal Joint, Left			
P Toe Phalangeal Joint, Right			
Q Toe Phalangeal Joint, Left			

Section	0	Medical and Surgical		
Body System	S	**Lower Joints**		
Operation	P	Removal: Taking out or off a device from a body part		

Body Part (Character 4)	Approach (Character 5)	Device (Character 6)	Qualifier (Character 7)
0 Lumbar Vertebral Joint **3** Lumbosacral Joint	**0** Open **3** Percutaneous **4** Percutaneous Endoscopic	**0** Drainage Device **3** Infusion Device **4** Internal Fixation Device **7** Autologous Tissue Substitute **8** Spacer **A** Interbody Fusion Device **J** Synthetic Substitute **K** Nonautologous Tissue Substitute	**Z** No Qualifier
0 Lumbar Vertebral Joint **3** Lumbosacral Joint	**X** External	**0** Drainage Device **3** Infusion Device **4** Internal Fixation Device	**Z** No Qualifier
2 Lumbar Vertebral Disc **4** Lumbosacral Disc	**0** Open **3** Percutaneous **4** Percutaneous Endoscopic	**0** Drainage Device **3** Infusion Device **7** Autologous Tissue Substitute **J** Synthetic Substitute **K** Nonautologous Tissue Substitute	**Z** No Qualifier

Continued on Next Page ▶

			Continued from ◀ Previous Page
2 Lumbar Vertebral Disc **4** Lumbosacral Disc	**X** External	**0** Drainage Device **3** Infusion Device	**Z** No Qualifier
5 Sacrococcygeal Joint **6** Coccygeal Joint **7** Sacroiliac Joint, Right **8** Sacroiliac Joint, Left	**0** Open **3** Percutaneous **4** Percutaneous Endoscopic	**0** Drainage Device **3** Infusion Device **4** Internal Fixation Device **7** Autologous Tissue Substitute **8** Spacer **J** Synthetic Substitute **K** Nonautologous Tissue Substitute	**Z** No Qualifier
5 Sacrococcygeal Joint **6** Coccygeal Joint **7** Sacroiliac Joint, Right **8** Sacroiliac Joint, Left	**X** External	**0** Drainage Device **3** Infusion Device **4** Internal Fixation Device	**Z** No Qualifier
9 Hip Joint, Right **B** Hip Joint, Left	**0** Open	**0** Drainage Device **3** Infusion Device **4** Internal Fixation Device **5** External Fixation Device **7** Autologous Tissue Substitute **8** Spacer **9** Liner **B** Resurfacing Device **J** Synthetic Substitute **K** Nonautologous Tissue Substitute	**Z** No Qualifier
9 Hip Joint, Right **B** Hip Joint, Left	**3** Percutaneous **4** Percutaneous Endoscopic	**0** Drainage Device **3** Infusion Device **4** Internal Fixation Device **5** External Fixation Device **7** Autologous Tissue Substitute **8** Spacer **J** Synthetic Substitute **K** Nonautologous Tissue Substitute	**Z** No Qualifier
9 Hip Joint, Right **B** Hip Joint, Lef	**X** Externl	**0** Drainage Device **3** Infusion Device **4** Internal Fixation Device **5** External Fixation Device	**Z** No Qualifier
A Hip Joint, Acetabular Surface, Right **E** Hip Joint, Acetabular Surface, Left **R** Hip Joint, Femoral Surface, Right **S** Hip Joint, Femoral Surface, Left **T** Knee Joint, Femoral Surface, Right **U** Knee Joint, Femoral Surface, Left	**0** Open **3** Percutaneous **4** Percutaneous Endoscopic	**J** Synthetic Substitute	**Z** No Qualifier Continued on Next Page ▶

			Continued from ◀ Previous Page
V Knee Joint, Tibial Surface, Right **W** Knee Joint			
C Knee Joint, Right **D** Knee Joint, Left	**0** Open	**0** Drainage Device **3** Infusion Device **4** Internal Fixation Device **5** External Fixation Device **7** Autologous Tissue Substitute **8** Spacer **9** Liner **K** Nonautologous Tissue Substitute	**Z** No Qualifier
C Knee Joint, Right **D** Knee Joint, Left	**0** Open	**J** Synthetic Substitute	**C** Patellar Surface **Z** No Qualifier
C Knee Joint, Right **D** Knee Joint, Left	**3** Percutaneous **4** Percutaneous Endoscopic	**0** Drainage Device **3** Infusion Device **4** Internal Fixation Device **5** External Fixation Device **7** Autologous Tissue Substitute **8** Spacer **K** Nonautologous Tissue Substitute	**Z** No Qualifier
C Knee Joint, Right **D** Knee Joint, Left	**3** Percutaneous **4** Percutaneous Endoscopic	**J** Synthetic Substitute	**C** Patellar Surface **Z** No Qualifier
C Knee Joint, Right **D** Knee Joint, Left	**X** External	**0** Drainage Device **3** Infusion Device **4** Internal Fixation Device **5** External Fixation Device	**Z** No Qualifier
F Ankle Joint, Right **G** Ankle Joint, Left **H** Tarsal Joint, Right **J** Tarsal Joint, Left **K** Metatarsal-Tarsal Joint, Right **L** Metatarsal-Tarsal Joint, Left **M** Metatarsal-Phalangeal Joint, Right **N** Metatarsal-Phalangeal Joint, Left **P** Toe Phalangeal Joint, Right **Q** Toe Phalangeal Joint, Left	**0** Open **3** Percutaneous **4** Percutaneous Endoscopic	**0** Drainage Device **3** Infusion Device **4** Internal Fixation Device **5** External Fixation Device **7** Autologous Tissue Substitute **8** Spacer **J** Synthetic Substitute **K** Nonautologous Tissue Substitute	**Z** No Qualifier
F Ankle Joint, Right **G** Ankle Joint, Left **H** Tarsal Joint, Right **J** Tarsal Joint, Left **K** Metatarsal-Tarsal Joint, Right **L** Metatarsal-Tarsal Joint, Left **M** Metatarsal-Phalangeal Joint, Right **N** Metatarsal-Phalangeal Joint, Left **P** Toe Phalangeal Joint, Right **Q** Toe Phalangeal Joint, Left	**X** External	**0** Drainage Device **3** Infusion Device **4** Internal Fixation Device **5** External Fixation Device	**Z** No Qualifier

Section	0	Medical and Surgical		
Body System	S	Lower Joints		
Operation	Q	Repair: Restoring, to the extent possible, a body part to its normal anatomic structure and function		

Body Part (Character 4)	Approach (Character 5)	Device (Character 6)	Qualifier (Character 7)
0 Lumbar Vertebral Joint	0 Open	Z No Device	Z No Qualifier
2 Lumbar Vertebral Disc	3 Percutaneous		
3 Lumbosacral Joint	4 Percutaneous Endoscopic		
4 Lumbosacral Disc	X External		
5 Sacrococcygeal Joint			
6 Coccygeal Joint			
7 Sacroiliac Joint, Right			
8 Sacroiliac Joint, Left			
9 Hip Joint, Right			
B Hip Joint, Left			
C Knee Joint, Right			
D Knee Joint, Left			
F Ankle Joint, Right			
G Ankle Joint, Left			
H Tarsal Joint, Right			
J Tarsal Joint, Left			
K Metatarsal-Tarsal Joint, Right			
L Metatarsal-Tarsal Joint, Left			
M Metatarsal-Phalangeal Joint, Right			
N Metatarsal-Phalangeal Joint, Left			
P Toe Phalangeal Joint, Right			
Q Toe Phalangeal Joint, Left			

Section	0	Medical and Surgical		
Body System	S	Lower Joints		
Operation	R	Replacement: Putting in or on biological or synthetic material that physically takes the place and/or function of all or a portion of a body part		

Body Part (Character 4)	Approach (Character 5)	Device (Character 6)	Qualifier (Character 7)
0 Lumbar Vertebral Joint	0 Open	7 Autologous Tissue Substitute	Z No Qualifier
2 Lumbar Vertebral Disc		J Synthetic Substitute	
3 Lumbosacral Joint		K Nonautologous Tissue Substitute	
4 Lumbosacral Disc			
5 Sacrococcygeal Joint			
6 Coccygeal Joint			
7 Sacroiliac Joint, Right			
8 Sacroiliac Joint, Left			
H Tarsal Joint, Right			
J Tarsal Joint, Left			
K Metatarsal-Tarsal Joint, Right			
L Metatarsal-Tarsal Joint, Left			
M Metatarsal-Phalangeal Joint, Right			
N Metatarsal-Phalangeal Joint, Left			
P Toe Phalangeal Joint, Right			
Q Toe Phalangeal Joint, Left			Continued on Next Page ▶

			Continued from ◀ **Previous Page**
9 Hip Joint, Right **B** Hip Joint, Left	**0** Open	**1** Synthetic Substitute, Metal **2** Synthetic Substitute, Metal on Polyethylene **3** Synthetic Substitute, Ceramic **4** Synthetic Substitute, Ceramic on Polyethylene **J** Synthetic Substitute	**9** Cemented **A** Uncemented **Z** No Qualifier
9 Hip Joint, Right **B** Hip Joint, Left	**0** Open	**7** Autologous Tissue Substitute **K** Nonautologous Tissue Substitute	**Z** No Qualifier
A Hip Joint, Acetabular Surface, Right **E** Hip Joint, Acetabular Surface, Left	**0** Open	**0** Synthetic Substitute, Polyethylene **1** Synthetic Substitute, Metal **3** Synthetic Substitute, Ceramic **J** Synthetic Substitute	**9** Cemented **A** Uncemented **Z** No Qualifier
A Hip Joint, Acetabular Surface, Right **E** Hip Joint, Acetabular Surface, Left	**0** Open	**7** Autologous Tissue Substitute **K** Nonautologous Tissue Substitute	**Z** No Qualifier
C Knee Joint, Right **D** Knee Joint, Left	**0** Open	**7** Autologous Tissue Substitute **K** Nonautologous Tissue Substitute	**Z** No Qualifier
C Knee Joint, Right **D** Knee Joint, Left	**0** Open	**J** Synthetic Substitute **L** Synthetic Substitute, Unicondylar	**9** Cemented **A** Uncemented **Z** No Qualifier
F Ankle Joint, Right **G** Ankle Joint, Left **T** Knee Joint, Femoral Surface, Right **U** Knee Joint, Femoral Surface, Left **V** Knee Joint, Tibial Surface, Right **W** Knee Joint, Tibial Surface, Left	**0** Open	**7** Autologous Tissue Substitute **K** Nonautologous Tissue Substitute	**Z** No Qualifier
F Ankle Joint, Right **G** Ankle Joint, Left **T** Knee Joint, Femoral Surface, Right **U** Knee Joint, Femoral Surface, Left **V** Knee Joint, Tibial Surface, Right **W** Knee Joint, Tibial Surface, Left	**0** Open	**J** Synthetic Substitute	**9** Cemented **A** Uncemented **Z** No Qualifier
R Hip Joint, Femoral Surface, Right **S** Hip Joint, Femoral Surface, Left	**0** Open	**1** Synthetic Substitute, Metal **3** Synthetic Substitute, Ceramic **J** Synthetic Substitute	**9** Cemented **A** Uncemented **Z** No Qualifier **Continued on** **Next Page ▶**

			Continued from ◀ Previous Page
R Hip Joint, Femoral Surface, Right S Hip Joint, Femoral Surface, Left	0 Open	7 Autologous Tissue Substitute K Nonautologous Tissue Substitute	Z No Qualifier

Section	0	Medical and Surgical	
Body System	S	Lower Joints	
Operation	S	Reposition: Moving to its normal location, or other suitable location, all or a portion of a body part	

Body Part (Character 4)	Approach (Character 5)	Device (Character 6)	Qualifier (Character 7)
0 Lumbar Vertebral Joint 3 Lumbosacral Joint 5 Sacrococcygeal Joint 6 Coccygeal Joint 7 Sacroiliac Joint, Right 8 Sacroiliac Joint, Left	0 Open 3 Percutaneous 4 Percutaneous Endoscopic X External	4 Internal Fixation Device Z No Device	Z No Qualifier
9 Hip Joint, Right B Hip Joint, Left C Knee Joint, Right D Knee Joint, Left F Ankle Joint, Right G Ankle Joint, Left H Tarsal Joint, Right J Tarsal Joint, Left K Metatarsal-Tarsal Joint, Right L Metatarsal-Tarsal Joint, Left M Metatarsal-Phalangeal Joint, Right N Metatarsal-Phalangeal Joint, Left P Toe Phalangeal Joint, Right Q Toe Phalangeal Joint, Left	0 Open 3 Percutaneous 4 Percutaneous Endoscopic X External	4 Internal Fixation Device 5 External Fixation Device Z No Device	Z No Qualifier

Section	0	Medical and Surgical	
Body System	S	Lower Joints	
Operation	T	Resection: Cutting out or off, without replacement, all of a body part	

Body Part (Character 4)	Approach (Character 5)	Device (Character 6)	Qualifier (Character 7)
2 Lumbar Vertebral Disc 4 Lumbosacral Disc 5 Sacrococcygeal Joint 6 Coccygeal Joint 7 Sacroiliac Joint, Right 8 Sacroiliac Joint, Left 9 Hip Joint, Right B Hip Joint, Left C Knee Joint, Right D Knee Joint, Left F Ankle Joint, Right G Ankle Joint, Left H Tarsal Joint, Right J Tarsal Joint, Left	0 Open	Z No Device	Z No Qualifier

Continued on Next Page ▶

Body Part (Character 4)	Approach (Character 5)	Device (Character 6)	Qualifier (Character 7)
K Metatarsal-Tarsal Joint, Right L Metatarsal-Tarsal Joint, Left M Metatarsal-Phalangeal Joint, Right N Metatarsal-Phalangeal Joint, Left P Toe Phalangeal Joint, Right Q Toe Phalangeal Joint, Left			Continued from ◀ Previous Page

Section	0	Medical and Surgical
Body System	S	Lower Joints
Operation	U	Supplement: Putting in or on biological or synthetic material that physically reinforces and/or augments the function of a portion of a body part

Body Part (Character 4)	Approach (Character 5)	Device (Character 6)	Qualifier (Character 7)
0 Lumbar Vertebral Joint 2 Lumbar Vertebral Disc 3 Lumbosacral Joint 4 Lumbosacral Disc 5 Sacrococcygeal Joint 6 Coccygeal Joint 7 Sacroiliac Joint, Right 8 Sacroiliac Joint, Left F Ankle Joint, Right G Ankle Joint, Left H Tarsal Joint, Right J Tarsal Joint, Left K Metatarsal-Tarsal Joint, Right L Metatarsal-Tarsal Joint, Left M Metatarsal-Phalangeal Joint, Right N Metatarsal-Phalangeal Joint, Left P Toe Phalangeal Joint, Right Q Toe Phalangeal Joint, Left	0 Open 3 Percutaneous 4 Percutaneous Endoscopic	7 Autologous Tissue Substitute J Synthetic Substitute K Nonautologous Tissue Substitute	Z No Qualifier
9 Hip Joint, Right B Hip Joint, Left	0 Open	7 Autologous Tissue Substitute 9 Liner B Resurfacing Device J Synthetic Substitute K Nonautologous Tissue Substitute	Z No Qualifier
9 Hip Joint, Right B Hip Joint, Left	3 Percutaneous 4 Percutaneous Endoscopic	7 Autologous Tissue Substitute J Synthetic Substitute K Nonautologous Tissue Substitute	Z No Qualifier
A Hip Joint, Acetabular Surface, Right E Hip Joint, Acetabular Surface, Left R Hip Joint, Femoral Surface, Right S Hip Joint, Femoral Surface, Left	0 Open	9 Liner B Resurfacing Device	Z No Qualifier Continued on Next Page ▶

			Continued from ◀ Previous Page
C Knee Joint, Right **D** Knee Joint, Left	**0** Open	**7** Autologous Tissue Substitute **J** Synthetic Substitute **K** Nonautologous Tissue Substitute	**Z** No Qualifier
C Knee Joint, Right **D** Knee Joint, Left	**0** Open	**9** Liner	**C** Patellar Surface **Z** No Qualifier
C Knee Joint, Right **D** Knee Joint, Left	**3** Percutaneous **4** Percutaneous Endoscopic	**7** Autologous Tissue Substitute **J** Synthetic Substitute **K** Nonautologous Tissue Substitute	**Z** No Qualifier
T Knee Joint, Femoral Surface, Right **U** Knee Joint, Femoral Surface, Left **V** Knee Joint, Tibial Surface, Right **W** Knee Joint, Tibial Surface, Left	**0** Open	**9** Liner	**Z** No Qualifier

Section	0	Medical and Surgical
Body System	S	Lower Joints
Operation	W	Revision: Correcting, to the extent possible, a portion of a malfunctioning device or the position of a displaced device

Body Part (Character 4)	Approach (Character 5)	Device (Character 6)	Qualifier (Character 7)
0 Lumbar Vertebral Joint **3** Lumbosacral Joint	**0** Open **3** Percutaneous **4** Percutaneous Endoscopic **X** External	**0** Drainage Device **3** Infusion Device **4** Internal Fixation Device **7** Autologous Tissue Substitute **8** Spacer **A** Interbody Fusion Device **J** Synthetic Substitute **K** Nonautologous Tissue Substitute	**Z** No Qualifier
2 Lumbar Vertebral Disc **4** Lumbosacral Disc	**0** Open **3** Percutaneous **4** Percutaneous Endoscopic **X** External	**0** Drainage Device **3** Infusion Device **7** Autologous Tissue Substitute **J** Synthetic Substitute **K** Nonautologous Tissue Substitute	**Z** No Qualifier
5 Sacrococcygeal Joint **6** Coccygeal Joint **7** Sacroiliac Joint, Right **8** Sacroiliac Joint, Left	**0** Open **3** Percutaneous **4** Percutaneous Endoscopic **X** External	**0** Drainage Device **3** Infusion Device **4** Internal Fixation Device **7** Autologous Tissue Substitute **8** Spacer **J** Synthetic Substitute **K** Nonautologous Tissue Substitute	**Z** No Qualifier

Continued on Next Page ▶

			Continued from ◀ Previous Page
9 Hip Joint, Right **B** Hip Joint, Left	**0** Open	**0** Drainage Device **3** Infusion Device **4** Internal Fixation Device **5** External Fixation Device **7** Autologous Tissue Substitute **8** Spacer **9** Liner **B** Resurfacing Device **J** Synthetic Substitute **K** Nonautologous Tissue Substitute	**Z** No Qualifier

Section	0	Medical and Surgical
Body System	S	Lower Joints
Operation	W	Revision: Correcting, to the extent possible, a portion of a malfunctioning device or the position of a displaced device

Body Part (Character 4)	Approach (Character 5)	Device (Character 6)	Qualifier (Character 7)
9 Hip Joint, Right **B** Hip Joint, Left	**3** Percutaneous **4** Percutaneous Endoscopic **X** External	**0** Drainage Device **3** Infusion Device **4** Internal Fixation Device **5** External Fixation Device **7** Autologous Tissue Substitute **8** Spacer **J** Synthetic Substitute **K** Nonautologous Tissue Substitute	**Z** No Qualifier
A Hip Joint, Acetabular Surface, Right **E** Hip Joint, Acetabular Surface, Left **R** Hip Joint, Femoral Surface, Right **S** Hip Joint, Femoral Surface, Left **T** Knee Joint, Femoral Surface, Right **U** Knee Joint, Femoral Surface, Left **V** Knee Joint, Tibial Surface, Right **W** Knee Joint, Tibial Surface, Left	**0** Open **3** Percutaneous **4** Percutaneous Endoscopic **X** External	**J** Synthetic Substitute	**Z** No Qualifier
C Knee Joint, Right **D** Knee Joint, Left	**0** Open	**0** Drainage Device **3** Infusion Device **4** Internal Fixation Device **5** External Fixation Device **7** Autologous Tissue Substitute **8** Spacer **9** Liner **K** Nonautologous Tissue Substitute	**Z** No Qualifier Continued on Next Page ▶

			Continued from ◀ Previous Page
C Knee Joint, Right D Knee Joint, Left	0 Open	J Synthetic Substitute	C Patellar Surface Z No Qualifier
C Knee Joint, Right D Knee Joint, Left	3 Percutaneous 4 Percutaneous Endoscopic X External	0 Drainage Device 3 Infusion Device 4 Internal Fixation Device 5 External Fixation Device 7 Autologous Tissue Substitute 8 Spacer K Nonautologous Tissue Substitute	Z No Qualifier
C Knee Joint, Right D Knee Joint, Left	3 Percutaneous 4 Percutaneous Endoscopic X External	J Synthetic Substitute	C Patellar Surface Z No Qualifier
F Ankle Joint, Right G Ankle Joint, Left H Tarsal Joint, Right J Tarsal Joint, Left K Metatarsal-Tarsal Joint, Right L Metatarsal-Tarsal Joint, Left M Metatarsal-Phalangeal Joint, Right N Metatarsal-Phalangeal Joint, Left P Toe Phalangeal Joint, Right Q Toe Phalangeal Joint, Left	0 Open 3 Percutaneous 4 Percutaneous Endoscopic X External	0 Drainage Device 3 Infusion Device 4 Internal Fixation Device 5 External Fixation Device 7 Autologous Tissue Substitute 8 Spacer J Synthetic Substitute K Nonautologous Tissue Substitute	Z No Qualifier

Section	0	Medical and Surgical	
Body System	T	Urinary System	
Operation	1	Bypass: Altering the route of passage of the contents of a tubular body part	

Body Part (Character 4)	Approach (Character 5)	Device (Character 6)	Qualifier (Character 7)
3 Kidney Pelvis, Right 4 Kidney Pelvis, Left	0 Open 4 Percutaneous Endoscopic	7 Autologous Tissue Substitute J Synthetic Substitute K Nonautologous Tissue Substitute Z No Device	3 Kidney Pelvis, Right 4 Kidney Pelvis, Left 6 Ureter, Right 7 Ureter, Left 8 Colon 9 Colocutaneous A Ileum B Bladder C Ileocutaneous D Cutaneous
3 Kidney Pelvis, Right 4 Kidney Pelvis, Left	3 Percutaneous	J Synthetic Substitute	D Cutaneous
6 Ureter, Right 7 Ureter, Left 8 Ureters, Bilateral	0 Open 4 Percutaneous Endoscopic	7 Autologous Tissue Substitute J Synthetic Substitute K Nonautologous Tissue Substitute Z No Device	6 Ureter, Right 7 Ureter, Left 8 Colon 9 Colocutaneous A Ileum B Bladder C Ileocutaneous D Cutaneous
6 Ureter, Right 7 Ureter, Left 8 Ureters, Bilateral	3 Percutaneous	J Synthetic Substitute	D Cutaneous
B Bladder	0 Open 4 Percutaneous Endoscopic	7 Autologous Tissue Substitute J Synthetic Substitute K Nonautologous Tissue Substitute Z No Device	9 Colocutaneous C Ileocutaneous D Cutaneous
B Bladder	3 Percutaneous	J Synthetic Substitute	D Cutaneous

Section	0	Medical and Surgical	
Body System	T	Urinary System	
Operation	2	Change: Taking out or off a device from a body part and putting back an identical or similar device in or on the same body part without cutting or puncturing the skin or a mucous membrane	

Body Part (Character 4)	Approach (Character 5)	Device (Character 6)	Qualifier (Character 7)
5 Kidney 9 Ureter B Bladder D Urethra	X External	0 Drainage Device Y Other Device	Z No Qualifier

Section	0	Medical and Surgical		
Body System	T	Urinary System		
Operation	5	Destruction: Physical eradication of all or a portion of a body part by the direct use of energy, force, or a destructive agent		

Body Part Character 4	Approach Character 5	Device	Qualifier
0 Kidney, Right 1 Kidney, Left 3 Kidney Pelvis, Right 4 Kidney Pelvis, Left 6 Ureter, Right 7 Ureter, Left B Bladder C Bladder Neck	0 Open 3 Percutaneous 4 Percutaneous Endoscopic 7 Via Natural or Artificial Opening 8 Via Natural or Artificial Opening Endoscopic	Z No Device	Z No Qualifier
D Urethra	0 Open 3 Percutaneous 4 Percutaneous Endoscopic 7 Via Natural or Artificial Opening 8 Via Natural or Artificial Opening Endoscopic X External	Z No Device	Z No Qualifier

Section	0	Medical and Surgical		
Body System	T	Urinary System		
Operation	7	Dilation: Expanding an orifice or the lumen of a tubular body part		

Body Part (Character 4)	Approach (Character 5)	Device (Character 6)	Qualifier (Character 7)
3 Kidney Pelvis, Right 4 Kidney Pelvis, Left 6 Ureter, Right 7 Ureter, Left 8 Ureters, Bilateral B Bladder C Bladder Neck D Urethra	0 Open 3 Percutaneous 4 Percutaneous Endoscopic 7 Via Natural or Artificial Opening 8 Via Natural or Artificial Opening Endoscopic	D Intraluminal Device Z No Device	Z No Qualifier

Section	0	Medical and Surgical		
Body System	T	Urinary System		
Operation	8	Division: Cutting into a body part, without draining fluids and/or gases from the body part, in order to separate or transect a body part		

Body Part (Character 4)	Approach (Character 5)	Device (Character 6)	Qualifier (Character 7)
2 Kidneys, Bilateral C Bladder Neck	0 Open 3 Percutaneous 4 Percutaneous Endoscopic	Z No Device	Z No Qualifier

Section	0	Medical and Surgical		
Body System	T	Urinary System		
Operation	9	Drainage: Taking or letting out fluids and/or gases from a body part		

Body Part (Character 4)	Approach (Character 5)	Device (Character 6)	Qualifier (Character 7)
0 Kidney, Right 1 Kidney, Left 3 Kidney Pelvis, Right 4 Kidney Pelvis, Left 6 Ureter, Right	0 Open 3 Percutaneous 4 Percutaneous Endoscopic 7 Via Natural or Artificial Opening	0 Drainage Device	Z No Qualifier Continued on Next Page ▶

7 Ureter, Left **8** Ureters, Bilateral **B** Bladder **C** Bladder Neck	**8** Via Natural or Artificial Opening Endoscopic		Continued from ◀ Previous Page
0 Kidney, Right **1** Kidney, Left **3** Kidney Pelvis, Right **4** Kidney Pelvis, Left **6** Ureter, Right **7** Ureter, Left **8** Ureters, Bilateral **B** Bladder **C** Bladder Neck	**0** Open **3** Percutaneous **4** Percutaneous Endoscopic **7** Via Natural or Artificial Opening **8** Via Natural or Artificial Opening Endoscopic	**Z** No Device	**X** Diagnostic **Z** No Qualifier
D Urethra	**0** Open **3** Percutaneous **4** Percutaneous Endoscopic **7** Via Natural or Artificial Opening **8** Via Natural or Artificial Opening Endoscopic **X** External	**0** Drainage Device	**Z** No Qualifier
D Urethra	**0** Open **3** Percutaneous **4** Percutaneous Endoscopic **7** Via Natural or Artificial Opening **8** Via Natural or Artificial Opening Endoscopic **X** External	**Z** No Device	**X** Diagnostic **Z** No Qualifier

Section	0	Medical and Surgical	
Body System	**T**	**Urinary System**	
Operation	**B**	**Excision: Cutting out or off, without replacement, a portion of a body part**	
Body Part (Character 4)	**Approach (Character 5)**	**Device (Character 6)**	**Qualifier (Character 7)**
0 Kidney, Right **1** Kidney, Left **3** Kidney Pelvis, Right **4** Kidney Pelvis, Left **6** Ureter, Right **7** Ureter, Left **B** Bladder **C** Bladder Neck	**0** Open **3** Percutaneous **4** Percutaneous Endoscopic **7** Via Natural or Artificial Opening **8** Via Natural or Artificial Opening Endoscopic	**Z** No Device	**X** Diagnostic **Z** No Qualifier
D Urethra	**0** Open **3** Percutaneous **4** Percutaneous Endoscopic **7** Via Natural or Artificial Opening **8** Via Natural or Artificial Opening Endoscopic **X** External	**Z** No Device	**X** Diagnostic **Z** No Qualifier

Section	0	Medical and Surgical		
Body System	T	Urinary System		
Operation	C	Extirpation: Taking or cutting out solid matter from a body part		

Body Part (Character 4)	Approach (Character 5)	Device (Character 6)	Qualifier (Character 7)
0 Kidney, Right 1 Kidney, Left 3 Kidney Pelvis, Right 4 Kidney Pelvis, Left 6 Ureter, Right 7 Ureter, Left B Bladder C Bladder Neck	0 Open 3 Percutaneous 4 Percutaneous Endoscopic 7 Via Natural or Artificial Opening 8 Via Natural or Artificial Opening Endoscopic	Z No Device	Z No Qualifier
D Urethra	0 Open 3 Percutaneous 4 Percutaneous Endoscopic 7 Via Natural or Artificial Opening 8 Via Natural or Artificial Opening Endoscopic X External	Z No Device	Z No Qualifier

Section	0	Medical and Surgical		
Body System	T	Urinary System		
Operation	D	Extraction: Pulling or stripping out or off all or a portion of a body part by the use of force		

Body Part (Character 4)	Approach (Character 5)	Device (Character 6)	Qualifier (Character 7)
0 Kidney, Right 1 Kidney, Left	0 Open 3 Percutaneous 4 Percutaneous Endoscopic	Z No Device	Z No Qualifier

Section	0	Medical and Surgical		
Body System	T	Urinary System		
Operation	F	Fragmentation: Breaking solid matter in a body part into pieces		

Body Part (Character 4)	Approach (Character 5)	Device (Character 6)	Qualifier (Character 7)
3 Kidney Pelvis, Right 4 Kidney Pelvis, Left 6 Ureter, Right 7 Ureter, Left B Bladder C Bladder Neck D Urethra	0 Open 3 Percutaneous 4 Percutaneous Endoscopic 7 Via Natural or Artificial Opening 8 Via Natural or Artificial Opening Endoscopic X External	Z No Device	Z No Qualifier

Section	0	Medical and Surgical		
Body System	T	Urinary System		
Operation	H	Insertion: Putting in a nonbiological appliance that monitors, assists, performs, or prevents a physiological function but does not physically take the place of a body part		

Body Part (Character 4)	Approach (Character 5)	Device (Character 6)	Qualifier (Character 7)
5 Kidney	0 Open 3 Percutaneous 4 Percutaneous Endoscopic 7 Via Natural or Artificial Opening 8 Via Natural or Artificial Opening Endoscopic	2 Monitoring Device 3 Infusion Device	Z No Qualifier

Continued on Next Page ▶

			Continued from ◀ Previous Page
9 Ureter	**0** Open **3** Percutaneous **4** Percutaneous Endoscopic **7** Via Natural or Artificial Opening **8** Via Natural or Artificial Opening Endoscopic	**2** Monitoring Device **3** Infusion Device **M** Stimulator Lead	**Z** No Qualifier
B Bladder	**0** Open **3** Percutaneous **4** Percutaneous Endoscopic **7** Via Natural or Artificial Opening **8** Via Natural or Artificial Opening Endoscopic	**2** Monitoring Device **3** Infusion Device **L** Artificial Sphincter **M** Stimulator Lead	**Z** No Qualifier
C Bladder Neck	**0** Open **3** Percutaneous **4** Percutaneous Endoscopic **7** Via Natural or Artificial Opening **8** Via Natural or Artificial Opening Endoscopic	**L** Artificial Sphincter	**Z** No Qualifier
D Urethra	**0** Open **3** Percutaneous **4** Percutaneous Endoscopic **7** Via Natural or Artificial Opening **8** Via Natural or Artificial Opening Endoscopic **X** External	**2** Monitoring Device **3** Infusion Device **L** Artificial Sphincter	**Z** No Qualifier

Section	0	Medical and Surgical
Body System	T	Urinary System
Operation	J	Inspection: Visually and/or manually exploring a body part

Body Part (Character 4)	Approach (Character 5)	Device (Character 6)	Qualifier (Character 7)
5 Kidney **9** Ureter **B** Bladder **D** Urethra	**0** Open **3** Percutaneous **4** Percutaneous Endoscopic **7** Via Natural or Artificial Opening **8** Via Natural or Artificial Opening Endoscopic **X** External	**Z** No Device	**Z** No Qualifier

Section	0	Medical and Surgical
Body System	T	Urinary System
Operation	L	Occlusion: Completely closing an orifice or the lumen of a tubular body part

Body Part (Character 4)	Approach (Character 5)	Device (Character 6)	Qualifier (Character 7)
3 Kidney Pelvis, Right **4** Kidney Pelvis, Left **6** Ureter, Right **7** Ureter, Left **B** Bladder **C** Bladder Neck	**0** Open **3** Percutaneous **4** Percutaneous Endoscopic	**C** Extraluminal Device **D** Intraluminal Device **Z** No Device	**Z** No Qualifier

Continued on Next Page ▶

			Continued from ◀ Previous Page
3 Kidney Pelvis, Right 4 Kidney Pelvis, Left 6 Ureter, Right 7 Ureter, Left B Bladder C Bladder Neck	7 Via Natural or Artificial Opening 8 Via Natural or Artificial Opening Endoscopic	D Intraluminal Device Z No Device	Z No Qualifier
D Urethra	0 Open 3 Percutaneous 4 Percutaneous Endoscopic X External	C Extraluminal Device D Intraluminal Device Z No Device	Z No Qualifier
D Urethra	7 Via Natural or Artificial Opening 8 Via Natural or Artificial Opening Endoscopic	D Intraluminal Device Z No Device	Z No Qualifier

Section	0	Medical and Surgical	
Body System	T	Urinary System	
Operation	M	Reattachment Putting back in or on all or a portion of a separated body part to its normal location or other suitable location	

Body Part (Character 4)	Approach (Character 5)	Device (Character 6)	Qualifier (Character 7)
0 Kidney, Right 1 Kidney, Left 2 Kidneys, Bilateral 3 Kidney Pelvis, Right 4 Kidney Pelvis, Left 6 Ureter, Right 7 Ureter, Left 8 Ureters, Bilateral B Bladder C Bladder Neck D Urethra	0 Open 4 Percutaneous Endoscopic	Z No Device	Z No Qualifier

Section	0	Medical and Surgical	
Body System	T	Urinary System	
Operation	N	Release: Freeing a body part from an abnormal physical constraint by cutting or by the use of force	

Body Part (Character 4)	Approach (Character 5)	Device (Character 6)	Qualifier (Character 7)
0 Kidney, Right 1 Kidney, Left 3 Kidney Pelvis, Right 4 Kidney Pelvis, Left 6 Ureter, Right 7 Ureter, Left B Bladder C Bladder Neck	0 Open 3 Percutaneous 4 Percutaneous Endoscopic 7 Via Natural or Artificial Opening 8 Via Natural or Artificial Opening Endoscopic	Z No Device	Z No Qualifier
D Urethra	0 Open 3 Percutaneous 4 Percutaneous Endoscopic 7 Via Natural or Artificial Opening 8 Via Natural or Artificial Opening Endoscopic X External	Z No Device	Z No Qualifier

Section	0	Medical and Surgical
Body System	T	Urinary System
Operation	P	Removal: Taking out or off a device from a body part

Body Part (Character 4)	Approach (Character 5)	Device (Character 6)	Qualifier (Character 7)
5 Kidney	0 Open 3 Percutaneous 4 Percutaneous Endoscopic 7 Via Natural or Artificial Opening 8 Via Natural or Artificial Opening Endoscopic	0 Drainage Device 2 Monitoring Device 3 Infusion Device 7 Autologous Tissue Substitute C Extraluminal Device D Intraluminal Device J Synthetic Substitute K Nonautologous Tissue Substitute	Z No Qualifier
5 Kidney	X External	0 Drainage Device 2 Monitoring Device 3 Infusion Device D Intraluminal Device	Z No Qualifier
9 Ureter	0 Open 3 Percutaneous 4 Percutaneous Endoscopic 7 Via Natural or Artificial Opening 8 Via Natural or Artificial Opening Endoscopic	0 Drainage Device 2 Monitoring Device 3 Infusion Device 7 Autologous Tissue Substitute C Extraluminal Device D Intraluminal Device J Synthetic Substitute K Nonautologous Tissue Substitute M Stimulator Lead	Z No Qualifier
9 Ureter	X External	0 Drainage Device 2 Monitoring Device 3 Infusion Device D Intraluminal Device M Stimulator Lead	Z No Qualifier
B Bladder	0 Open 3 Percutaneous 4 Percutaneous Endoscopic 7 Via Natural or Artificial Opening 8 Via Natural or Artificial Opening Endoscopic	0 Drainage Device 2 Monitoring Device 3 Infusion Device 7 Autologous Tissue Substitute C Extraluminal Device D Intraluminal Device J Synthetic Substitute K Nonautologous Tissue Substitute L Artificial Sphincter M Stimulator Lead	Z No Qualifier
B Bladder	X External	0 Drainage Device 2 Monitoring Device 3 Infusion Device D Intraluminal Device L Artificial Sphincter M Stimulator Lead	Z No Qualifier
D Urethra	0 Open 3 Percutaneous 4 Percutaneous Endoscopic	0 Drainage Device 2 Monitoring Device 3 Infusion Device	Z No Qualifier

Continued on Next Page ▶

	7 Via Natural or Artificial Opening 8 Via Natural or Artificial Opening Endoscopic	7 Autologous Tissue Substitute C Extraluminal Device D Intraluminal Device J Synthetic Substitute K Nonautologous Tissue Substitute L Artificial Sphincter	Continued from ◀ Previous Page
D Urethra	X External	0 Drainage Device 2 Monitoring Device 3 Infusion Device D Intraluminal Device L Artificial Sphincter	Z No Qualifier

Section	0	Medical and Surgical	
Body System	T	Urinary System	
Operation	Q	Repair: Restoring, to the extent possible, a body part to its normal anatomic structure and function	

Body Part (Character 4)	Approach (Character 5)	Device (Character 6)	Qualifier (Character 7)
0 Kidney, Right 1 Kidney, Left 3 Kidney Pelvis, Right 4 Kidney Pelvis, Left 6 Ureter, Right 7 Ureter, Left B Bladder C Bladder Neck	0 Open 3 Percutaneous 4 Percutaneous Endoscopic 7 Via Natural or Artificial Opening 8 Via Natural or Artificial Opening Endoscopic	Z No Device	Z No Qualifier
D Urethra	0 Open 3 Percutaneous 4 Percutaneous Endoscopic 7 Via Natural or Artificial Opening 8 Via Natural or Artificial Opening Endoscopic X External	Z No Device	Z No Qualifier

Section	0	Medical and Surgical	
Body System	T	Urinary System	
Operation	R	Replacement: Putting in or on biological or synthetic material that physically takes the place and/or function of all or a portion of a body part	

Body Part (Character 4)	Approach (Character 5)	Device (Character 6)	Qualifier (Character 7)
3 Kidney Pelvis, Right 4 Kidney Pelvis, Left 6 Ureter, Right 7 Ureter, Left B Bladder C Bladder Neck	0 Open 4 Percutaneous Endoscopic 7 Via Natural or Artificial Opening 8 Via Natural or Artificial Opening Endoscopic	7 Autologous Tissue Substitute J Synthetic Substitute K Nonautologous Tissue Substitute	Z No Qualifier
D Urethra	0 Open 4 Percutaneous Endoscopic 7 Via Natural or Artificial Opening 8 Via Natural or Artificial Opening Endoscopic X External	7 Autologous Tissue Substitute J Synthetic Substitute K Nonautologous Tissue Substitute	Z No Qualifier

Section	0	Medical and Surgical
Body System	T	Urinary System
Operation	S	Reposition: Moving to its normal location, or other suitable location, all or a portion of a body part

Body Part (Character 4)	Approach (Character 5)	Device (Character 6)	Qualifier (Character 7)
0 Kidney, Right 1 Kidney, Left 2 Kidneys, Bilateral 3 Kidney Pelvis, Right 4 Kidney Pelvis, Left 6 Ureter, Right 7 Ureter, Left 8 Ureters, Bilateral B Bladder C Bladder Neck D Urethra	0 Open 4 Percutaneous Endoscopic	Z No Device	Z No Qualifier

Section	0	Medical and Surgical
Body System	T	Urinary System
Operation	T	Resection: Cutting out or off, without replacement, all of a body part

Body Part (Character 4)	Approach (Character 5)	Device (Character 6)	Qualifier (Character 7)
0 Kidney, Right 1 Kidney, Left 2 Kidneys, Bilateral	0 Open 4 Percutaneous Endoscopic	Z No Device	Z No Qualifier
3 Kidney Pelvis, Right 4 Kidney Pelvis, Left 6 Ureter, Right 7 Ureter, Left B Bladder C Bladder Neck D Urethra	0 Open 4 Percutaneous Endoscopic 7 Via Natural or Artificial Opening 8 Via Natural or Artificial Opening Endoscopic	Z No Device	Z No Qualifier

Section	0	Medical and Surgical
Body System	T	Urinary System
Operation	U	Supplement: Putting in or on biological or synthetic material that physically reinforces and/or augments the function of a portion of a body part

Body Part (Character 4)	Approach (Character 5)	Device (Character 6)	Qualifier (Character 7)
3 Kidney Pelvis, Right 4 Kidney Pelvis, Left 6 Ureter, Right 7 Ureter, Left B Bladder C Bladder Neck	0 Open 4 Percutaneous Endoscopic 7 Via Natural or Artificial Opening 8 Via Natural or Artificial Opening Endoscopic	7 Autologous Tissue Substitute J Synthetic Substitute K Nonautologous Tissue Substitute	Z No Qualifier
D Urethra	0 Open 4 Percutaneous Endoscopic 7 Via Natural or Artificial Opening 8 Via Natural or Artificial Opening Endoscopic X External	7 Autologous Tissue Substitute J Synthetic Substitute K Nonautologous Tissue Substitute	Z No Qualifier

Section	0	Medical and Surgical		
Body System	T	Urinary System		
Operation	V	Restriction: Partially closing an orifice or the lumen of a tubular body part		

Body Part (Character 4)	Approach (Character 5)	Device (Character 6)	Qualifier (Character 7)
3 Kidney Pelvis, Right 4 Kidney Pelvis, Left 6 Ureter, Right 7 Ureter, Left B Bladder C Bladder Neck	0 Open 3 Percutaneous 4 Percutaneous Endoscopic	C Extraluminal Device D Intraluminal Device Z No Device	Z No Qualifier
3 Kidney Pelvis, Right 4 Kidney Pelvis, Left 6 Ureter, Right 7 Ureter, Left B Bladder C Bladder Neck	7 Via Natural or Artificial Opening 8 Via Natural or Artificial Opening Endoscopic	D Intraluminal Device Z No Device	Z No Qualifier
D Urethra	0 Open 3 Percutaneous 4 Percutaneous Endoscopic	C Extraluminal Device D Intraluminal Device Z No Device	Z No Qualifier
D Urethra	7 Via Natural or Artificial Opening 8 Via Natural or Artificial Opening Endoscopic	D Intraluminal Device Z No Device	Z No Qualifier
D Urethra	X External	Z No Device	Z No Qualifier

Section	0	Medical and Surgical		
Body System	T	Urinary System		
Operation	W	Revision: Correcting, to the extent possible, a portion of a malfunctioning device or the position of a displaced device		

Body Part (Character 4)	Approach (Character 5)	Device (Character 6)	Qualifier (Character 7)
5 Kidney	0 Open 3 Percutaneous 4 Percutaneous Endoscopic 7 Via Natural or Artificial Opening 8 Via Natural or Artificial Opening Endoscopic X External	0 Drainage Device 2 Monitoring Device 3 Infusion Device 7 Autologous Tissue Substitute C Extraluminal Device D Intraluminal Device J Synthetic Substitute K Nonautologous Tissue Substitute	Z No Qualifier
9 Ureter	0 Open 3 Percutaneous 4 Percutaneous Endoscopic 7 Via Natural or Artificial Opening 8 Via Natural or Artificial Opening Endoscopic X External	0 Drainage Device 2 Monitoring Device 3 Infusion Device 7 Autologous Tissue Substitute C Extraluminal Device D Intraluminal Device J Synthetic Substitute K Nonautologous Tissue Substitute M Stimulator Lead	Z No Qualifier
B Bladder	0 Open 3 Percutaneous 4 Percutaneous Endoscopic	0 Drainage Device 2 Monitoring Device 3 Infusion Device 7 Autologous Tissue	Z No Qualifier **Continued on Next Page ▶**

	7 Via Natural or Artificial Opening 8 Via Natural or Artificial Opening Endoscopic X External	Substitute C Extraluminal Device D Intraluminal Device J Synthetic Substitute K Nonautologous Tissue Substitute L Artificial Sphincter M Stimulator Lead	Continued from ◀ Previous Page
D Urethra	0 Open 3 Percutaneous 4 Percutaneous Endoscopic 7 Via Natural or Artificial Opening 8 Via Natural or Artificial Opening Endoscopic X External	0 Drainage Device 2 Monitoring Device 3 Infusion Device 7 Autologous Tissue Substitute C Extraluminal Device D Intraluminal Device J Synthetic Substitute K Nonautologous Tissue Substitute L Artificial Sphincter	Z No Qualifier

Section	0	Medical and Surgical
Body System	T	Urinary System
Operation	Y	Transplantation: Putting in or on all or a portion of a living body part taken from another individual or animal to physically take the place and/or function of all or a portion of a similar body part

Body Part (Character 4)	Approach (Character 5)	Device (Character 6)	Qualifier (Character 7)
0 Kidney, Right 1 Kidney, Left	0 Open	Z No Device	0 Allogeneic 1 Syngeneic 2 Zooplastic

Section	0	Medical and Surgical		
Body System	U	Female Reproductive System		
Operation	1	Bypass: Altering the route of passage of the contents of a tubular body part		
Body Part (Character 4)		**Approach (Character 5)**	**Device (Character 6)**	**Qualifier (Character 7)**
5 Fallopian Tube, Right 6 Fallopian Tube, Left		0 Open 4 Percutaneous Endoscopic	7 Autologous Tissue Substitute J Synthetic Substitute K Nonautologous Tissue Substitute Z No Device	5 Fallopian Tube, Right 6 Fallopian Tube, Left 9 Uterus

Section	0	Medical and Surgical		
Body System	U	Female Reproductive System		
Operation	2	Change: Taking out or off a device from a body part and putting back an identical or similar device in or on the same body part without cutting or puncturing the skin or a mucous membrane		
Body Part (Character 4)		**Approach (Character 5)**	**Device (Character 6)**	**Qualifier (Character 7)**
3 Ovary 8 Fallopian Tube M Vulva		X External	0 Drainage Device Y Other Device	Z No Qualifier
D Uterus and Cervix		X External	0 Drainage Device H Contraceptive Device Y Other Device	Z No Qualifier
H Vagina and Cul-de-sac		X External	0 Drainage Device G Intraluminal Device, Pessary Y Other Device	Z No Qualifier

Section	0	Medical and Surgical		
Body System	U	Female Reproductive System		
Operation	5	Destruction: Physical eradication of all or a portion of a body part by the direct use of energy, force, or a destructive agent		
Body Part (Character 4)		**Approach (Character 5)**	**Device (Character 6)**	**Qualifier (Character 7)**
0 Ovary, Right 1 Ovary, Left 2 Ovaries, Bilateral 4 Uterine Supporting Structure		0 Open 3 Percutaneous 4 Percutaneous Endoscopic	Z No Device	Z No Qualifier
5 Fallopian Tube, Right 6 Fallopian Tube, Left 7 Fallopian Tubes, Bilateral 9 Uterus B Endometrium C Cervix F Cul-de-sac		0 Open 3 Percutaneous 4 Percutaneous Endoscopic 7 Via Natural or Artificial Opening 8 Via Natural or Artificial Opening Endoscopic	Z No Device	Z No Qualifier
G Vagina K Hymen		0 Open 3 Percutaneous 4 Percutaneous Endoscopic 7 Via Natural or Artificial Opening 8 Via Natural or Artificial Opening Endoscopic X External	Z No Device	Z No Qualifier
J Clitoris L Vestibular Gland M Vulva		0 Open X External	Z No Device	Z No Qualifier

Section	0	Medical and Surgical		
Body System	U	Female Reproductive System		
Operation	7	Dilation: Expanding an orifice or the lumen of a tubular body part		

Body Part (Character 4)	Approach (Character 5)	Device (Character 6)	Qualifier (Character 7)
5 Fallopian Tube, Right 6 Fallopian Tube, Left 7 Fallopian Tubes, Bilateral 9 Uterus C Cervix G Vagina	0 Open 3 Percutaneous 4 Percutaneous Endoscopic 7 Via Natural or Artificial Opening 8 Via Natural or Artificial Opening Endoscopic	D Intraluminal Device Z No Device	Z No Qualifier
K Hymen	0 Open 3 Percutaneous 4 Percutaneous Endoscopic 7 Via Natural or Artificial Opening 8 Via Natural or Artificial Opening Endoscopic X External	D Intraluminal Device Z No Device	Z No Qualifier

Section	0	Medical and Surgical		
Body System	U	Female Reproductive System		
Operation	8	Division: Cutting into a body part, without draining fluids and/or gases from the body part, in order to separate or transect a body part		

Body Part (Character 4)	Approach (Character 5)	Device (Character 6)	Qualifier (Character 7)
0 Ovary, Right 1 Ovary, Left 2 Ovaries, Bilateral 4 Uterine Supporting Structure	0 Open 3 Percutaneous 4 Percutaneous Endoscopic	Z No Device	Z No Qualifier
K Hymen	7 Via Natural or Artificial Opening 8 Via Natural or Artificial Opening Endoscopic X External	Z No Device	Z No Qualifier

Section	0	Medical and Surgical		
Body System	U	Female Reproductive System		
Operation	9	Drainage: Taking or letting out fluids and/or gases from a body part		

Body Part (Character 4)	Approach (Character 5)	Device (Character 6)	Qualifier (Character 7)
0 Ovary, Right 1 Ovary, Left 2 Ovaries, Bilateral	0 Open 3 Percutaneous 4 Percutaneous Endoscopic	0 Drainage Device	Z No Qualifier
0 Ovary, Right 1 Ovary, Left 2 Ovaries, Bilateral	0 Open 3 Percutaneous 4 Percutaneous Endoscopic	Z No Device	X Diagnostic Z No Qualifier
0 Ovary, Right 1 Ovary, Left 2 Ovaries, Bilateral	X External	Z No Device	Z No Qualifier
4 Uterine Supporting Structure	0 Open 3 Percutaneous 4 Percutaneous Endoscopic	0 Drainage Device	Z No Qualifier
4 Uterine Supporting Structure	0 Open 3 Percutaneous 4 Percutaneous Endoscopic	Z No Device	X Diagnostic Z No Qualifier

Continued on Next Page ▶

			Continued from ◄ Previous Page
5 Fallopian Tube, Right **6** Fallopian Tube, Left **7** Fallopian Tubes, Bilateral **9** Uterus **C** Cervix **F** Cul-de-sac	**0** Open **3** Percutaneous **4** Percutaneous Endoscopic **7** Via Natural or Artificial Opening **8** Via Natural or Artificial Opening Endoscopic	**0** Drainage Device	**Z** No Qualifier
5 Fallopian Tube, Right **6** Fallopian Tube, Left **7** Fallopian Tubes, Bilateral **9** Uterus **C** Cervix **F** Cul-de-sac	**0** Open **3** Percutaneous **4** Percutaneous Endoscopic **7** Via Natural or Artificial Opening **8** Via Natural or Artificial Opening Endoscopic	**Z** No Device	**X** Diagnostic **Z** No Qualifier
G Vagina **K** Hymen	**0** Open **3** Percutaneous **4** Percutaneous Endoscopic **7** Via Natural or Artificial Opening **8** Via Natural or Artificial Opening Endoscopic **X** External	**0** Drainage Device	**Z** No Qualifier
G Vagina **K** Hymen	**0** Open **3** Percutaneous **4** Percutaneous Endoscopic **7** Via Natural or Artificial Opening **8** Via Natural or Artificial Opening Endoscopic **X** External	**Z** No Device	**X** Diagnostic **Z** No Qualifier
J Clitoris **L** Vestibular Gland **M** Vulva	**0** Open **X** External	**0** Drainage Device	**Z** No Qualifier
J Clitoris **L** Vestibular Gland **M** Vulva	**0** Open **X** External	**Z** No Device	**X** Diagnostic **Z** No Qualifier

Section	0	Medical and Surgical	
Body System	U	Female Reproductive System	
Operation	B	Excision: Cutting out or off, without replacement, a portion of a body part	
Body Part (Character 4)	**Approach (Character 5)**	**Device (Character 6)**	**Qualifier (Character 7)**
0 Ovary, Right **1** Ovary, Left **2** Ovaries, Bilateral **4** Uterine Supporting Structure **5** Fallopian Tube, Right **6** Fallopian Tube, Left **7** Fallopian Tubes, Bilateral **9** Uterus **C** Cervix **F** Cul-de-sac	**0** Open **3** Percutaneous **4** Percutaneous Endoscopic **7** Via Natural or Artificial Opening **8** Via Natural or Artificial Opening Endoscopic	**Z** No Device	**X** Diagnostic **Z** No Qualifier

Continued on Next Page ►

			Continued from ◀ Previous Page
G Vagina **K** Hymen	**0** Open **3** Percutaneous **4** Percutaneous Endoscopic **7** Via Natural or Artificial Opening **8** Via Natural or Artificial Opening Endoscopic **X** External	**Z** No Device	**X** Diagnostic **Z** No Qualifier
J Clitoris **L** Vestibular Gland **M** Vulva	**0** Open **X** External	**Z** No Device	**X** Diagnostic **Z** No Qualifier

Section	0	Medical and Surgical	
Body System	**U**	**Female Reproductive System**	
Operation	**C**	**Extirpation: Taking or cutting out solid matter from a body part**	

Body Part (Character 4)	Approach (Character 5)	Device (Character 6)	Qualifier (Character 7)
0 Ovary, Right **1** Ovary, Left **2** Ovaries, Bilateral **4** Uterine Supporting Structure	**0** Open **3** Percutaneous **4** Percutaneous Endoscopic	**Z** No Device	**Z** No Qualifier
5 Fallopian Tube, Right **6** Fallopian Tube, Left **7** Fallopian Tubes, Bilateral **9** Uterus **B** Endometrium **C** Cervix **F** Cul-de-sac	**0** Open **3** Percutaneous **4** Percutaneous Endoscopic **7** Via Natural or Artificial Opening **8** Via Natural or Artificial Opening Endoscopic	**Z** No Device	**Z** No Qualifier
G Vagina **K** Hymen	**0** Open **3** Percutaneous **4** Percutaneous Endoscopic **7** Via Natural or Artificial Opening **8** Via Natural or Artificial Opening Endoscopic **X** External	**Z** No Device	**Z** No Qualifier
J Clitoris **L** Vestibular Gland **M** Vulva	**0** Open **X** External	**Z** No Device	**Z** No Qualifier

Section	0	Medical and Surgical	
Body System	**U**	**Female Reproductive System**	
Operation	**D**	**Extraction: Pulling or stripping out or off all or a portion of a body part by the use of force**	

Body Part (Character 4)	Approach (Character 5)	Device (Character 6)	Qualifier (Character 7)
B Endometrium	**7** Via Natural or Artificial Opening **8** Via Natural or Artificial Opening Endoscopic	**Z** No Device	**X** Diagnostic **Z** No Qualifier
N Ova	**0** Open **3** Percutaneous **4** Percutaneous Endoscopic	**Z** No Device	**Z** No Qualifier

Section	0	Medical and Surgical		
Body System	U	Female Reproductive System		
Operation	F	Fragmentation: Breaking solid matter in a body part into pieces		

Body Part (Character 4)	Approach (Character 5)	Device (Character 6)	Qualifier (Character 7)
5 Fallopian Tube, Right 6 Fallopian Tube, Left 7 Fallopian Tubes, Bilateral 9 Uterus	0 Open 3 Percutaneous 4 Percutaneous Endoscopic 7 Via Natural or Artificial Opening 8 Via Natural or Artificial Opening Endoscopic X External	Z No Device	Z No Qualifier

Section	0	Medical and Surgical		
Body System	U	Female Reproductive System		
Operation	H	Insertion: Putting in a nonbiological appliance that monitors, assists, performs, or prevents a physiological function but does not physically take the place of a body part		

Body Part (Character 4)	Approach (Character 5)	Device (Character 6)	Qualifier (Character 7)
3 Ovary	0 Open 3 Percutaneous 4 Percutaneous Endoscopic	3 Infusion Device	Z No Qualifier
8 Fallopian Tube D Uterus and Cervix H Vagina and Cul-de-sac	0 Open 3 Percutaneous 4 Percutaneous Endoscopic 7 Via Natural or Artificial Opening 8 Via Natural or Artificial Opening Endoscopic	3 Infusion Device	Z No Qualifier
9 Uterus	7 Via Natural or Artificial Opening 8 Via Natural or Artificial Opening Endoscopic	H Contraceptive Device	Z No Qualifier
C Cervix	0 Open 3 Percutaneous 4 Percutaneous Endoscopic	1 Radioactive Element	Z No Qualifier
C Cervix	7 Via Natural or Artificial Opening 8 Via Natural or Artificial Opening Endoscopic	1 Radioactive Element H Contraceptive Device	Z No Qualifier
F Cul-de-sac	7 Via Natural or Artificial Opening 8 Via Natural or Artificial Opening Endoscopic	G Intraluminal Device, Pessary	Z No Qualifier
G Vagina	0 Open 3 Percutaneous 4 Percutaneous Endoscopic X External	1 Radioactive Element	Z No Qualifier
G Vagina	7 Via Natural or Artificial Opening 8 Via Natural or Artificial Opening Endoscopic	1 Radioactive Element G Intraluminal Device, Pessary	Z No Qualifier

Section	0	Medical and Surgical		
Body System	U	Female Reproductive System		
Operation	J	Inspection: Visually and/or manually exploring a body part		

Body Part (Character 4)	Approach (Character 5)	Device (Character 6)	Qualifier (Character 7)
3 Ovary	0 Open 3 Percutaneous 4 Percutaneous Endoscopic X External	Z No Device	Z No Qualifier
8 Fallopian Tube D Uterus and Cervix H Vagina and Cul-de-sac	0 Open 3 Percutaneous 4 Percutaneous Endoscopic 7 Via Natural or Artificial Opening 8 Via Natural or Artificial Opening Endoscopic X External	Z No Device	Z No Qualifier
M Vulva	0 Open X External	Z No Device	Z No Qualifier

Section	0	Medical and Surgical		
Body System	U	Female Reproductive System		
Operation	L	Occlusion: Completely closing an orifice or the lumen of a tubular body part		

Body Part (Character 4)	Approach (Character 5)	Device (Character 6)	Qualifier (Character 7)
5 Fallopian Tube, Right 6 Fallopian Tube, Left 7 Fallopian Tubes, Bilateral	0 Open 3 Percutaneous 4 Percutaneous Endoscopic	C Extraluminal Device D Intraluminal Device Z No Device	Z No Qualifier
5 Fallopian Tube, Right 6 Fallopian Tube, Left 7 Fallopian Tubes, Bilateral	7 Via Natural or Artificial Opening 8 Via Natural or Artificial Opening Endoscopic	D Intraluminal Device Z No Device	Z No Qualifier
F Cul-de-sac G Vagina	7 Via Natural or Artificial Opening 8 Via Natural or Artificial Opening Endoscopic	D Intraluminal Device Z No Device	Z No Qualifier

Section	0	Medical and Surgical		
Body System	U	Female Reproductive System		
Operation	M	Reattachment Putting back in or on all or a portion of a separated body part to its normal location or other suitable location		

Body Part (Character 4)	Approach (Character 5)	Device (Character 6)	Qualifier (Character 7)
0 Ovary, Right 1 Ovary, Left 2 Ovaries, Bilateral 4 Uterine Supporting Structure 5 Fallopian Tube, Right 6 Fallopian Tube, Left 7 Fallopian Tubes, Bilateral 9 Uterus C Cervix F Cul-de-sac G Vagina	0 Open 4 Percutaneous Endoscopic	Z No Device	Z No Qualifier
J Clitoris M Vulva	X External	Z No Device	Z No Qualifier
K Hymen	0 Open 4 Percutaneous Endoscopic X External	Z No Device	Z No Qualifier

Section	0	Medical and Surgical		
Body System	U	Female Reproductive System		
Operation	N	Release: Freeing a body part from an abnormal physical constraint by cutting or by the use of force		

Body Part (Character 4)	Approach (Character 5)	Device (Character 6)	Qualifier (Character 7)
0 Ovary, Right 1 Ovary, Left 2 Ovaries, Bilateral 4 Uterine Supporting Structure	0 Open 3 Percutaneous 4 Percutaneous Endoscopic	Z No Device	Z No Qualifier
5 Fallopian Tube, Right 6 Fallopian Tube, Left 7 Fallopian Tubes, Bilateral 9 Uterus C Cervix F Cul-de-sac	0 Open 3 Percutaneous 4 Percutaneous Endoscopic 7 Via Natural or Artificial Opening 8 Via Natural or Artificial Opening Endoscopic	Z No Device	Z No Qualifier
G Vagina K Hymen	0 Open 3 Percutaneous 4 Percutaneous Endoscopic 7 Via Natural or Artificial Opening 8 Via Natural or Artificial Opening Endoscopic X External	Z No Device	Z No Qualifier
J Clitoris L Vestibular Gland M Vulva	0 Open X External	Z No Device	Z No Qualifier

Section	0	Medical and Surgical		
Body System	U	Female Reproductive System		
Operation	P	Removal: Taking out or off a device from a body part		

Body Part (Character 4)	Approach (Character 5)	Device (Character 6)	Qualifier (Character 7)
3 Ovary	0 Open 3 Percutaneous 4 Percutaneous Endoscopic X External	0 Drainage Device 3 Infusion Device	Z No Qualifier
8 Fallopian Tube	0 Open 3 Percutaneous 4 Percutaneous Endoscopic 7 Via Natural or Artificial Opening 8 Via Natural or Artificial Opening Endoscopic	0 Drainage Device 3 Infusion Device 7 Autologous Tissue Substitute C Extraluminal Device D Intraluminal Device J Synthetic Substitute K Nonautologous Tissue Substitute	Z No Qualifier
8 Fallopian Tube	X External	0 Drainage Device 3 Infusion Device D Intraluminal Device	Z No Qualifier
D Uterus and Cervix	0 Open 3 Percutaneous 4 Percutaneous Endoscopic 7 Via Natural or Artificial Opening 8 Via Natural or Artificial Opening Endoscopic	0 Drainage Device 1 Radioactive Element 3 Infusion Device 7 Autologous Tissue Substitute C Extraluminal Device D Intraluminal Device	Z No Qualifier

Continued on Next Page ▶

		H Contraceptive Device J Synthetic Substitute K Nonautologous Tissue Substitute	Continued from ◀ Previous Page
D Uterus and Cervix	X External	0 Drainage Device 3 Infusion Device D Intraluminal Device H Contraceptive Device	Z No Qualifier
H Vagina and Cul-de-sac	0 Open 3 Percutaneous 4 Percutaneous Endoscopic 7 Via Natural or Artificial Opening 8 Via Natural or Artificial Opening Endoscopic	0 Drainage Device 1 Radioactive Element 3 Infusion Device 7 Autologous Tissue Substitute D Intraluminal Device J Synthetic Substitute K Nonautologous Tissue Substitute	Z No Qualifier
H Vagina and Cul-de-sac	X External	0 Drainage Device 1 Radioactive Element 3 Infusion Device D Intraluminal Device	Z No Qualifier
M Vulva	0 Open	0 Drainage Device 7 Autologous Tissue Substitute J Synthetic Substitute K Nonautologous Tissue Substitute	Z No Qualifier
M Vulva	X External	0 Drainage Device	Z No Qualifier

Section	0	Medical and Surgical	
Body System	U	Female Reproductive System	
Operation	Q	Repair: Restoring, to the extent possible, a body part to its normal anatomic structure and function	

Body Part (Character 4)	Approach (Character 5)	Device (Character 6)	Qualifier (Character 7)
0 Ovary, Right 1 Ovary, Left 2 Ovaries, Bilateral 4 Uterine Supporting Structure	0 Open 3 Percutaneous 4 Percutaneous Endoscopic	Z No Device	Z No Qualifier
5 Fallopian Tube, Right 6 Fallopian Tube, Left 7 Fallopian Tubes, Bilateral 9 Uterus C Cervix F Cul-de-sac	0 Open 3 Percutaneous 4 Percutaneous Endoscopic 7 Via Natural or Artificial Opening 8 Via Natural or Artificial Opening Endoscopic	Z No Device	Z No Qualifier
G Vagina K Hymen	0 Open 3 Percutaneous 4 Percutaneous Endoscopic 7 Via Natural or Artificial Opening 8 Via Natural or Artificial Opening Endoscopic X External	Z No Device	Z No Qualifier
J Clitoris L Vestibular Gland M Vulva	0 Open X External	Z No Device	Z No Qualifier

Section	0	Medical and Surgical		
Body System	U	Female Reproductive System		
Operation	S	Reposition: Moving to its normal location, or other suitable location, all or a portion of a body part		

Body Part (Character 4)	Approach (Character 5)	Device (Character 6)	Qualifier (Character 7)
0 Ovary, Right 1 Ovary, Left 2 Ovaries, Bilateral 4 Uterine Supporting Structure 5 Fallopian Tube, Right 6 Fallopian Tube, Left 7 Fallopian Tubes, Bilateral C Cervix F Cul-de-sac	0 Open 4 Percutaneous Endoscopic	Z No Device	Z No Qualifier
9 Uterus G Vagina	0 Open 4 Percutaneous Endoscopic X External	Z No Device	Z No Qualifier

Section	0	Medical and Surgical		
Body System	U	Female Reproductive System		
Operation	T	Resection: Cutting out or off, without replacement, all of a body part		

Body Part (Character 4)	Approach (Character 5)	Device (Character 6)	Qualifier (Character 7)
0 Ovary, Right 1 Ovary, Left 2 Ovaries, Bilateral 5 Fallopian Tube, Right 6 Fallopian Tube, Left 7 Fallopian Tubes, Bilateral 9 Uterus	0 Open 4 Percutaneous Endoscopic 7 Via Natural or Artificial Opening 8 Via Natural or Artificial Opening Endoscopic F Via Natural or Artificial Opening With Percutaneous Endoscopic Assistance	Z No Device	Z No Qualifier
4 Uterine Supporting Structure C Cervix F Cul-de-sac G Vagina	0 Open 4 Percutaneous Endoscopic 7 Via Natural or Artificial Opening 8 Via Natural or Artificial Opening Endoscopic	Z No Device	Z No Qualifier
J Clitoris L Vestibular Gland M Vulva	0 Open X External	Z No Device	Z No Qualifier
K Hymen	0 Open 4 Percutaneous Endoscopic 7 Via Natural or Artificial Opening 8 Via Natural or Artificial Opening Endoscopic X External	Z No Device	Z No Qualifier

Section	0	Medical and Surgical		
Body System	U	Female Reproductive System		
Operation	U	Supplement: Putting in or on biological or synthetic material that physically reinforces and/or augments the function of a portion of a body part		

Body Part (Character 4)	Approach (Character 5)	Device (Character 6)	Qualifier (Character 7)
4 Uterine Supporting Structure	0 Open 4 Percutaneous Endoscopic	7 Autologous Tissue Substitute J Synthetic Substitute K Nonautologous Tissue Substitute	Z No Qualifier
5 Fallopian Tube, Right 6 Fallopian Tube, Left 7 Fallopian Tubes, Bilateral F Cul-de-sac	0 Open 4 Percutaneous Endoscopic 7 Via Natural or Artificial Opening 8 Via Natural or Artificial Opening Endoscopic	7 Autologous Tissue Substitute J Synthetic Substitute K Nonautologous Tissue Substitute	Z No Qualifier
G Vagina K Hymen	0 Open 4 Percutaneous Endoscopic 7 Via Natural or Artificial Opening 8 Via Natural or Artificial Opening Endoscopic X External	7 Autologous Tissue Substitute J Synthetic Substitute K Nonautologous Tissue Substitute	Z No Qualifier
J Clitoris M Vulva	0 Open X External	7 Autologous Tissue Substitute J Synthetic Substitute K Nonautologous Tissue Substitute	Z No Qualifier

Section	0	Medical and Surgical		
Body System	U	Female Reproductive System		
Operation	V	Restriction: Partially closing an orifice or the lumen of a tubular body part		

Body Part (Character 4)	Approach (Character 5)	Device (Character 6)	Qualifier (Character 7)
C Cervix	0 Open 3 Percutaneous 4 Percutaneous Endoscopic	C Extraluminal Device D Intraluminal Device Z No Device	Z No Qualifier
C Cervix	7 Via Natural or Artificial Opening 8 Via Natural or Artificial Opening Endoscopic	D Intraluminal Device Z No Device	Z No Qualifier

Section	0	Medical and Surgical		
Body System	U	Female Reproductive System		
Operation	W	Revision: Correcting, to the extent possible, a portion of a malfunctioning device or the position of a displaced device		

Body Part (Character 4)	Approach (Character 5)	Device (Character 6)	Qualifier (Character 7)
3 Ovary	0 Open 3 Percutaneous 4 Percutaneous Endoscopic X External	0 Drainage Device 3 Infusion Device	Z No Qualifier
8 Fallopian Tube	0 Open 3 Percutaneous 4 Percutaneous Endoscopic 7 Via Natural or Artificial Opening	0 Drainage Device 3 Infusion Device 7 Autologous Tissue Substitute C Extraluminal Device D Intraluminal Device	Z No Qualifier **Continued on Next Page ▶**

	8 Via Natural or Artificial Opening Endoscopic X External	J Synthetic Substitute K Nonautologous Tissue Substitute	**Continued from ◀ Previous Page**
D Uterus and Cervix	0 Open 3 Percutaneous 4 Percutaneous Endoscopic 7 Via Natural or Artificial Opening 8 Via Natural or Artificial Opening Endoscopic	0 Drainage Device 1 Radioactive Element 3 Infusion Device 7 Autologous Tissue Substitute C Extraluminal Device D Intraluminal Device H Contraceptive Device J Synthetic Substitute K Nonautologous Tissue Substitute	Z No Qualifier
D Uterus and Cervix	X External	0 Drainage Device 3 Infusion Device 7 Autologous Tissue Substitute C Extraluminal Device D Intraluminal Device H Contraceptive Device J Synthetic Substitute K Nonautologous Tissue Substitute	Z No Qualifier
H Vagina and Cul-de-sac	0 Open 3 Percutaneous 4 Percutaneous Endoscopic 7 Via Natural or Artificial Opening 8 Via Natural or Artificial Opening Endoscopic	0 Drainage Device 1 Radioactive Element 3 Infusion Device 7 Autologous Tissue Substitute D Intraluminal Device J Synthetic Substitute K Nonautologous Tissue Substitute	Z No Qualifier
H Vagina and Cul-de-sac	X External	0 Drainage Device 3 Infusion Device 7 Autologous Tissue Substitute D Intraluminal Device J Synthetic Substitute K Nonautologous Tissue Substitute	Z No Qualifier
M Vulva	0 Open X External	0 Drainage Device 7 Autologous Tissue Substitute J Synthetic Substitute K Nonautologous Tissue Substitute	Z No Qualifier

Section	0	Medical and Surgical
Body System	U	Female Reproductive System
Operation	Y	Transplantation: Putting in or on all or a portion of a living body part taken from another individual or animal to physically take the place and/or function of all or a portion of a similar body part

Body Part (Character 4)	Approach (Character 5)	Device (Character 6)	Qualifier (Character 7)
0 Ovary, Right	0 Open	Z No Device	0 Allogeneic
1 Ovary, Left			1 Syngeneic
			2 Zooplastic

Section	0	Medical and Surgical		
Body System	V	Male Reproductive System		
Operation	1	Bypass: Altering the route of passage of the contents of a tubular body part		

Body Part (Character 4)	Approach (Character 5)	Device (Character 6)	Qualifier (Character 7)
N Vas Deferens, Right P Vas Deferens, Left Q Vas Deferens, Bilateral	0 Open 4 Percutaneous Endoscopic	7 Autologous Tissue Substitute J Synthetic Substitute K Nonautologous Tissue Substitute Z No Device	J Epididymis, Right K Epididymis, Left N Vas Deferens, Right P Vas Deferens, Left

Section	0	Medical and Surgical		
Body System	V	Male Reproductive System		
Operation	2	Change: Taking out or off a device from a body part and putting back an identical or similar device in or on the same body part without cutting or puncturing the skin or a mucous membrane		

Body Part (Character 4)	Approach (Character 5)	Device (Character 6)	Qualifier (Character 7)
4 Prostate and Seminal Vesicles 8 Scrotum and Tunica Vaginalis D Testis M Epididymis and Spermatic Cord R Vas Deferens 5 Penis	X External	0 Drainage Device Y Other Device	Z No Qualifier

Section	0	Medical and Surgical		
Body System	V	Male Reproductive System		
Operation	5	Destruction: Physical eradication of all or a portion of a body part by the direct use of energy, force, or a destructive agent		

Body Part (Character 4)	Approach (Character 5)	Device (Character 6)	Qualifier (Character 7)
0 Prostate	0 Open 3 Percutaneous 4 Percutaneous Endoscopic 7 Via Natural or Artificial Opening 8 Via Natural or Artificial Opening Endoscopic	Z No Device	Z No Qualifier
1 Seminal Vesicle, Right 2 Seminal Vesicle, Left 3 Seminal Vesicles, Bilateral 6 Tunica Vaginalis, Right 7 Tunica Vaginalis, Left 9 Testis, Right B Testis, Left C Testes, Bilateral F Spermatic Cord, Right G Spermatic Cord, Left H Spermatic Cords, Bilateral J Epididymis, Right K Epididymis, Left L Epididymis, Bilateral N Vas Deferens, Right	0 Open 3 Percutaneous 4 Percutaneous Endoscopic	Z No Device	Z No Qualifier

Continued on Next Page ▶

			Continued from ◀ Previous Page
P Vas Deferens, Left **Q** Vas Deferens, Bilateral			
5 Scrotum **S** Penis **T** Prepuce	**0** Open **3** Percutaneous **4** Percutaneous Endoscopic **X** External	**Z** No Device	**Z** No Qualifier

Section	0	Medical and Surgical	
Body System	V	Male Reproductive System	
Operation	7	Dilation: Expanding an orifice or the lumen of a tubular body part	

Body Part (Character 4)	Approach (Character 5)	Device (Character 6)	Qualifier (Character 7)
N Vas Deferens, Right **P** Vas Deferens, Left **Q** Vas Deferens, Bilateral	**0** Open **3** Percutaneous **4** Percutaneous Endoscopic	**D** Intraluminal Device **Z** No Device	**Z** No Qualifier

Section	0	Medical and Surgical	
Body System	V	Male Reproductive System	
Operation	9	Drainage: Taking or letting out fluids and/or gases from a body part	

Body Part (Character 4)	Approach (Character 5)	Device (Character 6)	Qualifier (Character 7)
0 Prostate	**0** Open **3** Percutaneous **4** Percutaneous Endoscopic **7** Via Natural or Artificial Opening **8** Via Natural or Artificial Opening Endoscopic	**0** Drainage Device	**Z** No Qualifier
0 Prostate	**0** Open **3** Percutaneous **4** Percutaneous Endoscopic **7** Via Natural or Artificial Opening **8** Via Natural or Artificial Opening Endoscopic	**Z** No Device	**X** Diagnostic **Z** No Qualifier
1 Seminal Vesicle, Right **2** Seminal Vesicle, Left **3** Seminal Vesicles, Bilateral **6** Tunica Vaginalis, Right **7** Tunica Vaginalis, Left **9** Testis, Right **B** Testis, Left **C** Testes, Bilateral **F** Spermatic Cord, Right **G** Spermatic Cord, Left **H** Spermatic Cords, Bilateral **J** Epididymis, Right **K** Epididymis, Left **L** Epididymis, Bilateral **N** Vas Deferens, Right **P** Vas Deferens, Left **Q** Vas Deferens, Bilateral	**0** Open **3** Percutaneous **4** Percutaneous Endoscopic	**0** Drainage Device	**Z** No Qualifier
1 Seminal Vesicle, Right **2** Seminal Vesicle, Left **3** Seminal Vesicles, Bilateral **6** Tunica Vaginalis, Right	**0** Open **3** Percutaneous **4** Percutaneous Endoscopic	**Z** No Device	**X** Diagnostic **Z** No Qualifier

Continued on Next Page ▶

			Continued from ◀ Previous Page
7 Tunica Vaginalis, Left **9** Testis, Right **B** Testis, Left **C** Testes, Bilateral **F** Spermatic Cord, Right **G** Spermatic Cord, Left **H** Spermatic Cords, Bilateral **J** Epididymis, Right **K** Epididymis, Left **L** Epididymis, Bilateral **N** Vas Deferens, Right **P** Vas Deferens, Left **Q** Vas Deferens, Bilateral			
5 Scrotum **S** Penis **T** Prepuce	**0** Open **3** Percutaneous **4** Percutaneous Endoscopic **X** External	**0** Drainage Device	**Z** No Qualifier
5 Scrotum **S** Penis **T** Prepuce	**0** Open **3** Percutaneous **4** Percutaneous Endoscopic **X** External	**Z** No Device	**X** Diagnostic **Z** No Qualifier

Section	0	Medical and Surgical
Body System	V	Male Reproductive System
Operation	B	Excision: Cutting out or off, without replacement, a portion of a body part

Body Part (Character 4)	Approach (Character 5)	Device (Character 6)	Qualifier (Character 7)
0 Prostate	**0** Open **3** Percutaneous **4** Percutaneous Endoscopic **7** Via Natural or Artificial Opening **8** Via Natural or Artificial Opening Endoscopic	**Z** No Device	**X** Diagnostic **Z** No Qualifier
1 Seminal Vesicle, Right **2** Seminal Vesicle, Left **3** Seminal Vesicles, Bilateral **6** Tunica Vaginalis, Right **7** Tunica Vaginalis, Left **9** Testis, Right **B** Testis, Left **C** Testes, Bilateral **F** Spermatic Cord, Right **G** Spermatic Cord, Left **H** Spermatic Cords, Bilateral **J** Epididymis, Right **K** Epididymis, Left **L** Epididymis, Bilateral **N** Vas Deferens, Right **P** Vas Deferens, Left **Q** Vas Deferens, Bilateral	**0** Open **3** Percutaneous **4** Percutaneous Endoscopic	**Z** No Device	**X** Diagnostic **Z** No Qualifier
5 Scrotum **S** Penis **T** Prepuce	**0** Open **3** Percutaneous **4** Percutaneous Endoscopic **X** External	**Z** No Device	**X** Diagnostic **Z** No Qualifier

Section	0	Medical and Surgical
Body System	V	Male Reproductive System
Operation	C	Extirpation: Taking or cutting out solid matter from a body part

Body Part (Character 4)	Approach (Character 5)	Device (Character 6)	Qualifier (Character 7)
0 Prostate	**0** Open **3** Percutaneous **4** Percutaneous Endoscopic **7** Via Natural or Artificial Opening **8** Via Natural or Artificial Opening Endoscopic	**Z** No Device	**Z** No Qualifier
1 Seminal Vesicle, Right **2** Seminal Vesicle, Left **3** Seminal Vesicles, Bilateral **6** Tunica Vaginalis, Right **7** Tunica Vaginalis, Left **9** Testis, Right **B** Testis, Left **C** Testes, Bilateral **F** Spermatic Cord, Right **G** Spermatic Cord, Left **H** Spermatic Cords, Bilateral **J** Epididymis, Right **K** Epididymis, Left **L** Epididymis, Bilateral **N** Vas Deferens, Right **P** Vas Deferens, Left **Q** Vas Deferens, Bilateral	**0** Open **3** Percutaneous **4** Percutaneous Endoscopic	**Z** No Device	**Z** No Qualifier
5 Scrotum **S** Penis **T** Prepuce	**0** Open **3** Percutaneous **4** Percutaneous Endoscopic **X** External	**Z** No Device	**Z** No Qualifier

Section	0	Medical and Surgical
Body System	V	Male Reproductive System
Operation	H	Insertion: Putting in a nonbiological appliance that monitors, assists, performs, or prevents a physiological function but does not physically take the place of a body part

Body Part (Character 4)	Approach (Character 5)	Device (Character 6)	Qualifier (Character 7)
0 Prostate	**0** Open **3** Percutaneous **4** Percutaneous Endoscopic **7** Via Natural or Artificial Opening **8** Via Natural or Artificial Opening Endoscopic	**1** Radioactive Element	**Z** No Qualifier
4 Prostate and Seminal Vesicles **8** Scrotum and Tunica Vaginalis **D** Testis **M** Epididymis and Spermatic Cord **R** Vas Deferens	**0** Open **3** Percutaneous **4** Percutaneous Endoscopic **7** Via Natural or Artificial Opening **8** Via Natural or Artificial Opening Endoscopic	**3** Infusion Device	**Z** No Qualifier

Continued on Next Page ▶

			Continued from ◀ Previous Page
S Penis	**0** Open **3** Percutaneous **4** Percutaneous Endoscopic **X** External	**3** Infusion Device	**Z** No Qualifier

Section	0	Medical and Surgical
Body System	V	Male Reproductive System
Operation	J	Inspection: Visually and/or manually exploring a body part

Body Part (Character 4)	Approach (Character 5)	Device (Character 6)	Qualifier (Character 7)
4 Prostate and Seminal Vesicles **8** Scrotum and Tunica Vaginalis **D** Testis **M** Epididymis and Spermatic Cord **R** Vas Deferens **5** Penis	**0** Open **3** Percutaneous **4** Percutaneous Endoscopic **X** External	**Z** No Device	**Z** No Qualifier

Section	0	Medical and Surgical
Body System	V	Male Reproductive System
Operation	L	Occlusion: Completely closing an orifice or the lumen of a tubular body part

Body Part (Character 4)	Approach (Character 5)	Device (Character 6)	Qualifier (Character 7)
F Spermatic Cord, Right **G** Spermatic Cord, Left **H** Spermatic Cords, Bilateral **N** Vas Deferens, Right **P** Vas Deferens, Left **Q** Vas Deferens, Bilateral	**0** Open **3** Percutaneous **4** Percutaneous Endoscopic	**C** Extraluminal Device **D** Intraluminal Device **Z** No Device	**Z** No Qualifier

Section	0	Medical and Surgical
Body System	V	Male Reproductive System
Operation	M	Reattachment Putting back in or on all or a portion of a separated body part to its normal location or other suitable location

Body Part (Character 4)	Approach (Character 5)	Device (Character 6)	Qualifier (Character 7)
5 Scrotum **S** Penis	**X** External	**Z** No Device	**Z** No Qualifier
6 Tunica Vaginalis, Right **7** Tunica Vaginalis, Left **9** Testis, Right **B** Testis, Left **C** Testes, Bilateral **F** Spermatic Cord, Right **G** Spermatic Cord, Left **H** Spermatic Cords, Bilateral	**0** Open **4** Percutaneous Endoscopic	**Z** No Device	**Z** No Qualifier

Section	0	Medical and Surgical	
Body System	V	Male Reproductive System	
Operation	N	Release: Freeing a body part from an abnormal physical constraint by cutting or by the use of force	

Body Part (Character 4)	Approach (Character 5)	Device (Character 6)	Qualifier (Character 7)
0 Prostate	**0** Open **3** Percutaneous **4** Percutaneous Endoscopic **7** Via Natural or Artificial Opening **8** Via Natural or Artificial Opening Endoscopic	**Z** No Device	**Z** No Qualifier
1 Seminal Vesicle, Right **2** Seminal Vesicle, Left **3** Seminal Vesicles, Bilateral **6** Tunica Vaginalis, Right **7** Tunica Vaginalis, Left **9** Testis, Right **B** Testis, Left **C** Testes, Bilateral **F** Spermatic Cord, Right **G** Spermatic Cord, Left **H** Spermatic Cords, Bilateral **J** Epididymis, Right **K** Epididymis, Left **L** Epididymis, Bilateral **N** Vas Deferens, Right **P** Vas Deferens, Left **Q** Vas Deferens, Bilateral	**0** Open **3** Percutaneous **4** Percutaneous Endoscopic	**Z** No Device	**Z** No Qualifier
5 Scrotum **S** Penis **T** Prepuce	**0** Open **3** Percutaneous **4** Percutaneous Endoscopic **X** External	**Z** No Device	**Z** No Qualifier

Section	0	Medical and Surgical	
Body System	V	Male Reproductive System	
Operation	P	Removal: Taking out or off a device from a body part	

Body Part (Character 4)	Approach (Character 5)	Device (Character 6)	Qualifier (Character 7)
4 Prostate and Seminal Vesicles	**0** Open **3** Percutaneous **4** Percutaneous Endoscopic **7** Via Natural or Artificial Opening **8** Via Natural or Artificial Opening Endoscopic	**0** Drainage Device **1** Radioactive Element **3** Infusion Device **7** Autologous Tissue Substitute **J** Synthetic Substitute **K** Nonautologous Tissue Substitute	**Z** No Qualifier
4 Prostate and Seminal Vesicles	**X** External	**0** Drainage Device **1** Radioactive Element **3** Infusion Device	**Z** No Qualifier
8 Scrotum and Tunica Vaginalis **D** Testis **S** Penis	**0** Open **3** Percutaneous **4** Percutaneous Endoscopic **7** Via Natural or Artificial Opening	**0** Drainage Device **3** Infusion Device **7** Autologous Tissue Substitute **J** Synthetic Substitute	**Z** No Qualifier **Continued on Next Page ▶**

	8 Via Natural or Artificial Opening Endoscopic	**K** Nonautologous Tissue Substitute	**Continued from** ◀ **Previous Page**
8 Scrotum and Tunica Vaginalis **D** Testis **S** Penis	**X** External	**0** Drainage Device **3** Infusion Device	**Z** No Qualifier
M Epididymis and Spermatic Cord	**0** Open **3** Percutaneous **4** Percutaneous Endoscopic **7** Via Natural or Artificial Opening **8** Via Natural or Artificial Opening Endoscopic	**0** Drainage Device **3** Infusion Device **7** Autologous Tissue Substitute **C** Extraluminal Device **J** Synthetic Substitute **K** Nonautologous Tissue Substitute	**Z** No Qualifier
M Epididymis and Spermatic Cord	**X** External	**0** Drainage Device **3** Infusion Device	**Z** No Qualifier
R Vas Deferens	**0** Open **3** Percutaneous **4** Percutaneous Endoscopic **7** Via Natural or Artificial Opening **8** Via Natural or Artificial Opening Endoscopic	**0** Drainage Device **3** Infusion Device **7** Autologous Tissue Substitute **C** Extraluminal Device **D** Intraluminal Device **J** Synthetic Substitute **K** Nonautologous Tissue Substitute	**Z** No Qualifier
R Vas Deferens	**X** External	**0** Drainage Device **3** Infusion Device **D** Intraluminal Device	**Z** No Qualifier

Section	0	Medical and Surgical
Body System	**V**	**Male Reproductive System**
Operation	**Q**	**Repair: Restoring, to the extent possible, a body part to its normal anatomic structure and function**

Body Part (Character 4)	Approach (Character 5)	Device (Character 6)	Qualifier (Character 7)
0 Prostate	**0** Open **3** Percutaneous **4** Percutaneous Endoscopic **7** Via Natural or Artificial Opening **8** Via Natural or Artificial Opening Endoscopic	**Z** No Device	**Z** No Qualifier
1 Seminal Vesicle, Right **2** Seminal Vesicle, Left **3** Seminal Vesicles, Bilateral **6** Tunica Vaginalis, Right **7** Tunica Vaginalis, Left **9** Testis, Right **B** Testis, Left **C** Testes, Bilateral **F** Spermatic Cord, Right **G** Spermatic Cord, Left **H** Spermatic Cords, Bilateral **J** Epididymis, Right **K** Epididymis, Left	**0** Open **3** Percutaneous **4** Percutaneous Endoscopic	**Z** No Device	**Z** No Qualifier **Continued on Next Page** ▶

L Epididymis, Bilateral N Vas Deferens, Right P Vas Deferens, Left Q Vas Deferens, Bilateral			Continued from ◀ Previous Page
5 Scrotum S Penis T Prepuce	0 Open 3 Percutaneous 4 Percutaneous Endoscopic X External	Z No Device	Z No Qualifier

Section	0	Medical and Surgical
Body System	V	Male Reproductive System
Operation	R	Replacement: Putting in or on biological or synthetic material that physically takes the place and/or function of all or a portion of a body part

Body Part (Character 4)	Approach (Character 5)	Device (Character 6)	Qualifier (Character 7)
9 Testis, Right B Testis, Left C Testes, Bilateral	0 Open	J Synthetic Substitute	Z No Qualifier

Section	0	Medical and Surgical
Body System	V	Male Reproductive System
Operation	S	Reposition: Moving to its normal location, or other suitable location, all or a portion of a body part

Body Part (Character 4)	Approach (Character 5)	Device (Character 6)	Qualifier (Character 7)
9 Testis, Right B Testis, Left C Testes, Bilateral F Spermatic Cord, Right G Spermatic Cord, Left H Spermatic Cords, Bilateral	0 Open 3 Percutaneous 4 Percutaneous Endoscopic	Z No Device	Z No Qualifier

Section	0	Medical and Surgical
Body System	V	Male Reproductive System
Operation	T	Resection: Cutting out or off, without replacement, all of a body part

Body Part (Character 4)	Approach (Character 5)	Device (Character 6)	Qualifier (Character 7)
0 Prostate	0 Open 4 Percutaneous Endoscopic 7 Via Natural or Artificial Opening 8 Via Natural or Artificial Opening Endoscopic	Z No Device	Z No Qualifier
1 Seminal Vesicle, Right 2 Seminal Vesicle, Left 3 Seminal Vesicles, Bilateral 6 Tunica Vaginalis, Right 7 Tunica Vaginalis, Left 9 Testis, Right B Testis, Left C Testes, Bilateral F Spermatic Cord, Right G Spermatic Cord, Left H Spermatic Cords, Bilateral J Epididymis, Right K Epididymis, Left L Epididymis, Bilateral	0 Open 4 Percutaneous Endoscopic	Z No Device	Z No Qualifier Continued on Next Page ▶

N Vas Deferens, Right P Vas Deferens, Left Q Vas Deferens, Bilateral			Continued from ◀ Previous Page
5 Scrotum S Penis T Prepuce	0 Open 4 Percutaneous Endoscopic X External	Z No Device	Z No Qualifier

Section	0	Medical and Surgical	
Body System	V	Male Reproductive System	
Operation	U	Supplement: Putting in or on biological or synthetic material that physically reinforces and/or augments the function of a portion of a body part	

Body Part (Character 4)	Approach (Character 5)	Device (Character 6)	Qualifier (Character 7)
1 Seminal Vesicle, Right 2 Seminal Vesicle, Left 3 Seminal Vesicles, Bilateral 6 Tunica Vaginalis, Right 7 Tunica Vaginalis, Left F Spermatic Cord, Right G Spermatic Cord, Left H Spermatic Cords, Bilateral J Epididymis, Right K Epididymis, Left L Epididymis, Bilateral N Vas Deferens, Right P Vas Deferens, Left Q Vas Deferens, Bilateral	0 Open 4 Percutaneous Endoscopic	7 Autologous Tissue Substitute J Synthetic Substitute K Nonautologous Tissue Substitute	Z No Qualifier
5 Scrotum S Penis T Prepuce	0 Open 4 Percutaneous Endoscopic X External	7 Autologous Tissue Substitute J Synthetic Substitute K Nonautologous Tissue Substitute	Z No Qualifier
9 Testis, Right B Testis, Left C Testes, Bilateral	0 Open	7 Autologous Tissue Substitute J Synthetic Substitute K Nonautologous Tissue Substitute	Z No Qualifier

Section	0	Medical and Surgical	
Body System	V	Male Reproductive System	
Operation	W	Revision: Correcting, to the extent possible, a portion of a malfunctioning device or the position of a displaced device	

Body Part (Character 4)	Approach (Character 5)	Device (Character 6)	Qualifier (Character 7)
4 Prostate and Seminal Vesicles 8 Scrotum and Tunica Vaginalis D Testis 5 Penis	0 Open 3 Percutaneous 4 Percutaneous Endoscopic 7 Via Natural or Artificial Opening 8 Via Natural or Artificial Opening Endoscopic X External	0 Drainage Device 3 Infusion Device 7 Autologous Tissue Substitute J Synthetic Substitute K Nonautologous Tissue Substitute	Z No Qualifier
M Epididymis and Spermatic Cord	0 Open 3 Percutaneous 4 Percutaneous Endoscopic 7 Via Natural or Artificial Opening	0 Drainage Device 3 Infusion Device 7 Autologous Tissue Substitute C Extraluminal Device	Z No Qualifier Continued on Next Page ▶

	8 Via Natural or Artificial Opening Endoscopic **X** External	**J** Synthetic Substitute **K** Nonautologous Tissue Substitute	**Continued from ◀ Previous Page**
R Vas Deferens	**0** Open **3** Percutaneous **4** Percutaneous Endoscopic **7** Via Natural or Artificial Opening **8** Via Natural or Artificial Opening Endoscopic **X** External	**0** Drainage Device **3** Infusion Device **7** Autologous Tissue Substitute **C** Extraluminal Device **D** Intraluminal Device **J** Synthetic Substitute **K** Nonautologous Tissue Substitute	**Z** No Qualifier

Section	0	Medical and Surgical			
Body System	W	Anatomical Regions, General			
Operation	0	Alteration: Modifying the anatomic structure of a body part without affecting the function of the body part			

Body Part (Character 4)	Approach (Character 5)	Device (Character 6)	Qualifier (Character 7)
0 Head 2 Face 4 Upper Jaw 5 Lower Jaw 6 Neck 8 Chest Wall F Abdominal Wall K Upper Back L Lower Back M Perineum, Male N Perineum, Female	0 Open 3 Percutaneous 4 Percutaneous Endoscopic	7 Autologous Tissue Substitute J Synthetic Substitute K Nonautologous Tissue Substitute Z No Device	Z No Qualifier

Section	0	Medical and Surgical			
Body System	W	Anatomical Regions, General			
Operation	1	Bypass: Altering the route of passage of the contents of a tubular body part			

Body Part (Character 4)	Approach (Character 5)	Device (Character 6)	Qualifier (Character 7)
1 Cranial Cavity	0 Open	J Synthetic Substitute	9 Pleural Cavity, Right B Pleural Cavity, Left G Peritoneal Cavity J Pelvic Cavity
9 Pleural Cavity, Right B Pleural Cavity, Left G Peritoneal Cavity J Pelvic Cavity	0 Open 4 Percutaneous Endoscopic	J Synthetic Substitute	4 Cutaneous 9 Pleural Cavity, Right B Pleural Cavity, Left G Peritoneal Cavity J Pelvic Cavity Y Lower Vein
9 Pleural Cavity, Right B Pleural Cavity, Left G Peritoneal Cavity J Pelvic Cavity	3 Percutaneous	J Synthetic Substitute	4 Cutaneous

Section	0	Medical and Surgical			
Body System	W	Anatomical Regions, General			
Operation	2	Change: Taking out or off a device from a body part and putting back an identical or similar device in or on the same body part without cutting or puncturing the skin or a mucous membrane			

Body Part (Character 4)	Approach (Character 5)	Device (Character 6)	Qualifier (Character 7)
0 Head 1 Cranial Cavity 2 Face 4 Upper Jaw 5 Lower Jaw 6 Neck 8 Chest Wall 9 Pleural Cavity, Right B Pleural Cavity, Left C Mediastinum D Pericardial Cavity F Abdominal Wall	X External	0 Drainage Device Y Other Device	Z No Qualifier

Continued on Next Page ▶

G Peritoneal Cavity H Retroperitoneum J Pelvic Cavity K Upper Back L Lower Back M Perineum, Male N Perineum, Female			Continued from ◄ Previous Page

Section	0	Medical and Surgical		
Body System	W	Anatomical Regions, General		
Operation	3	Control: Stopping, or attempting to stop, postprocedural or other acute bleeding		

Body Part (Character 4)	Approach (Character 5)	Device (Character 6)	Qualifier (Character 7)
0 Head 1 Cranial Cavity 2 Face 4 Upper Jaw 5 Lower Jaw 6 Neck 8 Chest Wall 9 Pleural Cavity, Right B Pleural Cavity, Left C Mediastinum D Pericardial Cavity F Abdominal Wall G Peritoneal Cavity H Retroperitoneum J Pelvic Cavity K Upper Back L Lower Back M Perineum, Male N Perineum, Female	0 Open 3 Percutaneous 4 Percutaneous Endoscopic	Z No Device	Z No Qualifier
3 Oral Cavity and Throat	0 Open 3 Percutaneous 4 Percutaneous Endoscopic 7 Via Natural or Artificial Opening 8 Via Natural or Artificial Opening Endoscopic X External	Z No Device	Z No Qualifier
P Gastrointestinal Tract Q Respiratory Tract R Genitourinary Tract	0 Open 3 Percutaneous 4 Percutaneous Endoscopic 7 Via Natural or Artificial Opening 8 Via Natural or Artificial Opening Endoscopic	Z No Device	Z No Qualifier

Section	0	Medical and Surgical		
Body System	W	Anatomical Regions, General		
Operation	4	Creation: Putting in or on biological or synthetic material to form a new body part that to the extent possible replicates the anatomic structure or function of an absent body part		

Body Part (Character 4)	Approach (Character 5)	Device (Character 6)	Qualifier (Character 7)
M Perineum, Male	0 Open	7 Autologous Tissue Substitute J Synthetic Substitute K Nonautologous Tissue Substitute Z No Device	0 Vagina
N Perineum, Female	0 Open	7 Autologous Tissue Substitute J Synthetic Substitute K Nonautologous Tissue Substitute Z No Device	1 Penis

Section	0	Medical and Surgical		
Body System	W	Anatomical Regions, General		
Operation	8	Division: Cutting into a body part, without draining fluids and/or gases from the body part, in order to separate or transect a body part		

Body Part (Character 4)	Approach (Character 5)	Device (Character 6)	Qualifier (Character 7)
N Perineum, Female	X External	Z No Device	Z No Qualifier

Section	0	Medical and Surgical		
Body System	W	Anatomical Regions, General		
Operation	9	Drainage: Taking or letting out fluids and/or gases from a body part		

Body Part (Character 4)	Approach (Character 5)	Device (Character 6)	Qualifier (Character 7)
0 Head 1 Cranial Cavity 2 Face 3 Oral Cavity and Throat 4 Upper Jaw 5 Lower Jaw 6 Neck 8 Chest Wall 9 Pleural Cavity, Right B Pleural Cavity, Left C Mediastinum D Pericardial Cavity F Abdominal Wall G Peritoneal Cavity H Retroperitoneum J Pelvic Cavity K Upper Back L Lower Back M Perineum, Male N Perineum, Female	0 Open 3 Percutaneous 4 Percutaneous Endoscopic	0 Drainage Device	Z No Qualifier
0 Head 1 Cranial Cavity 2 Face 3 Oral Cavity and Throat	0 Open 3 Percutaneous 4 Percutaneous Endoscopic	Z No Device	X Diagnostic Z No Qualifier Continued on Next Page ▶

			Continued from
4 Upper Jaw			◀ Previous Page
5 Lower Jaw			
6 Neck			
8 Chest Wall			
9 Pleural Cavity, Right			
B Pleural Cavity, Left			
C Mediastinum			
D Pericardial Cavity			
F Abdominal Wall			
G Peritoneal Cavity			
H Retroperitoneum			
J Pelvic Cavity			
K Upper Back			
L Lower Back			
M Perineum, Male			
N Perineum, Female			

Section	0	Medical and Surgical	
Body System	W	Anatomical Regions, General	
Operation	B	Excision: Cutting out or off, without replacement, a portion of a body part	

Body Part (Character 4)	Approach (Character 5)	Device (Character 6)	Qualifier (Character 7)
0 Head 2 Face 4 Upper Jaw 5 Lower Jaw 8 Chest Wall K Upper Back L Lower Back M Perineum, Male N Perineum, Female	0 Open 3 Percutaneous 4 Percutaneous Endoscopic X External	Z No Device	X Diagnostic Z No Qualifier
6 Neck F Abdominal Wall	0 Open 3 Percutaneous 4 Percutaneous Endoscopic	Z No Device	X Diagnostic Z No Qualifier
6 Neck F Abdominal Wall	X External	Z No Device	2 Stoma X Diagnostic Z No Qualifier
C Mediastinum H Retroperitoneum	0 Open 3 Percutaneous 4 Percutaneous Endoscopic	Z No Device	X Diagnostic Z No Qualifier

Section	0	Medical and Surgical	
Body System	W	Anatomical Regions, General	
Operation	C	Extirpation: Taking or cutting out solid matter from a body part	

Body Part (Character 4)	Approach (Character 5)	Device (Character 6)	Qualifier (Character 7)
1 Cranial Cavity 3 Oral Cavity and Throat 9 Pleural Cavity, Right B Pleural Cavity, Left C Mediastinum D Pericardial Cavity G Peritoneal Cavity J Pelvic Cavity	0 Open 3 Percutaneous 4 Percutaneous Endoscopic X External	Z No Device	Z No Qualifier
P Gastrointestinal Tract Q Respiratory Tract	0 Open 3 Percutaneous	Z No Device	Z No Qualifier **Continued on Next Page ▶**

| R Genitourinary Tract | 4 Percutaneous Endoscopic
7 Via Natural or Artificial Opening
8 Via Natural or Artificial Opening Endoscopic
X External | | Continued from
◀ Previous Page |

Section	0	Medical and Surgical
Body System	W	Anatomical Regions, General
Operation	F	Fragmentation: Breaking solid matter in a body part into pieces

Body Part (Character 4)	Approach (Character 5)	Device (Character 6)	Qualifier (Character 7)
1 Cranial Cavity 3 Oral Cavity and Throat 9 Pleural Cavity, Right B Pleural Cavity, Left C Mediastinum D Pericardial Cavity G Peritoneal Cavity J Pelvic Cavity	0 Open 3 Percutaneous 4 Percutaneous Endoscopic X External	Z No Device	Z No Qualifier
P Gastrointestinal Tract Q Respiratory Tract R Genitourinary Tract	0 Open 3 Percutaneous 4 Percutaneous Endoscopic 7 Via Natural or Artificial Opening 8 Via Natural or Artificial Opening Endoscopic X External	Z No Device	Z No Qualifier

Section	0	Medical and Surgical
Body System	W	Anatomical Regions, General
Operation	H	Insertion: Putting in a nonbiological appliance that monitors, assists, performs, or prevents a physiological function but does not physically take the place of a body part

Body Part (Character 4)	Approach (Character 5)	Device (Character 6)	Qualifier (Character 7)
0 Head 1 Cranial Cavity 2 Face 3 Oral Cavity and Throat 4 Upper Jaw 5 Lower Jaw 6 Neck 8 Chest Wall 9 Pleural Cavity, Right B Pleural Cavity, Left C Mediastinum D Pericardial Cavity F Abdominal Wall G Peritoneal Cavity H Retroperitoneum J Pelvic Cavity K Upper Back L Lower Back M Perineum, Male N Perineum, Female	0 Open 3 Percutaneous 4 Percutaneous Endoscopic	1 Radioactive Element 3 Infusion Device Y Other Device	Z No Qualifier
P Gastrointestinal Tract Q Respiratory Tract R Genitourinary Tract	0 Open 3 Percutaneous 4 Percutaneous Endoscopic	1 Radioactive Element 3 Infusion Device Y Other Device	Z No Qualifier Continued on Next Page ▶

	7 Via Natural or Artificial Opening 8 Via Natural or Artificial Opening Endoscopic		Continued from ◀ Previous Page

Section	0	Medical and Surgical		
Body System	W	Anatomical Regions, General		
Operation	J	Inspection: Visually and/or manually exploring a body part		

Body Part (Character 4)	Approach (Character 5)	Device (Character 6)	Qualifier (Character 7)
0 Head 2 Face 3 Oral Cavity and Throat 4 Upper Jaw 5 Lower Jaw 6 Neck 8 Chest Wall F Abdominal Wall K Upper Back L Lower Back M Perineum, Male N Perineum, Female	0 Open 3 Percutaneous 4 Percutaneous Endoscopic X External	Z No Device	Z No Qualifier
1 Cranial Cavity 9 Pleural Cavity, Right B Pleural Cavity, Left C Mediastinum D Pericardial Cavity G Peritoneal Cavity H Retroperitoneum J Pelvic Cavity	0 Open 3 Percutaneous 4 Percutaneous Endoscopic	Z No Device	Z No Qualifier
P Gastrointestinal Tract Q Respiratory Tract R Genitourinary Tract	0 Open 3 Percutaneous 4 Percutaneous Endoscopic 7 Via Natural or Artificial Opening 8 Via Natural or Artificial Opening Endoscopic	Z No Device	Z No Qualifier

Section	0	Medical and Surgical		
Body System	W	Anatomical Regions, General		
Operation	M	Reattachment Putting back in or on all or a portion of a separated body part to its normal location or other suitable location		

Body Part (Character 4)	Approach (Character 5)	Device (Character 6)	Qualifier (Character 7)
2 Face 4 Upper Jaw 5 Lower Jaw 6 Neck 8 Chest Wall F Abdominal Wall K Upper Back L Lower Back M Perineum, Male N Perineum, Female	0 Open	Z No Device	Z No Qualifier

Section	0	Medical and Surgical
Body System	W	Anatomical Regions, General
Operation	P	Removal: Taking out or off a device from a body part

Body Part (Character 4)	Approach (Character 5)	Device (Character 6)	Qualifier (Character 7)
0 Head 2 Face 4 Upper Jaw 5 Lower Jaw 6 Neck 8 Chest Wall C Mediastinum F Abdominal Wall K Upper Back L Lower Back M Perineum, Male N Perineum, Female	0 Open 3 Percutaneous 4 Percutaneous Endoscopic X External	0 Drainage Device 1 Radioactive Element 3 Infusion Device 7 Autologous Tissue Substitute J Synthetic Substitute K Nonautologous Tissue Substitute Y Other Device	Z No Qualifier
1 Cranial Cavity 9 Pleural Cavity, Right B Pleural Cavity, Left G Peritoneal Cavity J Pelvic Cavity	0 Open 3 Percutaneous 4 Percutaneous Endoscopic	0 Drainage Device 1 Radioactive Element 3 Infusion Device J Synthetic Substitute Y Other Device	Z No Qualifier
1 Cranial Cavity 9 Pleural Cavity, Right B Pleural Cavity, Left G Peritoneal Cavity J Pelvic Cavity	X External	0 Drainage Device 1 Radioactive Element 3 Infusion Device	Z No Qualifier
D Pericardial Cavity H Retroperitoneum	0 Open 3 Percutaneous 4 Percutaneous Endoscopic	0 Drainage Device 1 Radioactive Element 3 Infusion Device Y Other Device	Z No Qualifier
D Pericardial Cavity H Retroperitoneum	X External	0 Drainage Device 1 Radioactive Element 3 Infusion Device	Z No Qualifier
P Gastrointestinal Tract Q Respiratory Tract R Genitourinary Tract	0 Open 3 Percutaneous 4 Percutaneous Endoscopic 7 Via Natural or Artificial Opening 8 Via Natural or Artificial Opening Endoscopic X External	1 Radioactive Element 3 Infusion Device Y Other Device	Z No Qualifier

Section	0	Medical and Surgical		
Body System	W	Anatomical Regions, General		
Operation	Q	Repair: Restoring, to the extent possible, a body part to its normal anatomic structure and function		

Body Part (Character 4)	Approach (Character 5)	Device (Character 6)	Qualifier (Character 7)
0 Head 2 Face 4 Upper Jaw 5 Lower Jaw 8 Chest Wall K Upper Back L Lower Back M Perineum, Male N Perineum, Female	0 Open 3 Percutaneous 4 Percutaneous Endoscopic X External	Z No Device	Z No Qualifier
6 Neck F Abdominal Wall	0 Open 3 Percutaneous 4 Percutaneous Endoscopic	Z No Device	Z No Qualifier
6 Neck F Abdominal Wall	X External	Z No Device	2 Stoma Z No Qualifier
C Mediastinum	0 Open 3 Percutaneous 4 Percutaneous Endoscopic	Z No Device	Z No Qualifier

Section	0	Medical and Surgical		
Body System	W	Anatomical Regions, General		
Operation	U	Supplement: Putting in or on biological or synthetic material that physically reinforces and/or augments the function of a portion of a body part		

Body Part (Character 4)	Approach (Character 5)	Device (Character 6)	Qualifier (Character 7)
0 Head 2 Face 4 Upper Jaw 5 Lower Jaw 6 Neck 8 Chest Wall C Mediastinum F Abdominal Wall K Upper Back L Lower Back M Perineum, Male N Perineum, Female	0 Open 4 Percutaneous Endoscopic	7 Autologous Tissue Substitute J Synthetic Substitute K Nonautologous Tissue Substitute	Z No Qualifier

Section	0	Medical and Surgical		
Body System	W	Anatomical Regions, General		
Operation	W	Revision: Correcting, to the extent possible, a portion of a malfunctioning device or the position of a displaced device		

Body Part (Character 4)	Approach (Character 5)	Device (Character 6)	Qualifier (Character 7)
0 Head 2 Face 4 Upper Jaw 5 Lower Jaw 6 Neck 8 Chest Wall C Mediastinum F Abdominal Wall	0 Open 3 Percutaneous 4 Percutaneous Endoscopic X External	0 Drainage Device 1 Radioactive Element 3 Infusion Device 7 Autologous Tissue Substitute J Synthetic Substitute K Nonautologous Tissue Substitute	Z No Qualifier

Continued on Next Page ▶

		Y Other Device	Continued from ◀ Previous Page
K Upper Back L Lower Back M Perineum, Male N Perineum, Female			
1 Cranial Cavity 9 Pleural Cavity, Right B Pleural Cavity, Left G Peritoneal Cavity J Pelvic Cavity	0 Open 3 Percutaneous 4 Percutaneous Endoscopic X External	0 Drainage Device 1 Radioactive Element 3 Infusion Device J Synthetic Substitute Y Other Device	Z No Qualifier
D Pericardial Cavity H Retroperitoneum	0 Open 3 Percutaneous 4 Percutaneous Endoscopic X External	0 Drainage Device 1 Radioactive Element 3 Infusion Device Y Other Device	Z No Qualifier
P Gastrointestinal Tract Q Respiratory Tract R Genitourinary Tract	0 Open 3 Percutaneous 4 Percutaneous Endoscopic 7 Via Natural or Artificial Opening 8 Via Natural or Artificial Opening Endoscopic X External	1 Radioactive Element 3 Infusion Device Y Other Device	Z No Qualifier

Section	0	Medical and Surgical
Body System	W	Anatomical Regions, General
Operation	Y	Transplantation: Putting in or on all or a portion of a living body part taken from another individual or animal to physically take the place and/or function of all or a portion of a similar body part

Body Part (Character 4)	Approach (Character 5)	Device (Character 6)	Qualifier (Character 7)
2 Face	0 Open	Z No Device	0 Allogeneic 1 Syngeneic

Section	0	Medical and Surgical
Body System	X	Anatomical Regions, Upper Extremities
Operation	0	Alteration: Modifying the anatomic structure of a body part without affecting the function of the body part

Body Part (Character 4)	Approach (Character 5)	Device (Character 6)	Qualifier (Character 7)
2 Shoulder Region, Right 3 Shoulder Region, Left 4 Axilla, Right 5 Axilla, Left 6 Upper Extremity, Right 7 Upper Extremity, Left 8 Upper Arm, Right 9 Upper Arm, Left B Elbow Region, Right C Elbow Region, Left D Lower Arm, Right F Lower Arm, Left G Wrist Region, Right H Wrist Region, Left	0 Open 3 Percutaneous 4 Percutaneous Endoscopic	7 Autologous Tissue Substitute J Synthetic Substitute K Nonautologous Tissue Substitute Z No Device	Z No Qualifier

Section	0	Medical and Surgical
Body System	X	Anatomical Regions, Upper Extremities
Operation	2	Change: Taking out or off a device from a body part and putting back an identical or similar device in or on the same body part without cutting or puncturing the skin or a mucous membrane

Body Part (Character 4)	Approach (Character 5)	Device (Character 6)	Qualifier (Character 7)
6 Upper Extremity, Right 7 Upper Extremity, Left	X External	0 Drainage Device Y Other Device	Z No Qualifier

Section	0	Medical and Surgical
Body System	X	Anatomical Regions, Upper Extremities
Operation	3	Control: Stopping, or attempting to stop, postprocedural or other acute bleeding

Body Part (Character 4)	Approach (Character 5)	Device (Character 6)	Qualifier (Character 7)
2 Shoulder Region, Right 3 Shoulder Region, Left 4 Axilla, Right 5 Axilla, Left 6 Upper Extremity, Right 7 Upper Extremity, Left 8 Upper Arm, Right 9 Upper Arm, Left B Elbow Region, Right C Elbow Region, Left D Lower Arm, Right F Lower Arm, Left G Wrist Region, Right H Wrist Region, Left J Hand, Right K Hand, Left	0 Open 3 Percutaneous 4 Percutaneous Endoscopic	Z No Device	Z No Qualifier

Section	0	Medical and Surgical		
Body System	X	Anatomical Regions, Upper Extremities		
Operation	6	Detachment: Cutting off all or a portion of the upper or lower extremities		

Body Part (Character 4)	Approach (Character 5)	Device (Character 6)	Qualifier (Character 7)
0 Forequarter, Right **1** Forequarter, Left **2** Shoulder Region, Right **3** Shoulder Region, Left **B** Elbow Region, Right **C** Elbow Region, Left	**0** Open	**Z** No Device	**Z** No Qualifier
8 Upper Arm, Right **9** Upper Arm, Left **D** Lower Arm, Right **F** Lower Arm, Left	**0** Open	**Z** No Device	**1** High **2** Mid **3** Low
J Hand, Right **K** Hand, Left	**0** Open	**Z** No Device	**0** Complete **4** Complete 1st Ray **5** Complete 2nd Ray **6** Complete 3rd Ray **7** Complete 4th Ray **8** Complete 5th Ray **9** Partial 1st Ray **B** Partial 2nd Ray **C** Partial 3rd Ray **D** Partial 4th Ray **F** Partial 5th Ray
L Thumb, Right **M** Thumb, Left **N** Index Finger, Right **P** Index Finger, Left **Q** Middle Finger, Right **R** Middle Finger, Left **S** Ring Finger, Right **T** Ring Finger, Left **V** Little Finger, Right **W** Little Finger, Left	**0** Open	**Z** No Device	**0** Complete **1** High **2** Mid **3** Low

Section	0	Medical and Surgical		
Body System	X	Anatomical Regions, Upper Extremities		
Operation	9	Drainage: Taking or letting out fluids and/or gases from a body part		

Body Part (Character 4)	Approach (Character 5)	Device (Character 6)	Qualifier (Character 7)
2 Shoulder Region, Right **3** Shoulder Region, Left **4** Axilla, Right **5** Axilla, Left **6** Upper Extremity, Right **7** Upper Extremity, Left **8** Upper Arm, Right **9** Upper Arm, Left **B** Elbow Region, Right **C** Elbow Region, Left **D** Lower Arm, Right **F** Lower Arm, Left **G** Wrist Region, Right **H** Wrist Region, Left	**0** Open **3** Percutaneous **4** Percutaneous Endoscopic	**0** Drainage Device	**Z** No Qualifier

Continued on Next Page ▶

			Continued from ◄ Previous Page
J Hand, Right **K** Hand, Left			
2 Shoulder Region, Right **3** Shoulder Region, Left **4** Axilla, Right **5** Axilla, Left **6** Upper Extremity, Right **7** Upper Extremity, Left **8** Upper Arm, Right **9** Upper Arm, Left **B** Elbow Region, Right **C** Elbow Region, Left **D** Lower Arm, Right **F** Lower Arm, Left **G** Wrist Region, Right **H** Wrist Region, Left **J** Hand, Right **K** Hand, Left	**0** Open **3** Percutaneous **4** Percutaneous Endoscopic	**Z** No Device	**X** Diagnostic **Z** No Qualifier

Section	0	Medical and Surgical
Body System	X	Anatomical Regions, Upper Extremities
Operation	B	Excision: Cutting out or off, without replacement, a portion of a body part

Body Part (Character 4)	Approach (Character 5)	Device (Character 6)	Qualifier (Character 7)
2 Shoulder Region, Right **3** Shoulder Region, Left **4** Axilla, Right **5** Axilla, Left **6** Upper Extremity, Right **7** Upper Extremity, Left **8** Upper Arm, Right **9** Upper Arm, Left **B** Elbow Region, Right **C** Elbow Region, Left **D** Lower Arm, Right **F** Lower Arm, Left **G** Wrist Region, Right **H** Wrist Region, Left **J** Hand, Right **K** Hand, Left	**0** Open **3** Percutaneous **4** Percutaneous Endoscopic	**Z** No Device	**X** Diagnostic **Z** No Qualifier

Section	0	Medical and Surgical
Body System	X	Anatomical Regions, Upper Extremities
Operation	H	Insertion: Putting in a nonbiological appliance that monitors, assists, performs, or prevents a physiological function but does not physically take the place of a body part

Body Part (Character 4)	Approach (Character 5)	Device (Character 6)	Qualifier (Character 7)
2 Shoulder Region, Right **3** Shoulder Region, Left **4** Axilla, Right **5** Axilla, Left **6** Upper Extremity, Right **7** Upper Extremity, Left **8** Upper Arm, Right **9** Upper Arm, Left **B** Elbow Region, Right	**0** Open **3** Percutaneous **4** Percutaneous Endoscopic	**1** Radioactive Element **3** Infusion Device **Y** Other Device	**Z** No Qualifier Continued on Next Page ►

C Elbow Region, Left **D** Lower Arm, Right **F** Lower Arm, Left **G** Wrist Region, Right **H** Wrist Region, Left **J** Hand, Right **K** Hand, Left			**Continued from** ◀ **Previous Page**

Section	0	Medical and Surgical		
Body System	X	Anatomical Regions, Upper Extremities		
Operation	J	Inspection: Visually and/or manually exploring a body part		

Body Part (Character 4)	Approach (Character 5)	Device (Character 6)	Qualifier (Character 7)
2 Shoulder Region, Right **3** Shoulder Region, Left **4** Axilla, Right **5** Axilla, Left **6** Upper Extremity, Right **7** Upper Extremity, Left **8** Upper Arm, Right **9** Upper Arm, Left **B** Elbow Region, Right **C** Elbow Region, Left **D** Lower Arm, Right **F** Lower Arm, Left **G** Wrist Region, Right **H** Wrist Region, Left **J** Hand, Right **K** Hand, Left	**0** Open **3** Percutaneous **4** Percutaneous Endoscopic **X** External	**Z** No Device	**Z** No Qualifier

Section	0	Medical and Surgical		
Body System	X	Anatomical Regions, Upper Extremities		
Operation	M	Reattachment Putting back in or on all or a portion of a separated body part to its normal location or other suitable location		

Body Part (Character 4)	Approach (Character 5)	Device (Character 6)	Qualifier (Character 7)
0 Forequarter, Right **1** Forequarter, Left **2** Shoulder Region, Right **3** Shoulder Region, Left **4** Axilla, Right **5** Axilla, Left **6** Upper Extremity, Right **7** Upper Extremity, Left **8** Upper Arm, Right **9** Upper Arm, Left **B** Elbow Region, Right **C** Elbow Region, Left **D** Lower Arm, Right **F** Lower Arm, Left **G** Wrist Region, Right **H** Wrist Region, Left **J** Hand, Right **K** Hand, Left **L** Thumb, Right **M** Thumb, Left	**0** Open	**Z** No Device	**Z** No Qualifier *(see navigation below)*

Continued on
Next Page ▶

			Continued from ◀ Previous Page
N Index Finger, Right			
P Index Finger, Left			
Q Middle Finger, Right			
R Middle Finger, Left			
S Ring Finger, Right			
T Ring Finger, Left			
V Little Finger, Right			
W Little Finger, Left			

Section	0	Medical and Surgical		
Body System	X	Anatomical Regions, Upper Extremities		
Operation	P	Removal: Taking out or off a device from a body part		

Body Part (Character 4)	Approach (Character 5)	Device (Character 6)	Qualifier (Character 7)
6 Upper Extremity, Right	0 Open	0 Drainage Device	Z No Qualifier
7 Upper Extremity, Left	3 Percutaneous	1 Radioactive Element	
	4 Percutaneous Endoscopic	3 Infusion Device	
	X External	7 Autologous Tissue Substitute	
		J Synthetic Substitute	
		K Nonautologous Tissue Substitute	
		Y Other Device	

Section	0	Medical and Surgical		
Body System	X	Anatomical Regions, Upper Extremities		
Operation	Q	Repair: Restoring, to the extent possible, a body part to its normal anatomic structure and function		

Body Part (Character 4)	Approach (Character 5)	Device (Character 6)	Qualifier (Character 7)
2 Shoulder Region, Right	0 Open	Z No Device	Z No Qualifier
3 Shoulder Region, Left	3 Percutaneous		
4 Axilla, Right	4 Percutaneous Endoscopic		
5 Axilla, Left	X External		
6 Upper Extremity, Right			
7 Upper Extremity, Left			
8 Upper Arm, Right			
9 Upper Arm, Left			
B Elbow Region, Right			
C Elbow Region, Left			
D Lower Arm, Right			
F Lower Arm, Left			
G Wrist Region, Right			
H Wrist Region, Left			
J Hand, Right			
K Hand, Left			
L Thumb, Right			
M Thumb, Left			
N Index Finger, Right			
P Index Finger, Left			
Q Middle Finger, Right			
R Middle Finger, Left			
S Ring Finger, Right			
T Ring Finger, Left			
V Little Finger, Right			
W Little Finger, Left			

Section	0	Medical and Surgical			
Body System	X	Anatomical Regions, Upper Extremities			
Operation	R	Replacement: Putting in or on biological or synthetic material that physically takes the place and/or function of all or a portion of a body part			

Body Part (Character 4)	Approach (Character 5)	Device (Character 6)	Qualifier (Character 7)
L Thumb, Right M Thumb, Left		0 Open 4 Percutaneous Endoscopic	7 Autologous Tissue Substitute

Section	0	Medical and Surgical			
Body System	X	Anatomical Regions, Upper Extremities			
Operation	U	Supplement: Putting in or on biological or synthetic material that physically reinforces and/or augments the function of a portion of a body part			

Body Part (Character 4)	Approach (Character 5)	Device (Character 6)	Qualifier (Character 7)
2 Shoulder Region, Right 3 Shoulder Region, Left 4 Axilla, Right 5 Axilla, Left 6 Upper Extremity, Right 7 Upper Extremity, Left 8 Upper Arm, Right 9 Upper Arm, Left B Elbow Region, Right C Elbow Region, Left D Lower Arm, Right F Lower Arm, Left G Wrist Region, Right H Wrist Region, Left J Hand, Right K Hand, Left L Thumb, Right M Thumb, Left N Index Finger, Right P Index Finger, Left Q Middle Finger, Right R Middle Finger, Left S Ring Finger, Right T Ring Finger, Left V Little Finger, Right W Little Finger, Left	0 Open 4 Percutaneous Endoscopic	7 Autologous Tissue Substitute J Synthetic Substitute K Nonautologous Tissue Substitute	Z No Qualifier

Section	0	Medical and Surgical			
Body System	X	Anatomical Regions, Upper Extremities			
Operation	W	Revision: Correcting, to the extent possible, a portion of a malfunctioning device or the position of a displaced device			

Body Part (Character 4)	Approach (Character 5)	Device (Character 6)	Qualifier (Character 7)
6 Upper Extremity, Right 7 Upper Extremity, Left	0 Open 3 Percutaneous 4 Percutaneous Endoscopic X External	0 Drainage Device 3 Infusion Device 7 Autologous Tissue Substitute J Synthetic Substitute K Nonautologous Tissue Substitute Y Other Device	Z No Qualifier

Section	0	Medical and Surgical			
Body System	X	Anatomical Regions, Upper Extremities			
Operation	X	Transfer: Moving, without taking out, all or a portion of a body part to another location to take over the function of all or a portion of a body part			

Body Part (Character 4)	Approach (Character 5)	Device (Character 6)	Qualifier (Character 7)
N Index Finger, Right	**0** Open	**Z** No Device	**L** Thumb, Right
P Index Finger, Left	**0** Open	**Z** No Device	**M** Thumb, Left

Section	0	Medical and Surgical			
Body System	X	Anatomical Regions, Upper Extremities			
Operation	Y	Transplantation: Putting in or on all or a portion of a living body part taken from another individual or animal to physically take the place and/or function of all or a portion of a similar body part			

Body Part (Character 4)	Approach (Character 5)	Device (Character 6)	Qualifier (Character 7)
J Hand, Right	**0** Open	**Z** No Device	**0** Allogeneic
K Hand, Lef			**1** Syngeneic

Section	0	Medical and Surgical		
Body System	Y	Anatomical Regions, Lower Extremities		
Operation	0	Alteration: Modifying the anatomic structure of a body part without affecting the function of the body part		

Body Part (Character 4)	Approach (Character 5)	Device (Character 6)	Qualifier (Character 7)
0 Buttock, Right	0 Open	7 Autologous Tissue Substitute	Z No Qualifier
1 Buttock, Left	3 Percutaneous	J Synthetic Substitute	
9 Lower Extremity, Right	4 Percutaneous Endoscopic	K Nonautologous Tissue Substitute	
B Lower Extremity, Left		Z No Device	
C Upper Leg, Right			
D Upper Leg, Left			
F Knee Region, Right			
G Knee Region, Left			
H Lower Leg, Right			
J Lower Leg, Left			
K Ankle Region, Right			
L Ankle Region, Left			

Section	0	Medical and Surgical		
Body System	Y	Anatomical Regions, Lower Extremities		
Operation	2	Change: Taking out or off a device from a body part and putting back an identical or similar device in or on the same body part without cutting or puncturing the skin or a mucous membrane		

Body Part (Character 4)	Approach (Character 5)	Device (Character 6)	Qualifier (Character 7)
9 Lower Extremity, Right	X External	0 Drainage Device	Z No Qualifier
B Lower Extremity, Left		Y Other Device	

Section	0	Medical and Surgical		
Body System	Y	Anatomical Regions, Lower Extremities		
Operation	3	Control: Stopping, or attempting to stop, postprocedural or other acute bleeding		

Body Part (Character 4)	Approach (Character 5)	Device (Character 6)	Qualifier (Character 7)
0 Buttock, Right	0 Open	Z No Device	Z No Qualifier
1 Buttock, Left	3 Percutaneous		
5 Inguinal Region, Right	4 Percutaneous Endoscopic		
6 Inguinal Region, Left			
7 Femoral Region, Right			
8 Femoral Region, Left			
9 Lower Extremity, Right			
B Lower Extremity, Left			
C Upper Leg, Right			
D Upper Leg, Left			
F Knee Region, Right			
G Knee Region, Left			
H Lower Leg, Right			
J Lower Leg, Left			
K Ankle Region, Right			
L Ankle Region, Left			
M Foot, Right			
N Foot, Left			

Section	0	Medical and Surgical		
Body System	Y	Anatomical Regions, Lower Extremities		
Operation	6	Detachment: Cutting off all or a portion of the upper or lower extremities		

Body Part (Character 4)	Approach (Character 5)	Device (Character 6)	Qualifier (Character 7)
2 Hindquarter, Right 3 Hindquarter, Left 4 Hindquarter, Bilateral 7 Femoral Region, Right 8 Femoral Region, Left F Knee Region, Right G Knee Region, Left	0 Open	Z No Device	Z No Qualifier
C Upper Leg, Right D Upper Leg, Left H Lower Leg, Right J Lower Leg, Left	0 Open	Z No Device	1 High 2 Mid 3 Low
M Foot, Right N Foot, Left	0 Open	Z No Device	0 Complete 4 Complete 1st Ray 5 Complete 2nd Ray 6 Complete 3rd Ray 7 Complete 4th Ray 8 Complete 5th Ray 9 Partial 1st Ray B Partial 2nd Ray C Partial 3rd Ray D Partial 4th Ray F Partial 5th Ray
P 1st Toe, Right Q 1st Toe, Left R 2nd Toe, Right S 2nd Toe, Left T 3rd Toe, Right U 3rd Toe, Left V 4th Toe, Right W 4th Toe, Left X 5th Toe, Right Y 5th Toe, Left	0 Open	Z No Device	0 Complete 1 High 2 Mid 3 Low

Section	0	Medical and Surgical		
Body System	Y	Anatomical Regions, Lower Extremities		
Operation	9	Drainage: Taking or letting out fluids and/or gases from a body part		

Body Part (Character 4)	Approach (Character 5)	Device (Character 6)	Qualifier (Character 7)
0 Buttock, Right 1 Buttock, Left 5 Inguinal Region, Right 6 Inguinal Region, Left 7 Femoral Region, Right 8 Femoral Region, Left 9 Lower Extremity, Right B Lower Extremity, Left C Upper Leg, Right D Upper Leg, Left F Knee Region, Right G Knee Region, Left H Lower Leg, Right	0 Open 3 Percutaneous 4 Percutaneous Endoscopic	0 Drainage Device	Z No Qualifier

Continued on Next Page ▶

			Continued from ◀ Previous Page
J Lower Leg, Left **K** Ankle Region, Right **L** Ankle Region, Left **M** Foot, Right **N** Foot, Left			
0 Buttock, Right **1** Buttock, Left **5** Inguinal Region, Right **6** Inguinal Region, Left **7** Femoral Region, Right **8** Femoral Region, Left **9** Lower Extremity, Right **B** Lower Extremity, Left **C** Upper Leg, Right **D** Upper Leg, Left **F** Knee Region, Right **G** Knee Region, Left **H** Lower Leg, Right **J** Lower Leg, Left **K** Ankle Region, Right **L** Ankle Region, Left **M** Foot, Right **N** Foot, Left	**0** Open **3** Percutaneous **4** Percutaneous Endoscopic	**Z** No Device	**X** Diagnostic **Z** No Qualifier

Section	0	Medical and Surgical	
Body System	Y	Anatomical Regions, Lower Extremities	
Operation	B	Excision: Cutting out or off, without replacement, a portion of a body part	
Body Part (Character 4)	**Approach (Character 5)**	**Device (Character 6)**	**Qualifier (Character 7)**
0 Buttock, Right **1** Buttock, Left **5** Inguinal Region, Right **6** Inguinal Region, Left **7** Femoral Region, Right **8** Femoral Region, Left **9** Lower Extremity, Right **B** Lower Extremity, Left **C** Upper Leg, Right **D** Upper Leg, Left **F** Knee Region, Right **G** Knee Region, Left **H** Lower Leg, Right **J** Lower Leg, Left **K** Ankle Region, Right **L** Ankle Region, Left **M** Foot, Right **N** Foot, Left	**0** Open **3** Percutaneous **4** Percutaneous Endoscopic	**Z** No Device	**X** Diagnostic **Z** No Qualifier

Section	0	Medical and Surgical		
Body System	Y	Anatomical Regions, Lower Extremities		
Operation	H	Insertion: Putting in a nonbiological appliance that monitors, assists, performs, or prevents a physiological function but does not physically take the place of a body part		

Body Part (Character 4)	Approach (Character 5)	Device (Character 6)	Qualifier (Character 7)
0 Buttock, Right	0 Open	1 Radioactive Element	Z No Qualifier
1 Buttock, Left	3 Percutaneous	3 Infusion Device	
5 Inguinal Region, Right	4 Percutaneous Endoscopic	Y Other Device	
6 Inguinal Region, Left			
7 Femoral Region, Right			
8 Femoral Region, Left			
9 Lower Extremity, Right			
B Lower Extremity, Left			
C Upper Leg, Right			
D Upper Leg, Left			
F Knee Region, Right			
G Knee Region, Left			
H Lower Leg, Right			
J Lower Leg, Left			
K Ankle Region, Right			
L Ankle Region, Left			
M Foot, Right			
N Foot, Left			

Section	0	Medical and Surgical		
Body System	Y	Anatomical Regions, Lower Extremities		
Operation	J	Inspection: Visually and/or manually exploring a body part		

Body Part (Character 4)	Approach (Character 5)	Device (Character 6)	Qualifier (Character 7)
0 Buttock, Right	0 Open	Z No Device	Z No Qualifier
1 Buttock, Left	3 Percutaneous		
5 Inguinal Region, Right	4 Percutaneous Endoscopic		
6 Inguinal Region, Left	X External		
7 Femoral Region, Right			
8 Femoral Region, Left			
9 Lower Extremity, Right			
A Inguinal Region, Bilateral			
B Lower Extremity, Left			
C Upper Leg, Right			
D Upper Leg, Left			
E Femoral Region, Bilateral			
F Knee Region, Right			
G Knee Region, Left			
H Lower Leg, Right			
J Lower Leg, Left			
K Ankle Region, Right			
L Ankle Region, Left			
M Foot, Right			
N Foot, Left			

Section	0	Medical and Surgical		
Body System	Y	Anatomical Regions, Lower Extremities		
Operation	M	Reattachment Putting back in or on all or a portion of a separated body part to its normal location or other suitable location		

Body Part (Character 4)	Approach (Character 5)	Device (Character 6)	Qualifier (Character 7)
0 Buttock, Right	0 Open	Z No Device	Z No Qualifier
1 Buttock, Left			
2 Hindquarter, Right			
3 Hindquarter, Left			
4 Hindquarter, Bilateral			
5 Inguinal Region, Right			
6 Inguinal Region, Left			
7 Femoral Region, Right			
8 Femoral Region, Left			
9 Lower Extremity, Right			
B Lower Extremity, Left			
C Upper Leg, Right			
D Upper Leg, Left			
F Knee Region, Right			
G Knee Region, Left			
H Lower Leg, Right			
J Lower Leg, Left			
K Ankle Region, Right			
L Ankle Region, Left			
M Foot, Right			
N Foot, Left			
P 1st Toe, Right			
Q 1st Toe, Left			
R 2nd Toe, Right			
S 2nd Toe, Left			
T 3rd Toe, Right			
U 3rd Toe, Left			
V 4th Toe, Right			
W 4th Toe, Left			
X 5th Toe, Right			
Y 5th Toe, Left			

Section	0	Medical and Surgical		
Body System	Y	Anatomical Regions, Lower Extremities		
Operation	P	Removal: Taking out or off a device from a body part		

Body Part (Character 4)	Approach (Character 5)	Device (Character 6)	Qualifier (Character 7)
9 Lower Extremity, Right	0 Open	0 Drainage Device	Z No Qualifier
B Lower Extremity, Left	3 Percutaneous	1 Radioactive Element	
	4 Percutaneous Endoscopic	3 Infusion Device	
	X External	7 Autologous Tissue Substitute	
		J Synthetic Substitute	
		K Nonautologous Tissue Substitute	
		Y Other Device	

Section	0	Medical and Surgical		
Body System	Y	Anatomical Regions, Lower Extremities		
Operation	Q	Repair: Restoring, to the extent possible, a body part to its normal anatomic structure and function		

Body Part (Character 4)	Approach (Character 5)	Device (Character 6)	Qualifier (Character 7)
0 Buttock, Right	0 Open	Z No Device	Z No Qualifier
1 Buttock, Left	3 Percutaneous		
5 Inguinal Region, Right	4 Percutaneous Endoscopic		
6 Inguinal Region, Left	X External		
7 Femoral Region, Right			
8 Femoral Region, Left			
9 Lower Extremity, Right			
A Inguinal Region, Bilateral			
B Lower Extremity, Left			
C Upper Leg, Right			
D Upper Leg, Left			
E Femoral Region, Bilateral			
F Knee Region, Right			
G Knee Region, Left			
H Lower Leg, Right			
J Lower Leg, Left			
K Ankle Region, Right			
L Ankle Region, Left			
M Foot, Right			
N Foot, Left			
P 1st Toe, Right			
Q 1st Toe, Left			
R 2nd Toe, Right			
S 2nd Toe, Left			
T 3rd Toe, Right			
U 3rd Toe, Left			
V 4th Toe, Right			
W 4th Toe, Left			
X 5th Toe, Right			
Y 5th Toe, Left			

Section	0	Medical and Surgical		
Body System	Y	Anatomical Regions, Lower Extremities		
Operation	U	Supplement: Putting in or on biological or synthetic material that physically reinforces and/or augments the function of a portion of a body part		

Body Part (Character 4)	Approach (Character 5)	Device (Character 6)	Qualifier (Character 7)
0 Buttock, Right	0 Open	7 Autologous Tissue Substitute	Z No Qualifier
1 Buttock, Left	4 Percutaneous Endoscopic	J Synthetic Substitute	
5 Inguinal Region, Right		K Nonautologous Tissue Substitute	
6 Inguinal Region, Left			
7 Femoral Region, Right			
8 Femoral Region, Left			
9 Lower Extremity, Right			
A Inguinal Region, Bilateral			
B Lower Extremity, Left			
C Upper Leg, Right			
D Upper Leg, Left			
E Femoral Region, Bilateral			
F Knee Region, Right			

Continued on Next Page ▶

			Continued from ◀ Previous Page
G Knee Region, Left			
H Lower Leg, Right			
J Lower Leg, Left			
K Ankle Region, Right			
L Ankle Region, Left			
M Foot, Right			
N Foot, Left			
P 1st Toe, Right			
Q 1st Toe, Left			
R 2nd Toe, Right			
S 2nd Toe, Left			
T 3rd Toe, Right			
U 3rd Toe, Left			
V 4th Toe, Right			
W 4th Toe, Left			
X 5th Toe, Right			
Y 5th Toe, Left			

Section	0	Medical and Surgical
Body System	Y	Anatomical Regions, Lower Extremities
Operation	W	Revision: Correcting, to the extent possible, a portion of a malfunctioning device or the position of a displaced device

Body Part (Character 4)	Approach (Character 5)	Device (Character 6)	Qualifier (Character 7)
9 Lower Extremity, Right	**0** Open	**0** Drainage Device	**Z** No Qualifier
B Lower Extremity, Left	**3** Percutaneous	**3** Infusion Device	
	4 Percutaneous Endoscopic	**7** Autologous Tissue Substitute	
	X External	**J** Synthetic Substitute	
		K Nonautologous Tissue Substitute	
		Y Other Device	

Section	1	Obstetrics		
Body System	0	Pregnancy		
Operation	2	Change: Taking out or off a device from a body part and putting back an identical or similar device in or on the same body part without cutting or puncturing the skin or a mucous membrane		

Body Part (Character 4)	Approach (Character 5)	Device (Character 6)	Qualifier (Character 7)
0 Products of Conception	7 Via Natural or Artificial Opening	3 Monitoring Electrode Y Other Device	Z No Qualifier

Section	1	Obstetrics		
Body System	0	Pregnancy		
Operation	9	Drainage: Taking or letting out fluids and/or gases from a body part		

Body Part (Character 4)	Approach (Character 5)	Device (Character 6)	Qualifier (Character 7)
0 Products of Conception	0 Open 3 Percutaneous 4 Percutaneous Endoscopic 7 Via Natural or Artificial Opening 8 Via Natural or Artificial Opening Endoscopic	Z No Device	9 Fetal Blood A Fetal Cerebrospinal Fluid B Fetal Fluid, Other C Amniotic Fluid, Therapeutic D Fluid, Other U Amniotic Fluid, Diagnostic

Section	1	Obstetrics		
Body System	0	Pregnancy		
Operation	A	Abortion: Artificially terminating a pregnancy		

Body Part (Character 4)	Approach (Character 5)	Device (Character 6)	Qualifier (Character 7)
0 Products of Conception	0 Open 3 Percutaneous 4 Percutaneous Endoscopic 8 Via Natural or Artificial Opening Endoscopic	Z No Device	Z No Qualifier
0 Products of Conception	7 Via Natural or Artificial Opening	Z No Device	6 Vacuum W Laminaria X Abortifacient Z No Qualifier

Section	1	Obstetrics		
Body System	0	Pregnancy		
Operation	D	Extraction: Pulling or stripping out or off all or a portion of a body part by the use of force		

Body Part (Character 4)	Approach (Character 5)	Device (Character 6)	Qualifier (Character 7)
0 Products of Conception	0 Open	Z No Device	0 Classical 1 Low Cervical 2 Extraperitoneal
0 Products of Conception	7 Via Natural or Artificial Opening	Z No Device	3 Low Forceps 4 Mid Forceps 5 High Forceps 6 Vacuum 7 Internal Version 8 Other
1 Products of Conception, Retained 2 Products of Conception, Ectoplc	7 Via Natural or Artificial Opening 8 Via Natural or Artificial Opening Endoscopic	Z No Device	Z No Qualifier

Section	1	Obstetrics		
Body System	0	Pregnancy		
Operation	E	Delivery: Assisting the passage of the products of conception from the genital canal		

Body Part (Character 4)	Approach (Character 5)	Device (Character 6)	Qualifier (Character 7)
0 Products of Conception	X External	Z No Device	Z No Qualifier

Section	1	Obstetrics		
Body System	0	Pregnancy		
Operation	H	Insertion: Putting in a nonbiological appliance that monitors, assists, performs, or prevents a physiological function but does not physically take the place of a body part		

Body Part (Character 4)	Approach (Character 5)	Device (Character 6)	Qualifier (Character 7)
0 Products of Conception	0 Open 7 Via Natural or Artificial Opening	3 Monitoring Electrode Y Other Device	Z No Qualifier

Section	1	Obstetrics		
Body System	0	Pregnancy		
Operation	J	Inspection: Visually and/or manually exploring a body part		

Body Part (Character 4)	Approach (Character 5)	Device (Character 6)	Qualifier (Character 7)
0 Products of Conception 1 Products of Conception, Retained 2 Products of Conception, Ectopic	0 Open 3 Percutaneous 4 Percutaneous Endoscopic 7 Via Natural or Artificial Opening 8 Via Natural or Artificial Opening Endoscopic X External	Z No Device	Z No Qualifier

Section	1	Obstetrics		
Body System	0	Pregnancy		
Operation	P	Removal: Taking out or off a device from a body part, region or orifice		

Body Part (Character 4)	Approach (Character 5)	Device (Character 6)	Qualifier (Character 7)
0 Products of Conception	0 Open 7 Via Natural or Artificial Opening	3 Monitoring Electrode Y Other Device	Z No Qualifier

Section	1	Obstetrics		
Body System	0	Pregnancy		
Operation	Q	Repair: Restoring, to the extent possible, a body part to its normal anatomic structure and function		

Body Part (Character 4)	Approach (Character 5)	Device (Character 6)	Qualifier (Character 7)
0 Products of Conception	0 Open 3 Percutaneous 4 Percutaneous Endoscopic 7 Via Natural or Artificial Opening 8 Via Natural or Artificial Opening Endoscopic	Y Other Device Z No Device	E Nervous System F Cardiovascular System G Lymphatics and Hemic H Eye J Ear, Nose and Sinus K Respiratory System L Mouth and Throat M Gastrointestinal System N Hepatobiliary and Pancreas P Endocrine System Q Skin **Continued on Next Page ▶**

			Continued from ◀ Previous Page
			R Musculoskeletal System
			S Urinary System
			T Female Reproductive System
			V Male Reproductive System
			Y Other Body System

Section	1	Obstetrics	
Body System	0	Pregnancy	
Operation	S	Reposition: Moving to its normal location, or other suitable location, all or a portion of a body part	

Body Part (Character 4)	Approach (Character 5)	Device (Character 6)	Qualifier (Character 7)
0 Products of Conception	7 Via Natural or Artificial Opening X External	Z No Device	Z No Qualifier
2 Products of Conception, Ectopic	0 Open 3 Percutaneous 4 Percutaneous Endoscopic 7 Via Natural or Artificial Opening 8 Via Natural or Artificial Opening Endoscopic	Z No Device	Z No Qualifier

Section	1	Obstetrics	
Body System	0	Pregnancy	
Operation	T	Resection: Cutting out or off, without replacement, all of a body part	

Body Part (Character 4)	Approach (Character 5)	Device (Character 6)	Qualifier (Character 7)
2 Products of Conception, Ectopic	0 Open 3 Percutaneous 4 Percutaneous Endoscopic 7 Via Natural or Artificial Opening 8 Via Natural or Artificial Opening Endoscopic	Z No Device	Z No Qualifier

Section	1	Obstetrics	
Body System	0	Pregnancy	
Operation	Y	Transplantation: Putting in or on all or a portion of a living body part taken from another individual or animal to physically take the place and/or function of all or a portion of a similar body part	

Body Part (Character 4)	Approach (Character 5)	Device (Character 6)	Qualifier (Character 7)
0 Products of Conception	3 Percutaneous 4 Percutaneous Endoscopic 7 Via Natural or Artificial Opening	Z No Device	E Nervous System F Cardiovascular System G Lymphatics and Hemic H Eye J Ear, Nose and Sinus K Respiratory System L Mouth and Throat M Gastrointestinal System

Continued on Next Page ▶

			Continued from ◀ Previous Page
			N Hepatobiliary and Pancreas **P** Endocrine System **Q** Skin **R** Musculoskeletal System **S** Urinary System **T** Female Reproductive System **V** Male Reproductive System **Y** Other Body System

Section	2	Placement
Body System	W	Anatomical Regions
Operation	0	Change: Taking out or off a device from a body part and putting back an identical or similar device in or on the same body part without cutting or puncturing the skin or a mucous membrane

Body Region (Character 4)	Approach (Character 5)	Device (Character 6)	Qualifier (Character 7)
0 Head	X External	0 Traction Apparatus	Z No Qualifier
2 Neck		1 Splint	
3 Abdominal Wall		2 Cast	
4 Chest Wall		3 Brace	
5 Back		4 Bandage	
6 Inguinal Region, Right		5 Packing Material	
7 Inguinal Region, Left		6 Pressure Dressing	
8 Upper Extremity, Right		7 Intermittent Pressure Device	
9 Upper Extremity, Left		Y Other Device	
A Upper Arm, Right			
B Upper Arm, Left			
C Lower Arm, Right			
D Lower Arm, Left			
E Hand, Right			
F Hand, Left			
G Thumb, Right			
H Thumb, Left			
J Finger, Right			
K Finger, Left			
L Lower Extremity, Right			
M Lower Extremity, Left			
N Upper Leg, Right			
P Upper Leg, Left			
Q Lower Leg, Right			
R Lower Leg, Left			
S Foot, Right			
T Foot, Left			
U Toe, Right			
V Toe, Left			
1 Face	X External	0 Traction Apparatus	Z No Qualifier
		1 Splint	
		2 Cast	
		3 Brace	
		4 Bandage	
		5 Packing Material	
		6 Pressure Dressing	
		7 Intermittent Pressure Device	
		9 Wire	
		Y Other Device	

Section	2	Placement		
Body System	W	Anatomical Regions		
Operation	1	Compression: Putting pressure on a body region		

Body Region (Character 4)	Approach (Character 5)	Device (Character 6)	Qualifier (Character 7)
0 Head	X External	6 Pressure Dressing	Z No Qualifier
1 Face		7 Intermittent Pressure Device	
2 Neck			
3 Abdominal Wall			
4 Chest Wall			
5 Back			
6 Inguinal Region, Right			
7 Inguinal Region, Left			
8 Upper Extremity, Right			
9 Upper Extremity, Left			
A Upper Arm, Right			
B Upper Arm, Left			
C Lower Arm, Right			
D Lower Arm, Left			
E Hand, Right			
F Hand, Left			
G Thumb, Right			
H Thumb, Left			
J Finger, Right			
K Finger, Left			
L Lower Extremity, Right			
M Lower Extremity, Left			
N Upper Leg, Right			
P Upper Leg, Left			
Q Lower Leg, Right			
R Lower Leg, Left			
S Foot, Right			
T Foot, Left			
U Toe, Right			
V Toe, Left			

Section	2	Placement		
Body System	W	Anatomical Regions		
Operation	2	Dressing: Putting material on a body region for protection		

Body Region (Character 4)	Approach (Character 5)	Device (Character 6)	Qualifier (Character 7)
0 Head	X External	4 Bandage	Z No Qualifier
1 Face			
2 Neck			
3 Abdominal Wall			
4 Chest Wall			
5 Back			
6 Inguinal Region, Right			
7 Inguinal Region, Left			
8 Upper Extremity, Right			
9 Upper Extremity, Left			
A Upper Arm, Right			
B Upper Arm, Left			
C Lower Arm, Right			
D Lower Arm, Left			
E Hand, Right			

Continued on Next Page ▶

F Hand, Left			**Continued from** ◀ **Previous Page**
G Thumb, Right			
H Thumb, Left			
J Finger, Right			
K Finger, Left			
L Lower Extremity, Right			
M Lower Extremity, Left			
N Upper Leg, Right			
P Upper Leg, Left			
Q Lower Leg, Right			
R Lower Leg, Left			
S Foot, Right			
T Foot, Left			
U Toe, Right			
V Toe, Left			

Section	2	Placement	
Body System	W	Anatomical Regions	
Operation	3	Immobilization: Limiting or preventing motion of a body region	

Body Region (Character 4)	Approach (Character 5)	Device (Character 6)	Qualifier (Character 7)
0 Head	X External	1 Splint	Z No Qualifier
2 Neck		2 Cast	
3 Abdominal Wall		3 Brace	
4 Chest Wall		Y Other Device	
5 Back			
6 Inguinal Region, Right			
7 Inguinal Region, Left			
8 Upper Extremity, Right			
9 Upper Extremity, Left			
A Upper Arm, Right			
B Upper Arm, Left			
C Lower Arm, Right			
D Lower Arm, Left			
E Hand, Right			
F Hand, Left			
G Thumb, Right			
H Thumb, Left			
J Finger, Right			
K Finger, Left			
L Lower Extremity, Right			
M Lower Extremity, Left			
N Upper Leg, Right			
P Upper Leg, Left			
Q Lower Leg, Right			
R Lower Leg, Left			
S Foot, Right			
T Foot, Left			
U Toe, Right			
V Toe, Left			
1 Face	X External	1 Splint	Z No Qualifier
		2 Cast	
		3 Brace	
		9 Wire	
		Y Other Device	

Section	2	Placement		
Body System	W	Anatomical Regions		
Operation	4	Packing: Putting material in a body region or orifice		

Body Region (Character 4)	Approach (Character 5)	Device (Character 6)	Qualifier (Character 7)
0 Head	X External	5 Packing Material	Z No Qualifier
1 Face			
2 Neck			
3 Abdominal Wall			
4 Chest Wall			
5 Back			
6 Inguinal Region, Right			
7 Inguinal Region, Left			
8 Upper Extremity, Right			
9 Upper Extremity, Left			
A Upper Arm, Right			
B Upper Arm, Left			
C Lower Arm, Right			
D Lower Arm, Left			
E Hand, Right			
F Hand, Left			
G Thumb, Right			
H Thumb, Left			
J Finger, Right			
K Finger, Left			
L Lower Extremity, Right			
M Lower Extremity, Left			
N Upper Leg, Right			
P Upper Leg, Left			
Q Lower Leg, Right			
R Lower Leg, Left			
S Foot, Right			
T Foot, Left			
U Toe, Right			
V Toe, Left			

Section	2	Placement		
Body System	W	Anatomical Regions		
Operation	5	Removal: Taking out or off a device from a body part		

Body Region (Character 4)	Approach (Character 5)	Device (Character 6)	Qualifier (Character 7)
0 Head	X External	0 Traction Apparatus	Z No Qualifier
2 Neck		1 Splint	
3 Abdominal Wall		2 Cast	
4 Chest Wall		3 Brace	
5 Back		4 Bandage	
6 Inguinal Region, Right		5 Packing Material	
7 Inguinal Region, Left		6 Pressure Dressing	
8 Upper Extremity, Right		7 Intermittent Pressure Device	
9 Upper Extremity, Left		Y Other Device	
A Upper Arm, Right			
B Upper Arm, Left			
C Lower Arm, Right			
D Lower Arm, Left			
E Hand, Right			
F Hand, Left			**Continued on Next Page ▶**

G Thumb, Right H Thumb, Left J Finger, Right K Finger, Left L Lower Extremity, Right M Lower Extremity, Left N Upper Leg, Right P Upper Leg, Left Q Lower Leg, Right R Lower Leg, Left S Foot, Right T Foot, Left U Toe, Right V Toe, Left			**Continued from** ◀ **Previous Page**
1 Face	X External	0 Traction Apparatus 1 Splint 2 Cast 3 Brace 4 Bandage 5 Packing Material 6 Pressure Dressing 7 Intermittent Pressure Device 9 Wire Y Other Device	Z No Qualifier

Section	2	Placement	
Body System	W	Anatomical Regions	
Operation	6	Traction: Exerting a pulling force on a body region in a distal direction	

Body Region (Character 4)	Approach (Character 5)	Device (Character 6)	Qualifier (Character 7)
0 Head 1 Face 2 Neck 3 Abdominal Wall 4 Chest Wall 5 Back 6 Inguinal Region, Right 7 Inguinal Region, Left 8 Upper Extremity, Right 9 Upper Extremity, Left A Upper Arm, Right B Upper Arm, Left C Lower Arm, Right D Lower Arm, Left E Hand, Right F Hand, Left G Thumb, Right H Thumb, Left J Finger, Right K Finger, Left L Lower Extremity, Right M Lower Extremity, Left N Upper Leg, Right P Upper Leg, Left	X External	0 Traction Apparatus Z No Device	Z No Qualifier **Continued on** **Next Page** ▶

Q Lower Leg, Right **R** Lower Leg, Left **S** Foot, Right **T** Foot, Left **U** Toe, Right **V** Toe, Left			Continued from ◀ Previous Page

Section	2	Placement	
Body System	Y	Anatomical Orifices	
Operation	0	Change: Taking out or off a device from a body part and putting back an identical or similar device in or on the same body part without cutting or puncturing the skin or a mucous membrane	

Body Region (Character 4)	Approach (Character 5)	Device (Character 6)	Qualifier (Character 7)
0 Mouth and Pharynx **1** Nasal **2** Ear **3** Anorectal **4** Female Genital Tract **5** Urethra	**X** External	**5** Packing Material	**Z** No Qualifier

Section	2	Placement	
Body System	Y	Anatomical Orifices	
Operation	4	Packing: Putting material in a body region or orifice	

Body Region (Character 4)	Approach (Character 5)	Device (Character 6)	Qualifier (Character 7)
0 Mouth and Pharynx **1** Nasal **2** Ear **3** Anorectal **4** Female Genital Tract **5** Urethra	**X** External	**5** Packing Material	**Z** No Qualifier

Section	2	Placement	
Body System	Y	Anatomical Orifices	
Operation	5	Removal: Taking out or off a device from a body part	

Body Region (Character 4)	Approach (Character 5)	Device (Character 6)	Qualifier (Character 7)
0 Mouth and Pharynx **1** Nasal **2** Ear **3** Anorectal **4** Female Genital Tract **5** Urethra	**X** External	**5** Packing Material	**Z** No Qualifier

Section	3	Administration
Body System	0	Circulatory
Operation	2	Transfusion: Putting in blood or blood products

Body System/Region (Character 4)	Approach (Character 5)	Substance (Character 6)	Qualifier (Character 7)
3 Peripheral Vein 4 Central Vein	0 Open 3 Percutaneous	A Stem Cells, Embryonic	Z No Qualifier
3 Peripheral Vein 4 Central Vein	0 Open 3 Percutaneous	G Bone Marrow X Stem Cells, Cord Blood Y Stem Cells, Hematopoietic	0 Autologous 2 Allogeneic, Related 3 Allogeneic, Unrelated 4 Allogeneic, Unspecified
3 Peripheral Vein 4 Central Vein	0 Open 3 Percutaneous	H Whole Blood J Serum Albumin K Frozen Plasma L Fresh Plasma M Plasma Cryoprecipitate N Red Blood Cells P Frozen Red Cells Q White Cells R Platelets S Globulin T Fibrinogen V Antihemophilic Factors W Factor IX	0 Autologous 1 Nonautologous
5 Peripheral Artery 6 Central Artery	0 Open 3 Percutaneous	G Bone Marrow H Whole Blood J Serum Albumin K Frozen Plasma L Fresh Plasma M Plasma Cryoprecipitate N Red Blood Cells P Frozen Red Cells Q White Cells R Platelets S Globulin T Fibrinogen V Antihemophilic Factors W Factor IX X Stem Cells, Cord Blood Y Stem Cells, Hematopoietic	0 Autologous 1 Nonautologous
7 Products of Conception, Circulatory	3 Percutaneous 7 Via Natural or Artificial Opening	H Whole Blood J Serum Albumin K Frozen Plasma L Fresh Plasma M Plasma Cryoprecipitate N Red Blood Cells P Frozen Red Cells Q White Cells R Platelets S Globulin T Fibrinogen V Antihemophilic Factors W Factor IX	1 Nonautologous
8 Vein	0 Open 3 Percutaneous	B 4-Factor Prothrombin Complex Concentrate	1 Nonautologous

509

Section	3	Administration		
Body System	C	Indwelling Device		
Operation	1	Irrigation: Putting in or on a cleansing substance		

Body System/Region (Character 4)	Approach (Character 5)	Substance (Character 6)	Qualifier (Character 7)
Z None	X External	8 Irrigating Substance	Z No Qualifier

Section	3	Administration		
Body System	E	Physiological Systems and Anatomical Regions		
Operation	0	Introduction: Putting in or on a therapeutic, diagnostic, nutritional, physiological, or prophylactic substance except blood or blood products		

Body System/Region (Character 4)	Approach (Character 5)	Substance (Character 6)	Qualifier (Character 7)
0 Skin and Mucous Membranes	X External	0 Antineoplastic	5 Other Antineoplastic M Monoclonal Antibody
0 Skin and Mucous Membranes	X External	2 Anti-infective	8 Oxazolidinones 9 Other Anti-infective
0 Skin and Mucous Membranes	X External	3 Anti-inflammatory 4 Serum, Toxoid and Vaccine B Local Anesthetic K Other Diagnostic Substance M Pigment N Analgesics, Hypnotics, Sedatives T Destructive Agent	Z No Qualifier
0 Skin and Mucous Membranes	X External	G Other Therapeutic Substance	C Other Substance
1 Subcutaneous Tissue	0 Open	2 Anti-infective	A Anti-Infective Envelope
1 Subcutaneous Tissue	3 Percutaneous	0 Antineoplastic	5 Other Antineoplastic M Monoclonal Antibody
1 Subcutaneous Tissue	3 Percutaneous	2 Anti-infective	8 Oxazolidinones 9 Other Anti-infective A Anti-Infective Envelope
1 Subcutaneous Tissue	3 Percutaneous	3 Anti-inflammatory 4 Serum, Toxoid and Vaccine 6 Nutritional Substance 7 Electrolytic and Water Balance Substance B Local Anesthetic H Radioactive Substance K Other Diagnostic Substance N Analgesics, Hypnotics, Sedatives T Destructive Agent	Z No Qualifier
1 Subcutaneous Tissue	3 Percutaneous	G Other Therapeutic Substance	C Other Substance
1 Subcutaneous Tissue	3 Percutaneous	V Hormone	G Insulin J Other Hormone
2 Muscle	3 Percutaneous	0 Antineoplastic	5 Other Antineoplastic M Monoclonal Antibody
2 Muscle	3 Percutaneous	2 Anti-infective	8 Oxazolidinones 9 Other Anti-infective

Continued on Next Page ▶

			Continued from ◀ Previous Page
2 Muscle	**3** Percutaneous	**3** Anti-inflammatory **4** Serum, Toxoid and Vaccine **6** Nutritional Substance **7** Electrolytic and Water Balance Substance **B** Local Anesthetic **H** Radioactive Substance **K** Other Diagnostic Substance **N** Analgesics, Hypnotics, Sedatives **T** Destructive Agent	**Z** No Qualifier
2 Muscle	**3** Percutaneous	**G** Other Therapeutic Substance	**C** Other Substance
3 Peripheral Vein	**0** Open	**0** Antineoplastic	**2** High-dose Interleukin-2 **3** Low-dose Interleukin-2 **5** Other Antineoplastic **M** Monoclonal Antibody **P** Clofarabine
3 Peripheral Vein	**0** Open	**1** Thrombolytic	**6** Recombinant Human-activated Protein C **7** Other Thrombolytic
3 Peripheral Vein	**0** Open	**2** Anti-infective	**8** Oxazolidinones **9** Other Anti-infective
3 Peripheral Vein	**0** Open	**3** Anti-inflammatory **4** Serum, Toxoid and Vaccine **6** Nutritional Substance **7** Electrolytic and Water Balance Substance **F** Intracirculatory Anesthetic **H** Radioactive Substance **K** Other Diagnostic Substance **N** Analgesics, Hypnotics, Sedatives **P** Platelet Inhibitor **R** Antiarrhythmic **T** Destructive Agent **X** Vasopressor	**Z** No Qualifier
3 Peripheral Vein	**0** Open	**G** Other Therapeutic Substance	**C** Other Substance **N** Blood Brain Barrier Disruption
3 Peripheral Vein	**0** Open	**U** Pancreatic Islet Cells	**0** Autologous **1** Nonautologous
3 Peripheral Vein	**0** Open	**V** Hormone	**G** Insulin **H** Human B-Type Natriuretic Peptide **J** Other Hormone

Continued on Next Page ▶

			Continued from ◄ Previous Page
3 Peripheral Vein	**0** Open	**W** Immunotherapeutic	**K** Immunostimulator **L** Immunosuppressive
3 Peripheral Vein	**3** Percutaneous	**0** Antineoplastic	**2** High-dose Interleukin-2 **3** Low-dose Interleukin-2 **5** Other Antineoplastic **M** Monoclonal Antibody **P** Clofarabine
3 Peripheral Vein	**3** Percutaneous	**1** Thrombolytic	**6** Recombinant Human-activated Protein C **7** Other Thrombolytic
3 Peripheral Vein	**3** Percutaneous	**2** Anti-infective	**8** Oxazolidinones **9** Other Anti-infective
3 Vein	**3** Percutaneous	**3** Anti-inflammatory **4** Serum, Toxoid and Vaccine **6** Nutritional Substance **7** Electrolytic and Water Balance Substance **F** Intracirculatory Anesthetic **H** Radioactive Substance **K** Other Diagnostic Substance **N** Analgesics, Hypnotics, Sedatives **P** Platelet Inhibitor **R** Antiarrhythmic **T** Destructive Agent **X** Vasopressor	**Z** No Qualifier
3 Peripheral Vein	**3** Percutaneous	**G** Other Therapeutic Substance	**C** Other Substance **N** Blood Brain Barrier Disruption **Q** Glucarpidase
3 Peripheral Vein	**3** Percutaneous	**U** Pancreatic Islet Cells	**0** Autologous **1** Nonautologous
3 Peripheral Vein	**3** Percutaneous	**V** Hormone	**G** Insulin **H** Human B-Type Natriuretic Peptide **J** Other Hormone
3 Peripheral Vein	**3** Percutaneous	**W** Immunotherapeutic	**K** Immunostimulator **L** Immunosuppressive
4 Central Vein	**0** Open	**0** Antineoplastic	**2** High-dose Interleukin-2 **3** Low-dose Interleukin-2 **5** Other Antineoplastic **M** Monoclonal Antibody **P** Clofarabine
4 Central Vein	**0** Open	**1** Thrombolytic	**6** Recombinant Human-activated Protein C **7** Other Thrombolytic

Continued on Next Page ▶

			Continued from ◄ Previous Page
4 Central Vein	**0** Open	**2** Anti-infective	**8** Oxazolidinones **9** Other Anti-infective
4 Central Vein	**0** Open	**3** Anti-inflammatory **4** Serum, Toxoid and Vaccine **6** Nutritional Substance **7** Electrolytic and Water Balance Substance **F** Intracirculatory Anesthetic **H** Radioactive Substance **K** Other Diagnostic Substance **N** Analgesics, Hypnotics, Sedatives **P** Platelet Inhibitor **R** Antiarrhythmic **T** Destructive Agent **X** Vasopressor	**Z** No Qualifier
4 Central Vein	**0** Open	**G** Other Therapeutic Substance	**C** Other Substance **N** Blood Brain Barrier Disruption
4 Central Vein	**0** Open	**V** Hormone	**G** Insulin **H** Human B-Type Natriuretic Peptide **J** Other Hormone
4 Central Vein	**0** Open	**W** Immunotherapeutic	**K** Immunostimulator **L** Immunosuppressive
4 Central Vein	**3** Percutaneous	**0** Antineoplastic	**2** High-dose Interleukin-2 **3** Low-dose Interleukin-2 **5** Other Antineoplastic **M** Monoclonal Antibody **P** Clofarabine
4 Central Vein	**3** Percutaneous	**1** Thrombolytic	**6** Recombinant Human-activated Protein C **7** Other Thrombolytic
4 Central Vein	**3** Percutaneous	**2** Anti-infective	**8** Oxazolidinones **9** Other Anti-infective
4 Central Vein	**3** Percutaneous	**3** Anti-inflammatory **4** Serum, Toxoid and Vaccine **6** Nutritional Substance **7** Electrolytic and Water Balance Substance **F** Intracirculatory Anesthetic **H** Radioactive Substance **K** Other Diagnostic Substance **N** Analgesics, Hypnotics, Sedatives **P** Platelet Inhibitor **R** Antiarrhythmic **T** Destructive Agent **X** Vasopressor	**Z** No Qualifier Continued on Next Page ▶

			Continued from ◀ Previous Page
4 Central Vein	3 Percutaneous	G Other Therapeutic Substance	C Other Substance N Blood Brain Barrier Disruption Q Glucarpidase
4 Central Vein	3 Percutaneous	V Hormone	G Insulin H Human B- Type Natriuretic Peptide J Other Hormone
4 Central Vein	3 Percutaneous	W Immunotherapeutic	K Immunostimulator L Immunosuppressive
5 Peripheral Artery 6 Central Artery	0 Open 3 Percutaneous	0 Antineoplastic	2 High-dose Interleukin-2 3 Low-dose Interleukin-2 5 Other Antineoplastic M Monoclonal Antibody P Clofarabine
5 Peripheral Artery 6 Central Artery	0 Open 3 Percutaneous	1 Thrombolytic	6 Recombinant Human- activated Protein C 7 Other Thrombolytic
5 Peripheral Artery 6 Central Artery	0 Open 3 Percutaneous	2 Anti-infective	8 Oxazolidinones 9 Other Anti-infective
5 Peripheral Artery 6 Central Artery	0 Open 3 Percutaneous	3 Anti-inflammatory 4 Serum, Toxoid and Vaccine 6 Nutritional Substance 7 Electrolytic and Water Balance Substance F Intracirculatory Anesthetic H Radioactive Substance K Other Diagnostic Substance N Analgesics, Hypnotics, Sedatives P Platelet Inhibitor R Antiarrhythmic T Destructive Agent X Vasopressor	Z No Qualifier
5 Peripheral Artery 6 Central Artery	0 Open 3 Percutaneous	G Other Therapeutic Substance	C Other Substance N Blood Brain Barrier Disruption
5 Peripheral Artery 6 Central Artery	0 Open 3 Percutaneous	V Hormone	G Insulin H Human B- Type Natriuretic Peptide J Other Hormone
5 Peripheral Artery 6 Central Artery	0 Open 3 Percutaneous	W Immunotherapeutic	K Immunostimulator L Immunosuppressive
7 Coronary Artery 8 Heart	0 Open 3 Percutaneous	1 Thrombolytic	6 Recombinant Human- activated Protein C 7 Other Thrombolytic
7 Coronary Artery 8 Heart	0 Open 3 Percutaneous	G Other Therapeutic Substance	C Other Substance

Continued on
Next Page ▶

			Continued from ◀ Previous Page
7 Coronary Artery **8** Heart	**0** Open **3** Percutaneous	**K** Other Diagnostic Substance **P** Platelet Inhibitor	**Z** No Qualifier
9 Nose	**3** Percutaneous **7** Via Natural or Artificial Opening **X** External	**0** Antineoplastic	**5** Other Antineoplastic **M** Monoclonal Antibody
9 Nose	**3** Percutaneous **7** Via Natural or Artificial Opening **X** External	**2** Anti-infective	**8** Oxazolidinones **9** Other Anti-infective
9 Nose	**3** Percutaneous **7** Via Natural or Artificial Opening **X** External	**3** Anti-inflammatory **4** Serum, Toxoid and Vaccine **B** Local Anesthetic **H** Radioactive Substance **K** Other Diagnostic Substance **N** Analgesics, Hypnotics, Sedatives **T** Destructive Agent	**Z** No Qualifier
9 Nose	**3** Percutaneous **7** Via Natural or Artificial Opening **X** External	**G** Other Therapeutic Substance	**C** Other Substance
A Bone Marrow	**3** Percutaneous	**0** Antineoplastic	**5** Other Antineoplastic **M** Monoclonal Antibody
A Bone Marrow	**3** Percutaneous	**G** Other Therapeutic Substance	**C** Other Substance
B Ear	**3** Percutaneous **7** Via Natural or Artificial Opening **X** External	**0** Antineoplastic	**4** Liquid Brachytherapy Radioisotope **5** Other Antineoplastic **M** Monoclonal Antibody
B Ear	**3** Percutaneous **7** Via Natural or Artificial Opening **X** External	**2** Anti-infective	**8** Oxazolidinones **9** Other Anti-infective
B Ear	**3** Percutaneous **7** Via Natural or Artificial Opening **X** External	**3** Anti-inflammatory **B** Local Anesthetic **H** Radioactive Substance **K** Other Diagnostic Substance **N** Analgesics, Hypnotics, Sedatives **T** Destructive Agent	**Z** No Qualifier
B Ear	**3** Percutaneous **7** Via Natural or Artificial Opening **X** External	**G** Other Therapeutic Substance	**C** Other Substance
C Eye	**3** Percutaneous **7** Via Natural or Artificial Opening **X** External	**0** Antineoplastic	**4** Liquid Brachytherapy Radioisotope **5** Other Antineoplastic **Continued on Next Page ▶**

515

			Continued from ◀ Previous Page
			M Monoclonal Antibody
C Eye	**3** Percutaneous **7** Via Natural or Artificial Opening **X** External	**2** Anti-infective	**8** Oxazolidinones **9** Other Anti-infective
C Eye	**3** Percutaneous **7** Via Natural or Artificial Opening **X** External	**3** Anti-inflammatory **B** Local Anesthetic **H** Radioactive Substance **K** Other Diagnostic Substance **M** Pigment **N** Analgesics, Hypnotics, Sedatives **T** Destructive Agent	**Z** No Qualifier
C Eye	**3** Percutaneous **7** Via Natural or Artificial Opening **X** External	**G** Other Therapeutic Substance	**C** Other Substance
C Eye	**3** Percutaneous **7** Via Natural or Artificial Opening **X** External	**S** Gas	**F** Other Gas
D Mouth and Pharynx	**3** Percutaneous **7** Via Natural or Artificial Opening **X** External	**0** Antineoplastic	**4** Liquid Brachytherapy Radioisotope **5** Other Antineoplastic **M** Monoclonal Antibody
D Mouth and Pharynx	**3** Percutaneous **7** Via Natural or Artificial Opening **X** External	**2** Anti-infective	**8** Oxazolidinones **9** Other Anti-infective
D Mouth and Pharynx	**3** Percutaneous **7** Via Natural or Artificial Opening **X** External	**3** Anti-inflammatory **4** Serum, Toxoid and Vaccine **6** Nutritional Substance **7** Electrolytic and Water Balance Substance **B** Local Anesthetic **H** Radioactive Substance **K** Other Diagnostic Substance **N** Analgesics, Hypnotics, Sedatives **R** Antiarrhythmic **T** Destructive Agent	**Z** No Qualifier
D Mouth and Pharynx	**3** Percutaneous **7** Via Natural or Artificial Opening **X** External	**G** Other Therapeutic Substance	**C** Other Substance
E Products of Conception **G** Upper GI **H** Lower GI **K** Genitourinary Tract **N** Male Reproductive	**3** Percutaneous **7** Via Natural or Artificial Opening **8** Via Natural or Artificial Opening Endoscopic	**0** Antineoplastic	**4** Liquid Brachytherapy Radioisotope **5** Other Antineoplastic **M** Monoclonal Antibody **Continued on Next Page ▶**

			Continued from ◄ Previous Page
E Products of Conception G Upper GI H Lower GI K Genitourinary Tract N Male Reproductive	3 Percutaneous 7 Via Natural or Artificial Opening 8 Via Natural or Artificial Opening Endoscopic	2 Anti-infective	8 Oxazolidinones 9 Other Anti-infective
E Products of Conception G Upper GI H Lower GI K Genitourinary Tract N Male Reproductive	3 Percutaneous 7 Via Natural or Artificial Opening 8 Via Natural or Artificial Opening Endoscopic	3 Anti-inflammatory 6 Nutritional Substance 7 Electrolytic and Water Balance Substance B Local Anesthetic H Radioactive Substance K Other Diagnostic Substance N Analgesics, Hypnotics, Sedatives T Destructive Agent	Z No Qualifier
E Products of Conception G Upper GI H Lower GI K Genitourinary Tract N Male Reproductive	3 Percutaneous 7 Via Natural or Artificial Opening 8 Via Natural or Artificial Opening Endoscopic	G Other Therapeutic Substance	C Other Substance
E Products of Conception G Upper GI H Lower GI K Genitourinary Tract N Male Reproductive	3 Percutaneous 7 Via Natural or Artificial Opening 8 Via Natural or Artificial Opening Endoscopic	S Gas	F Other Gas
F Respiratory Tract	3 Percutaneous	0 Antineoplastic	4 Liquid Brachytherapy Radioisotope 5 Other Antineoplastic M Monoclonal Antibody
F Respiratory Tract	3 Percutaneous	2 Anti-infective	8 Oxazolidinones 9 Other Anti-infective
F Respiratory Tract	3 Percutaneous	3 Anti-inflammatory 6 Nutritional Substance 7 Electrolytic and Water Balance Substance B Local Anesthetic H Radioactive Substance K Other Diagnostic Substance N Analgesics, Hypnotics, Sedatives T Destructive Agent	Z No Qualifier
F Respiratory Tract	3 Percutaneous	G Other Therapeutic Substance	C Other Substance
F Respiratory Tract	3 Percutaneous	S Gas	D Nitric Oxide F Other Gas
F Respiratory Tract	7 Via Natural or Artificial Opening 8 Via Natural or Artificial Opening Endoscopic	0 Antineoplastic	4 Liquid Brachytherapy Radioisotope 5 Other Antineoplastic M Monoclonal Antibody
			Continued on Next Page ►

			Continued from ◀ Previous Page
F Respiratory Tract	**7** Via Natural or Artificial Opening **8** Via Natural or Artificial Opening Endoscopic	**2** Anti-infective	**8** Oxazolidinones **9** Other Anti-infective
F Respiratory Tract	**7** Via Natural or Artificial Opening **8** Via Natural or Artificial Opening Endoscopic	**3** Anti-inflammatory **6** Nutritional Substance **7** Electrolytic and Water Balance Substance **B** Local Anesthetic **D** Inhalation Anesthetic **H** Radioactive Substance **K** Other Diagnostic Substance **N** Analgesics, Hypnotics, Sedatives **T** Destructive Agent	**Z** No Qualifier
F Respiratory Tract	**7** Via Natural or Artificial Opening **8** Via Natural or Artificial Opening Endoscopic	**G** Other Therapeutic Substance	**C** Other Substance
F Respiratory Tract	**7** Via Natural or Artificial Opening **8** Via Natural or Artificial Opening Endoscopic	**S** Gas	**D** Nitric Oxide **F** Other Gas
J Biliary and Pancreatic Tract	**3** Percutaneous **7** Via Natural or Artificial Opening **8** Via Natural or Artificial Opening Endoscopic	**0** Antineoplastic	**4** Liquid Brachytherapy Radioisotope **5** Other Antineoplastic **M** Monoclonal Antibody
J Biliary and Pancreatic Tract	**3** Percutaneous **7** Via Natural or Artificial Opening **8** Via Natural or Artificial Opening Endoscopic	**2** Anti-infective	**8** Oxazolidinones **9** Other Anti-infective
J Biliary and Pancreatic Tract	**3** Percutaneous **7** Via Natural or Artificial Opening **8** Via Natural or Artificial Opening Endoscopic	**3** Anti-inflammatory **6** Nutritional Substance **7** Electrolytic and Water Balance Substance **B** Local Anesthetic **H** Radioactive Substance **K** Other Diagnostic Substance **N** Analgesics, Hypnotics, Sedatives **T** Destructive Agent	**Z** No Qualifier
J Biliary and Pancreatic Tract	**3** Percutaneous **7** Via Natural or Artificial Opening **8** Via Natural or Artificial Opening Endoscopic	**G** Other Therapeutic Substance	**C** Other Substance
J Biliary and Pancreatic Tract	**3** Percutaneous **7** Via Natural or Artificial Opening **8** Via Natural or Artificial Opening Endoscopic	**S** Gas	**F** Other Gas

Continued on Next Page ▶

			Continued from ◀ Previous Page
J Biliary and Pancreatic Tract	**3** Percutaneous **7** Via Natural or Artificial Opening **8** Via Natural or Artificial Opening Endoscopic	**U** Pancreatic Islet Cells	**0** Autologous **1** Nonautologous
L Pleural Cavity **M** Peritoneal Cavity	**0** Open	**5** Adhesion Barrier	**Z** No Qualifier
L Pleural Cavity **M** Peritoneal Cavity	**3** Percutaneous	**0** Antineoplastic	**4** Liquid Brachytherapy Radioisotope **5** Other Antineoplastic **M** Monoclonal Antibody
L Pleural Cavity **M** Peritoneal Cavity	**3** Percutaneous	**2** Anti-infective	**8** Oxazolidinones **9** Other Anti-infective
L Pleural Cavity **M** Peritoneal Cavity	**3** Percutaneous	**3** Anti-inflammatory **6** Nutritional Substance **7** Electrolytic and Water Balance Substance **B** Local Anesthetic **H** Radioactive Substance **K** Other Diagnostic Substance **N** Analgesics, Hypnotics, Sedatives **T** Destructive Agent	**Z** No Qualifier
L Pleural Cavity **M** Peritoneal Cavity	**3** Percutaneous	**G** Other Therapeutic Substance	**C** Other Substance
L Pleural Cavity **M** Peritoneal Cavity	**3** Percutaneous	**S** Gas	**F** Other Gas
L Pleural Cavity **M** Peritoneal Cavity	**7** Via Natural or Artificial Opening	**0** Antineoplastic	**4** Liquid Brachytherapy Radioisotope **5** Other Antineoplastic **M** Monoclonal Antibody
L Pleural Cavity **M** Peritoneal Cavity	**7** Via Natural or Artificial Opening	**S** Gas	**F** Other Gas
P Female Reproductive	**0** Open	**5** Adhesion Barrier	**Z** No Qualifier
P Female Reproductive	**3** Percutaneous **7** Via Natural or Artificial Opening	**0** Antineoplastic	**4** Liquid Brachytherapy Radioisotope **5** Other Antineoplastic **M** Monoclonal Antibody
P Female Reproductive	**3** Percutaneous **7** Via Natural or Artificial Opening	**2** Anti-infective	**8** Oxazolidinones **9** Other Anti-infective
P Female Reproductive	**3** Percutaneous **7** Via Natural or Artificial Opening	**3** Anti-inflammatory **6** Nutritional Substance **7** Electrolytic and Water Balance Substance **B** Local Anesthetic **H** Radioactive Substance **K** Other Diagnostic Substance **L** Sperm **N** Analgesics, Hypnotics, Sedatives **T** Destructive Agent	**Z** No Qualifier

Continued on Next Page ▶

			Continued from ◀ Previous Page
P Female Reproductive	**3** Percutaneous **7** Via Natural or Artificial Opening	**G** Other Therapeutic Substance	**C** Other Substance
P Female Reproductive	**3** Percutaneous **7** Via Natural or Artificial Opening	**Q** Fertilized Ovum	**0** Autologous **1** Nonautologous
P Female Reproductive	**3** Percutaneous **7** Via Natural or Artificial Opening	**S** Gas	**F** Other Gas
P Female Reproductive	**8** Via Natural or Artificial Opening Endoscopic	**0** Antineoplastic	**4** Liquid Brachytherapy Radioisotope **5** Other Antineoplastic **M** Monoclonal Antibody
P Female Reproductive	**8** Via Natural or Artificial Opening Endoscopic	**2** Anti-infective	**8** Oxazolidinones **9** Other Anti-infective
P Female Reproductive	**8** Via Natural or Artificial Opening Endoscopic	**3** Anti-inflammatory **6** Nutritional Substance **7** Electrolytic and Water Balance Substance **B** Local Anesthetic **H** Radioactive Substance **K** Other Diagnostic Substance **N** Analgesics, Hypnotics, Sedatives **T** Destructive Agent	**Z** No Qualifier
P Female Reproductive	**8** Via Natural or Artificial Opening Endoscopic	**G** Other Therapeutic Substance	**C** Other Substance
P Female Reproductive	**8** Via Natural or Artificial Opening Endoscopic	**S** Gas	**F** Other Gas
Q Cranial Cavity and Brain	**0** Open **3** Percutaneous	**0** Antineoplastic	**4** Liquid Brachytherapy Radioisotope **5** Other Antineoplastic **M** Monoclonal Antibody
Q Cranial Cavity and Brain	**0** Open **3** Percutaneous	**2** Anti-infective	**8** Oxazolidinones **9** Other Anti-infective
Q Cranial Cavity and Brain	**0** Open **3** Percutaneous	**3** Anti-inflammatory **6** Nutritional Substance **7** Electrolytic and Water Balance Substance **A** Stem Cells, Embryonic **B** Local Anesthetic **H** Radioactive Substance **K** Other Diagnostic Substance **N** Analgesics, Hypnotics, Sedatives **T** Destructive Agent	**Z** No Qualifier
Q Cranial Cavity and Brain	**0** Open **3** Percutaneous	**E** Stem Cells, Somatic	**0** Autologous **1** Nonautologous
Q Cranial Cavity and Brain	**0** Open **3** Percutaneous	**G** Other Therapeutic Substance	**C** Other Substance

Continued on Next Page ▶

			Continued from ◀ Previous Page
Q Cranial Cavity and Brain	**0** Open **3** Percutaneous	**S** Gas	**F** Other Gas
Q Cranial Cavity and Brain	**7** Via Natural or Artificial Opening	**0** Antineoplastic	**4** Liquid Brachytherapy Radioisotope **5** Other Antineoplastic **M** Monoclonal Antibody
Q Cranial Cavity and Brain	**7** Via Natural or Artificial Opening	**S** Gas	**F** Other Gas
R Spinal Canal	**0** Open	**A** Stem Cells, Embryonic	**Z** No Qualifier
R Spinal Canal	**0** Open	**E** Stem Cells, Somatic	**0** Autologous **1** Nonautologous
R Spinal Canal	**3** Percutaneous	**0** Antineoplastic	**2** High-dose Interleukin-2 **3** Low-dose Interleukin-2 **4** Liquid Brachytherapy Radioisotope **5** Other Antineoplastic **M** Monoclonal Antibody
R Spinal Canal	**3** Percutaneous	**2** Anti-infective	**8** Oxazolidinones **9** Other Anti-infective
R Spinal Canal	**3** Percutaneous	**3** Anti-inflammatory **6** Nutritional Substance **7** Electrolytic and Water Balance Substance **A** Stem Cells, Embryonic **B** Local Anesthetic **C** Regional Anesthetic **H** Radioactive Substance **K** Other Diagnostic Substance **N** Analgesics, Hypnotics, Sedatives **T** Destructive Agent	**Z** No Qualifier
R Spinal Canal	**3** Percutaneous	**E** Stem Cells, Somatic	**0** Autologous **1** Nonautologous
R Spinal Canal	**3** Percutaneous	**G** Other Therapeutic Substance	**C** Other Substance
R Spinal Canal	**3** Percutaneous	**S** Gas	**F** Other Gas
R Spinal Canal	**7** Via Natural or Artificial Opening	**S** Gas	**F** Other Gas
S Epidural Space	**3** Percutaneous	**0** Antineoplastic	**2** High-dose Interleukin-2 **3** Low-dose Interleukin-2 **4** Liquid Brachytherapy Radioisotope **5** Other Antineoplastic **M** Monoclonal Antibody
S Epidural Space	**3** Percutaneous	**2** Anti-infective	**8** Oxazolidinones **9** Other Anti-infective
S Epidural Space	**3** Percutaneous	**3** Anti-inflammatory **6** Nutritional Substance **7** Electrolytic and Water Balance Substance **B** Local Anesthetic **C** Regional Anesthetic	**Z** No Qualifier

Continued on Next Page ▶

		H Radioactive Substance K Other Diagnostic Substance N Analgesics, Hypnotics, Sedatives T Destructive Agent	Continued from ◀ Previous Page
S Epidural Space	**3** Percutaneous	**G** Other Therapeutic Substance	**C** Other Substance
S Epidural Space	**3** Percutaneous	**S** Gas	**F** Other Gas
S Epidural Space	**7** Via Natural or Artificial Opening	**S** Gas	**F** Other Gas
T Peripheral Nerves and Plexi **X** Cranial Nerves	**3** Percutaneous	**3** Anti-inflammatory **B** Local Anesthetic **C** Regional Anesthetic **T** Destructive Agent	**Z** No Qualifier
T Peripheral Nerves and Plexi **X** Cranial Nerves	**3** Percutaneous	**G** Other Therapeutic Substance	**C** Other Substance
U Joints	**0** Open	**2** Anti-infective	**8** Oxazolidinones **9** Other Anti-infective
U Joints	**0** Open	**G** Other Therapeutic Substance	**B** Recombinant Bone Morphogenetic Protein
U Joints	**3** Percutaneous	**0** Antineoplastic	**4** Liquid Brachytherapy Radioisotope **5** Other Antineoplastic **M** Monoclonal Antibody
U Joints	**3** Percutaneous	**2** Anti-infective	**8** Oxazolidinones **9** Other Anti-infective
U Joints	**3** Percutaneous	**3** Anti-inflammatory **6** Nutritional Substance **7** Electrolytic and Water Balance Substance **B** Local Anesthetic **H** Radioactive Substance **K** Other Diagnostic Substance **N** Analgesics, Hypnotics, Sedatives **T** Destructive Agent	**Z** No Qualifier
U Joints	**3** Percutaneous	**G** Other Therapeutic Substance	**B** Recombinant Bone Morphogenetic Protein **C** Other Substance
U Joints	**3** Percutaneous	**S** Gas	**F** Other Gas
V Bones	**0** Open	**G** Other Therapeutic Substance	**B** Recombinant Bone Morphogenetic Protein
V Bones	**3** Percutaneous	**0** Antineoplastic	**5** Other Antineoplastic **M** Monoclonal Antibody
V Bones	**3** Percutaneous	**2** Anti-infective	**8** Oxazolidinones **9** Other Anti-infective
V Bones	**3** Percutaneous	**3** Anti-inflammatory **6** Nutritional Substance **7** Electrolytic and Water Balance Substance **B** Local Anesthetic **H** Radioactive Substance	**Z** No Qualifier

Continued on Next Page ▶

		K Other Diagnostic Substance N Analgesics, Hypnotics, Sedatives T Destructive Agent	Continued from ◀ Previous Page
V Bones	3 Percutaneous	G Other Therapeutic Substance	B Recombinant Bone Morphogenetic Protein C Other Substance
W Lymphatics	3 Percutaneous	0 Antineoplastic	5 Other Antineoplastic M Monoclonal Antibody
W Lymphatics	3 Percutaneous	2 Anti-infective	8 Oxazolidinones 9 Other Anti-infective
W Lymphatics	3 Percutaneous	3 Anti-inflammatory 6 Nutritional Substance 7 Electrolytic and Water Balance Substance B Local Anesthetic H Radioactive Substance K Other Diagnostic Substance N Analgesics, Hypnotics, Sedatives T Destructive Agent	Z No Qualifier
W Lymphatics	3 Percutaneous	G Other Therapeutic Substance	C Other Substance
Y Pericardial Cavity	3 Percutaneous	0 Antineoplastic	4 Liquid Brachytherapy Radioisotope 5 Other Antineoplastic M Monoclonal Antibody
Y Pericardial Cavity	3 Percutaneous	2 Anti-infective	8 Oxazolidinones 9 Other Anti-infective
Y Pericardial Cavity	3 Percutaneous	3 Anti-inflammatory 6 Nutritional Substance 7 Electrolytic and Water Balance Substance B Local Anesthetic H Radioactive Substance K Other Diagnostic Substance N Analgesics, Hypnotics, Sedatives T Destructive Agent	Z No Qualifier
Y Pericardial Cavity	3 Percutaneous	G Other Therapeutic Substance	C Other Substance
Y Pericardial Cavity	3 Percutaneous	S Gas	F Other Gas
Y Pericardial Cavity	7 Via Natural or Artificial Opening	0 Antineoplastic	4 Liquid Brachytherapy Radioisotope 5 Other Antineoplastic M Monoclonal Antibody
Y Pericardial Cavity	7 Via Natural or Artificial Opening	S Gas	F Other Gas

Section	3	Administration		
Body System	E	Physiological Systems and Anatomical Regions		
Operation	1	Irrigation: Putting in or on a cleansing substance		

Body System/Region (Character 4)	Approach (Character 5)	Substance (Character 6)	Qualifier (Character 7)
0 Skin and Mucous Membranes **C** Eye	**3** Percutaneous **X** External	**8** Irrigating Substance	**X** Diagnostic **Z** No Qualifier
9 Nose **B** Ear **F** Respiratory Tract **G** Upper GI **H** Lower GI **J** Biliary and Pancreatic Tract **K** Genitourinary Tract **N** Male Reproductive **P** Female Reproductive	**3** Percutaneous **7** Via Natural or Artificial Opening **8** Via Natural or Artificial Opening Endoscopic	**8** Irrigating Substance	**X** Diagnostic **Z** No Qualifier
L Pleural Cavity **Q** Cranial Cavity and Brain **R** Spinal Canal **S** Epidural Space **U** Joints **Y** Pericardial Cavity	**3** Percutaneous	**8** Irrigating Substance	**X** Diagnostic **Z** No Qualifier
M Peritoneal Cavity	**3** Percutaneous	**8** Irrigating Substance	**X** Diagnostic **Z** No Qualifier
M Peritoneal Cavity	**3** Percutaneous	**9** Dialysate	**Z** No Qualifier

Section	4	Measurement and Monitoring
Body System	A	Physiological Systems
Operation	0	Measurement: Determining the level of a physiological or physical function at a point in time

Body System (Character 4)	Approach (Character 5)	Function/Device (Character 6)	Qualifier (Character 7)
0 Central Nervous	0 Open	2 Conductivity 4 Electrical Activity B Pressure	Z No Qualifier
0 Central Nervous	3 Percutaneous	4 Electrical Activity	Z No Qualifier
0 Central Nervous	3 Percutaneous	B Pressure K Temperature R Saturation	D Intracranial
0 Central Nervous	7 Via Natural or Artificial Opening	B Pressure K Temperature R Saturation	D Intracranial
0 Central Nervous	X External	2 Conductivity 4 Electrical Activity	Z No Qualifier
1 Peripheral Nervous	0 Open 3 Percutaneous X External	2 Conductivity	9 Sensory B Motor
1 Peripheral Nervous	0 Open 3 Percutaneous X External	4 Electrical Activity	Z No Qualifier
2 Cardiac	0 Open 3 Percutaneous	4 Electrical Activity 9 Output C Rate F Rhythm H Sound P Action Currents	Z No Qualifier
2 Cardiac	0 Open 3 Percutaneous	N Sampling and Pressure	6 Right Heart 7 Left Heart 8 Bilateral
2 Cardiac	X External	4 Electrical Activity	A Guidance Z No Qualifier
2 Cardiac	X External	9 Output C Rate F Rhythm H Sound P Action Currents	Z No Qualifier
2 Cardiac	X External	M Total Activity	4 Stress
3 Arterial	0 Open 3 Percutaneous	5 Flow J Pulse	1 Peripheral 3 Pulmonary C Coronary
3 Arterial	0 Open 3 Percutaneous	B Pressure	1 Peripheral 3 Pulmonary C Coronary F Other Thoracic
3 Arterial	0 Open 3 Percutaneous	H Sound R Saturation	1 Peripheral
3 Arterial	X External	5 Flow B Pressure H Sound J Pulse R Saturation	1 Peripheral

Continued on Next Page ▶

			Continued from ◀ Previous Page
4 Venous	**0** Open **3** Percutaneous	**5** Flow **B** Pressure **J** Pulse	**0** Central **1** Peripheral **2** Portal **3** Pulmonary
4 Venous	**0** Open **3** Percutaneous	**R** Saturation	**1** Peripheral
4 Venous	**X** External	**5** Flow **B** Pressure **J** Pulse **R** Saturation	**1** Peripheral
5 Circulatory	**X** External	**L** Volume	**Z** No Qualifier
6 Lymphatic	**0** Open **3** Percutaneous	**5** Flow **B** Pressure	**Z** No Qualifier
7 Visual	**X** External	**0** Acuity **7** Mobility **B** Pressure	**Z** No Qualifier
8 Olfactory	**X** External	**0** Acuity	**Z** No Qualifier
9 Respiratory	**7** Via Natural or Artificial Opening **8** Via Natural or Artificial Opening Endoscopic **X** External	**1** Capacity **5** Flow **C** Rate **D** Resistance **L** Volume **M** Total Activity	**Z** No Qualifier
B Gastrointestinal	**7** Via Natural or Artificial Opening **8** Via Natural or Artificial Opening Endoscopic	**8** Motility **B** Pressure **G** Secretion	**Z** No Qualifier
C Biliary	**3** Percutaneous **4** Percutaneous Endoscopic **7** Via Natural or Artificial Opening **8** Via Natural or Artificial Opening Endoscopic	**5** Flow **B** Pressure	**Z** No Qualifier
D Urinary	**7** Via Natural or Artificial Opening	**3** Contractility **5** Flow **B** Pressure **D** Resistance **L** Volume	**Z** No Qualifier
F Musculoskeletal	**3** Percutaneous **X** External	**3** Contractility	**Z** No Qualifier
H Products of Conception, Cardiac	**7** Via Natural or Artificial Opening **8** Via Natural or Artificial Opening Endoscopic **X** External	**4** Electrical Activity **C** Rate **F** Rhythm **H** Sound	**Z** No Qualifier
J Products of Conception, Nervous	**7** Via Natural or Artificial Opening **8** Via Natural or Artificial Opening Endoscopic **X** External	**2** Conductivity **4** Electrical Activity **B** Pressure	**Z** No Qualifier
Z None	**7** Via Natural or Artificial Opening	**6** Metabolism **K** Temperature	**Z** No Qualifier
Z None	**X** External	**6** Metabolism **K** Temperature **Q** Sleep	**Z** No Qualifier

Section	4	Measurement and Monitoring
Body System	A	Physiological Systems
Operation	1	Monitoring Determining the level of a physiological or physical function repetitively over a period of time

Body System (Character 4)	Approach (Character 5)	Function/Device (Character 6)	Qualifier (Character 7)
0 Central Nervous	0 Open	2 Conductivity B Pressure	Z No Qualifier
0 Central Nervous	0 Open	4 Electrical Activity	G Intraoperative Z No Qualifier
0 Central Nervous	3 Percutaneous	4 Electrical Activity	G Intraoperative Z No Qualifier
0 Central Nervous	3 Percutaneous	B Pressure K Temperature R Saturation	D Intracranial
0 Central Nervous	7 Via Natural or Artificial Opening	B Pressure K Temperature R Saturation	D Intracranial
0 Central Nervous	X External	2 Conductivity	Z No Qualifier
0 Central Nervous	X External	4 Electrical Activity	G Intraoperative Z No Qualifier
1 Peripheral Nervous	0 Open 3 Percutaneous X External	2 Conductivity	9 Sensory B Motor
1 Peripheral Nervous	0 Open 3 Percutaneous X External	4 Electrical Activity	G Intraoperative Z No Qualifier
2 Cardiac	0 Open 3 Percutaneous	4 Electrical Activity 9 Output C Rate F Rhythm H Sound	Z No Qualifier
2 Cardiac	X External	4 Electrical Activity	5 Ambulatory Z No Qualifier
2 Cardiac	X External	9 Output C Rate F Rhythm H Sound	Z No Qualifier
2 Cardiac	X External	M Total Activity	4 Stress
2 Cardiac	X External	S Vascular Perfusion	H Indocyanine Green Dye
3 Arterial	0 Open 3 Percutaneous	5 Flow B Pressure J Pulse	1 Peripheral 3 Pulmonary C Coronary
3 Arterial	0 Open 3 Percutaneous	H Sound R Saturation	1 Peripheral
3 Arterial	X External	5 Flow B Pressure H Sound J Pulse R Saturation	1 Peripheral

Continued on Next Page ▶

			Continued from ◀ Previous Page
4 Venous	**0** Open **3** Percutaneous	**5** Flow **B** Pressure **J** Pulse	**0** Central **1** Peripheral **2** Portal **3** Pulmonary
4 Venous	**0** Open **3** Percutaneous	**R** Saturation	**0** Central **2** Portal **3** Pulmonary
4 Venous	**X** External	**5** Flow **B** Pressure **J** Pulse	**1** Peripheral
6 Lymphatic	**0** Open **3** Percutaneous	**5** Flow **B** Pressure	**Z** No Qualifier
9 Respiratory	**7** Via Natural or Artificial Opening **X** External	**1** Capacity **5** Flow **C** Rate **D** Resistance **L** Volume	**Z** No Qualifier
B Gastrointestinal	**7** Via Natural or Artificial Opening **8** Via Natural or Artificial Opening Endoscopic	**8** Motility **B** Pressure **G** Secretion	**Z** No Qualifier
B Gastrointestinal	**X** External	**S** Vascular Perfusion	**H** Indocyanine Green Dye
D Urinary	**7** Via Natural or Artificial Opening	**3** Contractility **5** Flow **B** Pressure **D** Resistance **L** Volume	**Z** No Qualifier
G Skin and Breast	**X** External	**S** Vascular Perfusion	**H** Indocyanine Green Dye
H Products of Conception, Cardiac	**7** Via Natural or Artificial Opening **8** Via Natural or Artificial Opening Endoscopic **X** External	**4** Electrical Activity **C** Rate **F** Rhythm **H** Sound	**Z** No Qualifier
J Products of Conception, Nervous	**7** Via Natural or Artificial Opening **8** Via Natural or Artificial Opening Endoscopic **X** External	**2** Conductivity **4** Electrical Activity **B** Pressure	**Z** No Qualifier
Z None	**7** Via Natural or Artificial Opening	**K** Temperature	**Z** No Qualifier
Z None	**X** External	**K** Temperature **Q** Sleep	**Z** No Qualifier

Section	4	Measurement and Monitoring
Body System	B	Physiological Devices
Operation	0	Measurement: Determining the level of a physiological or physical function at a point in time

Body System (Character 4)	Approach (Character 5)	Function/Device (Character 6)	Qualifier (Character 7)
0 Central Nervous **1** Peripheral Nervous **F** Musculoskeletal	**X** External	**V** Stimulator	**Z** No Qualifier
2 Cardiac	**X** External	**S** Pacemaker **T** Defibrillator	**Z** No Qualifier
9 Respiratory	**X** External	**S** Pacemaker	**Z** No Qualifier

Section	5	Extracorporeal Assistance and Performance	
Body System	A	Physiological Systems	
Operation	0	Assistance: Taking over a portion of a physiological function by extracorporeal means	

Body System (Character 4)	Duration (Character 5)	Function (Character 6)	Qualifier (Character 7)
2 Cardiac	1 Intermittent 2 Continuous	1 Output	0 Balloon Pump 5 Pulsatile Compression 6 Other Pump D Impeller Pump
5 Circulatory	1 Intermittent 2 Continuous	2 Oxygenation	1 Hyperbaric C Supersaturated
9 Respiratory	3 Less than 24 Consecutive Hours 4 24-96 Consecutive Hours 5 Greater than 96 Consecutive Hours	5 Ventilation	7 Continuous Positive Airway Pressure 8 Intermittent Positive Airway Pressure 9 Continuous Negative Airway Pressure B Intermittent Negative Airway Pressure Z No Qualifier

Section	5	Extracorporeal Assistance and Performance	
Body System	A	Physiological Systems	
Operation	1	Performance: Completely taking over a physiological function by extracorporeal means	

Body System (Character 4)	Duration (Character 5)	Function (Character 6)	Qualifier (Character 7)
2 Cardiac	0 Single	1 Output	2 Manual
2 Cardiac	1 Intermittent	3 Pacing	Z No Qualifier
2 Cardiac	2 Continuous	1 Output 3 Pacing	Z No Qualifier
5 Circulatory	2 Continuous	2 Oxygenation	3 Membrane
9 Respiratory	0 Single	5 Ventilation	4 Nonmechanical
9 Respiratory	3 Less than 24 Consecutive Hours 4 24-96 Consecutive Hours 5 Greater than 96 Consecutive Hours	5 Ventilation	Z No Qualifier
C Biliary D Urinary	0 Single 6 Multiple	0 Filtration	Z No Qualifier

Section	5	Extracorporeal Assistance and Performance	
Body System	A	Physiological Systems	
Operation	2	Restoration: Returning, or attempting to return, a physiological function to its original state by extracorporeal means	

Body System (Character 4)	Duration (Character 5)	Function (Character 6)	Qualifier (Character 7)
2 Cardiac	0 Single	4 Rhythm	Z No Qualifier

Section	6	Extracorporeal Therapies		
Body System	A	Physiological Systems		
Operation	0	Atmospheric Control: Extracorporeal control of atmospheric pressure and composition		
Body System (Character 4)		**Duration (Character 5)**	**Qualifier (Character 6)**	**Qualifier (Character 7)**
Z None		0 Single 1 Multiple	Z No Qualifier	Z No Qualifier

Section	6	Extracorporeal Therapies		
Body System	A	Physiological Systems		
Operation	1	Decompression: Extracorporeal elimination of undissolved gas from body fluids		
Body System (Character 4)		**Duration (Character 5)**	**Qualifier (Character 6)**	**Qualifier (Character 7)**
5 Circulatory		0 Single 1 Multiple	Z No Qualifier	Z No Qualifier

Section	6	Extracorporeal Therapies		
Body System	A	Physiological Systems		
Operation	2	Electromagnetic Therapy: Extracorporeal treatment by electromagnetic rays		
Body System (Character 4)		**Duration (Character 5)**	**Qualifier (Character 6)**	**Qualifier (Character 7)**
1 Urinary 2 Central Nervous		0 Single 1 Multiple	Z No Qualifier	Z No Qualifier

Section	6	Extracorporeal Therapies		
Body System	A	Physiological Systems		
Operation	3	Hyperthermia: Extracorporeal raising of body temperature		
Body System (Character 4)		**Duration (Character 5)**	**Qualifier (Character 6)**	**Qualifier (Character 7)**
Z None		0 Single 1 Multiple	Z No Qualifier	Z No Qualifier

Section	6	Extracorporeal Therapies		
Body System	A	Physiological Systems		
Operation	4	Extracorporeal Therapies Physiological Systems Hypothermia: Extracorporeal lowering of body temperature		
Body System (Character 4)		**Duration (Character 5)**	**Qualifier (Character 6)**	**Qualifier (Character 7)**
Z None		0 Single 1 Multiple	Z No Qualifier	Z No Qualifier

Section	6	Extracorporeal Therapies		
Body System	A	Physiological Systems		
Operation	5	Pheresis: Extracorporeal separation of blood products		
Body System (Character 4)		**Duration (Character 5)**	**Qualifier (Character 6)**	**Qualifier (Character 7)**
5 Circulatory		0 Single 1 Multiple	Z No Qualifier	0 Erythrocytes 1 Leukocytes 2 Platelets 3 Plasma T Stem Cells, Cord Blood V Stem Cells, Hematopoietic

Section	6	Extracorporeal Therapies		
Body System	A	Physiological Systems		
Operation	6	Phototherapy: Extracorporeal treatment by light rays		
Body System (Character 4)		**Duration (Character 5)**	**Qualifier (Character 6)**	**Qualifier (Character 7)**
0 Skin 5 Circulatory		0 Single 1 Multiple	Z No Qualifier	Z No Qualifier

Section	6	Extracorporeal Therapies		
Body System	A	Physiological Systems		
Operation	7	Ultrasound Therapy: Extracorporeal treatment by ultrasound		

Body System (Character 4)	Duration (Character 5)	Qualifier (Character 6)	Qualifier (Character 7)
5 Circulatory	0 Single 1 Multiple	Z No Qualifier	4 Head and Neck Vessels 5 Heart 6 Peripheral Vessels 7 Other Vessels Z No Qualifier

Section	6	Extracorporeal Therapies		
Body System	A	Physiological Systems		
Operation	8	Ultraviolet Light Therapy: Extracorporeal treatment by ultraviolet light		

Body System (Character 4)	Duration (Character 5)	Qualifier (Character 6)	Qualifier (Character 7)
0 Skin	0 Single 1 Multiple	Z No Qualifier	Z No Qualifier

Section	6	Extracorporeal Therapies		
Body System	A	Physiological Systems		
Operation	9	Shock Wave Therapy: Extracorporeal treatment by shock waves		

Body System (Character 4)	Duration (Character 5)	Qualifier (Character 6)	Qualifier (Character 7)
3 Musculoskeletal	0 Single 1 Multiple	Z No Qualifier	Z No Qualifier

Section	6	Extracorporeal Therapies		
Body System	A	Physiological Systems		
Operation	B	Perfusion: Extracorporeal treatment by diffusion of therapeutic fluid		

Body System (Character 4)	Duration (Character 5)	Qualifier (Character 6)	Qualifier (Character 7)
5 Circulatory B Respiratory System F Hepatobiliary System and Pancreas T Urinary System	0 Single	B Donor Organ	Z No Qualifier

Section	7	Osteopathic		
Body System	W	Anatomical Regions		
Operation	0	Treatment: Manual treatment to eliminate or alleviate somatic dysfunction and related disorders		

Body Region (Character 4)	Approach (Character 5)	Method (Character 6)	Qualifier (Character 7)
0 Head	X External	0 Articulatory-Raising	Z None
1 Cervical		1 Fascial Release	
2 Thoracic		2 General Mobilization	
3 Lumbar		3 High Velocity-Low Amplitude	
4 Sacrum		4 Indirect	
5 Pelvis		5 Low Velocity-High Amplitude	
6 Lower Extremities		6 Lymphatic Pump	
7 Upper Extremities		7 Muscle Energy-Isometric	
8 Rib Cage		8 Muscle Energy-Isotonic	
9 Abdomen		9 Other Method	

Section	8	Other Procedures	
Body System	C	Indwelling Device	
Operation	0	Other Procedures: Methodologies which attempt to remediate or cure a disorder or disease	

Body Region (Character 4)	Approach (Character 5)	Method (Character 6)	Qualifier (Character 7)
1 Nervous System	X External	6 Collection	J Cerebrospinal Fluid L Other Fluid
2 Circulatory System	X External	6 Collection	K Blood L Other Fluid

Section	8	Other Procedures	
Body System	E	Physiological Systems and Anatomical Regions	
Operation	0	Other Procedures: Methodologies which attempt to remediate or cure a disorder or disease	

Body Region (Character 4)	Approach (Character 5)	Method (Character 6)	Qualifier (Character 7)
1 Nervous System U Female Reproductive System	X External	Y Other Method	7 Examination
2 Circulatory System	3 Percutaneous	D Near Infrared Spectroscopy	Z No Qualifier
9 Head and Neck Region W Trunk Region	0 Open 3 Percutaneous 4 Percutaneous Endoscopic 7 Via Natural or Artificial Opening 8 Via Natural or Artificial Opening Endoscopic	C Robotic Assisted Procedure	Z No Qualifier
9 Head and Neck Region W Trunk Region	X External	B Computer Assisted Procedure	F With Fluoroscopy G With Computerized Tomography H With Magnetic Resonance Imaging Z No Qualifier
9 Head and Neck Region W Trunk Region	X External	C Robotic Assisted Procedure	Z No Qualifier
9 Head and Neck Region W Trunk Region	X External	Y Other Method	8 Suture Removal
H Integumentary System and Breast	3 Percutaneous	0 Acupuncture	0 Anesthesia Z No Qualifier
H Integumentary System and Breast	X External	6 Collection	2 Breast Milk
H Integumentary System and Breast	X External	Y Other Method	9 Piercing
K Musculoskeletal System	X External	1 Therapeutic Massage	Z No Qualifier
K Musculoskeletal System	X External	Y Other Method	7 Examination
V Male Reproductive System	X External	1 Therapeutic Massage	C Prostate D Rectum
V Male Reproductive System	X External	6 Collection	3 Sperm
X Upper Extremity Y Lower Extremity	0 Open 3 Percutaneous 4 Percutaneous Endoscopic	C Robotic Assisted Procedure	Z No Qualifier

Continued on Next Page ▶

			Continued from ◀ Previous Page
X Upper Extremity **Y** Lower Extremity	**X** External	**B** Computer Assisted Procedure	**F** With Fluoroscopy **G** With Computerized Tomography **H** With Magnetic Resonance Imaging **Z** No Qualifier
X Upper Extremity **Y** Lower Extremity	**X** External	**C** Robotic Assisted Procedure	**Z** No Qualifier
X Upper Extremity **Y** Lower Extremity	**X** External	**Y** Other Method	**8** Suture Removal
Z None	**X** External	**Y** Other Method	**1** In Vitro Fertilization **4** Yoga Therapy **5** Meditation **6** Isolation

Section	9	Chiropractic
Body System	W	Anatomical Regions
Operation	B	Manipulation: Manual procedure that involves a directed thrust to move a joint past the physiological range of motion, without exceeding the anatomical limit

Body Region (Character 4)	Approach (Character 5)	Method (Character 6)	Qualifier (Character 7)
0 Head	X External	B Non-Manual	Z None
1 Cervical		C Indirect Visceral	
2 Thoracic		D Extra-Articular	
3 Lumbar		F Direct Visceral	
4 Sacrum		G Long Lever Specific Contact	
5 Pelvis		H Short Lever Specific Contact	
6 Lower Extremities		J Long and Short Lever Specific Contact	
7 Upper Extremities		K Mechanically Assisted	
8 Rib Cage		L Other Method	
9 Abdomen			

Section	B	Imaging		
Body System	0	Central Nervous System		
Type	0	Plain Radiography: Planar display of an image developed from the capture of external ionizing radiation on photographic or photoconductive plate		
Body Part (Character 4)		**Contrast (Character 5)**	**Qualifier (Character 6)**	**Qualifier (Character 7)**
B Spinal Cord		0 High Osmolar 1 Low Osmolar Y Other Contrast Z None	Z None	Z None

Section	B	Imaging		
Body System	0	Central Nervous System		
Type	1	Fluoroscopy: Single plane or bi-plane real time display of an image developed from the capture of external ionizing radiation on a fluorescent screen. The image may also be stored by either digital or analog means		
Body Part (Character 4)		**Contrast (Character 5)**	**Qualifier (Character 6)**	**Qualifier (Character 7)**
B Spinal Cord		0 High Osmolar 1 Low Osmolar Y Other Contrast Z None	Z None	Z None

Section	B	Imaging		
Body System	0	Central Nervous System		
Type	2	Computerized Tomography (CT Scan): Computer reformatted digital display of multiplanar images developed from the capture of multiple exposures of external ionizing radiation		
Body Part (Character 4)		**Contrast (Character 5)**	**Qualifier (Character 6)**	**Qualifier (Character 7)**
0 Brain 7 Cisterna 8 Cerebral Ventricle(s) 9 Sella Turcica/Pituitary Gland B Spinal Cord		0 High Osmolar 1 Low Osmolar Y Other Contrast	0 Unenhanced and Enhanced Z None	Z None
0 Brain 7 Cisterna 8 Cerebral Ventricle(s) 9 Sella Turcica/Pituitary Gland B Spinal Cord		Z None	Z None	Z None

Section	B	Imaging		
Body System	0	Central Nervous System		
Type	3	Magnetic Resonance Imaging (MRI): Computer reformatted digital display of multiplanar images developed from the capture of radiofrequency signals emitted by nuclei in a body site excited within a magnetic field		
Body Part (Character 4)		**Contrast (Character 5)**	**Qualifier (Character 6)**	**Qualifier (Character 7)**
0 Brain 9 Sella Turcica/Pituitary Gland B Spinal Cord C Acoustic Nerves		Y Other Contrast	0 Unenhanced and Enhanced Z None	Z None
0 Brain 9 Sella Turcica/Pituitary Gland B Spinal Cord C Acoustic Nerves		Z None	Z None	Z None

Section	B	Imaging		
Body System	0	Central Nervous System		
Type	4	Ultrasonography: Real time display of images of anatomy or flow information developed from the capture of reflected and attenuated high frequency sound waves		
Body Part (Character 4)	**Contrast (Character 5)**		**Qualifier (Character 6)**	**Qualifier (Character 7)**
0 Brain	Z None		Z None	Z None
B Spinal Cord				

Section	B	Imaging		
Body System	2	Heart		
Type	0	Plain Radiography: Planar display of an image developed from the capture of external ionizing radiation on photographic or photoconductive plate		
Body Part (Character 4)	**Contrast (Character 5)**		**Qualifier (Character 6)**	**Qualifier (Character 7)**
0 Coronary Artery, Single	0 High Osmolar		Z None	Z None
1 Coronary Arteries, Multiple	1 Low Osmolar			
2 Coronary Artery Bypass Graft, Single	Y Other Contrast			
3 Coronary Artery Bypass Grafts, Multiple				
4 Heart, Right				
5 Heart, Left				
6 Heart, Right and Left				
7 Internal Mammary Bypass Graft, Right				
8 Internal Mammary Bypass Graft, Left				
F Bypass Graft, Other				

Section	B	Imaging		
Body System	2	Heart		
Type	1	Fluoroscopy: Single plane or bi-plane real time display of an image developed from the capture of external ionizing radiation on a fluorescent screen. The image may also be stored by either digital or analog means		
Body Part (Character 4)	**Contrast (Character 5)**		**Qualifier (Character 6)**	**Qualifier (Character 7)**
0 Coronary Artery, Single	0 High Osmolar		1 Laser	0 Intraoperative
1 Coronary Arteries, Multiple	1 Low Osmolar			
2 Coronary Artery Bypass Graft, Single	Y Other Contrast			
3 Coronary Artery Bypass Grafts, Multiple				
0 Coronary Artery, Single	0 High Osmolar		Z None	Z None
1 Coronary Arteries, Multiple	1 Low Osmolar			
2 Coronary Artery Bypass Graft, Single	Y Other Contrast			
3 Coronary Artery Bypass Grafts, Multiple				
4 Heart, Right	0 High Osmolar		Z None	Z None
5 Heart, Left	1 Low Osmolar			
6 Heart, Right and Left	Y Other Contrast			
7 Internal Mammary Bypass Graft, Right				
8 Internal Mammary Bypass Graft, Left				
F Bypass Graft, Other				

Section	B	Imaging		
Body System	2	Heart		
Type	2	Computerized Tomography (CT Scan): Computer reformatted digital display of multiplanar images developed from the capture of multiple exposures of external ionizing radiation		

Body Part (Character 4)	Contrast (Character 5)	Qualifier (Character 6)	Qualifier (Character 7)
1 Coronary Arteries, Multiple 3 Coronary Artery Bypass Grafts, Multiple 6 Heart, Right and Left	0 High Osmolar 1 Low Osmolar Y Other Contrast	0 Unenhanced and Enhanced Z None	Z None
1 Coronary Arteries, Multiple 3 Coronary Artery Bypass Grafts, Multiple 6 Heart, Right and Left	Z None	2 Intravascular Optical Coherence Z None	Z None

Section	B	Imaging		
Body System	2	Heart		
Type	3	Magnetic Resonance Imaging (MRI): Computer reformatted digital display of multiplanar images developed from the capture of radiofrequency signals emitted by nuclei in a body site excited within a magnetic field		

Body Part (Character 4)	Contrast (Character 5)	Qualifier (Character 6)	Qualifier (Character 7)
1 Coronary Arteries, Multiple 3 Coronary Artery Bypass Grafts, Multiple 6 Heart, Right and Left	Y Other Contrast	0 Unenhanced and Enhanced Z None	Z None
1 Coronary Arteries, Multiple 3 Coronary Artery Bypass Grafts, Multiple 6 Heart, Right and Left	Z None	Z None	Z None

Section	B	Imaging		
Body System	2	Heart		
Type	4	Ultrasonography: Real time display of images of anatomy or flow information developed from the capture of reflected and attenuated high frequency sound waves		

Body Part (Character 4)	Contrast (Character 5)	Qualifier (Character 6)	Qualifier (Character 7)
0 Coronary Artery, Single 1 Coronary Arteries, Multiple 4 Heart, Right 5 Heart, Left 6 Heart, Right and Left B Heart with Aorta C Pericardium D Pediatric Heart	Y Other Contrast	Z None	Z None
0 Coronary Artery, Single 1 Coronary Arteries, Multiple 4 Heart, Right 5 Heart, Left 6 Heart, Right and Left B Heart with Aorta C Pericardium D Pediatric Heart	Z None	Z None	3 Intravascular 4 Transesophageal Z None

Section	B	Imaging		
Body System	3	Upper Arteries		
Type	0	Plain Radiography: Planar display of an image developed from the capture of external ionizing radiation on photographic or photoconductive plate		

Body Part (Character 4)	Contrast (Character 5)	Qualifier (Character 6)	Qualifier (Character 7)
0 Thoracic Aorta	0 High Osmolar	Z None	Z None
1 Brachiocephalic-Subclavian Artery, Right	1 Low Osmolar		
2 Subclavian Artery, Left	Y Other Contrast		
3 Common Carotid Artery, Right	Z None		
4 Common Carotid Artery, Left			
5 Common Carotid Arteries, Bilateral			
6 Internal Carotid Artery, Right			
7 Internal Carotid Artery, Left			
8 Internal Carotid Arteries, Bilateral			
9 External Carotid Artery, Right			
B External Carotid Artery, Left			
C External Carotid Arteries, Bilateral			
D Vertebral Artery, Right			
F Vertebral Artery, Left			
G Vertebral Arteries, Bilateral			
H Upper Extremity Arteries, Right			
J Upper Extremity Arteries, Left			
K Upper Extremity Arteries, Bilateral			
L Intercostal and Bronchial Arteries			
M Spinal Arteries			
N Upper Arteries, Other			
P Thoraco-Abdominal Aorta			
Q Cervico-Cerebral Arch			
R Intracranial Arteries			
S Pulmonary Artery, Right			
T Pulmonary Artery, Left			

Section	B	Imaging		
Body System	3	Upper Arteries		
Type	1	Fluoroscopy: Single plane or bi-plane real time display of an image developed from the capture of external ionizing radiation on a fluorescent screen. The image may also be stored by either digital or analog means		

Body Part (Character 4)	Contrast (Character 5)	Qualifier (Character 6)	Qualifier (Character 7)
0 Thoracic Aorta	0 High Osmolar	1 Laser	0 Intraoperative
1 Brachiocephalic-Subclavian Artery, Right	1 Low Osmolar		
2 Subclavian Artery, Left	Y Other Contrast		
3 Common Carotid Artery, Right			
4 Common Carotid Artery, Left			
5 Common Carotid Arteries,			

Continued on Next Page ▶

Bilateral			**Continued from** ◀ **Previous Page**
6 Internal Carotid Artery, Right			
7 Internal Carotid Artery, Left			
8 Internal Carotid Arteries, Bilateral			
9 External Carotid Artery, Right			
B External Carotid Artery, Left			
C External Carotid Arteries, Bilateral			
D Vertebral Artery, Right			
F Vertebral Artery, Left			
G Vertebral Arteries, Bilateral			
H Upper Extremity Arteries, Right			
J Upper Extremity Arteries, Left			
K Upper Extremity Arteries, Bilateral			
L Intercostal and Bronchial Arteries			
M Spinal Arteries			
N Upper Arteries, Other			
P Thoraco-Abdominal Aorta			
Q Cervico-Cerebral Arch			
R Intracranial Arteries			
S Pulmonary Artery, Right			
T Pulmonary Artery, Left			
0 Thoracic Aorta	**0** High Osmolar	**Z** None	**Z** None
1 Brachiocephalic-Subclavian Artery, Right	**1** Low Osmolar		
2 Subclavian Artery, Left	**Y** Other Contrast		
3 Common Carotid Artery, Right			
4 Common Carotid Artery, Left			
5 Common Carotid Arteries, Bilateral			
6 Internal Carotid Artery, Right			
7 Internal Carotid Artery, Left			
8 Internal Carotid Arteries, Bilateral			
9 External Carotid Artery, Right			
B External Carotid Artery, Left			
C External Carotid Arteries, Bilateral			
D Vertebral Artery, Right			
F Vertebral Artery, Left			
G Vertebral Arteries, Bilateral			
H Upper Extremity Arteries, Right			
J Upper Extremity Arteries, Left			
K Upper Extremity Arteries, Bilateral			
L Intercostal and Bronchial Arteries			
M Spinal Arteries			**Continued on** **Next Page** ▶

N Upper Arteries, Other			**Continued from** ◀ **Previous Page**
P Thoraco-Abdominal Aorta			
Q Cervico-Cerebral Arch			
R Intracranial Arteries			
S Pulmonary Artery, Right			
T Pulmonary Artery, Left			
0 Thoracic Aorta	Z None	Z None	Z None
1 Brachiocephalic-Subclavian Artery, Right			
2 Subclavian Artery, Left			
3 Common Carotid Artery, Right			
4 Common Carotid Artery, Left			
5 Common Carotid Arteries, Bilateral			
6 Internal Carotid Artery, Right			
7 Internal Carotid Artery, Left			
8 Internal Carotid Arteries, Bilateral			
9 External Carotid Artery, Right			
B External Carotid Artery, Left			
C External Carotid Arteries, Bilateral			
D Vertebral Artery, Right			
F Vertebral Artery, Left			
G Vertebral Arteries, Bilateral			
H Upper Extremity Arteries, Right			
J Upper Extremity Arteries, Left			
K Upper Extremity Arteries, Bilateral			
L Intercostal and Bronchial Arteries			
M Spinal Arteries			
N Upper Arteries, Other			
P Thoraco-Abdominal Aorta			
Q Cervico-Cerebral Arch			
R Intracranial Arteries			
S Pulmonary Artery, Right			
T Pulmonary Artery, Left			

Section	B	Imaging	
Body System	3	Upper Arteries	
Type	2	Computerized Tomography (CT Scan): Computer reformatted digital display of multiplanar images developed from the capture of multiple exposures of external ionizing radiation	

Body Part (Character 4)	Contrast (Character 5)	Qualifier (Character 6)	Qualifier (Character 7)
0 Thoracic Aorta	0 High Osmolar	Z None	Z None
5 Common Carotid Arteries, Bilateral	1 Low Osmolar		
	Y Other Contrast		
8 Internal Carotid Arteries, Bilateral			
G Vertebral Arteries, Bilateral			**Continued on Next Page ▶**
R Intracranial Arteries			

S Pulmonary Artery, Right T Pulmonary Artery, Left			Continued from ◀ Previous Page
0 Thoracic Aorta 5 Common Carotid Arteries, Bilateral 8 Internal Carotid Arteries, Bilateral G Vertebral Arteries, Bilateral R Intracranial Arteries S Pulmonary Artery, Right T Pulmonary Artery, Left	Z None	2 Intravascular Optical Coherence Z None	Z None

Section	B	Imaging
Body System	3	Upper Arteries
Type	3	Magnetic Resonance Imaging (MRI): Computer reformatted digital display of multiplanar images developed from the capture of radiofrequency signals emitted by nuclei in a body site excited within a magnetic field

Body Part (Character 4)	Contrast (Character 5)	Qualifier (Character 6)	Qualifier (Character 7)
0 Thoracic Aorta 5 Common Carotid Arteries, Bilateral 8 Internal Carotid Arteries, Bilateral G Vertebral Arteries, Bilateral H Upper Extremity Arteries, Right J Upper Extremity Arteries, Left K Upper Extremity Arteries, Bilateral M Spinal Arteries Q Cervico-Cerebral Arch R Intracranial Arteries	Y Other Contrast	0 Unenhanced and Enhanced Z None	Z None
0 Thoracic Aorta 5 Common Carotid Arteries, Bilateral 8 Internal Carotid Arteries, Bilateral G Vertebral Arteries, Bilateral H Upper Extremity Arteries, Right J Upper Extremity Arteries, Left K Upper Extremity Arteries, Bilateral M Spinal Arteries Q Cervico-Cerebral Arch R Intracranial Arteries	Z None	Z None	Z None

Section	B	Imaging		
Body System	3	Upper Arteries		
Type	4	Ultrasonography: Real time display of images of anatomy or flow information developed from the capture of reflected and attenuated high frequency sound waves		

Body Part (Character 4)	Contrast (Character 5)	Qualifier (Character 6)	Qualifier (Character 7)
0 Thoracic Aorta	Z None	Z None	3 Intravascular
1 Brachiocephalic-Subclavian Artery, Right			Z None
2 Subclavian Artery, Left			
3 Common Carotid Artery, Right			
4 Common Carotid Artery, Left			
5 Common Carotid Arteries, Bilateral			
6 Internal Carotid Artery, Right			
7 Internal Carotid Artery, Left			
8 Internal Carotid Arteries, Bilateral			
H Upper Extremity Arteries, Right			
J Upper Extremity Arteries, Left			
K Upper Extremity Arteries, Bilateral			
R Intracranial Arteries			
S Pulmonary Artery, Right			
T Pulmonary Artery, Left			
V Ophthalmic Arteries			

Section	B	Imaging		
Body System	4	Lower Arteries		
Type	0	Plain Radiography: Planar display of an image developed from the capture of external ionizing radiation on photographic or photoconductive plate		

Body Part (Character 4)	Contrast (Character 5)	Qualifier (Character 6)	Qualifier (Character 7)
0 Abdominal Aorta	0 High Osmolar	Z None	Z None
2 Hepatic Artery	1 Low Osmolar		
3 Splenic Arteries	Y Other Contrast		
4 Superior Mesenteric Artery			
5 Inferior Mesenteric Artery			
6 Renal Artery, Right			
7 Renal Artery, Left			
8 Renal Arteries, Bilateral			
9 Lumbar Arteries			
B Intra-Abdominal Arteries, Other			
C Pelvic Arteries			
D Aorta and Bilateral Lower Extremity Arteries			
F Lower Extremity Arteries, Right			
G Lower Extremity Arteries, Left			
J Lower Arteries, Other			
M Renal Artery Transplant			

Section	B	Imaging
Body System	4	Lower Arteries
Type	1	Fluoroscopy: Single plane or bi-plane real time display of an image developed from the capture of external ionizing radiation on a fluorescent screen. The image may also be stored by either digital or analog means

Body Part (Character 4)	Contrast (Character 5)	Qualifier (Character 6)	Qualifier (Character 7)
0 Abdominal Aorta 2 Hepatic Artery 3 Splenic Arteries 4 Superior Mesenteric Artery 5 Inferior Mesenteric Artery 6 Renal Artery, Right 7 Renal Artery, Left 8 Renal Arteries, Bilateral 9 Lumbar Arteries B Intra-Abdominal Arteries, Other C Pelvic Arteries D Aorta and Bilateral Lower Extremity Arteries F Lower Extremity Arteries, Right G Lower Extremity Arteries, Left J Lower Arteries, Other	0 High Osmolar 1 Low Osmolar Y Other Contrast	1 Laser	0 Intraoperative
0 Abdominal Aorta 2 Hepatic Artery 3 Splenic Arteries 4 Superior Mesenteric Artery 5 Inferior Mesenteric Artery 6 Renal Artery, Right 7 Renal Artery, Left 8 Renal Arteries, Bilateral 9 Lumbar Arteries B Intra-Abdominal Arteries, Other C Pelvic Arteries D Aorta and Bilateral Lower Extremity Arteries F Lower Extremity Arteries, Right G Lower Extremity Arteries, Left J Lower Arteries, Other	0 High Osmolar 1 Low Osmolar Y Other Contrast	Z None	Z None
0 Abdominal Aorta 2 Hepatic Artery 3 Splenic Arteries 4 Superior Mesenteric Artery 5 Inferior Mesenteric Artery 6 Renal Artery, Right 7 Renal Artery, Left 8 Renal Arteries, Bilateral 9 Lumbar Arteries B Intra-Abdominal Arteries, Other C Pelvic Arteries	Z None	Z None	Z None

Continued on Next Page ▶

D Aorta and Bilateral Lower Extremity Arteries			Continued from ◀ Previous Page
F Lower Extremity Arteries, Right			
G Lower Extremity Arteries, Left			
J Lower Arteries, Other			

Section	B	Imaging		
Body System	4	Lower Arteries		
Type	2	Computerized Tomography (CT Scan): Computer reformatted digital display of multiplanar images developed from the capture of multiple exposures of external ionizing radiation		

Body Part (Character 4)	Contrast (Character 5)	Qualifier (Character 6)	Qualifier (Character 7)
0 Abdominal Aorta 1 Celiac Artery 4 Superior Mesenteric Artery 8 Renal Arteries, Bilateral C Pelvic Arteries F Lower Extremity Arteries, Right G Lower Extremity Arteries, Left H Lower Extremity Arteries, Bilateral M Renal Artery Transplant	0 High Osmolar 1 Low Osmolar Y Other Contrast	Z None	Z None
0 Abdominal Aorta 1 Celiac Artery 4 Superior Mesenteric Artery 8 Renal Arteries, Bilateral C Pelvic Arteries F Lower Extremity Arteries, Right G Lower Extremity Arteries, Left H Lower Extremity Arteries, Bilateral M Renal Artery Transplant	Z None	2 Intravascular Optical Coherence Z None	Z None

Section	B	Imaging		
Body System	4	Lower Arteries		
Type	3	Magnetic Resonance Imaging (MRI): Computer reformatted digital display of multiplanar images developed from the capture of radiofrequency signals emitted by nuclei in a body site excited within a magnetic field		

Body Part (Character 4)	Contrast (Character 5)	Qualifier (Character 6)	Qualifier (Character 7)
0 Abdominal Aorta 1 Celiac Artery 4 Superior Mesenteric Artery 8 Renal Arteries, Bilateral C Pelvic Arteries F Lower Extremity Arteries, Right G Lower Extremity Arteries, Left H Lower Extremity Arteries, Bilateral	Y Other Contrast	0 Unenhanced and Enhanced Z None	Z None

Continued on Next Page ▶

			Continued from ◀ Previous Page
0 Abdominal Aorta **1** Celiac Artery **4** Superior Mesenteric Artery **8** Renal Arteries, Bilateral **C** Pelvic Arteries **F** Lower Extremity Arteries, Right **G** Lower Extremity Arteries, Left **H** Lower Extremity Arteries, Bilateral	**Z** None	**Z** None	**Z** None

Section	B	Imaging
Body System	4	Lower Arteries
Type	4	Ultrasonography: Real time display of images of anatomy or flow information developed from the capture of reflected and attenuated high frequency sound waves

Body Part (Character 4)	Contrast (Character 5)	Qualifier (Character 6)	Qualifier (Character 7)
0 Abdominal Aorta **4** Superior Mesenteric Artery **5** Inferior Mesenteric Artery **6** Renal Artery, Right **7** Renal Artery, Left **8** Renal Arteries, Bilateral **B** Intra-Abdominal Arteries, Other **F** Lower Extremity Arteries, Right **G** Lower Extremity Arteries, Left **H** Lower Extremity Arteries, Bilateral **K** Celiac and Mesenteric Arteries **L** Femoral Artery **N** Penile Arteries	**Z** None	**Z** None	**3** Intravascular **Z** None

Section	B	Imaging
Body System	5	Veins
Type	0	Plain Radiography: Planar display of an image developed from the capture of external ionizing radiation on photographic or photoconductive plate

Body Part (Character 4)	Contrast (Character 5)	Qualifier (Character 6)	Qualifier (Character 7)
0 Epidural Veins **1** Cerebral and Cerebellar Veins **2** Intracranial Sinuses **3** Jugular Veins, Right **4** Jugular Veins, Left **5** Jugular Veins, Bilateral **6** Subclavian Vein, Right **7** Subclavian Vein, Left **8** Superior Vena Cava **9** Inferior Vena Cava **B** Lower Extremity Veins, Right	**0** High Osmolar **1** Low Osmolar **Y** Other Contrast	**Z** None	**Z** None Continued on Next Page ▶

			Continued from ◀ Previous Page
C Lower Extremity Veins, Left			
D Lower Extremity Veins, Bilateral			
F Pelvic (Iliac) Veins, Right			
G Pelvic (Iliac) Veins, Left			
H Pelvic (Iliac) Veins, Bilateral			
J Renal Vein, Right			
K Renal Vein, Left			
L Renal Veins, Bilateral			
M Upper Extremity Veins, Right			
N Upper Extremity Veins, Left			
P Upper Extremity Veins, Bilateral			
Q Pulmonary Vein, Right			
R Pulmonary Vein, Left			
S Pulmonary Veins, Bilateral			
T Portal and Splanchnic Veins			
V Veins, Other			
W Dialysis Shunt/Fistula			

Section	B	Imaging
Body System	5	Veins
Type	1	Fluoroscopy: Single plane or bi-plane real time display of an image developed from the capture of external ionizing radiation on a fluorescent screen. The image may also be stored by either digital or analog means

Body Part (Character 4)	Contrast (Character 5)	Qualifier (Character 6)	Qualifier (Character 7)
0 Epidural Veins	0 High Osmolar	Z None	A Guidance
1 Cerebral and Cerebellar Veins	1 Low Osmolar		Z None
2 Intracranial Sinuses	Y Other Contrast		
3 Jugular Veins, Right	Z None		
4 Jugular Veins, Left			
5 Jugular Veins, Bilateral			
6 Subclavian Vein, Right			
7 Subclavian Vein, Left			
8 Superior Vena Cava			
9 Inferior Vena Cava			
B Lower Extremity Veins, Right			
C Lower Extremity Veins, Left			
D Lower Extremity Veins, Bilateral			
F Pelvic (Iliac) Veins, Right			
G Pelvic (Iliac) Veins, Left			
H Pelvic (Iliac) Veins, Bilateral			
J Renal Vein, Right			
K Renal Vein, Left			
L Renal Veins, Bilateral			
M Upper Extremity Veins, Right			
N Upper Extremity Veins, Left			
P Upper Extremity Veins, Bilateral			
Q Pulmonary Vein, Right			Continued on Next Page ▶

R Pulmonary Vein, Left S Pulmonary Veins, Bilateral T Portal and Splanchnic Veins V Veins, Other W Dialysis Shunt/Fistula			Continued from ◀ Previous Page

Section	B	Imaging
Body System	5	Veins
Type	2	Computerized Tomography (CT Scan): Computer reformatted digital display of multiplanar images developed from the capture of multiple exposures of external ionizing radiation

Body Part (Character 4)	Contrast (Character 5)	Qualifier (Character 6)	Qualifier (Character 7)
2 Intracranial Sinuses 8 Superior Vena Cava 9 Inferior Vena Cava F Pelvic (Iliac) Veins, Right G Pelvic (Iliac) Veins, Left H Pelvic (Iliac) Veins, Bilateral J Renal Vein, Right K Renal Vein, Left L Renal Veins, Bilateral Q Pulmonary Vein, Right R Pulmonary Vein, Left S Pulmonary Veins, Bilateral T Portal and Splanchnic Veins	0 High Osmolar 1 Low Osmolar Y Other Contrast	0 Unenhanced and Enhanced Z None	Z None
2 Intracranial Sinuses 8 Superior Vena Cava 9 Inferior Vena Cava F Pelvic (Iliac) Veins, Right G Pelvic (Iliac) Veins, Left H Pelvic (Iliac) Veins, Bilateral J Renal Vein, Right K Renal Vein, Left L Renal Veins, Bilateral Q Pulmonary Vein, Right R Pulmonary Vein, Left S Pulmonary Veins, Bilateral T Portal and Splanchnic Veins	Z None	2 Intravascular Optical Coherence Z None	Z None

Section	B	Imaging
Body System	5	Veins
Type	3	Magnetic Resonance Imaging (MRI): Computer reformatted digital display of multiplanar images developed from the capture of radiofrequency signals emitted by nuclei in a body site excited within a magnetic field

Body Part (Character 4)	Contrast (Character 5)	Qualifier (Character 6)	Qualifier (Character 7)
1 Cerebral and Cerebellar Veins 2 Intracranial Sinuses 5 Jugular Veins, Bilateral 8 Superior Vena Cava 9 Inferior Vena Cava B Lower Extremity Veins, Right C Lower Extremity Veins, Left D Lower Extremity Veins, Bilateral	Y Other Contrast	0 Unenhanced and Enhanced Z None	Z None

Continued on Next Page ▶

H Pelvic (Iliac) Veins, Bilateral L Renal Veins, Bilateral M Upper Extremity Veins, Right N Upper Extremity Veins, Left P Upper Extremity Veins, Bilateral S Pulmonary Veins, Bilateral T Portal and Splanchnic Veins V Veins, Other			Continued from ◀ Previous Page
1 Cerebral and Cerebellar Veins 2 Intracranial Sinuses 5 Jugular Veins, Bilateral 8 Superior Vena Cava 9 Inferior Vena Cava B Lower Extremity Veins, Right C Lower Extremity Veins, Left D Lower Extremity Veins, Bilateral H Pelvic (Iliac) Veins, Bilateral L Renal Veins, Bilateral M Upper Extremity Veins, Right N Upper Extremity Veins, Left P Upper Extremity Veins, Bilateral S Pulmonary Veins, Bilateral T Portal and Splanchnic Veins V Veins, Other	Z None	Z None	Z None

Section	B	Imaging	
Body System	5	Veins	
Type	4	Ultrasonography: Real time display of images of anatomy or flow information developed from the capture of reflected and attenuated high frequency sound waves	

Body Part (Character 4)	Contrast (Character 5)	Qualifier (Character 6)	Qualifier (Character 7)
3 Jugular Veins, Right 4 Jugular Veins, Left 6 Subclavian Vein, Right 7 Subclavian Vein, Left 8 Superior Vena Cava 9 Inferior Vena Cava B Lower Extremity Veins, Right C Lower Extremity Veins, Left D Lower Extremity Veins, Bilateral J Renal Vein, Right K Renal Vein, Left L Renal Veins, Bilateral M Upper Extremity Veins, Right N Upper Extremity Veins, Left P Upper Extremity Veins, Bilateral T Portal and Splanchnic Veins	Z None	Z None	3 Intravascular A Guidance Z None

Section	B	Imaging		
Body System	7	Lymphatic System		
Type	0	Plain Radiography: Planar display of an image developed from the capture of external ionizing radiation on photographic or photoconductive plate		
Body Part (Character 4)		**Contrast (Character 5)**	**Qualifier (Character 6)**	**Qualifier (Character 7)**
0 Abdominal/Retroperitoneal Lymphatics, Unilateral 1 Abdominal/Retroperitoneal Lymphatics, Bilateral 4 Lymphatics, Head and Neck 5 Upper Extremity Lymphatics, Right 6 Upper Extremity Lymphatics, Left 7 Upper Extremity Lymphatics, Bilateral 8 Lower Extremity Lymphatics, Right 9 Lower Extremity Lymphatics, Left B Lower Extremity Lymphatics, Bilateral C Lymphatics, Pelvic		0 High Osmolar 1 Low Osmolar Y Other Contrast	Z None	Z None

Section	B	Imaging		
Body System	8	Eye		
Type	0	Plain Radiography: Planar display of an image developed from the capture of external ionizing radiation on photographic or photoconductive plate		
Body Part (Character 4)		**Contrast (Character 5)**	**Qualifier (Character 6)**	**Qualifier (Character 7)**
0 Lacrimal Duct, Right 1 Lacrimal Duct, Left 2 Lacrimal Ducts, Bilateral		0 High Osmolar 1 Low Osmolar Y Other Contrast	Z None	Z None
3 Optic Foramina, Right 4 Optic Foramina, Left 5 Eye, Right 6 Eye, Left 7 Eyes, Bilateral		Z None	Z None	Z None

Section	B	Imaging		
Body System	8	Eye		
Type	2	Computerized Tomography (CT Scan): Computer reformatted digital display of multiplanar images developed from the capture of multiple exposures of external ionizing radiation		
Body Part (Character 4)		**Contrast (Character 5)**	**Qualifier (Character 6)**	**Qualifier (Character 7)**
5 Eye, Right 6 Eye, Left 7 Eyes, Bilateral		0 High Osmolar 1 Low Osmolar Y Other Contrast	0 Unenhanced and Enhanced Z None	Z None
5 Eye, Right 6 Eye, Left 7 Eyes, Bilateral		Z None	Z None	Z None

Section	B	Imaging		
Body System	8	Eye		
Type	3	Magnetic Resonance Imaging (MRI): Computer reformatted digital display of multiplanar images developed from the capture of radiofrequency signals emitted by nuclei in a body site excited within a magnetic field		

Body Part (Character 4)	Contrast (Character 5)	Qualifier (Character 6)	Qualifier (Character 7)
5 Eye, Right 6 Eye, Left 7 Eyes, Bilateral	Y Other Contrast	0 Unenhanced and Enhanced Z None	Z None
5 Eye, Right 6 Eye, Left 7 Eyes, Bilateral	Z None	Z None	Z None

Section	B	Imaging		
Body System	8	Eye		
Type	4	Ultrasonography: Real time display of images of anatomy or flow information developed from the capture of reflected and attenuated high frequency sound waves		

Body Part (Character 4)	Contrast (Character 5)	Qualifier (Character 6)	Qualifier (Character 7)
5 Eye, Right 6 Eye, Left 7 Eyes, Bilateral		Z None	Z None

Section	B	Imaging		
Body System	9	Ear, Nose, Mouth and Throat		
Type	0	Plain Radiography: Planar display of an image developed from the capture of external ionizing radiation on photographic or photoconductive plate		

Body Part (Character 4)	Contrast (Character 5)	Qualifier (Character 6)	Qualifier (Character 7)
2 Paranasal Sinuses F Nasopharynx/Oropharynx H Mastoids	Z None	Z None	Z None
4 Parotid Gland, Right 5 Parotid Gland, Left 6 Parotid Glands, Bilateral 7 Submandibular Gland, Right 8 Submandibular Gland, Left 9 Submandibular Glands, Bilateral B Salivary Gland, Right C Salivary Gland, Left D Salivary Glands, Bilateral	0 High Osmolar 1 Low Osmolar Y Other Contrast	Z None	Z None

Section	B	Imaging		
Body System	9	Ear, Nose, Mouth and Throat		
Type	1	Fluoroscopy: Single plane or bi-plane real time display of an image developed from the capture of external ionizing radiation on a fluorescent screen. The image may also be stored by either digital or analog means		

Body Part (Character 4)	Contrast (Character 5)	Qualifier (Character 6)	Qualifier (Character 7)
G Pharynx and Epiglottis J Larynx	Y Other Contrast Z None	Z None	Z None

Section	B	Imaging		
Body System	9	Ear, Nose, Mouth and Throat		
Type	2	Computerized Tomography (CT Scan): Computer reformatted digital display of multiplanar images developed from the capture of multiple exposures of external ionizing radiation		

Body Part (Character 4)	Contrast (Character 5)	Qualifier (Character 6)	Qualifier (Character 7)
0 Ear 2 Paranasal Sinuses 6 Parotid Glands, Bilateral 9 Submandibular Glands, Bilateral D Salivary Glands, Bilateral F Nasopharynx/Oropharynx J Larynx	0 High Osmolar 1 Low Osmolar Y Other Contrast	0 Unenhanced and Enhanced Z None	Z None
0 Ear 2 Paranasal Sinuses 6 Parotid Glands, Bilateral 9 Submandibular Glands, Bilateral D Salivary Glands, Bilateral F Nasopharynx/Oropharynx J Larynx	Z None	Z None	Z None

Section	B	Imaging		
Body System	9	Ear, Nose, Mouth and Throat		
Type	3	Magnetic Resonance Imaging (MRI): Computer reformatted digital display of multiplanar images developed from the capture of radiofrequency signals emitted by nuclei in a body site excited within a magnetic field		

Body Part (Character 4)	Contrast (Character 5)	Qualifier (Character 6)	Qualifier (Character 7)
0 Ear 2 Paranasal Sinuses 6 Parotid Glands, Bilateral 9 Submandibular Glands, Bilateral D Salivary Glands, Bilateral F Nasopharynx/Oropharynx J Larynx	Y Other Contrast	0 Unenhanced and Enhanced Z None	Z None
0 Ear 2 Paranasal Sinuses 6 Parotid Glands, Bilateral 9 Submandibular Glands, Bilateral D Salivary Glands, Bilateral F Nasopharynx/Oropharynx J Larynx	Z None	Z None	Z None

Section	B	Imaging		
Body System	B	Respiratory System		
Type	0	Plain Radiography: Planar display of an image developed from the capture of external ionizing radiation on photographic or photoconductive plate		

Body Part (Character 4)	Contrast (Character 5)	Qualifier (Character 6)	Qualifier (Character 7)
7 Tracheobronchial Tree, Right 8 Tracheobronchial Tree, Left 9 Tracheobronchial Trees, Bilateral	Y Other Contrast	Z None	Z None
D Upper Airways	Z None	Z None	Z None

Section	B	Imaging		
Body System	B	Respiratory System		
Type	1	Fluoroscopy: Single plane or bi-plane real time display of an image developed from the capture of external ionizing radiation on a fluorescent screen. The image may also be stored by either digital or analog means		

Body Part (Character 4)	Contrast (Character 5)	Qualifier (Character 6)	Qualifier (Character 7)
2 Lung, Right 3 Lung, Left 4 Lungs, Bilateral 6 Diaphragm C Mediastinum D Upper Airways	Z None	Z None	Z None
7 Tracheobronchial Tree, Right 8 Tracheobronchial Tree, Left 9 Tracheobronchial Trees, Bilateral	Y Other Contrast	Z None	Z None

Section	B	Imaging		
Body System	B	Respiratory System		
Type	2	Computerized Tomography (CT Scan): Computer reformatted digital display of multiplanar images developed from the capture of multiple exposures of external ionizing radiation		

Body Part (Character 4)	Contrast (Character 5)	Qualifier (Character 6)	Qualifier (Character 7)
4 Lungs, Bilateral 7 Tracheobronchial Tree, Right 8 Tracheobronchial Tree, Left 9 Tracheobronchial Trees, Bilateral F Trachea/Airways	0 High Osmolar 1 Low Osmolar Y Other Contrast	0 Unenhanced and Enhanced Z None	Z None
4 Lungs, Bilateral 7 Tracheobronchial Tree, Right 8 Tracheobronchial Tree, Left 9 Tracheobronchial Trees, Bilateral F Trachea/Airways	Z None	Z None	Z None

Section	B	Imaging		
Body System	B	Respiratory System		
Type	3	Magnetic Resonance Imaging (MRI): Computer reformatted digital display of multiplanar images developed from the capture of radiofrequency signals emitted by nuclei in a body site excited within a magnetic field		

Body Part (Character 4)	Contrast (Character 5)	Qualifier (Character 6)	Qualifier (Character 7)
G Lung Apices	Y Other Contrast	0 Unenhanced and Enhanced Z None	Z None
G Lung Apices	Z None	Z None	Z None

Section	B	Imaging		
Body System	B	Respiratory System		
Type	4	Ultrasonography: Real time display of images of anatomy or flow information developed from the capture of reflected and attenuated high frequency sound waves		

Body Part (Character 4)	Contrast (Character 5)	Qualifier (Character 6)	Qualifier (Character 7)
B Pleura C Mediastinum	Z None	Z None	Z None

Section	B	Imaging		
Body System	D	Gastrointestinal System		
Type	1	Fluoroscopy: Single plane or bi-plane real time display of an image developed from the capture of external ionizing radiation on a fluorescent screen. The image may also be stored by either digital or analog means		
Body Part (Character 4)		**Contrast (Character 5)**	**Qualifier (Character 6)**	**Qualifier (Character 7)**
1 Esophagus 2 Stomach 3 Small Bowel 4 Colon 5 Upper GI 6 Upper GI and Small Bowel 9 Duodenum B Mouth/Oropharynx		Y Other Contrast Z None	Z None	Z None

Section	B	Imaging		
Body System	D	Gastrointestinal System		
Type	2	Computerized Tomography (CT Scan): Computer reformatted digital display of multiplanar images developed from the capture of multiple exposures of external ionizing radiation		
Body Part (Character 4)		**Contrast (Character 5)**	**Qualifier (Character 6)**	**Qualifier (Character 7)**
4 Colon		0 High Osmolar 1 Low Osmolar Y Other Contrast	0 Unenhanced and Enhanced Z None	Z None
4 Colon		Z None	Z None	Z None

Section	B	Imaging		
Body System	D	Gastrointestinal System		
Type	4	Ultrasonography: Real time display of images of anatomy or flow information developed from the capture of reflected and attenuated high frequency sound waves		
Body Part (Character 4)		**Contrast (Character 5)**	**Qualifier (Character 6)**	**Qualifier (Character 7)**
1 Esophagus 2 Stomach 7 Gastrointestinal Tract 8 Appendix 9 Duodenum C Rectum		Z None	Z None	Z None

Section	B	Imaging		
Body System	F	Hepatobiliary System and Pancreas		
Type	0	Plain Radiography: Planar display of an image developed from the capture of external ionizing radiation on photographic or photoconductive plate		
Body Part (Character 4)		**Contrast (Character 5)**	**Qualifier (Character 6)**	**Qualifier (Character 7)**
0 Bile Ducts 3 Gallbladder and Bile Ducts C Hepatobiliary System, All		0 High Osmolar 1 Low Osmolar Y Other Contrast	Z None	Z None

Section	B	Imaging		
Body System	F	Hepatobiliary System and Pancreas		
Type	1	Fluoroscopy: Single plane or bi-plane real time display of an image developed from the capture of external ionizing radiation on a fluorescent screen. The image may also be stored by either digital or analog means		

Body Part (Character 4)	Contrast (Character 5)	Qualifier (Character 6)	Qualifier (Character 7)
0 Bile Ducts 1 Biliary and Pancreatic Ducts 2 Gallbladder 3 Gallbladder and Bile Ducts 4 Gallbladder, Bile Ducts and Pancreatic Ducts 8 Pancreatic Ducts	0 High Osmolar 1 Low Osmolar Y Other Contrast	Z None	Z None

Section	B	Imaging		
Body System	F	Hepatobiliary System and Pancreas		
Type	2	Computerized Tomography (CT Scan): Computer reformatted digital display of multiplanar images developed from the capture of multiple exposures of external ionizing radiation		

Body Part (Character 4)	Contrast (Character 5)	Qualifier (Character 6)	Qualifier (Character 7)
5 Liver 6 Liver and Spleen 7 Pancreas C Hepatobiliary System, All	0 High Osmolar 1 Low Osmolar Y Other Contrast	0 Unenhanced and Enhanced Z None	Z None
5 Liver 6 Liver and Spleen 7 Pancreas C Hepatobiliary System, All	Z None	Z None	Z None

Section	B	Imaging		
Body System	F	Hepatobiliary System and Pancreas		
Type	3	Magnetic Resonance Imaging (MRI): Computer reformatted digital display of multiplanar images developed from the capture of radiofrequency signals emitted by nuclei in a body site excited within a magnetic field		

Body Part (Character 4)	Contrast (Character 5)	Qualifier (Character 6)	Qualifier (Character 7)
5 Liver 6 Liver and Spleen 7 Pancreas	Y Other Contrast	0 Unenhanced and Enhanced Z None	Z None
5 Liver 6 Liver and Spleen 7 Pancreas	Z None	Z None	Z None

Section	B	Imaging		
Body System	F	Hepatobiliary System and Pancreas		
Type	4	Ultrasonography: Real time display of images of anatomy or flow information developed from the capture of reflected and attenuated high frequency sound waves		

Body Part (Character 4)	Contrast (Character 5)	Qualifier (Character 6)	Qualifier (Character 7)
0 Bile Ducts 2 Gallbladder 3 Gallbladder and Bile Ducts 5 Liver 6 Liver and Spleen 7 Pancreas C Hepatobiliary System, All	Z None	Z None	Z None

Section	B	Imaging		
Body System	G	Endocrine System		
Type	2	Computerized Tomography (CT Scan): Computer reformatted digital display of multiplanar images developed from the capture of multiple exposures of external ionizing radiation		

Body Part (Character 4)	Contrast (Character 5)	Qualifier (Character 6)	Qualifier (Character 7)
2 Adrenal Glands, Bilateral 3 Parathyroid Glands 4 Thyroid Gland	0 High Osmolar 1 Low Osmolar Y Other Contrast	0 Unenhanced and Enhanced Z None	Z None
2 Adrenal Glands, Bilateral 3 Parathyroid Glands 4 Thyroid Gland	Z None	Z None	Z None

Section	B	Imaging		
Body System	G	Endocrine System		
Type	3	Magnetic Resonance Imaging (MRI): Computer reformatted digital display of multiplanar images developed from the capture of radiofrequency signals emitted by nuclei in a body site excited within a magnetic field		

Body Part (Character 4)	Contrast (Character 5)	Qualifier (Character 6)	Qualifier (Character 7)
2 Adrenal Glands, Bilateral 3 Parathyroid Glands 4 Thyroid Gland	Y Other Contrast	0 Unenhanced and Enhanced Z None	Z None
2 Adrenal Glands, Bilateral 3 Parathyroid Glands 4 Thyroid Gland	Z None	Z None	Z None

Section	B	Imaging		
Body System	G	Endocrine System		
Type	4	Ultrasonography: Real time display of images of anatomy or flow information developed from the capture of reflected and attenuated high frequency sound waves		

Body Part (Character 4)	Contrast (Character 5)	Qualifier (Character 6)	Qualifier (Character 7)
0 Adrenal Gland, Right 1 Adrenal Gland, Left 2 Adrenal Glands, Bilateral 3 Parathyroid Glands 4 Thyroid Gland	Z None	Z None	Z None

Section	B	Imaging		
Body System	H	Skin, Subcutaneous Tissue and Breast		
Type	0	Plain Radiography: Planar display of an image developed from the capture of external ionizing radiation on photographic or photoconductive plate		

Body Part (Character 4)	Contrast (Character 5)	Qualifier (Character 6)	Qualifier (Character 7)
0 Breast, Right 1 Breast, Left 2 Breasts, Bilateral	Z None	Z None	Z None
3 Single Mammary Duct, Right 4 Single Mammary Duct, Left 5 Multiple Mammary Ducts, Right 6 Multiple Mammary Ducts, Left	0 High Osmolar 1 Low Osmolar Y Other Contrast Z None	Z None	Z None

Section	B	Imaging		
Body System	H	Skin, Subcutaneous Tissue and Breast		
Type	3	Magnetic Resonance Imaging (MRI): Computer reformatted digital display of multiplanar images developed from the capture of radiofrequency signals emitted by nuclei in a body site excited within a magnetic field		

Body Part (Character 4)	Contrast (Character 5)	Qualifier (Character 6)	Qualifier (Character 7)
0 Breast, Right 1 Breast, Left 2 Breasts, Bilateral D Subcutaneous Tissue, Head/Neck F Subcutaneous Tissue, Upper Extremity G Subcutaneous Tissue, Thorax H Subcutaneous Tissue, Abdomen and Pelvis J Subcutaneous Tissue, Lower Extremity	Y Other Contrast	0 Unenhanced and Enhanced Z None	Z None
0 Breast, Right 1 Breast, Left 2 Breasts, Bilateral D Subcutaneous Tissue, Head/Neck F Subcutaneous Tissue, Upper Extremity G Subcutaneous Tissue, Thorax H Subcutaneous Tissue, Abdomen and Pelvis J Subcutaneous Tissue, Lower Extremity	Z None	Z None	Z None

Section	B	Imaging		
Body System	H	Skin, Subcutaneous Tissue and Breast		
Type	4	Ultrasonography: Real time display of images of anatomy or flow information developed from the capture of reflected and attenuated high frequency sound waves		

Body Part (Character 4)	Contrast (Character 5)	Qualifier (Character 6)	Qualifier (Character 7)
0 Breast, Right 1 Breast, Left 2 Breasts, Bilateral 7 Extremity, Upper 8 Extremity, Lower 9 Abdominal Wall B Chest Wall C Head and Neck	Z None	Z None	Z None

Section	B	Imaging			
Body System	L	Connective Tissue			
Type	3	Magnetic Resonance Imaging (MRI): Computer reformatted digital display of multiplanar images developed from the capture of radiofrequency signals emitted by nuclei in a body site excited within a magnetic field			

Body Part (Character 4)	Contrast (Character 5)	Qualifier (Character 6)	Qualifier (Character 7)
0 Connective Tissue, Upper Extremity 1 Connective Tissue, Lower Extremity 2 Tendons, Upper Extremity 3 Tendons, Lower Extremity	Y Other Contrast	0 Unenhanced and Enhanced Z None	Z None
0 Connective Tissue, Upper Extremity 1 Connective Tissue, Lower Extremity 2 Tendons, Upper Extremity 3 Tendons, Lower Extremity	Z None	Z None	Z None

Section	B	Imaging			
Body System	L	Connective Tissue			
Type	4	Ultrasonography: Real time display of images of anatomy or flow information developed from the capture of reflected and attenuated high frequency sound waves			

Body Part (Character 4)	Contrast (Character 5)	Qualifier (Character 6)	Qualifier (Character 7)
0 Connective Tissue, Upper Extremity 1 Connective Tissue, Lower Extremity 2 Tendons, Upper Extremity 3 Tendons, Lower Extremity	Z None	Z None	Z None

Section	B	Imaging			
Body System	N	Skull and Facial Bones			
Type	0	Plain Radiography: Planar display of an image developed from the capture of external ionizing radiation on photographic or photoconductive plate			

Body Part (Character 4)	Contrast (Character 5)	Qualifier (Character 6)	Qualifier (Character 7)
0 Skull 1 Orbit, Right 2 Orbit, Left 3 Orbits, Bilateral 4 Nasal Bones 5 Facial Bones 6 Mandible B Zygomatic Arch, Right C Zygomatic Arch, Left D Zygomatic Arches, Bilateral G Tooth, Single H Teeth, Multiple J Teeth, All	Z None	Z None	Z None
7 Temporomandibular Joint, Right 8 Temporomandibular Joint, Left 9 Temporomandibular Joints, Bilateral	0 High Osmolar 1 Low Osmolar Y Other Contrast Z None	Z None	Z None

Section	B	Imaging
Body System	N	Skull and Facial Bones
Type	1	Fluoroscopy: Single plane or bi-plane real time display of an image developed from the capture of external ionizing radiation on a fluorescent screen. The image may also be stored by either digital or analog means

Body Part (Character 4)	Contrast (Character 5)	Qualifier (Character 6)	Qualifier (Character 7)
7 Temporomandibular Joint, Right 8 Temporomandibular Joint, Left 9 Temporomandibular Joints, Bilateral	0 High Osmolar 1 Low Osmolar Y Other Contrast Z None	Z None	Z None

Section	B	Imaging
Body System	N	Skull and Facial Bones
Type	2	Computerized Tomography (CT Scan): Computer reformatted digital display of multiplanar images developed from the capture of multiple exposures of external ionizing radiation

Body Part (Character 4)	Contrast (Character 5)	Qualifier (Character 6)	Qualifier (Character 7)
0 Skull 3 Orbits, Bilateral 5 Facial Bones 6 Mandible 9 Temporomandibular Joints, Bilateral F Temporal Bones	0 High Osmolar 1 Low Osmolar Y Other Contrast Z None	Z None	Z None

Section	B	Imaging
Body System	N	Skull and Facial Bones
Type	3	Magnetic Resonance Imaging (MRI): Computer reformatted digital display of multiplanar images developed from the capture of radiofrequency signals emitted by nuclei in a body site excited within a magnetic field

Body Part (Character 4)	Contrast (Character 5)	Qualifier (Character 6)	Qualifier (Character 7)
9 Temporomandibular Joints, Bilateral	Y Other Contrast Z None	Z None	Z None

Section	B	Imaging
Body System	P	Non-Axial Upper Bones
Type	0	Plain Radiography: Planar display of an image developed from the capture of external ionizing radiation on photographic or photoconductive plate

Body Part (Character 4)	Contrast (Character 5)	Qualifier (Character 6)	Qualifier (Character 7)
0 Sternoclavicular Joint, Right 1 Sternoclavicular Joint, Left 2 Sternoclavicular Joints, Bilateral 3 Acromioclavicular Joints, Bilateral 4 Clavicle, Right 5 Clavicle, Left 6 Scapula, Right 7 Scapula, Left A Humerus, Right B Humerus, Left E Upper Arm, Right F Upper Arm, Left J Forearm, Right K Forearm, Left	Z None	Z None	Z None

Continued on Next Page ▶

N Hand, Right **P** Hand, Left **R** Finger(s), Right **S** Finger(s), Left **X** Ribs, Right **Y** Ribs, Left			Continued from ◀ Previous Page
8 Shoulder, Right **9** Shoulder, Left **C** Hand/Finger Joint, Right **D** Hand/Finger Joint, Left **G** Elbow, Right **H** Elbow, Left **L** Wrist, Right **M** Wrist, Left	**0** High Osmolar **1** Low Osmolar **Y** Other Contrast **Z** None	**Z** None	**Z** None

Section	B	Imaging
Body System	P	Non-Axial Upper Bones
Type	1	Fluoroscopy: Single plane or bi-plane real time display of an image developed from the capture of external ionizing radiation on a fluorescent screen. The image may also be stored by either digital or analog means

Body Part (Character 4)	Contrast (Character 5)	Qualifier (Character 6)	Qualifier (Character 7)
0 Sternoclavicular Joint, Right **1** Sternoclavicular Joint, Left **2** Sternoclavicular Joints, Bilateral **3** Acromioclavicular Joints, Bilateral **4** Clavicle, Right **5** Clavicle, Left **6** Scapula, Right **7** Scapula, Left **A** Humerus, Right **B** Humerus, Left **E** Upper Arm, Right **F** Upper Arm, Left **J** Forearm, Right **K** Forearm, Left **N** Hand, Right **P** Hand, Left **R** Finger(s), Right **S** Finger(s), Left **X** Ribs, Right **Y** Ribs, Left	**Z** None	**Z** None	**Z** None
8 Shoulder, Right **9** Shoulder, Left **L** Wrist, Right **M** Wrist, Left	**0** High Osmolar **1** Low Osmolar **Y** Other Contrast **Z** None	**Z** None	**Z** None
C Hand/Finger Joint, Right **D** Hand/Finger Joint, Left **G** Elbow, Right **H** Elbow, Left	**0** High Osmolar **1** Low Osmolar **Y** Other Contrast	**Z** None	**Z** None

Section	B	Imaging		
Body System	P	Non-Axial Upper Bones		
Type	2	Computerized Tomography (CT Scan): Computer reformatted digital display of multiplanar images developed from the capture of multiple exposures of external ionizing radiation		

Body Part (Character 4)	Contrast (Character 5)	Qualifier (Character 6)	Qualifier (Character 7)
0 Sternoclavicular Joint, Right 1 Sternoclavicular Joint, Left W Thorax	0 High Osmolar 1 Low Osmolar Y Other Contrast	Z None	Z None
2 Sternoclavicular Joints, Bilateral 3 Acromioclavicular Joints, Bilateral 4 Clavicle, Right 5 Clavicle, Left 6 Scapula, Right 7 Scapula, Left 8 Shoulder, Right 9 Shoulder, Left A Humerus, Right B Humerus, Left E Upper Arm, Right F Upper Arm, Left G Elbow, Right H Elbow, Left J Forearm, Right K Forearm, Left L Wrist, Right M Wrist, Left N Hand, Right P Hand, Left Q Hands and Wrists, Bilateral R Finger(s), Right S Finger(s), Left T Upper Extremity, Right U Upper Extremity, Left V Upper Extremities, Bilateral X Ribs, Right Y Ribs, Left	0 High Osmolar 1 Low Osmolar Y Other Contrast Z None	Z None	Z None
C Hand/Finger Joint, Right D Hand/Finger Joint, Left	Z None	Z None	Z None

Section	B	Imaging		
Body System	P	Non-Axial Upper Bones		
Type	3	Magnetic Resonance Imaging (MRI): Computer reformatted digital display of multiplanar images developed from the capture of radiofrequency signals emitted by nuclei in a body site excited within a magnetic field		

Body Part (Character 4)	Contrast (Character 5)	Qualifier (Character 6)	Qualifier (Character 7)
8 Shoulder, Right 9 Shoulder, Left C Hand/Finger Joint, Right D Hand/Finger Joint, Left E Upper Arm, Right F Upper Arm, Left G Elbow, Right H Elbow, Left	Y Other Contrast	0 Unenhanced and Enhanced Z None	Z None

Continued on Next Page ▶

J Forearm, Right K Forearm, Left L Wrist, Right M Wrist, Left			Continued from ◄ Previous Page
8 Shoulder, Right 9 Shoulder, Left C Hand/Finger Joint, Right D Hand/Finger Joint, Left E Upper Arm, Right F Upper Arm, Left G Elbow, Right H Elbow, Left J Forearm, Right K Forearm, Left L Wrist, Right M Wrist, Left	Z None	Z None	Z None

Section	B	Imaging	
Body System	P	Non-Axial Upper Bones	
Type	4	Ultrasonography: Real time display of images of anatomy or flow information developed from the capture of reflected and attenuated high frequency sound waves	

Body Part (Character 4)	Contrast (Character 5)	Qualifier (Character 6)	Qualifier (Character 7)
8 Shoulder, Right 9 Shoulder, Left G Elbow, Right H Elbow, Left L Wrist, Right M Wrist, Left N Hand, Right P Hand, Left	Z None	Z None	1 Densitometry Z None

Section	B	Imaging	
Body System	Q	Non-Axial Lower Bones	
Type	0	Plain Radiography: Planar display of an image developed from the capture of external ionizing radiation on photographic or photoconductive plate	

Body Part (Character 4)	Contrast (Character 5)	Qualifier (Character 6)	Qualifier (Character 7)
0 Hip, Right 1 Hip, Left	0 High Osmolar 1 Low Osmolar Y Other Contrast	Z None	Z None
0 Hip, Right 1 Hip, Left	Z None	Z None	1 Densitometry Z None
3 Femur, Right 4 Femur, Left	Z None	Z None	1 Densitometry Z None
7 Knee, Right 8 Knee, Left G Ankle, Right H Ankle, Left	0 High Osmolar 1 Low Osmolar Y Other Contrast Z None	Z None	Z None
D Lower Leg, Right F Lower Leg, Left J Calcaneus, Right K Calcaneus, Left L Foot, Right M Foot, Left P Toe(s), Right	Z None	Z None	Z None Continued on Next Page ►

Q Toe(s), Left V Patella, Right W Patella, Left			Continued from ◀ Previous Page
X Foot/Toe Joint, Right Y Foot/Toe Joint, Left	0 High Osmolar 1 Low Osmolar Y Other Contrast	Z None	Z None

Section	B	Imaging
Body System	Q	Non-Axial Lower Bones
Type	1	Fluoroscopy: Single plane or bi-plane real time display of an image developed from the capture of external ionizing radiation on a fluorescent screen. The image may also be stored by either digital or analog means

Body Part (Character 4)	Contrast (Character 5)	Qualifier (Character 6)	Qualifier (Character 7)
0 Hip, Right 1 Hip, Left 7 Knee, Right 8 Knee, Left G Ankle, Right H Ankle, Left X Foot/Toe Joint, Right Y Foot/Toe Joint, Left	0 High Osmolar 1 Low Osmolar Y Other Contrast Z None	Z None	Z None
3 Femur, Right 4 Femur, Left D Lower Leg, Right F Lower Leg, Left J Calcaneus, Right K Calcaneus, Left L Foot, Right M Foot, Left P Toe(s), Right Q Toe(s), Left V Patella, Right W Patella, Left	Z None	Z None	Z None

Section	B	Imaging
Body System	Q	Non-Axial Lower Bones
Type	2	Computerized Tomography (CT Scan): Computer reformatted digital display of multiplanar images developed from the capture of multiple exposures of external ionizing radiation

Body Part (Character 4)	Contrast (Character 5)	Qualifier (Character 6)	Qualifier (Character 7)
0 Hip, Right 1 Hip, Left 3 Femur, Right 4 Femur, Left 7 Knee, Right 8 Knee, Left D Lower Leg, Right F Lower Leg, Left G Ankle, Right H Ankle, Left J Calcaneus, Right K Calcaneus, Left L Foot, Right M Foot, Left P Toe(s), Right	0 High Osmolar 1 Low Osmolar Y Other Contrast Z None	Z None	Z None Continued on Next Page ▶

			Continued from ◀ Previous Page
Q Toe(s), Left **R** Lower Extremity, Right **S** Lower Extremity, Left **V** Patella, Right **W** Patella, Left **X** Foot/Toe Joint, Right **Y** Foot/Toe Joint, Left			
B Tibia/Fibula, Right **C** Tibia/Fibula, Left	**0** High Osmolar **1** Low Osmolar **Y** Other Contrast	**Z** None	**Z** None

Section	B	Imaging
Body System	Q	**Non-Axial Lower Bones**
Type	3	**Magnetic Resonance Imaging (MRI): Computer reformatted digital display of multiplanar images developed from the capture of radiofrequency signals emitted by nuclei in a body site excited within a magnetic field**

Body Part (Character 4)	Contrast (Character 5)	Qualifier (Character 6)	Qualifier (Character 7)
0 Hip, Right **1** Hip, Left **3** Femur, Right **4** Femur, Left **7** Knee, Right **8** Knee, Left **D** Lower Leg, Right **F** Lower Leg, Left **G** Ankle, Right **H** Ankle, Left **J** Calcaneus, Right **K** Calcaneus, Left **L** Foot, Right **M** Foot, Left **P** Toe(s), Right **Q** Toe(s), Left **V** Patella, Right **W** Patella, Left	**Y** Other Contrast	**0** Unenhanced and Enhanced **Z** None	**Z** None
0 Hip, Right **1** Hip, Left **3** Femur, Right **4** Femur, Left **7** Knee, Right **8** Knee, Left **D** Lower Leg, Right **F** Lower Leg, Left **G** Ankle, Right **H** Ankle, Left **J** Calcaneus, Right **K** Calcaneus, Left **L** Foot, Right **M** Foot, Left **P** Toe(s), Right **Q** Toe(s), Left **V** Patella, Right **W** Patella, Left	**Z** None	**Z** None	**Z** None

Section	B	Imaging		
Body System	Q	Non-Axial Lower Bones		
Type	4	Ultrasonography: Real time display of images of anatomy or flow information developed from the capture of reflected and attenuated high frequency sound waves		

Body Part (Character 4)	Contrast (Character 5)	Qualifier (Character 6)	Qualifier (Character 7)
0 Hip, Right 1 Hip, Left 2 Hips, Bilateral 7 Knee, Right 8 Knee, Left 9 Knees, Bilateral	Z None	Z None	Z None

Section	B	Imaging		
Body System	R	Axial Skeleton, Except Skull and Facial Bones		
Type	0	Plain Radiography: Planar display of an image developed from the capture of external ionizing radiation on photographic or photoconductive plate		

Body Part (Character 4)	Contrast (Character 5)	Qualifier (Character 6)	Qualifier (Character 7)
0 Cervical Spine 7 Thoracic Spine 9 Lumbar Spine G Whole Spine	Z None	Z None	1 Densitometry Z None
1 Cervical Disc(s) 2 Thoracic Disc(s) 3 Lumbar Disc(s) 4 Cervical Facet Joint(s) 5 Thoracic Facet Joint(s) 6 Lumbar Facet Joint(s) D Sacroiliac Joints	0 High Osmolar 1 Low Osmolar Y Other Contrast Z None	Z None	Z None
8 Thoracolumbar Joint B Lumbosacral Joint C Pelvis F Sacrum and Coccyx H Sternum	Z None	Z None	Z None

Section	B	Imaging		
Body System	R	Axial Skeleton, Except Skull and Facial Bones		
Type	1	Fluoroscopy: Single plane or bi-plane real time display of an image developed from the capture of external ionizing radiation on a fluorescent screen. The image may also be stored by either digital or analog means		

Body Part (Character 4)	Contrast (Character 5)	Qualifier (Character 6)	Qualifier (Character 7)
0 Cervical Spine 1 Cervical Disc(s) 2 Thoracic Disc(s) 3 Lumbar Disc(s) 4 Cervical Facet Joint(s) 5 Thoracic Facet Joint(s) 6 Lumbar Facet Joint(s) 7 Thoracic Spine 8 Thoracolumbar Joint 9 Lumbar Spine B Lumbosacral Joint C Pelvis D Sacroiliac Joints F Sacrum and Coccyx G Whole Spine H Sternum	0 High Osmolar 1 Low Osmolar Y Other Contrast Z None	Z None	Z None

Section	B	Imaging
Body System	R	Axial Skeleton, Except Skull and Facial Bones
Type	2	Computerized Tomography (CT Scan): Computer reformatted digital display of multiplanar images developed from the capture of multiple exposures of external ionizing radiation

Body Part (Character 4)	Contrast (Character 5)	Qualifier (Character 6)	Qualifier (Character 7)
0 Cervical Spine 7 Thoracic Spine 9 Lumbar Spine C Pelvis D Sacroiliac Joints F Sacrum and Coccyx	0 High Osmolar 1 Low Osmolar Y Other Contrast Z None	Z None	Z None

Section	B	Imaging
Body System	R	Axial Skeleton, Except Skull and Facial Bones
Type	3	Magnetic Resonance Imaging (MRI): Computer reformatted digital display of multiplanar images developed from the capture of radiofrequency signals emitted by nuclei in a body site excited within a magnetic field

Body Part (Character 4)	Contrast (Character 5)	Qualifier (Character 6)	Qualifier (Character 7)
0 Cervical Spine 1 Cervical Disc(s) 2 Thoracic Disc(s) 3 Lumbar Disc(s) 7 Thoracic Spine 9 Lumbar Spine C Pelvis F Sacrum and Coccyx	Y Other Contrast	0 Unenhanced and Enhanced Z None	Z None
0 Cervical Spine 1 Cervical Disc(s) 2 Thoracic Disc(s) 3 Lumbar Disc(s) 7 Thoracic Spine 9 Lumbar Spine C Pelvis F Sacrum and Coccyx	Z None	Z None	Z None

Section	B	Imaging
Body System	R	Axial Skeleton, Except Skull and Facial Bones
Type	4	Ultrasonography: Real time display of images of anatomy or flow information developed from the capture of reflected and attenuated high frequency sound waves

Body Part (Character 4)	Contrast (Character 5)	Qualifier (Character 6)	Qualifier (Character 7)
0 Cervical Spine 7 Thoracic Spine 9 Lumbar Spine F Sacrum and Coccyx	Z None	Z None	Z None

Section	B	Imaging
Body System	T	Urinary System
Type	0	Plain Radiography: Planar display of an image developed from the capture of external ionizing radiation on photographic or photoconductive plate

Body Part (Character 4)	Contrast (Character 5)	Qualifier (Character 6)	Qualifier (Character 7)
0 Bladder 1 Kidney, Right 2 Kidney, Left 3 Kidneys, Bilateral	0 High Osmolar 1 Low Osmolar Y Other Contrast Z None	Z None	Z None **Continued on Next Page ▶**

4 Kidneys, Ureters and Bladder **5** Urethra **6** Ureter, Right **7** Ureter, Left **8** Ureters, Bilateral **B** Bladder and Urethra **C** Ileal Diversion Loop			Continued from ◀ Previous Page

Section	B	Imaging	
Body System	T	Urinary System	
Type	1	Fluoroscopy: Single plane or bi-plane real time display of an image developed from the capture of external ionizing radiation on a fluorescent screen. The image may also be stored by either digital or analog means	

Body Part (Character 4)	Contrast (Character 5)	Qualifier (Character 6)	Qualifier (Character 7)
0 Bladder **1** Kidney, Right **2** Kidney, Left **3** Kidneys, Bilateral **4** Kidneys, Ureters and Bladder **5** Urethra **6** Ureter, Right **7** Ureter, Left **B** Bladder and Urethra **C** Ileal Diversion Loop **D** Kidney, Ureter and Bladder, Right **F** Kidney, Ureter and Bladder, Left **G** Ileal Loop, Ureters and Kidneys	**0** High Osmolar **1** Low Osmolar **Y** Other Contrast **Z** None	**Z** None	**Z** None

Section	B	Imaging	
Body System	T	Urinary System	
Type	2	Computerized Tomography (CT Scan): Computer reformatted digital display of multiplanar images developed from the capture of multiple exposures of external ionizing radiation	

Body Part (Character 4)	Contrast (Character 5)	Qualifier (Character 6)	Qualifier (Character 7)
0 Bladder **1** Kidney, Right **2** Kidney, Left **3** Kidneys, Bilateral **9** Kidney Transplant	**0** High Osmolar **1** Low Osmolar **Y** Other Contrast	**0** Unenhanced and Enhanced **Z** None	**Z** None
0 Bladder **1** Kidney, Right **2** Kidney, Left **3** Kidneys, Bilateral **9** Kidney Transplant	**Z** None	**Z** None	**Z** None

Section	B	Imaging
Body System	T	Urinary System
Type	3	Magnetic Resonance Imaging (MRI): Computer reformatted digital display of multiplanar images developed from the capture of radiofrequency signals emitted by nuclei in a body site excited within a magnetic field

Body Part (Character 4)	Contrast (Character 5)	Qualifier (Character 6)	Qualifier (Character 7)
0 Bladder 1 Kidney, Right 2 Kidney, Left 3 Kidneys, Bilateral 9 Kidney Transplant	Y Other Contrast	0 Unenhanced and Enhanced Z None	Z None
0 Bladder 1 Kidney, Right 2 Kidney, Left 3 Kidneys, Bilateral 9 Kidney Transplant	Z None	Z None	Z None

Section	B	Imaging
Body System	T	Urinary System
Type	4	Ultrasonography: Real time display of images of anatomy or flow information developed from the capture of reflected and attenuated high frequency sound waves

Body Part (Character 4)	Contrast (Character 5)	Qualifier (Character 6)	Qualifier (Character 7)
0 Bladder 1 Kidney, Right 2 Kidney, Left 3 Kidneys, Bilateral 5 Urethra 6 Ureter, Right 7 Ureter, Left 8 Ureters, Bilateral 9 Kidney Transplant J Kidneys and Bladder	Z None	Z None	Z None

Section	B	Imaging
Body System	U	Female Reproductive System
Type	0	Plain Radiography: Planar display of an image developed from the capture of external ionizing radiation on photographic or photoconductive plate

Body Part (Character 4)	Contrast (Character 5)	Qualifier (Character 6)	Qualifier (Character 7)
0 Fallopian Tube, Right 1 Fallopian Tube, Left 2 Fallopian Tubes, Bilateral 6 Uterus 8 Uterus and Fallopian Tubes 9 Vagina	0 High Osmolar 1 Low Osmolar Y Other Contrast	Z None	Z None

Section	B	Imaging
Body System	U	Female Reproductive System
Type	1	Fluoroscopy: Single plane or bi-plane real time display of an image developed from the capture of external ionizing radiation on a fluorescent screen. The image may also be stored by either digital or analog means

Body Part (Character 4)	Contrast (Character 5)	Qualifier (Character 6)	Qualifier (Character 7)
0 Fallopian Tube, Right 1 Fallopian Tube, Left 2 Fallopian Tubes, Bilateral 6 Uterus 8 Uterus and Fallopian Tubes 9 Vagina	0 High Osmolar 1 Low Osmolar Y Other Contrast Z None	Z None	Z None

Section	B	Imaging		
Body System	U	Female Reproductive System		
Type	3	Magnetic Resonance Imaging (MRI): Computer reformatted digital display of multiplanar images developed from the capture of radiofrequency signals emitted by nuclei in a body site excited within a magnetic field		

Body Part (Character 4)	Contrast (Character 5)	Qualifier (Character 6)	Qualifier (Character 7)
3 Ovary, Right 4 Ovary, Left 5 Ovaries, Bilateral 6 Uterus 9 Vagina B Pregnant Uterus C Uterus and Ovaries	Y Other Contrast	0 Unenhanced and Enhanced Z None	Z None
3 Ovary, Right 4 Ovary, Left 5 Ovaries, Bilateral 6 Uterus 9 Vagina B Pregnant Uterus C Uterus and Ovaries	Z None	Z None	Z None

Section	B	Imaging		
Body System	U	Female Reproductive System		
Type	4	Ultrasonography: Real time display of images of anatomy or flow information developed from the capture of reflected and attenuated high frequency sound waves		

Body Part (Character 4)	Contrast (Character 5)	Qualifier (Character 6)	Qualifier (Character 7)
0 Fallopian Tube, Right 1 Fallopian Tube, Left 2 Fallopian Tubes, Bilateral 3 Ovary, Right 4 Ovary, Left 5 Ovaries, Bilateral 6 Uterus C Uterus and Ovaries	Y Other Contrast Z None	Z None	Z None

Section	B	Imaging		
Body System	V	Male Reproductive System		
Type	0	Plain Radiography: Planar display of an image developed from the capture of external ionizing radiation on photographic or photoconductive plate		

Body Part (Character 4)	Contrast (Character 5)	Qualifier (Character 6)	Qualifier (Character 7)
0 Corpora Cavernosa 1 Epididymis, Right 2 Epididymis, Left 3 Prostate 5 Testicle, Right 6 Testicle, Left 8 Vasa Vasorum	0 High Osmolar 1 Low Osmolar Y Other Contrast	Z None	Z None

Section	B	Imaging
Body System	V	Male Reproductive System
Type	1	Fluoroscopy: Single plane or bi-plane real time display of an image developed from the capture of external ionizing radiation on a fluorescent screen. The image may also be stored by either digital or analog means

Body Part (Character 4)	Contrast (Character 5)	Qualifier (Character 6)	Qualifier (Character 7)
0 Corpora Cavernosa 8 Vasa Vasorum	0 High Osmolar 1 Low Osmolar Y Other Contrast Z None	Z None	Z None

Section	B	Imaging
Body System	V	Male Reproductive System
Type	2	Computerized Tomography (CT Scan): Computer reformatted digital display of multiplanar images developed from the capture of multiple exposures of external ionizing radiation

Body Part (Character 4)	Contrast (Character 5)	Qualifier (Character 6)	Qualifier (Character 7)
3 Prostate	0 High Osmolar 1 Low Osmolar Y Other Contrast	0 Unenhanced and Enhanced Z None	Z None
3 Prostate	Z None	Z None	Z None

Section	B	Imaging
Body System	V	Male Reproductive System
Type	3	Magnetic Resonance Imaging (MRI): Computer reformatted digital display of multiplanar images developed from the capture of radiofrequency signals emitted by nuclei in a body site excited within a magnetic field

Body Part (Character 4)	Contrast (Character 5)	Qualifier (Character 6)	Qualifier (Character 7)
0 Corpora Cavernosa 3 Prostate 4 Scrotum 5 Testicle, Right 6 Testicle, Left 7 Testicles, Bilateral	Y Other Contrast	0 Unenhanced and Enhanced Z None	Z None
0 Corpora Cavernosa 3 Prostate 4 Scrotum 5 Testicle, Right 6 Testicle, Left 7 Testicles, Bilateral	Z None	Z None	Z None

Section	B	Imaging
Body System	V	Male Reproductive System
Type	4	Ultrasonography: Real time display of images of anatomy or flow information developed from the capture of reflected and attenuated high frequency sound waves

Body Part (Character 4)	Contrast (Character 5)	Qualifier (Character 6)	Qualifier (Character 7)
4 Scrotum 9 Prostate and Seminal Vesicles B Penis	Z None	Z None	Z None

Section	B	Imaging
Body System	W	Anatomical Regions
Type	0	Plain Radiography: Planar display of an image developed from the capture of external ionizing radiation on photographic or photoconductive plate

Body Part (Character 4)	Contrast (Character 5)	Qualifier (Character 6)	Qualifier (Character 7)
0 Abdomen **1** Abdomen and Pelvis **3** Chest **B** Long Bones, All **C** Lower Extremity **J** Upper Extremity **K** Whole Body **L** Whole Skeleton **M** Whole Body, Infant	**Z** None	**Z** None	**Z** None

Section	B	Imaging
Body System	W	Anatomical Regions
Type	1	Fluoroscopy: Single plane or bi-plane real time display of an image developed from the capture of external ionizing radiation on a fluorescent screen. The image may also be stored by either digital or analog means

Body Part (Character 4)	Contrast (Character 5)	Qualifier (Character 6)	Qualifier (Character 7)
1 Abdomen and Pelvis **9** Head and Neck **C** Lower Extremity **J** Upper Extremity	**0** High Osmolar **1** Low Osmolar **Y** Other Contrast **Z** None	**Z** None	**Z** None

Section	B	Imaging
Body System	W	Anatomical Regions
Type	2	Computerized Tomography (CT Scan): Computer reformatted digital display of multiplanar images developed from the capture of multiple exposures of external ionizing radiation

Body Part (Character 4)	Contrast (Character 5)	Qualifier (Character 6)	Qualifier (Character 7)
0 Abdomen **1** Abdomen and Pelvis **4** Chest and Abdomen **5** Chest, Abdomen and Pelvis **8** Head **9** Head and Neck **F** Neck **G** Pelvic Region	**0** High Osmolar **1** Low Osmolar **Y** Other Contrast	**0** Unenhanced and Enhanced **Z** None	**Z** None
0 Abdomen **1** Abdomen and Pelvis **4** Chest and Abdomen **5** Chest, Abdomen and Pelvis **8** Head **9** Head and Neck **F** Neck **G** Pelvic Region	**Z** None	**Z** None	**Z** None

Section	B	Imaging		
Body System	W	Anatomical Regions		
Type	3	Magnetic Resonance Imaging (MRI): Computer reformatted digital display of multiplanar images developed from the capture of radiofrequency signals emitted by nuclei in a body site excited within a magnetic field		
Body Part (Character 4)	**Contrast (Character 5)**	**Qualifier (Character 6)**	**Qualifier (Character 7)**	
0 Abdomen 8 Head F Neck G Pelvic Region H Retroperitoneum P Brachial Plexus	Y Other Contrast	0 Unenhanced and Enhanced Z None	Z None	
0 Abdomen 8 Head F Neck G Pelvic Region H Retroperitoneum P Brachial Plexus	Z None	Z None	Z None	
3 Chest	Y Other Contrast	0 Unenhanced and Enhanced Z None	Z None	

Section	B	Imaging		
Body System	W	Anatomical Regions		
Type	4	Ultrasonography: Real time display of images of anatomy or flow information developed from the capture of reflected and attenuated high frequency sound waves		
Body Part (Character 4)	**Contrast (Character 5)**	**Qualifier (Character 6)**	**Qualifier (Character 7)**	
0 Abdomen 1 Abdomen and Pelvis F Neck G Pelvic Region	Z None	Z None	Z None	

Section	B	Imaging		
Body System	Y	Fetus and Obstetrical		
Type	3	Magnetic Resonance Imaging (MRI): Computer reformatted digital display of multiplanar images developed from the capture of radiofrequency signals emitted by nuclei in a body site excited within a magnetic field		
Body Part (Character 4)	**Contrast (Character 5)**	**Qualifier (Character 6)**	**Qualifier (Character 7)**	
0 Fetal Head 1 Fetal Heart 2 Fetal Thorax 3 Fetal Abdomen 4 Fetal Spine 5 Fetal Extremities 6 Whole Fetus	Y Other Contrast	0 Unenhanced and Enhanced Z None	Z None	
0 Fetal Head 1 Fetal Heart 2 Fetal Thorax 3 Fetal Abdomen 4 Fetal Spine 5 Fetal Extremities 6 Whole Fetus	Z None	Z None	Z None	

Section	B	Imaging		
Body System	Y	Fetus and Obstetrical		
Type	4	Ultrasonography: Real time display of images of anatomy or flow information developed from the capture of reflected and attenuated high frequency sound waves		

Body Part (Character 4)	Contrast (Character 5)	Qualifier (Character 6)	Qualifier (Character 7)
7 Fetal Umbilical Cord 8 Placenta 9 First Trimester, Single Fetus B First Trimester, Multiple Gestation C Second Trimester, Single Fetus D Second Trimester, Multiple Gestation F Third Trimester, Single Fetus G Third Trimester, Multiple Gestation	Z None	Z None	Z None

Section	C	Nuclear Medicine
Body System	0	Central Nervous System
Type	1	Planar Nuclear Medicine Imaging: Introduction of radioactive materials into the body for single plane display of images developed from the capture of radioactive emissions

Body Part (Character 4)	Radionuclide (Character 5)	Qualifier (Character 6)	Qualifier (Character 7)
0 Brain	1 Technetium 99m (Tc-99m) Y Other Radionuclide	Z None	Z None
5 Cerebrospinal Fluid	D Indium 111 (In-111) Y Other Radionuclide	Z None	Z None
Y Central Nervous System	Y Other Radionuclide	Z None	Z None

Section	C	Nuclear Medicine
Body System	0	Central Nervous System
Type	2	Tomographic (Tomo) Nuclear Medicine Imaging: Introduction of radioactive materials into the body for three dimensional display of images developed from the capture of radioactive emissions

Body Part (Character 4)	Radionuclide (Character 5)	Qualifier (Character 6)	Qualifier (Character 7)
0 Brain	1 Technetium 99m (Tc-99m) F Iodine 123 (I-123) S Thallium 201 (Tl-201) Y Other Radionuclide	Z None	Z None
5 Cerebrospinal Fluid	D Indium 111 (In-111) Y Other Radionuclide	Z None	Z None
Y Central Nervous System	Y Other Radionuclide	Z None	Z None

Section	C	Nuclear Medicine
Body System	0	Central Nervous System
Type	3	Positron Emission Tomographic (PET) Imaging: Introduction of radioactive materials into the body for three dimensional display of images developed from the simultaneous capture, 180 degrees apart, of radioactive emissions

Body Part (Character 4)	Radionuclide (Character 5)	Qualifier (Character 6)	Qualifier (Character 7)
0 Brain	B Carbon 11 (C-11) K Fluorine 18 (F-18) M Oxygen 15 (O-15) Y Other Radionuclide	Z None	Z None
Y Central Nervous System	Y Other Radionuclide	Z None	Z None

Section	C	Nuclear Medicine
Body System	0	Central Nervous System
Type	5	Nonimaging Nuclear Medicine Probe: Introduction of radioactive materials into the body for the study of distribution and fate of certain substances by the detection of radioactive emissions; or, alternatively, measurement of absorption of radioactive emissions from an external source

Body Part (Character 4)	Radionuclide (Character 5)	Qualifier (Character 6)	Qualifier (Character 7)
0 Brain	V Xenon 133 (Xe-133) Y Other Radionuclide	Z None	Z None
Y Central Nervous System	Y Other Radionuclide	Z None	Z None

Section	C	Nuclear Medicine		
Body System	2	Heart		
Type	1	Planar Nuclear Medicine Imaging: Introduction of radioactive materials into the body for single plane display of images developed from the capture of radioactive emissions		

Body Part (Character 4)	Radionuclide (Character 5)	Qualifier (Character 6)	Qualifier (Character 7)
6 Heart, Right and Left	1 Technetium 99m (Tc-99m) Y Other Radionuclide	Z None	Z None
G Myocardium	1 Technetium 99m (Tc-99m) D Indium 111 (In-111) S Thallium 201 (Tl-201) Y Other Radionuclide Z None	Z None	Z None
Y Heart	Y Other Radionuclide	Z None	Z None

Section	C	Nuclear Medicine		
Body System	2	Heart		
Type	2	Tomographic (Tomo) Nuclear Medicine Imaging: Introduction of radioactive materials into the body for three dimensional display of images developed from the capture of radioactive emissions		

Body Part (Character 4)	Radionuclide (Character 5)	Qualifier (Character 6)	Qualifier (Character 7)
6 Heart, Right and Left	1 Technetium 99m (Tc-99m) Y Other Radionuclide	Z None	Z None
G Myocardium	1 Technetium 99m (Tc-99m) D Indium 111 (In-111) K Fluorine 18 (F-18) S Thallium 201 (Tl-201) Y Other Radionuclide Z None	Z None	Z None
Y Heart	Y Other Radionuclide	Z None	Z None

Section	C	Nuclear Medicine		
Body System	2	Heart		
Type	3	Positron Emission Tomographic (PET) Imaging: Introduction of radioactive materials into the body for three dimensional display of images developed from the simultaneous capture, 180·degrees apart, of radioactive emissions		

Body Part (Character 4)	Radionuclide (Character 5)	Qualifier (Character 6)	Qualifier (Character 7)
G Myocardium	K Fluorine 18 (F-18) M Oxygen 15 (O-15) Q Rubidium 82 (Rb-82) R Nitrogen 13 (N-13) Y Other Radionuclide	Z None	Z None
Y Heart	Y Other Radionuclide	Z None	Z None

Section	C	Nuclear Medicine		
Body System	2	Heart		
Type	5	Nonimaging Nuclear Medicine Probe: Introduction of radioactive materials into the body for the study of distribution and fate of certain substances by the detection of radioactive emissions; or, alternatively, measurement of absorption of radioactive emissions from an external source		

Body Part (Character 4)	Radionuclide (Character 5)	Qualifier (Character 6)	Qualifier (Character 7)
6 Heart, Right and Left	1 Technetium 99m (Tc-99m) Y Other Radionuclide	Z None	Z None
Y Heart	Y Other Radionuclide	Z None	Z None

Section	C	Nuclear Medicine		
Body System	5	Veins		
Type	1	Planar Nuclear Medicine Imaging: Introduction of radioactive materials into the body for single plane display of images developed from the capture of radioactive emissions		

Body Part (Character 4)	Radionuclide (Character 5)	Qualifier (Character 6)	Qualifier (Character 7)
B Lower Extremity Veins, Right C Lower Extremity Veins, Left D Lower Extremity Veins, Bilateral N Upper Extremity Veins, Right P Upper Extremity Veins, Left Q Upper Extremity Veins, Bilateral R Central Veins	1 Technetium 99m (Tc-99m) Y Other Radionuclide	Z None	Z None
Y Veins	Y Other Radionuclide	Z None	Z None

Section	C	Nuclear Medicine		
Body System	7	Lymphatic and Hematologic System		
Type	1	Planar Nuclear Medicine Imaging: Introduction of radioactive materials into the body for single plane display of images developed from the capture of radioactive emissions		

Body Part (Character 4)	Radionuclide (Character 5)	Qualifier (Character 6)	Qualifier (Character 7)
0 Bone Marrow	1 Technetium 99m (Tc-99m) D Indium 111 (In-111) Y Other Radionuclide	Z None	Z None
2 Spleen 5 Lymphatics, Head and Neck D Lymphatics, Pelvic J Lymphatics, Head K Lymphatics, Neck L Lymphatics, Upper Chest M Lymphatics, Trunk N Lymphatics, Upper Extremity P Lymphatics, Lower Extremity	1 Technetium 99m (Tc-99m) Y Other Radionuclide	Z None	Z None
3 Blood	D Indium 111 (In-111) Y Other Radionuclide	Z None	Z None
Y Lymphatic and Hematologic System	Y Other Radionuclide	Z None	Z None

Section	C	Nuclear Medicine		
Body System	7	Lymphatic and Hematologic System		
Type	2	Tomographic (Tomo) Nuclear Medicine Imaging: Introduction of radioactive materials into the body for three dimensional display of images developed from the capture of radioactive emissions		

Body Part (Character 4)	Radionuclide (Character 5)	Qualifier (Character 6)	Qualifier (Character 7)
2 Spleen	1 Technetium 99m (Tc-99m) Y Other Radionuclide	Z None	Z None
Y Lymphatic and Hematologic System	Y Other Radionuclide	Z None	Z None

Section	C	Nuclear Medicine		
Body System	7	Lymphatic and Hematologic System		
Type	5	Nonimaging Nuclear Medicine Probe: Introduction of radioactive materials into the body for the study of distribution and fate of certain substances by the detection of radioactive emissions; or, alternatively, measurement of absorption of radioactive emissions from an external source		

Body Part (Character 4)	Radionuclide (Character 5)	Qualifier (Character 6)	Qualifier (Character 7)
5 Lymphatics, Head and Neck **D** Lymphatics, Pelvic **J** Lymphatics, Head **K** Lymphatics, Neck **L** Lymphatics, Upper Chest **M** Lymphatics, Trunk **N** Lymphatics, Upper Extremity **P** Lymphatics, Lower Extremity	**1** Technetium 99m (Tc-99m) **Y** Other Radionuclide	**Z** None	**Z** None
Y Lymphatic and Hematologic System	**Y** Other Radionuclide	**Z** None	**Z** None

Section	C	Nuclear Medicine		
Body System	7	Lymphatic and Hematologic System		
Type	6	Nonimaging Nuclear Medicine Assay: Introduction of radioactive materials into the body for the study of body fluids and blood elements, by the detection of radioactive emissions		

Body Part (Character 4)	Radionuclide (Character 5)	Qualifier (Character 6)	Qualifier (Character 7)
3 Blood	**1** Technetium 99m (Tc-99m) **7** Cobalt 58 (Co-58) **C** Cobalt 57 (Co-57) **D** Indium 111 (In-111) **H** Iodine 125 (I-125) **W** Chromium (Cr-51) **Y** Other Radionuclide	**Z** None	**Z** None
Y Lymphatic and Hematologic System	**Y** Other Radionuclide	**Z** None	**Z** None

Section	C	Nuclear Medicine		
Body System	8	Eye		
Type	1	Planar Nuclear Medicine Imaging: Introduction of radioactive materials into the body for single plane display of images developed from the capture of radioactive emissions		

Body Part (Character 4)	Radionuclide (Character 5)	Qualifier (Character 6)	Qualifier (Character 7)
9 Lacrimal Ducts, Bilateral	**1** Technetium 99m (Tc-99m) **Y** Other Radionuclide	**Z** None	**Z** None
Y Eye	**Y** Other Radionuclide	**Z** None	**Z** None

Section	C	Nuclear Medicine		
Body System	9	Ear, Nose, Mouth and Throat		
Type	1	Planar Nuclear Medicine Imaging: Introduction of radioactive materials into the body for single plane display of images developed from the capture of radioactive emissions		

Body Part Character 4	Radionuclide	Qualifier	Qualifier
B Salivary Glands, Bilateral	**1** Technetium 99m (Tc-99m) **Y** Other Radionuclide	**Z** None	**Z** None
Y Ear, Nose, Mouth and Throat	**Y** Other Radionuclide	**Z** None	**Z** None

Section	C	Nuclear Medicine		
Body System	B	Respiratory System		
Type	1	Planar Nuclear Medicine Imaging: Introduction of radioactive materials into the body for single plane display of images developed from the capture of radioactive emissions		

Body Part (Character 4)	Radionuclide (Character 5)	Qualifier (Character 6)	Qualifier (Character 7)
2 Lungs and Bronchi	1 Technetium 99m (Tc-99m) 9 Krypton (Kr-81m) T Xenon 127 (Xe-127) V Xenon 133 (Xe-133) Y Other Radionuclide	Z None	Z None
Y Respiratory System	Y Other Radionuclide	Z None	Z None

Section	C	Nuclear Medicine		
Body System	B	Respiratory System		
Type	2	Tomographic (Tomo) Nuclear Medicine Imaging: Introduction of radioactive materials into the body for three dimensional display of images developed from the capture of radioactive emissions		

Body Part (Character 4)	Radionuclide (Character 5)	Qualifier (Character 6)	Qualifier (Character 7)
2 Lungs and Bronchi	1 Technetium 99m (Tc-99m) 9 Krypton (Kr-81m) Y Other Radionuclide	Z None	Z None
Y Respiratory System	Y Other Radionuclide	Z None	Z None

Section	C	Nuclear Medicine		
Body System	B	Respiratory System		
Type	3	Positron Emission Tomographic (PET) Imaging: Introduction of radioactive materials into the body for three dimensional display of images developed from the simultaneous capture, 180 degrees apart, of radioactive emissions		

Body Part (Character 4)	Radionuclide (Character 5)	Qualifier (Character 6)	Qualifier (Character 7)
2 Lungs and Bronchi	K Fluorine 18 (F-18) Y Other Radionuclide	Z None	Z None
Y Respiratory System	Y Other Radionuclide	Z None	Z None

Section	C	Nuclear Medicine		
Body System	D	Gastrointestinal System		
Type	1	Planar Nuclear Medicine Imaging: Introduction of radioactive materials into the body for single plane display of images developed from the capture of radioactive emissions		

Body Part (Character 4)	Radionuclide (Character 5)	Qualifier (Character 6)	Qualifier (Character 7)
5 Upper Gastrointestinal Tract 7 Gastrointestinal Tract	1 Technetium 99m (Tc-99m) D Indium 111 (In-111) Y Other Radionuclide	Z None	Z None
Y Digestive System	Y Other Radionuclide	Z None	Z None

Section	C	Nuclear Medicine		
Body System	D	Gastrointestinal System		
Type	2	Tomographic (Tomo) Nuclear Medicine Imaging: Introduction of radioactive materials into the body for three dimensional display of images developed from the capture of radioactive emissions		

Body Part (Character 4)	Radionuclide (Character 5)	Qualifier (Character 6)	Qualifier (Character 7)
7 Gastrointestinal Tract	1 Technetium 99m (Tc-99m) D Indium 111 (In-111) Y Other Radionuclide	Z None	Z None
Y Digestive System	Y Other Radionuclide	Z None	Z None

Section	C	Nuclear Medicine		
Body System	F	Hepatobiliary System and Pancreas		
Type	1	Planar Nuclear Medicine Imaging: Introduction of radioactive materials into the body for single plane display of images developed from the capture of radioactive emissions		

Body Part (Character 4)	Radionuclide (Character 5)	Qualifier (Character 6)	Qualifier (Character 7)
4 Gallbladder 5 Liver 6 Liver and Spleen C Hepatobiliary System, All	1 Technetium 99m (Tc-99m) Y Other Radionuclide	Z None	Z None
Y Hepatobiliary System and Pancreas	Y Other Radionuclide	Z None	Z None

Section	C	Nuclear Medicine		
Body System	F	Hepatobiliary System and Pancreas		
Type	2	Tomographic (Tomo) Nuclear Medicine Imaging: Introduction of radioactive materials into the body for three dimensional display of images developed from the capture of radioactive emissions		

Body Part (Character 4)	Radionuclide (Character 5)	Qualifier (Character 6)	Qualifier (Character 7)
4 Gallbladder 5 Liver 6 Liver and Spleen	1 Technetium 99m (Tc-99m) Y Other Radionuclide	Z None	Z None
Y Hepatobiliary System and Pancreas	Y Other Radionuclide	Z None	Z None

Section	C	Nuclear Medicine		
Body System	G	Endocrine System		
Type	1	Planar Nuclear Medicine Imaging: Introduction of radioactive materials into the body for single plane display of images developed from the capture of radioactive emissions		

Body Part (Character 4)	Radionuclide (Character 5)	Qualifier (Character 6)	Qualifier (Character 7)
1 Parathyroid Glands	1 Technetium 99m (Tc-99m) S Thallium 201 (Tl-201) Y Other Radionuclide	Z None	Z None
2 Thyroid Gland	1 Technetium 99m (Tc-99m) F Iodine 123 (I-123) G Iodine 131 (I-131) Y Other Radionuclide	Z None	Z None
4 Adrenal Glands, Bilateral	G Iodine 131 (I-131) Y Other Radionuclide	Z None	Z None
Y Endocrine System	Y Other Radionuclide	Z None	Z None

Section	C	Nuclear Medicine		
Body System	G	Endocrine System		
Type	2	Tomographic (Tomo) Nuclear Medicine Imaging: Introduction of radioactive materials into the body for three dimensional display of images developed from the capture of radioactive emissions		

Body Part (Character 4)	Radionuclide (Character 5)	Qualifier (Character 6)	Qualifier (Character 7)
1 Parathyroid Glands	1 Technetium 99m (Tc-99m) S Thallium 201 (Tl-201) Y Other Radionuclide	Z None	Z None
Y Endocrine System	Y Other Radionuclide	Z None	Z None

Section	C	Nuclear Medicine		
Body System	G	Endocrine System		
Type	4	Nonimaging Nuclear Medicine Uptake: Introduction of radioactive materials into the body for measurements of organ function, from the detection of radioactive emissions		

Body Part (Character 4)	Radionuclide (Character 5)	Qualifier (Character 6)	Qualifier (Character 7)
2 Thyroid Gland	1 Technetium 99m (Tc-99m) F Iodine 123 (I-123) G Iodine 131 (I-131) Y Other Radionuclide	Z None	Z None
Y Endocrine System	Y Other Radionuclide	Z None	Z None

Section	C	Nuclear Medicine		
Body System	H	Skin, Subcutaneous Tissue and Breast		
Type	1	Planar Nuclear Medicine Imaging: Introduction of radioactive materials into the body for single plane display of images developed from the capture of radioactive emissions		

Body Part (Character 4)	Radionuclide (Character 5)	Qualifier (Character 6)	Qualifier (Character 7)
0 Breast, Right 1 Breast, Left 2 Breasts, Bilateral	1 Technetium 99m (Tc-99m) S Thallium 201 (Tl-201) Y Other Radionuclide	Z None	Z None
Y Skin, Subcutaneous Tissue and Breast	Y Other Radionuclide	Z None	Z None

Section	C	Nuclear Medicine		
Body System	H	Skin, Subcutaneous Tissue and Breast		
Type	2	Tomographic (Tomo) Nuclear Medicine Imaging: Introduction of radioactive materials into the body for three dimensional display of images developed from the capture of radioactive emissions		

Body Part (Character 4)	Radionuclide (Character 5)	Qualifier (Character 6)	Qualifier (Character 7)
0 Breast, Right 1 Breast, Left 2 Breasts, Bilateral	1 Technetium 99m (Tc-99m) S Thallium 201 (Tl-201) Y Other Radionuclide	Z None	Z None
Y Skin, Subcutaneous Tissue and Breast	Y Other Radionuclide	Z None	Z None

Section	C	Nuclear Medicine		
Body System	P	Musculoskeletal System		
Type	1	Planar Nuclear Medicine Imaging: Introduction of radioactive materials into the body for single plane display of images developed from the capture of radioactive emissions		

Body Part (Character 4)	Radionuclide (Character 5)	Qualifier (Character 6)	Qualifier (Character 7)
1 Skull 4 Thorax 5 Spine 6 Pelvis 7 Spine and Pelvis 8 Upper Extremity, Right 9 Upper Extremity, Left B Upper Extremities, Bilateral C Lower Extremity, Right D Lower Extremity, Left F Lower Extremities, Bilateral Z Musculoskeletal System, All	1 Technetium 99m (Tc-99m) Y Other Radionuclide	Z None	Z None
Y Musculoskeletal System, Other	Y Other Radionuclide	Z None	Z None

Section	C	Nuclear Medicine		
Body System	P	Musculoskeletal System		
Type	2	Tomographic (Tomo) Nuclear Medicine Imaging: Introduction of radioactive materials into the body for three dimensional display of images developed from the capture of radioactive emissions		

Body Part (Character 4)	Radionuclide (Character 5)	Qualifier (Character 6)	Qualifier (Character 7)
1 Skull 2 Cervical Spine 3 Skull and Cervical Spine 4 Thorax 6 Pelvis 7 Spine and Pelvis 8 Upper Extremity, Right 9 Upper Extremity, Left B Upper Extremities, Bilateral C Lower Extremity, Right D Lower Extremity, Left F Lower Extremities, Bilateral G Thoracic Spine H Lumbar Spine J Thoracolumbar Spine	1 Technetium 99m (Tc-99m) Y Other Radionuclide	Z None	Z None
Y Musculoskeletal System, Other	Y Other Radionuclide	Z None	Z None

Section	C	Nuclear Medicine		
Body System	P	Musculoskeletal System		
Type	5	Nonimaging Nuclear Medicine Probe: Introduction of radioactive materials into the body for the study of distribution and fate of certain substances by the detection of radioactive emissions; or, alternatively, measurement of absorption of radioactive emissions from an external source		

Body Part (Character 4)	Radionuclide (Character 5)	Qualifier (Character 6)	Qualifier (Character 7)
5 Spine N Upper Extremities P Lower Extremities	Z None	Z None	Z None
Y Musculoskeletal System, Other	Y Other Radionuclide	Z None	Z None

Section	C	Nuclear Medicine		
Body System	T	Urinary System		
Type	1	Planar Nuclear Medicine Imaging: Introduction of radioactive materials into the body for single plane display of images developed from the capture of radioactive emissions		

Body Part (Character 4)	Radionuclide (Character 5)	Qualifier (Character 6)	Qualifier (Character 7)
3 Kidneys, Ureters and Bladder	1 Technetium 99m (Tc-99m) F Iodine 123 (I-123) G Iodine 131 (I-131) Y Other Radionuclide	Z None	Z None
H Bladder and Ureters	1 Technetium 99m (Tc-99m) Y Other Radionuclide	Z None	Z None
Y Urinary System	Y Other Radionuclide	Z None	Z None

Section	C	Nuclear Medicine		
Body System	T	Urinary System		
Type	2	Tomographic (Tomo) Nuclear Medicine Imaging: Introduction of radioactive materials into the body for three dimensional display of images developed from the capture of radioactive emissions		

Body Part (Character 4)	Radionuclide (Character 5)	Qualifier (Character 6)	Qualifier (Character 7)
3 Kidneys, Ureters and Bladder	1 Technetium 99m (Tc-99m) Y Other Radionuclide	Z None	Z None
Y Urinary System	Y Other Radionuclide	Z None	Z None

Section	C	Nuclear Medicine		
Body System	T	Urinary System		
Type	6	Nonimaging Nuclear Medicine Assay: Introduction of radioactive materials into the body for the study of body fluids and blood elements, by the detection of radioactive emissions		

Body Part (Character 4)	Radionuclide (Character 5)	Qualifier (Character 6)	Qualifier (Character 7)
3 Kidneys, Ureters and Bladder	1 Technetium 99m (Tc-99m) F Iodine 123 (I-123) G Iodine 131 (I-131) H Iodine 125 (I-125) Y Other Radionuclide	Z None	Z None
Y Urinary System	Y Other Radionuclide	Z None	Z None

Section	C	Nuclear Medicine		
Body System	V	Male Reproductive System		
Type	1	Planar Nuclear Medicine Imaging: Introduction of radioactive materials into the body for single plane display of images developed from the capture of radioactive emissions		

Body Part (Character 4)	Radionuclide (Character 5)	Qualifier (Character 6)	Qualifier (Character 7)
9 Testicles, Bilateral	1 Technetium 99m (Tc-99m) Y Other Radionuclide	Z None	Z None
Y Male Reproductive System	Y Other Radionuclide	Z None	Z None

Section	C	Nuclear Medicine		
Body System	W	Anatomical Regions		
Type	1	Planar Nuclear Medicine Imaging: Introduction of radioactive materials into the body for single plane display of images developed from the capture of radioactive emissions		

Body Part (Character 4)	Radionuclide (Character 5)	Qualifier (Character 6)	Qualifier (Character 7)
0 Abdomen 1 Abdomen and Pelvis 4 Chest and Abdomen 6 Chest and Neck B Head and Neck D Lower Extremity J Pelvic Region M Upper Extremity N Whole Body	1 Technetium 99m (Tc-99m) D Indium 111 (In-111) F Iodine 123 (I-123) G Iodine 131 (I-131) L Gallium 67 (Ga-67) S Thallium 201 (Tl-201) Y Other Radionuclide	Z None	Z None
3 Chest	1 Technetium 99m (Tc-99m) D Indium 111 (In-111) F Iodine 123 (I-123) G Iodine 131 (I-131) K Fluorine 18 (F-18) L Gallium 67 (Ga-67) S Thallium 201 (Tl-201) Y Other Radionuclide	Z None	Z None
Y Anatomical Regions, Multiple	Y Other Radionuclide	Z None	Z None
Z Anatomical Region, Other	Z None	Z None	Z None

Section	C	Nuclear Medicine		
Body System	W	Anatomical Regions		
Type	2	Tomographic (Tomo) Nuclear Medicine Imaging: Introduction of radioactive materials into the body for three dimensional display of images developed from the capture of radioactive emissions		

Body Part (Character 4)	Radionuclide (Character 5)	Qualifier (Character 6)	Qualifier (Character 7)
0 Abdomen 1 Abdomen and Pelvis 3 Chest 4 Chest and Abdomen 6 Chest and Neck B Head and Neck D Lower Extremity J Pelvic Region M Upper Extremity	1 Technetium 99m (Tc-99m) D Indium 111 (In-111) F Iodine 123 (I-123) G Iodine 131 (I-131) K Fluorine 18 (F-18) L Gallium 67 (Ga-67) S Thallium 201 (Tl-201) Y Other Radionuclide	Z None	Z None
Y Anatomical Regions, Multiple	Y Other Radionuclide	Z None	Z None

Section	C	Nuclear Medicine		
Body System	W	Anatomical Regions		
Type	3	Positron Emission Tomographic (PET) Imaging: Introduction of radioactive materials into the body for three dimensional display of images developed from the simultaneous capture, 180 degrees apart, of radioactive emissions		

Body Part (Character 4)	Radionuclide (Character 5)	Qualifier (Character 6)	Qualifier (Character 7)
N Whole Body	Y Other Radionuclide	Z None	Z None

Section	C	Nuclear Medicine		
Body System	W	Anatomical Regions		
Type	5	Nonimaging Nuclear Medicine Probe: Introduction of radioactive materials into the body for the study of distribution and fate of certain substances by the detection of radioactive emissions; or, alternatively, measurement of absorption of radioactive emissions from an external source		

Body Part (Character 4)	Radionuclide (Character 5)	Qualifier (Character 6)	Qualifier (Character 7)
0 Abdomen 1 Abdomen and Pelvis 3 Chest 4 Chest and Abdomen 6 Chest and Neck B Head and Neck D Lower Extremity J Pelvic Region M Upper Extremity	1 Technetium 99m (Tc-99m) D Indium 111 (In-111) Y Other Radionuclide	Z None	Z None

Section	C	Nuclear Medicine		
Body System	W	Anatomical Regions		
Type	7	Systemic Nuclear Medicine Therapy: Introduction of unsealed radioactive materials into the body for treatment		

Body Part (Character 4)	Radionuclide (Character 5)	Qualifier (Character 6)	Qualifier (Character 7)
0 Abdomen 3 Chest	N Phosphorus 32 (P-32) Y Other Radionuclide	Z None	Z None
G Thyroid	G Iodine 131 (I-131) Y Other Radionuclide	Z None	Z None
N Whole Body	8 Samarium 153 (Sm-153) G Iodine 131 (I-131) N Phosphorus 32 (P-32) P Strontium 89 (Sr-89) Y Other Radionuclide	Z None	Z None
Y Anatomical Regions, Multiple	Y Other Radionuclide	Z None	Z None

Section	D	Radiation Therapy		
Body System	0	Central and Peripheral Nervous System		
Modality	0	Beam Radiation		
Treatment Site (Character 4)	**Modality Qualifier (Character 5)**		**Isotope (Character 6)**	**Qualifier (Character 7)**
0 Brain 1 Brain Stem 6 Spinal Cord 7 Peripheral Nerve	0 Photons <1 MeV 1 Photons 1 - 10 MeV 2 Photons >10 MeV 4 Heavy Particles (Protons, Ions) 5 Neutrons 6 Neutron Capture		Z None	Z None
0 Brain 1 Brain Stem 6 Spinal Cord 7 Peripheral Nerve	3 Electrons		Z None	0 Intraoperative Z None

Section	D	Radiation Therapy		
Body System	0	Central and Peripheral Nervous System		
Modality	1	Brachytherapy		
Treatment Site (Character 4)	**Modality Qualifier (Character 5)**		**Isotope (Character 6)**	**Qualifier (Character 7)**
0 Brain 1 Brain Stem 6 Spinal Cord 7 Peripheral Nerve	9 High Dose Rate (HDR) B Low Dose Rate (LDR)		7 Cesium 137 (Cs-137) 8 Iridium 192 (Ir-192) 9 Iodine 125 (I-125) B Palladium 103 (Pd-103) C Californium 252 (Cf-252) Y Other Isotope	Z None

Section	D	Radiation Therapy		
Body System	0	Central and Peripheral Nervous System		
Modality	2	Stereotactic Radiosurgery		
Treatment Site (Character 4)	**Modality Qualifier (Character 5)**		**Isotope (Character 6)**	**Qualifier (Character 7)**
0 Brain 1 Brain Stem 6 Spinal Cord 7 Peripheral Nerve	D Stereotactic Other Photon Radiosurgery H Stereotactic Particulate Radiosurgery J Stereotactic Gamma Beam Radiosurgery		Z None	Z None

Section	D	Radiation Therapy		
Body System	0	Central and Peripheral Nervous System		
Modality	Y	Other Radiation		
Treatment Site (Character 4)	**Modality Qualifier (Character 5)**		**Isotope (Character 6)**	**Qualifier (Character 7)**
0 Brain 1 Brain Stem 6 Spinal Cord 7 Peripheral Nerve	7 Contact Radiation 8 Hyperthermia F Plaque Radiation K Laser Interstitial Thermal Therapy		Z None	Z None

Section	D	Radiation Therapy		
Body System	7	Lymphatic and Hematologic System		
Modality	0	Beam Radiation		
Treatment Site (Character 4)	**Modality Qualifier (Character 5)**		**Isotope (Character 6)**	**Qualifier (Character 7)**
0 Bone Marrow 1 Thymus 2 Spleen 3 Lymphatics, Neck 4 Lymphatics, Axillary 5 Lymphatics, Thorax 6 Lymphatics, Abdomen 7 Lymphatics, Pelvis 8 Lymphatics, Inguinal	0 Photons <1 MeV 1 Photons 1 - 10 MeV 2 Photons >10 MeV 4 Heavy Particles (Protons, Ions) 5 Neutrons 6 Neutron Capture		Z None	Z None
0 Bone Marrow 1 Thymus 2 Spleen 3 Lymphatics, Neck 4 Lymphatics, Axillary 5 Lymphatics, Thorax 6 Lymphatics, Abdomen 7 Lymphatics, Pelvis 8 Lymphatics, Inguinal	3 Electrons		Z None	0 Intraoperative Z None

Section	D	Radiation Therapy		
Body System	7	Lymphatic and Hematologic System		
Modality	1	Brachytherapy		
Treatment Site (Character 4)	**Modality Qualifier (Character 5)**		**Isotope (Character 6)**	**Qualifier (Character 7)**
0 Bone Marrow 1 Thymus 2 Spleen 3 Lymphatics, Neck 4 Lymphatics, Axillary 5 Lymphatics, Thorax 6 Lymphatics, Abdomen 7 Lymphatics, Pelvis 8 Lymphatics, Inguinal	9 High Dose Rate (HDR) B Low Dose Rate (LDR)		7 Cesium 137 (Cs-137) 8 Iridium 192 (Ir-192) 9 Iodine 125 (I-125) B Palladium 103 (Pd-103) C Californium 252 (Cf-252) Y Other Isotope	Z None

Section	D	Radiation Therapy		
Body System	7	Lymphatic and Hematologic System		
Modality	2	Stereotactic Radiosurgery		
Treatment Site (Character 4)	**Modality Qualifier (Character 5)**		**Isotope (Character 6)**	**Qualifier (Character 7)**
0 Bone Marrow 1 Thymus 2 Spleen 3 Lymphatics, Neck 4 Lymphatics, Axillary 5 Lymphatics, Thorax 6 Lymphatics, Abdomen 7 Lymphatics, Pelvis 8 Lymphatics, Inguinal	D Stereotactic Other Photon Radiosurgery H Stereotactic Particulate Radiosurgery J Stereotactic Gamma Beam Radiosurgery		Z None	Z None

Section	D	Radiation Therapy			
Body System	7	Lymphatic and Hematologic System			
Modality	Y	Other Radiation			
Treatment Site (Character 4)		Modality Qualifier (Character 5)	Isotope (Character 6)	Qualifier (Character 7)	
0 Bone Marrow 1 Thymus 2 Spleen 3 Lymphatics, Neck 4 Lymphatics, Axillary 5 Lymphatics, Thorax 6 Lymphatics, Abdomen 7 Lymphatics, Pelvis 8 Lymphatics, Inguinal		8 Hyperthermia F Plaque Radiation	Z None	Z None	

Section	D	Radiation Therapy			
Body System	8	Eye			
Modality	0	Beam Radiation			
Treatment Site (Character 4)		Modality Qualifier (Character 5)	Isotope (Character 6)	Qualifier (Character 7)	
0 Eye		0 Photons <1 MeV 1 Photons 1 - 10 MeV 2 Photons >10 MeV 4 Heavy Particles (Protons, Ions) 5 Neutrons 6 Neutron Capture	Z None	Z None	
0 Eye		3 Electrons	Z None	0 Intraoperative Z None	

Section	D	Radiation Therapy			
Body System	8	Eye			
Modality	1	Brachytherapy			
Treatment Site (Character 4)		Modality Qualifier (Character 5)	Isotope (Character 6)	Qualifier (Character 7)	
0 Eye		9 High Dose Rate (HDR) B Low Dose Rate (LDR)	7 Cesium 137 (Cs-137) 8 Iridium 192 (Ir-192) 9 Iodine 125 (I-125) B Palladium 103 (Pd-103) C Californium 252 (Cf-252) Y Other Isotope	Z None	

Section	D	Radiation Therapy			
Body System	8	Eye			
Modality	2	Stereotactic Radiosurgery			
Treatment Site (Character 4)		Modality Qualifier (Character 5)	Isotope (Character 6)	Qualifier (Character 7)	
0 Eye		D Stereotactic Other Photon Radiosurgery H Stereotactic Particulate Radiosurgery J Stereotactic Gamma Beam Radiosurgery	Z None	Z None	

Section	D	Radiation Therapy			
Body System	8	Eye			
Modality	Y	Other Radiation			

Treatment Site (Character 4)	Modality Qualifier (Character 5)	Isotope (Character 6)	Qualifier (Character 7)
0 Eye	7 Contact Radiation 8 Hyperthermia F Plaque Radiation	Z None	Z None

Section	D	Radiation Therapy			
Body System	9	Ear, Nose, Mouth and Throat			
Modality	0	Beam Radiation			

Treatment Site (Character 4)	Modality Qualifier (Character 5)	Isotope (Character 6)	Qualifier (Character 7)
0 Ear 1 Nose 3 Hypopharynx 4 Mouth 5 Tongue 6 Salivary Glands 7 Sinuses 8 Hard Palate 9 Soft Palate B Larynx D Nasopharynx F Oropharynx	0 Photons <1 MeV 1 Photons 1 - 10 MeV 2 Photons >10 MeV 4 Heavy Particles (Protons, Ions) 5 Neutrons 6 Neutron Capture	Z None	Z None
0 Ear 1 Nose 3 Hypopharynx 4 Mouth 5 Tongue 6 Salivary Glands 7 Sinuses 8 Hard Palate 9 Soft Palate B Larynx D Nasopharynx F Oropharynx	3 Electrons	Z None	0 Intraoperative Z None

Section	D	Radiation Therapy			
Body System	9	Ear, Nose, Mouth and Throat			
Modality	1	Brachytherapy			

Treatment Site (Character 4)	Modality Qualifier (Character 5)	Isotope (Character 6)	Qualifier (Character 7)
0 Ear 1 Nose 3 Hypopharynx 4 Mouth 5 Tongue 6 Salivary Glands 7 Sinuses 8 Hard Palate 9 Soft Palate B Larynx D Nasopharynx F Oropharynx	9 High Dose Rate (HDR) B Low Dose Rate (LDR)	7 Cesium 137 (Cs-137) 8 Iridium 192 (Ir-192) 9 Iodine 125 (I-125) B Palladium 103 (Pd-103) C Californium 252 (Cf-252) Y Other Isotope	Z None

Section	D	Radiation Therapy			
Body System	9	Ear, Nose, Mouth and Throat			
Modality	2	Stereotactic Radiosurgery			

Treatment Site (Character 4)	Modality Qualifier (Character 5)	Isotope (Character 6)	Qualifier (Character 7)

0 Ear
1 Nose
4 Mouth
5 Tongue
6 Salivary Glands
7 Sinuses
8 Hard Palate
9 Soft Palate
B Larynx
C Pharynx
D Nasopharynx
	D Stereotactic Other Photon
	   Radiosurgery
	H Stereotactic Particulate
	   Radiosurgery
	J Stereotactic Gamma Beam
	   Radiosurgery
		Z None	Z None

Section	D	Radiation Therapy			
Body System	9	Ear, Nose, Mouth and Throat			
Modality	Y	Other Radiation			

Treatment Site (Character 4)	Modality Qualifier (Character 5)	Isotope (Character 6)	Qualifier (Character 7)
0 Ear 1 Nose 5 Tongue 6 Salivary Glands 7 Sinuses 8 Hard Palate 9 Soft Palate	7 Contact Radiation 8 Hyperthermia F Plaque Radiation	Z None	Z None
3 Hypopharynx F Oropharynx	7 Contact Radiation 8 Hyperthermia	Z None	Z None
4 Mouth B Larynx D Nasopharynx	7 Contact Radiation 8 Hyperthermia C Intraoperative Radiation Therapy (IORT) F Plaque Radiation	Z None	Z None
C Pharynx	C Intraoperative Radiation Therapy (IORT) F Plaque Radiation	Z None	Z None

Section	D	Radiation Therapy			
Body System	B	Respiratory System			
Modality	0	Beam Radiation			

Treatment Site (Character 4)	Modality Qualifier (Character 5)	Isotope (Character 6)	Qualifier (Character 7)
0 Trachea 1 Bronchus 2 Lung 5 Pleura 6 Mediastinum 7 Chest Wall 8 Diaphragm	0 Photons <1 MeV 1 Photons 1 - 10 MeV 2 Photons >10 MeV 4 Heavy Particles (Protons, Ions) 5 Neutrons 6 Neutron Capture	Z None	Z None
0 Trachea 1 Bronchus 2 Lung 5 Pleura 6 Mediastinum 7 Chest Wall 8 Diaphragm	3 Electrons	Z None	0 Intraoperative Z None

Section	D	Radiation Therapy			
Body System	B	Respiratory System			
Modality	1	Brachytherapy			

Treatment Site (Character 4)	Modality Qualifier (Character 5)	Isotope (Character 6)	Qualifier (Character 7)
0 Trachea 1 Bronchus 2 Lung 5 Pleura 6 Mediastinum 7 Chest Wall 8 Diaphragm	9 High Dose Rate (HDR) B Low Dose Rate (LDR)	7 Cesium 137 (Cs-137) 8 Iridium 192 (Ir-192) 9 Iodine 125 (I-125) B Palladium 103 (Pd-103) C Californium 252 (Cf-252) Y Other Isotope	Z None

Section	D	Radiation Therapy			
Body System	B	Respiratory System			
Modality	2	Stereotactic Radiosurgery			

Treatment Site (Character 4)	Modality Qualifier (Character 5)	Isotope (Character 6)	Qualifier (Character 7)
0 Trachea 1 Bronchus 2 Lung 5 Pleura 6 Mediastinum 7 Chest Wall 8 Diaphragm	D Stereotactic Other Photon Radiosurgery H Stereotactic Particulate Radiosurgery J Stereotactic Gamma Beam Radiosurgery	Z None	Z None

Section	D	Radiation Therapy			
Body System	B	Respiratory System			
Modality	Y	Other Radiation			

Treatment Site (Character 4)	Modality Qualifier (Character 5)	Isotope (Character 6)	Qualifier (Character 7)
0 Trachea 1 Bronchus 2 Lung 5 Pleura 6 Mediastinum 7 Chest Wall 8 Diaphragm	7 Contact Radiation 8 Hyperthermia F Plaque Radiation K Laser Interstitial Thermal Therapy	Z None	Z None

Section	D	Radiation Therapy			
Body System	D	Gastrointestinal System			
Modality	0	Beam Radiation			

Treatment Site (Character 4)	Modality Qualifier (Character 5)	Isotope (Character 6)	Qualifier (Character 7)
0 Esophagus 1 Stomach 2 Duodenum 3 Jejunum 4 Ileum 5 Colon 7 Rectum	0 Photons <1 MeV 1 Photons 1 - 10 MeV 2 Photons >10 MeV 4 Heavy Particles (Protons, Ions) 5 Neutrons 6 Neutron Capture	Z None	Z None
0 Esophagus 1 Stomach 2 Duodenum 3 Jejunum 4 Ileum 5 Colon 7 Rectum	3 Electrons	Z None	0 Intraoperative Z None

Section	D	Radiation Therapy			
Body System	D	Gastrointestinal System			
Modality	1	Brachytherapy			

Treatment Site (Character 4)	Modality Qualifier (Character 5)	Isotope (Character 6)	Qualifier (Character 7)
0 Esophagus 1 Stomach 2 Duodenum 3 Jejunum 4 Ileum 5 Colon 7 Rectum	9 High Dose Rate (HDR) B Low Dose Rate (LDR)	7 Cesium 137 (Cs-137) 8 Iridium 192 (Ir-192) 9 Iodine 125 (I-125) B Palladium 103 (Pd-103) C Californium 252 (Cf-252) Y Other Isotope	Z None

Section	D	Radiation Therapy			
Body System	D	Gastrointestinal System			
Modality	2	Stereotactic Radiosurgery			

Treatment Site (Character 4)	Modality Qualifier (Character 5)	Isotope (Character 6)	Qualifier (Character 7)
0 Esophagus 1 Stomach 2 Duodenum 3 Jejunum 4 Ileum 5 Colon 7 Rectum	D Stereotactic Other Photon Radiosurgery H Stereotactic Particulate Radiosurgery J Stereotactic Gamma Beam Radiosurgery	Z None	Z None

Section	D	Radiation Therapy			
Body System	D	Gastrointestinal System			
Modality	Y	Other Radiation			

Treatment Site (Character 4)	Modality Qualifier (Character 5)	Isotope (Character 6)	Qualifier (Character 7)
0 Esophagus	7 Contact Radiation 8 Hyperthermia F Plaque Radiation K Laser Interstitial Thermal Therapy	Z None	Z None
1 Stomach 2 Duodenum 3 Jejunum 4 Ileum 5 Colon 7 Rectum	7 Contact Radiation 8 Hyperthermia C Intraoperative Radiation Therapy (IORT) F Plaque Radiation K Laser Interstitial Thermal Therapy	Z None	Z None
8 Anus	C Intraoperative Radiation Therapy (IORT) F Plaque Radiation K Laser Interstitial Thermal Therapy	Z None	Z None

Section	D	Radiation Therapy
Body System	F	Hepatobiliary System and Pancreas
Modality	0	Beam Radiation

Treatment Site (Character 4)	Modality Qualifier (Character 5)	Isotope (Character 6)	Qualifier (Character 7)
0 Liver 1 Gallbladder 2 Bile Ducts 3 Pancreas	0 Photons <1 MeV 1 Photons 1 - 10 MeV 2 Photons >10 MeV 4 Heavy Particles (Protons, Ions) 5 Neutrons 6 Neutron Capture	Z None	Z None
0 Liver 1 Gallbladder 2 Bile Ducts 3 Pancreas	3 Electrons	Z None	0 Intraoperative Z None

Section	D	Radiation Therapy
Body System	F	Hepatobiliary System and Pancreas
Modality	1	Brachytherapy

Treatment Site (Character 4)	Modality Qualifier (Character 5)	Isotope (Character 6)	Qualifier (Character 7)
0 Liver 1 Gallbladder 2 Bile Ducts 3 Pancreas	9 High Dose Rate (HDR) B Low Dose Rate (LDR)	7 Cesium 137 (Cs-137) 8 Iridium 192 (Ir-192) 9 Iodine 125 (I-125) B Palladium 103 (Pd-103) C Californium 252 (Cf-252) Y Other Isotope	Z None

Section	D	Radiation Therapy
Body System	F	Hepatobiliary System and Pancreas
Modality	2	Stereotactic Radiosurgery

Treatment Site (Character 4)	Modality Qualifier (Character 5)	Isotope (Character 6)	Qualifier (Character 7)
0 Liver 1 Gallbladder 2 Bile Ducts 3 Pancreas	D Stereotactic Other Photon Radiosurgery H Stereotactic Particulate Radiosurgery J Stereotactic Gamma Beam Radiosurgery	Z None	Z None

Section	D	Radiation Therapy
Body System	F	Hepatobiliary System and Pancreas
Modality	Y	Other Radiation

Treatment Site (Character 4)	Modality Qualifier (Character 5)	Isotope (Character 6)	Qualifier (Character 7)
0 Liver 1 Gallbladder 2 Bile Ducts 3 Pancreas	7 Contact Radiation 8 Hyperthermia C Intraoperative Radiation Therapy (IORT) F Plaque Radiation K Laser Interstitial Thermal Therapy	Z None	Z None

Section	D	Radiation Therapy		
Body System	G	Endocrine System		
Modality	0	Beam Radiation		
Treatment Site (Character 4)	**Modality Qualifier (Character 5)**		**Isotope (Character 6)**	**Qualifier (Character 7)**
0 Pituitary Gland **1** Pineal Body **2** Adrenal Glands **4** Parathyroid Glands **5** Thyroid	**0** Photons <1 MeV **1** Photons 1 - 10 MeV **2** Photons >10 MeV **5** Neutrons **6** Neutron Capture		**Z** None	**Z** None
0 Pituitary Gland **1** Pineal Body **2** Adrenal Glands **4** Parathyroid Glands **5** Thyroid	**3** Electrons		**Z** None	**0** Intraoperative **Z** None

Section	D	Radiation Therapy		
Body System	G	Endocrine System		
Modality	1	Brachytherapy		
Treatment Site (Character 4)	**Modality Qualifier (Character 5)**		**Isotope (Character 6)**	**Qualifier (Character 7)**
0 Pituitary Gland **1** Pineal Body **2** Adrenal Glands **4** Parathyroid Glands **5** Thyroid	**9** High Dose Rate (HDR) **B** Low Dose Rate (LDR)		**7** Cesium 137 (Cs-137) **8** Iridium 192 (Ir-192) **9** Iodine 125 (I-125) **B** Palladium 103 (Pd-103) **C** Californium 252 (Cf-252) **Y** Other Isotope	**Z** None

Section	D	Radiation Therapy		
Body System	G	Endocrine System		
Modality	2	Stereotactic Radiosurgery		
Treatment Site (Character 4)	**Modality Qualifier (Character 5)**		**Isotope (Character 6)**	**Qualifier (Character 7)**
0 Pituitary Gland **1** Pineal Body **2** Adrenal Glands **4** Parathyroid Glands **5** Thyroid	**D** Stereotactic Other Photon Radiosurgery **H** Stereotactic Particulate Radiosurgery **J** Stereotactic Gamma Beam Radiosurgery		**Z** None	**Z** None

Section	D	Radiation Therapy		
Body System	G	Endocrine System		
Modality	Y	Other Radiation		
Treatment Site (Character 4)	**Modality Qualifier (Character 5)**		**Isotope (Character 6)**	**Qualifier (Character 7)**
0 Pituitary Gland **1** Pineal Body **2** Adrenal Glands **4** Parathyroid Glands **5** Thyroid	**7** Contact Radiation **8** Hyperthermia **F** Plaque Radiation **K** Laser Interstitial Thermal Therapy		**Z** None	**Z** None

Section	D	Radiation Therapy		
Body System	H	Skin		
Modality	0	Beam Radiation		
Treatment Site (Character 4)		Modality Qualifier (Character 5)	Isotope (Character 6)	Qualifier (Character 7)
2 Skin, Face 3 Skin, Neck 4 Skin, Arm 6 Skin, Chest 7 Skin, Back 8 Skin, Abdomen 9 Skin, Buttock B Skin, Leg		0 Photons <1 MeV 1 Photons 1 - 10 MeV 2 Photons >10 MeV 4 Heavy Particles (Protons, Ions) 5 Neutrons 6 Neutron Capture	Z None	Z None
2 Skin, Face 3 Skin, Neck 4 Skin, Arm 6 Skin, Chest 7 Skin, Back 8 Skin, Abdomen 9 Skin, Buttock B Skin, Leg		3 Electrons	Z None	0 Intraoperative Z None

Section	D	Radiation Therapy		
Body System	H	Skin		
Modality	Y	Other Radiation		
Treatment Site (Character 4)		Modality Qualifier (Character 5)	Isotope (Character 6)	Qualifier (Character 7)
2 Skin, Face 3 Skin, Neck 4 Skin, Arm 6 Skin, Chest 7 Skin, Back 8 Skin, Abdomen 9 Skin, Buttock B Skin, Leg		7 Contact Radiation 8 Hyperthermia F Plaque Radiation	Z None	Z None
5 Skin, Hand C Skin, Foot		F Plaque Radiation	Z None	Z None

Section	D	Radiation Therapy		
Body System	M	Breast		
Modality	0	Beam Radiation		
Treatment Site (Character 4)		Modality Qualifier (Character 5)	Isotope (Character 6)	Qualifier (Character 7)
0 Breast, Left 1 Breast, Right		0 Photons <1 MeV 1 Photons 1 - 10 MeV 2 Photons >10 MeV 4 Heavy Particles (Protons, Ions) 5 Neutrons 6 Neutron Capture	Z None	Z None
0 Breast, Left 1 Breast, Right		3 Electrons	Z None	0 Intraoperative Z None

Section	D	Radiation Therapy			
Body System	M	Breast			
Modality	1	Brachytherapy			
Treatment Site (Character 4)		Modality Qualifier (Character 5)	Isotope (Character 6)	Qualifier (Character 7)	
0 Breast, Left 1 Breast, Right		9 High Dose Rate (HDR) B Low Dose Rate (LDR)	7 Cesium 137 (Cs-137) 8 Iridium 192 (Ir-192) 9 Iodine 125 (I-125) B Palladium 103 (Pd-103) C Californium 252 (Cf-252) Y Other Isotope	Z None	

Section	D	Radiation Therapy			
Body System	M	Breast			
Modality	2	Stereotactic Radiosurgery			
Treatment Site (Character 4)		Modality Qualifier (Character 5)	Isotope (Character 6)	Qualifier (Character 7)	
0 Breast, Left 1 Breast, Right		D Stereotactic Other Photon Radiosurgery H Stereotactic Particulate Radiosurgery J Stereotactic Gamma Beam Radiosurgery	Z None	Z None	

Section	D	Radiation Therapy			
Body System	M	Breast			
Modality	Y	Other Radiation			
Treatment Site (Character 4)		Modality Qualifier (Character 5)	Isotope (Character 6)	Qualifier (Character 7)	
0 Breast, Left 1 Breast, Right		7 Contact Radiation 8 Hyperthermia F Plaque Radiation K Laser Interstitial Thermal Therapy	Z None	Z None	

Section	D	Radiation Therapy			
Body System	P	Musculoskeletal System			
Modality	0	Beam Radiation			
Treatment Site (Character 4)		Modality Qualifier (Character 5)	Isotope (Character 6)	Qualifier (Character 7)	
0 Skull 2 Maxilla 3 Mandible 4 Sternum 5 Rib(s) 6 Humerus 7 Radius/Ulna 8 Pelvic Bones 9 Femur B Tibia/Fibula C Other Bone		0 Photons <1 MeV 1 Photons 1 - 10 MeV 2 Photons >10 MeV 4 Heavy Particles (Protons, Ions) 5 Neutrons 6 Neutron Capture	Z None	Z None	
0 Skull 2 Maxilla 3 Mandible 4 Sternum 5 Rib(s) 6 Humerus		3 Electrons	Z None	0 Intraoperative Z None	

Continued on Next Page ▶

7 Radius/Ulna 8 Pelvic Bones 9 Femur B Tibia/Fibula C Other Bone			Continued from ◄ Previous Page

Section	D	Radiation Therapy
Body System	P	Musculoskeletal System
Modality	Y	Other Radiation

Treatment Site (Character 4)	Modality Qualifier (Character 5)	Isotope (Character 6)	Qualifier (Character 7)
0 Skull 2 Maxilla 3 Mandible 4 Sternum 5 Rib(s) 6 Humerus 7 Radius/Ulna 8 Pelvic Bones 9 Femur B Tibia/Fibula C Other Bone	7 Contact Radiation 8 Hyperthermia F Plaque Radiation	Z None	Z None

Section	D	Radiation Therapy
Body System	T	Urinary System
Modality	0	Beam Radiation

Treatment Site (Character 4)	Modality Qualifier (Character 5)	Isotope (Character 6)	Qualifier (Character 7)
0 Kidney 1 Ureter 2 Bladder 3 Urethra	0 Photons <1 MeV 1 Photons 1 - 10 MeV 2 Photons >10 MeV 4 Heavy Particles (Protons, Ions) 5 Neutrons 6 Neutron Capture	Z None	Z None
0 Kidney 1 Ureter 2 Bladder 3 Urethra	3 Electrons	Z None	0 Intraoperative Z None

Section	D	Radiation Therapy
Body System	T	Urinary System
Modality	1	Brachytherapy

Treatment Site (Character 4)	Modality Qualifier (Character 5)	Isotope (Character 6)	Qualifier (Character 7)
0 Kidney 1 Ureter 2 Bladder 3 Urethra	9 High Dose Rate (HDR) B Low Dose Rate (LDR)	7 Cesium 137 (Cs-137) 8 Iridium 192 (Ir-192) 9 Iodine 125 (I-125) B Palladium 103 (Pd-103) C Californium 252 (Cf-252) Y Other Isotope	Z None

Section	D	Radiation Therapy		
Body System	T	Urinary System		
Modality	2	Stereotactic Radiosurgery		
Treatment Site (Character 4)	**Modality Qualifier (Character 5)**		**Isotope (Character 6)**	**Qualifier (Character 7)**

0 Kidney
1 Ureter
2 Bladder
3 Urethra
	D Stereotactic Other Photon
	   Radiosurgery
	H Stereotactic Particulate
	   Radiosurgery
	J Stereotactic Gamma Beam
	   Radiosurgery
			Z None	Z None

Section	D	Radiation Therapy		
Body System	T	Urinary System		
Modality	Y	Other Radiation		
Treatment Site (Character 4)	**Modality Qualifier (Character 5)**		**Isotope (Character 6)**	**Qualifier (Character 7)**
0 Kidney 1 Ureter 2 Bladder 3 Urethra	7 Contact Radiation 8 Hyperthermia C Intraoperative Radiation Therapy (IORT) F Plaque Radiation		Z None	Z None

Section	D	Radiation Therapy		
Body System	U	Female Reproductive System		
Modality	0	Beam Radiation		
Treatment Site (Character 4)	**Modality Qualifier (Character 5)**		**Isotope (Character 6)**	**Qualifier (Character 7)**
0 Ovary 1 Cervix 2 Uterus	0 Photons <1 MeV 1 Photons 1 - 10 MeV 2 Photons >10 MeV 4 Heavy Particles (Protons, Ions) 5 Neutrons 6 Neutron Capture		Z None	Z None
0 Ovary 1 Cervix 2 Uterus	3 Electrons		Z None	0 Intraoperative Z None

Section	D	Radiation Therapy		
Body System	U	Female Reproductive System		
Modality	1	Brachytherapy		
Treatment Site (Character 4)	**Modality Qualifier (Character 5)**		**Isotope (Character 6)**	**Qualifier (Character 7)**

0 Ovary
1 Cervix
2 Uterus
	9 High Dose Rate (HDR)
	B Low Dose Rate (LDR)
			7 Cesium 137 (Cs-137)
			8 Iridium 192 (Ir-192)
			9 Iodine 125 (I-125)
			B Palladium 103 (Pd-
			   103)
			C Californium 252 (Cf-
			   252)
			Y Other Isotope
				Z None

Section	D	Radiation Therapy			
Body System	U	Female Reproductive System			
Modality	2	Stereotactic Radiosurgery			

Treatment Site (Character 4)	Modality Qualifier (Character 5)	Isotope (Character 6)	Qualifier (Character 7)
0 Ovary 1 Cervix 2 Uterus	D Stereotactic Other Photon Radiosurgery H Stereotactic Particulate Radiosurgery J Stereotactic Gamma Beam Radiosurgery	Z None	Z None

Section	D	Radiation Therapy			
Body System	U	Female Reproductive System			
Modality	Y	Other Radiation			

Treatment Site (Character 4)	Modality Qualifier (Character 5)	Isotope (Character 6)	Qualifier (Character 7)
0 Ovary 1 Cervix 2 Uterus	7 Contact Radiation 8 Hyperthermia C Intraoperative Radiation Therapy (IORT) F Plaque Radiation	Z None	Z None

Section	D	Radiation Therapy			
Body System	V	Male Reproductive System			
Modality	0	Male Reproductive System 0 Beam Radiation			

Treatment Site (Character 4)	Modality Qualifier (Character 5)	Isotope (Character 6)	Qualifier (Character 7)
0 Prostate 1 Testis	0 Photons <1 MeV 1 Photons 1 - 10 MeV 2 Photons >10 MeV 4 Heavy Particles (Protons, Ions) 5 Neutrons 6 Neutron Capture	Z None	Z None
0 Prostate 1 Testis	3 Electrons	Z None	0 Intraoperative Z None

Section	D	Radiation Therapy			
Body System	V	Male Reproductive System			
Modality	1	Brachytherapy			

Treatment Site (Character 4)	Modality Qualifier (Character 5)	Isotope (Character 6)	Qualifier (Character 7)
0 Prostate 1 Testis	9 High Dose Rate (HDR) B Low Dose Rate (LDR)	7 Cesium 137 (Cs-137) 8 Iridium 192 (Ir-192) 9 Iodine 125 (I-125) B Palladium 103 (Pd-103) C Californium 252 (Cf-252) Y Other Isotope	Z None

Section	D	Radiation Therapy			
Body System	V	Male Reproductive System			
Modality	2	Stereotactic Radiosurgery			

Treatment Site (Character 4)	Modality Qualifier (Character 5)	Isotope (Character 6)	Qualifier (Character 7)
0 Prostate 1 Testis	D Stereotactic Other Photon Radiosurgery H Stereotactic Particulate Radiosurgery J Stereotactic Gamma Beam Radiosurgery	Z None	Z None

Section	D	Radiation Therapy		
Body System	V	Male Reproductive System		
Modality	Y	Other Radiation		

Treatment Site (Character 4)	Modality Qualifier (Character 5)	Isotope (Character 6)	Qualifier (Character 7)
0 Prostate	7 Contact Radiation 8 Hyperthermia C Intraoperative Radiation Therapy (IORT) F Plaque Radiation K Laser Interstitial Thermal Therapy	Z None	Z None
1 Testis	7 Contact Radiation 8 Hyperthermia F Plaque Radiation	Z None	Z None

Section	D	Radiation Therapy		
Body System	W	Anatomical Regions		
Modality	0	Beam Radiation		

Treatment Site (Character 4)	Modality Qualifier (Character 5)	Isotope (Character 6)	Qualifier (Character 7)
1 Head and Neck 2 Chest 3 Abdomen 4 Hemibody 5 Whole Body 6 Pelvic Region	0 Photons <1 MeV 1 Photons 1 - 10 MeV 2 Photons >10 MeV 4 Heavy Particles (Protons, Ions) 5 Neutrons 6 Neutron Capture	Z None	Z None
1 Head and Neck 2 Chest 3 Abdomen 4 Hemibody 5 Whole Body 6 Pelvic Region	3 Electrons	Z None	0 Intraoperative Z None

Section	D	Radiation Therapy		
Body System	W	Anatomical Regions		
Modality	1	Brachytherapy		

Treatment Site (Character 4)	Modality Qualifier (Character 5)	Isotope (Character 6)	Qualifier (Character 7)
1 Head and Neck 2 Chest 3 Abdomen 6 Pelvic Region	9 High Dose Rate (HDR) B Low Dose Rate (LDR)	7 Cesium 137 (Cs-137) 8 Iridium 192 (Ir-192) 9 Iodine 125 (I-125) B Palladium 103 (Pd-103) C Californium 252 (Cf-252) Y Other Isotope	Z None

Section	D	Radiation Therapy		
Body System	W	Anatomical Regions		
Modality	2	Stereotactic Radiosurgery		

Treatment Site (Character 4)	Modality Qualifier (Character 5)	Isotope (Character 6)	Qualifier (Character 7)
1 Head and Neck 2 Chest 3 Abdomen 6 Pelvic Region	D Stereotactic Other Photon Radiosurgery H Stereotactic Particulate Radiosurgery J Stereotactic Gamma Beam Radiosurgery	Z None	Z None

Section	D	Radiation Therapy			
Body System	W	Anatomical Regions			
Modality	Y	Other Radiation			

Treatment Site (Character 4)	Modality Qualifier (Character 5)	Isotope (Character 6)	Qualifier (Character 7)
1 Head and Neck 2 Chest 3 Abdomen 4 Hemibody 6 Pelvic Region	7 Contact Radiation 8 Hyperthermia F Plaque Radiation	Z None	Z None
5 Whole Body	7 Contact Radiation 8 Hyperthermia F Plaque Radiation	Z None	Z None
5 Whole Body	G Isotope Administration	D Iodine 131 (I-131) F Phosphorus 32 (P-32) G Strontium 89 (Sr-89) H Strontium 90 (Sr-90) Y Other Isotope	Z None

Section	F	Physical Rehabilitation and Diagnostic Audiology		
Section Qualifier	0	Rehabilitation		
Type	0	Speech Assessment: Measurement of speech and related functions		

Body System/Region (Character 4)	Type Qualifier (Character 5)	Equipment (Character 6)	Qualifier (Character 7)
3 Neurological System - Whole Body	G Communicative/Cognitive Integration Skills	K Audiovisual M Augmentative / Alternative Communication P Computer Y Other Equipment Z None	Z None
Z None	0 Filtered Speech 3 Staggered Spondaic Word Q Performance Intensity Phonetically Balanced Speech Discrimination R Brief Tone Stimuli S Distorted Speech T Dichotic Stimuli V Temporal Ordering of Stimuli W Masking Patterns	1 Audiometer 2 Sound Field / Booth K Audiovisual Z None	Z None
Z None	1 Speech Threshold 2 Speech/Word Recognition	1 Audiometer 2 Sound Field / Booth 9 Cochlear Implant K Audiovisual Z None	Z None
Z None	4 Sensorineural Acuity Level	1 Audiometer 2 Sound Field / Booth Z None	Z None
Z None	5 Synthetic Sentence Identification	1 Audiometer 2 Sound Field / Booth 9 Cochlear Implant K Audiovisual	Z None
Z None	6 Speech and/or Language Screening 7 Nonspoken Language 8 Receptive/Expressive Language C Aphasia G Communicative/Cognitive Integration Skills L Augmentative/Alternative Communication System	K Audiovisual M Augmentative / Alternative Communication P Computer Y Other Equipment Z None	Z None
Z None	9 Articulation/Phonology	K Audiovisual P Computer Q Speech Analysis Y Other Equipment Z None	Z None

Section	F	Physical Rehabilitation and Diagnostic Audiology		
Section Qualifier	0	Rehabilitation		
Type	0	Speech Assessment: Measurement of speech and related functions		

Body System/Region (Character 4)	Type Qualifier (Character 5)	Equipment (Character 6)	Qualifier (Character 7)
Z None	B Motor Speech	K Audiovisual N Biosensory Feedback P Computer Q Speech Analysis T Aerodynamic Function Y Other Equipment Z None	Z None
Z None	D Fluency	K Audiovisual N Biosensory Feedback P Computer Q Speech Analysis S Voice Analysis T Aerodynamic Function Y Other Equipment Z None	Z None
Z None	F Voice	K Audiovisual N Biosensory Feedback P Computer S Voice Analysis T Aerodynamic Function Y Other Equipment Z None	Z None
Z None	H Bedside Swallowing and Oral Function P Oral Peripheral Mechanism	Y Other Equipment Z None	Z None
Z None	J Instrumental Swallowing and Oral Function	T Aerodynamic Function W Swallowing Y Other Equipment	Z None
Z None	K Orofacial Myofunctional	K Audiovisual P Computer Y Other Equipment Z None	Z None
Z None	M Voice Prosthetic	K Audiovisual P Computer S Voice Analysis V Speech Prosthesis Y Other Equipment Z None	Z None
Z None	N Non-invasive Instrumental Status	N Biosensory Feedback P Computer Q Speech Analysis S Voice Analysis T Aerodynamic Function Y Other Equipment	Z None
Z None	X Other Specified Central Auditory Processing	Z None	Z None

Section	F	Physical Rehabilitation and Diagnostic Audiology		
Section Qualifier	0	Rehabilitation		
Type	1	Motor and/or Nerve Function Assessment: Measurement of motor, nerve, and related functions		

Body System/Region (Character 4)	Type Qualifier (Character 5)	Equipment (Character 6)	Qualifier (Character 7)
0 Neurological System - Head and Neck **1** Neurological System - Upper Back /Upper Extremity **2** Neurological System - Lower Back /Lower Extremity **3** Neurological System - Whole Body	**0** Muscle Performance	**E** Orthosis **F** Assistive, Adaptive, Supportive or Protective **U** Prosthesis **Y** Other Equipment **Z** None	**Z** None
0 Neurological System - Head and Neck **1** Neurological System - Upper Back /Upper Extremity **2** Neurological System - Lower Back /Lower Extremity **3** Neurological System - Whole Body	**1** Integumentary Integrity **3** Coordination/Dexterity **4** Motor Function **G** Reflex Integrity	**Z** None	**Z** None
0 Neurological System - Head and Neck **1** Neurological System - Upper Back /Upper Extremity **2** Neurological System - Lower Back /Lower Extremity **3** Neurological System - Whole Body	**5** Range of Motion and Joint Integrity **6** Sensory Awareness/Processing/ Integrity	**Y** Other Equipment **Z** None	**Z** None
D Integumentary System - Head and Neck **F** Integumentary System - Upper Back /Upper Extremity **G** Integumentary System - Lower Back /Lower Extremity **H** Integumentary System - Whole Body **J** Musculoskeletal System - Head and Neck **K** Musculoskeletal System - Upper Back /Upper Extremity **L** Musculoskeletal System - Lower Back /Lower Extremity **M** Musculoskeletal System - Whole Body	**0** Muscle Performance	**E** Orthosis **F** Assistive, Adaptive, Supportive or Protective **U** Prosthesis **Y** Other Equipment **Z** None	**Z** None
D Integumentary System - Head and Neck **F** Integumentary System - Upper Back /Upper Extremity **G** Integumentary System - Lower Back /Lower Extremity **H** Integumentary System - Whole Body **J** Musculoskeletal System - Head and Neck **K** Musculoskeletal System - Upper Back /Upper Extremity **L** Musculoskeletal System - Lower Back /Lower Extremity **M** Musculoskeletal System - Whole Body	**1** Integumentary Integrity	**Z** None	**Z** None **Continued on Next Page ▶**

			Continued from ◀ Previous Page
D Integumentary System - Head and Neck **F** Integumentary System - Upper Back /Upper Extremity **G** Integumentary System - Lower Back /Lower Extremity **H** Integumentary System - Whole Body **J** Musculoskeletal System - Head and Neck **K** Musculoskeletal System - Upper Back /Upper Extremity **L** Musculoskeletal System - Lower Back /Lower Extremity **M** Musculoskeletal System - Whole Body	**5** Range of Motion and Joint Integrity **6** Sensory Awareness/ Processing/ Integrity	**Y** Other Equipment **Z** None	**Z** None
N Genitourinary System	**0** Muscle Performance	**E** Orthosis **F** Assistive, Adaptive, Supportive or Protective **U** Prosthesis **Y** Other Equipment **Z** None	**Z** None
Z None	**2** Visual Motor Integration	**K** Audiovisual **M** Augmentative / Alternative Communication **N** Biosensory Feedback **P** Computer **Q** Speech Analysis **S** Voice Analysis **Y** Other Equipment **Z** None	**Z** None
Z None	**7** Facial Nerve Function	**7** Electrophysiologic	**Z** None
Z None	**9** Somatosensory Evoked Potentials	**J** Somatosensory	**Z** None
Z None	**B** Bed Mobility **C** Transfer **F** Wheelchair Mobility	**E** Orthosis **F** Assistive, Adaptive, Supportive or Protective **U** Prosthesis **Z** None	**Z** None
Z None	**D** Gait and/or Balance	**E** Orthosis **F** Assistive, Adaptive, Supportive or Protective **U** Prosthesis **Y** Other Equipment **Z** None	**Z** None

Section	F	Physical Rehabilitation and Diagnostic Audiology		
Section Qualifier	0	Rehabilitation		
Type	2	Activities of Daily Living Assessment: Measurement of functional level for activities of daily living		

Body System/Region (Character 4)	Type Qualifier (Character 5)	Equipment (Character 6)	Qualifier (Character 7)
0 Neurological System - Head and Neck	**9** Cranial Nerve Integrity **D** Neuromotor Development	**Y** Other Equipment **Z** None	**Z** None
1 Neurological System - Upper Back /Upper Extremity **2** Neurological System - Lower Back /Lower Extremity **3** Neurological System - Whole Body	**D** Neuromotor Development	**Y** Other Equipment **Z** None	**Z** None
4 Circulatory System - Head and Neck **5** Circulatory System - Upper Back / Upper Extremity **6** Circulatory System - Lower Back / Lower Extremity **8** Respiratory System - Head and Neck **9** Respiratory System - Upper Back /Upper Extremity **B** Respiratory System - Lower Back /Lower Extremity	**G** Ventilation, Respiration and Circulation	**C** Mechanical **G** Aerobic Endurance and Conditioning **Y** Other Equipment **Z** None	**Z** None
7 Circulatory System - Whole Body **C** Respiratory System - Whole Body	**7** Aerobic Capacity and Endurance	**E** Orthosis **G** Aerobic Endurance and Conditioning **U** Prosthesis **Y** Other Equipment **Z** None	**Z** None
7 Circulatory System - Whole Body **C** Respiratory System - Whole Body	**G** Ventilation, Respiration and Circulation	**C** Mechanical **G** Aerobic Endurance and Conditioning **Y** Other Equipment **Z** None	**Z** None
Z None	**0** Bathing/Showering **1** Dressing **3** Grooming/Personal Hygiene **4** Home Management	**E** Orthosis **F** Assistive, Adaptive, Supportive or Protective **U** Prosthesis **Z** None	**Z** None
Z None	**2** Feeding/Eating **8** Anthropometric Characteristics **F** Pain	**Y** Other Equipment **Z** None	**Z** None
Z None	**5** Perceptual Processing	**K** Audiovisual **M** Augmentative / Alternative Communication **N** Biosensory Feedback **P** Computer **Q** Speech Analysis **S** Voice Analysis **Y** Other Equipment **Z** None	**Z** None

Continued on Next Page ▶

			Continued from ◀ Previous Page
Z None	6 Psychosocial Skills	Z None	Z None
Z None	B Environmental, Home and Work Barriers C Ergonomics and Body Mechanics	E Orthosis F Assistive, Adaptive, Supportive or Protective U Prosthesis Y Other Equipment Z None	Z None
Z None	H Vocational Activities and Functional Community or Work Reintegration Skills	E Orthosis F Assistive, Adaptive, Supportive or Protective G Aerobic Endurance and Conditioning U Prosthesis Y Other Equipment Z None	Z None

Section	F	Physical Rehabilitation and Diagnostic Audiology
Section Qualifier	0	Rehabilitation
Type	6	Speech Treatment: Application of techniques to improve, augment, or compensate for speech and related functional impairment

Body System/Region (Character 4)	Type Qualifier (Character 5)	Equipment (Character 6)	Qualifier (Character 7)
3 Neurological System - Whole Body	6 Communicative/Cognitive Integration Skills	K Audiovisual M Augmentative / Alternative Communication P Computer Y Other Equipment Z None	Z None
Z None	0 Nonspoken Language 3 Aphasia 6 Communicative/Cognitive Integration Skills	K Audiovisual M Augmentative / Alternative Communication P Computer Y Other Equipment Z None	Z None
Z None	1 Speech-Language Pathology and Related Disorders Counseling 2 Speech-Language Pathology and Related Disorders Prevention	K Audiovisual Z None	Z None
Z None	4 Articulation/Phonology	K Audiovisual P Computer Q Speech Analysis T Aerodynamic Function Y Other Equipment Z None	Z None
Z None	5 Aural Rehabilitation	K Audiovisual L Assistive Listening M Augmentative / Alternative Communication N Biosensory Feedback P Computer	Z None

Continued on Next Page ▶

		Q Speech Analysis **S** Voice Analysis **Y** Other Equipment **Z** None	**Continued from** ◀ **Previous Page**
Z None	**7** Fluency	**4** Electroacoustic Immittance / Acoustic Reflex **K** Audiovisual **N** Biosensory Feedback **Q** Speech Analysis **5** Voice Analysis **T** Aerodynamic Function **Y** Other Equipment **Z** None	**Z** None
Z None	**8** Motor Speech	**K** Audiovisual **N** Biosensory Feedback **P** Computer **Q** Speech Analysis **S** Voice Analysis **T** Aerodynamic Function **Y** Other Equipment **Z** None	**Z** None
Z None	**9** Orofacial Myofunctional	**K** Audiovisual **P** Computer **Y** Other Equipment **Z** None	**Z** None
Z None	**B** Receptive/Expressive Language	**K** Audiovisual **L** Assistive Listening **M** Augmentative / Alternative Communication **P** Computer **Y** Other Equipment **Z** None	**Z** None
Z None	**C** Voice	**K** Audiovisual **N** Biosensory Feedback **P** Computer **S** Voice Analysis **T** Aerodynamic Function **V** Speech Prosthesis **Y** Other Equipment **Z** None	**Z** None
Z None	**D** Swallowing Dysfunction	**M** Augmentative / Alternative Communication **T** Aerodynamic Function **V** Speech Prosthesis **Y** Other Equipment **Z** None	**Z** None

Section	F	Physical Rehabilitation and Diagnostic Audiology		
Section Qualifier	0	Rehabilitation		
Type	7	Motor Treatment: Exercise or activities to increase or facilitate motor function		

Body System/Region (Character 4)	Type Qualifier (Character 5)	Equipment (Character 6)	Qualifier (Character 7)
0 Neurological System - Head and Neck 1 Neurological System - Upper Back /Upper Extremity 2 Neurological System - Lower Back /Lower Extremity 3 Neurological System - Whole Body D Integumentary System - Head and Neck F Integumentary System - Upper Back /Upper Extremity G Integumentary System - Lower Back /Lower Extremity H Integumentary System - Whole Body J Musculoskeletal System - Head and Neck K Musculoskeletal System - Upper Back /Upper Extremity L Musculoskeletal System - Lower Back /Lower Extremity M Musculoskeletal System - Whole Body	0 Range of Motion and Joint Mobility 1 Muscle Performance 2 Coordination/Dexterity 3 Motor Function	E Orthosis F Assistive, Adaptive, Supportive or Protective U Prosthesis Y Other Equipment Z None	Z None
0 Neurological System - Head and Neck 1 Neurological System - Upper Back /Upper Extremity 2 Neurological System - Lower Back /Lower Extremity 3 Neurological System - Whole Body D Integumentary System - Head and Neck F Integumentary System - Upper Back /Upper Extremity G Integumentary System - Lower Back /Lower Extremity H Integumentary System - Whole Body J Musculoskeletal System - Head and Neck K Musculoskeletal System - Upper Back /Upper Extremity L Musculoskeletal System - Lower Back /Lower Extremity M Musculoskeletal System - Whole Body	6 Therapeutic Exercise	B Physical Agents C Mechanical D Electrotherapeutic E Orthosis F Assistive, Adaptive, Supportive or Protective G Aerobic Endurance and Conditioning H Mechanical or Electromechanical U Prosthesis Y Other Equipment Z None	Z None
4 Circulatory System - Head and Neck 5 Circulatory System - Upper Back / Upper Extremity 6 Circulatory System - Lower Back / Lower Extremity 7 Circulatory System - Whole Body	6 Therapeutic Exercise	B Physical Agents C Mechanical D Electrotherapeutic E Orthosis F Assistive, Adaptive, Supportive or Protective G Aerobic Endurance and Conditioning	Z None

Continued on Next Page ▶

8 Respiratory System - Head and Neck **9** Respiratory System - Upper Back /Upper Extremity **B** Respiratory System - Lower Back /Lower Extremity **C** Respiratory System - Whole Body		**H** Mechanical or Electromechanical **U** Prosthesis **Y** Other Equipment **Z** None	**Continued from** ◀ **Previous Page**
N Genitourinary System	**1** Muscle Performance	**E** Orthosis **F** Assistive, Adaptive, Supportive or Protective **U** Prosthesis **Y** Other Equipment **Z** None	**Z** None
N Genitourinary System	**6** Therapeutic Exercise	**B** Physical Agents **C** Mechanical **D** Electrotherapeutic **E** Orthosis **F** Assistive, Adaptive, Supportive or Protective **G** Aerobic Endurance and Conditioning **H** Mechanical or Electromechanical **U** Prosthesis **Y** Other Equipment **Z** None	**Z** None
Z None	**4** Wheelchair Mobility	**D** Electrotherapeutic **E** Orthosis **F** Assistive, Adaptive, Supportive or Protective **U** Prosthesis **Y** Other Equipment **Z** None	**Z** None
Z None	**5** Bed Mobility	**C** Mechanical **E** Orthosis **F** Assistive, Adaptive, Supportive or Protective **U** Prosthesis **Y** Other Equipment **Z** None	**Z** None
Z None	**8** Transfer Training	**C** Mechanical **D** Electrotherapeutic **E** Orthosis **F** Assistive, Adaptive, Supportive or Protective **U** Prosthesis **Y** Other Equipment **Z** None	**Z** None
Z None	**9** Gait Training/Functional Ambulation	**C** Mechanical **D** Electrotherapeutic **E** Orthosis **F** Assistive, Adaptive, Supportive or Protective **G** Aerobic Endurance and Conditioning **U** Prosthesis **Y** Other Equipment **Z** None	**Z** None

Section	F	Physical Rehabilitation and Diagnostic Audiology
Section Qualifier	0	Rehabilitation
Type	8	Activities of Daily Living Treatment: Exercise or activities to facilitate functional competence for activities of daily living

Body System/Region (Character 4)	Type Qualifier (Character 5)	Equipment (Character 6)	Qualifier (Character 7)
D Integumentary System - Head and Neck F Integumentary System - Upper Back /Upper Extremity G Integumentary System - Lower Back /Lower Extremity H Integumentary System - Whole Body J Musculoskeletal System - Head and Neck K Musculoskeletal System - Upper Back /Upper Extremity L Musculoskeletal System - Lower Back /Lower Extremity M Musculoskeletal System - Whole Body	5 Wound Management	B Physical Agents C Mechanical D Electrotherapeutic E Orthosis F Assistive, Adaptive, Supportive or Protective U Prosthesis Y Other Equipment Z None	Z None
Z None	0 Bathing/Showering Techniques 1 Dressing Techniques 2 Grooming/Personal Hygiene	E Orthosis F Assistive, Adaptive, Supportive or Protective U Prosthesis Y Other Equipment Z None	Z None
Z None	3 Feeding/Eating	C Mechanical D Electrotherapeutic E Orthosis F Assistive, Adaptive, Supportive or Protective U Prosthesis Y Other Equipment Z None	Z None
Z None	4 Home Management	D Electrotherapeutic E Orthosis F Assistive, Adaptive, Supportive or Protective U Prosthesis Y Other Equipment Z None	Z None
Z None	6 Psychosocial Skills	Z None	Z None
Z None	7 Vocational Activities and Functional Community or Work Reintegration Skills	B Physical Agents C Mechanical D Electrotherapeutic E Orthosis F Assistive, Adaptive, Supportive or Protective G Aerobic Endurance and Conditioning U Prosthesis Y Other Equipment Z None	Z None

Section	F	Physical Rehabilitation and Diagnostic Audiology		
Section Qualifier	0	Rehabilitation		
Type	9	Hearing Treatment: Application of techniques to improve, augment, or compensate for hearing and related functional impairment		
Body System/Region (Character 4)	**Type Qualifier (Character 5)**		**Equipment (Character 6)**	**Qualifier (Character 7)**
Z None	0 Hearing and Related Disorders Counseling 1 Hearing and Related Disorders Prevention		K Audiovisual Z None	Z None
Z None	2 Auditory Processing		K Audiovisual L Assistive Listening P Computer Y Other Equipment Z None	Z None
Z None	3 Cerumen Management		X Cerumen Management Z None	Z None

Section	F	Physical Rehabilitation and Diagnostic Audiology		
Section Qualifier	0	Rehabilitation		
Type	B	Cochlear Implant Treatment: Application of techniques to improve the communication abilities of individuals with cochlear implant		
Body System/Region (Character 4)	**Type Qualifier (Character 5)**		**Equipment (Character 6)**	**Qualifier (Character 7)**
Z None	0 Cochlear Implant Rehabilitation		1 Audiometer 2 Sound Field / Booth 9 Cochlear Implant K Audiovisual P Computer Y Other Equipment	Z None

Section	F	Physical Rehabilitation and Diagnostic Audiology		
Section Qualifier	0	Rehabilitation		
Type	C	Vestibular Treatment: Application of techniques to improve, augment, or compensate for vestibular and related functional impairment		
Body System/Region (Character 4)	**Type Qualifier (Character 5)**		**Equipment (Character 6)**	**Qualifier (Character 7)**
3 Neurological System - Whole Body H Integumentary System - Whole Body M Musculoskeletal System - Whole Body	3 Postural Control		E Orthosis F Assistive, Adaptive, Supportive or Protective U Prosthesis Y Other Equipment Z None	Z None
Z None	0 Vestibular		8 Vestibular / Balance Z None	Z None
Z None	1 Perceptual Processing 2 Visual Motor Integration		K Audiovisual L Assistive Listening N Biosensory Feedback P Computer Q Speech Analysis S Voice Analysis T Aerodynamic Function Y Other Equipment Z None	Z None

Section	F	Physical Rehabilitation and Diagnostic Audiology		
Section Qualifier	0	Rehabilitation		
Type	D	Device Fitting: Fitting of a device designed to facilitate or support achievement of a\ higher level of function		

Body System/Region (Character 4)	Type Qualifier (Character 5)	Equipment (Character 6)	Qualifier (Character 7)
Z None	0 Tinnitus Masker	5 Hearing Aid Selection / Fitting /Test Z None	Z None
Z None	1 Monaural Hearing Aid 2 Binaural Hearing Aid 5 Assistive Listening Device	1 Audiometer 2 Sound Field /Booth 5 Hearing Aid Selection / Fitting /Test K Audiovisual L Assistive Listening Z None	Z None
Z None	3 Augmentative/Alternative Communication System	M Augmentative / Alternative Communication	Z None
Z None	4 Voice Prosthetic	S Voice Analysis V Speech Prosthesis	Z None
Z None	6 Dynamic Orthosis 7 Static Orthosis 8 Prosthesis 9 Assistive, Adaptive, Supportive or Protective Devices	E Orthosis F Assistive, Adaptive, Supportive or Protective U Prosthesis Z None	Z None

Section	F	Physical Rehabilitation and Diagnostic Audiology		
Section Qualifier	0	Rehabilitation		
Type	F	Caregiver Training: Training in activities to support patient's optimal level of function		

Body System/Region (Character 4)	Type Qualifier (Character 5)	Equipment (Character 6)	Qualifier (Character 7)
Z None	0 Bathing/Showering Technique 1 Dressing 2 Feeding and Eating 3 Grooming/Personal Hygiene 4 Bed Mobility 5 Transfer 6 Wheelchair Mobility 7 Therapeutic Exercise 8 Airway Clearance Techniques 9 Wound Management B Vocational Activities and Functional Community or Work Reintegration Skills C Gait Training/Functional Ambulation D Application, Proper Use and Care of Devices F Application, Proper Use and Care of Orthoses G Application, Proper Use and Care of Prosthesis H Home Management	E Orthosis F Assistive, Adaptive, Supportive or Protective U Prosthesis Z None	Z None

Continued on Next Page ►

			Continued from ◀ Previous Page
Z None	J Communication Skills	K Audiovisual L Assistive Listening M Augmentative / Alternative Communication P Computer Z None	Z None

Section	F	Physical Rehabilitation and Diagnostic Audiology		
Section Qualifier	1	Diagnostic Audiology		
Type	3	Hearing Assessment: Measurement of hearing and related functions		

Body System/Region (Character 4)	Type Qualifier (Character 5)	Equipment (Character 6)	Qualifier (Character 7)
Z None	0 Hearing Screening	0 Occupational Hearing 1 Audiometer 2 Sound Field / Booth 3 Tympanometer 8 Vestibular / Balance 9 Cochlear Implant Z None	Z None
Z None	1 Pure Tone Audiometry, Air 2 Pure Tone Audiometry, Air and Bone	0 Occupational Hearing 1 Audiometer 2 Sound Field / Booth Z None	Z None
Z None	3 Bekesy Audiometry 6 Visual Reinforcement Audiometry 9 Short Increment Sensitivity Index B Stenger C Pure Tone Stenger	1 Audiometer 2 Sound Field / Booth Z None	Z None
Z None	4 Conditioned Play Audiometry 5 Select Picture Audiometry	1 Audiometer 2 Sound Field / Booth K Audiovisual Z None	Z None
Z None	7 Alternate Binaural or Monaural Loudness Balance	1 Audiometer K Audiovisual Z None	Z None
Z None	8 Tone Decay D Tympanometry F Eustachian Tube Function G Acoustic Reflex Patterns H Acoustic Reflex Threshold J Acoustic Reflex Decay	3 Tympanometer 4 Electroacoustic Immittance / Acoustic Reflex Z None	Z None
Z None	K Electrocochleography L Auditory Evoked Potentials	7 Electrophysiologic Z None	Z None
Z None	M Evoked Otoacoustic Emissions, Screening N Evoked Otoacoustic Emissions, Diagnostic	6 Otoacoustic Emission (OAE) Z None	Z None

Section	F	Physical Rehabilitation and Diagnostic Audiology
Section Qualifier	1	Diagnostic Audiology
Type	3	Hearing Assessment: Measurement of hearing and related functions

Body System/Region (Character 4)	Type Qualifier (Character 5)	Equipment (Character 6)	Qualifier (Character 7)
Z None	P Aural Rehabilitation Status	1 Audiometer 2 Sound Field / Booth 4 Electroacoustic Immittance / Acoustic Reflex 9 Cochlear Implant K Audiovisual L Assistive Listening P Computer Z None	Z None
Z None	Q Auditory Processing	K Audiovisual P Computer Y Other Equipment Z None	Z None

Section	F	Physical Rehabilitation and Diagnostic Audiology
Section Qualifier	1	Diagnostic Audiology
Type	4	Hearing Aid Assessment: Measurement of the appropriateness and/or effectiveness of a hearing device

Body System/Region (Character 4)	Type Qualifier (Character 5)	Equipment (Character 6)	Qualifier (Character 7)
Z None	0 Cochlear Implant	1 Audiometer 2 Sound Field /Booth 3 Tympanometer 4 Electroacoustic Immittance / Acoustic Reflex 5 Hearing Aid Selection / Fitting /Test 7 Electrophysiologic 9 Cochlear Implant K Audiovisual L Assistive Listening P Computer Y Other Equipment Z None	Z None
Z None	1 Ear Canal Probe Microphone 6 Binaural Electroacoustic Hearing Aid Check 8 Monaural Electroacoustic Hearing Aid Check	5 Hearing Aid Selection / Fitting / Test Z None	Z None
Z None	2 Monaural Hearing Aid 3 Binaural Hearing Aid	1 Audiometer 2 Sound Field /Booth 3 Tympanometer 4 Electroacoustic Immittance / Acoustic Reflex 5 Hearing Aid Selection / Fitting /Test K Audiovisual L Assistive Listening P Computer Z None	Z None

Continued on Next Page ▶

			<div align="right">Continued from ◀ Previous Page</div>
Z None	4 Assistive Listening System/Device Selection	1 Audiometer 2 Sound Field /Booth 3 Tympanometer 4 Electroacoustic Immittance /Acoustic Reflex K Audiovisual L Assistive Listening Z None	Z None
Z None	5 Sensory Aids	1 Audiometer 2 Sound Field / Booth 3 Tympanometer 4 Electroacoustic Immittance /Acoustic Reflex 5 Hearing Aid Selection / Fitting /Test K Audiovisual L Assistive Listening Z None	Z None
Z None	7 Ear Protector Attenuation	0 Occupational Hearing Z None	Z None

Section	F	Physical Rehabilitation and Diagnostic Audiology	
Section Qualifier	1	Diagnostic Audiology	
Type	5	Vestibular Assessment: Measurement of the vestibular system and related functions	

Body System/Region (Character 4)	Type Qualifier (Character 5)	Equipment (Character 6)	Qualifier (Character 7)
Z None	0 Bithermal, Binaural Caloric Irrigation 1 Bithermal, Monaural Caloric Irrigation 2 Unithermal Binaural Screen 3 Oscillating Tracking 4 Sinusoidal Vertical Axis Rotational 5 Dix-Hallpike Dynamic 6 Computerized Dynamic Posturography	8 Vestibular /Balance Z None	Z None
Z None	7 Tinnitus Masker	5 Hearing Aid Selection / Fitting /Test Z None	Z None

Section	G	Mental Health		
Body System	Z	None		
Type	1	Psychological Tests: The administration and interpretation of standardized psychological tests and measurement instruments for the assessment of psychological function		
Qualifier (Character 4)		**Qualifier (Character 5)**	**Qualifier (Character 6)**	**Qualifier (Character 7)**
0 Developmental **1** Personality and Behavioral **2** Intellectual and Psychoeducational **3** Neuropsychological **4** Neurobehavioral and Cognitive Status		**Z** None	**Z** None	**Z** None

Section	G	Mental Health		
Body System	Z	None		
Type	2	Crisis Intervention: Treatment of a traumatized, acutely disturbed or distressed individual for the purpose of short-term stabilization		
Qualifier (Character 4)		**Qualifier (Character 5)**	**Qualifier (Character 6)**	**Qualifier (Character 7)**
Z None		**Z** None	**Z** None	**Z** None

Section	G	Mental Health		
Body System	Z	None		
Type	3	Medication Management: Monitoring and adjusting the use of medications for the treatment of a mental health disorder		
Qualifier (Character 4)		**Qualifier (Character 5)**	**Qualifier (Character 6)**	**Qualifier (Character 7)**
Z None		**Z** None	**Z** None	**Z** None

Section	G	Mental Health		
Body System	Z	None		
Type	5	Individual Psychotherapy: Treatment of an individual with a mental health disorder by behavioral, cognitive, psychoanalytic, psychodynamic or psychophysiological means to improve functioning or well-being		
Qualifier (Character 4)		**Qualifier (Character 5)**	**Qualifier (Character 6)**	**Qualifier (Character 7)**
0 Interactive **1** Behavioral **2** Cognitive **3** Interpersonal **4** Psychoanalysis **5** Psychodynamic **6** Supportive **8** Cognitive-Behavioral **9** Psychophysiological		**Z** None	**Z** None	**Z** None

Section	G	Mental Health		
Body System	Z	None		
Type	6	Counseling: The application of psychological methods to treat an individual with normal developmental issues and psychological problems in order to increase function, improve well-being, alleviate distress, maladjustment or resolve crises		
Qualifier (Character 4)		**Qualifier (Character 5)**	**Qualifier (Character 6)**	**Qualifier (Character 7)**
0 Educational **1** Vocational **3** Other Counseling		**Z** None	**Z** None	**Z** None

Section	G	Mental Health		
Body System	Z	None		
Type	7	Family Psychotherapy: Treatment that includes one or more family members of an individual with a mental health disorder by behavioral, cognitive, psychoanalytic, psychodynamic or psychophysiological means to improve functioning or well-being		
Qualifier (Character 4)	**Qualifier (Character 5)**	**Qualifier (Character 6)**	**Qualifier (Character 7)**
2 Other Family Psychotherapy	Z None	Z None	Z None

Section	G	Mental Health		
Body System	Z	None		
Type	B	Electroconvulsive Therapy: The application of controlled electrical voltages to treat a mental health disorder		
Qualifier (Character 4)	**Qualifier (Character 5)**	**Qualifier (Character 6)**	**Qualifier (Character 7)**
0 Unilateral-Single Seizure 1 Unilateral-Multiple Seizure 2 Bilateral-Single Seizure 3 Bilateral-Multiple Seizure 4 Other Electroconvulsive Therapy	Z None	Z None	Z None

Section	G	Mental Health		
Body System	Z	None		
Type	C	Biofeedback: Provision of information from the monitoring and regulating of physiological processes in conjunction with cognitive-behavioral techniques to improve patient functioning or well-being		
Qualifier (Character 4)	**Qualifier (Character 5)**	**Qualifier (Character 6)**	**Qualifier (Character 7)**
9 Other Biofeedback	Z None	Z None	Z None

Section	G	Mental Health		
Body System	Z	None		
Type	F	Hypnosis: Induction of a state of heightened suggestibility by auditory, visual and tactile techniques to elicit an emotional or behavioral response		
Qualifier (Character 4)	**Qualifier (Character 5)**	**Qualifier (Character 6)**	**Qualifier (Character 7)**
Z None	Z None	Z None	Z None

Section	G	Mental Health		
Body System	Z	None		
Type	G	Narcosynthesis: Administration of intravenous barbiturates in order to release suppressed or repressed thoughts		
Qualifier (Character 4)	**Qualifier (Character 5)**	**Qualifier (Character 6)**	**Qualifier (Character 7)**
Z None	Z None	Z None	Z None

Section	G	Mental Health		
Body System	Z	None		
Type	H	Group Psychotherapy: Treatment of two or more individuals with a mental health disorder by behavioral, cognitive, psychoanalytic, psychodynamic or psychophysiological means to improve functioning or well-being		
Qualifier (Character 4)	**Qualifier (Character 5)**	**Qualifier (Character 6)**	**Qualifier (Character 7)**
Z None	Z None	Z None	Z None

Section	G	Mental Health		
Body System	Z	None		
Type	J	Light Therapy: Application of specialized light treatments to improve functioning or well-being		
Qualifier (Character 4)	**Qualifier (Character 5)**	**Qualifier (Character 6)**	**Qualifier (Character 7)**
Z None	Z None	Z None	Z None

Section	H	Substance Abuse Treatment		
Body System	Z	None		
Type	2	Detoxification Services: Detoxification from alcohol and/or drugs		
Qualifier (Character 4)		**Qualifier (Character 5)**	**Qualifier (Character 6)**	**Qualifier (Character 7)**
Z None		Z None	Z None	Z None

Section	H	Substance Abuse Treatment		
Body System	Z	None		
Type	3	Individual Counseling: The application of psychological methods to treat an individual with addictive behavior		
Qualifier (Character 4)		**Qualifier (Character 5)**	**Qualifier (Character 6)**	**Qualifier (Character 7)**
0 Cognitive 1 Behavioral 2 Cognitive-Behavioral 3 12-Step 4 Interpersonal 5 Vocational 6 Psychoeducation 7 Motivational Enhancement 8 Confrontational 9 Continuing Care B Spiritual C Pre/Post-Test Infectious Disease		Z None	Z None	Z None

Section	H	Substance Abuse Treatment		
Body System	Z	None		
Type	4	Group Counseling: The application of psychological methods to treat two or more individuals with addictive behavior		
Qualifier (Character 4)		**Qualifier (Character 5)**	**Qualifier (Character 6)**	**Qualifier (Character 7)**
0 Cognitive 1 Behavioral 2 Cognitive-Behavioral 3 12-Step 4 Interpersonal 5 Vocational 6 Psychoeducation 7 Motivational Enhancement 8 Confrontational 9 Continuing Care B Spiritual C Pre/Post-Test Infectious Disease		Z None	Z None	Z None

Section	H	Substance Abuse Treatment		
Body System	Z	None		
Type	5	Individual Psychotherapy: Treatment of an individual with addictive behavior by behavioral, cognitive, psychoanalytic, psychodynamic or psychophysiological means		
Qualifier (Character 4)		**Qualifier (Character 5)**	**Qualifier (Character 6)**	**Qualifier (Character 7)**
0 Cognitive 1 Behavioral 2 Cognitive-Behavioral 3 12-Step 4 Interpersonal		Z None	Z None	Z None

Continued on Next Page ▶

623

5 Interactive 6 Psychoeducation 7 Motivational Enhancement 8 Confrontational 9 Supportive B Psychoanalysis C Psychodynamic D Psychophysiological			Continued from ◄ Previous Page

Section	H	Substance Abuse Treatment	
Body System	Z	None	
Type	6	Family Counseling: The application of psychological methods that includes one or more family members to treat an individual with addictive behavior	
Qualifier (Character 4)	**Qualifier (Character 5)**	**Qualifier (Character 6)**	**Qualifier (Character 7)**
3 Other Family Counseling	Z None	Z None	Z None

Section	H	Substance Abuse Treatment	
Body System	Z	None	
Type	8	Medication Management: Monitoring and adjusting the use of replacement medications for the treatment of addiction	
Qualifier (Character 4)	**Qualifier (Character 5)**	**Qualifier (Character 6)**	**Qualifier (Character 7)**
0 Nicotine Replacement 1 Methadone Maintenance 2 Levo-alpha-acetyl-methadol (LAAM) 3 Antabuse 4 Naltrexone 5 Naloxone 6 Clonidine 7 Bupropion 8 Psychiatric Medication 9 Other Replacement Medication	Z None	Z None	Z None

Section	H	Substance Abuse Treatment	
Body System	Z	None	
Type	9	Pharmacotherapy: The use of replacement medications for the treatment of addiction	
Qualifier (Character 4)	**Qualifier (Character 5)**	**Qualifier (Character 6)**	**Qualifier (Character 7)**
0 Nicotine Replacement 1 Methadone Maintenance 2 Levo-alpha-acetyl-methadol (LAAM) 3 Antabuse 4 Naltrexone 5 Naloxone 6 Clonidine 7 Bupropion 8 Psychiatric Medication 9 Other Replacement Medication	Z None	Z None	Z None

Section	X	New Technology		
Body System	2	Cardiovascular System		
Type	A	Assistance : Taking over a portion of a physiological function by extracorporeal means		

Body Part	Approach	Device/Substance/Technology	Qualifier
5 Innominate Artery and Left Common Carotid Artery	3 Percutaneous	1 Cerebral Embolic Filtration, Dual Filter	2 New Technology Group 2

Section	X	New Technology		
Body System	2	Cardiovascular System		
Type	C	Extirpation: Taking or cutting out solid matter from a body part		

Body Part	Approach	Device/Substance/Technology	Qualifier
0 Coronary Artery, One Artery 1 Coronary Artery, Two Arteries 2 Coronary Artery, Three Arteries 3 Coronary Artery, Four or More Arteries	3 Percutaneous	6 Orbital Atherectomy Technology	1 New Technology Group 1

Section	X	New Technology		
Body System	2	Joints		
Type	R	Replacement: Putting in or on biological or synthetic material that physically takes the place and/or function of all or a portion of a body part		

Body Part	Approach	Device/Substance/Technology	Qualifier
F Aortic Valve	0 Open 3 Percutaneous 4 Percutaneous Endoscopic	3 Zooplastic Tissue, Rapid Deployment Technique	2 New Technology Group 2

Section	X	New Technology		
Body System	H	Skin, Subcutaneous Tissue, Fascia and Breast		
Type	R	Replacement: Putting in or on biological or synthetic material that physically takes the place and/or function of all or a portion of a body part		

Body Part	Approach	Device/Substance/Technology	Qualifier
P Skin	X External	L Skin Substitute, Porcine Liver Derived	2 New Technology Group 2

Section	X	New Technology		
Body System	N	Bones		
Type	S	Replacement: Putting in or on biological or synthetic material that physically takes the place and/or function of all or a portion of a body part		

Body Part	Approach	Device/Substance/Technology	Qualifier
0 Lumbar Vertebra 3 Cervical Vertebra 4 Thoracic Vertebra	0 Open 4 Percutaneous Endoscopic	3 Magnetically Controlled Growth Rod(s)	2 New Technology Group 2

Section	X	New Technology		
Body System	R	Joints		
Type	G	Fusion: Joining together portions of an articular body part rendering the articular body part immobile		

Body Part	Approach	Device/Substance/Technology	Qualifier
0 Occipital-cervical Joint **1** Cervical Vertebral Joint **2** Cervical Vertebral Joints, 2 or more **4** Cervicothoracic Vertebral Joint **6** Thoracic Vertebral Joint **7** Thoracic Vertebral Joints, 2 to 7 **8** Thoracic Vertebral Joints, 8 or more **A** Thoracolumbar Vertebral Joint **B** Lumbar Vertebral Joint **C** Lumbar Vertebral Joints, 2 or more **D** Lumbosacral Joint	**0** Open	**9** Interbody Fusion Device, Nanotextured Surface	**2** New Technology Group 2

Section	X	New Technology		
Body System	W	Anatomical Regions		
Type	0	Introduction: Putting in or on a therapeutic, diagnostic, nutritional, physiological, or prophylactic substance except blood or blood products		

Body Part	Approach	Device/Substance/Technology	Qualifier
3 Peripheral Vein	3 Percutaneous	**2** Ceftazidime-Avibactam Anti-infective **3** Idarucizumab, Dabigatran Reversal Agent **4** Isavuconazole Anti-infective **5** Blinatumomab Antineoplastic Immunotherapy	**1** New Technology Group 1
3 Peripheral Vein	3 Percutaneous	**7** Andexanet Alfa, Factor Xa Inhibitor Reversal Agent **9** Defibrotide Sodium Anticoagulant	**2** New Technology Group 2
4 Central Vein	3 Percutaneous	**2** Ceftazidime-Avibactam Anti-infective **3** Idarucizumab, Dabigatran Reversal Agent **4** Isavuconazole Anti-infective **5** Blinatumomab Antineoplastic Immunotherapy	**1** New Technology Group 1
4 Central Vein	3 Percutaneous	**7** Andexanet Alfa, Factor Xa Inhibitor Reversal Agent **9** Defibrotide Sodium Anticoagulant	**2** New Technology Group 2
D Mouth and Pharynx	X External	**8** Uridine Triacetate	**2** New Technology Group 2

A

Abdominal aortic plexus *use* Nerve, Abdominal Sympathetic

Abdominal esophagus *use* Esophagus, Lower

Abdominohysterectomy
  see Resection, Cervix **0UTC**
  see Resection, Uterus **0UT9**

Abdominoplasty
  see Alteration, Abdominal Wall **0W0F**
  see Repair, Abdominal Wall **0WQF**
  see Supplement, Abdominal Wall **0WUF**

Abductor hallucis muscle
  use Muscle, Foot, Right
  use Muscle, Foot, Left

AbioCor® Total Replacement Heart *use* Synthetic Substitute

Ablation *see* Destruction

Abortion
  Products of Conception **10A0**
  Abortifacient **10A07ZX**
  Laminaria **10A07ZW**
  Vacuum **10A07Z6**

Abrasion *see* Extraction

Accessory cephalic vein
  use Vein, Cephalic, Right
  use Vein, Cephalic, Left

Accessory obturator nerve *use* Nerve, Lumbar Plexus

Accessory phrenic nerve *use* Nerve, Phrenic

Accessory spleen *use* Spleen

Acellular Hydrated Dermis *use* Nonautologous Tissue Substitute

Acetabular cup *use* Liner in Lower Joints

Acetabulectomy
  see Excision, Lower Bones **0QB**
  see Resection, Lower Bones **0QT**

Acetabulofemoral joint
  use Joint, Hip, Right
  use Joint, Hip, Left

Acetabuloplasty
  see Repair, Lower Bones **0QQ**
  see Replacement, Lower Bones **0QR**
  see Supplement, Lower Bones **0QU**

Achilles tendon
  use Tendon, Lower Leg, Left
  use Tendon, Lower Leg, Right

Achillorrhaphy *see* Repair, Tendons **0LQ**

Achillotenotomy, achillotomy
  see Division, Tendons **0L8**
  see Drainage, Tendons **0L9**

Acromioclavicular ligament
  use Bursa and Ligament, Shoulder, Left
  use Bursa and Ligament, Shoulder, Right

Acromion (process)
  use Scapula, Left
  use Scapula, Right

Acromionectomy
  see Excision, Upper Joints **0RB**
  see Resection, Upper Joints **0RT**

Acromioplasty
  see Repair, Upper Joints **0RQ**
  see Replacement, Upper Joints **0RR**
  see Supplement, Upper Joints **0RU**

Activa PC neurostimulator *use* Stimulator Generator, Multiple Array in **0JH**

Activa RC neurostimulator *use* Stimulator Generator, Multiple Array Rechargeable in **0JH**

Activa SC neurostimulator *use* Stimulator Generator, Single Array in **0JH**

Activities of Daily Living Assessment F02

Activities of Daily Living Treatment F08

ACUITY™ Steerable Lead
  use Cardiac Lead, Defibrillator in **02H**
  use Cardiac Lead, Pacemaker in **02H**

Acupuncture
  Breast
    Anesthesia **8E0H300**
    No Qualifier **8E0H30Z**
  Integumentary System
    Anesthesia **8E0H300**
    No Qualifier **8E0H30Z**

Adductor brevis muscle
  use Muscle, Upper Leg, Left
  use Muscle, Upper Leg, Right

Adductor hallucis muscle
  use Muscle, Foot, Left
  use Muscle, Foot, Right

Adductor longus muscle
  use Muscle, Upper Leg, Right
  use Muscle, Upper Leg, Left

Adductor magnus muscle
  use Muscle, Upper Leg, Right
  use Muscle, Upper Leg, Left

Adenohypophysis *use* Gland, Pituitary

Adenoidectomy
  see Excision, Adenoids **0CBQ**
  see Resection, Adenoids **0CTQ**

Adenoidotomy *see* Drainage, Adenoids **0C9Q**

Adhesiolysis *see* Release

Administration
  Blood products *see* Transfusion
  Other substance *see* Introduction of substance in or on

Adrenalectomy
  see Excision, Endocrine System **0GB**
  see Resection, Endocrine System **0GT**

Adrenalorrhaphy *see* Repair, Endocrine System **0GQ**

Adrenalotomy *see* Drainage, Endocrine System **0G9**

Advancement
  see Reposition
  see Transfer

AFX(R) Endovascular AAA System *use* Intraluminal Device

Alar ligament of axis *use* Bursa and Ligament, Head and Neck

Alimentation *see* Introduction of substance in or on

Alteration
  Abdominal Wall **0W0F**
  Ankle Region
    Left **0Y0L**
    Right **0Y0K**
  Arm
    Lower
      Left **0X0F**
      Right **0X0D**
    Upper
      Left **0X09**
      Right **0X08**

Alteration *(continued)*
  Axilla
    Left **0X05**
    Right **0X04**
  Back
    Lower **0W0L**
    Upper **0W0K**
  Breast
    Bilateral **0H0V**
    Left **0H0U**
    Right **0H0T**
  Buttock
    Left **0Y01**
    Right **0Y00**
  Chest Wall **0W08**
  Ear
    Bilateral **0902**
    Left **0901**
    Right **0900**
  Elbow Region
    Left **0X0C**
    Right **0X0B**
  Extremity
    Lower
      Left **0Y0B**
      Right **0Y09**
    Upper
      Left **0X07**
      Right **0X06**
  Eyelid
    Lower
      Left **080R**
      Right **080Q**
    Upper
      Left **080P**
      Right **080N**
  Face **0W02**
  Head **0W00**
  Jaw
    Lower **0W05**
    Upper **0W04**
  Knee Region
    Left **0Y0G**
    Right **0Y0F**
  Leg
    Lower
      Left **0Y0J**
      Right **0Y0H**
    Upper
      Left **0Y0D**
      Right **0Y0C**
  Lip
    Lower **0C01X**
    Upper **0C00X**
  Neck **0W06**
  Nose **090K**
  Perineum
    Female **0W0N**
    Male **0W0M**
  Shoulder Region
    Left **0X03**
    Right **0X02**
  Subcutaneous Tissue and Fascia
    Abdomen **0J08**
    Back **0J07**
    Buttock **0J09**

Alteration *(continued)*
    Chest **0J06**
    Face **0J01**
    Lower Arm
        Left **0J0H**
        Right **0J0G**
    Lower Leg
        Left **0J0P**
        Right **0J0N**
    Neck
        Anterior **0J04**
        Posterior **0J05**
    Upper Arm
        Left **0J0F**
        Right **0J0D**
    Upper Leg
        Left **0J0M**
        Right **0J0L**
    Wrist Region
        Left **0X0H**
        Right **0X0G**
Alveolar process of mandible
    use Mandible, Left
    use Mandible, Right
Alveolar process of maxilla
    use Maxilla, Right
    use Maxilla, Left
Alveolectomy
    see Excision, Head and Facial Bones **0NB**
    see Resection, Head and Facial Bones **0NT**
Alveoloplasty
    see Repair, Head and Facial Bones **0NQ**
    see Replacement, Head and Facial Bones **0NR**
    see Supplement, Head and Facial Bones **0NU**
Alveolotomy
    see Division, Head and Facial Bones **0N8**
    see Drainage, Head and Facial Bones **0N9**
Ambulatory cardiac monitoring 4A12X45
Amniocentesis *see* Drainage, Products of Conception **1090**
Amnioinfusion *see* Introduction of substance in or on, Products of Conception **3E0E**
Amnioscopy 10J08ZZ
Amniotomy *see* Drainage, Products of Conception **1090**
AMPLATZER® Muscular VSD Occluder
    use Synthetic Substitute
Amputation *see* Detachment
AMS 800® Urinary Control System *use* Artificial Sphincter in Urinary System
Anal orifice *use* Anus
Analog radiography *see* Plain Radiography
Analog radiology *see* Plain Radiography
Anastomosis *see* Bypass
Anatomical snuffbox
    use Muscle, Lower Arm and Wrist, Left
    use Muscle, Lower Arm and Wrist, Right
Andexanet Alfa, Factor Xa Inhibitor Reversal Agent XW0
AneuRx® AAA Advantage® *use* Intraluminal Device
Angiectomy
    see Excision, Heart and Great Vessels **02B**
    see Excision, Upper Arteries **03B**
    see Excision, Lower Arteries **04B**

Angiectomy *(continued)*
    see Excision, Upper Veins **05B**
    see Excision, Lower Veins **06B**
Angiocardiography
    Combined right and left heart *see* Fluoroscopy, Heart, Right and Left **B216**
    Left Heart *see* Fluoroscopy, Heart, Left **B215**
    Right Heart *see* Fluoroscopy, Heart, Right **B214**
    SPY system intravascular fluorescence *see* Monitoring, Physiological Systems **4A1**
Angiography
    see Plain Radiography, Heart **B20**
    see Fluoroscopy, Heart **B21**
Angioplasty
    see Dilation, Heart and Great Vessels **027**
    see Repair, Heart and Great Vessels **02Q**
    see Replacement, Heart and Great Vessels **02R**
    see Dilation, Lower Arteries **047**
    see Dilation, Upper Arteries **037**
    see Repair, Lower Arteries **04Q**
    see Repair, Upper Arteries **03Q**
    see Replacement, Lower Arteries **04R**
    see Replacement, Upper Arteries **03R**
    see Supplement, Heart and Great Vessels **02U**
Angioplasty *(continued)*
    see Supplement, Lower Arteries **04U**
    see Supplement, Upper Arteries **03U**
Angiorrhaphy
    see Repair, Heart and Great Vessels **02Q**
    see Repair, Upper Arteries **03Q**
    see Repair, Lower Arteries **04Q**
Angioscopy
    02JY4ZZ
    03JY4ZZ
    04JY4ZZ
Angiotripsy
    see Occlusion, Upper Arteries **03L**
    see Occlusion, Lower Arteries **04L**
Angular artery *use* Artery, Face
Angular vein
    use Vein, Face, Left
    use Vein, Face, Right
Annular ligament
    use Bursa and Ligament, Elbow, Left
    use Bursa and Ligament, Elbow, Right
Annuloplasty
    see Repair, Heart and Great Vessels **02Q**
    see Supplement, Heart and Great Vessels **02U**
Annuloplasty ring *use* Synthetic Substitute
Anoplasty
    see Repair, Anus **0DQQ**
    see Supplement, Anus **0DUQ**
Anorectal junction *use* Rectum
Anoscopy 0DJD8ZZ
Ansa cervicalis *use* Nerve, Cervical Plexus
Antabuse therapy HZ93ZZZ
Antebrachial fascia
    use Subcutaneous Tissue and Fascia, Lower Arm, Left
    use Subcutaneous Tissue and Fascia, Lower Arm, Right

Anterior (pectoral) lymph node
    use Lymphatic, Axillary, Right
    use Lymphatic, Axillary, Left
Anterior cerebral artery *use* Artery, Intracranial
Anterior cerebral vein *use* Vein, Intracranial
Anterior choroidal artery *use* Artery, Intracranial
Anterior circumflex humeral artery
    use Artery, Axillary, Left
    use Artery, Axillary, Right
Anterior communicating artery *use* Artery, Intracranial
Anterior cruciate ligament (ACL)
    use Bursa and Ligament, Knee, Left
    use Bursa and Ligament, Knee, Right
Anterior crural nerve *use* Nerve, Femoral
Anterior facial vein
    use Vein, Face, Left
    use Vein, Face, Right
Anterior intercostal artery
    use Artery, Internal Mammary, Right
    use Artery, Internal Mammary, Left
Anterior interosseous nerve *use* Nerve, Median
Anterior lateral malleolar artery
    use Artery, Anterior Tibial, Right
    use Artery, Anterior Tibial, Left
Anterior lingual gland *use* Gland, Minor Salivary
Anterior medial malleolar artery
    use Artery, Anterior Tibial, Right
    use Artery, Anterior Tibial, Left
Anterior spinal artery
    use Artery, Vertebral, Right
    use Artery, Vertebral, Left
Anterior tibial recurrent artery
    use Artery, Anterior Tibial, Right
    use Artery, Anterior Tibial, Left
Anterior ulnar recurrent artery
    use Artery, Ulnar, Right
Anterior ulnar recurrent artery
    use Artery, Ulnar, Left
Anterior vagal trunk *use* Nerve, Vagus
Anterior vertebral muscle
    use Muscle, Neck, Left
    use Muscle, Neck, Right
Antihelix
    use Ear, External, Bilateral
    use Ear, External, Left
    use Ear, External, Right
Antitragus
    use Ear, External, Bilateral
    use Ear, External, Right
    use Ear, External, Left
Antrostomy *see* Drainage, Ear, Nose, Sinus **099**
Antrotomy *see* Drainage, Ear, Nose, Sinus **099**
Antrum of Highmore
    use Sinus, Maxillary, Left
    use Sinus, Maxillary, Right
Aortic annulus *use* Valve, Aortic
Aortic arch *use* Thoracic Aorta, Ascending/Arch
Aortic intercostal artery *use* Upper Artery

Aortography
  see Fluoroscopy, Lower Arteries **B41** #
  see Fluoroscopy, Upper Arteries **B31**
  see Plain Radiography, Lower Arteries **B40**
  see Plain Radiography, Upper Arteries **B30**
Aortoplasty
  see Repair, Aorta, Abdominal **04Q0**
  see Repair, Aorta, Thoracic, Descending **02QW**
  see Repair, Aorta, Thoracic, Ascending/Arch **02QX**
  see Replacement, Aorta, Abdominal **04R0**
  see Replacement, Aorta, Thoracic, Descending **02RW**
  see Replacement, Aorta, Thoracic, Ascending/Arch **02RX**
  see Supplement, Aorta, Abdominal **04U0**
  see Supplement, Aorta, Thoracic, Descending **02UW**
  see Supplement, Aorta, Thoracic, Ascending/Arch **02UX**
Apical (subclavicular) lymph node
  use Lymphatic, Axillary, Left
  use Lymphatic, Axillary, Right
Apneustic center *use* Pons
Appendectomy
  see Excision, Appendix **0DBJ**
  see Resection, Appendix **0DTJ**
Appendicolysis *see* Release, Appendix **0DNJ**
Appendicotomy *see* Drainage, Appendix **0D9J**
Application *see* Introduction of substance in or on
Aquapheresis 6A550Z3
Aqueduct of Sylvius *use* Cerebral Ventricle
Aqueous humor
  use Anterior Chamber, Right
  use Anterior Chamber, Left
Arachnoid mater, intracranial *use* Cerebral Meninges
Arachnoid mater, spinal *use* Spinal Meninges
Arcuate artery
  use Artery, Foot, Left
  use Artery, Foot, Right
Areola *use* Nipple, Left
  use Nipple, Right
AROM (artificial rupture of membranes) 10907ZC
Arterial canal (duct) *use* Artery, Pulmonary, Left
Arterial pulse tracing *see* Measurement, Arterial **4A03**
Arteriectomy
  see Excision, Heart and Great Vessels **02B**
  see Excision, Lower Arteries **04B**
  see Excision, Upper Arteries **03B**
Arteriography
  see Fluoroscopy, Heart **B21**
  see Fluoroscopy, Lower Arteries **B41**
  see Fluoroscopy, Upper Arteries **B31**
  see Plain Radiography, Heart **B20**
  see Plain Radiography, Lower Arteries **B40**
  see Plain Radiography, Upper Arteries **B30**
Arterioplasty
  see Repair, Heart and Great Vessels **02Q**
  see Replacement, Heart and Great Vessels **02R**
  see Repair, Lower Arteries **04Q**

Arterioplasty *(continued)*
  see Repair, Upper Arteries **03Q**
  see Replacement, Lower Arteries **04R**
  see Replacement, Upper Arteries **03R**
  see Supplement, Heart and Great Vessels **02U**
  see Supplement, Lower Arteries **04U**
  see Supplement, Upper Arteries **03U**
Arteriorrhaphy
  see Repair, Heart and Great Vessels **02Q**
  see Repair, Upper Arteries **03Q**
  see Repair, Lower Arteries **04Q**
Arterioscopy
  see Inspection, Great Vessel **02JY**
  see Inspection, Artery, Upper **03JY**
  see Inspection, Artery, Lower **04JY**
Arthrectomy
  see Excision, Lower Joints **0SB**
  see Excision, Upper Joints **0RB**
  see Resection, Lower Joints **0ST**
  see Resection, Upper Joints **0RT**
Arthrocentesis
  see Drainage, Lower Joints **0S9**
  see Drainage, Upper Joints **0R9**
Arthrodesis
Arthrodesis
  see Fusion, Lower Joints **0SG**
  see Fusion, Upper Joints **0RG**
Arthrography
  see Plain Radiography, Skull and Facial Bones **BN0**
  see Plain Radiography, Non-Axial Upper Bones **BP0**
  see Plain Radiography, Non-Axial Lower Bones **BQ0**
Arthrolysis
  see Release, Lower Joints **0SN**
  see Release, Upper Joints **0RN**
Arthropexy
  see Repair, Lower Joints **0SQ**
  see Repair, Upper Joints **0RQ**
  see Reposition, Lower Joints **0SS**
  see Reposition, Upper Joints **0RS**
Arthroplasty
  see Repair, Lower Joints **0SQ**
  see Repair, Upper Joints **0RQ**
  see Replacement, Lower Joints **0SR**
Arthroplasty *(continued)*
  see Replacement, Upper Joints **0RR**
  see Supplement, Lower Joints **0SU**
  see Supplement, Upper Joints **0RU**
Arthroscopy
  see Inspection, Lower Joints **0SJ**
  see Inspection, Upper Joints **0RJ**
Arthrotomy
  see Drainage, Lower Joints **0S9**
  see Drainage, Upper Joints **0R9**
Artificial anal sphincter (AAS) *use* Artificial Sphincter in Gastrointestinal System
Artificial bowel sphincter (neosphincter) *use* Artificial Sphincter in Gastrointestinal System
Artificial Sphincter
  Insertion of device in
    Anus **0DHQ**
    Bladder **0THB**

Artificial Sphincter *(continued)*
    Bladder Neck **0THC**
    Urethra **0THD**
  Removal of device from
    Anus **0DPQ**
    Bladder **0TPB**
    Urethra **0TPD**
  Revision of device in
    Anus **0DWQ**
    Bladder **0TWB**
    Urethra **0TWD**
Artificial urinary sphincter (AUS) *use* Artificial Sphincter in Urinary System
Aryepiglottic fold *use* Larynx
Arytenoid cartilage *use* Larynx
Arytenoid muscle
  use Muscle, Neck, Left
  use Muscle, Neck, Right
Arytenoidectomy *see* Excision, Larynx **0CBS**
Arytenoidopexy *see* Repair, Larynx **0CQS**
Ascending aorta *use* Thoracic Aorta, Ascending/Arch
Ascending palatine artery *use* Artery, Face
Ascending pharyngeal artery
  use Artery, External Carotid, Left
  use Artery, External Carotid, Right
Aspiration, fine needle
  fluid or gas *see* Drainage
  tissue *see* Excision
Assessment
  Activities of daily living *see* Activities of Daily Living Assessment, Rehabilitation **F02**
  Hearing aid *see* Hearing Aid Assessment, Diagnostic Audiology **F14**
  Hearing *see* Hearing Assessment, Diagnostic Audiology **F13**
  intravascular perfusion, using indocyanine green (ICG) dye see Monitoring, Physiological Systems **4A1**
  Motor function *see* Motor Function Assessment, Rehabilitation **F01**
  Nerve function *see* Motor Function Assessment, Rehabilitation **F01**
  Speech *see* Speech Assessment, Rehabilitation **F00**
  Vestibular *see* Vestibular Assessment, Diagnostic Audiology **F15**
  Vocational *see* Activities of Daily Living Treatment, Rehabilitation **F08**
Assistance
  Cardiac
    Continuous
      Balloon Pump **5A02210**
      Impeller Pump **5A0221D**
      Other Pump **5A02216**
      Pulsatile Compression **5A02215**
    Intermittent
      Balloon Pump **5A02110**
      Impeller Pump **5A0211D**
      Other Pump **5A02116**
      Pulsatile Compression **5A02115**
  Circulatory
    Continuous
      Hyperbaric **5A05221**
      Supersaturated **5A0522C**

Assistance *(continued)*
  Intermittent
    Hyperbaric **5A05121**
    Supersaturated **5A0512C**
  Respiratory
    24-96 Consecutive Hours
      Continuous Negative Airway Pressure **5A09459**
      Continuous Positive Airway Pressure **5A09457**
      Intermittent Negative Airway Pressure **5A0945B**
      Intermittent Positive Airway Pressure **5A09458**
      No Qualifier **5A0945Z**
    Greater than 96 Consecutive Hours
      Continuous Negative Airway Pressure **5A09559**
      Continuous Positive Airway Pressure **5A09557**
      Intermittent Negative Airway Pressure **5A0955B**
      Intermittent Positive Airway Pressure **5A09558**
      No Qualifier **5A0955Z**
    Less than 24 Consecutive Hours
      Continuous Negative Airway Pressure **5A09359**
      Continuous Positive Airway Pressure **5A09357**
      Intermittent Negative Airway Pressure **5A0935B**
      Intermittent Positive Airway Pressure **5A09358**
      No Qualifier **5A0935Z**
Assurant (Cobalt) stent *use* Intraluminal Device
Atherectomy
  see Extirpation, Heart and Great Vessels **02C**
  see Extirpation, Upper Arteries **03C**
  see Extirpation, Lower Arteries **04C**
Atlantoaxial joint *use* Joint, Cervical Vertebral
Atmospheric Control 6A0Z
Atrioseptoplasty
  see Repair, Heart and Great Vessels **02Q**
  see Replacement, Heart and Great Vessels **02R**
  see Supplement, Heart and Great Vessels **02U**
Atrioventricular node *use* Conduction Mechanism
Atrium dextrum cordis *use* Atrium, Right
Atrium pulmonale *use* Atrium, Left
Attain Ability® lead
  use Cardiac Lead, Pacemaker in **02H**
  use Cardiac Lead, Defibrillator in **02H**
Attain StarFix® (OTW) lead
  use Cardiac Lead, Defibrillator in **02H**
  use Cardiac Lead, Pacemaker in **02H**
Audiology, diagnostic
  see Hearing Assessment, Diagnostic Audiology **F13**
  see Hearing Aid Assessment, Diagnostic Audiology **F14**

Audiology, diagnostic *(continued)*
  see Vestibular Assessment, Diagnostic Audiology **F15**
Audiometry *see* Hearing Assessment, Diagnostic Audiology **F13**
Auditory tube
  use Eustachian Tube, Right
  use Eustachian Tube, Left
Auerbach's (myenteric) plexus *use* Nerve, Abdominal Sympathetic
Auricle
  use Ear, External, Left
  use Ear, External, Bilateral
  use Ear, External, Right
Auricularis muscle *use* Muscle, Head
Autograft *use* Autologous Tissue Substitute
Autologous artery graft
  use Autologous Arterial Tissue in Lower Arteries
  use Autologous Arterial Tissue in Upper Veins
  use Autologous Arterial Tissue in Lower Veins
  use Autologous Arterial Tissue in Heart and Great Vessels
Autologous artery graft
  use Autologous Arterial Tissue in Upper Arteries
Autologous vein graft
  use Autologous Venous Tissue in Heart and Great Vessels
  use Autologous Venous Tissue in Lower Arteries
  use Autologous Venous Tissue in Lower Veins
  use Autologous Venous Tissue in Upper Arteries
  use Autologous Venous Tissue in Upper Veins
Autotransfusion *see* Transfusion
Autotransplant
  Adrenal tissue *see* Reposition, Endocrine System **0GS**
  Kidney *see* Reposition, Urinary System **0TS**
  Pancreatic tissue *see* Reposition, Pancreas **0FSG**
  Parathyroid tissue *see* Reposition, Endocrine System **0GS**
  Thyroid tissue *see* Reposition, Endocrine System **0GS**
  Tooth *see* Reattachment, Mouth and Throat **0CM**
Avulsion *see* Extraction
Axial Lumbar Interbody Fusion System *use* Interbody Fusion Device in Lower Joints
AxiaLIF® System *use* Interbody Fusion Device in Lower Joints
Axillary fascia
  use Subcutaneous Tissue and Fascia, Upper Arm, Left
  use Subcutaneous Tissue and Fascia, Upper Arm, Right
Axillary nerve *use* Nerve, Brachial Plexus

B

BAK/C® Interbody Cervical Fusion System
  use Interbody Fusion Device in Upper Joints
BAL (bronchial alveolar lavage), diagnostic
  see Drainage, Respiratory System **0B9**
Balanoplasty
  see Repair, Penis **0VQS**
  see Supplement, Penis **0VUS**
Balloon Pump
  Continuous, Output **5A02210**
  Intermittent, Output **5A02110**
Bandage, Elastic *see* Compression
Banding *see* Restriction
Bard® Composix® (E/X)(LP) mesh *use* Synthetic Substitute
Bard® Composix® Kugel® patch *use* Synthetic Substitute
Bard® Dulex™ mesh *use* Synthetic Substitute
Bard® Ventralex™ hernia patch *use* Synthetic Substitute
Barium swallow *see* Fluoroscopy, Gastrointestinal System **BD1**
Baroreflex Activation Therapy® (BAT®)
  use Stimulator Lead in Upper Arteries
  use Cardiac Rhythm Related Device in Subcutaneous Tissue and Fascia
Bartholin's (greater vestibular) gland *use* Gland, Vestibular
Basal (internal) cerebral vein *use* Vein, Intracranial
Basal metabolic rate (BMR) *see* Measurement, Physiological Systems **4A0Z**
Basal nuclei *use* Basal Ganglia
Base of Tongue *use* Pharynx
Basilar artery *use* Artery, Intracranial
Basis pontis *use* Pons
Beam Radiation
  Abdomen **DW03**
    Intraoperative **DW033Z0**
  Adrenal Gland **DG02**
    Intraoperative **DG023Z0**
  Bile Ducts **DF02**
    Intraoperative **DF023Z0**
  Bladder **DT02**
    Intraoperative **DT023Z0**
  Bone
    Other **DP0C**
    Intraoperative **DP0C3Z0**
  Bone Marrow **D700**
    Intraoperative **D7003Z0**
  Brain **D000**
    Intraoperative **D0003Z0**
  Brain Stem **D001**
    Intraoperative **D0013Z0**
  Breast
    Left **DM00**
      Intraoperative **DM003Z0**
    Right **DM01**
      Intraoperative **DM013Z0**
  Bronchus **DB01**
    Intraoperative **DB013Z0**
  Cervix **DU01**
    Intraoperative **DU013Z0**
  Chest **DW02**
    Intraoperative **DW023Z0**
  Chest Wall **DB07**
    Intraoperative **DB073Z0**

Beam Radiation *(continued)*
  Colon **DD05**
    Intraoperative **DD053Z0**
  Diaphragm **DB08**
    Intraoperative **DB083Z0**
  Duodenum **DD02**
    Intraoperative **DD023Z0**
  Ear **D900#**
    Intraoperative **D9003Z0**
  Esophagus **DD00**
    Intraoperative **DD003Z0**
  Eye **D800**
    Intraoperative **D8003Z0**
  Femur **DP09**
    Intraoperative **DP093Z0**
  Fibula **DP0B**
    Intraoperative **DP0B3Z0**
  Gallbladder **DF01**
    Intraoperative **DF013Z0**
  Gland
    Adrenal **DG02**
      Intraoperative **DG023Z0**
    Parathyroid **DG04**
      Intraoperative **DG043Z0**
    Pituitary **DG00**
      Intraoperative **DG003Z0**
    Thyroid **DG05**
      Intraoperative **DG053Z0**
  Glands
    Salivary **D906**
    Intraoperative **D9063Z0**
  Head and Neck **DW01**
    Intraoperative **DW013Z0**
  Hemibody **DW04**
    Intraoperative **DW043Z0**
  Humerus **DP06**
    Intraoperative **DP063Z0**
  Hypopharynx **D903**
    Intraoperative **D9033Z0**
  Ileum **DD04**
    Intraoperative **DD043Z0**
  Jejunum **DD03**
    Intraoperative **DD033Z0**
  Kidney **DT00**
    Intraoperative **DT003Z0**
  Larynx **D90B**
    Intraoperative **D90B3Z0**
  Liver **DF00**
    Intraoperative **DF003Z0**
  Lung **DB02**
    Intraoperative **DB023Z0**
  Lymphatics
    Abdomen **D706**
      Intraoperative **D7063Z0**
    Axillary **D704**
      Intraoperative **D7043Z0**
    Inguinal **D708**
      Intraoperative **D7083Z0**
    Neck **D703**
      Intraoperative **D7033Z0**
    Pelvis **D707**
      Intraoperative **D7073Z0**
    Thorax **D705**
      Intraoperative **D7053Z0**
  Mandible **DP03**
    Intraoperative **DP033Z0**

Beam Radiation *(continued)*
  Maxilla **DP02**
    Intraoperative **DP023Z0**
  Mediastinum **DB06**
    Intraoperative **DB063Z0**
  Mouth **D904**
    Intraoperative **D9043Z0**
  Nasopharynx **D90D**
    Intraoperative **D90D3Z0**
  Neck and Head **DW01**
    Intraoperative **DW013Z0**
  Nerve
    Peripheral **D007**
    Intraoperative **D0073Z0**
  Nose **D901**
    Intraoperative **D9013Z0**
  Oropharynx **D90F**
    Intraoperative **D90F3Z0**
  Ovary **DU00**
    Intraoperative **DU003Z0**
  Palate
    Hard **D908**
      Intraoperative **D9083Z0**
    Soft **D909**
      Intraoperative **D9093Z0**
  Pancreas **DF03**
    Intraoperative **DF033Z0**
  Parathyroid Gland **DG04**
    Intraoperative **DG043Z0**
  Pelvic Bones **DP08**
    Intraoperative **DP083Z0**
  Pelvic Region **DW06**
    Intraoperative **DW063Z0**
  Pineal Body **DG01**
    Intraoperative **DG013Z0**
  Pituitary Gland **DG00**
    Intraoperative **DG003Z0**
  Pleura **DB05**
    Intraoperative **DB053Z0**
  Prostate **DV00**
    Intraoperative **DV003Z0**
  Radius **DP07**
    Intraoperative **DP073Z0**
  Rectum **DD07**
    Intraoperative **DD073Z0**
  Rib **DP05**
    Intraoperative **DP053Z0**
  Sinuses **D907**
    Intraoperative **D9073Z0**
  Skin
    Abdomen **DH08**
      Intraoperative **DH083Z0**
    Arm **DH04**
      Intraoperative **DH043Z0**
    Back **DH07**
      Intraoperative **DH073Z0**
    Buttock **DH09**
      Intraoperative **DH093Z0**
    Chest **DH06**
      Intraoperative **DH063Z0**
    Face **DH02**
      Intraoperative **DH023Z0**
    Leg **DH0B**
      Intraoperative **DH0B3Z0**
Beam Radiation *(continued)*
    Neck **DH03**

Beam Radiation *(continued)*
      Intraoperative **DH033Z0**
  Skull **DP00**
    Intraoperative **DP003Z0**
  Spinal Cord **D006**
    Intraoperative **D0063Z0**
  Spleen **D702**
    Intraoperative **D7023Z0**
  Sternum **DP04**
    Intraoperative **DP043Z0**
  Stomach **DD01**
    Intraoperative **DD013Z0**
  Testis **DV01**
    Intraoperative **DV013Z0**
  Thymus **D701**
    Intraoperative **D7013Z0**
  Thyroid Gland **DG05**
    Intraoperative **DG053Z0**
  Tibia **DP0B**
    Intraoperative **DP0B3Z0**
  Tongue **D905**
    Intraoperative **D9053Z0**
  Trachea **DB00**
    Intraoperative **DB003Z0**
  Ulna **DP07**
    Intraoperative **DP073Z0**
  Ureter **DT01**
    Intraoperative **DT013Z0**
  Urethra **DT03**
    Intraoperative **DT033Z0**
  Uterus **DU02**
    Intraoperative **DU023Z0**
  Whole Body **DW05**
    Intraoperative **DW053Z0**
Berlin Heart Ventricular Assist Device *use* Implantable Heart Assist System in Heart and Great Vessels
Biceps brachii muscle
  use Muscle, Upper Arm, Right
  use Muscle, Upper Arm, Left
Biceps femoris muscle
  use Muscle, Upper Leg, Right
  use Muscle, Upper Leg, Left
Bicipital aponeurosis
  use Subcutaneous Tissue and Fascia, Lower Arm, Left
  use Subcutaneous Tissue and Fascia, Lower Arm, Right
Bicuspid valve *use* Valve, Mitral
Bililite therapy *see* Ultraviolet Light Therapy, Skin **6A80**
Bioactive embolization coil(s) *use* Intraluminal Device, Bioactive in Upper Arteries
Biofeedback GZC9ZZZ
Biopsy
  see Drainage with qualifier Diagnostic
  see Excision with qualifier Diagnostic
  Bone Marrow *see* Extraction with qualifier Diagnostic
BiPAP *see* Assistance, Respiratory **5A09**
Bisection *see* Division
Biventricular external heart assist system
  use External Heart Assist System in Heart and Great Vessels
Blepharectomy
  see Excision, Eye **08B**
  see Resection, Eye **08T**

Blepharoplasty
  see Repair, Eye **08Q**
  see Replacement, Eye **08R**
  see Reposition, Eye **08S**
  see Supplement, Eye **08U**
Blepharorrhaphy see Repair, Eye **08Q**
Blepharotomy see Drainage, Eye **089**
Blinatumomab Antineoplastic Immunotherapy XW0
Block, Nerve, anesthetic injection 3E0T3CZ
Blood glucose monitoring system use Monitoring Device
Blood pressure see Measurement, Arterial **4A03**
BMR (basal metabolic rate) see Measurement, Physiological Systems **4A0Z**
Body of femur
  use Femoral Shaft, Right
  use Femoral Shaft, Left
Body of fibula
  use Fibula, Right
  use Fibula, Left
Bone anchored hearing device
  use Hearing Device, Bone Conduction in **09H**
  use Hearing Device in Head and Facial Bones
Bone bank bone graft use Nonautologous Tissue Substitute
Bone Growth Stimulator
  Insertion of device in
    Bone
      Facial **0NHW**
      Lower **0QHY**
      Nasal **0NHB**
      Upper **0PHY**
    Skull **0NH0**
  Removal of device from
    Bone
      Facial **0NPW**
      Lower **0QPY**
      Nasal **0NPB**
      Upper **0PPY**
    Skull **0NP0**
  Revision of device in
    Facial **0NWW**
    Lower **0QWY**
    Nasal **0NWB**
    Upper **0PWY**
    Skull **0NW0**
Bone marrow transplant see Transfusion, Circulatory **302**
Bone screw (interlocking)(lag)(pedicle)(recessed)
  use Internal Fixation Device in Head and Facial Bones
  use Internal Fixation Device in Lower Bones
  use Internal Fixation Device in Upper Bones
Bony labyrinth
  use Ear, Inner, Left
  use Ear, Inner, Right
Bony orbit
  use Orbit, Right
  use Orbit, Left
Bony vestibule
  use Ear, Inner, Right
  use Ear, Inner, Left

Botallo's duct use Artery, Pulmonary, Left
Bovine pericardial valve use Zooplastic Tissue in Heart and Great Vessels
Bovine pericardium graft use Zooplastic Tissue in Heart and Great Vessels
BP (blood pressure) see Measurement, Arterial **4A03**
Brachial (lateral) lymph node
  use Lymphatic, Axillary, Left
  use Lymphatic, Axillary, Right
Brachialis muscle
  use Muscle, Upper Arm, Left
  use Muscle, Upper Arm, Right
Brachiocephalic artery use Artery, Innominate
Brachiocephalic trunk use Artery, Innominate
Brachiocephalic vein
  use Vein, Innominate, Left
  use Vein, Innominate, Right
Brachioradialis muscle
  use Muscle, Lower Arm and Wrist, Left
  use Muscle, Lower Arm and Wrist, Right
Brachytherapy
  Abdomen **DW13**
  Adrenal Gland **DG12**
  Bile Ducts **DF12**
  Bladder **DT12**
  Bone Marrow **D710**
  Brain **D010**
  Brain Stem **D011**
  Breast
    Left **DM10**
    Right **DM11**
  Bronchus **DB11**
  Cervix **DU11**
  Chest **DW12**
  Chest Wall **DB17**
  Colon **DD15**
  Diaphragm **DB18**
  Duodenum **DD12**
  Ear **D910**
  Esophagus **DD10**
  Eye **D810**
  Gallbladder **DF11** Gland
    Adrenal **DG12**
    Parathyroid **DG14**
    Pituitary **DG10**
    Thyroid **DG15**
  Glands, Salivary **D916**
  Head and Neck **DW11**
  Hypopharynx **D913**
  Ileum **DD14**
  Jejunum **DD13**
  Kidney **DT10**
  Larynx **D91B**
  Liver **DF10**
  Lung **DB12**
  Lymphatics
    Abdomen **D716**
    Axillary **D714**
    Inguinal **D718**
    Neck **D713**
    Pelvis **D717**
    Thorax **D715**
  Mediastinum **DB16**
  Mouth **D914**

Brachytherapy *(continued)*
  Nasopharynx **D91D**
  Neck and Head **DW11**
  Nerve, Peripheral **D017**
  Nose **D911**
  Oropharynx **D91F**
  Ovary **DU10**
  Palate
    Hard **D918**
    Soft **D919**
  Pancreas **DF13**
  Parathyroid Gland **DG14**
  Pelvic Region **DW16**
  Pineal Body **DG11**
  Pituitary Gland **DG10**
  Pleura **DB15**
  Prostate **DV10**
  Rectum **DD17**
  Sinuses **D917**
  Spinal Cord **D016**
  Spleen **D712**
  Stomach **DD11**
  Testis **DV11**
  Thymus **D711**
  Thyroid Gland **DG15**
  Tongue **D915**
  Trachea **DB10**
  Ureter **DT11**
  Urethra **DT13**
  Uterus **DU12**
Brachytherapy seeds use Radioactive Element
Broad ligament use Uterine Supporting Structure
Bronchial artery use Upper Artery
Bronchography
  see Plain Radiography, Respiratory System **BB0**
  see Fluoroscopy, Respiratory System **BB1**
Bronchoplasty
  see Repair, Respiratory System **0BQ**
  see Supplement, Respiratory System **0BU**
Bronchorrhaphy see Repair, Respiratory System **0BQ**
Bronchoscopy 0BJ08ZZ
Bronchotomy see Drainage, Respiratory System **0B9**
Bronchus Intermedius use Main Bronchus, Right
BRYAN® Cervical Disc System use Synthetic Substitute
Buccal gland use Buccal Mucosa
Buccinator lymph node use Lymphatic, Head
Buccinator muscle use Muscle, Facial
Buckling, scleral with implant see Supplement, Eye **08U**
Bulbospongiosus muscle use Muscle, Perineum
Bulbourethral (Cowper's) gland use Urethra
Bundle of His use Conduction Mechanism
Bundle of Kent use Conduction Mechanism
Bunionectomy see Excision, Lower Bones **0QB**
Bursectomy
  see Excision, Bursae and Ligaments **0MB**
  see Resection, Bursae and Ligaments **0MT**
Bursocentesis see Drainage, Bursae and Ligaments **0M9**

Bursography
  see Plain Radiography, Non-Axial Upper Bones **BP0**
  see Plain Radiography, Non-Axial Lower Bones **BQ0**
Bursotomy
  see Division, Bursae and Ligaments **0M8**
  see Drainage, Bursae and Ligaments **0M9**
BVS 5000 Ventricular Assist Device *use* External Heart Assist System in Heart and Great Vessels
Bypass
  Anterior Chamber
    Left **08133**
    Right **08123**
  Aorta
    Abdominal **0410**
    Ascending/Arch **021X**
    Descending **021W**
    Thoracic
  Artery
    Axillary
      Left **03160**
      Right **03150**
    Brachial
      Left **03180**
      Right **03170**
    Common Carotid
      Left **031J0**
      Right **031H0**
    Common Iliac
      Left **041D**
      Right **041C**
    Coronary
      Four or More Arteries **0213**
      One Artery **0210**
      Three Arteries **0212**
      Two Arteries **0211**
    External Carotid
      Left **031N0**
      Right **031M0**
    External Iliac
      Left **041J**
      Right **041H**
    Femoral
      Left **041L**
      Right **041K**
    Innominate **03120**
    Internal Carotid
      Left **031L0**
      Right **031K0**
    Internal Iliac
      Left **041F**
      Right **041E**
    Intracranial **031G0**
    Popliteal
      Left **041N**
      Right **041M**
    Pulmonary
      Left **021R**
      Right **021Q**
    Pulmonary Trunk **021P**
    Radial
      Left **031C0**
      Right **031B0**
    Splenic **0414**

Bypass *(continued)*
    Subclavian
      Left **03140**
      Right **03130**
    Temporal
      Left **031T0**
      Right **031S0**
    Ulnar
      Left **031A0**
      Right **03190**
  Atrium
    Left **0217**
    Right **0216**
  Bladder **0T1B**
  Cavity, Cranial **0W110J**
  Cecum **0D1H**
  Cerebral Ventricle **0016**
  Colon
    Ascending **0D1K**
    Descending **0D1M**
    Sigmoid **0D1N**
    Transverse **0D1L**
  Duct
    Common Bile **0F19**
    Cystic **0F18**
    Hepatic
      Left **0F16**
      Right **0F15**
    Lacrimal
      Left **081Y**
      Right **081X**
    Pancreatic **0F1D**
      Accessory **0F1F**
  Duodenum **0D19**
  Ear
    Left **091E0**
    Right **091D0**
  Esophagus **0D15**
    Lower **0D13**
    Middle **0D12**
    Upper **0D11**
  Fallopian Tube
    Left **0U16**
    Right **0U15**
  Gallbladder **0F14**
  Ileum **0D1B**
  Jejunum **0D1A**
  Kidney Pelvis
    Left **0T14**
    Right **0T13**
  Pancreas **0F1G**
  Pelvic Cavity **0W1J**
  Peritoneal Cavity **0W1G**
  Pleural Cavity
    Left **0W1B**
    Right **0W19**
  Spinal Canal **001U**
  Stomach **0D16**
  Trachea **0B11**
  Ureter
    Left **0T17**
    Right **0T16**
  Ureters, Bilateral **0T18**
  Vas Deferens
    Bilateral **0V1Q**
    Left **0V1P**

Bypass *(continued)*
    Right **0V1N**
  Vein
    Axillary
      Left **0518**
      Right **0517**
    Azygos **0510**
    Basilic
      Left **051C**
      Right **051B**
    Brachial
      Left **051A**
      Right **0519**
    Cephalic
      Left **051F**
      Right **051D**
    Colic **0617**
    Common Iliac
      Left **061D**
      Right **061C**
    Esophageal **0613**
    External Iliac
      Left **061G**
      Right **061F**
    External Jugular
      Left **051Q**
      Right **051P**
    Face
      Left **051V**
      Right **051T**
    Femoral
      Left **061N**
      Right **061M**
    Foot
      Left **061V**
      Right **061T**
    Gastric **0612**
    Greater Saphenous
      Left **061Q**
      Right **061P**
    Hand
      Left **051H**
      Right **051G**
    Hemiazygos **0511**
    Hepatic **0614**
    Hypogastric
      Left **061J**
      Right **061H**
    Inferior Mesenteric **0616**
    Innominate
      Left **0514**
      Right **0513**
    Internal Jugular
      Left **051N**
      Right **051M**
    Intracranial **051L**
    Lesser Saphenous
      Left **061S**
      Right **061R**
    Portal **0618**
    Renal
      Left **061B**
      Right **0619**
    Splenic **0611**
    Subclavian
      Left **0516**

Bypass *(continued)*
    Right **0515**
    Superior Mesenteric **0615**
    Vertebral
        Left **051S**
        Right **051R**
    Vena Cava
        Inferior **0610**
        Superior **021V**
    Ventricle
        Left **021L**
        Right **021K**
Bypass, cardiopulmonary 5A1221Z

C

Caesarean section *see* Extraction, Products of Conception **10D0**
Calcaneocuboid joint
    use Joint, Tarsal, Left
    use Joint, Tarsal, Right
Calcaneocuboid ligament
    use Bursa and Ligament, Foot, Right
    use Bursa and Ligament, Foot, Left
Calcaneofibular ligament
    use Bursa and Ligament, Ankle, Left
    use Bursa and Ligament, Ankle, Right
Calcaneus
    use Tarsal, Right
    use Tarsal, Left
Cannulation
    see Bypass
    see Dilation
    see Drainage
    see Irrigation
Canthorrhaphy *see* Repair, Eye **08Q**
Canthotomy *see* Release, Eye **08N**
Capitate bone
    use Carpal, Left
    use Carpal, Right
Capsulectomy, lens *see* Excision, Eye **08B**
Capsulorrhaphy, joint
    see Repair, Upper Joints **0RQ**
    see Repair, Lower Joints **0SQ**
Cardia *use* Esophagogastric Junction
Cardiac contractility modulation lead *use* Cardiac Lead in Heart and Great Vessels
Cardiac event recorder *use* Monitoring Device
Cardiac Lead
    Defibrillator
        Atrium
            Left **02H7**
            Right **02H6**
        Pericardium **02HN**
        Vein, Coronary **02H4**
        Ventricle
            Left **02HL**
            Right **02HK**
    Insertion of device in
        Atrium
            Left **02H7**
            Right **02H6**
        Pericardium **02HN**
        Vein, Coronary **02H4**
        Ventricle

Cardiac Lead *(continued)*
        Left **02HL**
        Right **02HK**
    Pacemaker
        Atrium
            Left **02H7**
            Right **02H6**
        Pericardium **02HN**
        Vein, Coronary **02H4**
        Ventricle
            Left **02HL**
            Right **02HK**
    Removal of device from, Heart **02PA**
    Revision of device in, Heart **02WA**
Cardiac plexus *use* Nerve, Thoracic Sympathetic
Cardiac Resynchronization Defibrillator Pulse Generator
    Abdomen **0JH8**
    Chest **0JH6**
Cardiac Resynchronization Pacemaker Pulse Generator
    Abdomen **0JH8**
    Chest **0JH6**
Cardiac resynchronization therapy (CRT) lead
    use Cardiac Lead, Pacemaker in **02H**
    use Cardiac Lead, Defibrillator in **02H**
Cardiac Rhythm Related Device
    Insertion of device in
        Abdomen **0JH8**
        Chest **0JH6**
    Removal of device from, Subcutaneous Tissue and Fascia, Trunk **0JPT**
    Revision of device in, Subcutaneous Tissue and Fascia, Trunk **0JWT**
Cardiocentesis *see* Drainage, Pericardial Cavity **0W9D**
Cardioesophageal junction *use* Esophagogastric Junction
Cardiolysis *see* Release, Heart and Great Vessels **02N**
CardioMEMS® pressure sensor *use* Monitoring Device, Pressure Sensor in **02H**
Cardiomyotomy *see* Division, Esophagogastric Junction **0D84**
Cardioplegia *see* Introduction of substance in or on, Heart **3E08**
Cardiorrhaphy *see* Repair, Heart and Great Vessels **02Q**
Cardioversion 5A2204Z
Caregiver Training F0FZ
Caroticotympanic artery
    use Artery, Internal Carotid, Right
    use Artery, Internal Carotid, Left
Carotid (artery) sinus (baroreceptor) lead
    use Stimulator Lead in Upper Arteries
Carotid glomus
    use Carotid Bodies, Bilateral
    use Carotid Body, Right
    use Carotid Body, Left
Carotid sinus
    use Artery, Internal Carotid, Left
    use Artery, Internal Carotid, Right
Carotid sinus nerve *use* Nerve, Glossopharyngeal

Carotid WALLSTENT® Monorail® Endoprosthesis *use* Intraluminal Device
Carpectomy
    see Excision, Upper Bones **0PB**
    see Resection, Upper Bones **0PT**
Carpometacarpal (CMC) joint
    use Joint, Metacarpocarpal, Left
    use Joint, Metacarpocarpal, Right
Carpometacarpal ligament
    use Bursa and Ligament, Hand, Left
    use Bursa and Ligament, Hand, Right
Casting *see* Immobilization
CAT scan *see* Computerized Tomography (CT Scan)
Catheterization
    see Dilation
    see Drainage
    see Irrigation
    see Insertion of device in
    Heart *see* Measurement, Cardiac **4A02**
    Umbilical vein, for infusion **06H033T**
Cauda equina *use* Spinal Cord, Lumbar
Cauterization   *see* Destruction
    see Repair
Cavernous plexus *use* Nerve, Head and Neck Sympathetic
Cecectomy
    see Excision, Cecum **0DBH**
    see Resection, Cecum **0DTH**
Cecocolostomy
    see Bypass, Gastrointestinal System **0D1**
    see Drainage, Gastrointestinal System **0D9**
Cecopexy
    see Repair, Cecum **0DQH**
    see Reposition, Cecum **0DSH**
Cecoplication *see* Restriction, Cecum **0DVH**
Cecorrhaphy *see* Repair, Cecum **0DQH**
Cecostomy
    see Bypass, Cecum **0D1H**
    see Drainage, Cecum **0D9H**
Cecotomy *see* Drainage, Cecum **0D9H**
Ceftazidime-Avibactam Anti-Infective XW0
Celiac (solar) plexus *use* Nerve, Abdominal Sympathetic
Celiac ganglion *use* Nerve, Abdominal Sympathetic
Celiac lymph node *use* Lymphatic, Aortic
Celiac trunk *use* Artery, Celiac
Central axillary lymph node
    use Lymphatic, Axillary, Left
    use Lymphatic, Axillary, Right
Central venous pressure *see* Measurement, Venous **4A04**
Centrimag® Blood Pump *use* Intraluminal Device
Cephalogram BN00ZZZ
Ceramic on ceramic bearing surface *use* Synthetic Substitute, Ceramic in **0SR**
Cerebral Embolic Filtration, Dual Filter X2A5312
Cerclage *see* Restriction
Cerebral aqueduct (Sylvius) *use* Cerebral Ventricle
Cerebrum *use* Brain
Cervical esophagus *use* Esophagus, Upper
Cervical facet joint
    use Joint, Cervical Vertebral

Cervical facet joint *(continued)*
  use Joint, Cervical Vertebral, 2 or more
Cervical ganglion *use* Nerve, Head and Neck
  Sympathetic
Cervical interspinous ligament *use* Bursa and
  Ligament, Head and Neck
Cervical intertransverse ligament *use* Bursa
  and Ligament, Head and Neck
Cervical ligamentum flavum *use* Bursa and
  Ligament, Head and Neck
Cervical lymph node
  use Lymphatic, Neck, Right
  use Lymphatic, Neck, Left
Cervicectomy
  see Excision, Cervix 0UBC
  see Resection, Cervix 0UTC
Cervicothoracic facet joint *use* Joint,
  Cervicothoracic Vertebral
Cesarean section *see* Extraction, Products of
  Conception 10D0
Change device in
  Abdominal Wall **0W2FX**
  Back
    Lower **0W2LX**
    Upper **0W2KX**
  Bladder **0T2BX**
  Bone
    Facial **0N2WX**
    Lower **0Q2YX**
    Nasal **0N2BX**
    Upper **0P2YX**
  Bone Marrow **072TX**
  Brain **0020X**
  Breast
    Left **0H2UX**
    Right **0H2TX**
  Bursa and Ligament
    Lower **0M2YX**
    Upper **0M2XX**
  Cavity, Cranial **0W21X**
  Chest Wall **0W28X**
  Cisterna Chyli **072LX**
  Diaphragm **0B2TX**
  Duct
    Hepatobiliary **0F2BX**
    Pancreatic **0F2DX**
  Ear
    Left **092JX**
    Right **092HX**
  Epididymis and Spermatic Cord **0V2MX**
  Extremity
    Lower
      Left **0Y2BX**
      Right **0Y29X**
    Upper
      Left **0X27X**
      Right **0X26X**
  Eye
    Left **0821X**
    Right **0820X**
  Face **0W22X**
  Fallopian Tube **0U28X**
  Gallbladder **0F24X**
  Gland
    Adrenal **0G25X**
    Endocrine **0G2SX**

Change device in *(continued)*
  Pituitary **0G20X**
  Salivary **0C2AX**
  Head **0W20X**
  Intestinal Tract
    Lower **0D2DXUZ**
    Upper **0D20XUZ**
  Jaw
    Lower **0W25X**
    Upper **0W24X**
  Joint
    Lower **0S2YX**
    Upper **0R2YX**
  Kidney **0T25X**
  Larynx **0C2SX**
  Liver **0F20X**
  Lung
    Left **0B2LX**
    Right **0B2KX**
  Lymphatic **072NX**
    Thoracic Duct **072KX**
  Mediastinum **0W2CX**
  Mesentery **0D2VX**
  Mouth and Throat **0C2YX**
  Muscle
    Lower **0K2YX**
    Upper **0K2XX**
  Neck **0W26X**
  Nerve
    Cranial **002EX**
    Peripheral **012YX**
  Nose **092KX**
  Omentum **0D2UX**
  Ovary **0U23X**
  Pancreas **0F2GX**
  Parathyroid Gland **0G2RX**
  Pelvic Cavity **0W2JX**
  Penis **0V2SX**
  Pericardial Cavity **0W2DX**
  Perineum
    Female **0W2NX**
    Male **0W2MX**
  Peritoneal Cavity **0W2GX**
  Peritoneum **0D2WX**
  Pineal Body **0G21X**
  Pleura **0B2QX**
  Pleural Cavity
    Left **0W2BX**
    Right **0W29X**
  Products of Conception **10207**
  Prostate and Seminal Vesicles **0V24X**
  Retroperitoneum **0W2HX**
  Scrotum and Tunica Vaginalis **0V28X**
  Sinus **092YX**
  Skin **0H2PX**
  Skull **0N20X**
  Spinal Canal **002UX**
  Spleen **072PX**
  Subcutaneous Tissue and Fascia
    Head and Neck **0J2SX**
    Lower Extremity **0J2WX**
    Trunk **0J2TX**
    Upper Extremity **0J2VX**
  Tendon
    Lower **0L2YX**
    Upper **0L2XX**

Change device in *(continued)*
  Testis **0V2DX**
  Thymus **072MX**
  Thyroid Gland **0G2KX**
  Trachea **0B21**
  Tracheobronchial Tree **0B20X**
  Ureter **0T29X**
  Urethra **0T2DX**
  Uterus and Cervix **0U2DXHZ**
  Vagina and Cul-de-sac **0U2HXGZ**
  Vas Deferens **0V2RX**
  Vulva **0U2MX**
Change device in or on
  Abdominal Wall **2W03X**
  Anorectal **2Y03X5Z**
  Arm
    Lower
      Left **2W0DX**
      Right **2W0CX**
    Upper
      Left **2W0BX**
      Right **2W0AX**
  Back **2W05X**
  Chest Wall **2W04X**
  Ear **2Y02X5Z**
  Extremity
    Lower
      Left **2W0MX**
      Right **2W0LX**
    Upper
      Left **2W09X**
      Right **2W08X**
  Face **2W01X**
  Finger
    Left **2W0KX**
    Right **2W0JX**
  Foot
    Left **2W0TX**
    Right **2W0SX**
  Genital Tract, Female **2Y04X5Z**
  Hand
    Left **2W0FX**
    Right **2W0EX**
  Head **2W00X**
  Inguinal Region
    Left **2W07X**
    Right **2W06X**
  Leg
    Lower
      Left **2W0RX**
      Right **2W0QX**
    Upper
      Left **2W0PX**
      Right **2W0NX**
  Mouth and Pharynx **2Y00X5Z**
  Nasal **2Y01X5Z**
  Neck **2W02X**
  Thumb
    Left **2W0HX**
    Right **2W0GX**
  Toe
    Left **2W0VX**
    Right **2W0UX**
  Urethra **2Y05X5Z**
Chemoembolization *see* Introduction of
  substance in or on

Chemosurgery, Skin 3E00XTZ

Chemothalamectomy *see* Destruction, Thalamus 0059

Chemotherapy, Infusion for cancer *see* Introduction of substance in or on

Chest x-ray *see* Plain Radiography, Chest BW03

Chiropractic Manipulation
  Abdomen 9WB9X
  Cervical 9WB1X
  Extremities
    Lower 9WB6X
    Upper 9WB7X
  Head 9WB0X
  Lumbar 9WB3X
  Pelvis 9WB5X
  Rib Cage 9WB8X
  Sacrum 9WB4X
  Thoracic 9WB2X

Choana *use* Nasopharynx

Cholangiogram
  see Plain Radiography, Hepatobiliary System and Pancreas BF0
  see Fluoroscopy, Hepatobiliary System and Pancreas BF1

Cholecystectomy
  see Excision, Gallbladder 0FB4
  see Resection, Gallbladder 0FT4

Cholecystojejunostomy
  see Bypass, Hepatobiliary System and Pancreas 0F1
  see Drainage, Hepatobiliary System and Pancreas 0F9

Cholecystopexy
  see Repair, Gallbladder 0FQ4
  see Reposition, Gallbladder 0FS4

Cholecystoscopy 0FJ44ZZ

Cholecystostomy
  see Drainage, Gallbladder 0F94
  see Bypass, Gallbladder 0F14

Cholecystotomy *see* Drainage, Gallbladder 0F94

Choledochectomy
  see Excision, Hepatobiliary System and Pancreas 0FB
  see Resection, Hepatobiliary System and Pancreas 0FT

Choledocholithotomy *see* Extirpation, Duct, Common Bile 0FC9

Choledochoplasty
  see Repair, Hepatobiliary System and Pancreas 0FQ
  see Replacement, Hepatobiliary System and Pancreas 0FR
  see Supplement, Hepatobiliary System and Pancreas 0FU

Choledochoscopy 0FJB8ZZ

Choledochotomy *see* Drainage, Hepatobiliary System and Pancreas 0F9

Cholelithotomy *see* Extirpation, Hepatobiliary System and Pancreas 0FC

Chondrectomy
  see Excision, Upper Joints 0RB
  see Excision, Lower Joints 0SB
  Knee *see* Excision, Lower Joints 0SB
  Semilunar cartilage *see* Excision, Lower Joints 0SB

Chondroglossus muscle *use* Muscle, Tongue, Palate, Pharynx

Chorda tympani *use* Nerve, Facial

Chordotomy *see* Division, Central Nervous System 008

Choroid plexus *use* Cerebral Ventricle

Choroidectomy
  see Excision, Eye 08B
  see Resection, Eye 08T

Circumcision 0VTTXZZ

Ciliary body
  use Eye, Right
  use Eye, Left

Ciliary ganglion *use* Nerve, Head and Neck Sympathetic

Circle of Willis *use* Artery, Intracranial

Circumflex iliac artery
  use Artery, Femoral, Right
  use Artery, Femoral, Left

Clamp and rod internal fixation system (CRIF)
  use Internal Fixation Device in Upper Bones
  use Internal Fixation Device in Lower Bones

Clamping *see* Occlusion

Claustrum *use* Basal Ganglia

Claviculectomy
  see Excision, Upper Bones 0PB
  see Resection, Upper Bones 0PT

Claviculotomy
  see Division, Upper Bones 0P8
  see Drainage, Upper Bones 0P9

Clipping, aneurysm *see* Restriction using Extraluminal Device

Clitorectomy, clitoridectomy
  see Excision, Clitoris 0UBJ
  see Resection, Clitoris 0UTJ

Closure
  see Occlusion
  see Repair

Clysis *see* Introduction of substance in or on

Coagulation *see* Destruction

CoAxia NeuroFlo catheter *use* Intraluminal Device

Cobalt/chromium head and polyethylene socket *use* Synthetic Substitute, Metal on Polyethylene in 0SR

Cobalt/chromium head and socket *use* Synthetic Substitute, Metal in 0SR

Coccygeal body *use* Coccygeal Glomus

Coccygeus muscle
  use Muscle, Trunk, Left
  use Muscle, Trunk, Right

Cochlea
  use Ear, Inner, Left
  use Ear, Inner, Right

Cochlear implant (CI), multiple channel (electrode) *use* Hearing Device, Multiple Channel Cochlear Prosthesis in 09H

Cochlear implant (CI), single channel (electrode) *use* Hearing Device, Single Channel Cochlear Prosthesis in 09H

Cochlear Implant Treatment F0BZ0

Cochlear nerve *use* Nerve, Acoustic

COGNIS® CRT-D *use* Cardiac Resynchronization Defibrillator Pulse Generator in 0JH

Colectomy
  see Excision, Gastrointestinal System 0DB
  see Resection, Gastrointestinal System 0DT

Collapse *see* Occlusion

Collection from
  Breast, Breast Milk 8E0HX62
  Indwelling Device
    Circulatory System
      Blood 8C02X6K
      Other Fluid 8C02X6L
    Nervous System
      Cerebrospinal Fluid 8C01X6J
      Other Fluid 8C01X6L
  Integumentary System, Breast Milk 8E0HX62
  Reproductive System, Male, Sperm 8E0VX63

Colocentesis *see* Drainage, Gastrointestinal System 0D9

Colofixation
  see Repair, Gastrointestinal System 0DQ
  see Reposition, Gastrointestinal System 0DS

Cololysis *see* Release, Gastrointestinal System 0DN

Colonic Z-Stent® *use* Intraluminal Device

Colonoscopy 0DJD8ZZ

Colopexy
  see Repair, Gastrointestinal System 0DQ
  see Reposition, Gastrointestinal System 0DS

Coloplication *see* Restriction, Gastrointestinal System 0DV

Coloproctectomy
  see Excision, Gastrointestinal System 0DB
  see Resection, Gastrointestinal System 0DT

Coloproctostomy
  see Bypass, Gastrointestinal System 0D1
  see Drainage, Gastrointestinal System 0D9

Colopuncture *see* Drainage, Gastrointestinal System 0D9

Colorrhaphy *see* Repair, Gastrointestinal System 0DQ

Colostomy
  see Bypass, Gastrointestinal System 0D1
  see Drainage, Gastrointestinal System 0D9

Colpectomy
  see Excision, Vagina 0UBG
  see Resection, Vagina 0UTG

Colpocentesis *see* Drainage, Vagina 0U9G

Colpopexy
  see Repair, Vagina 0UQG
  see Reposition, Vagina 0USG

Colpoplasty
  see Repair, Vagina 0UQG
  see Supplement, Vagina 0UUG

Colporrhaphy *see* Repair, Vagina 0UQG

Colposcopy 0UJH8ZZ

Columella *use* Nose

Common digital vein
  use Vein, Foot, Right
  use Vein, Foot, Left

Common facial vein
  use Vein, Face, Left
  use Vein, Face, Right Common fibular nerve *use* Nerve, Peroneal

Common hepatic artery *use* Artery, Hepatic

Common iliac (subaortic) lymph node *use*
  Lymphatic, Pelvis
Common interosseous artery
  use Artery, Ulnar, Left
  use Artery, Ulnar, Right
Common peroneal nerve *use* Nerve, Peroneal
Complete (SE) stent *use* Intraluminal Device
Compression
  see Restriction
  Abdominal Wall **2W13X**
  Arm
    Lower
      Left **2W1DX**
      Right **2W1CX**
    Upper
      Left **2W1BX**
      Right **2W1AX**
  Back **2W15X**
  Chest Wall **2W14X**
  Extremity
    Lower
      Left **2W1MX**
      Right **2W1LX**
    Upper
      Left **2W19X**
      Right **2W18X**
  Face **2W11X**
  Finger
    Left **2W1KX**
    Right **2W1JX**
  Foot
    Left **2W1TX**
    Right **2W1SX**
  Hand
    Left **2W1FX**
    Right **2W1EX**
  Head **2W10X**
  Inguinal Region
    Left **2W17X**
    Right **2W16X**
  Leg
    Lower
      Left **2W1RX**
      Right **2W1QX**
    Upper
      Left **2W1PX**
      Right **2W1NX**
  Neck **2W12X**
  Thumb
    Left **2W1HX**
    Right **2W1GX**
  Toe
    Left **2W1VX**
    Right **2W1UX**
Computer Assisted Procedure
  Extremity
    Lower
      No Qualifier **8E0YXBZ**
      With Computerized Tomography
        8E0YXBG
      With Fluoroscopy **8E0YXBF**
      With Magnetic Resonance Imaging
        8E0YXBH
    Upper
      No Qualifier **8E0XXBZ**
      With Computerized Tomography

Computer Assisted Procedure *(continued)*
        8E0XXBG
      With Fluoroscopy **8E0XXBF**
      With Magnetic Resonance Imaging
        8E0XXBH
  Head and Neck Region
    No Qualifier **8E09XBZ**
    With Computerized Tomography
      8E09XBG
    With Fluoroscopy **8E09XBF**
    With Magnetic Resonance Imaging
      8E09XBH
  Trunk Region
    No Qualifier **8E0WXBZ**
    With Computerized Tomography
      8E0WXBG
    With Fluoroscopy **8E0WXBF**
    With Magnetic Resonance Imaging
      8E0WXBH
Computerized Tomography (CT Scan)
  Abdomen **BW20**
    Chest and Pelvis **BW25**
  Abdomen and Chest **BW24**
  Abdomen and Pelvis **BW21**
  Airway, Trachea **BB2F**
  Ankle
    Left **BQ2H**
    Right **BQ2G**
  Aorta
    Abdominal **B420**
      Intravascular Optical Coherence
        B420Z2Z
    Thoracic **B320**
      Intravascular Optical Coherence
        B320Z2Z
    Left **BP2F**
    Right **BP2E**
  Artery
    Celiac **B421**
      Intravascular Optical Coherence
        B421Z2Z
    Common Carotid
      Bilateral **B325**
      Intravascular Optical Coherence
        B325Z2Z
    Coronary
      Bypass Graft
        Multiple **B223**
          Intravascular Optical Coherence
            B223Z2Z
        Multiple **B221**
          Intravascular Optical Coherence
            B221Z2Z
    Internal Carotid
      Bilateral **B328**
      Intravascular Optical Coherence
        B328Z2Z
    Intracranial **B32R**
    Intravascular Optical Coherence
      B32RZ2Z
    Lower Extremity
      Bilateral **B42H**
        Intravascular Optical Coherence
          B42HZ2Z
      Left **B42G**
        Intravascular Optical Coherence

Computerized Tomography (CT Scan)
(continued)
          B42GZ2Z
      Right **B42F**
        Intravascular Optical Coherence
          B42FZ2Z
    Pelvic **B42C**
      Intravascular Optical Coherence
        B42CZ2Z
    Pulmonary
      Left **B32T**
        Intravascular Optical Coherence
          B32TZ2Z
      Right **B32S**
        Intravascular Optical Coherence
          B32SZ2Z
    Renal
      Bilateral **B428**
        Intravascular Optical Coherence
          B428Z2Z
      Transplant **B42M**
        Intravascular Optical Coherence
          B42MZ2Z
    Superior Mesenteric **B424**
      Intravascular Optical Coherence
        B424Z2Z
    Vertebral
      Bilateral **B32G**
        Intravascular Optical Coherence
          B32GZ2Z
  Bladder **BT20**
  Bone
    Facial **BN25**
    Temporal **BN2F**
  Brain **B020**
  Calcaneus
    Left **BQ2K**
    Right **BQ2J**
  Cerebral Ventricle **B028**
  Chest, Abdomen and Pelvis **BW25**
  Chest and Abdomen **BW24**
  Cisterna **B027**
  Clavicle
    Left **BP25**
    Right **BP24**
  Coccyx **BR2F**
  Colon **BD24**
  Ear **B920**
  Elbow
    Left **BP2H**
    Right **BP2G**
  Extremity
    Lower
      Left **BQ2S**
      Right **BQ2R**
    Upper
      Bilateral **BP2V**
      Left **BP2U**
      Right **BP2T**
  Eye
    Bilateral **B827**
    Left **B826**
    Right **B825**
  Femur
    Left **BQ24**
    Right **BQ23**

Computerized Tomography (CT Scan)
(continued)
- Fibula
  - Left **BQ2C**
  - Right **BQ2B**
- Finger
  - Left **BP2S**
  - Right **BP2R**
- Foot
  - Left **BQ2M**
  - Right **BQ2L**
- Forearm
  - Left **BP2K**
  - Right **BP2J**
- Gland
  - Adrenal, Bilateral **BG22**
  - Parathyroid **BG23**
  - Parotid, Bilateral **B926**
  - Salivary, Bilateral **B92D**
  - Submandibular, Bilateral **B929**
  - Thyroid **BG24**
- Hand
  - Left **BP2P**
  - Right **BP2N**
- Hands and Wrists, Bilateral **BP2Q**
- Head **BW28**
- Head and Neck **BW29**
- Heart
  - Right and Left **B226**
  - Intravascular Optical Coherence **B226Z2Z**
- Hepatobiliary System, All **BF2C**
- Hip
  - Left **BQ21**
  - Right **BQ20**
- Humerus
  - Left **BP2B**
  - Right **BP2A**
- Intracranial Sinus **B522**
  - Intravascular Optical Coherence **B522Z2Z**
- Joint
  - Acromioclavicular, Bilateral **BP23**
  - Finger
    - Left **BP2DZZZ**
    - Right **BP2CZZZ**
  - Foot
    - Left **BQ2Y**
    - Right **BQ2X**
  - Hand
    - Left **BP2DZZZ**
    - Right **BP2CZZZ**
  - Sacroiliac **BR2D**
  - Sternoclavicular
    - Bilateral **BP22**
    - Left **BP21**
    - Right **BP20**
  - Temporomandibular, Bilateral **BN29**
  - Toe
    - Left **BQ2Y**
    - Right **BQ2X**
- Kidney
  - Bilateral **BT23**
  - Left **BT22**
  - Right **BT21**
  - Transplant **BT29**

Computerized Tomography (CT Scan)
(continued)
- Knee
  - Left **BQ28**
  - Right **BQ27**
- Larynx **B92J**
- Leg
  - Left **BQ2F**
  - Right **BQ2D**
- Liver **BF25**
- Liver and Spleen **BF26**
- Lung, Bilateral **BB24**
- Mandible **BN26**
- Nasopharynx **B92F**
- Neck **BW2F**
- Neck and Head **BW29**
- Orbit, Bilateral **BN23**
- Oropharynx **B92F**
- Pancreas **BF27**
- Patella
  - Left **BQ2W**
  - Right **BQ2V**
- Pelvic Region **BW2G**
- Pelvis **BR2C**
  - Chest and Abdomen **BW25**
- Pelvis and Abdomen **BW21**
- Pituitary Gland **B029**
- Prostate **BV23**
- Ribs
  - Left **BP2Y**
  - Right **BP2X**
- Sacrum **BR2F**
- Scapula
  - Left **BP27**
  - Right **BP26**
- Sella Turcica **B029**
- Shoulder
  - Left **BP29**
  - Right **BP28**
- Sinus
  - Intracranial **B522**
  - Intravascular Optical Coherence **B522Z2Z**
  - Paranasal **B922**
- Skull **BN20**
- Spinal Cord **B02B**
- Spine
  - Cervical **BR20**
  - Lumbar **BR29**
  - Thoracic **BR27**
- Spleen and Liver **BF26**
- Thorax **BP2W**
- Tibia
  - Left **BQ2C**
  - Right **BQ2B**
- Toe
  - Left **BQ2Q**
  - Right **BQ2P**
- Trachea **BB2F**
- Tracheobronchial Tree
  - Bilateral **BB29**
  - Left **BB28**
  - Right **BB27**
- Vein
  - Pelvic (Iliac)
    - Left **B52G**

Computerized Tomography (CT Scan)
(continued)
- Intravascular Optical Coherence **B52GZ2Z**
  - Right **B52F**
    - Intravascular Optical Coherence **B52FZ2Z**
  - Pelvic (Iliac) Bilateral **B52H**
    - Intravascular Optical Coherence **B52HZ2Z**
  - Portal **B52T**
    - Intravascular Optical Coherence **B52TZ2Z**
  - Pulmonary
    - Bilateral **B52S**
      - Intravascular Optical Coherence **B52SZ2Z**
    - Left **B52R**
      - Intravascular Optical Coherence **B52RZ2Z**
    - Right **B52Q**
      - Intravascular Optical Coherence **B52QZ2Z**
  - Renal
    - Bilateral **B52L**
      - Intravascular Optical Coherence **B52LZ2Z**
    - Left **B52K**
      - Intravascular Optical Coherence **B52KZ2Z**
    - Right **B52J**
      - Intravascular Optical Coherence **B52JZ2Z**
  - Splanchnic **B52T**
    - Intravascular Optical Coherence **B52TZ2Z**
  - Vena Cava
    - Inferior **B529**
      - Intravascular Optical Coherence **B529Z2Z**
    - Superior **B528**
      - Intravascular Optical Coherence **B528Z2Z**
- Ventricle, Cerebral **B028**
- Wrist
  - Left **BP2M**
  - Right **BP2L**

Concerto II CRT-D *use* Cardiac Resynchronization Defibrillator Pulse Generator in **0JH**

Condylectomy
see Excision, Head and Facial Bones **0NB**
see Excision, Upper Bones **0PB**
see Excision, Lower Bones **0QB**

Condyloid process
use Mandible, Left
use Mandible, Right

Condylotomy
see Division, Head and Facial Bones **0N8**
see Division, Lower Bones **0Q8**
see Division, Upper Bones **0P8**
see Drainage, Head and Facial Bones **0N9**
see Drainage, Lower Bones **0Q9**
see Drainage, Upper Bones **0P9**

Condylysis
   see Release, Head and Facial Bones **0NN**
   see Release, Upper Bones **0PN**
   see Release, Lower Bones **0QN**
Conization, cervix *see* Excision, Cervix
Conjunctivoplasty
   see Repair, Eye **08Q**
   see Replacement, Eye **08R**
CONSERVE® PLUS Total Resurfacing Hip
  System *use* Resurfacing Device in Lower
  Joints
Construction
   Auricle, ear *see* Replacement, Ear, Nose,
   Sinus **09R**
   Ileal conduit *see* Bypass, Urinary System
   0T1
Consulta CRT-D *use* Cardiac
  Resynchronization Defibrillator Pulse
  Generator in **0JH**
Consulta CRT-P *use* Cardiac
  Resynchronization Pacemaker Pulse
  Generator in **0JH**
Contact Radiation
   Abdomen **DWY37ZZ**
   Adrenal Gland **DGY27ZZ**
   Bile Ducts **DFY27ZZ**
   Bladder **DTY27ZZ**
   Bone, Other **DPYC7ZZ**
   Brain **D0Y07ZZ**
   Brain Stem **D0Y17ZZ**
   Breast
     Left **DMY07ZZ**
     Right **DMY17ZZ**
   Bronchus **DBY17ZZ**
   Cervix **DUY17ZZ**
   Chest **DWY27ZZ**
   Chest Wall **DBY77ZZ**
   Colon **DDY57ZZ**
   Diaphragm **DBY87ZZ**
   Duodenum **DDY27ZZ**
   Ear **D9Y07ZZ**
   Esophagus **DDY07ZZ**
   Eye **D8Y07ZZ**
   Femur **DPY97ZZ**
   Fibula **DPYB7ZZ**
   Gallbladder **DFY17ZZ**
   Gland
     Adrenal **DGY27ZZ**
     Parathyroid **DGY47ZZ**
     Pituitary **DGY07ZZ**
     Thyroid **DGY57ZZ**
   Glands, Salivary **D9Y67ZZ**
   Head and Neck **DWY17ZZ**
   Hemibody **DWY47ZZ**
   Humerus **DPY67ZZ**
   Hypopharynx **D9Y37ZZ**
   Ileum **DDY47ZZ**
   Jejunum **DDY37ZZ**
   Kidney **DTY07ZZ**
   Larynx **D9YB7ZZ**
   Liver **DFY07ZZ**
   Lung **DBY27ZZ**
   Mandible **DPY37ZZ**
   Maxilla **DPY27ZZ**
   Mediastinum **DBY67ZZ**
   Mouth **D9Y47ZZ**

Contact Radiation *(continued)*
   Nasopharynx **D9YD7ZZ**
   Neck and Head **DWY17ZZ**
   Nerve, Peripheral **D0Y77ZZ**
   Nose **D9Y17ZZ**
   Oropharynx **D9YF7ZZ**
   Ovary **DUY07ZZ**
   Palate
     Hard **D9Y87ZZ**
     Soft **D9Y97ZZ**
   Pancreas **DFY37ZZ**
   Parathyroid Gland **DGY47ZZ**
   Pelvic Bones **DPY87ZZ**
   Pelvic Region **DWY67ZZ**
   Pineal Body **DGY17ZZ**
   Pituitary Gland **DGY07ZZ**
   Pleura **DBY57ZZ**
   Prostate **DVY07ZZ**
   Radius **DPY77ZZ**
   Rectum **DDY77ZZ**
   Rib **DPY57ZZ**
   Sinuses **D9Y77ZZ**
   Skin
     Abdomen **DHY87ZZ**
     Arm **DHY47ZZ**
     Back **DHY77ZZ**
     Buttock **DHY97ZZ**
     Chest **DHY67ZZ**
     Face **DHY27ZZ**
     Leg **DHYB7ZZ**
     Neck **DHY37ZZ**
   Skull **DPY07ZZ**
   Spinal Cord **D0Y67ZZ**
   Sternum **DPY47ZZ**
   Stomach **DDY17ZZ**
   Testis **DVY17ZZ**
   Thyroid Gland **DGY57ZZ**
   Tibia **DPYB7ZZ**
   Tongue **D9Y57ZZ**
   Trachea **DBY07ZZ**
   Ulna **DPY77ZZ**
   Ureter **DTY17ZZ**
   Urethra **DTY37ZZ**
   Uterus **DUY27ZZ**
   Whole Body **DWY57ZZ**
CONTAK RENEWAL® 3 RF (HE) CRT-D
  use Cardiac Resynchronization Defibrillator
  Pulse Generator in **0JH**
Contegra Pulmonary Valved Conduit *use*
  Zooplastic Tissue in Heart and Great Vessels
Continuous Glucose Monitoring (CGM)
  device *use* Monitoring Device
Continuous Negative Airway Pressure
  24-96 Consecutive Hours, Ventilation
  5A09459
  Greater than 96 Consecutive Hours,
  Ventilation **5A09559**
  Less than 24 Consecutive Hours, Ventilation
  5A09359
Continuous Positive Airway Pressure
  24-96 Consecutive Hours, Ventilation
  5A09457
  Greater than 96 Consecutive Hours,
  Ventilation **5A09557**
  Less than 24 Consecutive Hours, Ventilation
  5A09357

Contraceptive Device
  Change device in, Uterus and Cervix
  0U2DXHZ
  Insertion of device in
   Cervix **0UHC**
   Subcutaneous Tissue and Fascia
    Abdomen **0JH8**
    Chest **0JH6**
    Lower Arm
     Left **0JHH**
     Right **0JHG**
    Lower Leg
     Left **0JHP**
     Right **0JHN**
    Upper Arm
     Left **0JHF**
     Right **0JHD**
    Upper Leg
     Left **0JHM**
     Right **0JHL**
   Uterus **0UH9**
  Removal of device from
   Subcutaneous Tissue and Fascia
    Lower Extremity **0JPW**
    Trunk **0JPT**
    Upper Extremity **0JPV**
   Uterus and Cervix **0UPD**
  Revision of device in
   Subcutaneous Tissue and Fascia
    Lower Extremity **0JWW**
    Trunk **0JWT**
    Upper Extremity **0JWV**
   Uterus and Cervix **0UWD**
Contractility Modulation Device
  Abdomen **0JH8**
  Chest **0JH6**
Control bleeding in
  Abdominal Wall **0W3F**
  Ankle Region
   Left **0Y3L**
   Right **0Y3K**
  Arm
   Lower
    Left **0X3F**
    Right **0X3D**
   Upper
    Left **0X39**
    Right **0X38**
  Axilla
   Left **0X35**
   Right **0X34**
  Back
   Lower **0W3L**
   Upper **0W3K**
  Buttock
   Left **0Y31**
   Right **0Y30**
  Cavity, Cranial **0W31**
  Chest Wall **0W38**
  Elbow Region
   Left **0X3C**
   Right **0X3B**
  Extremity
   Lower
    Left **0Y3B**
    Right **0Y39**

Control bleeding in *(continued)*
  Upper
    Left **0X37**
    Right **0X36**
  Face **0W32**
  Femoral Region
    Left **0Y38**
    Right **0Y37**
  Foot
    Left **0Y3N**
    Right **0Y3M**
  Gastrointestinal Tract **0W3P**
  Genitourinary Tract **0W3R**
  Hand
    Left **0X3K**
    Right **0X3J**
  Head **0W30**
  Inguinal Region
    Left **0Y36**
    Right **0Y35**
  Jaw
    Lower **0W35**
    Upper **0W34**
  Knee Region
    Left **0Y3G**
    Right **0Y3F**
  Leg
    Lower
      Left **0Y3J**
      Right **0Y3H**
    Upper
      Left **0Y3D**
      Right **0Y3C**
  Mediastinum **0W3C**
  Neck **0W36**
  Oral Cavity and Throat **0W33**
  Pelvic Cavity **0W3J**
  Pericardial Cavity **0W3D**
  Perineum
    Female **0W3N**
    Male **0W3M**
  Peritoneal Cavity **0W3G**
  Pleural Cavity
    Left **0W3B**
    Right **0W39**
  Respiratory Tract **0W3Q**
  Retroperitoneum **0W3H**
  Shoulder Region
    Left **0X33**
    Right **0X32**
  Wrist Region
    Left **0X3H**
    Right **0X3G**
Conus arteriosus *use* Ventricle, Right
Conus medullaris *use* Spinal Cord, Lumbar
Conversion
  Cardiac rhythm **5A2204Z**
  Gastrostomy to jejunostomy feeding device
  see Insertion of device in, Jejunum **0DHA**
Cook Biodesign(R) Fistula Plug(s) *use*
  Nonautologous Tissue Substitute
Cook Biodesign(R) Hernia Graft(s) *use*
  Nonautologous Tissue Substitute
Cook Biodesign(R) Layered Graft(s) *use*
  Nonautologous Tissue Substitute

Cook Zenapro(tm) Layered Graft(s) *use*
  Nonautologous Tissue Substitute
Cook Zenith AAA Endovascular Graft
  use Intraluminal Device, Branched or
    Fenestrated, One or Two Arteries in **04V**
  use Intraluminal Device, Branched or
    Fenestrated, Three or More Arteries in
    04V
  use Intraluminal Device
Coracoacromial ligament
  use Bursa and Ligament, Shoulder, Left
  use Bursa and Ligament, Shoulder, Right
Coracobrachialis muscle
  use Muscle, Upper Arm, Left
  use Muscle, Upper Arm, Right
Coracoclavicular ligament
  use Bursa and Ligament, Shoulder, Left
  use Bursa and Ligament, Shoulder, Right
Coracohumeral ligament
  use Bursa and Ligament, Shoulder, Left
  use Bursa and Ligament, Shoulder, Right
Coracoid process
  use Scapula, Right
  use Scapula, Left
Cordotomy *see* Division, Central Nervous
  System **008**
Core needle biopsy *see* Excision with qualifier
  Diagnostic
CoreValve transcatheter aortic valve *use*
  Zooplastic Tissue in Heart and Great Vessels
Cormet Hip Resurfacing System *use*
  Resurfacing Device in Lower Joints
Corniculate cartilage *use* Larynx
CoRoent® XL *use* Interbody Fusion Device in
  Lower Joints
Coronary arteriography
  see Plain Radiography, Heart **B20**
  see Fluoroscopy, Heart **B21**
Corox (OTW) Bipolar Lead
  use Cardiac Lead, Pacemaker in **02H**
  use Cardiac Lead, Defibrillator in **02H**
Corpus callosum *use* Brain
Corpus cavernosum *use* Penis
Corpus spongiosum *use* Penis
Corpus striatum *use* Basal Ganglia
Corrugator supercilii muscle *use* Muscle,
  Facial
Cortical strip neurostimulator lead *use*
  Neurostimulator Lead in Central Nervous
  System
Costatectomy
  see Excision, Upper Bones **0PB**
  see Resection, Upper Bones **0PT**
Costectomy
  see Excision, Upper Bones **0PB**
  see Resection, Upper Bones **0PT**
Costocervical trunk
  use Artery, Subclavian, Left
  use Artery, Subclavian, Right
Costochondrectomy
  see Excision, Upper Bones **0PB**
  see Resection, Upper Bones **0PT**
Costoclavicular ligament
  use Bursa and Ligament, Shoulder, Left
  use Bursa and Ligament, Shoulder, Right

Costosternoplasty
  see Repair, Upper Bones **0PQ**
  see Replacement, Upper Bones **0PR**
  see Supplement, Upper Bones **0PU**
Costotomy
  see Division, Upper Bones **0P8**
  see Drainage, Upper Bones **0P9**
Costotransverse joint
  use Joint, Thoracic Vertebral
  use Joint, Thoracic Vertebral, 2 to 7
  use Joint, Thoracic Vertebral, 8 or more
Costotransverse ligament
  use Bursa and Ligament, Thorax, Right
  use Bursa and Ligament, Thorax, Left
Costovertebral joint
  use Joint, Thoracic Vertebral, 8 or more
  use Joint, Thoracic Vertebral, 2 to 7
  use Joint, Thoracic Vertebral
Costoxiphoid ligament
  use Bursa and Ligament, Thorax, Right
  use Bursa and Ligament, Thorax, Left
Counseling
  Family, for substance abuse, Other Family
  Counseling **HZ63ZZZ**
  Group
    12-Step **HZ43ZZZ**
    Behavioral **HZ41ZZZ**
    Cognitive **HZ40ZZZ**
    Cognitive-Behavioral **HZ42ZZZ**
    Confrontational **HZ48ZZZ**
    Continuing Care **HZ49ZZZ**
    Infectious Disease
      Post-Test **HZ4CZZZ**
      Pre-Test **HZ4CZZZ**
    Interpersonal **HZ44ZZZ**
    Motivational Enhancement **HZ47ZZZ**
    Psychoeducation **HZ46ZZZ**
    Spiritual **HZ4BZZZ**
    Vocational **HZ45ZZZ**
  Individual
    12-Step **HZ33ZZZ**
    Behavioral **HZ31ZZZ**
    Cognitive **HZ30ZZZ**
    Cognitive-Behavioral **HZ32ZZZ**
    Confrontational **HZ38ZZZ**
    Continuing Care **HZ39ZZZ**
    Infectious Disease
      Post-Test **HZ3CZZZ**
      Pre-Test **HZ3CZZZ**
    Interpersonal **HZ34ZZZ**
    Motivational Enhancement **HZ37ZZZ**
    Psychoeducation **HZ36ZZZ**
    Spiritual **HZ3BZZZ**
    Vocational **HZ35ZZZ**
  Mental Health Services
    Educational **GZ60ZZZ**
    Other Counseling **GZ63ZZZ**
    Vocational **GZ61ZZZ**
Countershock, cardiac 5A2204Z
Cowper's (bulbourethral) gland *use* Urethra
CPAP (continuous positive airway pressure)
  see Assistance, Respiratory **5A09**
Craniectomy
  see Excision, Head and Facial Bones **0NB**
  see Resection, Head and Facial Bones **0NT**

Cranioplasty
- *see* Repair, Head and Facial Bones **0NQ**
- *see* Replacement, Head and Facial Bones **0NR**
- *see* Supplement, Head and Facial Bones **0NU**

Craniotomy
- *see* Drainage, Central Nervous System **009**
- *see* Division, Head and Facial Bones **0N8**
- *see* Drainage, Head and Facial Bones **0N9**

Creation
- Perineum
  - Female **0W4N0**
  - Male **0W4M0**
- Valve
  - Aortic **024F0**
  - Mitral **024G0**
  - Tricuspid **024J0**

Cremaster muscle *use* Muscle, Perineum

Cribriform plate
- *use* Bone, Ethmoid, Left
- *use* Bone, Ethmoid, Right

Cricoid cartilage *use* Trachea

Cricoidectomy *see* Excision, Larynx **0CBS**

Cricothyroid artery
- *use* Artery, Thyroid, Left
- *use* Artery, Thyroid, Right

Cricothyroid muscle
- *use* Muscle, Neck, Right
- *use* Muscle, Neck, Left

Crisis Intervention GZ2ZZZZ

Crural fascia
- *use* Subcutaneous Tissue and Fascia, Upper Leg, Right
- *use* Subcutaneous Tissue and Fascia, Upper Leg, Left

Crushing, nerve
- Cranial *see* Destruction, Central Nervous System **005**
- Peripheral *see* Destruction, Peripheral Nervous System **015**

Cryoablation *see* Destruction

Cryotherapy *see* Destruction

Cryptorchidectomy
- *see* Excision, Male Reproductive System **0VB**
- *see* Resection, Male Reproductive System **0VT**

Cryptorchiectomy
- *see* Excision, Male Reproductive System **0VB**
- *see* Resection, Male Reproductive System **0VT**

Cryptotomy
- *see* Division, Gastrointestinal System **0D8**
- *see* Drainage, Gastrointestinal System **0D9**

CT scan *see* Computerized Tomography (CT Scan)

CT sialogram *see* Computerized Tomography (CT Scan), Ear, Nose, Mouth and Throat **B92**

Cubital lymph node
- *use* Lymphatic, Upper Extremity, Left
- *use* Lymphatic, Upper Extremity, Right

Cubital nerve *use* Nerve, Ulnar

Cuboid bone
- *use* Tarsal, Left
- *use* Tarsal, Right

Cuboideonavicular joint
- *use* Joint, Tarsal, Right
- *use* Joint, Tarsal, Left

Culdocentesis *see* Drainage, Cul-de-sac **0U9F**

Culdoplasty
- *see* Repair, Cul-de-sac **0UQF**
- *see* Supplement, Cul-de-sac **0UUF**

Culdoscopy 0UJH8ZZ

Culdotomy *see* Drainage, Cul-de-sac **0U9F**

Culmen *use* Cerebellum

Cultured epidermal cell autograft *use* Autologous Tissue Substitute

Cuneiform cartilage *use* Larynx

Cuneonavicular joint
- *use* Joint, Tarsal, Left
- *use* Joint, Tarsal, Right

Cuneonavicular ligament
- *use* Bursa and Ligament, Foot, Left
- *use* Bursa and Ligament, Foot, Right

Curettage
- *see* Excision
- *see* Extraction

Cutaneous (transverse) cervical nerve *use* Nerve, Cervical Plexus

CVP (central venous pressure) *see* Measurement, Venous **4A04**

Cyclodiathermy *see* Destruction, Eye **085**

Cyclophotocoagulation *see* Destruction, Eye **085**

CYPHER® Stent *use* Intraluminal Device, Drug-eluting in Heart and Great Vessels

Cystectomy
- *see* Excision, Bladder **0TBB**
- *see* Resection, Bladder **0TTB**

Cystocele repair *see* Repair, Subcutaneous Tissue and Fascia, Pelvic Region **0JQC**

Cystography
- *see* Plain Radiography, Urinary System **BT0**
- *see* Fluoroscopy, Urinary System **BT1**

Cystolithotomy *see* Extirpation, Bladder **0TCB**

Cystopexy
- *see* Repair, Bladder **0TQB**
- *see* Reposition, Bladder **0TSB**

Cystoplasty
- *see* Repair, Bladder **0TQB**
- *see* Replacement, Bladder **0TRB**
- *see* Supplement, Bladder **0TUB**

Cystorrhaphy *see* Repair, Bladder **0TQB**

Cystoscopy 0TJB8ZZ

Cystostomy *see* Bypass, Bladder **0T1B**

Cystostomy tube *use* Drainage Device

Cystotomy *see* Drainage, Bladder **0T9B**

Cystourethrography
- *see* Plain Radiography, Urinary System **BT0**
- *see* Fluoroscopy, Urinary System **BT1**

Cystourethroplasty
- *see* Repair, Urinary System **0TQ**
- *see* Replacement, Urinary System **0TR**
- *see* Supplement, Urinary System **0TU**

D

DBS lead *use* Neurostimulator Lead in Central Nervous System

DeBakey Left Ventricular Assist Device *use* Implantable Heart Assist System in Heart and Great Vessels

Debridement
- Excisional *see* Excision
- Non-excisional *see* Extraction

Decompression, Circulatory 6A15

Decortication, lung *see* Extraction, Respiratory System **0BD**

Deep brain neurostimulator lead *use* Neurostimulator Lead in Central Nervous System

Deep cervical fascia *use* Subcutaneous Tissue and Fascia, Neck, Anterior

Deep cervical vein
- *use* Vein, Vertebral, Left
- *use* Vein, Vertebral, Right

Deep circumflex iliac artery
- *use* Artery, External Iliac, Left
- *use* Artery, External Iliac, Right

Deep facial vein
- *use* Vein, Face, Left
- *use* Vein, Face, Right

Deep femoral (profunda femoris) vein
- *use* Vein, Femoral, Left
- *use* Vein, Femoral, Right

Deep femoral artery
- *use* Artery, Femoral, Right
- *use* Artery, Femoral, Left

Deep Inferior Epigastric Artery Perforator Flap
- Bilateral **0HRV077**
- Left **0HRU077**
- Right **0HRT077**

Deep palmar arch
- *use* Artery, Hand, Left
- *use* Artery, Hand, Right

Deep transverse perineal muscle *use* Muscle, Perineum

Deferential artery
- *use* Artery, Internal Iliac, Right
- *use* Artery, Internal Iliac, Left

Defibrillator Generator
- Abdomen **0JH8**
- Chest **0JH6**

Defibrotide Sodium Anticoagulant XW0

Defitelio *use* Defibrotide Sodium Anticoagulant

Delivery
- Cesarean *see* Extraction, Products of Conception **10D0**
- Forceps *see* Extraction, Products of Conception **10D0**
- Manually assisted **10E0XZZ**
- Products of Conception **10E0XZZ**
- Vacuum assisted *see* Extraction, Products of Conception **10D0**

Delta frame external fixator
- *use* External Fixation Device, Hybrid in **0PH**
- *use* External Fixation Device, Hybrid in **0PS**
- *use* External Fixation Device, Hybrid in **0QH**
- *use* External Fixation Device, Hybrid in **0QS**

Delta III Reverse shoulder prosthesis *use*
Synthetic Substitute, Reverse Ball and
Socket in **0RR**

Deltoid fascia
use Subcutaneous Tissue and Fascia, Upper
Arm, Right
use Subcutaneous Tissue and Fascia, Upper
Arm, Left

Deltoid ligament
use Bursa and Ligament, Ankle, Left
use Bursa and Ligament, Ankle, Right

Deltoid muscle
use Muscle, Shoulder, Left
use Muscle, Shoulder, Right

Deltopectoral (infraclavicular) lymph node
use Lymphatic, Upper Extremity, Right
use Lymphatic, Upper Extremity, Left

Denervation
Cranial nerve *see* Destruction, Central
Nervous System **005**
Peripheral nerve *see* Destruction, Peripheral
Nervous System **015**

Densitometry
Plain Radiography
Femur
Left **BQ04ZZ1**
Right **BQ03ZZ1**
Hip
Left **BQ01ZZ1**
Right **BQ00ZZ1**
Spine
Cervical **BR00ZZ1**
Lumbar **BR09ZZ1**
Thoracic **BR07ZZ1**
Whole **BR0GZZ1**
Ultrasonography
Elbow
Left **BP4HZZ1**
Right **BP4GZZ1**
Hand
Left **BP4PZZ1**
Right **BP4NZZ1**
Shoulder
Left **BP49ZZ1**
Right **BP48ZZ1**
Wrist
Left **BP4MZZ1**
Right **BP4LZZ1**

Denticulate (dentate) ligament *use* Spinal
Meninges

Depressor anguli oris muscle *use* Muscle,
Facial

Depressor labii inferioris muscle *use* Muscle,
Facial

Depressor septi nasi muscle *use* Muscle,
Facial

Depressor supercilii muscle *use* Muscle,
Facial

Dermabrasion *see* Extraction, Skin and Breast
0HD

Dermis *use* Skin

Descending genicular artery
use Artery, Femoral, Right
use Artery, Femoral, Left

Destruction
Acetabulum
Left **0Q55**

Destruction *(continued)*
Right **0Q54**
Adenoids **0C5Q**
Ampulla of Vater **0F5C**
Anal Sphincter **0D5R**
Anterior Chamber
Left **08533ZZ**
Right **08523ZZ**
Anus **0D5Q**
Aorta
Abdominal **0450**
Thoracic
Ascending/Arch **025X**
Descending **025W**
Aortic Body **0G5D**
Appendix **0D5J**
Artery
Anterior Tibial
Left **045Q**
Right **045P**
Axillary
Left **0356**
Right **0355**
Brachial
Left **0358**
Right **0357**
Celiac **0451**
Colic
Left **0457**
Middle **0458**
Right **0456**
Common Carotid
Left **035J**
Right **035H**
Common Iliac
Left **045D**
Right **045C**
External Carotid
Left **035N**
Right **035M**
External Iliac
Left **045J**
Right **045H**
Face **035R**
Femoral
Left **045L**
Right **045K**
Foot
Left **045W**
Right **045V**
Gastric **0452**
Hand
Left **035F**
Right **035D**
Hepatic **0453**
Inferior Mesenteric **045B**
Innominate **0352**
Internal Carotid
Left **035L**
Right **035K**
Internal Iliac
Left **045F**
Right **045E**
Internal Mammary
Left **0351**
Right **0350**

Destruction *(continued)*
Intracranial **035G**
Lower **045Y**
Peroneal
Left **045U**
Right **045T**
Popliteal
Left **045N**
Right **045M**
Posterior Tibial
Left **045S**
Right **045R**
Pulmonary
Left **025R**
Right **025Q**
Pulmonary Trunk **025P**
Radial
Left **035C**
Right **035B**
Renal
Left **045A**
Right **0459**
Splenic **0454**
Subclavian
Left **0354**
Right **0353**
Superior Mesenteric **0455**
Temporal
Left **035T**
Right **035S**
Thyroid
Left **035V**
Right **035U**
Ulnar
Left **035A**
Right **0359**
Upper **035Y**
Vertebral
Left **035Q**
Right **035P**
Atrium
Left **0257**
Right **0256**
Auditory Ossicle
Left **095A0ZZ**
Right **09590ZZ**
Basal Ganglia **0058**
Bladder **0T5B**
Bladder Neck **0T5C**
Bone
Ethmoid
Left **0N5G**
Right **0N5F**
Frontal
Left **0N52**
Right **0N51**
Hyoid **0N5X**
Lacrimal
Left **0N5J**
Right **0N5H**
Nasal **0N5B**
Occipital
Left **0N58**
Right **0N57**
Palatine
Left **0N5L**

Destruction *(continued)*
Right 0N5K
Parietal
Left 0N54
Right 0N53
Pelvic
Left 0Q53
Right 0Q52
Sphenoid
Left 0N5D
Right 0N5C
Temporal
Left 0N56
Right 0N55
Zygomatic
Left 0N5N
Right 0N5M
Brain 0050
Breast
Bilateral 0H5V
Left 0H5U
Right 0H5T
Bronchus
Lingula 0B59
Lower Lobe
Left 0B5B
Right 0B56
Main
Left 0B57
Right 0B53
Middle Lobe, Right 0B55
Upper Lobe
Left 0B58
Right 0B54
Buccal Mucosa 0C54
Bursa and Ligament
Abdomen
Left 0M5J
Right 0M5H
Ankle
Left 0M5R
Right 0M5Q
Elbow
Left 0M54
Right 0M53
Foot
Left 0M5T
Right 0M5S
Hand
Left 0M58
Right 0M57
Head and Neck 0M50
Hip
Left 0M5M
Right 0M5L
Knee
Left 0M5P
Right 0M5N
Lower Extremity
Left 0M5W
Right 0M5V
Perineum 0M5K
Shoulder
Left 0M52
Right 0M51
Thorax

Destruction *(continued)*
Left 0M5G
Right 0M5F
Trunk
Left 0M5D
Right 0M5C
Upper Extremity
Left 0M5B
Right 0M59
Wrist
Left 0M56
Right 0M55
Carina 0B52
Carotid Bodies, Bilateral 0G58
Carotid Body
Left 0G56
Right 0G57
Carpal
Left 0P5N
Right 0P5M
Cecum 0D5H
Cerebellum 005C
Cerebral Hemisphere 0057
Cerebral Meninges 0051
Cerebral Ventricle 0056
Cervix 0U5C
Chordae Tendineae 0259
Choroid
Left 085B
Right 085A
Cisterna Chyli 075L
Clavicle
Left 0P5B
Right 0P59
Clitoris 0U5J
Coccygeal Glomus 0G5B
Coccyx 0Q5S
Colon
Ascending 0D5K
Descending 0D5M
Sigmoid 0D5N
Transverse 0D5L
Conduction Mechanism 0258
Conjunctiva
Left 085TXZZ
Right 085SXZZ
Cord
Bilateral 0V5H
Left 0V5G
Right 0V5F
Cornea
Left 0859XZZ
Right 0858XZZ
Cul-de-sac 0U5F
Diaphragm
Left 0B5S
Right 0B5R
Disc
Cervical Vertebral 0R53
Cervicothoracic Vertebral 0R55
Lumbar Vertebral 0S52
Lumbosacral 0S54
Thoracic Vertebral 0R59
Thoracolumbar Vertebral 0R5B
Duct
Common Bile 0F59

Destruction *(continued)*
Cystic 0F58
Hepatic
Left 0F56
Right 0F55
Lacrimal
Left 085Y
Right 085X
Pancreatic 0F5D
Accessory 0F5F
Parotid
Left 0C5C
Right 0C5B
Duodenum 0D59
Dura Mater 0052
Ear
External
Left 0951
Right 0950
External Auditory Canal
Left 0954
Right 0953
Inner
Left 095E0ZZ
Right 095D0ZZ
Middle
Left 09560ZZ
Right 09550ZZ
Endometrium 0U5B
Epididymis
Bilateral 0V5L
Left 0V5K
Right 0V5J
Epiglottis 0C5R
Esophagogastric Junction 0D54
Esophagus 0D55
Lower 0D53
Middle 0D52
Upper 0D51
Eustachian Tube
Left 095G
Right 095F
Eye
Left 0851XZZ
Right 0850XZZ
Eyelid
Lower
Left 085R
Right 085Q
Upper
Left 085P
Right 085N
Fallopian Tube
Left 0U56
Right 0U55
Fallopian Tubes, Bilateral 0U57
Femoral Shaft
Left 0Q59
Right 0Q58
Femur
Lower
Left 0Q5C
Right 0Q5B
Upper
Left 0Q57
Right 0Q56

Destruction *(continued)*
Fibula
  Left **0Q5K**
  Right **0Q5J**
Finger Nail **0H5QXZZ**
Gallbladder **0F54**
Gingiva
  Lower **0C56**
  Upper **0C55**
Gland
  Adrenal
    Bilateral **0G54**
    Left **0G52**
    Right **0G53**
  Lacrimal
    Left **085W**
    Right **085V**
  Minor Salivary **0C5J**
  Parotid
    Left **0C59**
    Right **0C58**
  Pituitary **0G50**
  Sublingual
    Left **0C5F**
    Right **0C5D**
  Submaxillary
    Left **0C5H**
    Right **0C5G**
  Vestibular **0U5L**
Glenoid Cavity
  Left **0P58**
  Right **0P57**
Glomus Jugulare **0G5C**
Humeral Head
  Left **0P5D**
  Right **0P5C**
Humeral Shaft
  Left **0P5G**
  Right **0P5F**
Hymen **0U5K**
Hypothalamus **005A**
Ileocecal Valve **0D5C**
Ileum **0D5B**
Intestine
  Large **0D5E**
    Left **0D5G**
    Right **0D5F**
  Small **0D58**
Iris
  Left **085D3ZZ**
  Right **085C3ZZ**
Jejunum **0D5A**
Joint
  Acromioclavicular
    Left **0R5H**
    Right **0R5G**
  Ankle
    Left **0S5G**
    Right **0S5F**
  Carpal
    Left **0R5R**
    Right **0R5Q**
  Cervical Vertebral **0R51**
  Cervicothoracic Vertebral **0R54**
  Coccygeal **0S56**
  Elbow

Destruction *(continued)*
    Left **0R5M**
    Right **0R5L**
  Finger Phalangeal
    Left **0R5X**
    Right **0R5W**
  Hip
    Left **0S5B**
    Right **0S59**
  Knee
    Left **0S5D**
    Right **0S5C**
  Lumbar Vertebral **0S50**
  Lumbosacral **0S53**
  Metacarpocarpal
    Left **0R5T**
    Right **0R5S**
  Metacarpophalangeal
    Left **0R5V**
    Right **0R5U**
  Metatarsal-Phalangeal
    Left **0S5N**
    Right **0S5M**
  Metatarsal-Tarsal
    Left **0S5L**
    Right **0S5K**
  Occipital-cervical **0R50**
  Sacrococcygeal **0S55**
  Sacroiliac
    Left **0S58**
    Right **0S57**
  Shoulder
    Left **0R5K**
    Right **0R5J**
  Sternoclavicular
    Left **0R5F**
    Right **0R5E**
  Tarsal
    Left **0S5J**
    Right **0S5H**
  Temporomandibular
    Left **0R5D**
    Right **0R5C**
  Thoracic Vertebral **0R56**
  Thoracolumbar Vertebral **0R5A**
  Toe Phalangeal
    Left **0S5Q**
    Right **0S5P**
  Wrist
    Left **0R5P**
    Right **0R5N**
Kidney
  Left **0T51**
  Right **0T50**
Kidney Pelvis
  Left **0T54**
  Right **0T53**
Larynx **0C5S**
Lens
  Left **085K3ZZ**
  Right **085J3ZZ**
Lip
  Lower **0C51**
  Upper **0C50**
Liver **0F50**
  Left Lobe **0F52**

Destruction *(continued)*
  Right Lobe **0F51**
Lung
  Bilateral **0B5M**
  Left **0B5L**
  Lower Lobe
    Left **0B5J**
    Right **0B5F**
  Middle Lobe, Right **0B5D**
  Right **0B5K**
  Upper Lobe
    Left **0B5G**
    Right **0B5C**
Lung Lingula **0B5H**
Lymphatic
  Aortic **075D**
  Axillary
    Left **0756**
    Right **0755**
  Head **0750**
  Inguinal
    Left **075J**
    Right **075H**
  Internal Mammary
    Left **0759**
    Right **0758**
  Lower Extremity
    Left **075G**
    Right **075F**
  Mesenteric **075B**
  Neck
    Left **0752**
    Right **0751**
  Pelvis **075C**
  Thoracic Duct **075K**
  Thorax **0757**
  Upper Extremity
    Left **0754**
    Right **0753**
Mandible
  Left **0N5V**
  Right **0N5T**
Maxilla
  Left **0N5S**
  Right **0N5R**
Medulla Oblongata **005D**
Mesentery **0D5V**
Metacarpal
  Left **0P5Q**
  Right **0P5P**
Metatarsal
  Left **0Q5P**
  Right **0Q5N**
Muscle
  Abdomen
    Left **0K5L**
    Right **0K5K**
  Extraocular
    Left **085M**
    Right **085L**
  Facial **0K51**
  Foot
    Left **0K5W**
    Right **0K5V**
  Hand
    Left **0K5D**

Destruction *(continued)*
    Right **0K5C**
    Head **0K50**
    Hip
        Left **0K5P**
        Right **0K5N**
    Lower Arm and Wrist
        Left **0K5B**
        Right **0K59**
    Lower Leg
        Left **0K5T**
        Right **0K5S**
    Neck
        Left **0K53**
        Right **0K52**
    Papillary **025D**
    Perineum **0K5M**
    Shoulder
        Left **0K56**
        Right **0K55**
    Thorax
        Left **0K5J**
        Right **0K5H**
    Tongue, Palate, Pharynx **0K54**
    Trunk
        Left **0K5G**
        Right **0K5F**
    Upper Arm
        Left **0K58**
        Right **0K57**
    Upper Leg
        Left **0K5R**
        Right **0K5Q**
  Nasopharynx **095N**
  Nerve
    Abdominal Sympathetic **015M**
    Abducens **005L**
    Accessory **005R**
    Acoustic **005N**
    Brachial Plexus **0153**
    Cervical **0151**
    Cervical Plexus **0150**
    Facial **005M**
    Femoral **015D**
    Glossopharyngeal **005P**
    Head and Neck Sympathetic **015K**
    Hypoglossal **005S**
    Lumbar **015B**
    Lumbar Plexus **0159**
    Lumbar Sympathetic **015N**
    Lumbosacral Plexus **015A**
    Median **0155**
    Oculomotor **005H**
    Olfactory **005F**
    Optic **005G**
    Peroneal **015H**
    Phrenic **0152**
    Pudendal **015C**
    Radial **0156**
    Sacral **015R**
    Sacral Plexus **015Q**
    Sacral Sympathetic **015P**
    Sciatic **015F**
    Thoracic **0158**
    Thoracic Sympathetic **015L**
    Tibial **015G**

Destruction *(continued)*
    Trigeminal **005K**
    Trochlear **005J**
    Ulnar **0154**
    Vagus **005Q**
  Nipple
    Left **0H5X**
    Right **0H5W**
  Nose **095K**
  Omentum
    Greater **0D5S**
    Lesser **0D5T**
  Orbit
    Left **0N5Q**
    Right **0N5P**
  Ovary
    Bilateral **0U52**
    Left **0U51**
    Right **0U50**
  Palate
    Hard **0C52**
    Soft **0C53**
  Pancreas **0F5G**
  Para-aortic Body **0G59**
  Paraganglion Extremity **0G5F**
  Parathyroid Gland **0G5R**
    Inferior
        Left **0G5P**
        Right **0G5N**
    Multiple **0G5Q**
    Superior
        Left **0G5M**
        Right **0G5L**
  Patella
    Left **0Q5F**
    Right **0Q5D**
  Penis **0V5S**
  Pericardium **025N**
  Peritoneum **0D5W**
  Phalanx
    Finger
        Left **0P5V**
        Right **0P5T**
    Thumb
        Left **0P5S**
        Right **0P5R**
    Toe
        Left **0Q5R**
        Right **0Q5Q**
  Pharynx **0C5M**
  Pineal Body **0G51**
  Pleura
    Left **0B5P**
    Right **0B5N**
  Pons **005B**
  Prepuce **0V5T**
  Prostate **0V50**
  Radius
    Left **0P5J**
    Right **0P5H**
  Rectum **0D5P**
  Retina
    Left **085F3ZZ**
    Right **085E3ZZ**
  Retinal Vessel
    Left **085H3ZZ**

Destruction *(continued)*
    Right **085G3ZZ**
  Rib
    Left **0P52**
    Right **0P51**
  Sacrum **0Q51**
  Scapula
    Left **0P56**
    Right **0P55**
  Sclera
    Left **0857XZZ**
    Right **0856XZZ**
  Scrotum **0V55**
  Septum
    Atrial **0255**
    Nasal **095M**
    Ventricular **025M**
  Sinus
    Accessory **095P**
    Ethmoid
        Left **095V**
        Right **095U**
    Frontal
        Left **095T**
        Right **095S**
    Mastoid
        Left **095C**
        Right **095B**
    Maxillary
        Left **095R**
        Right **095Q**
    Sphenoid
        Left **095X**
        Right **095W**
  Skin
    Abdomen **0H57XZ**
    Back **0H56XZ**
    Buttock **0H58XZ**
    Chest **0H55XZ**
    Ear
        Left **0H53XZ**
        Right **0H52XZ**
    Face **0H51XZ**
    Foot
        Left **0H5NXZ**
        Right **0H5MXZ**
    Genitalia **0H5AXZ**
    Hand
        Left **0H5GXZ**
        Right **0H5FXZ**
    Lower Arm
        Left **0H5EXZ**
        Right **0H5DXZ**
    Lower Leg
        Left **0H5LXZ**
        Right **0H5KXZ**
    Neck **0H54XZ**
    Perineum **0H59XZ**
    Scalp **0H50XZ**
    Upper Arm
        Left **0H5CXZ**
        Right **0H5BXZ**
    Upper Leg
        Left **0H5JXZ**
        Right **0H5HXZ**
  Skull **0N50**

Destruction *(continued)*

Spinal Cord
  Cervical **005W**
  Lumbar **005Y**
  Thoracic **005X**
Spinal Meninges **005T**
Spleen **075P**
Sternum **0P50**
Stomach **0D56**
  Pylorus **0D57**
Subcutaneous Tissue and Fascia
  Abdomen **0J58**
  Back **0J57**
  Buttock **0J59**
  Chest **0J56**
  Face **0J51**
  Foot
    Left **0J5R**
    Right **0J5Q**
  Hand
    Left **0J5K**
    Right **0J5J**
  Lower Arm
    Left **0J5H**
    Right **0J5G**
  Lower Leg
    Left **0J5P**
    Right **0J5N**
  Neck
    Anterior **0J54**
    Posterior **0J55**
  Pelvic Region **0J5C**
  Perineum **0J5B**
  Scalp **0J50**
  Upper Arm
    Left **0J5F**
    Right **0J5D**
  Upper Leg
    Left **0J5M**
    Right **0J5L**
Tarsal
  Left **0Q5M**
  Right **0Q5L**
Tendon
  Abdomen
    Left **0L5G**
    Right **0L5F**
  Ankle
    Left **0L5T**
    Right **0L5S**
  Foot
    Left **0L5W**
    Right **0L5V**
  Hand
    Left **0L58**
    Right **0L57**
  Head and Neck **0L50**
  Hip
    Left **0L5K**
    Right **0L5J**
  Knee
    Left **0L5R**
    Right **0L5Q**
  Lower Arm and Wrist
    Left **0L56**
    Right **0L55**

Destruction *(continued)*

Lower Leg
  Left **0L5P**
  Right **0L5N**
Perineum **0L5H**
Shoulder
  Left **0L52**
  Right **0L51**
Thorax
  Left **0L5D**
  Right **0L5C**
Trunk
  Left **0L5B**
  Right **0L59**
Upper Arm
  Left **0L54**
  Right **0L53**
Upper Leg
  Left **0L5M**
  Right **0L5L**
Testis
  Bilateral **0V5C**
  Left **0V5B**
  Right **0V59**
Thalamus **0059**
Thymus **075M**
Thyroid Gland **0G5K**
  Left Lobe **0G5G**
  Right Lobe **0G5H**
Tibia
  Left **0Q5H**
  Right **0Q5G**
Toe Nail **0H5RXZZ**
Tongue **0C57**
Tonsils **0C5P**
Tooth
  Lower **0C5X**
  Upper **0C5W**
Trachea **0B51**
Tunica Vaginalis
  Left **0V57**
  Right **0V56**
Turbinate, Nasal **095L**
Tympanic Membrane
  Left **0958**
  Right **0957**
Ulna
  Left **0P5L**
  Right **0P5K**
Ureter
  Left **0T57**
  Right **0T56**
Urethra **0T5D**
Uterine Supporting Structure **0U54**
Uterus **0U59**
Uvula **0C5N**
Vagina **0U5G**
Valve
  Aortic **025F**
  Mitral **025G**
  Pulmonary **025H**
  Tricuspid **025J**
Vas Deferens
  Bilateral **0V5Q**
  Left **0V5P**
  Right **0V5N**

Destruction *(continued)*

Vein
  Axillary
    Left **0558**
    Right **0557**
  Azygos **0550**
  Basilic
    Left **055C**
    Right **055B**
  Brachial
    Left **055A**
    Right **0559**
  Cephalic
    Left **055F**
    Right **055D**
  Colic **0657**
  Common Iliac
    Left **065D**
    Right **065C**
  Coronary **0254**
  Esophageal **0653**
  External Iliac
    Left **065G**
    Right **065F**
  External Jugular
    Left **055Q**
    Right **055P**
  Face
    Left **055V**
    Right **055T**
  Femoral
    Left **065N**
    Right **065M**
  Foot
    Left **065V**
    Right **065T**
  Gastric **0652**
  Greater Saphenous
    Left **065Q**
    Right **065P**
  Hand
    Left **055H**
    Right **055G**
  Hemiazygos **0551**
  Hepatic **0654**
  Hypogastric
    Left **065J**
    Right **065H**
  Inferior Mesenteric **0656**
  Innominate
    Left **0554**
    Right **0553**
  Internal Jugular
    Left **055N**
    Right **055M**
  Intracranial **055L**
  Lesser Saphenous
    Left **065S**
    Right **065R**
  Lower **065Y**
  Portal **0658**
  Pulmonary
    Left **025T**
    Right **025S**
  Renal
    Left **065B**

Destruction (*continued*)
   Right **0659**
   Splenic **0651**
   Subclavian
    Left **0556**
    Right **0555**
   Superior Mesenteric **0655**
   Upper **055Y**
   Vertebral
    Left **055S**
    Right **055R**
  Vena Cava
   Inferior **0650**
   Superior **025V**
  Ventricle
   Left **025L**
   Right **025K**
  Vertebra
   Cervical **0P53**
   Lumbar **0Q50**
   Thoracic **0P54**
  Vesicle
   Bilateral **0V53**
   Left **0V52**
   Right **0V51**
  Vitreous
   Left **08553ZZ**
   Right **08543ZZ**
  Vocal Cord
   Left **0C5V**
   Right **0C5T**
  Vulva **0U5M**
Detachment
  Arm
   Lower
    Left **0X6F0Z**
    Right **0X6D0Z**
   Upper
    Left **0X690Z**
    Right **0X680Z**
  Elbow Region
   Left **0X6C0ZZ**
   Right **0X6B0ZZ**
  Femoral Region
   Left **0Y680ZZ**
   Right **0Y670ZZ**
  Finger
   Index
    Left **0X6P0Z**
    Right **0X6N0Z**
   Little
    Left **0X6W0Z**
    Right **0X6V0Z**
   Middle
    Left **0X6R0Z**
    Right **0X6Q0Z**
   Ring
    Left **0X6T0Z**
    Right **0X6S0Z**
  Foot
   Left **0Y6N0Z**
   Right **0Y6M0Z**
  Forequarter
   Left **0X610ZZ**
   Right **0X600ZZ**
  Hand

Detachment (*continued*)
   Left **0X6K0Z**
   Right **0X6J0Z**
  Hindquarter
   Bilateral **0Y640ZZ**
   Left **0Y630ZZ**
   Right **0Y620ZZ**
  Knee Region
   Left **0Y6G0ZZ**
   Right **0Y6F0ZZ**
  Leg
   Lower
    Left **0Y6J0Z**
    Right **0Y6H0Z**
   Upper
    Left **0Y6D0Z**
    Right **0Y6C0Z**
  Shoulder Region
   Left **0X630ZZ**
   Right **0X620ZZ**
  Thumb
   Left **0X6M0Z**
   Right **0X6L0Z**
  Toe
   1st
    Left **0Y6Q0Z**
    Right **0Y6P0Z**
   2nd
    Left **0Y6S0Z**
    Right **0Y6R0Z**
   3rd
    Left **0Y6U0Z**
    Right **0Y6T0Z**
   4th
    Left **0Y6W0Z**
    Right **0Y6V0Z**
   5th
    Left **0Y6Y0Z**
    Right **0Y6X0Z**
Determination, Mental status GZ14ZZZ
Detorsion
 see Release
 see Reposition
Detoxification Services, for substance abuse HZ2ZZZZ
Device Fitting F0DZ
Diagnostic Audiology *see* Audiology, Diagnostic
Diagnostic imaging *see* Imaging, Diagnostic
Diagnostic radiology *see* Imaging, Diagnostic
Dialysis
 Hemodialysis **5A1D00Z**
 Peritoneal **3E1M39Z**
Diaphragma sellae *use* Dura Mater
Diaphragmatic pacemaker generator *use* Stimulator Generator in Subcutaneous Tissue and Fascia
Diaphragmatic Pacemaker Lead
 Insertion of device in
  Left **0BHS**
  Right **0BHR**
 Removal of device from, Diaphragm **0BPT**
 Revision of device in, Diaphragm **0BWT**
Digital radiography, plain *see* Plain Radiography

Dilation
 Ampulla of Vater **0F7C**
 Anus **0D7Q**
 Aorta
  Abdominal **0470**
  Thoracic
   Ascending/Arch **027X**
   Descending **027W**
 Artery
  Anterior Tibial
   Left **047Q**
   Right **047P**
  Axillary
   Left **0376**
   Right **0375**
  Brachial
   Left **0378**
   Right **0377**
  Celiac **0471**
  Colic
   Left **0477**
   Middle **0478**
   Right **0476**
  Common Carotid
   Left **037J**
   Right **037H**
  Common Iliac
   Left **047D**
   Right **047C**
  Coronary
   Four or More Arteries **0273**
   One Artery **0270**
   Three Arteries **0272**
   Two Arteries **0271**
  External Carotid
   Left **037N**
   Right **037M**
  External Iliac
   Left **047J**
   Right **047H**
  Face **037R**
  Femoral
   Left **047L**
   Right **047K**
  Foot
   Left **047W**
   Right **047V**
  Gastric **0472**
  Hand
   Left **037F**
   Right **037D**
  Hepatic **0473**
  Inferior Mesenteric **047B**
  Innominate **0372**
  Internal Carotid
   Left **037L**
   Right **037K**
  Internal Iliac
   Left **047F**
   Right **047E**
  Internal Mammary
   Left **0371**
   Right **0370**
  Intracranial **037G**
  Lower **047Y**
  Peroneal

Dilation *(continued)*
- Left **047U**
- Right **047T**
Popliteal
- Left **047N**
- Right **047M**
Posterior Tibial
- Left **047S**
- Right **047R**
Pulmonary
- Left **027R**
- Right **027Q**
Pulmonary Trunk **027P**
Radial
- Left **037C**
- Right **037B**
Renal
- Left **047A**
- Right **0479**
Splenic **0474**
Subclavian
- Left **0374**
- Right **0373**
Superior Mesenteric **0475**
Temporal

- Left **037T**
- Right **037S**
Thyroid
- Left **037V**
- Right **037U**
Ulnar
- Left **037A**
- Right **0379**
Upper **037Y**
Vertebral
- Left **037Q**
- Right **037P**
Bladder **0T7B**
Bladder Neck **0T7C**
Bronchus
- Lingula **0B79**
- Lower Lobe
  - Left **0B7B**
  - Right **0B76**
- Main
  - Left **0B77**
  - Right **0B73**
- Middle Lobe, Right **0B75**
- Upper Lobe
  - Left **0B78**
  - Right **0B74**
Carina **0B72**
Cecum **0D7H**
Cervix **0U7C**
Colon
- Ascending **0D7K**
- Descending **0D7M**
- Sigmoid **0D7N**
- Transverse **0D7L**
Duct
- Common Bile **0F79**
- Cystic **0F78**
- Hepatic
  - Left **0F76**
  - Right **0F75**

Dilation *(continued)*
Lacrimal
- Left **087Y**
- Right **087X**
Pancreatic **0F7D**
- Accessory **0F7F**
Parotid
- Left **0C7C**
- Right **0C7B**
Duodenum **0D79**
Esophagogastric Junction **0D74**
Esophagus **0D75**
- Lower **0D73**
- Middle **0D72**
- Upper **0D71**
Eustachian Tube
- Left **097G**
- Right **097F**
Fallopian Tube
- Left **0U76**
- Right **0U75**
Fallopian Tubes, Bilateral **0U77**
Hymen **0U7K**
Ileocecal Valve **0D7C**
Ileum **0D7B**
Intestine
- Large **0D7E**
  - Left **0D7G**
  - Right **0D7F**
- Small **0D78**
Jejunum **0D7A**
Kidney Pelvis
- Left **0T74**
- Right **0T73**
Larynx **0C7S**
Pharynx **0C7M**
Rectum **0D7P**
Stomach **0D76**
- Pylorus **0D77**
Trachea **0B71**
Ureter
- Left **0T77**
- Right **0T76**
Ureters, Bilateral **0T78**
Urethra **0T7D**
Uterus **0U79**
Vagina **0U7G**
Valve
- Aortic **027F**
- Mitral **027G**
- Pulmonary **027H**
- Tricuspid **027J**
Vas Deferens
- Bilateral **0V7Q**
- Left **0V7P**
- Right **0V7N**
Vein
- Axillary
  - Left **0578**
  - Right **0577**
- Azygos **0570**
- Basilic
  - Left **057C**
  - Right **057B**
- Brachial
  - Left **057A**

Dilation *(continued)*
- Right **0579**
- Cephalic
  - Left **057F**
  - Right **057D**
- Colic **0677**
- Common Iliac
  - Left **067D**
  - Right **067C**
- Esophageal **0673**
- External Iliac
  - Left **067G**
  - Right **067F**
- External Jugular
  - Left **057Q**
  - Right **057P**
- Face
  - Left **057V**
  - Right **057T**
- Femoral
  - Left **067N**
  - Right **067M**
- Foot
  - Left **067V**
  - Right **067T**
- Gastric **0672**
- Greater Saphenous
  - Left **067Q**
  - Right **067P**
- Hand
  - Left **057H**
  - Right **057G**
- Hemiazygos **0571**
- Hepatic **0674**
- Hypogastric
  - Left **067J**
  - Right **067H**
- Inferior Mesenteric **0676**
- Innominate
  - Left **0574**
  - Right **0573**
- Internal Jugular
  - Left **057N**
  - Right **057M**
- Intracranial **057L**
- Lesser Saphenous
  - Left **067S**
  - Right **067R**
- Lower **067Y**
- Portal **0678**
- Pulmonary
  - Left **027T**
  - Right **027S**
- Renal
  - Left **067B**
  - Right **0679**
- Splenic **0671**
- Subclavian
  - Left **0576**
  - Right **0575**
- Superior Mesenteric **0675**
- Upper **057Y**
- Vertebral
  - Left **057S**
  - Right **057R**
- Vena Cava

Dilation *(continued)*
  Inferior **0670**
  Superior **027V**
  Ventricle, Right **027K**
Direct Lateral Interbody Fusion (DLIF)
  device *use* Interbody Fusion Device in
  Lower Joints
Disarticulation *see* Detachment
Discectomy, diskectomy
  see Excision, Upper Joints **0RB**
  see Resection, Upper Joints **0RT**
  see Excision, Lower Joints **0SB**
  see Resection, Lower Joints **0ST**
Discography
  see Plain Radiography, Axial Skeleton,
  Except Skull and Facial Bones **BR0**
  see Fluoroscopy, Axial Skeleton, Except
  Skull and Facial Bones **BR1**
Distal humerus
  use Humeral Shaft, Right
  use Humeral Shaft, Left
Distal humerus, involving joint
  use Joint, Elbow, Right
  use Joint, Elbow, Left
Distal radioulnar joint
  use Joint, Wrist, Right
  use Joint, Wrist, Left
Diversion *see* Bypass
Diverticulectomy *see* Excision,
  Gastrointestinal System **0DB**
Division
  Acetabulum
    Left **0Q85**
    Right **0Q84**
  Anal Sphincter **0D8R**
  Basal Ganglia **0088**
  Bladder Neck **0T8C**
  Bone
    Ethmoid
      Left **0N8G**
      Right **0N8F**
    Frontal
      Left **0N82**
      Right **0N81**
    Hyoid **0N8X**
    Lacrimal
      Left **0N8J**
      Right **0N8H**
    Nasal **0N8B**
    Occipital
      Left **0N88**
      Right **0N87**
    Palatine
      Left **0N8L**
      Right **0N8K**
    Parietal
      Left **0N84**
      Right **0N83**
    Pelvic
      Left **0Q83**
      Right **0Q82**
    Sphenoid
      Left **0N8D**
      Right **0N8C**
    Temporal
      Left **0N86**

Division *(continued)*
      Right **0N85**
    Zygomatic
      Left **0N8N**
      Right **0N8M**
  Brain **0080**
  Bursa and Ligament
    Abdomen
      Left **0M8J**
      Right **0M8H**
    Ankle
      Left **0M8R**
      Right **0M8Q**
    Elbow
      Left **0M84**
      Right **0M83**
    Foot
      Left **0M8T**
      Right **0M8S**
    Hand
      Left **0M88**
      Right **0M87**
    Head and Neck **0M80**
    Hip
      Left **0M8M**
      Right **0M8L**
    Knee
      Left **0M8P**
      Right **0M8N**
    Lower Extremity
      Left **0M8W**
      Right **0M8V**
    Perineum **0M8K**
    Shoulder
      Left **0M82**
      Right **0M81**
    Thorax
      Left **0M8G**
      Right **0M8F**
    Trunk
      Left **0M8D**
      Right **0M8C**
    Upper Extremity
      Left **0M8B**
      Right **0M89**
    Wrist
      Left **0M86**
      Right **0M85**
  Carpal
    Left **0P8N**
    Right **0P8M**
  Cerebral Hemisphere **0087**
  Chordae Tendineae **0289**
  Clavicle
    Left **0P8B**
    Right **0P89**
  Coccyx **0Q8S**
  Conduction Mechanism **0288**
  Esophagogastric Junction **0D84**
  Femoral Shaft
    Left **0Q89**
    Right **0Q88**
  Femur
    Lower
      Left **0Q8C**
      Right **0Q8B**

Division *(continued)*
    Upper
      Left **0Q87**
      Right **0Q86**
  Fibula
    Left **0Q8K**
    Right **0Q8J**
  Gland, Pituitary **0G80**
  Glenoid Cavity
    Left **0P88**
    Right **0P87**
  Humeral Head
    Left **0P8D**
    Right **0P8C**
  Humeral Shaft
    Left **0P8G**
    Right **0P8F**
  Hymen **0U8K**
  Kidneys, Bilateral **0T82**
  Mandible
    Left **0N8V**
    Right **0N8T**
  Maxilla
    Left **0N8S**
    Right **0N8R**
  Metacarpal
    Left **0P8Q**
    Right **0P8P**
  Metatarsal
    Left **0Q8P**
    Right **0Q8N**
  Muscle
    Abdomen
      Left **0K8L**
      Right **0K8K**
    Facial **0K81**
    Foot
      Left **0K8W**
      Right **0K8V**
    Hand
      Left **0K8D**
      Right **0K8C**
    Head **0K80**
    Hip
      Left **0K8P**
      Right **0K8N**
    Lower Arm and Wrist
      Left **0K8B**
      Right **0K89**
    Lower Leg
      Left **0K8T**
      Right **0K8S**
    Neck
      Left **0K83**
      Right **0K82**
    Papillary **028D**
    Perineum **0K8M**
    Shoulder
      Left **0K86**
      Right **0K85**
    Thorax
      Left **0K8J**
      Right **0K8H**
    Tongue, Palate, Pharynx **0K84**
    Trunk
      Left **0K8G**

Division (continued)

    Right **0K8F**

  Upper Arm

    Left **0K88**

    Right **0K87**

  Upper Leg

    Left **0K8R**

    Right **0K8Q**

Nerve

  Abdominal Sympathetic **018M**

  Abducens **008L**

  Accessory **008R**

  Acoustic **008N**

  Brachial Plexus **0183**

  Cervical **0181**

  Cervical Plexus **0180**

  Facial **008M**

  Femoral **018D**

  Glossopharyngeal **008P**

  Head and Neck Sympathetic **018K**

  Hypoglossal **008S**

  Lumbar **018B**

  Lumbar Plexus **0189**

  Lumbar Sympathetic **018N**

  Lumbosacral Plexus **018A**

  Median **0185**

  Oculomotor **008H**

  Olfactory **008F**

  Optic **008G**

  Peroneal **018H**

  Phrenic **0182**

  Pudendal **018C**

  Radial **0186**

  Sacral **018R**

  Sacral Plexus **018Q**

  Sacral Sympathetic **018P**

  Sciatic **018F**

  Thoracic **0188**

  Thoracic Sympathetic **018L**

  Tibial **018G**

  Trigeminal **008K**

  Trochlear **008J**

  Ulnar **0184**

  Vagus **008Q**

Orbit

  Left **0N8Q**

  Right **0N8P**

Ovary

  Bilateral **0U82**

  Left **0U81**

  Right **0U80**

Pancreas **0F8G**

Patella

  Left **0Q8F**

  Right **0Q8D**

Perineum, Female **0W8NXZZ**

Phalanx

  Finger

    Left **0P8V**

    Right **0P8T**

  Thumb

    Left **0P8S**

    Right **0P8R**

  Toe

    Left **0Q8R**

    Right **0Q8Q**

Division (continued)

  Radius

    Left **0P8J**

    Right **0P8H**

  Rib

    Left **0P82**

    Right **0P81**

  Sacrum **0Q81**

  Scapula

    Left **0P86**

    Right **0P85**

  Skin

    Abdomen **0H87XZZ**

    Back **0H86XZZ**

    Buttock **0H88XZZ**

    Chest **0H85XZZ**

    Ear

      Left **0H83XZZ**

      Right **0H82XZZ**

    Face **0H81XZZ**

    Foot

      Left **0H8NXZZ**

      Right **0H8MXZZ**

    Genitalia **0H8AXZZ**

    Hand

      Left **0H8GXZZ**

      Right **0H8FXZZ**

    Lower Arm

      Left **0H8EXZZ**

      Right **0H8DXZZ**

    Lower Leg

      Left **0H8LXZZ**

      Right **0H8KXZZ**

    Neck **0H84XZZ**

    Perineum **0H89XZZ**

    Scalp **0H80XZZ**

    Upper Arm

      Left **0H8CXZZ**

      Right **0H8BXZZ**

    Upper Leg

      Left **0H8JXZZ**

      Right **0H8HXZZ**

  Skull **0N80**

  Spinal Cord

    Cervical **008W**

    Lumbar **008Y**

    Thoracic **008X**

  Sternum **0P80**

  Stomach, Pylorus **0D87**

  Subcutaneous Tissue and Fascia

    Abdomen **0J88**

    Back **0J87**

    Buttock **0J89**

    Chest **0J86**

    Face **0J81**

    Foot

      Left **0J8R**

      Right **0J8Q**

    Hand

      Left **0J8K**

      Right **0J8J**

    Head and Neck **0J8S**

    Lower Arm

      Left **0J8H**

      Right **0J8G**

    Lower Extremity **0J8W**

Division (continued)

  Lower Leg

    Left **0J8P**

    Right **0J8N**

  Neck

    Anterior **0J84**

    Posterior **0J85**

  Pelvic Region **0J8C**

  Perineum **0J8B**

  Scalp **0J80**

  Trunk **0J8T**

  Upper Arm

    Left **0J8F**

    Right **0J8D**

  Upper Extremity **0J8V**

  Upper Leg

    Left **0J8M**

    Right **0J8L**

  Tarsal

    Left **0Q8M**

    Right **0Q8L**

  Tendon

    Abdomen

      Left **0L8G**

      Right **0L8F**

    Ankle

      Left **0L8T**

      Right **0L8S**

    Foot

      Left **0L8W**

      Right **0L8V**

    Hand

      Left **0L88**

      Right **0L87**

    Head and Neck **0L80**

    Hip

      Left **0L8K**

      Right **0L8J**

    Knee

      Left **0L8R**

      Right **0L8Q**

    Lower Arm and Wrist

      Left **0L86**

      Right **0L85**

    Lower Leg

      Left **0L8P**

      Right **0L8N**

    Perineum **0L8H**

    Shoulder

      Left **0L82**

      Right **0L81**

    Thorax

      Left **0L8D**

      Right **0L8C**

    Trunk

      Left **0L8B**

      Right **0L89**

    Upper Arm

      Left **0L84**

      Right **0L83**

    Upper Leg

      Left **0L8M**

      Right **0L8L**

  Thyroid Gland Isthmus **0G8J**

  Tibia

    Left **0Q8H**

Division *(continued)*
    Right **0Q8G**
  Turbinate, Nasal **098L**
  Ulna
    Left **0P8L**
    Right **0P8K**
  Uterine Supporting Structure **0U84**
  Vertebra
    Cervical **0P83**
    Lumbar **0Q80**
    Thoracic **0P84**
Doppler study *see* Ultrasonography
Dorsal digital nerve *use* Nerve, Radial
Dorsal metacarpal vein
  use Vein, Hand, Left
  use Vein, Hand, Right
Dorsal metatarsal artery
  use Artery, Foot, Left
  use Artery, Foot, Right
Dorsal metatarsal vein
  use Vein, Foot, Right
  use Vein, Foot, Left
Dorsal scapular artery
  use Artery, Subclavian, Right
  use Artery, Subclavian, Left
Dorsal scapular nerve *use* Nerve, Brachial
  Plexus
Dorsal venous arch
  use Vein, Foot, Right
  use Vein, Foot, Left
Dorsalis pedis artery
  use Artery, Anterior Tibial, Right
  use Artery, Anterior Tibial, Left
Drainage
  Abdominal Wall **0W9F**
  Acetabulum
    Left **0Q95**
    Right **0Q94**
  Adenoids **0C9Q**
  Ampulla of Vater **0F9C**
  Anal Sphincter **0D9R**
  Ankle Region
    Left **0Y9L**
    Right **0Y9K**
  Anterior Chamber
    Left **0893**
    Right **0892**
  Anus **0D9Q**
  Aorta, Abdominal **0490**
  Aortic Body **0G9D**
  Appendix **0D9J**
  Arm
    Lower
      Left **0X9F**
      Right **0X9D**
    Upper
      Left **0X99**
      Right **0X98**
  Artery
    Anterior Tibial
      Left **049Q**
      Right **049P**
    Axillary
      Left **0396**
      Right **0395**
    Brachial

Drainage *(continued)*
      Left **0398**
      Right **0397**
    Celiac **0491**
    Colic
      Left **0497**
      Middle **0498**
      Right **0496**
    Common Carotid
      Left **039J**
      Right **039H**
    Common Iliac
      Left **049D**
      Right **049C**
    External Carotid
      Left **039N**
      Right **039M**
    External Iliac
      Left **049J**
      Right **049H**
    Face **039R**
    Femoral
      Left **049L**
      Right **049K**
    Foot
      Left **049W**
      Right **049V**
    Gastric **0492**
    Hand
      Left **039F**
      Right **039D**
    Hepatic **0493**
    Inferior Mesenteric **049B**
    Innominate **0392**
    Internal Carotid
      Left **039L**
      Right **039K**
    Internal Iliac
      Left **049F**
      Right **049E**
    Internal Mammary
      Left **0391**
      Right **0390**
    Intracranial **039G**
    Lower **049Y**
    Peroneal
      Left **049U**
      Right **049T**
    Popliteal
      Left **049N**
      Right **049M**
    Posterior Tibial
      Left **049S**
      Right **049R**
    Radial
      Left **039C**
      Right **039B**
    Renal
      Left **049A**
      Right **0499**
    Splenic **0494**
    Subclavian
      Left **0394**
      Right **0393**
    Superior Mesenteric **0495**
    Temporal

Drainage *(continued)*
      Left **039T**
      Right **039S**
    Thyroid
      Left **039V**
      Right **039U**
    Ulnar
      Left **039A**
      Right **0399**
    Upper **039Y**
    Vertebral
      Left **039Q**
      Right **039P**
  Auditory Ossicle
    Left **099A**
    Right **0999**
  Axilla
    Left **0X95**
    Right **0X94**
  Back
    Lower **0W9L**
    Upper **0W9K**
  Basal Ganglia **0098**
  Bladder **0T9B**
  Bladder Neck **0T9C**
  Bone
    Ethmoid
      Left **0N9G**
      Right **0N9F**
    Frontal
      Left **0N92**
      Right **0N91**
    Hyoid **0N9X**
    Lacrimal
      Left **0N9J**
      Right **0N9H**
    Nasal **0N9B**
    Occipital
      Left **0N98**
      Right **0N97**
    Palatine
      Left **0N9L**
      Right **0N9K**
    Parietal
      Left **0N94**
      Right **0N93**
    Pelvic
      Left **0Q93**
      Right **0Q92**
    Sphenoid
      Left **0N9D**
      Right **0N9C**
    Temporal
      Left **0N96**
      Right **0N95**
    Zygomatic
      Left **0N9N**
      Right **0N9M**
  Bone Marrow **079T**
  Brain **0090**
  Breast
    Bilateral **0H9V**
    Left **0H9U**
    Right **0H9T**
  Bronchus
    Lingula **0B99**

Drainage *(continued)*

Lower Lobe
 Left **0B9B**
 Right **0B96**
Main
 Left **0B97**
 Right **0B93**
Middle Lobe, Right **0B95**
Upper Lobe
 Left **0B98**
 Right **0B94**
Buccal Mucosa **0C94**
Bursa and Ligament
 Abdomen
  Left **0M9J**
  Right **0M9H**
 Ankle
  Left **0M9R**
  Right **0M9Q**
 Elbow
  Left **0M94**
  Right **0M93**
 Foot
  Left **0M9T**
  Right **0M9S**
 Hand
  Left **0M98**
  Right **0M97**
 Head and Neck **0M90**
 Hip
  Left **0M9M**
  Right **0M9L**
 Knee
  Left **0M9P**
  Right **0M9N**
 Lower Extremity
  Left **0M9W**
  Right **0M9V**
 Perineum **0M9K**
 Shoulder
  Left **0M92**
  Right **0M91**
 Thorax
  Left **0M9G**
  Right **0M9F**
 Trunk
  Left **0M9D**
  Right **0M9C**
 Upper Extremity
  Left **0M9B**
  Right **0M99**
 Wrist
  Left **0M96**
  Right **0M95**
Buttock
 Left **0Y91**
 Right **0Y90**
Carina **0B92**
Carotid Bodies, Bilateral **0G98**
Carotid Body
 Left **0G96**
 Right **0G97**
Carpal
 Left **0P9N**
 Right **0P9M**
Cavity, Cranial **0W91**

Drainage *(continued)*

Cecum **0D9H**
Cerebellum **009C**
Cerebral Hemisphere **0097**
Cerebral Meninges **0091**
Cerebral Ventricle **0096**
Cervix **0U9C**
Chest Wall **0W98**
Choroid
 Left **089B**
 Right **089A**
Cisterna Chyli **079L**
Clavicle
 Left **0P9B**
 Right **0P99**
Clitoris **0U9J**
Coccygeal Glomus **0G9B**
Coccyx **0Q9S**
Colon
 Ascending **0D9K**
 Descending **0D9M**
 Sigmoid **0D9N**
 Transverse **0D9L**
Conjunctiva
 Left **089T**
 Right **089S**
Cord
 Bilateral **0V9H**
 Left **0V9G**
 Right **0V9F**
Cornea
 Left **0899**
 Right **0898**
Cul-de-sac **0U9F**
Diaphragm
 Left **0B9S**
 Right **0B9R**
Disc
 Cervical Vertebral **0R93**
 Cervicothoracic Vertebral **0R95**
 Lumbar Vertebral **0S92**
 Lumbosacral **0S94**
 Thoracic Vertebral **0R99**
 Thoracolumbar Vertebral **0R9B**
Duct
 Common Bile **0F99**
 Cystic **0F98**
 Hepatic
  Left **0F96**
  Right **0F95**
 Lacrimal
  Left **089Y**
  Right **089X**
 Pancreatic **0F9D**
  Accessory **0F9F**
 Parotid
  Left **0C9C**
  Right **0C9B**
Duodenum **0D99**
Dura Mater **0092**
Ear
 External
  Left **0991**
  Right **0990**
 External Auditory Canal
  Left **0994**

Drainage *(continued)*

 Right **0993**
 Inner
  Left **099E**
  Right **099D**
 Middle
  Left **0996**
  Right **0995**
Elbow Region
 Left **0X9C**
 Right **0X9B**
Epididymis
 Bilateral **0V9L**
 Left **0V9K**
 Right **0V9J**
Epidural Space **0093**
Epiglottis **0C9R**
Esophagogastric Junction **0D94**
Esophagus **0D95**
 Lower **0D93**
 Middle **0D92**
 Upper **0D91**
Eustachian Tube
 Left **099G**
 Right **099F**
Extremity
 Lower
  Left **0Y9B**
  Right **0Y99**
 Upper
  Left **0X97**
  Right **0X96**
Eye
 Left **0891**
 Right **0890**
Eyelid
 Lower
  Left **089R**
  Right **089Q**
 Upper
  Left **089P**
  Right **089N**
Face **0W92**
Fallopian Tube
 Left **0U96**
 Right **0U95**
Fallopian Tubes, Bilateral **0U97**
Femoral Region
 Left **0Y98**
 Right **0Y97**
Femoral Shaft
 Left **0Q99**
 Right **0Q98**
Femur
 Lower
  Left **0Q9C**
  Right **0Q9B**
 Upper
  Left **0Q97**
  Right **0Q96**
Fibula
 Left **0Q9K**
 Right **0Q9J**
Finger Nail **0H9Q**
Foot
 Left **0Y9N**

Drainage *(continued)*
    Right **0Y9M**
  Gallbladder **0F94**
  Gingiva
    Lower **0C96**
    Upper **0C95**
  Gland
    Adrenal
      Bilateral **0G94**
      Left **0G92**
      Right **0G93**
    Lacrimal
      Left **089W**
      Right **089V**
    Minor Salivary **0C9J**
    Parotid
      Left **0C99**
      Right **0C98**
    Pituitary **0G90**
    Sublingual
      Left **0C9F**
      Right **0C9D**
    Submaxillary
      Left **0C9H**
      Right **0C9G**
    Vestibular **0U9L**
  Glenoid Cavity
    Left **0P98**
    Right **0P97**
  Glomus Jugulare **0G9C**
  Hand
    Left **0X9K**
    Right **0X9J**
  Head **0W90**
  Humeral Head
    Left **0P9D**
    Right **0P9C**
  Humeral Shaft
    Left **0P9G**
    Right **0P9F**
  Hymen **0U9K**
  Hypothalamus **009A**
  Ileocecal Valve **0D9C**
  Ileum **0D9B**
  Inguinal Region
    Left **0Y96**
    Right **0Y95**
  Intestine
    Large **0D9E**
      Left **0D9G**
      Right **0D9F**
    Small **0D98**
  Iris
    Left **089D**
    Right **089C**
  Jaw
    Lower **0W95**
    Upper **0W94**
  Jejunum **0D9A**
  Joint
    Acromioclavicular
      Left **0R9H**
      Right **0R9G**
    Ankle
      Left **0S9G**
      Right **0S9F**

Drainage *(continued)*
    Carpal
      Left **0R9R**
      Right **0R9Q**
    Cervical Vertebral **0R91**
    Cervicothoracic Vertebral **0R94**
    Coccygeal **0S96**
    Elbow
      Left **0R9M**
      Right **0R9L**
    Finger Phalangeal
      Left **0R9X**
      Right **0R9W**
    Hip
      Left **0S9B**
      Right **0S99**
    Knee
      Left **0S9D**
      Right **0S9C**
    Lumbar Vertebral **0S90**
    Lumbosacral **0S93**
    Metacarpocarpal
      Left **0R9T**
      Right **0R9S**
    Metacarpophalangeal
      Left **0R9V**
      Right **0R9U**
    Metatarsal-Phalangeal
      Left **0S9N**
      Right **0S9M**
    Metatarsal-Tarsal
      Left **0S9L**
      Right **0S9K**
    Occipital-cervical **0R90**
    Sacrococcygeal **0S95**
    Sacroiliac
      Left **0S98**
      Right **0S97**
    Shoulder
      Left **0R9K**
      Right **0R9J**
    Sternoclavicular
      Left **0R9F**
      Right **0R9E**
    Tarsal
      Left **0S9J**
      Right **0S9H**
    Temporomandibular
      Left **0R9D**
      Right **0R9C**
    Thoracic Vertebral **0R96**
    Thoracolumbar Vertebral **0R9A**
    Toe Phalangeal
      Left **0S9Q**
      Right **0S9P**
    Wrist
      Left **0R9P**
      Right **0R9N**
  Kidney
    Left **0T91**
    Right **0T90**
  Kidney Pelvis
    Left **0T94**
    Right **0T93**
  Knee Region
    Left **0Y9G**

Drainage *(continued)*
    Right **0Y9F**
  Larynx **0C9S**
  Leg
    Lower
      Left **0Y9J**
      Right **0Y9H**
    Upper
      Left **0Y9D**
      Right **0Y9C**
  Lens
    Left **089K**
    Right **089J**
  Lip
    Lower **0C91**
    Upper **0C90**
  Liver **0F90**
    Left Lobe **0F92**
    Right Lobe **0F91**
  Lung
    Bilateral **0B9M**
    Left **0B9L**
    Lower Lobe
      Left **0B9J**
      Right **0B9F**
    Middle Lobe, Right **0B9D**
    Right **0B9K**
    Upper Lobe
      Left **0B9G**
      Right **0B9C**
  Lung Lingula **0B9H**
  Lymphatic
    Aortic **079D**
    Axillary
      Left **0796**
      Right **0795**
    Head **0790**
    Inguinal
      Left **079J**
      Right **079H**
    Internal Mammary
      Left **0799**
      Right **0798**
    Lower Extremity
      Left **079G**
      Right **079F**
    Mesenteric **079B**
    Neck
      Left **0792**
      Right **0791**
    Pelvis **079C**
    Thoracic Duct **079K**
    Thorax **0797**
    Upper Extremity
      Left **0794**
      Right **0793**
  Mandible
    Left **0N9V**
    Right **0N9T**
  Maxilla
    Left **0N9S**
    Right **0N9R**
  Mediastinum **0W9C**
  Medulla Oblongata **009D**
  Mesentery **0D9V**
  Metacarpal

Drainage *(continued)*
　Left 0P9Q
　Right 0P9P
Metatarsal
　Left 0Q9P
　Right 0Q9N
Muscle
　Abdomen
　　Left 0K9L
　　Right 0K9K
　Extraocular
　　Left 089M
　　Right 089L
　Facial 0K91
　Foot
　　Left 0K9W
　　Right 0K9V
　Hand
　　Left 0K9D
　　Right 0K9C
　Head 0K90
　Hip
　　Left 0K9P
　　Right 0K9N
　Lower Arm and Wrist
　　Left 0K9B
　　Right 0K99
　Lower Leg
　　Left 0K9T
　　Right 0K9S
　Neck
　　Left 0K93
　　Right 0K92
　Perineum 0K9M
　Shoulder
　　Left 0K96
　　Right 0K95
　Thorax
　　Left 0K9J
　　Right 0K9H
　Tongue, Palate, Pharynx 0K94
　Trunk
　　Left 0K9G
　　Right 0K9F
　Upper Arm
　　Left 0K98
　　Right 0K97
　Upper Leg
　　Left 0K9R
　　Right 0K9Q
Nasopharynx 099N
Neck 0W96
Nerve
　Abdominal Sympathetic 019M
　Abducens 009L
　Accessory 009R
　Acoustic 009N
　Brachial Plexus 0193
　Cervical 0191
　Cervical Plexus 0190
　Facial 009M
　Femoral 019D
　Glossopharyngeal 009P
　Head and Neck Sympathetic 019K
　Hypoglossal 009S
　Lumbar 019B

Drainage *(continued)*
Lumbar Plexus 0199
Lumbar Sympathetic 019N
Lumbosacral Plexus 019A
Median 0195
Oculomotor 009H
Olfactory 009F
Optic 009G
Peroneal 019H
Phrenic 0192
Pudendal 019C
Radial 0196
Sacral 019R
Sacral Plexus 019Q
Sacral Sympathetic 019P
Sciatic 019F
Thoracic 0198
Thoracic Sympathetic 019L
Tibial 019G
Trigeminal 009K
Trochlear 009J
Ulnar 0194
Vagus 009Q
Nipple
　Left 0H9X
　Right 0H9W
Nose 099K
Omentum
　Greater 0D9S
　Lesser 0D9T
Oral Cavity and Throat 0W93
Orbit
　Left 0N9Q
　Right 0N9P
Ovary
　Bilateral 0U92
　Left 0U91
　Right 0U90
Palate
　Hard 0C92
　Soft 0C93
Pancreas 0F9G
Para-aortic Body 0G99
Paraganglion Extremity 0G9F
Parathyroid Gland 0G9R
　Inferior
　　Left 0G9P
　　Right 0G9N
　Multiple 0G9Q
　Superior
　　Left 0G9M
　　Right 0G9L
Patella
　Left 0Q9F
　Right 0Q9D
Pelvic Cavity 0W9J
Penis 0V9S
Pericardial Cavity 0W9D
Perineum
　Female 0W9N
　Male 0W9M
Peritoneal Cavity 0W9G
Peritoneum 0D9W
Phalanx
　Finger
　　Left 0P9V

Drainage *(continued)*
　Right 0P9T
Thumb
　Left 0P9S
　Right 0P9R
Toe
　Left 0Q9R
　Right 0Q9Q
Pharynx 0C9M
Pineal Body 0G91
Pleura
　Left 0B9P
　Right 0B9N
Pleural Cavity
　Left 0W9B
　Right 0W99
Pons 009B
Prepuce 0V9T
Products of Conception
　Amniotic Fluid
　　Diagnostic 1090
　　Therapeutic 1090
　Fetal Blood 1090
　Fetal Cerebrospinal Fluid 1090
　Fetal Fluid, Other 1090
　Fluid, Other 1090
Prostate 0V90
Radius
　Left 0P9J
　Right 0P9H
Rectum 0D9P
Retina
　Left 089F
　Right 089E
Retinal Vessel
　Left 089H
　Right 089G
Retroperitoneum 0W9H
Rib
　Left 0P92
　Right 0P91
Sacrum 0Q91
Scapula
　Left 0P96
　Right 0P95
Sclera
　Left 0897
　Right 0896
Scrotum 0V95
Septum, Nasal 099M
Shoulder Region
　Left 0X93
　Right 0X92
Sinus
　Accessory 099P
　Ethmoid
　　Left 099V
　　Right 099U
　Frontal
　　Left 099T
　　Right 099S
　Mastoid
　　Left 099C
　　Right 099B
　Maxillary
　　Left 099R

Right **099Q**
Sphenoid
  Left **099X**
  Right **099W**
Skin
  Abdomen **0H97**
  Back **0H96**
  Buttock **0H98**
  Chest **0H95**
  Ear
    Left **0H93**
    Right **0H92**
  Face **0H91**
  Foot
    Left **0H9N**
    Right **0H9M**
  Genitalia **0H9A**
  Hand
    Left **0H9G**
    Right **0H9F**
  Lower Arm
    Left **0H9E**
    Right **0H9D**
  Lower Leg
    Left **0H9L**
    Right **0H9K**
  Neck **0H94**
  Perineum **0H99**
  Scalp **0H90**
  Upper Arm
    Left **0H9C**
    Right **0H9B**
  Upper Leg
    Left **0H9J**
    Right **0H9H**
Skull **0N90**
Spinal Canal **009U**
Spinal Cord
  Cervical **009W**
  Lumbar **009Y**
  Thoracic **009X**
Spinal Meninges **009T**
Spleen **079P**
Sternum **0P90**
Stomach **0D96**
  Pylorus **0D97**
Subarachnoid Space **0095**
Subcutaneous Tissue and Fascia
  Abdomen **0J98**
  Back **0J97**
  Buttock **0J99**
  Chest **0J96**
  Face **0J91**
  Foot
    Left **0J9R**
    Right **0J9Q**
  Hand
    Left **0J9K**
    Right **0J9J**
  Lower Arm
    Left **0J9H**
    Right **0J9G**
  Lower Leg
    Left **0J9P**
    Right **0J9N**

Neck
  Anterior **0J94**
  Posterior **0J95**
Pelvic Region **0J9C**
Perineum **0J9B**
Scalp **0J90**
Upper Arm
  Left **0J9F**
  Right **0J9D**
Upper Leg
  Left **0J9M**
  Right **0J9L**
Subdural Space **0094**
Tarsal
  Left **0Q9M**
  Right **0Q9L**
Tendon
  Abdomen
    Left **0L9G**
    Right **0L9F**
  Ankle
    Left **0L9T**
    Right **0L9S**
  Foot
    Left **0L9W**
    Right **0L9V**
  Hand
    Left **0L98**
    Right **0L97**
  Head and Neck **0L90**
  Hip
    Left **0L9K**
    Right **0L9J**
  Knee
    Left **0L9R**
    Right **0L9Q**
  Lower Arm and Wrist
    Left **0L96**
    Right **0L95**
  Lower Leg
    Left **0L9P**
    Right **0L9N**
  Perineum **0L9H**
  Shoulder
    Left **0L92**
    Right **0L91**
  Thorax
    Left **0L9D**
    Right **0L9C**
  Trunk
    Left **0L9B**
    Right **0L99**
  Upper Arm
    Left **0L94**
    Right **0L93**
  Upper Leg
    Left **0L9M**
    Right **0L9L**
Testis
  Bilateral **0V9C**
  Left **0V9B**
  Right **0V99**
Thalamus **0099**
Thymus **079M**
Thyroid Gland **0G9K**

  Left Lobe **0G9G**
  Right Lobe **0G9H**
Tibia
  Left **0Q9H**
  Right **0Q9G**
Toe Nail **0H9R**
Tongue **0C97**
Tonsils **0C9P**
Tooth
  Lower **0C9X**
  Upper **0C9W**
Trachea **0B91**
Tunica Vaginalis
  Left **0V97**
  Right **0V96**
Turbinate, Nasal **099L**
Tympanic Membrane
  Left **0998**
  Right **0997**
Ulna
  Left **0P9L**
  Right **0P9K**
Ureter
  Left **0T97**
  Right **0T96**
Ureters, Bilateral **0T98**
Urethra **0T9D**
Uterine Supporting Structure **0U94**
Uterus **0U99**
Uvula **0C9N**
Vagina **0U9G**
Vas Deferens
  Bilateral **0V9Q**
  Left **0V9P**
  Right **0V9N**
Vein
  Axillary
    Left **0598**
    Right **0597**
  Azygos **0590**
  Basilic
    Left **059C**
    Right **059B**
  Brachial
    Left **059A**
    Right **0599**
  Cephalic
    Left **059F**
    Right **059D**
  Colic **0697**
  Common Iliac
    Left **069D**
    Right **069C**
  Esophageal **0693**
  External Iliac
    Left **069G**
    Right **069F**
  External Jugular
    Left **059Q**
    Right **059P**
  Face
    Left **059V**
    Right **059T**
  Femoral
    Left **069N**

Drainage *(continued)*
    Right **069M**
    Foot
      Left **069V**
      Right **069T**
    Gastric **0692**
    Greater Saphenous
      Left **069Q**
      Right **069P**
    Hand
      Left **059H**
      Right **059G**
    Hemiazygos **0591**
    Hepatic **0694**
    Hypogastric
      Left **069J**
      Right **069H**
    Inferior Mesenteric **0696**
    Innominate
      Left **0594**
      Right **0593**
    Internal Jugular
      Left **059N**
      Right **059M**
    Intracranial **059L**
    Lesser Saphenous
      Left **069S**
      Right **069R**
    Lower **069Y**
    Portal **0698**
    Renal
      Left **069B**
      Right **0699**
    Splenic **0691**
    Subclavian
      Left **0596**
      Right **0595**
    Superior Mesenteric **0695**
    Upper **059Y**
    Vertebral
      Left **059S**
      Right **059R**
    Vena Cava, Inferior **0690**
    Vertebra
      Cervical **0P93**
      Lumbar **0Q90**
      Thoracic **0P94**
    Vesicle
      Bilateral **0V93**
      Left **0V92**
      Right **0V91**
    Vitreous
      Left **0895**
      Right **0894**
    Vocal Cord
      Left **0C9V**
      Right **0C9T**
    Vulva **0U9M**
    Wrist Region
      Left **0X9H**
      Right **0X9G**
Dressing
    Abdominal Wall **2W23X4Z**
    Arm
      Lower
        Left **2W2DX4Z**

Dressing *(continued)*
      Right **2W2CX4Z**
      Upper
        Left **2W2BX4Z**
        Right **2W2AX4Z**
    Back **2W25X4Z**
    Chest Wall **2W24X4Z**
    Extremity
      Lower
        Left **2W2MX4Z**
        Right **2W2LX4Z**
      Upper
        Left **2W29X4Z**
        Right **2W28X4Z**
    Face **2W21X4Z**
    Finger
      Left **2W2KX4Z**
      Right **2W2JX4Z**
    Foot
      Left **2W2TX4Z**
      Right **2W2SX4Z**
    Hand
      Left **2W2FX4Z**
      Right **2W2EX4Z**
    Head **2W20X4Z**
    Inguinal Region
      Left **2W27X4Z**
      Right **2W26X4Z**
    Leg
      Lower
        Left **2W2RX4Z**
        Right **2W2QX4Z**
      Upper
        Left **2W2PX4Z**
        Right **2W2NX4Z**
    Neck **2W22X4Z**
    Thumb
      Left **2W2HX4Z**
      Right **2W2GX4Z**
    Toe
      Left **2W2VX4Z**
      Right **2W2UX4Z**
Driver stent (RX) (OTW) *use* Intraluminal Device
Drotrecogin alfa *see* Introduction of Recombinant Human-activated Protein C
Duct of Santorini *use* Duct, Pancreatic, Accessory
Duct of Wirsung *use* Duct, Pancreatic
Ductogram, mammary *see* Plain Radiography, Skin, Subcutaneous Tissue and Breast **BH0**
Ductography, mammary *see* Plain Radiography, Skin, Subcutaneous Tissue and Breast **BH0**
Ductus deferens
  use Vas Deferens, Left
  use Vas Deferens, Right
  use Vas Deferens
  use Vas Deferens, Bilateral
Duodenal ampulla *use* Ampulla of Vater
Duodenectomy
  see Excision, Duodenum **0DB9**
  see Resection, Duodenum **0DT9**
Duodenocholedochotomy *see* Drainage, Gallbladder **0F94**

Duodenocystostomy
  see Bypass, Gallbladder **0F14**
  see Drainage, Gallbladder **0F94**
Duodenoenterostomy
  see Bypass, Gastrointestinal System **0D1**
  see Drainage, Gastrointestinal System **0D9**
Duodenojejunal flexure *use* Jejunum
Duodenolysis *see* Release, Duodenum **0DN9**
Duodenorrhaphy *see* Repair, Duodenum **0DQ9**
Duodenostomy
  see Bypass, Duodenum **0D19**
  see Drainage, Duodenum **0D99**
Duodenotomy *see* Drainage, Duodenum **0D99**
DuraHeart Left Ventricular Assist System *use* Implantable Heart Assist System in Heart and Great Vessels
Dura mater, intracranial *use* Dura Mater
Dura mater, spinal *use* Spinal Meninges
Dural venous sinus *use* Vein, Intracranial
Durata® Defibrillation Lead *use* Cardiac Lead, Defibrillator in **02H**
Dynesys® Dynamic Stabilization System
  use Spinal Stabilization Device, Pedicle-Based in **0RH**
  use Spinal Stabilization Device, Pedicle-Based in **0SH**

E

E-Luminexx™ (Biliary)(Vascular) Stent *use* Intraluminal Device
Earlobe
  use Ear, External, Left
  use Ear, External, Bilateral
  use Ear, External, Right
Echocardiogram *see* Ultrasonography, Heart **B24**
Echography *see* Ultrasonography
ECMO *see* Performance, Circulatory **5A15**
EDWARDS INTUITY Elite valve system *use* Zooplastic Tissue, Rapid Deployment Technique in New Technology
EEG (electroencephalogram) *see* Measurement, Central Nervous **4A00**
EGD (esophagogastroduodenoscopy) **0DJ08ZZ**
Eighth cranial nerve *use* Nerve, Acoustic
Ejaculatory duct
  use Vas Deferens, Bilateral
  use Vas Deferens, Left
  use Vas Deferens, Right
  use Vas Deferens
EKG (electrocardiogram) *see* Measurement, Cardiac **4A02**
Electrical bone growth stimulator (EBGS)
  use Bone Growth Stimulator in Head and Facial Bones
  use Bone Growth Stimulator in Upper Bones
  use Bone Growth Stimulator in Lower Bones
Electrical muscle stimulation (EMS) lead *use* Stimulator Lead in Muscles
Electrocautery
  Destruction *see* Destruction
  Repair *see* Repair

Electroconvulsive Therapy
  Bilateral-Multiple Seizure **GZB3ZZZ**
  Bilateral-Single Seizure **GZB2ZZZ**
Electroconvulsive Therapy *(continued)*
  Electroconvulsive Therapy, Other
    GZB4ZZZ
  Unilateral-Multiple Seizure **GZB1ZZZ**
  Unilateral-Single Seizure **GZB0ZZZ**
Electroencephalogram (EEG) *see*
  Measurement, Central Nervous **4A00**
Electromagnetic Therapy
  Central Nervous **6A22**
  Urinary **6A21**
Electronic muscle stimulator lead *use*
  Stimulator Lead in Muscles
Electrophysiologic stimulation (EPS) *see*
  Measurement, Cardiac **4A02**
Electroshock therapy *see* Electroconvulsive
  Therapy
Elevation, bone fragments, skull *see*
  Reposition, Head and Facial Bones **0NS**
Eleventh cranial nerve *use* Nerve, Accessory
Embolectomy *see* Extirpation
Embolization
  see Occlusion
  see Restriction
Embolization coil(s) *use* Intraluminal Device
EMG (electromyogram) *see* Measurement,
  Musculoskeletal **4A0F**
Encephalon *use* Brain
Endarterectomy
  see Extirpation, Upper Arteries **03C**
  see Extirpation, Lower Arteries **04C**
**Endeavor® (III)(IV) (Sprint) Zotarolimus-
  eluting Coronary Stent System** *use*
  Intraluminal Device, Drug-eluting in Heart
  and Great Vessels
**Endologix AFX(R) Endovascular AAA
  System** *use* Intraluminal Device
EndoSure® sensor *use* Monitoring Device,
  Pressure Sensor in **02H**
**ENDOTAK RELIANCE® (G) Defibrillation
  Lead** *use* Cardiac Lead, Defibrillator in **02H**
Endotracheal tube (cuffed)(double-lumen)
  use Intraluminal Device, Endotracheal
  Airway in Respiratory System
Endurant® II AAA stent graft system *use*
  Intraluminal Device
Endurant® Endovascular Stent Graft *use*
  Intraluminal Device
Enlargement
  see Dilation
  see Repair
EnRhythm *use* Pacemaker, Dual Chamber in
  0JH
Enterorrhaphy *see* Repair, Gastrointestinal
  System **0DQ**
Enterra gastric neurostimulator *use*
  Stimulator Generator, Multiple Array in **0JH**
Enucleation
  Eyeball *see* Resection, Eye **08T**
  Eyeball with prosthetic implant *see*
    Replacement, Eye **08R**
Ependyma *use* Cerebral Ventricle
Epicel® cultured epidermal autograft *use*
  Autologous Tissue Substitute
Epic™ Stented Tissue Valve (aortic) *use*
  Zooplastic Tissue in Heart and Great Vessels

Epidermis *use* Skin
Epididymectomy
  see Excision, Male Reproductive System
    0VB
  see Resection, Male Reproductive System
    0VT
Epididymoplasty
  see Repair, Male Reproductive System **0VQ**
  see Supplement, Male Reproductive System
    0VU
Epididymorrhaphy *see* Repair, Male
  Reproductive System **0VQ**
Epididymotomy *see* Drainage, Male
  Reproductive System **0V9**
Epidural space, intracranial *use* Epidural
  space
Epidural space, spinal *use* Spinal Canal
Epiphysiodesis
  see Fusion, Upper Joints **0RG**
  see Fusion, Lower Joints **0SG**
Epiploic foramen *use* Peritoneum
Epiretinal Visual Prosthesis
  Left **08H105Z**
  Right **08H005Z**
Episiorrhaphy *see* Repair, Perineum, Female
  0WQN
Episiotomy *see* Division, Perineum, Female
  0W8N
Epithalamus *use* Thalamus
Epitrochlear lymph node
  use Lymphatic, Upper Extremity, Left
  use Lymphatic, Upper Extremity, Right
EPS (electrophysiologic stimulation) *see*
  Measurement, Cardiac **4A02**
Eptifibatide, infusion *see* Introduction of
  Platelet Inhibitor
**ERCP (endoscopic retrograde
  cholangiopancreatography)** *see*
  Fluoroscopy, Hepatobiliary System and
  Pancreas **BF1**
Erector spinae muscle
  use Muscle, Trunk, Left
  use Muscle, Trunk, Right
Esophageal artery *use* Upper Artery
Esophageal obturator airway (EOA) *use*
  Intraluminal Device, Airway in
  Gastrointestinal System
Esophageal plexus *use* Nerve, Thoracic
  Sympathetic
Esophagectomy
  see Excision, Gastrointestinal System **0DB**
  see Resection, Gastrointestinal System **0DT**
Esophagocoloplasty
  see Repair, Gastrointestinal System **0DQ**
  see Supplement, Gastrointestinal System
    0DU
Esophagoenterostomy
  see Bypass, Gastrointestinal System **0D1**
  see Drainage, Gastrointestinal System **0D9**
Esophagoesophagostomy
  see Bypass, Gastrointestinal System **0D1**
  see Drainage, Gastrointestinal System **0D9**
Esophagogastrectomy
  see Excision, Gastrointestinal System **0DB**
  see Resection, Gastrointestinal System **0DT**
Esophagogastroduodenoscopy (EGD)
  0DJ08ZZ

Esophagogastroplasty
  see Repair, Gastrointestinal System **0DQ**
  see Supplement, Gastrointestinal System
    0DU
Esophagogastroscopy 0DJ68ZZ
Esophagogastrostomy
  see Bypass, Gastrointestinal System **0D1**
  see Drainage, Gastrointestinal System **0D9**
Esophagojejunoplasty *see* Supplement,
  Gastrointestinal System **0DU**
Esophagojejunostomy
  see Drainage, Gastrointestinal System **0D9**
  see Bypass, Gastrointestinal System **0D1**
Esophagomyotomy *see* Division,
  Esophagogastric Junction **0D84**
Esophagoplasty
  see Repair, Gastrointestinal System **0DQ**
  see Replacement, Esophagus **0DR5**
  see Supplement, Gastrointestinal System
    0DU
Esophagoplication *see* Restriction,
  Gastrointestinal System **0DV**
Esophagorrhaphy *see* Repair, Gastrointestinal
  System **0DQ**
Esophagoscopy 0DJ08ZZ
Esophagotomy *see* Drainage, Gastrointestinal
  System **0D9**
Esteem® implantable hearing system *use*
  Hearing Device in Ear, Nose, Sinus
**ESWL (extracorporeal shock wave
  lithotripsy)** *see* Fragmentation
Ethmoidal air cell
  use Sinus, Ethmoid, Left
  use Sinus, Ethmoid, Right
Ethmoidectomy
  see Excision, Ear, Nose, Sinus **09B**
  see Resection, Ear, Nose, Sinus **09T**
  see Excision, Head and Facial Bones **0NB**
  see Resection, Head and Facial Bones **0NT**
Ethmoidotomy *see* Drainage, Ear, Nose, Sinus
  099
Evacuation
  Hematoma *see* Extirpation
  Other Fluid *see* Drainage
Everolimus-eluting coronary stent *use*
  Intraluminal Device, Drug-eluting in Heart
  and Great Vessels
Evisceration
  Eyeball *see* Resection, Eye **08T**
  Eyeball with prosthetic implant *see*
    Replacement, Eye **08R**
Ex-PRESS™ mini glaucoma shunt *use*
  Synthetic Substitute
Examination *see* Inspection
Exchange *see* Change device in
Excision
  Abdominal Wall **0WBF**
  Acetabulum
    Left **0QB5**
    Right **0QB4**
  Adenoids **0CBQ**
  Ampulla of Vater **0FBC**
  Anal Sphincter **0DBR**
  Ankle Region
    Left **0YBL**
    Right **0YBK**
  Anus **0DBQ**

Excision *(continued)*
- Right **0MBV**
- Perineum **0MBK**
- Shoulder
  - Left **0MB2**
  - Right **0MB1**
- Thorax
  - Left **0MBG**
  - Right **0MBF**
- Trunk
  - Left **0MBD**
  - Right **0MBC**
- Upper Extremity
  - Left **0MBB**
  - Right **0MB9**
- Wrist
  - Left **0MB6**
  - Right **0MB5**
- Buttock
  - Left **0YB1**
  - Right **0YB0**
- Carina **0BB2**
- Carotid Bodies, Bilateral **0GB8**
- Carotid Body
  - Left **0GB6**
  - Right **0GB7**
- Carpal
  - Left **0PBN**
  - Right **0PBM**
- Cecum **0DBH**
- Cerebellum **00BC**
- Cerebral Hemisphere **00B7**
- Cerebral Meninges **00B1**
- Cerebral Ventricle **00B6**
- Cervix **0UBC**
- Chest Wall **0WB8**
- Chordae Tendineae **02B9**
- Choroid
  - Left **08BB**
  - Right **08BA**
- Cisterna Chyli **07BL**
- Clavicle
  - Left **0PBB**
  - Right **0PB9**
- Clitoris **0UBJ**
- Coccygeal Glomus **0GBB**
- Coccyx **0QBS**
- Colon
  - Ascending **0DBK**
  - Descending **0DBM**
  - Sigmoid **0DBN**
  - Transverse **0DBL**
- Conduction Mechanism **02B8**
- Conjunctiva
  - Left **08BTXZ**
  - Right **08BSXZ**
- Cord
  - Bilateral **0VBH**
  - Left **0VBG**
  - Right **0VBF**
- Cornea
  - Left **08B9XZ**
  - Right **08B8XZ**
- Cul-de-sac **0UBF**
- Diaphragm
  - Left **0BBS**

Excision *(continued)*
- Right **0BBR**
- Disc
  - Cervical Vertebral **0RB3**
  - Cervicothoracic Vertebral **0RB5**
  - Lumbar Vertebral **0SB2**
  - Lumbosacral **0SB4**
  - Thoracic Vertebral **0RB9**
  - Thoracolumbar Vertebral **0RBB**
- Duct
  - Common Bile **0FB9**
  - Cystic **0FB8**
  - Hepatic
    - Left **0FB6**
    - Right **0FB5**
  - Lacrimal
    - Left **08BY**
    - Right **08BX**
  - Pancreatic **0FBD**
    - Accessory **0FBF**
  - Parotid
    - Left **0CBC**
    - Right **0CBB**
- Duodenum **0DB9**
- Dura Mater **00B2**
- Ear
  - External
    - Left **09B1**
    - Right **09B0**
  - External Auditory Canal
    - Left **09B4**
    - Right **09B3**
  - Inner
    - Left **09BE0Z**
    - Right **09BD0Z**
  - Middle
    - Left **09B60Z**
    - Right **09B50Z**
- Elbow Region
  - Left **0XBC**
  - Right **0XBB**
- Epididymis
  - Bilateral **0VBL**
  - Left **0VBK**
  - Right **0VBJ**
- Epiglottis **0CBR**
- Esophagogastric Junction **0DB4**
- Esophagus **0DB5**
  - Lower **0DB3**
  - Middle **0DB2**
  - Upper **0DB1**
- Eustachian Tube
  - Left **09BG**
  - Right **09BF**
- Extremity
  - Lower
    - Left **0YBB**
    - Right **0YB9**
  - Upper
    - Left **0XB7**
    - Right **0XB6**
- Eye
  - Left **08B1**
  - Right **08B0**
- Eyelid
  - Lower

Excision *(continued)*
- Left **08BR**
- Right **08BQ**
- Upper
  - Left **08BP**
  - Right **08BN**
- Face **0WB2**
- Fallopian Tube
  - Left **0UB6**
  - Right **0UB5**
- Fallopian Tubes, Bilateral **0UB7**
- Femoral Region
  - Left **0YB8**
  - Right **0YB7**
- Femoral Shaft
  - Left **0QB9**
  - Right **0QB8**
- Femur
  - Lower
    - Left **0QBC**
    - Right **0QBB**
  - Upper
    - Left **0QB7**
    - Right **0QB6**
- Fibula
  - Left **0QBK**
  - Right **0QBJ**
- Finger Nail **0HBQXZ**
- Foot
  - Left **0YBN**
  - Right **0YBM**
- Gallbladder **0FB4**
- Gingiva
  - Lower **0CB6**
  - Upper **0CB5**
- Gland
  - Adrenal
    - Bilateral **0GB4**
    - Left **0GB2**
    - Right **0GB3**
  - Lacrimal
    - Left **08BW**
    - Right **08BV**
  - Minor Salivary **0CBJ**
  - Parotid
    - Left **0CB9**
    - Right **0CB8**
  - Pituitary **0GB0**
  - Sublingual
    - Left **0CBF**
    - Right **0CBD**
  - Submaxillary
    - Left **0CBH**
    - Right **0CBG**
  - Vestibular **0UBL**
- Glenoid Cavity
  - Left **0PB8**
  - Right **0PB7**
- Glomus Jugulare **0GBC**
- Hand
  - Left **0XBK**
  - Right **0XBJ**
- Head **0WB0**
- Humeral Head
  - Left **0PBD**
  - Right **0PBC**

Excision *(continued)*
  Humeral Shaft
    Left **0PBG**
    Right **0PBF**
  Hymen **0UBK**
  Hypothalamus **00BA**
  Ileocecal Valve **0DBC**
  Ileum **0DBB**
  Inguinal Region
    Left **0YB6**
    Right **0YB5**
  Intestine
    Large **0DBE**
      Left **0DBG**
      Right **0DBF**
    Small **0DB8**
  Iris
    Left **08BD3Z**
    Right **08BC3Z**
  Jaw
    Lower **0WB5**
    Upper **0WB4**
  Jejunum **0DBA**
  Joint
    Acromioclavicular
      Left **0RBH**
      Right **0RBG**
    Ankle
      Left **0SBG**
      Right **0SBF**
    Carpal
      Left **0RBR**
      Right **0RBQ**
    Cervical Vertebral **0RB1**
    Cervicothoracic Vertebral **0RB4**
    Coccygeal **0SB6**
    Elbow
      Left **0RBM**
      Right **0RBL**
    Finger Phalangeal
      Left **0RBX**
      Right **0RBW**
    Hip
      Left **0SBB**
      Right **0SB9**
    Knee
      Left **0SBD**
      Right **0SBC**
    Lumbar Vertebral **0SB0**
    Lumbosacral **0SB3**
    Metacarpocarpal
      Left **0RBT**
      Right **0RBS**
    Metacarpophalangeal
      Left **0RBV**
      Right **0RBU**
    Metatarsal-Phalangeal
      Left **0SBN**
      Right **0SBM**
    Metatarsal-Tarsal
      Left **0SBL**
      Right **0SBK**
    Occipital-cervical **0RB0**
    Sacrococcygeal **0SB5**
    Sacroiliac
      Left **0SB8**

Excision *(continued)*
      Right **0SB7**
    Shoulder
      Left **0RBK**
      Right **0RBJ**
    Sternoclavicular
      Left **0RBF**
      Right **0RBE**
    Tarsal
      Left **0SBJ**
      Right **0SBH**
    Temporomandibular
      Left **0RBD**
      Right **0RBC**
    Thoracic Vertebral **0RB6**
    Thoracolumbar Vertebral **0RBA**
    Toe Phalangeal
      Left **0SBQ**
      Right **0SBP**
    Wrist
      Left **0RBP**
      Right **0RBN**
  Kidney
    Left **0TB1**
    Right **0TB0**
  Kidney Pelvis
    Left **0TB4**
    Right **0TB3**
  Knee Region
    Left **0YBG**
    Right **0YBF**
  Larynx **0CBS**
  Leg
    Lower
      Left **0YBJ**
      Right **0YBH**
    Upper
      Left **0YBD**
      Right **0YBC**
  Lens
    Left **08BK3Z**
    Right **08BJ3Z**
  Lip
    Lower **0CB1**
    Upper **0CB0**
  Liver **0FB0**
    Left Lobe **0FB2**
    Right Lobe **0FB1**
  Lung
    Bilateral **0BBM**
    Left **0BBL**
    Lower Lobe
      Left **0BBJ**
      Right **0BBF**
    Middle Lobe, Right **0BBD**
    Right **0BBK**
    Upper Lobe
      Left **0BBG**
      Right **0BBC**
  Lung Lingula **0BBH**
  Lymphatic
    Aortic **07BD**
    Axillary
      Left **07B6**
      Right **07B5**
    Head **07B0**

Excision *(continued)*
    Inguinal
      Left **07BJ**
      Right **07BH**
    Internal Mammary
      Left **07B9**
      Right **07B8**
    Lower Extremity
      Left **07BG**
      Right **07BF**
    Mesenteric **07BB**
    Neck
      Left **07B2**
      Right **07B1**
    Pelvis **07BC**
    Thoracic Duct **07BK**
    Thorax **07B7**
    Upper Extremity
      Left **07B4**
      Right **07B3**
  Mandible
    Left **0NBV**
    Right **0NBT**
  Maxilla
    Left **0NBS**
    Right **0NBR**
  Mediastinum **0WBC**
  Medulla Oblongata **00BD**
  Mesentery **0DBV**
  Metacarpal
    Left **0PBQ**
    Right **0PBP**
  Metatarsal
    Left **0QBP**
    Right **0QBN**
  Muscle
    Abdomen
      Left **0KBL**
      Right **0KBK**
    Extraocular
      Left **08BM**
      Right **08BL**
    Facial **0KB1**
    Foot
      Left **0KBW**
      Right **0KBV**
    Hand
      Left **0KBD**
      Right **0KBC**
    Head **0KB0**
    Hip
      Left **0KBP**
      Right **0KBN**
    Lower Arm and Wrist
      Left **0KBB**
      Right **0KB9**
    Lower Leg
      Left **0KBT**
      Right **0KBS**
    Neck
      Left **0KB3**
      Right **0KB2**
    Papillary **02BD**
    Perineum **0KBM**
    Shoulder
      Left **0KB6**

Right **0KB5**
Thorax
   Left **0KBJ**
   Right **0KBH**
Tongue, Palate, Pharynx **0KB4**
Trunk
   Left **0KBG**
   Right **0KBF**
Upper Arm
   Left **0KB8**
   Right **0KB7**
Upper Leg
   Left **0KBR**
   Right **0KBQ**
Nasopharynx **09BN**
Neck **0WB6**
Nerve
   Abdominal Sympathetic **01BM**
   Abducens **00BL**
   Accessory **00BR**
   Acoustic **00BN**
   Brachial Plexus **01B3**
   Cervical **01B1**
   Cervical Plexus **01B0**
   Facial **00BM**
   Femoral **01BD**
   Glossopharyngeal **00BP**
   Head and Neck Sympathetic **01BK**
   Hypoglossal **00BS**
   Lumbar **01BB**
   Lumbar Plexus **01B9**
   Lumbar Sympathetic **01BN**
   Lumbosacral Plexus **01BA**
   Median **01B5**
   Oculomotor **00BH**
   Olfactory **00BF**
   Optic **00BG**
   Peroneal **01BH**
   Phrenic **01B2**
   Pudendal **01BC**
   Radial **01B6**
   Sacral **01BR**
   Sacral Plexus **01BQ**
   Sacral Sympathetic **01BP**
   Sciatic **01BF**
   Thoracic **01B8**
   Thoracic Sympathetic **01BL**
   Tibial **01BG**
   Trigeminal **00BK**
   Trochlear **00BJ**
   Ulnar **01B4**
   Vagus **00BQ**
Nipple
   Left **0HBX**
   Right **0HBW**
Nose **09BK**
Omentum
   Greater **0DBS**
   Lesser **0DBT**
Orbit
   Left **0NBQ**
   Right **0NBP**
Ovary
   Bilateral **0UB2**
   Left **0UB1**

Right **0UB0**
Palate
   Hard **0CB2**
   Soft **0CB3**
Pancreas **0FBG**
Para-aortic Body **0GB9**
Paraganglion Extremity **0GBF**
Parathyroid Gland **0GBR**
   Inferior
      Left **0GBP**
      Right **0GBN**
   Multiple **0GBQ**
   Superior
      Left **0GBM**
      Right **0GBL**
Patella
   Left **0QBF**
   Right **0QBD**
Penis **0VBS**
Pericardium **02BN**
Perineum
   Female **0WBN**
   Male **0WBM**
Peritoneum **0DBW**
Phalanx
   Finger
      Left **0PBV**
      Right **0PBT**
   Thumb
      Left **0PBS**
      Right **0PBR**
   Toe
      Left **0QBR**
      Right **0QBQ**
Pharynx **0CBM**
Pineal Body **0GB1**
Pleura
   Left **0BBP**
   Right **0BBN**
Pons **00BB**
Prepuce **0VBT**
Prostate **0VB0**
Radius
   Left **0PBJ**
   Right **0PBH**
Rectum **0DBP**
Retina
   Left **08BF3Z**
   Right **08BE3Z**
Retroperitoneum **0WBH**
Rib
   Left **0PB2**
   Right **0PB1**
Sacrum **0QB1**
Scapula
   Left **0PB6**
   Right **0PB5**
Sclera
   Left **08B7XZ**
   Right **08B6XZ**
Scrotum **0VB5**
Septum
   Atrial **02B5**
   Nasal **09BM**
   Ventricular **02BM**

Shoulder Region
   Left **0XB3**
   Right **0XB2**
Sinus
   Accessory **09BP**
   Ethmoid
      Left **09BV**
      Right **09BU**
   Frontal
      Left **09BT**
      Right **09BS**
   Mastoid
      Left **09BC**
      Right **09BB**
   Maxillary
      Left **09BR**
      Right **09BQ**
   Sphenoid
      Left **09BX**
      Right **09BW**
Skin
   Abdomen **0HB7XZ**
   Back **0HB6XZ**
   Buttock **0HB8XZ**
   Chest **0HB5XZ**
   Ear
      Left **0HB3XZ**
      Right **0HB2XZ**
   Face **0HB1XZ**
   Foot
      Left **0HBNXZ**
      Right **0HBMXZ**
   Genitalia **0HBAXZ**
   Hand
      Left **0HBGXZ**
      Right **0HBFXZ**
   Lower Arm
      Left **0HBEXZ**
      Right **0HBDXZ**
   Lower Leg
      Left **0HBLXZ**
      Right **0HBKXZ**
   Neck **0HB4XZ**
   Perineum **0HB9XZ**
   Scalp **0HB0XZ**
   Upper Arm
      Left **0HBCXZ**
      Right **0HBBXZ**
   Upper Leg
      Left **0HBJXZ**
      Right **0HBHXZ**
Skull **0NB0**
Spinal Cord
   Cervical **00BW**
   Lumbar **00BY**
   Thoracic **00BX**
Spinal Meninges **00BT**
Spleen **07BP**
Sternum **0PB0**
Stomach **0DB6**
   Pylorus **0DB7**
Subcutaneous Tissue and Fascia
   Abdomen **0JB8**
   Back **0JB7**
   Buttock **0JB9**

Excision *(continued)*
   Chest **0JB6**
   Face **0JB1**
   Foot
     Left **0JBR**
     Right **0JBQ**
   Hand
     Left **0JBK**
     Right **0JBJ**
   Lower Arm
     Left **0JBH**
     Right **0JBG**
   Lower Leg
     Left **0JBP**
     Right **0JBN**
   Neck
     Anterior **0JB4**
     Posterior **0JB5**
   Pelvic Region **0JBC**
   Perineum **0JBB**
   Scalp **0JB0**
   Upper Arm
     Left **0JBF**
     Right **0JBD**
   Upper Leg
     Left **0JBM**
     Right **0JBL**
Tarsal
   Left **0QBM**
   Right **0QBL**
Tendon
   Abdomen
     Left **0LBG**
     Right **0LBF**
   Ankle
     Left **0LBT**
     Right **0LBS**
   Foot
     Left **0LBW**
     Right **0LBV**
   Hand
     Left **0LB8**
     Right **0LB7**
   Head and Neck **0LB0**
   Hip
     Left **0LBK**
     Right **0LBJ**
   Knee
     Left **0LBR**
     Right **0LBQ**
   Lower Arm and Wrist
     Left **0LB6**
     Right **0LB5**
   Lower Leg
     Left **0LBP**
     Right **0LBN**
   Perineum **0LBH**
   Shoulder
     Left **0LB2**
     Right **0LB1**
   Thorax
     Left **0LBD**
     Right **0LBC**
   Trunk
     Left **0LBB**
     Right **0LB9**

Excision *(continued)*
   Upper Arm
     Left **0LB4**
     Right **0LB3**
   Upper Leg
     Left **0LBM**
     Right **0LBL**
Testis
   Bilateral **0VBC**
   Left **0VBB**
   Right **0VB9**
Thalamus **00B9**
Thymus **07BM**
Thyroid Gland
   Left Lobe **0GBG**
   Right Lobe **0GBH**
Tibia
   Left **0QBH**
   Right **0QBG**
Toe Nail **0HBRXZ**
Tongue **0CB7**
Tonsils **0CBP**
Tooth
   Lower **0CBX**
   Upper **0CBW**
Trachea **0BB1**
Tunica Vaginalis
   Left **0VB7**
   Right **0VB6**
Turbinate, Nasal **09BL**
Tympanic Membrane
   Left **09B8**
   Right **09B7**
Ulna
   Left **0PBL**
   Right **0PBK**
Ureter
   Left **0TB7**
   Right **0TB6**
Urethra **0TBD**
Uterine Supporting Structure **0UB4**
Uterus **0UB9**
Uvula **0CBN**
Vagina **0UBG**
Valve
   Aortic **02BF**
   Mitral **02BG**
   Pulmonary **02BH**
   Tricuspid **02BJ**
Vas Deferens
   Bilateral **0VBQ**
   Left **0VBP**
   Right **0VBN**
Vein
   Axillary
     Left **05B8**
     Right **05B7**
   Azygos **05B0**
   Basilic
     Left **05BC**
     Right **05BB**
   Brachial
     Left **05BA**
     Right **05B9**
   Cephalic
     Left **05BF**

Excision *(continued)*
     Right **05BD**
   Colic **06B7**
   Common Iliac
     Left **06BD**
     Right **06BC**
   Coronary **02B4**
   Esophageal **06B3**
   External Iliac
     Left **06BG**
     Right **06BF**
   External Jugular
     Left **05BQ**
     Right **05BP**
   Face
     Left **05BV**
     Right **05BT**
   Femoral
     Left **06BN**
     Right **06BM**
   Foot
     Left **06BV**
     Right **06BT**
   Gastric **06B2**
   Greater Saphenous
     Left **06BQ**
     Right **06BP**
   Hand
     Left **05BH**
     Right **05BG**
   Hemiazygos **05B1**
   Hepatic **06B4**
   Hypogastric
     Left **06BJ**
     Right **06BH**
   Inferior Mesenteric **06B6**
   Innominate
     Left **05B4**
     Right **05B3**
   Internal Jugular
     Left **05BN**
     Right **05BM**
   Intracranial **05BL**
   Lesser Saphenous
     Left **06BS**
     Right **06BR**
   Lower **06BY**
   Portal **06B8**
   Pulmonary
     Left **02BT**
     Right **02BS**
   Renal
     Left **06BB**
     Right **06B9**
   Splenic **06B1**
   Subclavian
     Left **05B6**
     Right **05B5**
   Superior Mesenteric **06B5**
   Upper **05BY**
   Vertebral
     Left **05BS**
     Right **05BR**
   Vena Cava
     Inferior **06B0**
     Superior **02BV**

Excision *(continued)*
  Ventricle
    Left **02BL**
    Right **02BK**
  Vertebra
    Cervical **0PB3**
    Lumbar **0QB0**
    Thoracic **0PB4**
  Vesicle
    Bilateral **0VB3**
    Left **0VB2**
    Right **0VB1**
  Vitreous
    Left **08B53Z**
    Right **08B43Z**
  Vocal Cord
    Left **0CBV**
    Right **0CBT**
  Vulva **0UBM**
  Wrist Region
    Left **0XBH**
    Right **0XBG**
EXCLUDER(R) AAA Endoprosthesis
  use Intraluminal Device, Branched or Fenestrated, One or Two Arteries in 04V
  use Intraluminal Device, Branched or Fenestrated, Three or More Arteries in 04V
  use Intraluminal Device
EXCLUDER(R) IBE Endoprosthesis *use* Intraluminal Device, Branched or Fenestrated, One or Two Arteries in 04V
Exclusion, Left atrial appendage (LAA) *see* Occlusion, Atrium, Left **02L7**
Exercise, rehabilitation *see* Motor Treatment, Rehabilitation **F07**
Exploration *see* Inspection
Express® (LD) Premounted Stent System *use* Intraluminal Device
Express® Biliary SD Monorail® Premounted Stent System *use* Intraluminal Device
Express® SD Renal Monorail® Premounted Stent System *use* Intraluminal Device
Extensor carpi radialis muscle
  use Muscle, Lower Arm and Wrist, Left
  use Muscle, Lower Arm and Wrist, Right
Extensor carpi ulnaris muscle
  use Muscle, Lower Arm and Wrist, Left
  use Muscle, Lower Arm and Wrist, Right
Extensor digitorum brevis muscle
  use Muscle, Foot, Right
  use Muscle, Foot, Left
Extensor digitorum longus muscle
  use Muscle, Lower Leg, Left
  use Muscle, Lower Leg, Right
Extensor hallucis brevis muscle
  use Muscle, Foot, Right
  use Muscle, Foot, Left
Extensor hallucis longus muscle
  use Muscle, Lower Leg, Right
  use Muscle, Lower Leg, Left
External anal sphincter *use* Anal Sphincter
External auditory meatus
  use Ear, External Auditory Canal, Left
  use Ear, External Auditory Canal, Right

External fixator
  use External Fixation Device in Head and Facial Bones
  use External Fixation Device in Lower Bones
  use External Fixation Device in Lower Joints
  use External Fixation Device in Upper Bones
  use External Fixation Device in Upper Joints
External maxillary artery *use* Artery, Face
External naris *use* Nose
External oblique aponeurosis *use* Subcutaneous Tissue and Fascia, Trunk
External oblique muscle
  use Muscle, Abdomen, Left
  use Muscle, Abdomen, Right
External popliteal nerve *use* Nerve, Peroneal
External pudendal artery
  use Artery, Femoral, Right
  use Artery, Femoral, Left
External pudendal vein
  use Vein, Greater Saphenous, Right
  use Vein, Greater Saphenous, Left
External urethral sphincter *use* Urethra
Extirpation
  Acetabulum
    Left **0QC5**
    Right **0QC4**
  Adenoids **0CCQ**
  Ampulla of Vater **0FCC**
  Anal Sphincter **0DCR**
  Anterior Chamber
    Left **08C3**
    Right **08C2**
  Anus **0DCQ**
  Aorta
    Abdominal **04C0**
    Thoracic
      Ascending/Arch **02CX**
      Descending **02CW**
  Aortic Body **0GCD**
  Appendix **0DCJ**
  Artery
    Anterior Tibial
      Left **04CQ**
      Right **04CP**
    Axillary
      Left **03C6**
      Right **03C5**
    Brachial
      Left **03C8**
      Right **03C7**
    Celiac **04C1**
    Colic
      Left **04C7**
      Middle **04C8**
      Right **04C6**
    Common Carotid
      Left **03CJ**
      Right **03CH**
    Common Iliac
      Left **04CD**
      Right **04CC**
    Coronary
      Four or More Arteries **02C3**

Extirpation *(continued)*
    One Artery **02C0**
    Three Arteries **02C2**
    Two Arteries **02C1**
    External Carotid
      Left **03CN**
      Right **03CM**
    External Iliac
      Left **04CJ**
      Right **04CH**
    Face **03CR**
    Femoral
      Left **04CL**
      Right **04CK**
    Foot
      Left **04CW**
      Right **04CV**
    Gastric **04C2**
    Hand
      Left **03CF**
      Right **03CD**
    Hepatic **04C3**
    Inferior Mesenteric **04CB**
    Innominate **03C2**
    Internal Carotid
      Left **03CL**
      Right **03CK**
    Internal Iliac
      Left **04CF**
      Right **04CE**
    Internal Mammary
      Left **03C1**
      Right **03C0**
    Intracranial **03CG**
    Lower **04CY**
    Peroneal
      Left **04CU**
      Right **04CT**
    Popliteal
      Left **04CN**
      Right **04CM**
    Posterior Tibial
      Left **04CS**
      Right **04CR**
    Pulmonary
      Left **02CR**
      Right **02CQ**
    Pulmonary Trunk **02CP**
    Radial
      Left **03CC**
      Right **03CB**
    Renal
      Left **04CA**
      Right **04C9**
    Splenic **04C4**
    Subclavian
      Left **03C4**
      Right **03C3**
    Superior Mesenteric **04C5**
    Temporal
      Left **03CT**
      Right **03CS**
    Thyroid
      Left **03CV**
      Right **03CU**
    Ulnar

Left **03CA**
Right **03C9**
Upper **03CY**
Vertebral
  Left **03CQ**
  Right **03CP**
Atrium
  Left **02C7**
  Right **02C6**
Auditory Ossicle
  Left **09CA0ZZ**
  Right **09C90ZZ**
Basal Ganglia **00C8**
Bladder **0TCB**
Bladder Neck **0TCC**
Bone
  Ethmoid
    Left **0NCG**
    Right **0NCF**
  Frontal
    Left **0NC2**
    Right **0NC1**
  Hyoid **0NCX**
  Lacrimal
    Left **0NCJ**
    Right **0NCH**
  Nasal **0NCB**
  Occipital
    Left **0NC8**
    Right **0NC7**
  Palatine
    Left **0NCL**
    Right **0NCK**
  Parietal
    Left **0NC4**
    Right **0NC3**
  Pelvic
    Left **0QC3**
    Right **0QC2**
  Sphenoid
    Left **0NCD**
    Right **0NCC**
  Temporal
    Left **0NC6**
    Right **0NC5**
  Zygomatic
    Left **0NCN**
    Right **0NCM**
Brain **00C0**
Breast
  Bilateral **0HCV**
  Left **0HCU**
  Right **0HCT**
Bronchus
  Lingula **0BC9**
  Lower Lobe
    Left **0BCB**
    Right **0BC6**
  Main
    Left **0BC7**
    Right **0BC3**
  Middle Lobe, Right **0BC5**
  Upper Lobe
    Left **0BC8**
    Right **0BC4**

Buccal Mucosa **0CC4**
Bursa and Ligament
  Abdomen
    Left **0MCJ**
    Right **0MCH**
  Ankle
    Left **0MCR**
    Right **0MCQ**
  Elbow
    Left **0MC4**
    Right **0MC3**
  Foot
    Left **0MCT**
    Right **0MCS**
  Hand
    Left **0MC8**
    Right **0MC7**
  Head and Neck **0MC0**
  Hip
    Left **0MCM**
    Right **0MCL**
  Knee
    Left **0MCP**
    Right **0MCN**
  Lower Extremity
    Left **0MCW**
    Right **0MCV**
  Perineum **0MCK**
  Shoulder
    Left **0MC2**
    Right **0MC1**
  Thorax
    Left **0MCG**
    Right **0MCF**
  Trunk
    Left **0MCD**
    Right **0MCC**
  Upper Extremity
    Left **0MCB**
    Right **0MC9**
  Wrist
    Left **0MC6**
    Right **0MC5**
Carina **0BC2**
Carotid Bodies, Bilateral **0GC8**
Carotid Body
  Left **0GC6**
  Right **0GC7**
Carpal
  Left **0PCN**
  Right **0PCM**
Cavity, Cranial **0WC1**
Cecum **0DCH**
Cerebellum **00CC**
Cerebral Hemisphere **00C7**
Cerebral Meninges **00C1**
Cerebral Ventricle **00C6**
Cervix **0UCC**
Chordae Tendineae **02C9**
Choroid
  Left **08CB**
  Right **08CA**
Cisterna Chyli **07CL**
Clavicle
  Left **0PCB**

Right **0PC9**
Clitoris **0UCJ**
Coccygeal Glomus **0GCB**
Coccyx **0QCS**
Colon
  Ascending **0DCK**
  Descending **0DCM**
  Sigmoid **0DCN**
  Transverse **0DCL**
Conduction Mechanism **02C8**
Conjunctiva
  Left **08CTXZZ**
  Right **08CSXZZ**
Cord
  Bilateral **0VCH**
  Left **0VCG**
  Right **0VCF**
Cornea
  Left **08C9XZZ**
  Right **08C8XZZ**
Cul-de-sac **0UCF**
Diaphragm
  Left **0BCS**
  Right **0BCR**
Disc
  Cervical Vertebral **0RC3**
  Cervicothoracic Vertebral **0RC5**
  Lumbar Vertebral **0SC2**
  Lumbosacral **0SC4**
  Thoracic Vertebral **0RC9**
  Thoracolumbar Vertebral **0RCB**
Duct
  Common Bile **0FC9**
  Cystic **0FC8**
  Hepatic
    Left **0FC6**
    Right **0FC5**
  Lacrimal
    Left **08CY**
    Right **08CX**
  Pancreatic **0FCD**
    Accessory **0FCF**
  Parotid
    Left **0CCC**
    Right **0CCB**
Duodenum **0DC9**
Dura Mater **00C2**
Ear
  External
    Left **09C1**
    Right **09C0**
  External Auditory Canal
    Left **09C4**
    Right **09C3**
  Inner
    Left **09CE0ZZ**
    Right **09CD0ZZ**
  Middle
    Left **09C60ZZ**
    Right **09C50ZZ**
Endometrium **0UCB**
Epididymis
  Bilateral **0VCL**
  Left **0VCK**
  Right **0VCJ**

Extirpation *(continued)*
  Epidural Space **00C3**
  Epiglottis **0CCR**
  Esophagogastric Junction **0DC4**
  Esophagus **0DC5**
    Lower **0DC3**
    Middle **0DC2**
    Upper **0DC1**
  Eustachian Tube
    Left **09CG**
    Right **09CF**
  Eye
    Left **08C1XZZ**
    Right **08C0XZZ**
  Eyelid
    Lower
      Left **08CR**
      Right **08CQ**
    Upper
      Left **08CP**
      Right **08CN**
  Fallopian Tube
    Left **0UC6**
    Right **0UC5**
  Fallopian Tubes, Bilateral **0UC7**
  Femoral Shaft
    Left **0QC9**
    Right **0QC8**
  Femur
    Lower
      Left **0QCC**
      Right **0QCB**
    Upper
      Left **0QC7**
      Right **0QC6**
  Fibula
    Left **0QCK**
    Right **0QCJ**
  Finger Nail **0HCQXZZ**
  Gallbladder **0FC4**
  Gastrointestinal Tract **0WCP**
  Genitourinary Tract **0WCR**
  Gingiva
    Lower **0CC6**
    Upper **0CC5**
  Gland
    Adrenal
      Bilateral **0GC4**
      Left **0GC2**
      Right **0GC3**
    Lacrimal
      Left **08CW**
      Right **08CV**
    Minor Salivary **0CCJ**
    Parotid
      Left **0CC9**
      Right **0CC8**
    Pituitary **0GC0**
    Sublingual
      Left **0CCF**
      Right **0CCD**
    Submaxillary
      Left **0CCH**
      Right **0CCG**
    Vestibular **0UCL**
  Glenoid Cavity

  Left **0PC8**
  Right **0PC7**
  Glomus Jugulare **0GCC**
  Humeral Head
    Left **0PCD**
    Right **0PCC**
  Humeral Shaft
    Left **0PCG**
    Right **0PCF**
  Hymen **0UCK**
  Hypothalamus **00CA**
  Ileocecal Valve **0DCC**
  Ileum **0DCB**
  Intestine
    Large **0DCE**
      Left **0DCG**
      Right **0DCF**
    Small **0DC8**
  Iris
    Left **08CD**
    Right **08CC**
  Jejunum **0DCA**
  Joint
    Acromioclavicular
      Left **0RCH**
      Right **0RCG**
    Ankle
      Left **0SCG**
      Right **0SCF**
    Carpal
      Left **0RCR**
      Right **0RCQ**
    Cervical Vertebral **0RC1**
    Cervicothoracic Vertebral **0RC4**
    Coccygeal **0SC6**
    Elbow
      Left **0RCM**
      Right **0RCL**
    Finger Phalangeal
      Left **0RCX**
      Right **0RCW**
    Hip
      Left **0SCB**
      Right **0SC9**
    Knee
      Left **0SCD**
      Right **0SCC**
    Lumbar Vertebral **0SC0**
    Lumbosacral **0SC3**
    Metacarpocarpal
      Left **0RCT**
      Right **0RCS**
    Metacarpophalangeal
      Left **0RCV**
      Right **0RCU**
    Metatarsal-Phalangeal
      Left **0SCN**
      Right **0SCM**
    Metatarsal-Tarsal
      Left **0SCL**
      Right **0SCK**
    Occipital-cervical **0RC0**
    Sacrococcygeal **0SC5**
    Sacroiliac
      Left **0SC8**

    Right **0SC7**
  Shoulder
    Left **0RCK**
    Right **0RCJ**
  Sternoclavicular
    Left **0RCF**
    Right **0RCE**
  Tarsal
    Left **0SCJ**
    Right **0SCH**
  Temporomandibular
    Left **0RCD**
    Right **0RCC**
  Thoracic Vertebral **0RC6**
  Thoracolumbar Vertebral **0RCA**
  Toe Phalangeal
    Left **0SCQ**
    Right **0SCP**
  Wrist
    Left **0RCP**
    Right **0RCN**
  Kidney
    Left **0TC1**
    Right **0TC0**
  Kidney Pelvis
    Left **0TC4**
    Right **0TC3**
  Larynx **0CCS**
  Lens
    Left **08CK**
    Right **08CJ**
  Lip
    Lower **0CC1**
    Upper **0CC0**
  Liver **0FC0**
    Left Lobe **0FC2**
    Right Lobe **0FC1**
  Lung
    Bilateral **0BCM**
    Left **0BCL**
    Lower Lobe
      Left **0BCJ**
      Right **0BCF**
    Middle Lobe, Right **0BCD**
    Right **0BCK**
    Upper Lobe
      Left **0BCG**
      Right **0BCC**
  Lung Lingula **0BCH**
  Lymphatic
    Aortic **07CD**
    Axillary
      Left **07C6**
      Right **07C5**
    Head **07C0**
    Inguinal
      Left **07CJ**
      Right **07CH**
    Internal Mammary
      Left **07C9**
      Right **07C8**
    Lower Extremity
      Left **07CG**
      Right **07CF**
    Mesenteric **07CB**

Neck
    Left **07C2**
    Right **07C1**
Pelvis **07CC**
Thoracic Duct **07CK**
Thorax **07C7**
Upper Extremity
    Left **07C4**
    Right **07C3**
Mandible
    Left **0NCV**
    Right **0NCT**
Maxilla
    Left **0NCS**
    Right **0NCR**
Mediastinum **0WCC**
Medulla Oblongata **00CD**
Mesentery **0DCV**
Metacarpal
    Left **0PCQ**
    Right **0PCP**
Metatarsal
    Left **0QCP**
    Right **0QCN**
Muscle
  Abdomen
    Left **0KCL**
    Right **0KCK**
  Extraocular
    Left **08CM**
    Right **08CL**
  Facial **0KC1**
  Foot
    Left **0KCW**
    Right **0KCV**
  Hand
    Left **0KCD**
    Right **0KCC**
  Head **0KC0**
  Hip
    Left **0KCP**
    Right **0KCN**
  Lower Arm and Wrist
    Left **0KCB**
    Right **0KC9**
  Lower Leg
    Left **0KCT**
    Right **0KCS**
  Neck
    Left **0KC3**
    Right **0KC2**
  Papillary **02CD**
  Perineum **0KCM**
  Shoulder
    Left **0KC6**
    Right **0KC5**
  Thorax
    Left **0KCJ**
    Right **0KCH**
  Tongue, Palate, Pharynx **0KC4**
  Trunk
    Left **0KCG**
    Right **0KCF**
  Upper Arm
    Left **0KC8**

    Right **0KC7**
  Upper Leg
    Left **0KCR**
    Right **0KCQ**
Nasopharynx **09CN**
Nerve
  Abdominal Sympathetic **01CM**
  Abducens **00CL**
  Accessory **00CR**
  Acoustic **00CN**
  Brachial Plexus **01C3**
  Cervical **01C1**
  Cervical Plexus **01C0**
  Facial **00CM**
  Femoral **01CD**
  Glossopharyngeal **00CP**
  Head and Neck Sympathetic **01CK**
  Hypoglossal **00CS**
  Lumbar **01CB**
  Lumbar Plexus **01C9**
  Lumbar Sympathetic **01CN**
  Lumbosacral Plexus **01CA**
  Median **01C5**
  Oculomotor **00CH**
  Olfactory **00CF**
  Optic **00CG**
  Peroneal **01CH**
  Phrenic **01C2**
  Pudendal **01CC**
  Radial **01C6**
  Sacral **01CR**
  Sacral Plexus **01CQ**
  Sacral Sympathetic **01CP**
  Sciatic **01CF**
  Thoracic **01C8**
  Thoracic Sympathetic **01CL**
  Tibial **01CG**
  Trigeminal **00CK**
  Trochlear **00CJ**
  Ulnar **01C4**
  Vagus **00CQ**
Nipple
  Left **0HCX**
  Right **0HCW**
Nose **09CK**
Omentum
  Greater **0DCS**
  Lesser **0DCT**
Oral Cavity and Throat **0WC3**
Orbit
  Left **0NCQ**
  Right **0NCP**
Orbital Atherectomy Technology **X2C**
Ovary
  Bilateral **0UC2**
  Left **0UC1**
  Right **0UC0**
Palate
  Hard **0CC2**
  Soft **0CC3**
Pancreas **0FCG**
Para-aortic Body **0GC9**
Paraganglion Extremity **0GCF**
Parathyroid Gland **0GCR**
  Inferior

    Left **0GCP**
    Right **0GCN**
  Multiple **0GCQ**
  Superior
    Left **0GCM**
    Right **0GCL**
Patella
  Left **0QCF**
  Right **0QCD**
Pelvic Cavity **0WCJ**
Penis **0VCS**
Pericardial Cavity **0WCD**
Pericardium **02CN**
Peritoneal Cavity **0WCG**
Peritoneum **0DCW**
Phalanx
  Finger
    Left **0PCV**
    Right **0PCT**
  Thumb
    Left **0PCS**
    Right **0PCR**
  Toe
    Left **0QCR**
    Right **0QCQ**
Pharynx **0CCM**
Pineal Body **0GC1**
Pleura
  Left **0BCP**
  Right **0BCN**
Pleural Cavity
  Left **0WCB**
  Right **0WC9**
Pons **00CB**
Prepuce **0VCT**
Prostate **0VC0**
Radius
  Left **0PCJ**
  Right **0PCH**
Rectum **0DCP**
Respiratory Tract **0WCQ**
Retina
  Left **08CF**
  Right **08CE**
Retinal Vessel
  Left **08CH**
  Right **08CG**
Rib
  Left **0PC2**
  Right **0PC1**
Sacrum **0QC1**
Scapula
  Left **0PC6**
  Right **0PC5**
Sclera
  Left **08C7XZZ**
  Right **08C6XZZ**
Scrotum **0VC5**
Septum
  Atrial **02C5**
  Nasal **09CM**
  Ventricular **02CM**
Sinus
  Accessory **09CP**
  Ethmoid

Extirpation *(continued)*

    Left **09CV**

    Right **09CU**

  Frontal

    Left **09CT**

    Right **09CS**

  Mastoid

    Left **09CC**

    Right **09CB**

  Maxillary

    Left **09CR**

    Right **09CQ**

  Sphenoid

    Left **09CX**

    Right **09CW**

Skin

  Abdomen **0HC7XZZ**

  Back **0HC6XZZ**

  Buttock **0HC8XZZ**

  Chest **0HC5XZZ**

  Ear

    Left **0HC3XZZ**

    Right **0HC2XZZ**

  Face **0HC1XZZ**

  Foot

    Left **0HCNXZZ**

    Right **0HCMXZZ**

  Genitalia **0HCAXZZ**

  Hand

    Left **0HCGXZZ**

    Right **0HCFXZZ**

  Lower Arm

    Left **0HCEXZZ**

    Right **0HCDXZZ**

  Lower Leg

    Left **0HCLXZZ**

    Right **0HCKXZZ**

  Neck **0HC4XZZ**

  Perineum **0HC9XZZ**

  Scalp **0HC0XZZ**

  Upper Arm

    Left **0HCCXZZ**

    Right **0HCBXZZ**

  Upper Leg

    Left **0HCJXZZ**

    Right **0HCHXZZ**

Spinal Cord

  Cervical **00CW**

  Lumbar **00CY**

  Thoracic **00CX**

Spinal Meninges **00CT**

Spleen **07CP**

Sternum **0PC0**

Stomach **0DC6**

  Pylorus **0DC7**

Subarachnoid Space **00C5**

Subcutaneous Tissue and Fascia

  Abdomen **0JC8**

  Back **0JC7**

  Buttock **0JC9**

  Chest **0JC6**

  Face **0JC1**

  Foot

    Left **0JCR**

    Right **0JCQ**

  Hand

Extirpation *(continued)*

    Left **0JCK**

    Right **0JCJ**

  Lower Arm

    Left **0JCH**

    Right **0JCG**

  Lower Leg

    Left **0JCP**

    Right **0JCN**

  Neck

    Anterior **0JC4**

    Posterior **0JC5**

  Pelvic Region **0JCC**

  Perineum **0JCB**

  Scalp **0JC0**

  Upper Arm

    Left **0JCF**

    Right **0JCD**

  Upper Leg

    Left **0JCM**

    Right **0JCL**

Subdural Space **00C4**

Tarsal

  Left **0QCM**

  Right **0QCL**

Tendon

  Abdomen

    Left **0LCG**

    Right **0LCF**

  Ankle

    Left **0LCT**

    Right **0LCS**

  Foot

    Left **0LCW**

    Right **0LCV**

  Hand

    Left **0LC8**

    Right **0LC7**

  Head and Neck **0LC0**

  Hip

    Left **0LCK**

    Right **0LCJ**

  Knee

    Left **0LCR**

    Right **0LCQ**

  Lower Arm and Wrist

    Left **0LC6**

    Right **0LC5**

  Lower Leg

    Left **0LCP**

    Right **0LCN**

  Perineum **0LCH**

  Shoulder

    Left **0LC2**

    Right **0LC1**

  Thorax

    Left **0LCD**

    Right **0LCC**

  Trunk

    Left **0LCB**

    Right **0LC9**

  Upper Arm

    Left **0LC4**

    Right **0LC3**

  Upper Leg

    Left **0LCM**

Extirpation *(continued)*

    Right **0LCL**

Testis

  Bilateral **0VCC**

  Left **0VCB**

  Right **0VC9**

Thalamus **00C9**

Thymus **07CM**

Thyroid Gland **0GCK**

  Left Lobe **0GCG**

  Right Lobe **0GCH**

Tibia

  Left **0QCH**

  Right **0QCG**

Toe Nail **0HCRXZZ**

Tongue **0CC7**

Tonsils **0CCP**

Tooth

  Lower **0CCX**

  Upper **0CCW**

Trachea **0BC1**

Tunica Vaginalis

  Left **0VC7**

  Right **0VC6**

Turbinate, Nasal **09CL**

Tympanic Membrane

  Left **09C8**

  Right **09C7**

Ulna

  Left **0PCL**

  Right **0PCK**

Ureter

  Left **0TC7**

  Right **0TC6**

Urethra **0TCD**

Uterine Supporting Structure **0UC4**

Uterus **0UC9**

Uvula **0CCN**

Vagina **0UCG**

Valve

  Aortic **02CF**

  Mitral **02CG**

  Pulmonary **02CH**

  Tricuspid **02CJ**

Vas Deferens

  Bilateral **0VCQ**

  Left **0VCP**

  Right **0VCN**

Vein

  Axillary

    Left **05C8**

    Right **05C7**

  Azygos **05C0**

  Basilic

    Left **05CC**

    Right **05CB**

  Brachial

    Left **05CA**

    Right **05C9**

  Cephalic

    Left **05CF**

    Right **05CD**

  Colic **06C7**

  Common Iliac

    Left **06CD**

    Right **06CC**

Extirpation (continued)
Coronary 02C4
Esophageal 06C3
External Iliac
  Left 06CG
  Right 06CF
External Jugular
  Left 05CQ
  Right 05CP
Face
  Left 05CV
  Right 05CT
Femoral
  Left 06CN
  Right 06CM
Foot
  Left 06CV
  Right 06CT
Gastric 06C2
Greater Saphenous
  Left 06CQ
  Right 06CP
Hand
  Left 05CH
  Right 05CG
Hemiazygos 05C1
Hepatic 06C4
Hypogastric
  Left 06CJ
  Right 06CH
Inferior Mesenteric 06C6
Innominate
  Left 05C4
  Right 05C3
Internal Jugular
  Left 05CN
  Right 05CM
Intracranial 05CL
Lesser Saphenous
  Left 06CS
  Right 06CR
Lower 06CY
Portal 06C8
Pulmonary
  Left 02CT
  Right 02CS
Renal
  Left 06CB
  Right 06C9
Splenic 06C1
Subclavian
  Left 05C6
  Right 05C5
Superior Mesenteric 06C5
Upper 05CY
Vertebral
  Left 05CS
  Right 05CR
Vena Cava
  Inferior 06C0
  Superior 02CV
Ventricle
  Left 02CL
  Right 02CK
Vertebra
  Cervical 0PC3

Extirpation (continued)
Lumbar 0QC0
Thoracic 0PC4
Vesicle
  Bilateral 0VC3
  Left 0VC2
  Right 0VC1
Vitreous
  Left 08C5
  Right 08C4
Vocal Cord
  Left 0CCV
  Right 0CCT
Vulva 0UCM
Extracorporeal shock wave lithotripsy see
Fragmentation
Extracranial-intracranial bypass (EC-IC)
  see Bypass, Upper Arteries 031
Extraction
Auditory Ossicle
  Left 09DA0ZZ
  Right 09D90ZZ
Bone Marrow
  Iliac 07DR
  Sternum 07DQ
  Vertebral 07DS
Bursa and Ligament
  Abdomen
    Left 0MDJ
    Right 0MDH
  Ankle
    Left 0MDR
    Right 0MDQ
  Elbow
    Left 0MD4
    Right 0MD3
  Foot
    Left 0MDT
    Right 0MDS
  Hand
    Left 0MD8
    Right 0MD7
  Head and Neck 0MD0
  Hip
    Left 0MDM
    Right 0MDL
  Knee
    Left 0MDP
    Right 0MDN
  Lower Extremity
    Left 0MDW
    Right 0MDV
  Perineum 0MDK
  Shoulder
    Left 0MD2
    Right 0MD1
  Thorax
    Left 0MDG
    Right 0MDF
  Trunk
    Left 0MDD
    Right 0MDC
  Upper Extremity
    Left 0MDB
    Right 0MD9
  Wrist

Extraction (continued)
  Left 0MD6
  Right 0MD5
Cerebral Meninges 00D1
Cornea
  Left 08D9XZ
  Right 08D8XZ
Dura Mater 00D2
Endometrium 0UDB
Finger Nail 0HDQXZZ
Hair 0HDSXZZ
Kidney
  Left 0TD1
  Right 0TD0
Lens
  Left 08DK3ZZ
  Right 08DJ3ZZ
Nerve
  Abdominal Sympathetic 01DM
  Abducens 00DL
  Accessory 00DR
  Acoustic 00DN
  Brachial Plexus 01D3
  Cervical 01D1
  Cervical Plexus 01D0
  Facial 00DM
  Femoral 01DD
  Glossopharyngeal 00DP
  Head and Neck Sympathetic 01DK
  Hypoglossal 00DS
  Lumbar 01DB
  Lumbar Plexus 01D9
  Lumbar Sympathetic 01DN
  Lumbosacral Plexus 01DA
  Median 01D5
  Oculomotor 00DH
  Olfactory 00DF
  Optic 00DG
  Peroneal 01DH
  Phrenic 01D2
  Pudendal 01DC
  Radial 01D6
  Sacral 01DR
  Sacral Plexus 01DQ
  Sacral Sympathetic 01DP
  Sciatic 01DF
  Thoracic 01D8
  Thoracic Sympathetic 01DL
  Tibial 01DG
  Trigeminal 00DK
  Trochlear 00DJ
  Ulnar 01D4
  Vagus 00DQ
Ova 0UDN
Pleura
  Left 0BDP
  Right 0BDN
Products of Conception
  Classical 10D00Z0
  Ectopic 10D2
  Extraperitoneal 10D00Z2
  High Forceps 10D07Z5
  Internal Version 10D07Z7
  Low Cervical 10D00Z1
  Low Forceps 10D07Z3
  Mid Forceps 10D07Z4

Extraction *(continued)*
    Other **10D07Z8**
    Retained **10D1**
    Vacuum **10D07Z6**
  Septum, Nasal **09DM**
  Sinus
    Accessory **09DP**
    Ethmoid
      Left **09DV**
      Right **09DU**
    Frontal
      Left **09DT**
      Right **09DS**
    Mastoid
      Left **09DC**
      Right **09DB**
    Maxillary
      Left **09DR**
      Right **09DQ**
    Sphenoid
      Left **09DX**
      Right **09DW**
  Skin
    Abdomen **0HD7XZZ**
    Back **0HD6XZZ**
    Buttock **0HD8XZZ**
    Chest **0HD5XZZ**
    Ear
      Left **0HD3XZZ**
      Right **0HD2XZZ**
    Face **0HD1XZZ**
    Foot
      Left **0HDNXZZ**
      Right **0HDMXZZ**
    Genitalia **0HDAXZZ**
    Hand
      Left **0HDGXZZ**
      Right **0HDFXZZ**
    Lower Arm
      Left **0HDEXZZ**
      Right **0HDDXZZ**
    Lower Leg
      Left **0HDLXZZ**
      Right **0HDKXZZ**
    Neck **0HD4XZZ**
    Perineum **0HD9XZZ**
    Scalp **0HD0XZZ**
    Upper Arm
      Left **0HDCXZZ**
      Right **0HDBXZZ**
    Upper Leg
      Left **0HDJXZZ**
      Right **0HDHXZZ**
  Spinal Meninges **00DT**
  Subcutaneous Tissue and Fascia
    Abdomen **0JD8**
    Back **0JD7**
    Buttock **0JD9**
    Chest **0JD6**
    Face **0JD1**
    Foot
      Left **0JDR**
      Right **0JDQ**
    Hand
      Left **0JDK**
      Right **0JDJ**

Extraction *(continued)*
    Lower Arm
      Left **0JDH**
      Right **0JDG**
    Lower Leg
      Left **0JDP**
      Right **0JDN**
    Neck
      Anterior **0JD4**
      Posterior **0JD5**
    Pelvic Region **0JDC**
    Perineum **0JDB**
    Scalp **0JD0**
    Upper Arm
      Left **0JDF**
      Right **0JDD**
    Upper Leg
      Left **0JDM**
      Right **0JDL**
  Toe Nail **0HDRXZZ**
  Tooth
    Lower **0CDXXZ**
    Upper **0CDWXZ**
  Turbinate, Nasal **09DL**
  Tympanic Membrane
    Left **09D8**
    Right **09D7**
  Vein
    Basilic
      Left **05DC**
      Right **05DB**
    Brachial
      Left **05DA**
      Right **05D9**
    Cephalic
      Left **05DF**
      Right **05DD**
    Femoral
      Left **06DN**
      Right **06DM**
    Foot
      Left **06DV**
      Right **06DT**
    Greater Saphenous
      Left **06DQ**
      Right **06DP**
    Hand
      Left **05DH**
      Right **05DG**
    Lesser Saphenous
      Left **06DS**
      Right **06DR**
    Lower **06DY**
    Upper **05DY**
  Vocal Cord
    Left **0CDV**
    Right **0CDT**
Extradural space, intracranial *use* Epidural Space
Extradural space, spinal *use* Spinal Canal
EXtreme Lateral Interbody Fusion (XLIF) device *use* Interbody Fusion Device in Lower Joints

F

Face lift *see* Alteration, Face **0W02**
Facet replacement spinal stabilization device
  use Spinal Stabilization Device, Facet Replacement in **0RH**
  use Spinal Stabilization Device, Facet Replacement in **0SH**
Facial artery *use* Artery, Face
Factor Xa Inhibitor Reversal Agent, Andexanet Alfa *use* Andexanet Alfa, Factor Xa Inhibitor Reversal Agent
False vocal cord *use* Larynx
Falx cerebri *use* Dura Mater
Fascia lata
  use Subcutaneous Tissue and Fascia, Upper Leg, Left
  use Subcutaneous Tissue and Fascia, Upper Leg, Right
Fasciaplasty, fascioplasty
  see Repair, Subcutaneous Tissue and Fascia **0JQ**
  see Replacement, Subcutaneous Tissue and Fascia **0JR**
Fasciectomy *see* Excision, Subcutaneous Tissue and Fascia **0JB**
Fasciorrhaphy *see* Repair, Subcutaneous Tissue and Fascia **0JQ**
Fasciotomy
  see Division, Subcutaneous Tissue and Fascia **0J8**
  see Drainage, Subcutaneous Tissue and Fascia **0J9**
  see Release
Feeding Device
  Change device in
    Lower **0D2DXUZ**
    Upper **0D20XUZ**
  Insertion of device in
    Duodenum **0DH9**
    Esophagus **0DH5**
    Ileum **0DHB**
    Intestine, Small **0DH8**
    Jejunum **0DHA**
    Stomach **0DH6**
  Removal of device from
    Esophagus **0DP5**
    Intestinal Tract
      Lower **0DPD**
      Upper **0DP0**
    Stomach **0DP6**
  Revision of device in
    Intestinal Tract
      Lower **0DWD**
      Upper **0DW0**
    Stomach **0DW6**
Femoral head
  use Femur, Upper, Right
  use Femur, Upper, Left
  use Lymphatic, Lower Extremity, Left
  use Lymphatic, Lower Extremity, Right
Femoropatellar joint
  use Joint, Knee, Right
  use Joint, Knee, Right, Femoral Surface
  use Joint, Knee, Left
  use Joint, Knee, Left, Femoral Surface
Femorotibial joint
  use Joint, Knee, Right

Femorotibial joint *(continued)*
   use Joint, Knee, Right, Tibial Surface
   use Joint, Knee, Left
   use Joint, Knee, Left, Tibial Surface
Fibular artery
   use Artery, Peroneal, Right
   use Artery, Peroneal, Left
Fibularis brevis muscle
   use Muscle, Lower Leg, Left
   use Muscle, Lower Leg, Right
Fibularis longus muscle
   use Muscle, Lower Leg, Left
   use Muscle, Lower Leg, Right
Fifth cranial nerve *use* Nerve, Trigeminal
Filum terminale *use* Spinal Meninges
Fimbriectomy
   see Excision, Female Reproductive System **0UB**
   see Resection, Female Reproductive System **0UT**
Fine needle aspiration
   fluid or gas *see* Drainage
   tissue *see* Excision
First cranial nerve *use* Nerve, Olfactory
First intercostal nerve *use* Nerve, Brachial Plexus
Fistulization
   see Bypass
   see Drainage
   see Repair
Fitting
   Arch bars, for fracture reduction *see* Reposition, Mouth and Throat **0CS**
   Arch bars, for immobilization *see* Immobilization, Face **2W31**
   Artificial limb *see* Device Fitting, Rehabilitation **F0D**
   Hearing aid *see* Device Fitting, Rehabilitation **F0D**
   Ocular prosthesis **F0DZ8UZ**
   Prosthesis, limb *see* Device Fitting, Rehabilitation **F0D**
   Prosthesis, ocular **F0DZ8UZ**
Fixation, bone
   External, with fracture reduction *see* Reposition
   External, without fracture reduction *see* Insertion
   Internal, with fracture reduction *see* Reposition
   Internal, without fracture reduction *see* Insertion
FLAIR® Endovascular Stent Graft *use* Intraluminal Device
Flexible Composite Mesh *use* Synthetic Substitute
Flexor carpi radialis muscle
   use Muscle, Lower Arm and Wrist, Right
   use Muscle, Lower Arm and Wrist, Left
Flexor carpi ulnaris muscle
   use Muscle, Lower Arm and Wrist, Right
   use Muscle, Lower Arm and Wrist, Left
Flexor digitorum brevis muscle
   use Muscle, Foot, Left
   use Muscle, Foot, Right

Flexor digitorum longus muscle
   use Muscle, Lower Leg, Left
   use Muscle, Lower Leg, Right
Flexor hallucis brevis muscle
   use Muscle, Foot, Left
   use Muscle, Foot, Right
Flexor hallucis longus muscle
   use Muscle, Lower Leg, Right
   use Muscle, Lower Leg, Left
Flexor pollicis longus muscle
   use Muscle, Lower Arm and Wrist, Left
   use Muscle, Lower Arm and Wrist, Right
Fluoroscopy
   Abdomen and Pelvis **BW11**
   Airway, Upper **BB1DZZZ**
   Ankle
     Left **BQ1H**
     Right **BQ1G**
   Aorta
     Abdominal **B410**
       Laser, Intraoperative **B410**
     Thoracic **B310**
       Laser, Intraoperative **B310**
     Thoraco-Abdominal **B31P**
       Laser, Intraoperative **B31P**
   Aorta and Bilateral Lower Extremity Arteries **B41D**
     Laser, Intraoperative **B41D**
   Arm
     Left **BP1FZZZ**
     Right **BP1EZZZ**
   Artery
     Brachiocephalic-Subclavian
       Right **B311**
         Laser, Intraoperative **B311**
     Bronchial **B31L**
       Laser, Intraoperative **B31L**
     Bypass Graft, Other **B21F**
     Cervico-Cerebral Arch **B31Q**
       Laser, Intraoperative **B31Q**
     Common Carotid
       Bilateral **B315**
         Laser, Intraoperative **B315**
       Left **B314**
         Laser, Intraoperative **B314**
       Right **B313**
         Laser, Intraoperative **B313**
     Coronary
       Bypass Graft
         Multiple **B213**
         Laser, Intraoperative **B213**
         Single **B212**
       Laser, Intraoperative **B212**
         Multiple **B211**
           Laser, Intraoperative **B211**
         Single **B210**
           Laser, Intraoperative **B210**
     External Carotid
       Bilateral **B31C**
         Laser, Intraoperative **B31C**
       Left **B31B**
         Laser, Intraoperative **B31B**
       Right **B319**
         Laser, Intraoperative **B319**
     Hepatic **B412**
       Laser, Intraoperative **B412**

Fluoroscopy *(continued)*
     Inferior Mesenteric **B415**
       Laser, Intraoperative **B415**
     Intercostal **B31L**
       Laser, Intraoperative **B31L**
     Internal Carotid
       Bilateral **B318**
         Laser, Intraoperative **B318**
       Left **B317**
         Laser, Intraoperative **B317**
       Right **B316**
         Laser, Intraoperative **B316**
     Internal Mammary Bypass Graft
       Left **B218**
       Right **B217**
     Intra-Abdominal
       Other **B41B**
       Laser, Intraoperative **B41B**
     Intracranial **B31R**
       Laser, Intraoperative **B31R**
     Lower
       Other **B41J**
       Laser, Intraoperative **B41J**
     Lower Extremity
       Bilateral and Aorta **B41D**
         Laser, Intraoperative **B41D**
       Left **B41G**
         Laser, Intraoperative **B41G**
       Right **B41F**
         Laser, Intraoperative **B41F**
     Lumbar **B419**
       Laser, Intraoperative **B419**
     Pelvic **B41C**
       Laser, Intraoperative **B41C**
     Pulmonary
       Left **B31T**
         Laser, Intraoperative **B31T**
       Right **B31S**
         Laser, Intraoperative **B31S**
     Renal
       Bilateral **B418**
         Laser, Intraoperative **B418**
       Left **B417**
         Laser, Intraoperative **B417**
       Right **B416**
         Laser, Intraoperative **B416**
     Spinal **B31M**
       Laser, Intraoperative **B31M**
     Splenic **B413**
       Laser, Intraoperative **B413**
     Subclavian
       Left **B312**
       Laser, Intraoperative **B312**
     Superior Mesenteric **B414**
       Laser, Intraoperative **B414**
     Upper
       Other **B31N**
       Laser, Intraoperative **B31N**
     Upper Extremity
       Bilateral **B31K**
         Laser, Intraoperative **B31K**
       Left **B31J**
         Laser, Intraoperative **B31J**
       Right **B31H**
         Laser, Intraoperative **B31H**
     Vertebral

Fluoroscopy *(continued)*
- Bilateral **B31G**
  - Laser, Intraoperative **B31G**
- Left **B31F**
  - Laser, Intraoperative **B31F**
- Right **B31D**
  - Laser, Intraoperative **B31D**
- Bile Duct **BF10**
  - Pancreatic Duct and Gallbladder **BF14**
- Bile Duct and Gallbladder **BF13**
- Biliary Duct **BF11**
- Bladder **BT10**
  - Kidney and Ureter **BT14**
    - Left **BT1F**
    - Right **BT1D**
- Bladder and Urethra **BT1B**
- Bowel, Small **BD1**
- Calcaneus
  - Left **BQ1KZZZ**
  - Right **BQ1JZZZ**
- Clavicle
  - Left **BP15ZZZ**
  - Right **BP14ZZZ**
- Coccyx **BR1F**
- Colon **BD14**
- Corpora Cavernosa **BV10**
- Dialysis Fistula **B51W**
- Dialysis Shunt **B51W**
- Diaphragm **BB16ZZZ**
- Disc
  - Cervical **BR11**
  - Lumbar **BR13**
  - Thoracic **BR12**
- Duodenum **BD19**
- Elbow
  - Left **BP1H**
  - Right **BP1G**
- Epiglottis **B91G**
- Esophagus **BD11**
- Extremity
  - Lower **BW1C**
  - Upper **BW1J**
- Facet Joint
  - Cervical **BR14**
  - Lumbar **BR16**
  - Thoracic **BR15**
- Fallopian Tube
  - Bilateral **BU12**
  - Left **BU11**
  - Right **BU10**
- Fallopian Tube and Uterus **BU18**
- Femur
  - Left **BQ14ZZZ**
  - Right **BQ13ZZZ**
- Finger
  - Left **BP1SZZZ**
  - Right **BP1RZZZ**
- Foot
  - Left **BQ1MZZZ**
  - Right **BQ1LZZZ**
- Forearm
  - Left **BP1KZZZ**
  - Right **BP1JZZZ**
- Gallbladder **BF12**
  - Bile Duct and Pancreatic Duct **BF14**
- Gallbladder and Bile Duct **BF13**

Fluoroscopy *(continued)*
- Gastrointestinal, Upper **BD1**
- Hand
  - Left **BP1PZZZ**
  - Right **BP1NZZZ**
- Head and Neck **BW19**
- Heart
  - Left **B215**
  - Right **B214**
  - Right and Left **B216**
- Hip
  - Left **BQ11**
  - Right **BQ10**
- Humerus
  - Left **BP1BZZZ**
  - Right **BP1AZZZ**
- Ileal Diversion Loop **BT1C**
- Ileal Loop, Ureters and Kidney **BT1G**
- Intracranial Sinus **B512**
- Joint
  - Acromioclavicular, Bilateral **BP13ZZZ**
  - Finger
    - Left **BP1D**
    - Right **BP1C**
  - Foot
    - Left **BQ1Y**
    - Right **BQ1X**
  - Hand
    - Left **BP1D**
    - Right **BP1C**
  - Lumbosacral **BR1B**
  - Sacroiliac **BR1D**
  - Sternoclavicular
    - Bilateral **BP12ZZZ**
    - Left **BP11ZZZ**
    - Right **BP10ZZZ**
  - Temporomandibular
    - Bilateral **BN19**
    - Left **BN18**
    - Right **BN17**
  - Thoracolumbar **BR18**
  - Toe
    - Left **BQ1Y**
    - Right **BQ1X**
- Kidney
  - Bilateral **BT13**
  - Ileal Loop and Ureter **BT1G**
  - Left **BT12**
  - Right **BT11**
  - Ureter and Bladder **BT14**
    - Left **BT1F**
    - Right **BT1D**
- Knee
  - Left **BQ18**
  - Right **BQ17**
- Larynx **B91J**
- Laser intraoperative
  - *see* Fluoroscopy, Heart B21
  - *see* Fluoroscopy, Upper Arteries B31
  - *see* Fluoroscopy, Lower Arteries B41
- Leg
  - Left **BQ1FZZZ**
  - Right **BQ1DZZZ**
- Lung
  - Bilateral **BB14ZZZ**
  - Left **BB13ZZZ**

Fluoroscopy *(continued)*
- Right **BB12ZZZ**
- Mediastinum **BB1CZZZ**
- Mouth **BD1B**
- Neck and Head **BW19**
- Oropharynx **BD1B**
- Pancreatic Duct **BF1**
  - Gallbladder and Bile Duct **BF14**
- Patella
  - Left **BQ1WZZZ**
  - Right **BQ1VZZZ**
- Pelvis **BR1C**
- Pelvis and Abdomen **BW11**
- Pharynx **B91G**
- Ribs
  - Left **BP1YZZZ**
  - Right **BP1XZZZ**
- Sacrum **BR1F**
- Scapula
  - Left **BP17ZZZ**
  - Right **BP16ZZZ**
- Shoulder
  - Left **BP19**
  - Right **BP18**
- Sinus, Intracranial **B512**
- Spinal Cord **B01B**
- Spine
  - Cervical **BR10**
  - Lumbar **BR19**
  - Thoracic **BR17**
  - Whole **BR1G**
- Sternum **BR1H**
- Stomach **BD12**
- Toe
  - Left **BQ1QZZZ**
  - Right **BQ1PZZZ**
- Tracheobronchial Tree
  - Bilateral **BB19YZZ**
  - Left **BB18YZZ**
  - Right **BB17YZZ**
- Ureter
  - Ileal Loop and Kidney **BT1G**
  - Kidney and Bladder **BT14**
    - Left **BT1F**
    - Right **BT1D**
  - Left **BT17**
  - Right **BT16**
- Urethra **BT15**
- Urethra and Bladder **BT1B**
- Uterus **BU16**
- Uterus and Fallopian Tube **BU18**
- Vagina **BU19**
- Vasa Vasorum **BV18**
- Vein
  - Cerebellar **B511**
  - Cerebral **B511**
  - Epidural **B510**
  - Jugular
    - Bilateral **B515**
    - Left **B514**
    - Right **B513**
  - Lower Extremity
    - Bilateral **B51D**
    - Left **B51C**
    - Right **B51B**
  - Other **B51V**

Fluoroscopy (continued)
- Pelvic (Iliac)
  - Left **B51G**
  - Right **B51F**
- Pelvic (Iliac) Bilateral **B51H**
- Portal **B51T**
- Pulmonary
  - Bilateral **B51S**
  - Left **B51R**
  - Right **B51Q**
- Renal
  - Bilateral **B51L**
  - Left **B51K**
  - Right **B51J**
- Splanchnic **B51T**
- Subclavian
  - Left **B517**
  - Right **B516**
- Upper Extremity
  - Bilateral **B51P**
  - Left **B51N**
  - Right **B51M**
- Vena Cava
  - Inferior **B519**
  - Superior **B518**
- Wrist
  - Left **BP1M**
  - Right **BP1L**

Flushing see Irrigation
Foley catheter use Drainage Device
Foramen magnum
- use Bone, Occipital, Right
- use Bone, Occipital, Left

Foramen of Monro (intraventricular) use Cerebral Ventricle
Foreskin use Prepuce
Formula™ Balloon-Expandable Renal Stent System use Intraluminal Device
Fossa of Rosenmüller use Nasopharynx
Fourth cranial nerve use Nerve, Trochlear
Fourth ventricle use Cerebral Ventricle
Fovea
- use Retina, Right
- use Retina, Left

Fragmentation
- Ampulla of Vater **0FFC**
- Anus **0DFQ**
- Appendix **0DFJ**
- Bladder **0TFB**
- Bladder Neck **0TFC**
- Bronchus
  - Lingula **0BF9**
  - Lower Lobe
    - Left **0BFB**
    - Right **0BF6**
  - Main
    - Left **0BF7**
    - Right **0BF3**
  - Middle Lobe, Right **0BF5**
  - Upper Lobe
    - Left **0BF8**
    - Right **0BF4**
- Carina **0BF2**
- Cavity, Cranial **0WF1**
- Cecum **0DFH**
- Cerebral Ventricle **00F6**

Fragmentation (continued)
- Colon
  - Ascending **0DFK**
  - Descending **0DFM**
  - Sigmoid **0DFN**
  - Transverse **0DFL**
- Duct
  - Common Bile **0FF9**
  - Cystic **0FF8**
  - Hepatic
    - Left **0FF6**
    - Right **0FF5**
  - Pancreatic **0FFD**
    - Accessory **0FFF**
  - Parotid
    - Left **0CFC**
    - Right **0CFB**
- Duodenum **0DF9**
- Epidural Space **00F3**
- Esophagus **0DF5**
- Fallopian Tube
  - Left **0UF6**
  - Right **0UF5**
- Fallopian Tubes, Bilateral **0UF7**
- Gallbladder **0FF4**
- Gastrointestinal Tract **0WFP**
- Genitourinary Tract **0WFR**
- Ileum **0DFB**
- Intestine
  - Large **0DFE**
    - Left **0DFG**
    - Right **0DFF**
  - Small **0DF8**
- Jejunum **0DFA**
- Kidney Pelvis
  - Left **0TF4**
  - Right **0TF3**
- Mediastinum **0WFC**
- Oral Cavity and Throat **0WF3**
- Pelvic Cavity **0WFJ**
- Pericardial Cavity **0WFD**
- Pericardium **02FN**
- Peritoneal Cavity **0WFG**
- Pleural Cavity
  - Left **0WFB**
  - Right **0WF9**
- Rectum **0DFP**
- Respiratory Tract **0WFQ**
- Spinal Canal **00FU**
- Stomach **0DF6**
- Subarachnoid Space **00F5**
- Subdural Space **00F4**
- Trachea **0BF1**
- Ureter
  - Left **0TF7**
  - Right **0TF6**
- Urethra **0TFD**
- Uterus **0UF9**
- Vitreous
  - Left **08F5**
  - Right **08F4**

Freestyle (Stentless) Aortic Root Bioprosthesis use Zooplastic Tissue in Heart and Great Vessels

Frenectomy
- see Excision, Mouth and Throat **0CB**
- see Resection, Mouth and Throat **0CT**

Frenoplasty, frenuloplasty
- see Repair, Mouth and Throat **0CQ**
- see Replacement, Mouth and Throat **0CR**

Frenoplasty, frenuloplasty (continued)
- see Supplement, Mouth and Throat **0CU**

Frenotomy
- see Drainage, Mouth and Throat **0C9**
- see Release, Mouth and Throat **0CN**

Frenulotomy
- see Drainage, Mouth and Throat **0C9**
- see Release, Mouth and Throat **0CN**

Frenulum labii inferioris use Lip, Lower
Frenulum labii superioris use Lip, Upper
Frenulum linguae use Tongue
Frenulumectomy
- see Excision, Mouth and Throat **0CB**
- see Resection, Mouth and Throat **0CT**

Frontal lobe use Cerebral Hemisphere
Frontal vein
- use Vein, Face, Right
- use Vein, Face, Left

Fulguration see Destruction
Fundoplication, gastroesophageal see Restriction, Esophagogastric Junction **0DV4**
Fundus uteri use Uterus
Fusion
- Acromioclavicular
  - Left **0RGH**
  - Right **0RGG**
- Ankle
  - Left **0SGG**
  - Right **0SGF**
- Carpal
  - Left **0RGR**
  - Right **0RGQ**
  - Interbody Fusion Device, Nanotextured Surface **XRG2092**
  - Interbody Fusion Device, Nanotextured Surface **XRG1092**
- Cervical Vertebral **0RG1**
  - 2 or more **0RG2**
- Cervicothoracic Vertebral **0RG4**
  - Interbody Fusion Device, Nanotextured Surface **XRG4092**
- Coccygeal **0SG6**
- Elbow
  - Left **0RGM**
  - Right **0RGL**
- Finger Phalangeal
  - Left **0RGX**
  - Right **0RGW**
- Hip
  - Left **0SGB**
  - Right **0SG9**
- Knee
  - Left **0SGD**
  - Right **0SGC**
- Lumbar Vertebral **0SG0**
  - 2 or more **0SG1**
  - Interbody Fusion Device, Nanotextured Surface **XRGC092**
  - Interbody Fusion Device, Nanotextured Surface **XRGB092**

Fusion (continued)
  Lumbosacral **0SG3**
    Interbody Fusion Device, Nanotextured
    Surface **XRGD092**
  Metacarpocarpal
    Left **0RGT**
    Right **0RGS**
  Metacarpophalangeal
    Left **0RGV**
    Right **0RGU**
  Metatarsal-Phalangeal
    Left **0SGN**
    Right **0SGM**
  Metatarsal-Tarsal
    Left **0SGL**
    Right **0SGK**
  Occipital-cervical **0RG0**
    Interbody Fusion Device, Nanotextured
      Surface **XRG0092**
  Sacrococcygeal **0SG5**
  Sacroiliac
    Left **0SG8**
    Right **0SG7**
  Shoulder
    Left **0RGK**
    Right **0RGJ**
  Sternoclavicular
    Left **0RGF**
    Right **0RGE**
  Tarsal
    Left **0SGJ**
    Right **0SGH**
  Temporomandibular
    Left **0RGD**
    Right **0RGC**
  Thoracic Vertebral **0RG6**
    2 to 7 **0RG7**
      Interbody Fusion Device, Nanotextured
        Surface **XRG7092**
    8 or more **0RG8**
      Interbody Fusion Device,
        Nanotextured Surface **XRG8092**
      Interbody Fusion Device,
        Nanotextured Surface **XRG6092**
  Thoracolumbar Vertebral **0RGA**
  Toe Phalangeal
    Left **0SGQ**
    Right **0SGP**
  Wrist
    Left **0RGP**
    Right **0RGN**
Fusion screw (compression)(lag)(locking)
  use Internal Fixation Device in Upper
    Joints
  use Internal Fixation Device in Lower
    Joints

G

Gait training *see* Motor Treatment,
  Rehabilitation **F07**
Galea aponeurotica *use* Subcutaneous Tissue
  and Fascia, Scalp
Ganglion impar (ganglion of Walther) *use*
  Nerve, Sacral Sympathetic

Ganglionectomy
  Destruction of lesion *see* Destruction
  Excision of lesion *see* Excision
Gasserian ganglion *use* Nerve, Trigeminal
Gastrectomy
  Partial *see* Excision, Stomach **0DB6**
  Total *see* Resection, Stomach **0DT6**
Gastrectomy (continued)
  Vertical (sleeve) *see* Excision, Stomach
    0DB6
Gastric electrical stimulation (GES) lead *use*
  Stimulator Lead in Gastrointestinal System
Gastric lymph node *use* Lymphatic, Aortic
Gastric pacemaker lead *use* Stimulator Lead
  in Gastrointestinal System
Gastric plexus *use* Nerve, Abdominal
  Sympathetic
Gastrocnemius muscle
  use Muscle, Lower Leg, Left
  use Muscle, Lower Leg, Right
Gastrocolic ligament *use* Omentum, Greater
Gastrocolic omentum *use* Omentum, Greater
Gastrocolostomy
  see Bypass, Gastrointestinal System **0D1**
  see Drainage, Gastrointestinal System **0D9**
Gastroduodenal artery *use* Artery, Hepatic
Gastroduodenectomy
  see Excision, Gastrointestinal System **0DB**
  see Resection, Gastrointestinal System **0DT**
Gastroduodenoscopy 0DJ08ZZ
Gastroenteroplasty
  see Repair, Gastrointestinal System **0DQ**
  see Supplement, Gastrointestinal System
    0DU
Gastroenterostomy
  see Bypass, Gastrointestinal System **0D1**
  see Drainage, Gastrointestinal System **0D9**
Gastroesophageal (GE) junction *use*
  Esophagogastric Junction
Gastrogastrostomy
  see Bypass, Stomach **0D16**
  see Drainage, Stomach **0D96**
Gastrohepatic omentum *use* Omentum,
  Lesser
Gastrojejunostomy
  see Bypass, Stomach **0D16**
  see Drainage, Stomach **0D96**
Gastrolysis *see* Release, Stomach **0DN6**
Gastropexy
  see Repair, Stomach **0DQ6**
  see Reposition, Stomach **0DS6**
Gastrophrenic ligament *use* Omentum,
  Greater
Gastroplasty
  see Repair, Stomach **0DQ6**
  see Supplement, Stomach **0DU6**
Gastroplication *see* Restriction, Stomach
  0DV6
Gastropylorectomy *see* Excision,
  Gastrointestinal System **0DB**
Gastrorrhaphy *see* Repair, Stomach **0DQ6**
Gastroscopy 0DJ68ZZ
Gastrosplenic ligament *use* Omentum, Greater
Gastrostomy
  see Bypass, Stomach **0D16**
  see Drainage, Stomach **0D96**
Gastrotomy *see* Drainage, Stomach **0D96**

Gemellus muscle
  use Muscle, Hip, Left
  use Muscle, Hip, Right
Geniculate ganglion *use* Nerve, Facial
Geniculate nucleus *use* Thalamus
Genioglossus muscle *use* Muscle, Tongue,
  Palate, Pharynx
Genioplasty *see* Alteration, Jaw, Lower **0W05**
Genitofemoral nerve *use* Nerve, Lumbar
  Plexus
Gingivectomy *see* Excision, Mouth and Throat
  0CB
Gingivoplasty
  see Repair, Mouth and Throat **0CQ**
  see Replacement, Mouth and Throat **0CR**
  see Supplement, Mouth and Throat **0CU**
Glans penis *use* Prepuce
Glenohumeral joint
  use Joint, Shoulder, Left
  use Joint, Shoulder, Right
Glenohumeral ligament
  use Bursa and Ligament, Shoulder, Right
  use Bursa and Ligament, Shoulder, Left
Glenoid fossa (of scapula)
  use Glenoid Cavity, Left
  use Glenoid Cavity, Right
Glenoid ligament (labrum)
  use Shoulder Joint, Left
  use Shoulder Joint, Right
Globus pallidus *use* Basal Ganglia
Glomectomy
  see Excision, Endocrine System **0GB**
  see Resection, Endocrine System **0GT**
Glossectomy
  see Excision, Tongue **0CB7**
  see Resection, Tongue **0CT7**
Glossoepiglottic fold *use* Epiglottis
Glossopexy
  see Repair, Tongue **0CQ7**
  see Reposition, Tongue **0CS7**
Glossoplasty
  see Repair, Tongue **0CQ7**
  see Replacement, Tongue **0CR7**
  see Supplement, Tongue **0CU7**
Glossorrhaphy *see* Repair, Tongue **0CQ7**
Glossotomy *see* Drainage, Tongue **0C97**
Glottis *use* Larynx
Gluteal Artery Perforator Flap
  Bilateral **0HRV079**
  Left **0HRU079**
  Right **0HRT079**
Gluteal lymph node *use* Lymphatic, Pelvis
Gluteal vein
  use Vein, Hypogastric, Right
  use Vein, Hypogastric, Left
Gluteus maximus muscle
  use Muscle, Hip, Right
  use Muscle, Hip, Left
Gluteus medius muscle
  use Muscle, Hip, Right
  use Muscle, Hip, Left
Gluteus minimus muscle
  use Muscle, Hip, Left
  use Muscle, Hip, Right
GORE® DUALMESH® *use* Synthetic
  Substitute

GORE EXCLUDER(R) AAA Endoprosthesis
- *use* Intraluminal Device, Branched or Fenestrated, One or Two Arteries in 04V
- *use* Intraluminal Device, Branched or Fenestrated, Three or More Arteries in 04V
- *use* Intraluminal Device

GORE EXCLUDER(R) IBE Endoprosthesis
- *use* Intraluminal Device, Branched or Fenestrated, One or Two Arteries in 04V

GORE TAG(R) Thoracic Endoprosthesis
- *use* Intraluminal Device

Gracilis muscle
- *use* Muscle, Upper Leg, Left
- *use* Muscle, Upper Leg, Right

Graft
- *see* Replacement
- *see* Supplement

Great auricular nerve *use* Nerve, Cervical Plexus

Great cerebral vein *use* Vein, Intracranial

Great saphenous vein
- *use* Vein, Greater Saphenous, Left
- *use* Vein, Greater Saphenous, Right

Greater alar cartilage *use* Nose

Greater occipital nerve *use* Nerve, Cervical

Greater splanchnic nerve *use* Nerve, Thoracic Sympathetic

Greater superficial petrosal nerve *use* Nerve, Facial

Greater trochanter
- *use* Femur, Upper, Left
- *use* Femur, Upper, Right

Greater tuberosity
- *use* Humeral Head, Right
- *use* Humeral Head, Left

Greater vestibular (Bartholin's) gland *use* Gland, Vestibular

Greater wing
- *use* Bone, Sphenoid, Left
- *use* Bone, Sphenoid, Right

Guedel airway *use* Intraluminal Device, Airway in Mouth and Throat

Guidance, catheter placement
- EKG *see* Measurement, Physiological Systems **4A0**
- Fluoroscopy *see* Fluoroscopy, Veins **B51**
- Ultrasound *see* Ultrasonography, Veins **B54**

H

Hallux
- *use* Toe, 1st, Right
- *use* Toe, 1st, Left

Hamate bone
- *use* Carpal, Right
- *use* Carpal, Left

Hancock Bioprosthesis (aortic) (mitral) valve *use* Zooplastic Tissue in Heart and Great Vessels

Hancock Bioprosthetic Valved Conduit *use* Zooplastic Tissue in Heart and Great Vessels

Harvesting, stem cells *see* Pheresis, Circulatory **6A55**

Head of fibula
- *use* Fibula, Right
- *use* Fibula, Left

Hearing Aid Assessment F14Z

Hearing Assessment F13Z

Hearing Device
- Bone Conduction
  - Left **09HE**
  - Right **09HD**
- Insertion of device in
  - Left **0NH6[034]SZ**
  - Right **0NH5[034]SZ**
- Multiple Channel Cochlear Prosthesis
  - Left **09HE**
  - Right **09HD**
- Removal of device from, Skull **0NP0**
- Revision of device in, Skull **0NW0**
- Single Channel Cochlear Prosthesis
  - Left **09HE**
  - Right **09HD** Hearing Treatment **F09Z**

Heart Assist System
- External
  - Insertion of device in, Heart **02HA**
  - Removal of device from, Heart **02PA**
  - Revision of device in, Heart **02WA**
- Implantable
  - Insertion of device in, Heart **02HA**

Heart Assist System *(continued)*
  - Removal of device from, Heart **02PA**
  - Revision of device in, Heart **02WA**

HeartMate II® Left Ventricular Assist Device (LVAD) *use* Implantable Heart Assist System in Heart and Great Vessels

HeartMate XVE® Left Ventricular Assist Device (LVAD) *use* Implantable Heart Assist System in Heart and Great Vessels

HeartMate® implantable heart assist system *see* Insertion of device in, Heart **02HA**

Helix
- *use* Ear, External, Bilateral
- *use* Ear, External, Right
- *use* Ear, External, Left

Hematopoietic cell transplant (HCT) *see* Transfusion, Circulatory **302**

Hemicolectomy *see* Resection, Gastrointestinal System **0DT**

Hemicystectomy *see* Excision, Urinary System **0TB**

Hemigastrectomy *see* Excision, Gastrointestinal System **0DB**

Hemiglossectomy *see* Excision, Mouth and Throat **0CB**

Hemilaminectomy
- *see* Excision, Upper Bones **0PB**
- *see* Excision, Lower Bones **0QB**

Hemilaryngectomy *see* Excision, Larynx **0CBS**

Hemimandibulectomy *see* Excision, Head and Facial Bones **0NB**

Hemimaxillectomy *see* Excision, Head and Facial Bones **0NB**

Hemipylorectomy *see* Excision, Gastrointestinal System **0DB**

Hemispherectomy
- *see* Excision, Central Nervous System **00B**
- *see* Resection, Central Nervous System **00T**

Hemithyroidectomy
- *see* Resection, Endocrine System **0GT**
- *see* Excision, Endocrine System **0GB**

Hemodialysis 5A1D00Z

Hepatectomy
- *see* Excision, Hepatobiliary System and Pancreas **0FB**
- *see* Resection, Hepatobiliary System and Pancreas **0FT**

Hepatic artery proper *use* Artery, Hepatic

Hepatic flexure *use* Colon, Ascending

Hepatic lymph node *use* Lymphatic, Aortic

Hepatic plexus *use* Nerve, Abdominal Sympathetic

Hepatic portal vein *use* Vein, Portal

Hepaticoduodenostomy
- *see* Bypass, Hepatobiliary System and Pancreas **0F1**
- *see* Drainage, Hepatobiliary System and Pancreas **0F9**

Hepaticotomy *see* Drainage, Hepatobiliary System and Pancreas **0F9**

Hepatocholedochostomy *see* Drainage, Duct, Common Bile **0F99**

Hepatogastric ligament *use* Omentum, Lesser

Hepatopancreatic ampulla *use* Ampulla of Vater

Hepatopexy
- *see* Repair, Hepatobiliary System and Pancreas **0FQ**
- *see* Reposition, Hepatobiliary System and Pancreas **0FS**

Hepatorrhaphy *see* Repair, Hepatobiliary System and Pancreas **0FQ**

Hepatotomy *see* Drainage, Hepatobiliary System and Pancreas **0F9**

Herniorrhaphy
- *see* Repair, Anatomical Regions, General **0WQ**
- *see* Repair, Anatomical Regions, Lower Extremities **0YQ**
- with synthetic substitute
  - *see* Supplement, Anatomical Regions, General **0WU**

Herniorrhaphy *(continued)*
- *see* Supplement, Anatomical Regions, Lower Extremities **0YU**

Hip (joint) liner *use* Liner in Lower Joints

Holter monitoring 4A12X45

Holter valve ventricular shunt *use* Synthetic Substitute

Humeroradial joint
- *use* Joint, Elbow, Right
- *use* Joint, Elbow, Left

Humeroulnar joint
- *use* Joint, Elbow, Left
- *use* Joint, Elbow, Right

Humerus, distal
- *use* Humeral Shaft, Right
- *use* Humeral Shaft, Left

Hydrocelectomy *see* Excision, Male Reproductive System **0VB**

Hydrotherapy
- Assisted exercise in pool *see* Motor Treatment, Rehabilitation **F07**
- Whirlpool *see* Activities of Daily Living Treatment, Rehabilitation **F08**

Hymenectomy
  see Excision, Hymen **0UBK**
  see Resection, Hymen **0UTK**
Hymenoplasty
  see Repair, Hymen **0UQK**
  see Supplement, Hymen **0UUK**
Hymenorrhaphy *see* Repair, Hymen **0UQK**
Hymenotomy
  see Division, Hymen **0U8K**
  see Drainage, Hymen **0U9K**
Hyoglossus muscle *use* Muscle, Tongue,
  Palate, Pharynx
Hyoid artery
  use Artery, Thyroid, Right
  use Artery, Thyroid, Left
Hyperalimentation *see* Introduction of
  substance in or on
Hyperbaric oxygenation
  Decompression sickness treatment *see*
  Decompression, Circulatory **6A15**
  Wound treatment *see* Assistance,
  Circulatory **5A05**
Hyperthermia
  Radiation Therapy
    Abdomen **DWY38ZZ**
    Adrenal Gland **DGY28ZZ**
    Bile Ducts **DFY28ZZ**
    Bladder **DTY28ZZ**
    Bone, Other **DPYC8ZZ**
    Bone Marrow **D7Y08ZZ**
    Brain **D0Y08ZZ**
    Brain Stem **D0Y18ZZ**
    Breast
      Left **DMY08ZZ**
      Right **DMY18ZZ**
    Bronchus **DBY18ZZ**
    Cervix **DUY18ZZ**
    Chest **DWY28ZZ**
    Chest Wall **DBY78ZZ**
    Colon **DDY58ZZ**
    Diaphragm **DBY88ZZ**
    Duodenum **DDY28ZZ**
    Ear **D9Y08ZZ**
    Esophagus **DDY08ZZ**
    Eye **D8Y08ZZ**
    Femur **DPY98ZZ**
    Fibula **DPYB8ZZ**
    Gallbladder **DFY18ZZ**
    Gland
      Adrenal **DGY28ZZ**
      Parathyroid **DGY48ZZ**
      Pituitary **DGY08ZZ**
      Thyroid **DGY58ZZ**
    Glands, Salivary **D9Y68ZZ**
    Head and Neck **DWY18ZZ**
    Hemibody **DWY48ZZ**
    Humerus **DPY68ZZ**
    Hypopharynx **D9Y38ZZ**
    Ileum **DDY48ZZ**
    Jejunum **DDY38ZZ**
    Kidney **DTY08ZZ**
    Larynx **D9YB8ZZ**
    Liver **DFY08ZZ**
    Lung **DBY28ZZ**
    Lymphatics
      Abdomen **D7Y68ZZ**

Hyperthermia *(continued)*
    Axillary **D7Y48ZZ**
    Inguinal **D7Y88ZZ**
    Neck **D7Y38ZZ**
    Pelvis **D7Y78ZZ**
    Thorax **D7Y58ZZ**
  Mandible **DPY38ZZ**
  Maxilla **DPY28ZZ**
  Mediastinum **DBY68ZZ**
  Mouth **D9Y48ZZ**
  Nasopharynx **D9YD8ZZ**
  Neck and Head **DWY18ZZ**
  Nerve, Peripheral **D0Y78ZZ**
  Nose **D9Y18ZZ**
  Oropharynx **D9YF8ZZ**
  Ovary **DUY08ZZ**
  Palate
    Hard **D9Y88ZZ**
    Soft **D9Y98ZZ**
  Pancreas **DFY38ZZ**
  Parathyroid Gland **DGY48ZZ**
  Pelvic Bones **DPY88ZZ**
  Pelvic Region **DWY68ZZ**
  Pineal Body **DGY18ZZ**
  Pituitary Gland **DGY08ZZ**
  Pleura **DBY58ZZ**
  Prostate **DVY08ZZ**
  Radius **DPY78ZZ**
  Rectum **DDY78ZZ**
  Rib **DPY58ZZ**
  Sinuses **D9Y78ZZ**
  Skin
    Abdomen **DHY88ZZ**
    Arm **DHY48ZZ**
    Back **DHY78ZZ**
    Buttock **DHY98ZZ**
    Chest **DHY68ZZ**
    Face **DHY28ZZ**
    Leg **DHYB8ZZ**
    Neck **DHY38ZZ**
  Skull **DPY08ZZ**
  Spinal Cord **D0Y68ZZ**
  Spleen **D7Y28ZZ**
  Sternum **DPY48ZZ**
  Stomach **DDY18ZZ**
  Testis **DVY18ZZ**
  Thymus **D7Y18ZZ**
  Thyroid Gland **DGY58ZZ**
  Tibia **DPYB8ZZ**
  Tongue **D9Y58ZZ**
  Trachea **DBY08ZZ**
  Ulna **DPY78ZZ**
  Ureter **DTY18ZZ**
  Urethra **DTY38ZZ**
  Uterus **DUY28ZZ**
  Whole Body **DWY58ZZ**
  Whole Body **6A3Z**
Hypnosis GZFZZZZZ
Hypogastric artery
  use Artery, Internal Iliac, Right
  use Artery, Internal Iliac, Left
Hypopharynx *use* Pharynx
Hypophysectomy
  see Excision, Gland, Pituitary **0GB0**
  see Resection, Gland, Pituitary **0GT0**
Hypophysis *use* Gland, Pituitary

Hypothalamotomy *see* Destruction, Thalamus
  0059
Hypothenar muscle
  use Muscle, Hand, Right
  use Muscle, Hand, Left
Hypothermia, Whole Body 6A4Z
Hysterectomy
  supracervical *see* Resection, Uterus **0UT9**
  total
    see Resection, Cervix **0UTC**
    see Resection, Uterus **0UT9**
Hysterolysis *see* Release, Uterus **0UN9**
Hysteropexy
  see Repair, Uterus **0UQ9**
  see Reposition, Uterus **0US9**
Hysteroplasty *see* Repair, Uterus **0UQ9**
Hysterorrhaphy *see* Repair, Uterus **0UQ9**
Hysteroscopy 0UJD8ZZ
Hysterotomy *see* Drainage, Uterus **0U99**
Hysterotrachelectomy
  see Resection, Cervix **0UTC**
  see Resection, Uterus **0UT9**
Hysterotracheloplasty *see* Repair, Uterus
  0UQ9
Hysterotrachelorrhaphy *see* Repair, Uterus
  0UQ9

I

IABP (Intra-aortic balloon pump) *see*
  Assistance, Cardiac **5A02**
IAEMT (Intraoperative anesthetic effect
  monitoring and titration) *see* Monitoring,
  Central Nervous **4A10**
Idarucizumab, Dabigatran Reversal Agent
  XW0
Ileal artery *use* Artery, Superior Mesenteric
Ileectomy
  see Excision, Ileum **0DBB**
  see Resection, Ileum **0DTB**
Ileocolic artery *use* Artery, Superior
  Mesenteric
Ileocolic vein *use* Vein, Colic
Ileopexy
  see Repair, Ileum **0DQB**
  see Reposition, Ileum **0DSB**
Ileorrhaphy *see* Repair, Ileum **0DQB**
Ileoscopy 0DJD8ZZ
Ileostomy
  see Bypass, Ileum **0D1B**
  see Drainage, Ileum **0D9B**
Ileotomy *see* Drainage, Ileum **0D9B**
Ileoureterostomy *see* Bypass, Urinary System
  0T1
Iliac crest
  use Bone, Pelvic, Left
  use Bone, Pelvic, Right
Iliac fascia
  use Subcutaneous Tissue and Fascia, Upper
  Leg, Left
  use Subcutaneous Tissue and Fascia, Upper
  Leg, Right
Iliac lymph node *use* Lymphatic, Pelvis
Iliacus muscle
  use Muscle, Hip, Right
  use Muscle, Hip, Left

Iliofemoral ligament
  use Bursa and Ligament, Hip, Left
  use Bursa and Ligament, Hip, Right
Iliohypogastric nerve *use* Nerve, Lumbar Plexus
Ilioinguinal nerve *use* Nerve, Lumbar Plexus
Iliolumbar artery
  use Artery, Internal Iliac, Left
  use Artery, Internal Iliac, Right
Iliolumbar ligament
  use Bursa and Ligament, Trunk, Left
  use Bursa and Ligament, Trunk, Right
Iliotibial tract (band)
  use Subcutaneous Tissue and Fascia, Upper Leg, Right
  use Subcutaneous Tissue and Fascia, Upper Leg, Left
Ilium
  use Bone, Pelvic, Left
  use Bone, Pelvic, Right
Ilizarov external fixator
  use External Fixation Device, Ring in **0PH**
  use External Fixation Device, Ring in **0PS**
  use External Fixation Device, Ring in **0QH**
  use External Fixation Device, Ring in **0QS**
Ilizarov-Vecklich device
  use External Fixation Device, Limb Lengthening in **0PH**
  use External Fixation Device, Limb Lengthening in **0QH**
Imaging, diagnostic
  see Plain Radiography
  see Fluoroscopy
  see Computerized Tomography (CT Scan)
  see Magnetic Resonance Imaging (MRI)
  see Ultrasonography
Immobilization
  Abdominal Wall **2W33X**
  Arm
    Lower
      Left **2W3DX**
      Right **2W3CX**
    Upper
      Left **2W3BX**
      Right **2W3AX**
  Back **2W35X**
  Chest Wall **2W34X**
  Extremity
    Lower
      Left **2W3MX**
      Right **2W3LX**
    Upper
      Left **2W39X**
      Right **2W38X**
  Face **2W31X**
  Finger
    Left **2W3KX**
    Right **2W3JX**
  Foot
    Left **2W3TX**
    Right **2W3SX**
  Hand
    Left **2W3FX**
    Right **2W3EX**
  Head **2W30X**
  Inguinal Region

Immobilization *(continued)*
    Left **2W37X**
    Right **2W36X**
  Leg
    Lower
      Left **2W3RX**
      Right **2W3QX**
    Upper
      Left **2W3PX**
      Right **2W3NX**
  Neck **2W32X**
  Thumb
    Left **2W3HX**
    Right **2W3GX**
  Toe
    Left **2W3VX**
    Right **2W3UX**
Immunization *see* Introduction of Serum, Toxoid, and Vaccine
Immunotherapy *see* Introduction of Immunotherapeutic Substance
Immunotherapy, antineoplastic
  Interferon *see* Introduction of Low-dose Interleukin-2
  Interleukin-2, high-dose *see* Introduction of High-dose Interleukin-2
  Interleukin-2, low-dose *see* Introduction of Low-dose Interleukin-2
  Monoclonal antibody *see* Introduction of Monoclonal Antibody
  Proleukin, high-dose *see* Introduction of High-dose Interleukin-2
  Proleukin, low-dose *see* Introduction of Low-dose Interleukin-2
Impella® (2.5) (5.0) (LD) cardiac assist device *use* Intraluminal Device
Impeller Pump
  Continuous, Output **5A0221D**
  Intermittent, Output **5A0211D**
Implantable cardioverter-defibrillator (ICD) *use* Defibrillator Generator in **0JH**
Implantable drug infusion pump (anti-spasmodic)(chemotherapy)(pain) *use* Infusion Device, Pump in Subcutaneous Tissue and Fascia
Implantable glucose monitoring device *use* Monitoring Device
Implantable hemodynamic monitor (IHM) *use* Monitoring Device, Hemodynamic in **0JH**
Implantable hemodynamic monitoring system (IHMS) *use* Monitoring Device, Hemodynamic in **0JH**
Implantable Miniature Telescope™ (IMT) *use* Synthetic Substitute, Intraocular Telescope in **08R**
Implantation
  see Insertion
  see Replacement
Implanted (venous)(access) port *use* Vascular Access Device, Reservoir in Subcutaneous Tissue and Fascia
IMV (intermittent mandatory ventilation) *see* Assistance, Respiratory **5A09**
In Vitro Fertilization 8E0ZXY1
Incision, abscess *see* Drainage

Incudectomy
  see Excision, Ear, Nose, Sinus **09B**
  see Resection, Ear, Nose, Sinus **09T**
Incudopexy
  see Reposition, Ear, Nose, Sinus **09S**
  see Repair, Ear, Nose, Sinus **09Q**
Incus
  use Auditory Ossicle, Left
  use Auditory Ossicle, Right
Induction of labor
  Artificial rupture of membranes *see* Drainage, Pregnancy **109**
  Oxytocin *see* Introduction of Hormone
InDura, intrathecal catheter (1P) (spinal) *use* Infusion Device
Inferior cardiac nerve *use* Nerve, Thoracic Sympathetic
Inferior cerebellar vein *use* Vein, Intracranial
Inferior cerebral vein *use* Vein, Intracranial
Inferior epigastric artery
  use Artery, External Iliac, Right
  use Artery, External Iliac, Left
Inferior epigastric lymph node *use* Lymphatic, Pelvis
Inferior genicular artery
  use Artery, Popliteal, Left
  use Artery, Popliteal, Right
Inferior gluteal artery
  use Artery, Internal Iliac, Right
  use Artery, Internal Iliac, Left
Inferior gluteal nerve *use* Nerve, Sacral Plexus
Inferior hypogastric plexus *use* Nerve, Abdominal Sympathetic
Inferior labial artery *use* Artery, Face
Inferior longitudinal muscle *use* Muscle, Tongue, Palate, Pharynx
Inferior mesenteric ganglion *use* Nerve, Abdominal Sympathetic
Inferior mesenteric lymph node *use* Lymphatic, Mesenteric
Inferior mesenteric plexus *use* Nerve, Abdominal Sympathetic
Inferior oblique muscle
  use Muscle, Extraocular, Right
  use Muscle, Extraocular, Left
Inferior pancreaticoduodenal artery *use* Artery, Superior Mesenteric
Inferior phrenic artery *use* Aorta, Abdominal
Inferior rectus muscle
  use Muscle, Extraocular, Right
  use Muscle, Extraocular, Left
Inferior suprarenal artery
  use Artery, Renal, Left
  use Artery, Renal, Right
Inferior tarsal plate
  use Eyelid, Lower, Left
  use Eyelid, Lower, Right
Inferior thyroid vein
  use Vein, Innominate, Left
  use Vein, Innominate, Right
Inferior tibiofibular joint
  use Joint, Ankle, Left
  use Joint, Ankle, Right
Inferior turbinate *use* Turbinate, Nasal

Inferior ulnar collateral artery
  use Artery, Brachial, Left
  use Artery, Brachial, Right
Inferior vesical artery
  use Artery, Internal Iliac, Left
  use Artery, Internal Iliac, Right
Infraauricular lymph node *use* Lymphatic, Head
Infraclavicular (deltopectoral) lymph node
  use Lymphatic, Upper Extremity, Left
  use Lymphatic, Upper Extremity, Right
Infrahyoid muscle
  use Muscle, Neck, Left
  use Muscle, Neck, Right
Infraparotid lymph node *use* Lymphatic, Head
Infraspinatus fascia
  use Subcutaneous Tissue and Fascia, Upper Arm, Left
  use Subcutaneous Tissue and Fascia, Upper Arm, Right
Infraspinatus muscle
  use Muscle, Shoulder, Left
  use Muscle, Shoulder, Right
Infundibulopelvic ligament *use* Uterine Supporting Structure
Infusion *see* Introduction of substance in or on
Infusion Device
  Insertion of device in
    Abdomen **0JH8**
    Back **0JH7**
    Chest **0JH6**
    Lower Arm
      Left **0JHH**
      Right **0JHG**
    Lower Leg
      Left **0JHP**
      Right **0JHN**
    Trunk **0JHT**
    Upper Arm
      Left **0JHF**
      Right **0JHD**
    Upper Leg
      Left **0JHM**
      Right **0JHL**
  Removal of device from
    Lower Extremity **0JPW**
    Trunk **0JPT**
    Upper Extremity **0JPV**
  Revision of device in
    Lower Extremity **0JWW**
    Trunk **0JWT**
    Upper Extremity **0JWV**
Infusion, glucarpidase
  Central vein **3E043GQ**
  Peripheral vein **3E033GQ**
Inguinal canal
  use Inguinal Region, Right
  use Inguinal Region, Left
  use Inguinal Region, Bilateral
Inguinal triangle
  use Inguinal Region, Right
  use Inguinal Region, Bilateral
  use Inguinal Region, Left
Injection *see* Introduction of substance in or on

Injection reservoir, port *use* Vascular Access Device, Reservoir in Subcutaneous Tissue and Fascia
Injection reservoir, pump *use* Infusion Device, Pump in Subcutaneous Tissue and Fascia
Insemination, artificial 3E0P7LZ
Insertion
  Antimicrobial envelope *see* Introduction of Anti-infective
  Aqueous drainage shunt
    see Bypass, Eye **081**
    see Drainage, Eye **089**
  Products of Conception **10H0**
Insertion *(continued)*
  Spinal Stabilization Device
    see Insertion of device in, Upper Joints **0RH**
    see Insertion of device in, Lower Joints **0SH**
Insertion of device in
  Abdominal Wall **0WHF**
  Acetabulum
    Left **0QH5**
    Right **0QH4**
  Anal Sphincter **0DHR**
  Ankle Region
    Left **0YHL**
    Right **0YHK**
  Anus **0DHQ**
  Aorta
    Abdominal **04H0**
    Thoracic
      Ascending/Arch **02HX**
      Descending **02HW**
  Arm
    Lower
      Left **0XHF**
      Right **0XHD**
    Upper
      Left **0XH9**
      Right **0XH8**
  Artery
    Anterior Tibial
      Left **04HQ**
      Right **04HP**
    Axillary
      Left **03H6**
      Right **03H5**
    Brachial
      Left **03H8**
      Right **03H7**
    Celiac **04H1**
    Colic
      Left **04H7**
      Middle **04H8**
      Right **04H6**
    Common Carotid
      Left **03HJ**
      Right **03HH**
    Common Iliac
      Left **04HD**
      Right **04HC**
    External Carotid
      Left **03HN**
      Right **03HM**

Insertion of device in *(continued)*
    External Iliac
      Left **04HJ**
      Right **04HH**
    Face **03HR**
    Femoral
      Left **04HL**
      Right **04HK**
    Foot
      Left **04HW**
      Right **04HV**
    Gastric **04H2**
    Hand
      Left **03HF**
      Right **03HD**
    Hepatic **04H3**
    Inferior Mesenteric **04HB**
    Innominate **03H2**
    Internal Carotid
      Left **03HL**
      Right **03HK**
    Internal Iliac
      Left **04HF**
      Right **04HE**
    Internal Mammary
      Left **03H1**
      Right **03H0**
    Intracranial **03HG**
    Lower **04HY**
    Peroneal
      Left **04HU**
      Right **04HT**
    Popliteal
      Left **04HN**
      Right **04HM**
    Posterior Tibial
      Left **04HS**
      Right **04HR**
    Pulmonary
      Left **02HR**
      Right **02HQ**
    Pulmonary Trunk **02HP**
    Radial
      Left **03HC**
      Right **03HB**
    Renal
      Left **04HA**
      Right **04H9**
    Splenic **04H4**
    Subclavian
      Left **03H4**
      Right **03H3**
    Superior Mesenteric **04H5**
    Temporal
      Left **03HT**
      Right **03HS**
    Thyroid
      Left **03HV**
      Right **03HU**
    Ulnar
      Left **03HA**
      Right **03H9**
    Upper **03HY**
    Vertebral
      Left **03HQ**
      Right **03HP**

Atrium
  Left **02H7**
  Right **02H6**
Axilla
  Left **0XH5**
  Right **0XH4**
Back
  Lower **0WHL**
  Upper **0WHK**
Bladder **0THB**
Bladder Neck **0THC**
Bone
  Ethmoid
    Left **0NHG**
    Right **0NHF**
  Facial **0NHW**
  Frontal
    Left **0NH2**
    Right **0NH1**
  Hyoid **0NHX**
  Lacrimal
    Left **0NHJ**
    Right **0NHH**
  Lower **0QHY**
  Nasal **0NHB**
  Occipital
    Left **0NH8**
    Right **0NH7**
  Palatine
    Left **0NHL**
    Right **0NHK**
  Parietal
    Left **0NH4**
    Right **0NH3**
  Pelvic
    Left **0QH3**
    Right **0QH2**
  Sphenoid
    Left **0NHD**
    Right **0NHC**
  Temporal
    Left **0NH6**
    Right **0NH5**
  Upper **0PHY**
  Zygomatic
    Left **0NHN**
    Right **0NHM**
Brain **00H0**
Breast
  Bilateral **0HHV**
  Left **0HHU**
  Right **0HHT**
Bronchus
  Lingula **0BH9**
  Lower Lobe
    Left **0BHB**
    Right **0BH6**
  Main
    Left **0BH7**
    Right **0BH3**
  Middle Lobe, Right **0BH5**
  Upper Lobe
    Left **0BH8**
    Right **0BH4**
Buttock

  Left **0YH1**
  Right **0YH0**
Carpal
  Left **0PHN**
  Right **0PHM**
Cavity, Cranial **0WH1**
Cerebral Ventricle **00H6**
Cervix **0UHC**
Chest Wall **0WH8**
Cisterna Chyli **07HL**
Clavicle
  Left **0PHB**
  Right **0PH9**
Coccyx **0QHS**
Cul-de-sac **0UHF**
Diaphragm
  Left **0BHS**
  Right **0BHR**
Disc
  Cervical Vertebral **0RH3**
  Cervicothoracic Vertebral **0RH5**
  Lumbar Vertebral **0SH2**
  Lumbosacral **0SH4**
  Thoracic Vertebral **0RH9**
  Thoracolumbar Vertebral **0RHB**
Duct
  Hepatobiliary **0FHB**
  Pancreatic **0FHD**
Duodenum **0DH9**
Ear
  Left **09HE**
  Right **09HD**
Elbow Region
  Left **0XHC**
  Right **0XHB**
Epididymis and Spermatic Cord **0VHM**
Esophagus **0DH5**
Extremity
  Lower
    Left **0YHB**
    Right **0YH9**
  Upper
    Left **0XH7**
    Right **0XH6**
Eye
  Left **08H1**
  Right **08H0**
Face **0WH2**
Fallopian Tube **0UH8**
Femoral Region
  Left **0YH8**
  Right **0YH7**
Femoral Shaft
  Left **0QH9**
  Right **0QH8**
Femur
  Lower
    Left **0QHC**
    Right **0QHB**
  Upper
    Left **0QH7**
    Right **0QH6**
Fibula
  Left **0QHK**
  Right **0QHJ**

Foot
  Left **0YHN**
  Right **0YHM**
Gallbladder **0FH4**
Gastrointestinal Tract **0WHP**
Genitourinary Tract **0WHR**
Gland, Endocrine **0GHS**
Glenoid Cavity
  Left **0PH8**
  Right **0PH7**
Hand
  Left **0XHK**
  Right **0XHJ**
Head **0WH0**
Heart **02HA**
Humeral Head
  Left **0PHD**
  Right **0PHC**
Humeral Shaft
  Left **0PHG**
  Right **0PHF**
Ileum **0DHB**
Inguinal Region
  Left **0YH6**
  Right **0YH5**
Intestine
  Large **0DHE**
  Small **0DH8**
Jaw
  Lower **0WH5**
  Upper **0WH4**
Jejunum **0DHA**
Joint
  Acromioclavicular
    Left **0RHH**
    Right **0RHG**
  Ankle
    Left **0SHG**
    Right **0SHF**
  Carpal
    Left **0RHR**
    Right **0RHQ**
  Cervical Vertebral **0RH1**
  Cervicothoracic Vertebral **0RH4**
  Coccygeal **0SH6**
  Elbow
    Left **0RHM**
    Right **0RHL**
  Finger Phalangeal
    Left **0RHX**
    Right **0RHW**
  Hip
    Left **0SHB**
    Right **0SH9**
  Knee
    Left **0SHD**
    Right **0SHC**
  Lumbar Vertebral **0SH0**
  Lumbosacral **0SH3**
  Metacarpocarpal
    Left **0RHT**
    Right **0RHS**
  Metacarpophalangeal
    Left **0RHV**
    Right **0RHU**

Metatarsal-Phalangeal
   Left **0SHN**
   Right **0SHM**
Metatarsal-Tarsal
   Left **0SHL**
   Right **0SHK**
Occipital-cervical **0RH0**
Sacrococcygeal **0SH5**
Sacroiliac
   Left **0SH8**
   Right **0SH7**
Shoulder
   Left **0RHK**
   Right **0RHJ**
Sternoclavicular
   Left **0RHF**
   Right **0RHE**
Tarsal
   Left **0SHJ**
   Right **0SHH**
Temporomandibular
   Left **0RHD**
   Right **0RHC**
Thoracic Vertebral **0RH6**
Thoracolumbar Vertebral **0RHA**
Toe Phalangeal
   Left **0SHQ**
   Right **0SHP**
Wrist
   Left **0RHP**
   Right **0RHN**
Kidney **0TH5**
Knee Region
   Left **0YHG**
   Right **0YHF**
Leg
  Lower
    Left **0YHJ**
    Right **0YHH**
  Upper
    Left **0YHD**
    Right **0YHC**
Liver **0FH0**
  Left Lobe **0FH2**
  Right Lobe **0FH1**
Lung
   Left **0BHL**
   Right **0BHK**
Lymphatic **07HN**
  Thoracic Duct **07HK**
Mandible
   Left **0NHV**
   Right **0NHT**
Maxilla
   Left **0NHS**
   Right **0NHR**
Mediastinum **0WHC**
Metacarpal
   Left **0PHQ**
   Right **0PHP**
Metatarsal
   Left **0QHP**
   Right **0QHN**
Mouth and Throat **0CHY**
Muscle

  Lower **0KHY**
  Upper **0KHX**
Nasopharynx **09HN**
Neck **0WH6**
Nerve
  Cranial **00HE**
  Peripheral **01HY**
Nipple
   Left **0HHX**
   Right **0HHW**
Oral Cavity and Throat **0WH3**
Orbit
   Left **0NHQ**
   Right **0NHP**
Ovary **0UH3**
Pancreas **0FHG**
Patella
   Left **0QHF**
   Right **0QHD**
Pelvic Cavity **0WHJ**
Penis **0VHS**
Pericardial Cavity **0WHD**
Pericardium **02HN**
Perineum
  Female **0WHN**
  Male **0WHM**
Peritoneal Cavity **0WHG**
Phalanx
  Finger
    Left **0PHV**
    Right **0PHT**
  Thumb
    Left **0PHS**
    Right **0PHR**
  Toe
    Left **0QHR**
    Right **0QHQ**
Pleural Cavity
   Left **0WHB**
   Right **0WH9**
Prostate **0VH0**
Prostate and Seminal Vesicles **0VH4**
Radius
   Left **0PHJ**
   Right **0PHH**
Rectum **0DHP**
Respiratory Tract **0WHQ**
Retroperitoneum **0WHH**
Rib
   Left **0PH2**
   Right **0PH1**
Sacrum **0QH1**
Scapula
   Left **0PH6**
   Right **0PH5**
Scrotum and Tunica Vaginalis **0VH8**
Shoulder Region
   Left **0XH3**
   Right **0XH2**
Skull **0NH0**
Spinal Canal **00HU**
Spinal Cord **00HV**
Spleen **07HP**
Sternum **0PH0**
Stomach **0DH6**

Subcutaneous Tissue and Fascia
  Abdomen **0JH8**
  Back **0JH7**
  Buttock **0JH9**
  Chest **0JH6**
  Face **0JH1**
  Foot
    Left **0JHR**
    Right **0JHQ**
  Hand
    Left **0JHK**
    Right **0JHJ**
  Head and Neck **0JHS**
  Lower Arm
    Left **0JHH**
    Right **0JHG**
  Lower Extremity **0JHW**
  Lower Leg
    Left **0JHP**
    Right **0JHN**
  Neck
    Anterior **0JH4**
    Posterior **0JH5**
  Pelvic Region **0JHC**
  Perineum **0JHB**
  Scalp **0JH0**
  Trunk **0JHT**
  Upper Arm
    Left **0JHF**
    Right **0JHD**
  Upper Extremity **0JHV**
  Upper Leg
    Left **0JHM**
    Right **0JHL**
Tarsal
   Left **0QHM**
   Right **0QHL**
Testis **0VHD**
Thymus **07HM**
Tibia
   Left **0QHH**
   Right **0QHG**
Tongue **0CH7**
Trachea **0BH1**
Tracheobronchial Tree **0BH0**
Ulna
   Left **0PHL**
   Right **0PHK**
Ureter **0TH9**
Urethra **0THD**
Uterus **0UH9**
Uterus and Cervix **0UHD**
Vagina **0UHG**
Vagina and Cul-de-sac **0UHH**
Vas Deferens **0VHR**
Vein
  Axillary
    Left **05H8**
    Right **05H7**
  Azygos **05H0**
  Basilic
    Left **05HC**
    Right **05HB**
  Brachial
    Left **05HA**

Insertion of device in *(continued)*
- Right **05H9**
- Cephalic
  - Left **05HF**
  - Right **05HD**
- Colic **06H7**
- Common Iliac
  - Left **06HD**
  - Right **06HC**
- Coronary **02H4**
- Esophageal **06H3**
- External Iliac
  - Left **06HG**
  - Right **06HF**
- External Jugular
  - Left **05HQ**
  - Right **05HP**
- Face
  - Left **05HV**
  - Right **05HT**
- Femoral
  - Left **06HN**
  - Right **06HM**
- Foot
  - Left **06HV**
  - Right **06HT**
- Gastric **06H2**
- Greater Saphenous
  - Left **06HQ**
  - Right **06HP**
- Hand
  - Left **05HH**
  - Right **05HG**
- Hemiazygos **05H1**
- Hepatic **06H4**
- Hypogastric
  - Left **06HJ**
  - Right **06HH**
- Inferior Mesenteric **06H6**
- Innominate
  - Left **05H4**
  - Right **05H3**
- Internal Jugular
  - Left **05HN**
  - Right **05HM**
- Intracranial **05HL**
- Lesser Saphenous
  - Left **06HS**
  - Right **06HR**
- Lower **06HY**
- Portal **06H8**
- Pulmonary
  - Left **02HT**
  - Right **02HS**
- Renal
  - Left **06HB**
  - Right **06H9**
- Splenic **06H1**
- Subclavian
  - Left **05H6**
  - Right **05H5**
- Superior Mesenteric **06H5**
- Upper **05HY**
- Vertebral
  - Left **05HS**
  - Right **05HR**

Insertion of device in *(continued)*
- Vena Cava
  - Inferior **06H0**
  - Superior **02HV**
- Ventricle
  - Left **02HL**
  - Right **02HK**
- Vertebra
  - Cervical **0PH3**
  - Lumbar **0QH0**
  - Thoracic **0PH4**
- Wrist Region
  - Left **0XHH**
  - Right **0XHG**

Inspection
- Abdominal Wall **0WJF**
- Ankle Region
  - Left **0YJL**
  - Right **0YJK**
- Arm
  - Lower
    - Left **0XJF**
    - Right **0XJD**
  - Upper
    - Left **0XJ9**
    - Right **0XJ8**
- Artery
  - Lower **04JY**
  - Upper **03JY**
- Axilla
  - Left **0XJ5**
  - Right **0XJ4**
- Back
  - Lower **0WJL**
  - Upper **0WJK**
- Bladder **0TJB**
- Bone
  - Facial **0NJW**
  - Lower **0QJY**
  - Nasal **0NJB**
  - Upper **0PJY**
- Bone Marrow **07JT**
- Brain **00J0**
- Breast
  - Left **0HJU**
  - Right **0HJT**
- Bursa and Ligament
  - Lower **0MJY**
  - Upper **0MJX**
- Buttock
  - Left **0YJ1**
  - Right **0YJ0**
- Cavity, Cranial **0WJ1**
- Chest Wall **0WJ8**
- Cisterna Chyli **07JL**
- Diaphragm **0BJT**
- Disc
  - Cervical Vertebral **0RJ3**
  - Cervicothoracic Vertebral **0RJ5**
  - Lumbar Vertebral **0SJ2**
  - Lumbosacral **0SJ4**
  - Thoracic Vertebral **0RJ9**
  - Thoracolumbar Vertebral **0RJB**
- Duct
  - Hepatobiliary **0FJB**
  - Pancreatic **0FJD**

Inspection *(continued)*
- Ear
  - Inner
    - Left **09JE**
    - Right **09JD**
  - Left **09JJ**
  - Right **09JH**
- Elbow Region
  - Left **0XJC**
  - Right **0XJB**
- Epididymis and Spermatic Cord **0VJM**
- Extremity
  - Lower
    - Left **0YJB**
    - Right **0YJ9**
  - Upper
    - Left **0XJ7**
    - Right **0XJ6**
- Eye
  - Left **08J1XZZ**
  - Right **08J0XZZ**
- Face **0WJ2**
- Fallopian Tube **0UJ8**
- Femoral Region
  - Bilateral **0YJE**
  - Left **0YJ8**
  - Right **0YJ7**
- Finger Nail **0HJQXZZ**
- Foot
  - Left **0YJN**
  - Right **0YJM**
- Gallbladder **0FJ4**
- Gastrointestinal Tract **0WJP**
- Genitourinary Tract **0WJR**
- Gland
  - Adrenal **0GJ5**
  - Endocrine **0GJS**
  - Pituitary **0GJ0**
  - Salivary **0CJA**
- Great Vessel **02JY**
- Hand
  - Left **0XJK**
  - Right **0XJJ**
- Head **0WJ0**
- Heart **02JA**
- Inguinal Region
  - Bilateral **0YJA**
  - Left **0YJ6**
  - Right **0YJ5**
- Intestinal Tract
  - Lower **0DJD**
  - Upper **0DJ0**
- Jaw
  - Lower **0WJ5**
  - Upper **0WJ4**
- Joint
  - Acromioclavicular
    - Left **0RJH**
    - Right **0RJG**
  - Ankle
    - Left **0SJG**
    - Right **0SJF**
  - Carpal
    - Left **0RJR**
    - Right **0RJQ**
  - Cervical Vertebral **0RJ1**

Inspection *(continued)*
   Cervicothoracic Vertebral **0RJ4**
   Coccygeal **0SJ6**
   Elbow
      Left **0RJM**
      Right **0RJL**
   Finger Phalangeal
      Left **0RJX**
      Right **0RJW**
   Hip
      Left **0SJB**
      Right **0SJ9**
   Knee
      Left **0SJD**
      Right **0SJC**
   Lumbar Vertebral **0SJ0**
   Lumbosacral **0SJ3**
   Metacarpocarpal
      Left **0RJT**
      Right **0RJS**
   Metacarpophalangeal
      Left **0RJV**
      Right **0RJU**
   Metatarsal-Phalangeal
      Left **0SJN**
      Right **0SJM**
   Metatarsal-Tarsal
      Left **0SJL**
      Right **0SJK**
   Occipital-cervical **0RJ0**
   Sacrococcygeal **0SJ5**
   Sacroiliac
      Left **0SJ8**
      Right **0SJ7**
   Shoulder
      Left **0RJK**
      Right **0RJJ**
   Sternoclavicular
      Left **0RJF**
      Right **0RJE**
   Tarsal
      Left **0SJJ**
      Right **0SJH**
   Temporomandibular
      Left **0RJD**
      Right **0RJC**
   Thoracic Vertebral **0RJ6**
   Thoracolumbar Vertebral **0RJA**
   Toe Phalangeal
      Left **0SJQ**
      Right **0SJP**
   Wrist
      Left **0RJP**
      Right **0RJN**
  Kidney **0TJ5**
  Knee Region
    Left **0YJG**
    Right **0YJF**
  Larynx **0CJS**
  Leg
    Lower
      Left **0YJJ**
      Right **0YJH**
    Upper
      Left **0YJD**
      Right **0YJC**

Inspection *(continued)*
  Lens
    Left **08JKXZZ**
    Right **08JJXZZ**
  Liver **0FJ0**
  Lung
    Left **0BJL**
    Right **0BJK**
  Lymphatic **07JN**
    Thoracic Duct **07JK**
  Mediastinum **0WJC**
  Mesentery **0DJV**
  Mouth and Throat **0CJY**
  Muscle
    Extraocular
      Left **08JM**
      Right **08JL**
    Lower **0KJY**
    Upper **0KJX**
  Neck **0WJ6**
  Nerve
    Cranial **00JE**
    Peripheral **01JY**
  Nose **09JK**
  Omentum **0DJU**
  Oral Cavity and Throat **0WJ3**
  Ovary **0UJ3**
  Pancreas **0FJG**
  Parathyroid Gland **0GJR**
  Pelvic Cavity **0WJJ**
  Penis **0VJS**
  Pericardial Cavity **0WJD**
  Perineum
    Female **0WJN**
    Male **0WJM**
  Peritoneal Cavity **0WJG**
  Peritoneum **0DJW**
  Pineal Body **0GJ1**
  Pleura **0BJQ**
  Pleural Cavity
    Left **0WJB**
    Right **0WJ9**
  Products of Conception **10J0**
    Ectopic **10J2**
    Retained **10J1**
  Prostate and Seminal Vesicles **0VJ4**
  Respiratory Tract **0WJQ**
  Retroperitoneum **0WJH**
  Scrotum and Tunica Vaginalis **0VJ8**
  Shoulder Region
    Left **0XJ3**
    Right **0XJ2**
  Sinus **09JY**
  Skin **0HJPXZZ**
  Skull **0NJ0**
  Spinal Canal **00JU**
  Spinal Cord **00JV**
  Spleen **07JP**
  Stomach **0DJ6**
  Subcutaneous Tissue and Fascia
    Head and Neck **0JJS**
    Lower Extremity **0JJW**
    Trunk **0JJT**
    Upper Extremity **0JJV**
  Tendon
    Lower **0LJY**

Inspection *(continued)*
    Upper **0LJX**
  Testis **0VJD**
  Thymus **07JM**
  Thyroid Gland **0GJK**
  Toe Nail **0HJRXZZ**
  Trachea **0BJ1**
  Tracheobronchial Tree **0BJ0**
  Tympanic Membrane
    Left **09J8**
    Right **09J7**
  Ureter **0TJ9**
  Urethra **0TJD**
  Uterus and Cervix **0UJD**
  Vagina and Cul-de-sac **0UJH**
  Vas Deferens **0VJR**
  Vein
    Lower **06JY**
    Upper **05JY**
  Vulva **0UJM**
  Wrist Region
    Left **0XJH**
    Right **0XJG**
Instillation *see* Introduction of substance in or on
Insufflation *see* Introduction of substance in or on
Interatrial septum *use* Septum, Atrial
Interbody Fusion Device, Nanotextured Surface
  Cervical Vertebral **XRG1092**
    2 or more **XRG2092**
Interbody Fusion Device, Nanotextured Surface *(continued)*
  Cervicothoracic Vertebral **XRG4092**
  Lumbar Vertebral **XRGB092**
    2 or more **XRGC092**
  Lumbosacral **XRGD092**
  Occipital-cervical **XRG0092**
  Thoracic Vertebral **XRG6092**
    2 to 7 **XRG7092**
    8 or more **XRG8092**
  Thoracolumbar Vertebral **XRGA092**
Interbody fusion (spine) cage
  use Interbody Fusion Device in Upper Joints
  use Interbody Fusion Device in Lower Joints
Intercarpal joint
  use Joint, Carpal, Right
  use Joint, Carpal, Left
Intercarpal ligament
  use Bursa and Ligament, Hand, Right
  use Bursa and Ligament, Hand, Left
Interclavicular ligament
  use Bursa and Ligament, Shoulder, Right
  use Bursa and Ligament, Shoulder, Left
Intercostal lymph node *use* Lymphatic, Thorax
Intercostal muscle
  use Muscle, Thorax, Right
  use Muscle, Thorax, Left
Intercostal nerve *use* Nerve, Thoracic
Intercostobrachial nerve *use* Nerve, Thoracic
Intercuneiform joint
  use Joint, Tarsal, Right
  use Joint, Tarsal, Left

Intercuneiform ligament
  use Bursa and Ligament, Foot, Left
  use Bursa and Ligament, Foot, Right
Intermediate bronchus *use* Main Bronchus, Right
Intermediate cuneiform bone
  use Tarsal, Right
  use Tarsal, Left
Intermittent mandatory ventilation *see* Assistance, Respiratory **5A09**
Intermittent Negative Airway Pressure
  24-96 Consecutive Hours, Ventilation **5A0945B**
  Greater than 96 Consecutive Hours, Ventilation **5A0955B**
  Less than 24 Consecutive Hours, Ventilation **5A0935B**
Intermittent Positive Airway Pressure
  24-96 Consecutive Hours, Ventilation **5A09458**
  Greater than 96 Consecutive Hours, Ventilation **5A09558**
  Less than 24 Consecutive Hours, Ventilation **5A09358**
Intermittent positive pressure breathing *see* Assistance, Respiratory **5A09**
Internal (basal) cerebral vein *use* Vein, Intracranial
Internal anal sphincter *use* Anal Sphincter
Internal carotid artery, intracranial portion
  use Intracranial Artery
Internal carotid plexus *use* Nerve, Head and Neck Sympathetic
Internal iliac vein
  use Vein, Hypogastric, Right
  use Vein, Hypogastric, Left
Internal maxillary artery
  use Artery, External Carotid, Left
  use Artery, External Carotid, Right
Internal naris *use* Nose
Internal oblique muscle
  use Muscle, Abdomen, Right
  use Muscle, Abdomen, Left
Internal pudendal artery
  use Artery, Internal Iliac, Right
  use Artery, Internal Iliac, Left
Internal pudendal vein
  use Vein, Hypogastric, Right
  use Vein, Hypogastric, Left
Internal thoracic artery
  use Artery, Subclavian, Right
  use Artery, Subclavian, Left
  use Artery, Internal Mammary, Left
  use Artery, Internal Mammary, Right
Internal urethral sphincter *use* Urethra
Interphalangeal (IP) joint
  use Joint, Finger Phalangeal, Left
  use Joint, Toe Phalangeal, Right
  use Joint, Toe Phalangeal, Left
  use Joint, Finger Phalangeal, Right
Interphalangeal ligament
  use Bursa and Ligament, Hand, Left
  use Bursa and Ligament, Hand, Right
  use Bursa and Ligament, Foot, Right
  use Bursa and Ligament, Foot, Left

Interrogation, cardiac rhythm related device
  Interrogation only *see* Measurement, Cardiac **4B02**
  With cardiac function testing *see* Measurement, Cardiac **4A02**
Interruption *see* Occlusion
Interspinalis muscle
  use Head and Neck Bursa and Ligament
  use Muscle, Trunk, Right
  use Muscle, Trunk, Left
Interspinous ligament
  use Bursa and Ligament, Trunk, Right
  use Bursa and Ligament, Trunk, Left
Interspinous process spinal stabilization device
  use Spinal Stabilization Device, Interspinous Process in **0RH**
  use Spinal Stabilization Device, Interspinous Process in **0SH**
InterStim® Therapy lead *use* Neurostimulator Lead in Peripheral Nervous System
InterStim® Therapy neurostimulator *use* Stimulator Generator, Single Array in **0JH**
Intertransversarius muscle
  use Muscle, Trunk, Left
  use Muscle, Trunk, Right
Intertransverse ligament
  use Bursa and Ligament, Trunk, Right
  use Bursa and Ligament, Trunk, Left
Interventricular foramen (Monro) *use* Cerebral Ventricle
Interventricular septum *use* Septum, Ventricular
Intestinal lymphatic trunk *use* Cisterna Chyli
Intraluminal Device
  Airway
    Esophagus **0DH5**
    Mouth and Throat **0CHY**
    Nasopharynx **09HN**
  Bioactive
  Occlusion
    Common Carotid
      Left **03LJ**
      Right **03LH**
    External Carotid
      Left **03LN**
      Right **03LM**
    Internal Carotid
      Left **03LL**
      Right **03LK**
    Intracranial **03LG**
    Vertebral
      Left **03LQ**
      Right **03LP**
  Restriction
    Common Carotid
      Left **03VJ**
      Right **03VH**
    External Carotid
      Left **03VN**
      Right **03VM**
    Internal Carotid
      Left **03VL**
      Right **03VK**
    Intracranial **03VG**
    Vertebral

Intraluminal Device *(continued)*
    Left **03VQ**
    Right **03VP**
  Endobronchial Valve
    Lingula **0BH9**
    Lower Lobe
      Left **0BHB**
      Right **0BH6**
    Main
      Left **0BH7**
      Right **0BH3**
    Middle Lobe, Right **0BH5**
    Upper Lobe
      Left **0BH8**
      Right **0BH4**
  Endotracheal Airway
    Change device in, Trachea **0B21XEZ**
    Insertion of device in, Trachea **0BH1**
  Pessary
    Change device in, Vagina and Cul-de-sac **0U2HXGZ**
    Insertion of device in
      Cul-de-sac **0UHF**
      Vagina **0UHG**
Intramedullary (IM) rod (nail)
  use Internal Fixation Device, Intramedullary in Upper Bones
  use Internal Fixation Device, Intramedullary in Lower Bones
Intramedullary skeletal kinetic distractor (ISKD)
  use Internal Fixation Device, Intramedullary in Upper Bones
  use Internal Fixation Device, Intramedullary in Lower Bones
Intraocular Telescope
  Left **08RK30Z**
  Right **08RJ30Z**
Intraoperative Knee Replacement Sensor XR2
Intraoperative Radiation Therapy (IORT)
  Anus **DDY8CZZ**
  Bile Ducts **DFY2CZZ**
  Bladder **DTY2CZZ**
  Cervix **DUY1CZZ**
  Colon **DDY5CZZ**
  Duodenum **DDY2CZZ**
  Gallbladder **DFY1CZZ**
  Ileum **DDY4CZZ**
  Jejunum **DDY3CZZ**
  Kidney **DTY0CZZ**
  Larynx **D9YBCZZ**
  Liver **DFY0CZZ**
  Mouth **D9Y4CZZ**
  Nasopharynx **D9YDCZZ**
  Ovary **DUY0CZZ**
  Pancreas **DFY3CZZ**
  Pharynx **D9YCCZZ**
  Prostate **DVY0CZZ**
  Rectum **DDY7CZZ**
  Stomach **DDY1CZZ**
  Ureter **DTY1CZZ**
  Urethra **DTY3CZZ**
  Uterus **DUY2CZZ**
Intrauterine device (IUD) *use* Contraceptive Device in Female Reproductive System

Intravascular fluorescence angiography (IFA) see Monitoring, Physiological Systems 4A1

Introduction of substance in or on

Artery

Central **3E06**

Analgesics **3E06**

Anesthetic, Intracirculatory **3E06**

Anti-infective **3E06**

Anti-inflammatory **3E06**

Antiarrhythmic **3E06**

Antineoplastic **3E06**

Destructive Agent **3E06**

Diagnostic Substance, Other **3E06**

Electrolytic Substance **3E06**

Hormone **3E06**

Hypnotics **3E06**

Immunotherapeutic **3E06**

Nutritional Substance **3E06**

Platelet Inhibitor **3E06**

Radioactive Substance **3E06**

Sedatives **3E06**

Serum **3E06**

Thrombolytic **3E06**

Toxoid **3E06**

Vaccine **3E06**

Vasopressor **3E06**

Water Balance Substance **3E06**

Coronary **3E07**

Diagnostic Substance, Other **3E07**

Platelet Inhibitor **3E07**

Thrombolytic **3E07**

Peripheral **3E05**

Analgesics **3E05**

Anesthetic, Intracirculatory **3E05**

Anti-infective **3E05**

Anti-inflammatory **3E05**

Antiarrhythmic **3E05**

Antineoplastic **3E05**

Destructive Agent **3E05**

Diagnostic Substance, Other **3E05**

Electrolytic Substance **3E05**

Hormone **3E05**

Hypnotics **3E05**

Immunotherapeutic **3E05**

Nutritional Substance **3E05**

Platelet Inhibitor **3E05**

Radioactive Substance **3E05**

Sedatives **3E05**

Serum **3E05**

Thrombolytic **3E05**

Toxoid **3E05**

Vaccine **3E05**

Vasopressor **3E05**

Water Balance Substance **3E05**

Biliary Tract **3E0J**

Analgesics **3E0J**

Anesthetic, Local **3E0J**

Anti-infective **3E0J**

Anti-inflammatory **3E0J**

Antineoplastic **3E0J**

Destructive Agent **3E0J**

Diagnostic Substance, Other **3E0J**

Electrolytic Substance **3E0J**

Gas **3E0J**

Hypnotics **3E0J**

Introduction of substance (continued)

Islet Cells, Pancreatic **3E0J**

Nutritional Substance **3E0J**

Radioactive Substance **3E0J**

Sedatives **3E0J**

Water Balance Substance **3E0J**

Bone **3E0V**

Analgesics **3E0V3NZ**

Anesthetic, Local **3E0V3BZ**

Anti-infective **3E0V32**

Anti-inflammatory **3E0V33Z**

Antineoplastic **3E0V30**

Destructive Agent **3E0V3TZ**

Diagnostic Substance, Other **3E0V3KZ**

Electrolytic Substance **3E0V37Z**

Hypnotics **3E0V3NZ**

Nutritional Substance **3E0V36Z**

Radioactive Substance **3E0V3HZ**

Sedatives **3E0V3NZ**

Water Balance Substance **3E0V37Z**

Bone Marrow **3E0A3GC**

Antineoplastic **3E0A30**

Brain **3E0Q**

Analgesics **3E0Q**

Anesthetic, Local **3E0Q**

Anti-infective **3E0Q**

Anti-inflammatory **3E0Q**

Antineoplastic **3E0Q**

Destructive Agent **3E0Q**

Diagnostic Substance, Other **3E0Q**

Electrolytic Substance **3E0Q**

Gas **3E0Q**

Hypnotics **3E0Q**

Nutritional Substance **3E0Q**

Radioactive Substance **3E0Q**

Sedatives **3E0Q**

Stem Cells

Embryonic **3E0Q**

Somatic **3E0Q**

Water Balance Substance **3E0Q**

Cranial Cavity **3E0Q**

Analgesics **3E0Q**

Anesthetic, Local **3E0Q**

Anti-infective **3E0**

Anti-inflammatory **3E0Q**

Antineoplastic **3E0Q**

Destructive Agent **3E0Q**

Diagnostic Substance, Other **3E0Q**

Electrolytic Substance **3E0Q**

Gas **3E0Q**

Hypnotics **3E0Q**

Nutritional Substance **3E0Q**

Radioactive Substance **3E0Q**

Sedatives **3E0Q**

Stem Cells

Embryonic **3E0Q**

Somatic **3E0Q**

Water Balance Substance **3E0Q**

Ear **3E0B**

Analgesics **3E0B**

Anesthetic, Local **3E0B**

Anti-infective **3E0B**

Anti-inflammatory **3E0B**

Antineoplastic **3E0B**

Destructive Agent **3E0B**

Diagnostic Substance, Other **3E0B**

Introduction of substance (continued)

Hypnotics **3E0B**

Radioactive Substance **3E0B**

Sedatives **3E0B**

Epidural Space **3E0S3GC**

Analgesics **3E0S3NZ**

Anesthetic

Local **3E0S3BZ**

Regional **3E0S3CZ**

Anti-infective **3E0S32**

Anti-inflammatory **3E0S33Z**

Antineoplastic **3E0S30**

Destructive Agent **3E0S3TZ**

Diagnostic Substance, Other **3E0S3KZ**

Electrolytic Substance **3E0S37Z**

Gas **3E0S**

Hypnotics **3E0S3NZ**

Nutritional Substance **3E0S36Z**

Radioactive Substance **3E0S3HZ**

Sedatives **3E0S3NZ**

Water Balance Substance **3E0S37Z**

Eye **3E0C**

Analgesics **3E0C**

Anesthetic, Local **3E0C**

Anti-infective **3E0C**

Anti-inflammatory **3E0C**

Antineoplastic **3E0C**

Destructive Agent **3E0C**

Diagnostic Substance, Other **3E0C**

Gas **3E0C**

Hypnotics **3E0C**

Pigment **3E0C**

Radioactive Substance **3E0C**

Sedatives **3E0C**

Gastrointestinal Tract

Lower **3E0H**

Analgesics **3E0H**

Anesthetic, Local **3E0H**

Anti-infective **3E0H**

Anti-inflammatory **3E0H**

Antineoplastic **3E0H**

Destructive Agent **3E0H**

Diagnostic Substance, Other **3E0H**

Electrolytic Substance **3E0H**

Gas **3E0H**

Hypnotics **3E0H**

Nutritional Substance **3E0H**

Radioactive Substance **3E0H**

Sedatives **3E0H**

Water Balance Substance **3E0H**

Upper **3E0G**

Analgesics **3E0G**

Anesthetic, Local **3E0G**

Anti-infective **3E0G**

Anti-inflammatory **3E0G**

Antineoplastic **3E0G**

Destructive Agent **3E0G**

Diagnostic Substance, Other **3E0G**

Electrolytic Substance **3E0G**

Gas **3E0G**

Hypnotics **3E0G**

Nutritional Substance **3E0G**

Radioactive Substance **3E0G**

Sedatives **3E0G**

Water Balance Substance **3E0G**

Genitourinary Tract **3E0K**

Introduction of substance (*continued*)

- Analgesics **3E0K**
- Anesthetic, Local **3E0K**
- Anti-infective **3E0K**
- Anti-inflammatory **3E0K**
- Antineoplastic **3E0K**
- Destructive Agent **3E0K**
- Diagnostic Substance, Other **3E0K**
- Electrolytic Substance **3E0K**
- Gas **3E0K**
- Hypnotics **3E0K**
- Nutritional Substance **3E0K**
- Radioactive Substance **3E0K**
- Sedatives **3E0K**
- Water Balance Substance **3E0K**

Heart **3E08**
- Diagnostic Substance, Other **3E08**
- Platelet Inhibitor **3E08**
- Thrombolytic **3E08**

Joint **3E0U**
- Analgesics **3E0U3NZ**
- Anesthetic, Local **3E0U3BZ**
- Anti-infective **3E0U**
- Anti-inflammatory **3E0U33Z**
- Antineoplastic **3E0U30**
- Destructive Agent **3E0U3TZ**
- Diagnostic Substance, Other **3E0U3KZ**
- Electrolytic Substance **3E0U37Z**
- Gas **3E0U3SF**
- Hypnotics **3E0U3NZ**
- Nutritional Substance **3E0U36Z**
- Radioactive Substance **3E0U3HZ**
- Sedatives **3E0U3NZ**
- Water Balance Substance **3E0U37Z**

Lymphatic **3E0W3GC**
- Analgesics **3E0W3NZ**
- Anesthetic, Local **3E0W3BZ**
- Anti-infective **3E0W32**
- Anti-inflammatory **3E0W33Z**
- Antineoplastic **3E0W30**
- Destructive Agent **3E0W3TZ**
- Diagnostic Substance, Other **3E0W3KZ**
- Electrolytic Substance **3E0W37Z**
- Hypnotics **3E0W3NZ**
- Nutritional Substance **3E0W36Z**
- Radioactive Substance **3E0W3HZ**
- Sedatives **3E0W3NZ**
- Water Balance Substance **3E0W37Z**

Mouth **3E0D**
- Analgesics **3E0D**
- Anesthetic, Local **3E0D**
- Anti-infective **3E0D**
- Anti-inflammatory **3E0D**
- Antiarrhythmic **3E0D**
- Antineoplastic **3E0D**
- Destructive Agent **3E0D**
- Diagnostic Substance, Other **3E0D**
- Electrolytic Substance **3E0D**
- Hypnotics **3E0D**
- Nutritional Substance **3E0D**
- Radioactive Substance **3E0D**
- Sedatives **3E0D**
- Serum **3E0D**
- Toxoid **3E0D**
- Vaccine **3E0D**
- Water Balance Substance **3E0D**

Introduction of substance (*continued*)

Mucous Membrane **3E00XGC**
- Analgesics **3E00XNZ**
- Anesthetic, Local **3E00XBZ**
- Anti-infective **3E00X2**
- Anti-inflammatory **3E00X3Z**
- Antineoplastic **3E00X0**
- Destructive Agent **3E00XTZ**
- Diagnostic Substance, Other **3E00XKZ**
- Hypnotics **3E00XNZ**
- Pigment **3E00XMZ**
- Sedatives **3E00XNZ**
- Serum **3E00X4Z**
- Toxoid **3E00X4Z**
- Vaccine **3E00X4Z**

Muscle **3E023GC**
- Analgesics **3E023NZ**
- Anesthetic, Local **3E023BZ**
- Anti-infective **3E0232**
- Anti-inflammatory **3E0233Z**
- Antineoplastic **3E0230**
- Destructive Agent **3E023TZ**
- Diagnostic Substance, Other **3E023KZ**
- Electrolytic Substance **3E0237Z**
- Hypnotics **3E023NZ**
- Nutritional Substance **3E0236Z**
- Radioactive Substance **3E023HZ**
- Sedatives **3E023NZ**
- Serum **3E0234Z**
- Toxoid **3E0234Z**
- Vaccine **3E0234Z**
- Water Balance Substance **3E0237Z**

Nerve
- Cranial **3E0X3GC**
  - Anesthetic
    - Local **3E0X3BZ**
    - Regional **3E0X3CZ**
  - Anti-inflammatory **3E0X33Z**
  - Destructive Agent **3E0X3TZ**
- Peripheral **3E0T3GC**
  - Anesthetic
    - Local **3E0T3BZ**
    - Regional **3E0T3CZ**
  - Anti-inflammatory **3E0T33Z**
  - Destructive Agent **3E0T3TZ**
- Plexus **3E0T3GC**
  - Anesthetic
    - Local **3E0T3BZ**
    - Regional **3E0T3CZ**
  - Anti-inflammatory **3E0T33Z**
  - Destructive Agent **3E0T3TZ**

Nose **3E09**
- Analgesics **3E09**
- Anesthetic, Local **3E09**
- Anti-infective **3E09**
- Anti-inflammatory **3E09**
- Antineoplastic **3E09**
- Destructive Agent **3E09**
- Diagnostic Substance, Other **3E09**
- Hypnotics **3E09**
- Radioactive Substance **3E09**
- Sedatives **3E09**
- Serum **3E09**
- Toxoid **3E09**
- Vaccine **3E09**

Pancreatic Tract **3E0J**

Introduction of substance (*continued*)

- Analgesics **3E0J**
- Anesthetic, Local **3E0J**
- Anti-infective **3E0J**
- Anti-inflammatory **3E0J**
- Antineoplastic **3E0J**
- Destructive Agent **3E0J**
- Diagnostic Substance, Other **3E0J**
- Electrolytic Substance **3E0J**
- Gas **3E0J**
- Hypnotics **3E0J**
- Islet Cells, Pancreatic **3E0J**
- Nutritional Substance **3E0J**
- Radioactive Substance **3E0J**
- Sedatives **3E0J**
- Water Balance Substance **3E0J**

Pericardial Cavity **3E0Y3GC**
- Analgesics **3E0Y3NZ**
- Anesthetic, Local **3E0Y3BZ**
- Anti-infective **3E0Y32**
- Anti-inflammatory **3E0Y33Z**
- Antineoplastic **3E0Y**
- Destructive Agent **3E0Y3TZ**
- Diagnostic Substance, Other **3E0Y3KZ**
- Electrolytic Substance **3E0Y37Z**
- Gas **3E0Y**
- Hypnotics **3E0Y3NZ**
- Nutritional Substance **3E0Y36Z**
- Radioactive Substance **3E0Y3HZ**
- Sedatives **3E0Y3NZ**
- Water Balance Substance **3E0Y37Z**

Peritoneal Cavity **3E0M3GC**
- Adhesion Barrier **3E0M05Z**
- Analgesics **3E0M3NZ**
- Anesthetic, Local **3E0M3BZ**
- Anti-infective **3E0M32**
- Anti-inflammatory **3E0M33Z**
- Antineoplastic **3E0M**
- Destructive Agent **3E0M3TZ**
- Diagnostic Substance, Other **3E0M3KZ**
- Electrolytic Substance **3E0M37Z**
- Gas **3E0M**
- Hypnotics **3E0M3NZ**
- Nutritional Substance **3E0M36Z**
- Radioactive Substance **3E0M3HZ**
- Sedatives **3E0M3NZ**
- Water Balance Substance **3E0M37Z**

Pharynx **3E0D**
- Analgesics **3E0D**
- Anesthetic, Local **3E0D**
- Anti-infective **3E0D**
- Anti-inflammatory **3E0D**
- Antiarrhythmic **3E0D**
- Antineoplastic **3E0D**
- Destructive Agent **3E0D**
- Diagnostic Substance, Other **3E0D**
- Electrolytic Substance **3E0D**
- Hypnotics **3E0D**
- Nutritional Substance **3E0D**
- Radioactive Substance **3E0D**
- Sedatives **3E0D**
- Serum **3E0D**
- Toxoid **3E0D**
- Vaccine **3E0D**
- Water Balance Substance **3E0D**

Pleural Cavity **3E0L3GC**

Introduction of substance *(continued)*
  Adhesion Barrier **3E0L05Z**
  Analgesics **3E0L3NZ**
  Anesthetic, Local **3E0L3BZ**
  Anti-infective **3E0L32**
  Anti-inflammatory **3E0L33Z**
  Antineoplastic **3E0L**
  Destructive Agent **3E0L3TZ**
  Diagnostic Substance, Other **3E0L3KZ**
  Electrolytic Substance **3E0L37Z**
  Gas **3E0L**
  Hypnotics **3E0L3NZ**
  Nutritional Substance **3E0L36Z**
  Radioactive Substance **3E0L3HZ**
  Sedatives **3E0L3NZ**
  Water Balance Substance **3E0L37Z**
Products of Conception **3E0E**
  Analgesics **3E0E**
  Anesthetic, Local **3E0E**
  Anti-infective **3E0E**
  Anti-inflammatory **3E0E**
  Antineoplastic **3E0E**
  Destructive Agent **3E0E**
  Diagnostic Substance, Other **3E0E**
  Electrolytic Substance **3E0E**
  Gas **3E0E**
  Hypnotics **3E0E**
  Nutritional Substance **3E0E**
  Radioactive Substance **3E0E**
  Sedatives **3E0E**
  Water Balance Substance **3E0E**
Reproductive
  Female **3E0P**
    Adhesion Barrier **3E0P05Z**
    Analgesics **3E0P**
    Anesthetic, Local **3E0P**
    Anti-infective **3E0P**
    Anti-inflammatory **3E0P**
    Antineoplastic **3E0P**
    Destructive Agent **3E0P**
    Diagnostic Substance, Other **3E0P**
    Electrolytic Substance **3E0P**
    Gas **3E0P**
    Hypnotics **3E0P**
    Nutritional Substance **3E0P**
    Ovum, Fertilized **3E0P**
    Radioactive Substance **3E0P**
    Sedatives **3E0P**
    Sperm **3E0P**
    Water Balance Substance **3E0P**
  Male **3E0N**
    Analgesics **3E0N**
    Anesthetic, Local **3E0N**
    Anti-infective **3E0N**
    Anti-inflammatory **3E0N**
    Antineoplastic **3E0N**
    Destructive Agent **3E0N**
    Diagnostic Substance, Other **3E0N**
    Electrolytic Substance **3E0N**
    Gas **3E0N**
    Hypnotics **3E0N**
    Nutritional Substance **3E0N**
    Radioactive Substance **3E0N**
    Sedatives **3E0N**
    Water Balance Substance **3E0N**
Respiratory Tract **3E0F**

Introduction of substance *(continued)*
  Analgesics **3E0F**
  Anesthetic
    Inhalation **3E0F**
    Local **3E0F**
  Anti-infective **3E0F**
  Anti-inflammatory **3E0F**
  Antineoplastic **3E0F**
  Destructive Agent **3E0F**
  Diagnostic Substance, Other **3E0F**
  Electrolytic Substance **3E0F**
  Gas **3E0F**
  Hypnotics **3E0F**
  Nutritional Substance **3E0F**
  Radioactive Substance **3E0F**
  Sedatives **3E0F**
  Water Balance Substance **3E0F**
Skin **3E00XGC**
  Analgesics **3E00XNZ**
  Anesthetic, Local **3E00XBZ**
  Anti-infective **3E00X2**
  Anti-inflammatory **3E00X3Z**
  Antineoplastic **3E00X0**
  Destructive Agent **3E00XTZ**
  Diagnostic Substance, Other **3E00XKZ**
  Hypnotics **3E00XNZ**
  Pigment **3E00XMZ**
  Sedatives **3E00XNZ**
  Serum **3E00X4Z**
  Toxoid **3E00X4Z**
  Vaccine **3E00X4Z**
Spinal Canal **3E0R3GC**
  Analgesics **3E0R3NZ**
  Anesthetic
    Local **3E0R3BZ**
    Regional **3E0R3CZ**
  Anti-infective **3E0R32**
  Anti-inflammatory **3E0R33Z**
  Antineoplastic **3E0R30**
  Destructive Agent **3E0R3TZ**
  Diagnostic Substance, Other **3E0R3KZ**
  Electrolytic Substance **3E0R37Z**
  Gas **3E0R**
  Hypnotics **3E0R3NZ**
  Nutritional Substance **3E0R36Z**
  Radioactive Substance **3E0R3HZ**
  Sedatives **3E0R3NZ**
  Stem Cells
    Embryonic **3E0R**
    Somatic **3E0R**
  Water Balance Substance **3E0R37Z**
Subcutaneous Tissue **3E013GC**
  Analgesics **3E013NZ**
  Anesthetic, Local **3E013BZ**
  Anti-infective **3E01**
  Anti-inflammatory **3E0133Z**
  Antineoplastic **3E0130**
  Destructive Agent **3E013TZ**
  Diagnostic Substance, Other **3E013KZ**
  Electrolytic Substance **3E0137Z**
  Hormone **3E013V**
  Hypnotics **3E013NZ**
  Nutritional Substance **3E0136Z**
  Radioactive Substance **3E013HZ**
  Sedatives **3E013NZ**
  Serum **3E0134Z**

Introduction of substance *(continued)*
  Toxoid **3E0134Z**
  Vaccine **3E0134Z**
  Water Balance Substance **3E0137Z**
Vein
  Central **3E04**
    Analgesics **3E04**
    Anesthetic, Intracirculatory **3E04**
    Anti-infective **3E04**
    Anti-inflammatory **3E04**
    Antiarrhythmic **3E04**
    Antineoplastic **3E04**
    Destructive Agent **3E04**
    Diagnostic Substance, Other **3E04**
    Electrolytic Substance **3E04**
    Hormone **3E04**
    Hypnotics **3E04**
    Immunotherapeutic **3E04**
    Nutritional Substance **3E04**
    Platelet Inhibitor **3E04**
    Radioactive Substance **3E04**
    Sedatives **3E04**
    Serum **3E04**
    Thrombolytic **3E04**
    Toxoid **3E04**
    Vaccine **3E04**
    Vasopressor **3E04**
    Water Balance Substance **3E04**
  Peripheral **3E03**
    Analgesics **3E03**
    Anesthetic, Intracirculatory **3E03**
    Anti-infective **3E03**
    Anti-inflammatory **3E03**
    Antiarrhythmic **3E03**
    Antineoplastic **3E03**
    Destructive Agent **3E03**
    Diagnostic Substance, Other **3E03**
    Electrolytic Substance **3E03**
    Hormone **3E03**
    Hypnotics **3E03**
    Immunotherapeutic **3E03**
    Islet Cells, Pancreatic **3E03**
    Nutritional Substance **3E03**
    Platelet Inhibitor **3E03**
    Radioactive Substance **3E03**
    Sedatives **3E03**
    Serum **3E03**
    Thrombolytic **3E03**
    Toxoid **3E03**
    Vaccine **3E03**
    Vasopressor **3E03**
    Water Balance Substance **3E03**
Intubation
  Airway
    see Insertion of device in, Trachea **0BH1**
    see Insertion of device in, Mouth and Throat **0CHY**
Intubation *(continued)*
    see Insertion of device in, Esophagus **0DH5**
  Drainage device *see* Drainage
  Feeding Device *see* Insertion of device in, Gastrointestinal System **0DH**
INTUITY Elite valve system, EDWARDS
use Zooplastic Tissue, Rapid Deployment Technique in New Technology

IPPB (intermittent positive pressure breathing) *see* Assistance, Respiratory **5A09**
Iridectomy
 see Excision, Eye **08B**
 see Resection, Eye **08T**
Iridoplasty
 see Repair, Eye **08Q**
 see Replacement, Eye **08R**
 see Supplement, Eye **08U**
Iridotomy *see* Drainage, Eye **089**
Irrigation
 Biliary Tract, Irrigating Substance **3E1J**
 Brain, Irrigating Substance **3E1Q38Z**
 Cranial Cavity, Irrigating Substance **3E1Q38Z**
 Ear, Irrigating Substance **3E1B**
 Epidural Space, Irrigating Substance **3E1S38Z**
 Eye, Irrigating Substance **3E1C**
 Gastrointestinal Tract
  Lower, Irrigating Substance **3E1H**
  Upper, Irrigating Substance **3E1G**
 Genitourinary Tract, Irrigating Substance **3E1K**
 Irrigating Substance **3C1ZX8Z**
 Joint, Irrigating Substance **3E1U38Z**
 Mucous Membrane, Irrigating Substance **3E10**
 Nose, Irrigating Substance **3E19**
 Pancreatic Tract, Irrigating Substance **3E1J**
 Pericardial Cavity, Irrigating Substance **3E1Y38Z**
 Peritoneal Cavity
  Dialysate **3E1M39Z**
  Irrigating Substance **3E1M38Z**
 Pleural Cavity, Irrigating Substance **3E1L38Z**
 Reproductive
  Female, Irrigating Substance **3E1P**
  Male, Irrigating Substance **3E1N**
 Respiratory Tract, Irrigating Substance **3E1F**
 Skin, Irrigating Substance **3E10**
 Spinal Canal, Irrigating Substance **3E1R38Z**
Isavuconazole Anti-infective XW0
Ischiatic nerve *use* Nerve, Sciatic
Ischiocavernosus muscle *use* Muscle, Perineum
Ischiofemoral ligament
 use Bursa and Ligament, Hip, Left
 use Bursa and Ligament, Hip, Right
Ischium
 use Bone, Pelvic, Right
 use Bone, Pelvic, Left
Isolation 8E0ZXY6
Isotope Administration, Whole Body DWY5G
Itrel (3)(4) neurostimulator *use* Stimulator Generator, Single Array in **0JH**

J

Jejunal artery *use* Artery, Superior Mesenteric

Jejunectomy
 see Excision, Jejunum **0DBA**
 see Resection, Jejunum **0DTA**
Jejunocolostomy
 see Bypass, Gastrointestinal System **0D1**
 see Drainage, Gastrointestinal System **0D9**
Jejunopexy
 see Repair, Jejunum **0DQA**
 see Reposition, Jejunum **0DSA**
Jejunostomy
 see Bypass, Jejunum **0D1A**
 see Drainage, Jejunum **0D9A**
Jejunotomy *see* Drainage, Jejunum **0D9A**
Joint fixation plate
 use Internal Fixation Device in Upper Joints
 use Internal Fixation Device in Lower Joints
Joint liner (insert) *use* Liner in Lower Joints
Joint spacer (antibiotic)
 use Spacer in Upper Joints
 use Spacer in Lower Joints
Jugular body *use* Glomus Jugulare
Jugular lymph node
 use Lymphatic, Neck, Left
 use Lymphatic, Neck, Right

K

Kappa *use* Pacemaker, Dual Chamber in **0JH**
Keratectomy, kerectomy
 see Excision, Eye **08B**
 see Resection, Eye **08T**
Keratocentesis *see* Drainage, Eye **089**
Keratoplasty
 see Repair, Eye **08Q**
 see Replacement, Eye **08R**
 see Supplement, Eye **08U**
Keratotomy
 see Drainage, Eye **089**
 see Repair, Eye **08Q**
Kinetra® neurostimulator *use* Stimulator Generator, Multiple Array in **0JH**
Kirschner wire (K-wire)
 use Internal Fixation Device in Head and Facial Bones
 use Internal Fixation Device in Upper Bones
 use Internal Fixation Device in Lower Bones
 use Internal Fixation Device in Upper Joints
 use Internal Fixation Device in Lower Joints
Knee (implant) insert *use* Liner in Lower Joints
KUB x-ray *see* Plain Radiography, Kidney, Ureter and Bladder **BT04**
Küntscher nail
 use Internal Fixation Device, Intramedullary in Upper Bones
 use Internal Fixation Device, Intramedullary in Lower Bones

L

Labia majora *use* Vulva
Labia minora *use* Vulva
Labial gland
 use Lip, Upper
 use Lip, Lower

Labiectomy
 see Excision, Female Reproductive System **0UB**
Labiectomy *(continued)*
 see Resection, Female Reproductive System **0UT**
Lacrimal canaliculus
 use Duct, Lacrimal, Left
 use Duct, Lacrimal, Right
Lacrimal punctum
 use Duct, Lacrimal, Right
 use Duct, Lacrimal, Left
Lacrimal sac
 use Duct, Lacrimal, Right
 use Duct, Lacrimal, Left
Laminectomy
 see Excision, Upper Bones **0PB**
 see Excision, Lower Bones **0QB**
 see Release, Central Nervous System **00N**
 see Release, Peripheral Nervous System **01N**
Laminotomy
 see Drainage, Upper Joints **0R9**
 see Drainage, Lower Joints **0S9**
 see Release, Central Nervous System **00N**
 see Release, Peripheral Nervous System **01N**
 see Release, Upper Joints **0RN**
 see Release, Lower Joints **0SN**
LAP-BAND® adjustable gastric banding system *use* Extraluminal Device
Laparoscopy *see* Inspection
Laparotomy
 Drainage *see* Drainage, Peritoneal Cavity **0W9G**
 Exploratory *see* Inspection, Peritoneal Cavity **0WJG**
Laryngectomy
 see Excision, Larynx **0CBS**
 see Resection, Larynx **0CTS**
Laryngocentesis *see* Drainage, Larynx **0C9S**
Laryngogram *see* Fluoroscopy, Larynx **B91J**
Laryngopexy *see* Repair, Larynx **0CQS**
Laryngopharynx *use* Pharynx
Laryngoplasty
 see Repair, Larynx **0CQS**
 see Replacement, Larynx **0CRS**
 see Supplement, Larynx **0CUS**
Laryngorrhaphy *see* Repair, Larynx **0CQS**
Laryngoscopy 0CJS8ZZ
Laryngotomy *see* Drainage, Larynx **0C9S**
Laser Interstitial Thermal Therapy
 Adrenal Gland **DGY2KZZ**
 Anus **DDY8KZZ**
 Bile Ducts **DFY2KZZ**
 Brain **D0Y0KZZ**
 Brain Stem **D0Y1KZZ**
 Breast
  Left **DMY0KZZ**
  Right **DMY1KZZ**
 Bronchus **DBY1KZZ**
 Chest Wall **DBY7KZZ**
 Colon **DDY5KZZ**
 Diaphragm **DBY8KZZ**
 Duodenum **DDY2KZZ**
 Esophagus **DDY0KZZ**
 Gallbladder **DFY1KZZ**
 Gland

Laser Interstitial Thermal Therapy
(continued)
Adrenal **DGY2KZZ**
Parathyroid **DGY4KZZ**
Pituitary **DGY0KZZ**
Thyroid **DGY5KZZ**
Ileum **DDY4KZZ**
Jejunum **DDY3KZZ**
Liver **DFY0KZZ**
Lung **DBY2KZZ**
Mediastinum **DBY6KZZ**
Nerve, Peripheral **D0Y7KZZ**
Pancreas **DFY3KZZ**
Parathyroid Gland **DGY4KZZ**
Pineal Body **DGY1KZZ**
Pituitary Gland **DGY0KZZ**
Pleura **DBY5KZZ**
Prostate **DVY0KZZ**
Rectum **DDY7KZZ**
Spinal Cord **D0Y6KZZ**
Stomach **DDY1KZZ**
Thyroid Gland **DGY5KZZ**
Trachea **DBY0KZZ**
Lateral (brachial) lymph node
use Lymphatic, Axillary, Left
use Lymphatic, Axillary, Right
Lateral canthus
use Eyelid, Upper, Right
use Eyelid, Upper, Left
Lateral collateral ligament (LCL)
use Bursa and Ligament, Knee, Right
use Bursa and Ligament, Knee, Left
Lateral condyle of femur
use Femur, Lower, Right
use Femur, Lower, Left
Lateral condyle of tibia
use Tibia, Left
use Tibia, Right
Lateral cuneiform bone
use Tarsal, Right
use Tarsal, Left
Lateral epicondyle of femur
use Femur, Lower, Left
use Femur, Lower, Right
Lateral epicondyle of humerus
use Humeral Shaft, Right
use Humeral Shaft, Left
Lateral femoral cutaneous nerve *use* Nerve, Lumbar Plexus
Lateral malleolus
use Fibula, Right
use Fibula, Left
Lateral meniscus
use Joint, Knee, Left
use Joint, Knee, Right
Lateral nasal cartilage *use* Nose
Lateral plantar artery
use Artery, Foot, Left
use Artery, Foot, Right
Lateral plantar nerve *use* Nerve, Tibial
Lateral rectus muscle
use Muscle, Extraocular, Left
use Muscle, Extraocular, Right
Lateral sacral artery
use Artery, Internal Iliac, Left
use Artery, Internal Iliac, Right

Lateral sacral vein
use Vein, Hypogastric, Left
use Vein, Hypogastric, Right
Lateral sural cutaneous nerve *use* Nerve, Peroneal
Lateral tarsal artery
use Artery, Foot, Right
use Artery, Foot, Left
Lateral temporomandibular ligament *use* Bursa and Ligament, Head and Neck
Lateral thoracic artery
use Artery, Axillary, Left
use Artery, Axillary, Right
Latissimus dorsi muscle
use Muscle, Trunk, Left
use Muscle, Trunk, Right
Latissimus Dorsi Myocutaneous Flap
Bilateral **0HRV075**
Left **0HRU075**
Right **0HRT075**
Lavage
see Irrigation
bronchial alveolar, diagnostic *see* Drainage, Respiratory System **0B9**
Least splanchnic nerve *use* Nerve, Thoracic Sympathetic
Left ascending lumbar vein *use* Vein, Hemiazygos
Left atrioventricular valve *use* Valve, Mitral
Left auricular appendix *use* Atrium, Left
Left colic vein *use* Vein, Colic
Left coronary sulcus *use* Heart, Left
Left gastric artery *use* Artery, Gastric
Left gastroepiploic artery *use* Artery, Splenic
Left gastroepiploic vein *use* Vein, Splenic
Left inferior phrenic vein *use* Vein, Renal, Left
Left inferior pulmonary vein *use* Vein, Pulmonary, Left
Left jugular trunk *use* Lymphatic, Thoracic Duct
Left lateral ventricle *use* Cerebral Ventricle
Left ovarian vein *use* Vein, Renal, Left
Left second lumbar vein *use* Vein, Renal, Left
Left subclavian trunk *use* Lymphatic, Thoracic Duct
Left subcostal vein *use* Vein, Hemiazygos
Left superior pulmonary vein *use* Vein, Pulmonary, Left
Left suprarenal vein *use* Vein, Renal, Left
Left testicular vein *use* Vein, Renal, Left
Lengthening
Bone, with device *see* Insertion of Limb Lengthening Device
Muscle, by incision *see* Division, Muscles **0K8**
Tendon, by incision *see* Division, Tendons **0L8**
Leptomeninges, intracranial *use* Cerebral Meninges
Leptomeninges, spinal *use* Spinal Meninges
Lesser alar cartilage *use* Nose
Lesser occipital nerve *use* Nerve, Cervical Plexus
Lesser splanchnic nerve *use* Nerve, Thoracic Sympathetic

Lesser trochanter
use Femur, Upper, Right
use Femur, Upper, Left
Lesser tuberosity
use Humeral Head, Left
use Humeral Head, Right
Lesser wing
use Bone, Sphenoid, Right
use Bone, Sphenoid, Left
Leukopheresis, therapeutic *see* Pheresis, Circulatory **6A55**
Levator anguli oris muscle *use* Muscle, Facial
Levator ani muscle *use* Perineum Muscle
Levator labii superioris alaeque nasi muscle *use* Muscle, Facial
Levator labii superioris muscle *use* Muscle, Facial
Levator palpebrae superioris muscle
use Eyelid, Upper, Left
use Eyelid, Upper, Right
Levator scapulae muscle
use Muscle, Neck, Left
use Muscle, Neck, Right
Levator veli palatini muscle *use* Muscle, Tongue, Palate, Pharynx
Levatores costarum muscle
use Muscle, Thorax, Left
use Muscle, Thorax, Right
LifeStent® (Flexstar)(XL) Vascular Stent System *use* Intraluminal Device
Ligament of head of fibula
use Bursa and Ligament, Knee, Right
use Bursa and Ligament, Knee, Left
Ligament of the lateral malleolus
use Bursa and Ligament, Ankle, Left
use Bursa and Ligament, Ankle, Right
Ligamentum flavum
use Bursa and Ligament, Trunk, Left
use Bursa and Ligament, Trunk, Right
Ligation *see* Occlusion
Ligation, hemorrhoid *see* Occlusion, Lower Veins, Hemorrhoidal Plexus
Light Therapy GZJZZZZ
Liner
Removal of device from
Hip
Left **0SPB09Z**
Right **0SP909Z**
Knee
Left **0SPD09Z**
Right **0SPC09Z**
Revision of device in
Hip
Left **0SWB09Z**
Right **0SW909Z**
Knee
Left **0SWD09Z**
Right **0SWC09Z**
Supplement
Hip
Left **0SUB09Z**
Acetabular Surface **0SUE09Z**
Femoral Surface **0SUS09Z**
Right **0SU909Z**
Acetabular Surface **0SUA09Z**
Femoral Surface **0SUR09Z**

Liner *(continued)*
  Knee
    Left **0SUD09**
      Femoral Surface **0SUU09Z**
      Tibial Surface **0SUW09Z**
    Right **0SUC09**
      Femoral Surface **0SUT09Z**
      Tibial Surface **0SUV09Z**

Lingual artery
  use Artery, External Carotid, Right
  use Artery, External Carotid, Left

Lingual tonsil *use* Tongue

Lingulectomy, lung
  see Excision, Lung Lingula **0BBH**
  see Resection, Lung Lingula **0BTH**

Lithotripsy
  see Fragmentation
  with removal of fragments *see* Extirpation

LITT (laser interstitial thermal therapy) *see* Laser Interstitial Thermal Therapy

LIVIAN™ CRT-D *use* Cardiac Resynchronization Defibrillator Pulse Generator in **0JH**

Lobectomy
  see Excision, Central Nervous System **00B**
  see Excision, Respiratory System **0BB**
  see Resection, Respiratory System **0BT**
  see Excision, Hepatobiliary System and Pancreas **0FB**
  see Resection, Hepatobiliary System and Pancreas **0FT**

Lobectomy *(continued)*
  see Excision, Endocrine System **0GB**
  see Resection, Endocrine System **0GT**

Lobotomy *see* Division, Brain **0080**

Localization
  see Map
  see Imaging

Locus ceruleus *use* Pons

Long thoracic nerve *use* Nerve, Brachial Plexus

Loop ileostomy *see* Bypass, Ileum **0D1B**

Loop recorder, implantable *use* Monitoring Device

Lower GI series *see* Fluoroscopy, Colon **BD14**

Lumbar artery *use* Aorta, Abdominal

Lumbar facet joint
  use Joint, Lumbar Vertebral, 2 or more
  use Joint, Lumbar Vertebral

Lumbar ganglion *use* Nerve, Lumbar Sympathetic

Lumbar lymph node *use* Lymphatic, Aortic

Lumbar lymphatic trunk *use* Cisterna Chyli

Lumbar splanchnic nerve *use* Nerve, Lumbar Sympathetic

Lumbosacral facet joint *use* Joint, Lumbosacral

Lumbosacral trunk *use* Nerve, Lumbar

Lumpectomy *see* Excision

Lunate bone
  use Carpal, Left
  use Carpal, Right

Lunotriquetral ligament
  use Bursa and Ligament, Hand, Left
  use Bursa and Ligament, Hand, Right

Lymphadenectomy
  see Excision, Lymphatic and Hemic Systems **07B**
  see Resection, Lymphatic and Hemic Systems **07T**

Lymphadenotomy *see* Drainage, Lymphatic and Hemic Systems **079**

Lymphangiectomy
  see Excision, Lymphatic and Hemic Systems **07B**
  see Resection, Lymphatic and Hemic Systems **07T**

Lymphangiogram *see* Plain Radiography, Lymphatic System **B70**

Lymphangioplasty
  see Repair, Lymphatic and Hemic Systems **07Q**
  see Supplement, Lymphatic and Hemic Systems **07U**

Lymphangiorrhaphy *see* Repair, Lymphatic and Hemic Systems **07Q**

Lymphangiotomy *see* Drainage, Lymphatic and Hemic Systems **079**

Lysis *see* Release

M

Macula
  use Retina, Right
  use Retina, Left

MAGEC(R) Spinal Bracing and Distraction System *use* Magnetically Controlled Growth Rod(s) in New Technology

Magnet extraction, ocular foreign body *see* Extirpation, Eye **08C**

Magnetic Resonance Imaging (MRI)
  Abdomen **BW30**
  Ankle
    Left **BQ3H**
    Right **BQ3G**
  Aorta
    Abdominal **B430**
    Thoracic **B330**
  Arm
    Left **BP3F**
    Right **BP3E**
  Artery
    Celiac **B431**
    Cervico-Cerebral Arch **B33Q**
    Common Carotid, Bilateral **B335**
    Coronary
      Bypass Graft, Multiple **B233**
      Multiple **B231**
    Internal Carotid, Bilateral **B338**
    Intracranial **B33R**
    Lower Extremity
      Bilateral **B43H**
      Left **B43G**
      Right **B43F**
    Pelvic **B43C**
    Renal, Bilateral **B438**
    Spinal **B33M**
    Superior Mesenteric **B434**
    Upper Extremity
      Bilateral **B33K**
      Left **B33J**

Magnetic Resonance Imaging *(continued)*
      Right **B33H**
      Vertebral, Bilateral **B33G**
  Bladder **BT30**
  Brachial Plexus **BW3P**
  Brain **B030**
  Breast
    Bilateral **BH32**
    Left **BH31**
    Right **BH30**
  Calcaneus
    Left **BQ3K**
    Right **BQ3J**
  Chest **BW33Y**
  Coccyx **BR3F**
  Connective Tissue
    Lower Extremity **BL31**
    Upper Extremity **BL30**
  Corpora Cavernosa **BV30**
  Disc
    Cervical **BR31**
    Lumbar **BR33**
    Thoracic **BR32**
  Ear **B930**
  Elbow
    Left **BP3H**
    Right **BP3G**
  Eye
    Bilateral **B837**
    Left **B836**
    Right **B835**
  Femur
    Left **BQ34**
    Right **BQ33**
  Fetal Abdomen **BY33**
  Fetal Extremity **BY35**
  Fetal Head **BY30**
  Fetal Heart **BY31**
  Fetal Spine **BY34**
  Fetal Thorax **BY32**
  Fetus, Whole **BY36**
  Foot
    Left **BQ3M**
    Right **BQ3L**
  Forearm
    Left **BP3K**
    Right **BP3J**
  Gland
    Adrenal, Bilateral **BG32**
    Parathyroid **BG33**
    Parotid, Bilateral **B936**
    Salivary, Bilateral **B93D**
    Submandibular, Bilateral **B939**
    Thyroid **BG34**
  Head **BW38**
  Heart, Right and Left **B236**
  Hip
    Left **BQ31**
    Right **BQ30**
  Intracranial Sinus **B532**
  Joint
    Finger
      Left **BP3D**
      Right **BP3C**
    Hand
      Left **BP3D**

Magnetic Resonance Imaging (continued)
- Right **BP3C**
- Temporomandibular, Bilateral **BN39**
- Kidney
  - Bilateral **BT33**
  - Left **BT32**
  - Right **BT31**
  - Transplant **BT39**
- Knee
  - Left **BQ38**
  - Right **BQ37**
- Larynx **B93J**
- Leg
  - Left **BQ3F**
  - Right **BQ3D**
- Liver **BF35**
- Liver and Spleen **BF36**
- Lung Apices **BB3G**
- Nasopharynx **B93F**
- Neck **BW3F**
- Nerve
  - Acoustic **B03C**
  - Brachial Plexus **BW3P**
- Oropharynx **B93F**
- Ovary
  - Bilateral **BU35**
  - Left **BU34**
  - Right **BU33**
- Ovary and Uterus **BU3C**
- Pancreas **BF37**
- Patella
  - Left **BQ3W**
  - Right **BQ3V**
- Pelvic Region **BW3G**
- Pelvis **BR3C**
- Pituitary Gland **B039**
- Plexus, Brachial **BW3P**
- Prostate **BV33**
- Retroperitoneum **BW3H**
- Sacrum **BR3F**
- Scrotum **BV34**
- Sella Turcica **B039**
- Shoulder
  - Left **BP39**
  - Right **BP38**
- Sinus
  - Intracranial **B532**
  - Paranasal **B932**
- Spinal Cord **B03B**
- Spine
  - Cervical **BR30**
  - Lumbar **BR39**
  - Thoracic **BR37**
- Spleen and Liver **BF36**
- Subcutaneous Tissue
  - Abdomen **BH3H**
  - Extremity
    - Lower **BH3J**
    - Upper **BH3F**
  - Head **BH3D**
  - Neck **BH3D**
  - Pelvis **BH3H**
  - Thorax **BH3G**
- Tendon
  - Lower Extremity **BL33**
  - Upper Extremity **BL32**

Magnetic Resonance Imaging (continued)
- Testicle
  - Bilateral **BV37**
  - Left **BV36**
  - Right **BV35**
- Toe
  - Left **BQ3Q**
  - Right **BQ3P**
- Uterus **BU36**
  - Pregnant **BU3B**
- Uterus and Ovary **BU3C**
- Vagina **BU39**
- Vein
  - Cerebellar **B531**
  - Cerebral **B531**
  - Jugular, Bilateral **B535**
  - Lower Extremity
    - Bilateral **B53D**
    - Left **B53C**
    - Right **B53B**
  - Other **B53V**
  - Pelvic (Iliac) Bilateral **B53H**
  - Portal **B53T**
  - Pulmonary, Bilateral **B53S**
  - Renal, Bilateral **B53L**
  - Splanchnic **B53T**
  - Upper Extremity
    - Bilateral **B53P**
    - Left **B53N**
    - Right **B53M**
  - Vena Cava
    - Inferior **B539**
    - Superior **B538**
- Wrist
  - Left **BP3M**
  - Right **BP3L**

Magnetically Controlled Growth Rod(s)
- Cervical **XNS3**
- Lumbar **XNS0**
- Thoracic **XNS4**

Malleotomy see Drainage, Ear, Nose, Sinus **099**

Malleus
- *use* Auditory Ossicle, Right
- *use* Auditory Ossicle, Left

Mammaplasty, mammoplasty
- *see* Alteration, Skin and Breast **0H0**
- *see* Repair, Skin and Breast **0HQ**
- *see* Replacement, Skin and Breast **0HR**
- *see* Supplement, Skin and Breast **0HU**

Mammary duct
- *use* Breast, Bilateral
- *use* Breast, Right
- *use* Breast, Left

Mammary gland
- *use* Breast, Bilateral
- *use* Breast, Right
- *use* Breast, Left

Mammectomy
- *see* Excision, Skin and Breast **0HB**
- *see* Resection, Skin and Breast **0HT**

Mammillary body *use* Hypothalamus

Mammography *see* Plain Radiography, Skin, Subcutaneous Tissue and Breast **BH0**

Mammotomy *see* Drainage, Skin and Breast **0H9**

Mandibular nerve *use* Nerve, Trigeminal

Mandibular notch
- *use* Mandible, Right
- *use* Mandible, Left

Mandibulectomy
- *see* Excision, Head and Facial Bones **0NB**
- *see* Resection, Head and Facial Bones **0NT**

Manipulation
- Adhesions *see* Release
- Chiropractic *see* Chiropractic Manipulation

Manubrium *use* Sternum

Map
- Basal Ganglia **00K8**
- Brain **00K0**
- Cerebellum **00KC**
- Cerebral Hemisphere **00K7**
- Conduction Mechanism **02K8**
- Hypothalamus **00KA**
- Medulla Oblongata **00KD**
- Pons **00KB**
- Thalamus **00K9**

Mapping
- Doppler ultrasound *see* Ultrasonography
- Electrocardiogram only *see* Measurement, Cardiac **4A02**

Mark IV Breathing Pacemaker System *use* Stimulator Generator in Subcutaneous Tissue and Fascia

Marsupialization
- *see* Drainage
- *see* Excision

Massage, cardiac
- External **5A12012**
- Open **02QA0ZZ**

Masseter muscle *use* Muscle, Head

Masseteric fascia *use* Subcutaneous Tissue and Fascia, Face

Mastectomy
- *see* Excision, Skin and Breast **0HB**
- *see* Resection, Skin and Breast **0HT**

Mastoid (postauricular) lymph node
- *use* Lymphatic, Neck, Left
- *use* Lymphatic, Neck, Right

Mastoid air cells
- *use* Sinus, Mastoid, Left
- *use* Sinus, Mastoid, Right

Mastoid process
- *use* Bone, Temporal, Right
- *use* Bone, Temporal, Left

Mastoidectomy
- *see* Excision, Ear, Nose, Sinus **09B**
- *see* Resection, Ear, Nose, Sinus **09T**

Mastoidotomy *see* Drainage, Ear, Nose, Sinus **099**

Mastopexy
- *see* Reposition, Skin and Breast **0HS**
- *see* Repair, Skin and Breast **0HQ**

Mastotomy *see* Drainage, Skin and Breast **0H9**

Maxillary artery
- *use* Artery, External Carotid, Right
- *use* Artery, External Carotid, Left

Maxillary nerve *use* Nerve, Trigeminal

Maximo II DR (VR) *use* Defibrillator Generator in **0JH**

Maximo II DR CRT-D *use* Cardiac Resynchronization Defibrillator Pulse Generator in **0JH**

Measurement
- Arterial
  - Flow
    - Coronary **4A03**
    - Peripheral **4A03**
    - Pulmonary **4A03**
  - Pressure
    - Coronary **4A03**
    - Peripheral **4A03**
    - Pulmonary **4A03**
    - Thoracic, Other **4A03**
  - Pulse
    - Coronary **4A03**
    - Peripheral **4A03**
    - Pulmonary **4A03**
  - Saturation, Peripheral **4A03**
  - Sound, Peripheral **4A03**
- Biliary
  - Flow **4A0C**
  - Pressure **4A0C**
- Cardiac
  - Action Currents **4A02**
  - Defibrillator **4B02XTZ**
  - Electrical Activity **4A02**
    - Guidance **4A02X4A**
    - No Qualifier **4A02X4Z**
  - Output **4A02**
  - Pacemaker **4B02XSZ**
  - Rate **4A02**
  - Rhythm **4A02**
  - Sampling and Pressure
    - Bilateral **4A02**
    - Left Heart **4A02**
    - Right Heart **4A02**
  - Sound **4A02**
  - Total Activity, Stress **4A02XM4**
- Central Nervous
  - Conductivity **4A00**
  - Electrical Activity **4A00**
  - Pressure **4A000BZ**
    - Intracranial **4A00**
  - Saturation, Intracranial **4A00**
  - Stimulator **4B00XVZ**
  - Temperature, Intracranial **4A00**
- Circulatory, Volume **4A05XLZ**
- Gastrointestinal
  - Motility **4A0B**
  - Pressure **4A0B**
  - Secretion **4A0B**
- Lymphatic
  - Flow **4A06**
  - Pressure **4A06**
- Metabolism **4A0Z**
- Musculoskeletal
  - Contractility **4A0F**
  - Stimulator **4B0FXVZ**
- Olfactory, Acuity **4A08X0Z**
- Peripheral Nervous
  - Conductivity
    - Motor **4A01**
    - Sensory **4A01**
  - Electrical Activity **4A01**
  - Stimulator **4B01XVZ**
- Products of Conception
  - Cardiac
    - Electrical Activity **4A0H**

Measurement *(continued)*
- Rate **4A0H**
- Rhythm **4A0H**
- Sound **4A0H**
- Nervous
  - Conductivity **4A0J**
  - Electrical Activity **4A0J**
  - Pressure **4A0J**
- Respiratory
  - Capacity **4A09**
  - Flow **4A09**
  - Pacemaker **4B09XSZ**
  - Rate **4A09**
  - Resistance **4A09**
  - Total Activity **4A09**
  - Volume **4A09**
- Sleep **4A0ZXQZ**
- Temperature **4A0Z**
- Urinary
  - Contractility **4A0D73Z**
  - Flow **4A0D75Z**
  - Pressure **4A0D7BZ**
  - Resistance **4A0D7DZ**
  - Volume **4A0D7LZ**
- Venous
  - Flow
    - Central **4A04**
    - Peripheral **4A04**
    - Portal **4A04**
    - Pulmonary **4A04**
  - Pressure
    - Central **4A04**
    - Peripheral **4A04**
    - Portal **4A04**
    - Pulmonary **4A04**
  - Pulse
    - Central **4A04**
    - Peripheral **4A04**
    - Portal **4A04**
    - Pulmonary **4A04**
  - Saturation, Peripheral **4A04**
- Visual
  - Acuity **4A07X0Z**
  - Mobility **4A07X7Z**
  - Pressure **4A07XBZ**

Meatoplasty, urethra *see* Repair, Urethra **0TQD**

Meatotomy *see* Drainage, Urinary System **0T9**

Mechanical ventilation *see* Performance, Respiratory **5A19**

Medial canthus
- *use* Eyelid, Lower, Left
- *use* Eyelid, Lower, Right

Medial collateral ligament (MCL)
- *use* Bursa and Ligament, Knee, Left
- *use* Bursa and Ligament, Knee, Right

Medial condyle of femur
- *use* Femur, Lower, Left
- *use* Femur, Lower, Right

Medial condyle of tibia
- *use* Tibia, Left
- *use* Tibia, Right

Medial cuneiform bone
- *use* Tarsal, Left
- *use* Tarsal, Right

Medial epicondyle of femur
- *use* Femur, Lower, Left
- *use* Femur, Lower, Right

Medial epicondyle of humerus
- *use* Humeral Shaft, Left
- *use* Humeral Shaft, Right

Medial malleolus
- *use* Tibia, Left
- *use* Tibia, Right

Medial meniscus
- *use* Joint, Knee, Left
- *use* Joint, Knee, Right

Medial plantar artery
- *use* Artery, Foot, Left
- *use* Artery, Foot, Right

Medial plantar nerve *use* Nerve, Tibial

Medial popliteal nerve *use* Nerve, Tibial

Medial rectus muscle
- *use* Muscle, Extraocular, Left
- *use* Muscle, Extraocular, Right

Medial sural cutaneous nerve *use* Nerve, Tibial

Median antebrachial vein
- *use* Vein, Basilic, Left
- *use* Vein, Basilic, Right

Median cubital vein
- *use* Vein, Basilic, Left
- *use* Vein, Basilic, Right

Median sacral artery *use* Aorta, Abdominal

Mediastinal lymph node *use* Lymphatic, Thorax

Mediastinoscopy 0WJC4ZZ

Medication Management GZ3ZZZZ
- for substance abuse
  - Antabuse **HZ83ZZZ**
  - Bupropion **HZ87ZZZ**
  - Clonidine **HZ86ZZZ**
  - Levo-alpha-acetyl-methadol (LAAM) **HZ82ZZZ**
  - Methadone Maintenance **HZ81ZZZ**
  - Naloxone **HZ85ZZZ**
  - Naltrexone **HZ84ZZZ**
  - Nicotine Replacement **HZ80ZZZ**
  - Other Replacement Medication **HZ89ZZZ**
  - Psychiatric Medication **HZ88ZZZ**

Meditation 8E0ZXY5

Medtronic Endurant(R) II AAA stent graft system *use* Intraluminal Device

Meissner's (submucous) plexus *use* Nerve, Abdominal Sympathetic

Melody® transcatheter pulmonary valve *use* Zooplastic Tissue in Heart and Great Vessels

Membranous urethra *use* Urethra

Meningeorrhaphy
- *see* Repair, Cerebral Meninges **00Q1**
- *see* Repair, Spinal Meninges **00QT**

Meniscectomy, knee
- *see* Excision, Joint, Knee, Right **0SBC**
- *see* Excision, Joint, Knee, Left **0SBD**

Mental foramen
- *use* Mandible, Left
- *use* Mandible, Right

Mentalis muscle *use* Muscle, Facial

Mentoplasty *see* Alteration, Jaw, Lower **0W05**

Mesenterectomy *see* Excision, Mesentery **0DBV**

Mesenteriorrhaphy, mesenterorrhaphy *see* Repair, Mesentery **0DQV**

Mesenteriplication *see* Repair, Mesentery **0DQV**

Mesoappendix *use* Mesentery

Mesocolon *use* Mesentery

Metacarpal ligament
  use Bursa and Ligament, Hand, Left
  use Bursa and Ligament, Hand, Right

Metacarpophalangeal ligament
  use Bursa and Ligament, Hand, Left
  use Bursa and Ligament, Hand, Right

Metal on metal bearing surface *use* Synthetic Substitute, Metal in 0SR

Metatarsal ligament
  use Bursa and Ligament, Foot, Left
  use Bursa and Ligament, Foot, Right

Metatarsectomy
  see Excision, Lower Bones **0QB**
  see Resection, Lower Bones **0QT**

Metatarsophalangeal (MTP) joint
  use Joint, Metatarsal-Phalangeal, Left
  use Joint, Metatarsal-Phalangeal, Right

Metatarsophalangeal ligament
  use Bursa and Ligament, Foot, Left
  use Bursa and Ligament, Foot, Right

Metathalamus *use* Thalamus

Micro-Driver stent (RX) (OTW) *use* Intraluminal Device

MicroMed Heart Assist *use* Implantable Heart Assist System in Heart and Great Vessels

Micrus CERECYTE microcoil *use* Intraluminal Device, Bioactive in Upper Arteries

Midcarpal joint
  use Joint, Carpal, Right
  use Joint, Carpal, Left

Middle cardiac nerve *use* Nerve, Thoracic Sympathetic

Middle cerebral artery *use* Artery, Intracranial

Middle cerebral vein *use* Vein, Intracranial

Middle colic vein *use* Vein, Colic

Middle genicular artery
  use Artery, Popliteal, Left
  use Artery, Popliteal, Right

Middle hemorrhoidal vein
  use Vein, Hypogastric, Left
  use Vein, Hypogastric, Right

Middle rectal artery
  use Artery, Internal Iliac, Left
  use Artery, Internal Iliac, Right

Middle suprarenal artery *use* Aorta, Abdominal

Middle temporal artery
  use Artery, Temporal, Left
  use Artery, Temporal, Right

Middle turbinate *use* Turbinate, Nasal

MIRODERM(tm) Biologic Wound Matrix *use* Skin Substitute, Porcine Liver Derived in New Technology

MitraClip valve repair system *use* Synthetic Substitute

Mitral annulus *use* Valve, Mitral

Mitroflow® Aortic Pericardial Heart Valve *use* Zooplastic Tissue in Heart and Great Vessels

Mobilization, adhesions *see* Release

Molar gland *use* Buccal Mucosa

Monitoring
  Arterial
    Flow
      Coronary **4A13**
      Peripheral **4A13**
      Pulmonary **4A13**
    Pressure
      Coronary **4A13**
      Peripheral **4A13**
      Pulmonary **4A13**
    Pulse
      Coronary **4A13**
      Peripheral **4A13**
      Pulmonary **4A13**
    Saturation, Peripheral **4A13**
    Sound, Peripheral **4A13**
  Cardiac
    Electrical Activity **4A12**
      Ambulatory **4A12X45**
      No Qualifier **4A12X4Z**
    Output **4A12**
    Rate **4A12**
    Rhythm **4A12**
    Sound **4A12**
    Total Activity, Stress **4A12XM4**
    Vascular Perfusion, Indocyanine Green Dye **4A12XSH**
  Central Nervous
    Conductivity **4A10**
    Electrical Activity
      Intraoperative **4A10**
      No Qualifier **4A10**
    Pressure **4A100BZ**
      Intracranial **4A10**
    Saturation, Intracranial **4A10**
    Temperature, Intracranial **4A10**
  Gastrointestinal
    Motility **4A1B**
    Pressure **4A1B**
    Secretion **4A1B**
    Skin and Breast, Vascular Perfusion, Indocyanine Green Dye **4A1GXSH**
    Vascular Perfusion, Indocyanine Green Dye **4A1BXSH**
  Intraoperative Knee Replacement Sensor **XR2**
  Lymphatic
    Flow **4A16**
    Pressure **4A16**
  Peripheral Nervous
    Conductivity
      Motor **4A11**
      Sensory **4A11**
    Electrical Activity
      Intraoperative **4A11**
      No Qualifier **4A11**
  Products of Conception
    Cardiac
      Electrical Activity **4A1H**
      Rate **4A1H**
      Rhythm **4A1H**

Monitoring *(continued)*
      Sound **4A1H**
  Nervous
    Conductivity **4A1J**
    Electrical Activity **4A1J**
    Pressure **4A1J**
  Respiratory
    Capacity **4A19**
    Flow **4A19**
    Rate **4A19**
    Resistance **4A19**
    Volume **4A19**
  Sleep **4A1ZXQZ**
  Temperature **4A1Z**
  Urinary
    Contractility **4A1D73Z**
    Flow **4A1D75Z**
    Pressure **4A1D7BZ**
    Resistance **4A1D7DZ**
    Volume **4A1D7LZ**
  Venous
    Flow
      Central **4A14**
      Peripheral **4A14**
      Portal **4A14**
      Pulmonary **4A14**
    Pressure
      Central **4A14**
      Peripheral **4A14**
      Portal **4A14**
      Pulmonary **4A14**
    Pulse
      Central **4A14**
      Peripheral **4A14**
      Portal **4A14**
      Pulmonary **4A14**
    Saturation
      Central **4A14**
      Portal **4A14**
      Pulmonary **4A14**

Monitoring Device
  Abdomen **0JH8**
  Chest **0JH6**

Motor Function Assessment F01

Motor Treatment F07

MR Angiography
  see Magnetic Resonance Imaging (MRI), Heart **B23**
  see Magnetic Resonance Imaging (MRI), Upper Arteries **B33**
  see Magnetic Resonance Imaging (MRI), Lower Arteries **B43**

Multiple sleep latency test 4A0ZXQZ

Musculocutaneous nerve *use* Nerve, Brachial Plexus

Musculopexy
  see Repair, Muscles **0KQ**
  see Reposition, Muscles **0KS**

Musculophrenic artery
  use Artery, Internal Mammary, Left
  use Artery, Internal Mammary, Right

Musculoplasty
  see Repair, Muscles **0KQ**
  see Supplement, Muscles **0KU**

Musculorrhaphy *see* Repair, Muscles **0KQ**

Musculospiral nerve *use* Nerve, Radial

Myectomy
see Excision, Muscles **0KB**
see Resection, Muscles **0KT**
Myelencephalon use Medulla Oblongata
Myelogram
CT see Computerized Tomography (CT Scan), Central Nervous System **B02**
MRI see Magnetic Resonance Imaging (MRI), Central Nervous System **B03**
Myenteric (Auerbach's) plexus use Nerve, Abdominal Sympathetic
Myomectomy see Excision, Female Reproductive System **0UB**
Myometrium use Uterus
Myopexy
see Repair, Muscles **0KQ**
see Reposition, Muscles **0KS**
Myoplasty
see Repair, Muscles **0KQ**
see Supplement, Muscles **0KU**
Myorrhaphy see Repair, Muscles **0KQ**
Myoscopy see Inspection, Muscles **0KJ**
Myotomy
see Division, Muscles **0K8**
see Drainage, Muscles **0K9**
Myringectomy
see Excision, Ear, Nose, Sinus **09B**
see Resection, Ear, Nose, Sinus **09T**
Myringoplasty
see Repair, Ear, Nose, Sinus **09Q**
see Replacement, Ear, Nose, Sinus **09R**
see Supplement, Ear, Nose, Sinus **09U**
Myringostomy see Drainage, Ear, Nose, Sinus **099**
Myringotomy see Drainage, Ear, Nose, Sinus **099**

N

Nail bed
use Finger Nail
use Toe Nail
Nail plate
use Finger Nail
use Toe Nail
nanoLOCK(tm) interbody fusion device use Interbody Fusion Device, Nanotextured Surface in New Technology
Narcosynthesis GZGZZZZ
Nasal cavity use Nose
Nasal concha use Turbinate, Nasal
Nasalis muscle use Muscle, Facial
Nasolacrimal duct
use Duct, Lacrimal, Right
use Duct, Lacrimal, Left
Nasopharyngeal airway (NPA) use Intraluminal Device, Airway in Ear, Nose, Sinus
Navicular bone
use Tarsal, Left
use Tarsal, Right
Near Infrared Spectroscopy, Circulatory System 8E023DZ
Neck of femur
use Femur, Upper, Right
use Femur, Upper, Left

Neck of humerus (anatomical)(surgical)
use Humeral Head, Right
use Humeral Head, Left
Nephrectomy
see Excision, Urinary System **0TB**
see Resection, Urinary System **0TT**
Nephrolithotomy see Extirpation, Urinary System **0TC**
Nephrolysis see Release, Urinary System **0TN**
Nephropexy
see Repair, Urinary System **0TQ**
see Reposition, Urinary System **0TS**
Nephroplasty
see Repair, Urinary System **0TQ**
see Supplement, Urinary System **0TU**
Nephropyeloureterostomy
see Bypass, Urinary System **0T1**
see Drainage, Urinary System **0T9**
Nephrorrhaphy see Repair, Urinary System **0TQ**
Nephroscopy, transurethral 0TJ58ZZ
Nephrostomy
see Bypass, Urinary System **0T1**
see Drainage, Urinary System **0T9**
Nephrotomography
see Plain Radiography, Urinary System **BT0**
see Fluoroscopy, Urinary System **BT1**
Nephrotomy
see Drainage, Urinary System **0T9**
see Division, Urinary System **0T8**
Nerve conduction study
see Measurement, Central Nervous **4A00**
see Measurement, Peripheral Nervous **4A01**
Nerve Function Assessment F01
Nerve to the stapedius use Nerve, Facial
Neurectomy
see Excision, Central Nervous System **00B**
see Excision, Peripheral Nervous System **01B**
Neurexeresis
see Extraction, Central Nervous System **00D**
see Extraction, Peripheral Nervous System **01D**
Neurohypophysis use Gland, Pituitary
Neurolysis
see Release, Central Nervous System **00N**
see Release, Peripheral Nervous System **01N**
Neuromuscular electrical stimulation (NEMS) lead use Stimulator Lead in Muscles
Neurophysiologic monitoring see Monitoring, Central Nervous **4A10**
Neuroplasty
see Repair, Central Nervous System **00Q**
see Repair, Peripheral Nervous System **01Q**
see Supplement, Central Nervous System **00U**
see Supplement, Peripheral Nervous System **01U**
Neurorrhaphy
see Repair, Central Nervous System **00Q**
see Repair, Peripheral Nervous System **01Q**
Neurostimulator Generator
Insertion of device in, Skull **0NH00NZ**
Removal of device from, Skull **0NP00NZ**
Revision of device in, Skull **0NW00NZ**

Neurostimulator generator, multiple channel use Stimulator Generator, Multiple Array in **0JH**
Neurostimulator generator, multiple channel rechargeable use Stimulator Generator, Multiple Array Rechargeable in **0JH**
Neurostimulator generator, single channel use Stimulator Generator, Single Array in **0JH**
Neurostimulator generator, single channel rechargeable use Stimulator Generator, Single Array Rechargeable in **0JH**
Neurostimulator Lead
Insertion of device in
Brain **00H0**
Cerebral Ventricle **00H6**
Nerve
Cranial **00HE**
Peripheral **01HY**
Spinal Canal **00HU**
Spinal Cord **00HV**
Vein
Azygos **05H0**
Innominate
Left **05H4**
Right **05H3**
Removal of device from
Brain **00P0**
Cerebral Ventricle **00P6**
Nerve
Cranial **00PE**
Peripheral **01PY**
Spinal Canal **00PU**
Spinal Cord **00PV**
Vein
Azygos **05P0**
Innominate
Left **05P4**
Right **05P3**
Revision of device in
Brain **00W0**
Cerebral Ventricle **00W6**
Nerve
Cranial **00WE**
Peripheral **01WY**
Spinal Canal **00WU**
Spinal Cord **00WV**
Vein
Azygos **05W0**
Innominate
Left **05W4**
Right **05W3**
Neurotomy
see Division, Central Nervous System **008**
see Division, Peripheral Nervous System **018**
Neurotripsy
see Destruction, Central Nervous System **005**
see Destruction, Peripheral Nervous System **015**
Neutralization plate
use Internal Fixation Device in Head and Facial Bones
use Internal Fixation Device in Upper Bones
use Internal Fixation Device in Lower Bones

New Technology

Andexanet Alfa, Factor Xa Inhibitor
Reversal Agent **XW0**
Blinatumomab Antineoplastic
Immunotherapy **XW0**
Ceftazidime-Avibactam Anti-infective **XW0**
Cerebral Embolic Filtration, Dual Filter
X2A5312
Defibrotide Sodium Anticoagulant **XW0**
Fusion
Cervical Vertebral
2 or more, Interbody Fusion Device,
Nanotextured Surface **XRG2092**
Interbody Fusion Device,
Nanotextured Surface **XRG1092**
Cervicothoracic Vertebral, Interbody
Fusion Device, Nanotextured Surface
XRG4092
Lumbar Vertebral
2 or more, Interbody Fusion Device,
Nanotextured Surface **XRGC092**
Interbody Fusion Device,
Nanotextured Surface **XRGB092**
Lumbosacral, Interbody Fusion Device,
Nanotextured Surface **XRGD092**
Occipital-cervical, Interbody Fusion
Device, Nanotextured Surface
XRG0092
Thoracic Vertebral
2 to 7, Interbody Fusion Device,
Nanotextured Surface **XRG7092**
8 or more, Interbody Fusion Device,
Nanotextured Surface **XRG8092**
Interbody Fusion Device,
Nanotextured Surface **XRG6092**
Thoracolumbar Vertebral, Interbody
Fusion Device, Nanotextured
Surface **XRGA092**
Replacement
Skin Substitute, Porcine Liver Derived
XHRPXL2
Zooplastic Tissue, Rapid Deployment
Technique **X2RF**
Reposition
Cervical, Magnetically Controlled
Growth Rod(s) XNS3
Lumbar, Magnetically Controlled
Growth Rod(s) XNS0
Thoracic, Magnetically Controlled
Growth Rod(s) XNS4
Uridine Triacetate **XW0DX82**
Idarucizumab, Dabigatran Reversal Agent
XW0
Intraoperative Knee Replacement Sensor
XR2
New Technology (continued)
Isavuconazole Anti-infective **XW0**
Orbital Atherectomy Technology **X2C**
Ninth cranial nerve use Nerve,
Glossopharyngeal
Nitinol framed polymer mesh use Synthetic
Substitute
Non-tunneled central venous catheter use
Infusion Device

Nonimaging Nuclear Medicine Assay

Bladder, Kidneys and Ureters **CT63**
Blood **C763**
Kidneys, Ureters and Bladder **CT63**
Lymphatics and Hematologic System
C76YYZZ
Ureters, Kidneys and Bladder **CT63**
Urinary System **CT6YYZZ**

Nonimaging Nuclear Medicine Probe

Abdomen **CW50**
Abdomen and Chest **CW54**
Abdomen and Pelvis **CW51**
Brain **C050**
Central Nervous System **C05YYZZ**
Chest **CW53**
Chest and Abdomen **CW54**
Chest and Neck **CW56**
Extremity
Lower **CP5PZZZ**
Upper **CP5NZZZ**
Head and Neck **CW5B**
Heart **C25YYZZ**
Right and Left **C256**
Lymphatics
Head **C75J**
Head and Neck **C755**
Lower Extremity **C75P**
Neck **C75K**
Pelvic **C75D**
Trunk **C75M**
Upper Chest **C75L**
Upper Extremity **C75N**
Lymphatics and Hematologic System
C75YYZZ
Musculoskeletal System, Other **CP5YYZZ**
Neck and Chest **CW56**
Neck and Head **CW5B**
Pelvic Region **CW5J**
Pelvis and Abdomen **CW51**
Spine **CP55ZZZ**

Nonimaging Nuclear Medicine Uptake

Endocrine System **CG4YYZZ**
Gland, Thyroid **CG42**
Nostril use Nose
Novacor Left Ventricular Assist Device use
Implantable Heart Assist System in Heart
and Great Vessels
**Novation® Ceramic AHS® (Articulation
Hip System)** use Synthetic Substitute,
Ceramic in **0SR**
Nuclear medicine
see Planar Nuclear Medicine Imaging
see Tomographic (Tomo) Nuclear Medicine
Imaging
see Positron Emission Tomographic (PET)
Imaging
see Nonimaging Nuclear Medicine Uptake
see Nonimaging Nuclear Medicine Probe
Nuclear medicine (continued)
see Nonimaging Nuclear Medicine Assay
see Systemic Nuclear Medicine Therapy
Nuclear scintigraphy see Nuclear Medicine
Nutrition, concentrated substances
Enteral infusion 3E0G36Z
Parenteral (peripheral) infusion see
Introduction of Nutritional Substance

O

Obliteration see Destruction
Obturator artery
use Artery, Internal Iliac, Left
use Artery, Internal Iliac, Right
Obturator lymph node use Lymphatic, Pelvis
Obturator muscle
use Muscle, Hip, Left
use Muscle, Hip, Right
Obturator nerve use Nerve, Lumbar Plexus
Obturator vein
use Vein, Hypogastric, Left
use Vein, Hypogastric, Right
Obtuse margin use Heart, Left
Occipital artery
use Artery, External Carotid, Left
use Artery, External Carotid, Right
Occipital lobe use Cerebral Hemisphere
Occipital lymph node
use Lymphatic, Neck, Left
use Lymphatic, Neck, Right
Occipitofrontalis muscle use Muscle, Facial
Occlusion
Ampulla of Vater **0FLC**
Anus **0DLQ**
Aorta, Abdominal **04L0**
Artery
Anterior Tibial
Left **04LQ**
Right **04LP**
Axillary
Left **03L6**
Right **03L5**
Brachial
Left **03L8**
Right **03L7**
Celiac **04L1**
Colic
Left **04L7**
Middle **04L8**
Right **04L6**
Common Carotid
Left **03LJ**
Right **03LH**
Common Iliac
Left **04LD**
Right **04LC**
External Carotid
Left **03LN**
Right **03LM**
External Iliac
Left **04LJ**
Right **04LH**
Face **03LR**
Femoral
Left **04LL**
Right **04LK**
Foot
Left **04LW**
Right **04LV**
Gastric **04L2**
Hand
Left **03LF**
Right **03LD**
Hepatic **04L3**

Occlusion *(continued)*
    Left **06LJ**
    Right **06LH**
    Inferior Mesenteric **06L6**
    Innominate
        Left **05L4**
        Right **05L3**
    Internal Jugular
        Left **05LN**
        Right **05LM**
    Intracranial **05LL**
    Lesser Saphenous
        Left **06LS**
        Right **06LR**
    Lower **06LY**
    Portal **06L8**
    Pulmonary
        Left **02LT**
        Right **02LS**
    Renal
    Left **06LB**
        Right **06L9**
    Splenic **06L1**
    Subclavian
        Left **05L6**
        Right **05L5**
    Superior Mesenteric **06L5**
    Upper **05LY**
    Vertebral
        Left **05LS**
        Right **05LR**
    Vena Cava
        Inferior **06L0**
        Superior **02LV**
Occupational therapy *see* Activities of Daily Living Treatment, Rehabilitation **F08**
Odontectomy
  see Excision, Mouth and Throat **0CB**
  see Resection, Mouth and Throat **0CT**
Olecranon bursa
  use Bursa and Ligament, Elbow, Left
  use Bursa and Ligament, Elbow, Right
Olecranon process
  use Ulna, Left
  use Ulna, Right
Olfactory bulb *use* Nerve, Olfactory
Omentectomy, omentumectomy
  see Excision, Gastrointestinal System **0DB**
  see Resection, Gastrointestinal System **0DT**
Omentofixation *see* Repair, Gastrointestinal System **0DQ**
Omentoplasty
  see Repair, Gastrointestinal System **0DQ**
  see Replacement, Gastrointestinal System **0DR**
  see Supplement, Gastrointestinal System **0DU**
Omentorrhaphy *see* Repair, Gastrointestinal System **0DQ**
Omentotomy *see* Drainage, Gastrointestinal System **0D9**
Onychectomy
  see Excision, Skin and Breast **0HB**
  see Resection, Skin and Breast **0HT**

Onychoplasty
  see Repair, Skin and Breast **0HQ**
  see Replacement, Skin and Breast **0HR**
Onychotomy *see* Drainage, Skin and Breast **0H9**
Oophorectomy
  see Excision, Female Reproductive System **0UB**
  see Resection, Female Reproductive System **0UT**
Oophoropexy
  see Repair, Female Reproductive System **0UQ**
  see Reposition, Female Reproductive System **0US**
Oophoroplasty
  see Repair, Female Reproductive System **0UQ**
  see Supplement, Female Reproductive System **0UU**
Oophororrhaphy *see* Repair, Female Reproductive System **0UQ**
Oophorostomy *see* Drainage, Female Reproductive System **0U9**
Oophorotomy
  see Drainage, Female Reproductive System **0U9**
  see Division, Female Reproductive System **0U8**
Oophorrhaphy *see* Repair, Female Reproductive System **0UQ**
Ophthalmic artery *use* Intracranial Artery
Ophthalmic nerve *use* Nerve, Trigeminal
Ophthalmic vein *use* Vein, Intracranial
Opponensplasty
  Tendon replacement *see* Replacement, Tendons **0LR**
  Tendon transfer *see* Transfer, Tendons **0LX**
Optic chiasma *use* Nerve, Optic
Optic disc
  use Retina, Left
  use Retina, Right
Optic foramen
  use Bone, Sphenoid, Left
  use Bone, Sphenoid, Right
Optical coherence tomography, intravascular *see* Computerized Tomography (CT Scan)
Optimizer™ III implantable pulse generator *use* Contractility Modulation Device in **0JH**
Orbicularis oculi muscle
  use Eyelid, Upper, Left
  use Eyelid, Upper, Right
Orbicularis oris muscle *use* Muscle, Facial
Orbital Atherectomy Technology X2C
Orbital fascia *use* Subcutaneous Tissue and Fascia, Face
Orbital portion of ethmoid bone
  use Orbit, Left
  use Orbit, Right
Orbital portion of frontal bone
  use Orbit, Left
  use Orbit, Right
Orbital portion of lacrimal bone
  use Orbit, Left
  use Orbit, Right

Orbital portion of maxilla
  use Orbit, Left
  use Orbit, Right
Orbital portion of palatine bone
  use Orbit, Left
  use Orbit, Right
Orbital portion of sphenoid bone
  use Orbit, Left
  use Orbit, Right
Orbital portion of zygomatic bone
  use Orbit, Left
  use Orbit, Right
Orchectomy, orchidectomy, orchiectomy
  see Excision, Male Reproductive System **0VB**
  see Resection, Male Reproductive System **0VT**
Orchidoplasty, orchioplasty
  see Repair, Male Reproductive System **0VQ**
  see Replacement, Male Reproductive System **0VR**
  see Supplement, Male Reproductive System **0VU**
Orchidorrhaphy, orchiorrhaphy *see* Repair, Male Reproductive System **0VQ**
Orchidotomy, orchiotomy, orchotomy *see* Drainage, Male Reproductive System **0V9**
Orchiopexy
  see Repair, Male Reproductive System **0VQ**
  see Reposition, Male Reproductive System **0VS**
Oropharyngeal airway (OPA) *use* Intraluminal Device, Airway in Mouth and Throat
Oropharynx *use* Pharynx
Ossiculectomy
  see Excision, Ear, Nose, Sinus **09B**
  see Resection, Ear, Nose, Sinus **09T**
Ossiculotomy *see* Drainage, Ear, Nose, Sinus **099**
Ostectomy
  see Excision, Head and Facial Bones **0NB**
  see Excision, Lower Bones **0QB**
  see Excision, Upper Bones **0PB**
  see Resection, Head and Facial Bones **0NT**
Ostectomy *(continued)*
  see Resection, Lower Bones **0QT**
  see Resection, Upper Bones **0PT**
Osteoclasis
  see Division, Head and Facial Bones **0N8**
  see Division, Upper Bones **0P8**
  see Division, Lower Bones **0Q8**
Osteolysis
  see Release, Head and Facial Bones **0NN**
  see Release, Upper Bones **0PN**
  see Release, Lower Bones **0QN**
Osteopathic Treatment
  Abdomen **7W09X**
  Cervical **7W01X**
  Extremity
    Lower **7W06X**
    Upper **7W07X**
  Head **7W00X**
  Lumbar **7W03X**
  Pelvis **7W05X**
  Rib Cage **7W08X**

Osteopathic Treatment (continued)
  Sacrum **7W04X**
  Thoracic **7W02X**
Osteopexy
  see Repair, Head and Facial Bones **0NQ**
  see Repair, Lower Bones **0QQ**
  see Repair, Upper Bones **0PQ**
  see Reposition, Head and Facial Bones **0NS**
  see Reposition, Lower Bones **0QS**
  see Reposition, Upper Bones **0PS**
Osteoplasty
  see Repair, Head and Facial Bones **0NQ**
  see Replacement, Head and Facial Bones **0NR**
  see Repair, Lower Bones **0QQ**
  see Repair, Upper Bones **0PQ**
  see Replacement, Lower Bones **0QR**
  see Replacement, Upper Bones **0PR**
  see Supplement, Head and Facial Bones **0NU**
  see Supplement, Lower Bones **0QU**
  see Supplement, Upper Bones **0PU**
Osteorrhaphy
  see Repair, Head and Facial Bones **0NQ**
  see Repair, Upper Bones **0PQ**
  see Repair, Lower Bones **0QQ**
Osteotomy, ostotomy
  see Division, Head and Facial Bones **0N8**
  see Division, Lower Bones **0Q8**
  see Division, Upper Bones **0P8**
  see Drainage, Head and Facial Bones **0N9**
  see Drainage, Lower Bones **0Q9**
  see Drainage, Upper Bones **0P9**
Otic ganglion use Nerve, Head and Neck Sympathetic
Otoplasty
  see Repair, Ear, Nose, Sinus **09Q**
  see Replacement, Ear, Nose, Sinus **09R**
  see Supplement, Ear, Nose, Sinus **09U**
Otoscopy see Inspection, Ear, Nose, Sinus **09J**
Oval window
  use Ear, Middle, Left
  use Ear, Middle, Right
Ovarian artery use Aorta, Abdominal
Ovarian ligament use Uterine Supporting Structure
Ovariectomy
  see Excision, Female Reproductive System **0UB**
  see Resection, Female Reproductive System **0UT**
Ovariocentesis see Drainage, Female Reproductive System **0U9**
Ovariopexy
  see Repair, Female Reproductive System **0UQ**
Ovariopexy (continued)
  see Reposition, Female Reproductive System **0US**
Ovariotomy
  see Drainage, Female Reproductive System **0U9**
  see Division, Female Reproductive System **0U8**

Ovatio™ CRT-D use Cardiac Resynchronization Defibrillator Pulse Generator in **0JH**
Oversewing
  Gastrointestinal ulcer see Repair, Gastrointestinal System **0DQ**
  Pleural bleb see Repair, Respiratory System **0BQ**
Oviduct
  use Fallopian Tube, Right
  use Fallopian Tube, Left
Oxidized zirconium ceramic hip bearing surface use Synthetic Substitute, Ceramic on Polyethylene in **0SR**
Oximetry, Fetal pulse 10H073Z
Oxygenation
  Extracorporeal membrane (ECMO) see Assistance, Circulatory **5A05**
  Hyperbaric see Assistance, Circulatory **5A05**
  Supersaturated see Assistance, Circulatory **5A05**

P

Pacemaker
  Dual Chamber
    Abdomen **0JH8**
    Chest **0JH6**
      Intracardiac
      Insertion of device in
        Atrium
          Left **02H7**
          Right **02H6**
        Vein, Coronary **02H4**
        Ventricle
          Left **02HL**
          Right **02HK**
      Removal of device from, Heart **02PA**
      Revision of device in, Heart **02WA**
  Single Chamber
    Abdomen **0JH8**
    Chest **0JH6**
  Single Chamber Rate Responsive
    Abdomen **0JH8**
    Chest **0JH6**
Packing
  Abdominal Wall **2W43X5Z**
  Anorectal **2Y43X5Z**
  Arm
    Lower
      Left **2W4DX5Z**
      Right **2W4CX5Z**
    Upper
      Left **2W4BX5Z**
      Right **2W4AX5Z**
  Back **2W45X5Z**
  Chest Wall **2W44X5Z**
  Ear **2Y42X5Z**
  Extremity
    Lower
      Left **2W4MX5Z**
      Right **2W4LX5Z**
    Upper
      Left **2W49X5Z**
      Right **2W48X5Z**

Packing (continued)
  Face **2W41X5Z**
  Finger
    Left **2W4KX5Z**
    Right **2W4JX5Z**
  Foot
    Left **2W4TX5Z**
    Right **2W4SX5Z**
  Genital Tract, Female **2Y44X5Z**
  Hand
    Left **2W4FX5Z**
    Right **2W4EX5Z**
  Head **2W40X5Z**
  Inguinal Region
    Left **2W47X5Z**
    Right **2W46X5Z**
  Leg
    Lower
      Left **2W4RX5Z**
      Right **2W4QX5Z**
    Upper
      Left **2W4PX5Z**
      Right **2W4NX5Z**
  Mouth and Pharynx **2Y40X5Z**
  Nasal **2Y41X5Z**
  Neck **2W42X5Z**
  Thumb
    Left **2W4HX5Z**
    Right **2W4GX5Z**
  Toe
    Left **2W4VX5Z**
    Right **2W4UX5Z**
  Urethra **2Y45X5Z**
Paclitaxel-eluting coronary stent use Intraluminal Device, Drug-eluting in Heart and Great Vessels
Paclitaxel-eluting peripheral stent
  use Intraluminal Device, Drug-eluting in Upper Arteries
  use Intraluminal Device, Drug-eluting in Lower Arteries
Palatine gland use Buccal Mucosa
Palatine tonsil use Tonsils
Palatine uvula use Uvula
Palatoglossal muscle use Muscle, Tongue, Palate, Pharynx
Palatopharyngeal muscle use Muscle, Tongue, Palate, Pharynx
Palatoplasty
  see Repair, Mouth and Throat **0CQ**
  see Replacement, Mouth and Throat **0CR**
  see Supplement, Mouth and Throat **0CU**
Palatorrhaphy see Repair, Mouth and Throat **0CQ**
Palmar (volar) digital vein
  use Vein, Hand, Right
  use Vein, Hand, Left
Palmar (volar) metacarpal vein
  use Vein, Hand, Left
  use Vein, Hand, Right
Palmar cutaneous nerve
  use Nerve, Radial
  use Nerve, Median
Palmar fascia (aponeurosis)
  use Subcutaneous Tissue and Fascia, Hand, Left

Palmar fascia (aponeurosis) *(continued)*
  use Subcutaneous Tissue and Fascia, Hand, Right
Palmar interosseous muscle
  use Muscle, Hand, Left
  use Muscle, Hand, Right
Palmar ulnocarpal ligament
  use Bursa and Ligament, Wrist, Right
  use Bursa and Ligament, Wrist, Left
Palmaris longus muscle
  use Muscle, Lower Arm and Wrist, Left
  use Muscle, Lower Arm and Wrist, Right
Pancreatectomy
  see Excision, Pancreas **0FBG**
  see Resection, Pancreas **0FTG**
Pancreatic artery *use* Artery, Splenic
Pancreatic plexus *use* Nerve, Abdominal Sympathetic
Pancreatic vein *use* Vein, Splenic
Pancreaticoduodenostomy *see* Bypass, Hepatobiliary System and Pancreas **0F1**
Pancreaticosplenic lymph node *use* Lymphatic, Aortic
Pancreatogram, endoscopic retrograde *see* Fluoroscopy, Pancreatic Duct **BF18**
Pancreatolithotomy *see* Extirpation, Pancreas **0FCG**
Pancreatotomy
  see Drainage, Pancreas **0F9G**
  see Division, Pancreas **0F8G**
Panniculectomy
  see Excision, Skin, Abdomen **0HB7**
  see Excision, Abdominal Wall **0WBF**
Paraaortic lymph node *use* Lymphatic, Aortic
Paracentesis
  Eye *see* Drainage, Eye **089**
  Peritoneal Cavity *see* Drainage, Peritoneal Cavity **0W9G**
  Tympanum *see* Drainage, Ear, Nose, Sinus **099**
Pararectal lymph node *use* Lymphatic, Mesenteric
Parasternal lymph node *use* Lymphatic, Thorax
Parathyroidectomy
  see Excision, Endocrine System **0GB**
  see Resection, Endocrine System **0GT**
Paratracheal lymph node *use* Lymphatic, Thorax
Paraurethral (Skene's) gland *use* Gland, Vestibular
Parenteral nutrition, total *see* Introduction of Nutritional Substance
Parietal lobe *use* Cerebral Hemisphere
Parotid lymph node *use* Lymphatic, Head
Parotid plexus *use* Nerve, Facial
Parotidectomy
  see Excision, Mouth and Throat **0CB**
  see Resection, Mouth and Throat **0CT**
Pars flaccida
  use Tympanic Membrane, Right
  use Tympanic Membrane, Left
Partial joint replacement
  Hip *see* Replacement, Lower Joints **0SR**
  Knee *see* Replacement, Lower Joints **0SR**
  Shoulder *see* Replacement, Upper Joints **0RR**

Partially absorbable mesh *use* Synthetic Substitute
Patch, blood, spinal 3E0S3GC
Patellapexy
  see Repair, Lower Bones **0QQ**
  see Reposition, Lower Bones **0QS**
Patellofemoral joint
  use Joint, Knee, Right
  use Joint, Knee, Left
Patellofemoral joint *(continued)*
  use Joint, Knee, Right, Femoral Surface
  use Joint, Knee, Left, Femoral Surface
Patelloplasty
  see Repair, Lower Bones **0QQ**
  see Replacement, Lower Bones **0QR**
  see Supplement, Lower Bones **0QU**
Patellar ligament
  use Bursa and Ligament, Knee, Right
  use Bursa and Ligament, Knee, Left
Patellar tendon
  use Tendon, Knee, Left
  use Tendon, Knee, Right
Patellectomy
  see Excision, Lower Bones **0QB**
  see Resection, Lower Bones **0QT**
Pectineus muscle
  use Muscle, Upper Leg, Left
  use Muscle, Upper Leg, Right
Pectoral (anterior) lymph node
  use Lymphatic, Axillary, Right
  use Lymphatic, Axillary, Left
Pectoral fascia *use* Subcutaneous Tissue and Fascia, Chest
Pectoralis major muscle
  use Muscle, Thorax, Left
  use Muscle, Thorax, Right
Pectoralis minor muscle
  use Muscle, Thorax, Left
  use Muscle, Thorax, Right
Pedicle-based dynamic stabilization device
  use Spinal Stabilization Device, Pedicle-Based in **0RH**
  use Spinal Stabilization Device, Pedicle-Based in **0SH**
PEEP (positive end expiratory pressure) *see* Assistance, Respiratory **5A09**
PEG (percutaneous endoscopic gastrostomy) 0DH63UZ
PEJ (percutaneous endoscopic jejunostomy) 0DHA3UZ
Pelvic splanchnic nerve
  use Nerve, Abdominal Sympathetic
  use Nerve, Sacral Sympathetic
Penectomy
  see Excision, Male Reproductive System **0VB**
  see Resection, Male Reproductive System **0VT**
Penile urethra *use* Urethra
Perceval sutureless valve *use* Zooplastic Tissue, Rapid Deployment Technique in New Technology
Percutaneous endoscopic gastrojejunostomy (PEG/J) tube *use* Feeding Device in Gastrointestinal System

Percutaneous endoscopic gastrostomy (PEG) tube *use* Feeding Device in Gastrointestinal System
Percutaneous nephrostomy catheter *use* Drainage Device
Percutaneous transluminal coronary angioplasty (PTCA) *see* Dilation, Heart and Great Vessels **027**
Performance
  Biliary
    Multiple, Filtration **5A1C60Z**
    Single, Filtration **5A1C00Z**
  Cardiac
    Continuous
      Output **5A1221Z**
      Pacing **5A1223Z**
    Intermittent, Pacing **5A1213Z**
    Single, Output, Manual **5A12012**
  Circulatory, Continuous, Oxygenation, Membrane **5A15223**
  Respiratory
    24-96 Consecutive Hours, Ventilation **5A1945Z**
    Greater than 96 Consecutive Hours, Ventilation **5A1955Z**
    Less than 24 Consecutive Hours, Ventilation **5A1935Z**
    Single, Ventilation, Nonmechanical **5A19054**
  Urinary
    Multiple, Filtration **5A1D60Z**
    Single, Filtration **5A1D00Z**
Perfusion *see* Introduction of substance in or on
Perfusion, donor organ
  Heart **6AB50BZ**
  Kidney(s) **6ABT0BZ**
  Liver **6ABF0BZ**
  Lung(s) **6ABB0BZ**
Pericardiectomy
  see Excision, Pericardium **02BN**
  see Resection, Pericardium **02TN**
Pericardiocentesis *see* Drainage, Pericardial Cavity **0W9D**
Pericardiolysis *see* Release, Pericardium **02NN**
Pericardiophrenic artery
  use Artery, Internal Mammary, Left
  use Artery, Internal Mammary, Right
Pericardioplasty
  see Repair, Pericardium **02QN**
  see Replacement, Pericardium **02RN**
  see Supplement, Pericardium **02UN**
Pericardiorrhaphy *see* Repair, Pericardium **02QN**
Pericardiostomy *see* Drainage, Pericardial Cavity **0W9D**
Pericardiotomy *see* Drainage, Pericardial Cavity **0W9D**
Perimetrium *use* Uterus
Peripheral parenteral nutrition *see* Introduction of Nutritional Substance
Peripherally inserted central catheter (PICC) *use* Infusion Device
Peritoneal dialysis 3E1M39Z

Peritoneocentesis
  see Drainage, Peritoneum **0D9W**
  see Drainage, Peritoneal Cavity **0W9G**
Peritoneoplasty
  see Repair, Peritoneum **0DQW**
  see Replacement, Peritoneum **0DRW**
  see Supplement, Peritoneum **0DUW**
Peritoneoscopy 0DJW4ZZ
Peritoneotomy *see* Drainage, Peritoneum
  0D9W
Peritoneumectomy *see* Excision, Peritoneum
  0DBW
Peroneus brevis muscle
  use Muscle, Lower Leg, Left
  use Muscle, Lower Leg, Right
Peroneus longus muscle
  use Muscle, Lower Leg, Left
  use Muscle, Lower Leg, Right
Pessary ring *use* Intraluminal Device, Pessary
  in Female Reproductive System
PET scan *see* Positron Emission Tomographic
  (PET) Imaging
Petrous part of temporal bone
  use Bone, Temporal, Left
  use Bone, Temporal, Right
Phacoemulsification, lens
  With IOL implant *see* Replacement, Eye
    08R
  Without IOL implant *see* Extraction, Eye
    08D
Phalangectomy
  see Excision, Lower Bones **0QB**
  see Excision, Upper Bones **0PB**
  see Resection, Lower Bones **0QT**
  see Resection, Upper Bones **0PT**
Phallectomy
  see Excision, Penis **0VBS**
  see Resection, Penis **0VTS**
Phalloplasty
  see Repair, Penis **0VQS**
  see Supplement, Penis **0VUS**
Phallotomy *see* Drainage, Penis **0V9S**
Pharmacotherapy
  Antabuse **HZ93ZZZ**
  Bupropion **HZ97ZZZ**
  Clonidine **HZ96ZZZ**
  Levo-alpha-acetyl-methadol (LAAM)
    HZ92ZZZ
  Methadone Maintenance **HZ91ZZZ**
  Naloxone **HZ95ZZZ**
  Naltrexone **HZ94ZZZ**
  Nicotine Replacement **HZ90ZZZ**
  Psychiatric Medication **HZ98ZZZ**
  Replacement Medication, Other **HZ99ZZZ**
Pharyngeal constrictor muscle *use* Muscle,
  Tongue, Palate, Pharynx
Pharyngeal plexus *use* Nerve, Vagus
Pharyngeal recess *use* Nasopharynx
Pharyngeal tonsil *use* Adenoids
Pharyngogram *see* Fluoroscopy, Pharynx
  B91G
Pharyngoplasty
  see Repair, Mouth and Throat **0CQ**
  see Replacement, Mouth and Throat **0CR**
  see Supplement, Mouth and Throat **0CU**
Pharyngorrhaphy *see* Repair, Mouth and
  Throat **0CQ**

Pharyngotomy *see* Drainage, Mouth and
  Throat **0C9**
Pharyngotympanic tube
  use Eustachian Tube, Left
  use Eustachian Tube, Right
Pheresis
  Erythrocytes **6A55**
  Leukocytes **6A55**
  Plasma **6A55**
  Platelets **6A55**
  Stem Cells
    Cord Blood **6A55**
    Hematopoietic **6A55**
Phlebectomy
  see Excision, Lower Veins **06B**
  see Excision, Upper Veins **05B**
  see Extraction, Lower Veins **06D**
  see Extraction, Upper Veins **05D**
Phlebography
  see Plain Radiography, Veins **B50**
  Impedance **4A04X51**
Phleborrhaphy
  see Repair, Lower Veins **06Q**
  see Repair, Upper Veins **05Q**
Phlebotomy
  see Drainage, Lower Veins **069**
  see Drainage, Upper Veins **059**
Photocoagulation
  for Destruction *see* Destruction
  for Repair *see* Repair
Photopheresis, therapeutic *see* Phototherapy,
  Circulatory **6A65**
Phototherapy
  Circulatory **6A65**
  Skin **6A60**
Phrenectomy, phrenoneurectomy *see*
  Excision, Nerve, Phrenic **01B2**
Phrenemphraxis *see* Destruction, Nerve,
  Phrenic **0152**
Phrenic nerve stimulator generator *use*
  Stimulator Generator in Subcutaneous
  Tissue and Fascia
Phrenic nerve stimulator lead *use*
  Diaphragmatic Pacemaker Lead in
  Respiratory System
Phreniclasis *see* Destruction, Nerve, Phrenic
  0152
Phrenicoexeresis *see* Extraction, Nerve,
  Phrenic **01D2**
Phrenicotomy *see* Division, Nerve, Phrenic
  0182
Phrenicotripsy *see* Destruction, Nerve,
  Phrenic **0152**
Phrenoplasty
  see Repair, Respiratory System **0BQ**
  see Supplement, Respiratory System **0BU**
Phrenotomy *see* Drainage, Respiratory System
  0B9
Physiatry *see* Motor Treatment, Rehabilitation
  F07
Physical medicine *see* Motor Treatment,
  Rehabilitation **F07**
Physical therapy *see* Motor Treatment,
  Rehabilitation **F07**
PHYSIOMESH™ Flexible Composite Mesh
  use Synthetic Substitute
Pia mater, intracranial *use* Cerebral
  Meninges

Pia mater, spinal *use* Spinal Meninges
Pinealectomy
  see Excision, Pineal Body **0GB1**
  see Resection, Pineal Body **0GT1**
Pinealoscopy 0GJ14ZZ
Pinealotomy *see* Drainage, Pineal Body **0G91**
Pinna
  use Ear, External, Bilateral
  use Ear, External, Left
  use Ear, External, Right
Pipeline™ Embolization device (PED) *use*
  Intraluminal Device
Piriform recess (sinus) *use* Pharynx
Piriformis muscle
  use Muscle, Hip, Left
  use Muscle, Hip, Right
Pisiform bone
  use Carpal, Left
  use Carpal, Right
Pisohamate ligament
  use Bursa and Ligament, Hand, Left
  use Bursa and Ligament, Hand, Right
Pisometacarpal ligament
  use Bursa and Ligament, Hand, Left
  use Bursa and Ligament, Hand, Right
Pituitectomy
  see Excision, Gland, Pituitary **0GB0**
  see Resection, Gland, Pituitary **0GT0**
Plain film radiology *see* Plain Radiography
Plain radiography
  Abdomen **BW00ZZZ**
  Abdomen and Pelvis **BW01ZZZ**
  Abdominal Lymphatic
    Bilateral **B701**
    Unilateral **B700**
  Airway, Upper **BB0DZZZ**
  Ankle
    Left **BQ0H**
    Right **BQ0G**
  Aorta
    Abdominal **B400**
    Thoracic **B300**
    Thoraco-Abdominal **B30P**
  Aorta and Bilateral Lower Extremity
  Arteries **B40D**
  Arch
    Bilateral **BN0DZZZ**
    Left **BN0CZZZ**
    Right **BN0BZZZ**
  Arm
    Left **BP0FZZZ**
    Right **BP0EZZZ**
  Artery
    Brachiocephalic-Subclavian, Right **B301**
    Bronchial **B30L**
    Bypass Graft, Other **B20F**
    Cervico-Cerebral Arch **B30Q**
    Common Carotid
      Bilateral **B305**
      Left **B304**
      Right **B303**
    Coronary
      Bypass Graft
        Multiple **B203**
        Single **B202**
      Multiple **B201**

Plain radiography *(continued)*
Single **B200**
External Carotid
Bilateral **B30C**
Left **B30B**
Right **B309**
Hepatic **B402**
Inferior Mesenteric **B405**
Intercostal **B30L**
Internal Carotid
Bilateral **B308**
Left **B307**
Right **B306**
Internal Mammary Bypass Graft
Left **B208**
Right **B207**
Intra-Abdominal, Other **B40B**
Intracranial **B30R**
Lower, Other **B40J**
Lower Extremity
Bilateral and Aorta **B40D**
Left **B40G**
Right **B40F**
Lumbar **B409**
Pelvic **B40C**
Pulmonary
Left **B30T**
Right **B30S**
Renal
Bilateral **B408**
Left **B407**
Right **B406**
Transplant **B40M**
Spinal **B30M**
Splenic **B403**
Subclavian, Left **B302**
Superior Mesenteric **B404**
Upper, Other **B30N**
Upper Extremity
Bilateral **B30K**
Left **B30J**
Right **B30H**
Vertebral
Bilateral **B30G**
Left **B30F**
Right **B30D**
Bile Duct **BF00**
Bile Duct and Gallbladder **BF03**
Bladder **BT00**
Kidney and Ureter **BT04**
Bladder and Urethra **BT0B**
Bone
Facial **BN05ZZZ**
Nasal **BN04ZZZ**
Bones, Long, All **BW0BZZZ**
Breast
Bilateral **BH02ZZZ**
Left **BH01ZZZ**
Right **BH00ZZZ**
Calcaneus
Left **BQ0KZZZ**
Right **BQ0JZZZ**
Chest **BW03ZZZ**
Clavicle
Left **BP05ZZZ**
Right **BP04ZZZ**

Plain radiography *(continued)*
Coccyx **BR0FZZZ**
Corpora Cavernosa **BV00**
Dialysis Fistula **B50W**
Dialysis Shunt **B50W**
Disc
Cervical **BR01**
Lumbar **BR03**
Thoracic **BR02**
Duct
Lacrimal
Bilateral **B802**
Left **B801**
Right **B800**
Mammary
Multiple
Left **BH06**
Right **BH05**
Single
Left **BH04**
Right **BH03**
Elbow
Left **BP0H**
Right **BP0G**
Epididymis
Left **BV02**
Right **BV01**
Extremity
Lower **BW0CZZZ**
Upper **BW0JZZZ**
Eye
Bilateral **B807ZZZ**
Left **B806ZZZ**
Right **B805ZZZ**
Facet Joint
Cervical **BR04**
Lumbar **BR06**
Thoracic **BR05**
Fallopian Tube
Bilateral **BU02**
Left **BU01**
Right **BU00**
Fallopian Tube and Uterus **BU08**
Femur
Left, Densitometry **BQ04ZZ1**
Right, Densitometry **BQ03ZZ1**
Finger
Left **BP0SZZZ**
Right **BP0RZZZ**
Foot
Left **BQ0MZZZ**
Right **BQ0LZZZ**
Forearm
Left **BP0KZZZ**
Right **BP0JZZZ**
Gallbladder and Bile Duct **BF03**
Gland
Parotid
Bilateral **B906**
Left **B905**
Right **B904**
Salivary
Bilateral **B90D**
Left **B90C**
Right **B90B**
Submandibular

Plain radiography *(continued)*
Bilateral **B909**
Left **B908**
Right **B907**
Hand
Left **BP0PZZZ**
Right **BP0NZZZ**
Heart
Left **B205**
Right **B204**
Right and Left **B206**
Hepatobiliary System, All **BF0C**
Hip
Left **BQ01**
Densitometry **BQ01ZZ1**
Right **BQ00**
Densitometry **BQ00ZZ1Plain**
Humerus
Left **BP0BZZZ**
Right **BP0AZZZ**
Ileal Diversion Loop **BT0C**
Intracranial Sinus **B502**
Joint
Acromioclavicular, Bilateral **BP03ZZZ**
Finger
Left **BP0D**
Right **BP0C**
Foot
Left **BQ0Y**
Right **BQ0X**
Hand
Left **BP0D**
Right **BP0C**
Lumbosacral **BR0BZZZ**
Sacroiliac **BR0D**
Sternoclavicular
Bilateral **BP02ZZZ**
Left **BP01ZZZ**
Right **BP00ZZZ**
Temporomandibular
Bilateral **BN09**
Left **BN08**
Right **BN07**
Thoracolumbar **BR08ZZZ**
Toe
Left **BQ0Y**
Right **BQ0X**
Kidney
Bilateral **BT03**
Left **BT02**
Right **BT01**
Ureter and Bladder **BT04**
Knee
Left **BQ08**
Right **BQ07**
Leg
Left **BQ0FZZZ**
Right **BQ0DZZZ**
Lymphatic
Head **B704**
Lower Extremity
Bilateral **B70B**
Left **B709**
Right **B708**
Neck **B704**
Pelvic **B70C**

Plain radiography *(continued)*
    Upper Extremity
        Bilateral **B707**
        Left **B706**
        Right **B705**
    Mandible **BN06ZZZ**
    Mastoid **B90HZZZ**
    Nasopharynx **B90FZZZ**
    Optic Foramina
        Left **B804ZZZ**
        Right **B803ZZZ**
    Orbit
        Bilateral **BN03ZZZ**
        Left **BN02ZZZ**
        Right **BN01ZZZ**
    Oropharynx **B90FZZZ**
    Patella
        Left **BQ0WZZZ**
        Right **BQ0VZZZ**
    Pelvis **BR0CZZZ**
    Pelvis and Abdomen **BW01ZZZ**
    Prostate **BV03**
    Retroperitoneal Lymphatic
        Bilateral **B701**
    Ribs
        Left **BP0YZZZ**
    Right **BP0XZZZ**
    Sacrum **BR0FZZZ**
    Scapula
        Left **BP07ZZZ**
        Right **BP06ZZZ**
    Shoulder
        Left **BP09**
        Right **BP08**
    Sinus
        Intracranial **B502**
        Paranasal **B902ZZZ**
    Skull **BN00ZZZ**
    Spinal Cord **B00B**
    Spine
        Cervical, Densitometry **BR00ZZ1**
        Lumbar, Densitometry **BR09ZZ1**
        Thoracic, Densitometry **BR07ZZ1**
        Whole, Densitometry **BR0GZZ1**
    Sternum **BR0HZZZ**
    Teeth
        All **BN0JZZZ**
        Multiple **BN0HZZZ**
    Testicle
        Left **BV06**
        Right **BV05**
    Toe
        Left **BQ0QZZZ**
        Right **BQ0PZZZ**
    Tooth, Single **BN0GZZZ**
    Tracheobronchial Tree
        Bilateral **BB09YZZ**
        Left **BB08YZZ**
        Right **BB07YZZ**
    Ureter
        Bilateral **BT08**
        Kidney and Bladder **BT04**
        Left **BT07**
        Right **BT06**
    Urethra **BT05**
    Urethra and Bladder **BT0B**

Plain radiography *(continued)*
    Uterus **BU06**
    Uterus and Fallopian Tube **BU08**
    Vagina **BU09**
    Vasa Vasorum **BV08**
    Vein
        Cerebellar **B501**
        Cerebral **B501**
        Epidural **B500**
        Jugular
            Bilateral **B505**
            Left **B504**
            Right **B503**
        Lower Extremity
            Bilateral **B50D**
            Left **B50C**
            Right **B50B**
        Other **B50V**
        Pelvic (Iliac)
            Left **B50G**
            Right **B50F**
        Pelvic (Iliac) Bilateral **B50H**
        Portal **B50T**
        Pulmonary
            Bilateral **B50S**
            Left **B50R**
            Right **B50Q**
        Renal
            Bilateral **B50L**
            Left **B50K**
            Right **B50J**
        Splanchnic **B50T**
        Subclavian
            Left **B507**
            Right **B506**
        Upper Extremity
            Bilateral **B50P**
            Left **B50N**
            Right **B50M**
    Vena Cava
        Inferior **B509**
        Superior **B508**
    Whole Body **BW0KZZZ**
        Infant **BW0MZZZ**
    Whole Skeleton **BW0LZZZ**
    Wrist
        Left **BP0M**
        Right **BP0L**

Planar Nuclear Medicine Imaging
    Abdomen **CW10**
    Abdomen and Chest **CW14**
    Abdomen and Pelvis **CW11**
    Anatomical Regions, Multiple **CW1YYZZ**
    Bladder, Kidneys and Ureters **CT13**
    Bladder and Ureters **CT1H**
    Blood **C713**
    Bone Marrow **C710**
    Brain **C010**
    Breast **CH1YYZZ**
        Bilateral **CH12**
        Left **CH11**
        Right **CH10**
    Bronchi and Lungs **CB12**
    Central Nervous System **C01YYZZ**
    Cerebrospinal Fluid **C015**
    Chest **CW13**

Planar Nuclear Medicine Imaging
(continued)
    Chest and Abdomen **CW14**
    Chest and Neck **CW16**
    Digestive System **CD1YYZZ**
    Ducts, Lacrimal, Bilateral **C819**
    Ear, Nose, Mouth and Throat **C91YYZZ**
    Endocrine System **CG1YYZZ**
    Extremity
        Lower **CW1D**
            Bilateral **CP1F**
            Left **CP1D**
            Right **CP1C**
        Upper **CW1M**
            Bilateral **CP1B**
            Left **CP19**
            Right **CP18**
    Eye **C81YYZZ**
    Gallbladder **CF14**
    Gastrointestinal Tract **CD17**
        Upper **CD15**
    Gland
        Adrenal, Bilateral **CG14**
        Parathyroid **CG11**
        Thyroid **CG12**
    Glands, Salivary, Bilateral **C91B**
    Head and Neck **CW1B**
    Heart **C21YYZZ**
        Right and Left **C216**
    Hepatobiliary System, All **CF1C**
    Hepatobiliary System and Pancreas
        CF1YYZZ
    Kidneys, Ureters and Bladder **CT13**
    Liver **CF15**
    Liver and Spleen **CF16**
    Lungs and Bronchi **CB12**
    Lymphatics
        Head **C71J**
        Head and Neck **C715**
        Lower Extremity **C71P**
        Neck **C71K**
        Pelvic **C71D**
        Trunk **C71M**
        Upper Chest **C71L**
        Upper Extremity **C71N**
    Lymphatics and Hematologic System
        C71YYZZ
    Musculoskeletal System
        All **CP1Z**
        Other **CP1YYZZ**
    Myocardium **C21G**
    Neck and Chest **CW16**
    Neck and Head **CW1B**
    Pancreas and Hepatobiliary System
        CF1YYZZ
    Pelvic Region **CW1J**
    Pelvis **CP16**
    Pelvis and Abdomen **CW11**
    Pelvis and Spine **CP17**
    Reproductive System, Male **CV1YYZZ**
    Respiratory System **CB1YYZZ**
    Skin **CH1YYZZ**
    Skull **CP11**
    Spine **CP15**
    Spine and Pelvis **CP17**
    Spleen **C712**

Planar Nuclear Medicine Imaging
(continued)
  Spleen and Liver **CF16**
  Subcutaneous Tissue **CH1YYZZ**
  Testicles, Bilateral **CV19**
  Thorax **CP14**
  Ureters, Kidneys and Bladder **CT13**
  Ureters and Bladder **CT1H**
  Urinary System **CT1YYZZ**
  Veins **C51YYZZ**
    Central **C51R**
    Lower Extremity
      Bilateral **C51D**
      Left **C51C**
      Right **C51B**
    Upper Extremity
      Bilateral **C51Q**
      Left **C51P**
      Right **C51N**
  Whole Body **CW1N**
Plantar digital vein
  use Vein, Foot, Right
  use Vein, Foot, Left
Plantar fascia (aponeurosis)
  use Subcutaneous Tissue and Fascia, Foot, Left
  use Subcutaneous Tissue and Fascia, Foot, Right
Plantar metatarsal vein
  use Vein, Foot, Left
  use Vein, Foot, Right
Plantar venous arch
  use Vein, Foot, Left
  use Vein, Foot, Right
Plaque Radiation
  Abdomen **DWY3FZZ**
  Adrenal Gland **DGY2FZZ**
  Anus **DDY8FZZ**
  Bile Ducts **DFY2FZZ**
  Bladder **DTY2FZZ**
  Bone, Other **DPYCFZZ**
  Bone Marrow **D7Y0FZZ**
  Brain **D0Y0FZZ**
  Brain Stem **D0Y1FZZ**
  Breast
    Left **DMY0FZZ**
    Right **DMY1FZZ**
  Bronchus **DBY1FZZ**
  Cervix **DUY1FZZ**
  Chest **DWY2FZZ**
  Chest Wall **DBY7FZZ**
  Colon **DDY5FZZ**
  Diaphragm **DBY8FZZ**
  Duodenum **DDY2FZZ**
  Ear **D9Y0FZZ**
  Esophagus **DDY0FZZ**
  Eye **D8Y0FZZ**
  Femur **DPY9FZZ**
  Fibula **DPYBFZZ**
  Gallbladder **DFY1FZZ**
  Gland
    Adrenal **DGY2FZZ**
    Parathyroid **DGY4FZZ**
    Pituitary **DGY0FZZ**
    Thyroid **DGY5FZZ**
  Glands, Salivary **D9Y6FZZ**

Plaque Radiation *(continued)*
  Head and Neck **DWY1FZZ**
  Hemibody **DWY4FZZ**
  Humerus **DPY6FZZ**
  Ileum **DDY4FZZ**
  Jejunum **DDY3FZZ**
  Kidney **DTY0FZZ**
  Larynx **D9YBFZZ**
  Liver **DFY0FZZ**
  Lung **DBY2FZZ**
  Lymphatics
    Abdomen **D7Y6FZZ**
    Axillary **D7Y4FZZ**
    Inguinal **D7Y8FZZ**
    Neck **D7Y3FZZ**
    Pelvis **D7Y7FZZ**
    Thorax **D7Y5FZZ**
  Mandible **DPY3FZZ**
  Maxilla **DPY2FZZ**
  Mediastinum **DBY6FZZ**
  Mouth **D9Y4FZZ**
  Nasopharynx **D9YDFZZ**
  Neck and Head **DWY1FZZ**
  Nerve, Peripheral **D0Y7FZZ**
  Nose **D9Y1FZZ**
  Ovary **DUY0FZZ**
  Palate
    Hard **D9Y8FZZ**
    Soft **D9Y9FZZ**
  Pancreas **DFY3FZZ**
  Parathyroid Gland **DGY4FZZ**
  Pelvic Bones **DPY8FZZ**
  Pelvic Region **DWY6FZZ**
  Pharynx **D9YCFZZ**
  Pineal Body **DGY1FZZ**
  Pituitary Gland **DGY0FZZ**
  Pleura **DBY5FZZ**
  Prostate **DVY0FZZ**
  Radius **DPY7FZZ**
  Rectum **DDY7FZZ**
  Rib **DPY5FZZ**
  Sinuses **D9Y7FZZ**
  Skin
    Abdomen **DHY8FZZ**
    Arm **DHY4FZZ**
    Back **DHY7FZZ**
    Buttock **DHY9FZZ**
    Chest **DHY6FZZ**
    Face **DHY2FZZ**
    Foot **DHYCFZZ**
    Hand **DHY5FZZ**
    Leg **DHYBFZZ**
    Neck **DHY3FZZ**
  Skull **DPY0FZZ**
  Spinal Cord **D0Y6FZZ**
  Spleen **D7Y2FZZ**
  Sternum **DPY4FZZ**
  Stomach **DDY1FZZ**
  Testis **DVY1FZZ**
  Thymus **D7Y1FZZ**
  Thyroid Gland **DGY5FZZ**
  Tibia **DPYBFZZ**
  Tongue **D9Y5FZZ**
  Trachea **DBY0FZZ**
  Ulna **DPY7FZZ**
  Ureter **DTY1FZZ**

Plaque Radiation *(continued)*
  Urethra **DTY3FZZ**
  Uterus **DUY2FZZ**
  Whole Body **DWY5FZZ**
Plasmapheresis, therapeutic 6A550Z3
Plateletpheresis, therapeutic 6A550Z2
Platysma muscle
  use Muscle, Neck, Left
  use Muscle, Neck, Right
Pleurectomy
  see Excision, Respiratory System **0BB**
  see Resection, Respiratory System **0BT**
Pleurocentesis *see* Drainage, Anatomical Regions, General **0W9**
Pleurodesis, pleurosclerosis
  Chemical injection *see* Introduction of substance in or on, Pleural Cavity **3E0L**
  Surgical *see* Destruction, Respiratory System **0B5**
Pleurolysis *see* Release, Respiratory System **0BN**
Pleuroscopy 0BJQ4ZZ
Pleurotomy *see* Drainage, Respiratory System **0B9**
Plica semilunaris
  use Conjunctiva, Left
  use Conjunctiva, Right
Plication *see* Restriction
Pneumectomy
  see Excision, Respiratory System **0BB**
  see Resection, Respiratory System **0BT**
Pneumocentesis *see* Drainage, Respiratory System **0B9**
Pneumogastric nerve *use* Nerve, Vagus
Pneumolysis *see* Release, Respiratory System **0BN**
Pneumonectomy *see* Resection, Respiratory System **0BT**
Pneumonolysis *see* Release, Respiratory System **0BN**
Pneumonopexy
  see Repair, Respiratory System **0BQ**
  see Reposition, Respiratory System **0BS**
Pneumonorrhaphy *see* Repair, Respiratory System **0BQ**
Pneumonotomy *see* Drainage, Respiratory System **0B9**
Pneumotaxic center *use* Pons
Pneumotomy *see* Drainage, Respiratory System **0B9**
Pollicization *see* Transfer, Anatomical Regions, Upper Extremities **0XX**
Polyethylene socket *use* Synthetic Substitute, Polyethylene in **0SR**
Polymethylmethacrylate (PMMA) *use* Synthetic Substitute
Polypectomy, gastrointestinal *see* Excision, Gastrointestinal System **0DB**
Polypropylene mesh *use* Synthetic Substitute
Polysomnogram 4A1ZXQZ
Pontine tegmentum *use* Pons
Popliteal ligament
  use Bursa and Ligament, Knee, Right
  use Bursa and Ligament, Knee, Left
Popliteal lymph node
  use Lymphatic, Lower Extremity, Right
  use Lymphatic, Lower Extremity, Left

Popliteal vein
use Vein, Femoral, Right
use Vein, Femoral, Left
Popliteus muscle
use Muscle, Lower Leg, Right
use Muscle, Lower Leg, Left
Porcine (bioprosthetic) valve use Zooplastic Tissue in Heart and Great Vessels
Positive end expiratory pressure see Performance, Respiratory **5A19**
Positron Emission Tomographic (PET) Imaging
Brain **C030**
Bronchi and Lungs **CB32**
Central Nervous System **C03YYZZ**
Heart **C23YYZZ**
Lungs and Bronchi **CB32**
Myocardium **C23G**
Respiratory System **CB3YYZZ**
Whole Body **CW3NYZZ**
Positron emission tomography see Positron Emission Tomographic (PET) Imaging
Postauricular (mastoid) lymph node
use Lymphatic, Neck, Right
use Lymphatic, Neck, Left
Postcava use Vena Cava, Inferior
Posterior (subscapular) lymph node
use Lymphatic, Axillary, Left
use Lymphatic, Axillary, Right
Posterior auricular artery
use Artery, External Carotid, Right
use Artery, External Carotid, Left
Posterior auricular nerve use Nerve, Facial
Posterior auricular vein
use Vein, External Jugular, Left
use Vein, External Jugular, Right
Posterior cerebral artery use Artery, Intracranial
Posterior chamber
use Eye, Right
use Eye, Left
Posterior circumflex humeral artery
use Artery, Axillary, Right
use Artery, Axillary, Left
Posterior communicating artery use Artery, Intracranial
Posterior cruciate ligament (PCL)
use Bursa and Ligament, Knee, Right
use Bursa and Ligament, Knee, Left
Posterior facial (retromandibular) vein
use Vein, Face, Right
use Vein, Face, Left
Posterior femoral cutaneous nerve use Nerve, Sacral Plexus
Posterior inferior cerebellar artery (PICA) use Artery, Intracranial
Posterior interosseous nerve use Nerve, Radial
Posterior labial nerve use Nerve, Pudendal
Posterior scrotal nerve use Nerve, Pudendal
Posterior spinal artery
use Artery, Vertebral, Left
use Artery, Vertebral, Right
Posterior tibial recurrent artery
use Artery, Anterior Tibial, Right
use Artery, Anterior Tibial, Left

Posterior ulnar recurrent artery
use Artery, Ulnar, Left
use Artery, Ulnar, Right
Posterior vagal trunk use Nerve, Vagus
PPN (peripheral parenteral nutrition) see Introduction of Nutritional Substance
Preauricular lymph node use Lymphatic, Head
Precava use Vena Cava, Superior
Prepatellar bursa
use Bursa and Ligament, Knee, Right
use Bursa and Ligament, Knee, Left
Preputiotomy see Drainage, Male Reproductive System **0V9**
Pressure support ventilation see Performance, Respiratory **5A19**
PRESTIGE® Cervical Disc use Synthetic Substitute
Pretracheal fascia use Subcutaneous Tissue and Fascia, Neck, Anterior
Prevertebral fascia use Subcutaneous Tissue and Fascia, Neck, Posterior
PrimeAdvanced neurostimulator use Stimulator Generator, Multiple Array in **0JH**
Princeps pollicis artery
use Artery, Hand, Left
use Artery, Hand, Right
Probing, duct
Diagnostic see Inspection
Dilation see Dilation
PROCEED™ Ventral Patch use Synthetic Substitute
Procerus muscle use Muscle, Facial
Proctectomy
see Excision, Rectum **0DBP**
see Resection, Rectum **0DTP**
Proctoclysis see Introduction of substance in or on, Gastrointestinal Tract, Lower **3E0H**
Proctocolectomy
see Excision, Gastrointestinal System **0DB**
see Resection, Gastrointestinal System **0DT**
Proctocolpoplasty
see Repair, Gastrointestinal System **0DQ**
see Supplement, Gastrointestinal System **0DU**
Proctoperineoplasty
see Repair, Gastrointestinal System **0DQ**
see Supplement, Gastrointestinal System **0DU**
Proctoperineorrhaphy see Repair, Gastrointestinal System **0DQ**
Proctopexy
see Repair, Rectum **0DQP**
see Reposition, Rectum **0DSP**
Proctoplasty
see Repair, Rectum **0DQP**
see Supplement, Rectum **0DUP**
Proctorrhaphy see Repair, Rectum **0DQP**
Proctoscopy 0DJD8ZZ
Proctosigmoidectomy
see Excision, Gastrointestinal System **0DB**
see Resection, Gastrointestinal System **0DT**
Proctosigmoidoscopy 0DJD8ZZ
Proctostomy see Drainage, Rectum **0D9P**
Proctotomy see Drainage, Rectum **0D9P**
Prodisc-C use Synthetic Substitute **Prodisc-L** use Synthetic Substitute

Production, atrial septal defect see Excision, Septum, Atrial **02B5**
Profunda brachii
use Artery, Brachial, Right
use Artery, Brachial, Left
Profunda femoris (deep femoral) vein
use Vein, Femoral, Right
use Vein, Femoral, Left
PROLENE Polypropylene Hernia System (PHS) use Synthetic Substitute
Pronator quadratus muscle
use Muscle, Lower Arm and Wrist, Left
use Muscle, Lower Arm and Wrist, Right
Pronator teres muscle
use Muscle, Lower Arm and Wrist, Right
use Muscle, Lower Arm and Wrist, Left
Prostatectomy
see Excision, Prostate **0VB0**
see Resection, Prostate **0VT0**
Prostatic urethra use Urethra
Prostatomy, prostatotomy see Drainage, Prostate **0V90**
Protecta XT CRT-D use Cardiac Resynchronization Defibrillator Pulse Generator in **0JH**
Protecta XT DR (XT VR) use Defibrillator Generator in **0JH**
Protégé® RX Carotid Stent System use Intraluminal Device
Proximal radioulnar joint
use Joint, Elbow, Left
use Joint, Elbow, Right
Psoas muscle
use Muscle, Hip, Right
use Muscle, Hip, Left
PSV (pressure support ventilation) see Performance, Respiratory **5A19**
Psychoanalysis GZ54ZZZ
Psychological Tests
Cognitive Status **GZ14ZZZ**
Developmental **GZ10ZZZ**
Intellectual and Psychoeducational **GZ12ZZZ**
Neurobehavioral Status **GZ14ZZZ**
Neuropsychological **GZ13ZZZ**
Personality and Behavioral **GZ11ZZZ**
Psychotherapy
Family, Mental Health Services **GZ72ZZZ**
Group **GZHZZZZ**
Mental Health Services **GZHZZZZ**
Individual
see Psychotherapy, Individual, Mental Health Services
for substance abuse
12-Step **HZ53ZZZ**
Behavioral **HZ51ZZZ**
Cognitive **HZ50ZZZ**
Cognitive-Behavioral **HZ52ZZZ**
Confrontational **HZ58ZZZ**
Interactive **HZ55ZZZ**
Interpersonal **HZ54ZZZ**
Motivational Enhancement **HZ57ZZZ**
Psychoanalysis **HZ5BZZZ**
Psychodynamic **HZ5CZZZ**
Psychoeducation **HZ56ZZZ**

Psychotherapy *(continued)*
    Psychophysiological **HZ5DZZZ**
    Supportive **HZ59ZZZ**
  Mental Health Services
    Behavioral **GZ51ZZZ**
    Cognitive **GZ52ZZZ**
    Cognitive-Behavioral **GZ58ZZZ**
    Interactive **GZ50ZZZ**
    Interpersonal **GZ53ZZZ**
    Psychoanalysis **GZ54ZZZ**
    Psychodynamic **GZ55ZZZ**
    Psychophysiological **GZ59ZZZ**
    Supportive **GZ56ZZZ**
PTCA (percutaneous transluminal coronary angioplasty) *see* Dilation, Heart and Great Vessels **027**
Pterygoid muscle *use* Muscle, Head
Pterygoid process
  use Bone, Sphenoid, Right
  use Bone, Sphenoid, Left
Pterygopalatine (sphenopalatine) ganglion
  use Nerve, Head and Neck Sympathetic
Pubic ligament
  use Bursa and Ligament, Trunk, Right
  use Bursa and Ligament, Trunk, Left
Pubis
  use Bone, Pelvic, Right
  use Bone, Pelvic, Left
Pubofemoral ligament
  use Bursa and Ligament, Hip, Left
  use Bursa and Ligament, Hip, Right
Pudendal nerve *use* Nerve, Sacral Plexus
Pull-through, rectal *see* Resection, Rectum **0DTP**
Pulmoaortic canal *use* Artery, Pulmonary, Left
Pulmonary annulus *use* Valve, Pulmonary
Pulmonary artery wedge monitoring *see* Monitoring, Arterial **4A13**
Pulmonary plexus
  use Nerve, Vagus
  use Nerve, Thoracic Sympathetic
Pulmonic valve *use* Valve, Pulmonary
Pulpectomy *see* Excision, Mouth and Throat **0CB**
Pulverization *see* Fragmentation
Pulvinar *use* Thalamus
Pump reservoir *use* Infusion Device, Pump in Subcutaneous Tissue and Fascia
Punch biopsy *see* Excision with qualifier Diagnostic
Puncture *see* Drainage
Puncture, lumbar *see* Drainage, Spinal Canal **009U**
Pyelography
  see Plain Radiography, Urinary System **BT0**
  see Fluoroscopy, Urinary System **BT1**
Pyeloileostomy, urinary diversion *see* Bypass, Urinary System **0T1**
Pyeloplasty
  see Repair, Urinary System **0TQ**
  see Replacement, Urinary System **0TR**
  see Supplement, Urinary System **0TU**
Pyelorrhaphy *see* Repair, Urinary System **0TQ**
Pyeloscopy 0TJ58ZZ

Pyelostomy
  see Drainage, Urinary System **0T9**
  see Bypass, Urinary System **0T1**
Pyelotomy *see* Drainage, Urinary System **0T9**
Pylorectomy
  see Excision, Stomach, Pylorus **0DB7**
  see Resection, Stomach, Pylorus **0DT7**
Pyloric antrum *use* Stomach, Pylorus
Pyloric canal *use* Stomach, Pylorus
Pyloric sphincter *use* Stomach, Pylorus
Pylorodiosis *see* Dilation, Stomach, Pylorus **0D77**
Pylorogastrectomy
  see Excision, Gastrointestinal System **0DB**
  see Resection, Gastrointestinal System **0DT**
Pyloroplasty
  see Repair, Stomach, Pylorus **0DQ7**
  see Supplement, Stomach, Pylorus **0DU7**
Pyloroscopy 0DJ68ZZ
Pylorotomy *see* Drainage, Stomach, Pylorus **0D97**
Pyramidalis muscle
  use Muscle, Abdomen, Left
  use Muscle, Abdomen, Right

Q

Quadrangular cartilage *use* Septum, Nasal
Quadrant resection of breast *see* Excision, Skin and Breast **0HB**
Quadrate lobe *use* Liver
Quadratus femoris muscle
  use Muscle, Hip, Left
  use Muscle, Hip, Right
Quadratus lumborum muscle
  use Muscle, Trunk, Left
  use Muscle, Trunk, Right
Quadratus plantae muscle
  use Muscle, Foot, Left
  use Muscle, Foot, Right
Quadriceps (femoris)
  use Muscle, Upper Leg, Left
  use Muscle, Upper Leg, Right
Quarantine 8E0ZXY6

R

Radial collateral carpal ligament
  use Bursa and Ligament, Wrist, Right
  use Bursa and Ligament, Wrist, Left
Radial collateral ligament
  use Bursa and Ligament, Elbow, Left
  use Bursa and Ligament, Elbow, Right
Radial notch
  use Ulna, Left
  use Ulna, Right
Radial recurrent artery
  use Artery, Radial, Right
  use Artery, Radial, Left
Radial vein
  use Vein, Brachial, Right
  use Vein, Brachial, Left
Radialis indicis
  use Artery, Hand, Right
  use Artery, Hand, Left

Radiation Therapy
  see Beam Radiation
  see Brachytherapy
  see Stereotactic Radiosurgery
Radiation treatment *see* Radiation Therapy
Radiocarpal joint
  use Joint, Wrist, Left
  use Joint, Wrist, Right
Radiocarpal ligament
  use Bursa and Ligament, Wrist, Left
  use Bursa and Ligament, Wrist, Right
Radiography *see* Plain Radiography
Radiology, analog *see* Plain Radiography
Radiology, diagnostic *see* Imaging, Diagnostic
Radioulnar ligament
  use Bursa and Ligament, Wrist, Right
  use Bursa and Ligament, Wrist, Left
Range of motion testing *see* Motor Function Assessment, Rehabilitation **F01**
REALIZE® Adjustable Gastric Band *use* Extraluminal Device
Reattachment
  Abdominal Wall **0WMF0ZZ**
  Ampulla of Vater **0FMC**
  Ankle Region
    Left **0YML0ZZ**
    Right **0YMK0ZZ**
  Arm
    Lower
      Left **0XMF0ZZ**
      Right **0XMD0ZZ**
    Upper
      Left **0XM90ZZ**
      Right **0XM80ZZ**
  Axilla
    Left **0XM50ZZ**
    Right **0XM40ZZ**
  Back
    Lower **0WML0ZZ**
    Upper **0WMK0ZZ**
  Bladder **0TMB**
  Bladder Neck **0TMC**
  Breast
    Bilateral **0HMVXZZ**
    Left **0HMUXZZ**
    Right **0HMTXZZ**
  Bronchus
    Lingula **0BM90ZZ**
    Lower Lobe
      Left **0BMB0ZZ**
      Right **0BM60ZZ**
    Main
      Left **0BM70ZZ**
      Right **0BM30ZZ**
    Middle Lobe, Right **0BM50ZZ**
    Upper Lobe
      Left **0BM80ZZ**
      Right **0BM40ZZ**
  Bursa and Ligament
    Abdomen
      Left **0MMJ**
      Right **0MMH**
    Ankle
      Left **0MMR**
      Right **0MMQ**
    Elbow

Reattachment (*continued*)

- Left **0MM4**
- Right **0MM3**
- Foot
  - Left **0MMT**
  - Right **0MMS**
- Hand
  - Left **0MM8**
  - Right **0MM7**
- Head and Neck **0MM0**
- Hip
  - Left **0MMM**
  - Right **0MML**
- Knee
  - Left **0MMP**
  - Right **0MMN**
- Lower Extremity
  - Left **0MMW**
  - Right **0MMV**
- Perineum **0MMK**
- Shoulder
  - Left **0MM2**
  - Right **0MM1**
- Thorax
  - Left **0MMG**
  - Right **0MMF**
- Trunk
  - Left **0MMD**
  - Right **0MMC**
- Upper Extremity
  - Left **0MMB**
  - Right **0MM9**
- Wrist
  - Left **0MM6**
  - Right **0MM5**
- Buttock
  - Left **0YM10ZZ**
  - Right **0YM00ZZ**
- Carina **0BM20ZZ**
- Cecum **0DMH**
- Cervix **0UMC**
- Chest Wall **0WM80ZZ**
- Clitoris **0UMJXZZ**
- Colon
  - Ascending **0DMK**
  - Descending **0DMM**
  - Sigmoid **0DMN**
  - Transverse **0DML**
- Cord
  - Bilateral **0VMH**
  - Left **0VMG**
  - Right **0VMF**
- Cul-de-sac **0UMF**
- Diaphragm
  - Left **0BMS0ZZ**
  - Right **0BMR0ZZ**
- Duct
  - Common Bile **0FM9**
  - Cystic **0FM8**
  - Hepatic
    - Left **0FM6**
    - Right **0FM5**
  - Pancreatic **0FMD**
    - Accessory **0FMF**
- Duodenum **0DM9**
- Ear

Reattachment (*continued*)

- Left **09M1XZZ**
- Right **09M0XZZ**
- Elbow Region
  - Left **0XMC0ZZ**
  - Right **0XMB0ZZ**
- Esophagus **0DM5**
- Extremity
  - Lower
    - Left **0YMB0ZZ**
    - Right **0YM90ZZ**
  - Upper
    - Left **0XM70ZZ**
    - Right **0XM60ZZ**
- Eyelid
  - Lower
    - Left **08MRXZZ**
    - Right **08MQXZZ**
  - Upper
    - Left **08MPXZZ**
    - Right **08MNXZZ**
- Face **0WM20ZZ**
- Fallopian Tube
  - Left **0UM6**
  - Right **0UM5**
- Fallopian Tubes, Bilateral **0UM7**
- Femoral Region
  - Left **0YM80ZZ**
  - Right **0YM70ZZ**
- Finger
  - Index
    - Left **0XMP0ZZ**
    - Right **0XMN0ZZ**
  - Little
    - Left **0XMW0ZZ**
    - Right **0XMV0ZZ**
  - Middle
    - Left **0XMR0ZZ**
    - Right **0XMQ0ZZ**
  - Ring
    - Left **0XMT0ZZ**
    - Right **0XMS0ZZ**
- Foot
  - Left **0YMN0ZZ**
  - Right **0YMM0ZZ**
- Forequarter
  - Left **0XM10ZZ**
  - Right **0XM00ZZ**
- Gallbladder **0FM4**
- Gland
  - Left **0GM2**
  - Right **0GM3**
- Hand
  - Left **0XMK0ZZ**
  - Right **0XMJ0ZZ**
- Hindquarter
  - Bilateral **0YM40ZZ**
  - Left **0YM30ZZ**
  - Right **0YM20ZZ**
- Hymen **0UMK**
- Ileum **0DMB**
- Inguinal Region
  - Left **0YM60ZZ**
  - Right **0YM50ZZ**
- Intestine
  - Large **0DME**

Reattachment (*continued*)

- Left **0DMG**
- Right **0DMF**
- Small **0DM8**
- Jaw
  - Lower **0WM50ZZ**
  - Upper **0WM40ZZ**
- Jejunum **0DMA**
- Kidney
  - Left **0TM1**
  - Right **0TM0**
- Kidney Pelvis
  - Left **0TM4**
  - Right **0TM3**
- Kidneys, Bilateral **0TM2**
- Knee Region
  - Left **0YMG0ZZ**
  - Right **0YMF0ZZ**
- Leg
  - Lower
    - Left **0YMJ0ZZ**
    - Right **0YMH0ZZ**
  - Upper
    - Left **0YMD0ZZ**
    - Right **0YMC0ZZ**
- Lip
  - Lower **0CM10ZZ**
  - Upper **0CM00ZZ**
- Liver **0FM0**
  - Left Lobe **0FM2**
  - Right Lobe **0FM1**
- Lung
  - Left **0BML0ZZ**
  - Lower Lobe
    - Left **0BMJ0ZZ**
    - Right **0BMF0ZZ**
  - Middle Lobe, Right **0BMD0ZZ**
  - Right **0BMK0ZZ**
  - Upper Lobe
    - Left **0BMG0ZZ**
    - Right **0BMC0ZZ**
- Lung Lingula **0BMH0ZZ**
- Muscle
  - Abdomen
    - Left **0KML**
    - Right **0KMK**
  - Facial **0KM1**
  - Foot
    - Left **0KMW**
    - Right **0KMV**
  - Hand
    - Left **0KMD**
    - Right **0KMC**
  - Head **0KM0**
  - Hip
    - Left **0KMP**
    - Right **0KMN**
  - Lower Arm and Wrist
    - Left **0KMB**
    - Right **0KM9**
  - Lower Leg
    - Left **0KMT**
    - Right **0KMS**
  - Neck
    - Left **0KM3**
    - Right **0KM2**

Reattachment *(continued)*
- Perineum 0KMM
- Shoulder
  - Left 0KM6
  - Right 0KM5
- Thorax
  - Left 0KMJ
  - Right 0KMH
- Tongue, Palate, Pharynx 0KM4
- Trunk
  - Left 0KMG
  - Right 0KMF
- Upper Arm
  - Left 0KM8
  - Right 0KM7
- Upper Leg
  - Left 0KMR
  - Right 0KMQ
- Neck 0WM60ZZ
- Nipple
  - Left 0HMXXZZ
  - Right 0HMWXZZ
- Nose 09MKXZZ
- Ovary
  - Bilateral 0UM2
  - Left 0UM1
  - Right 0UM0
- Palate, Soft 0CM30ZZ
- Pancreas 0FMG
- Parathyroid Gland 0GMR
  - Inferior
    - Left 0GMP
    - Right 0GMN
  - Multiple 0GMQ
  - Superior
    - Left 0GMM
    - Right 0GML
- Penis 0VMSXZZ
- Perineum
  - Female 0WMN0ZZ
  - Male 0WMM0ZZ
- Rectum 0DMP
- Scrotum 0VM5XZZ
- Shoulder Region
  - Left 0XM30ZZ
  - Right 0XM20ZZ
- Skin
  - Abdomen 0HM7XZZ
  - Back 0HM6XZZ
  - Buttock 0HM8XZZ
  - Chest 0HM5XZZ
  - Ear
    - Left 0HM3XZZ
    - Right 0HM2XZZ
  - Face 0HM1XZZ
  - Foot
    - Left 0HMNXZZ
    - Right 0HMMXZZ
  - Genitalia 0HMAXZZ
  - Hand
    - Left 0HMGXZZ
    - Right 0HMFXZZ
  - Lower Arm
    - Left 0HMEXZZ
    - Right 0HMDXZZ
  - Lower Leg

Reattachment *(continued)*
- Left 0HMLXZZ
- Right 0HMKXZZ
- Neck 0HM4XZZ
- Perineum 0HM9XZZ
- Scalp 0HM0XZZ
- Upper Arm
  - Left 0HMCXZZ
  - Right 0HMBXZZ
- Upper Leg
  - Left 0HMJXZZ
  - Right 0HMHXZZ
- Stomach 0DM6
- Tendon
  - Abdomen
    - Left 0LMG
    - Right 0LMF
  - Ankle
    - Left 0LMT
    - Right 0LMS
  - Foot
    - Left 0LMW
    - Right 0LMV
  - Hand
    - Left 0LM8
    - Right 0LM7
  - Head and Neck 0LM0
  - Hip
    - Left 0LMK
    - Right 0LMJ
  - Knee
    - Left 0LMR
    - Right 0LMQ
  - Lower Arm and Wrist
    - Left 0LM6
    - Right 0LM5
  - Lower Leg
    - Left 0LMP
    - Right 0LMN
  - Perineum 0LMH
  - Shoulder
    - Left 0LM2
    - Right 0LM1
  - Thorax
    - Left 0LMD
    - Right 0LMC
  - Trunk
    - Left 0LMB
    - Right 0LM9
  - Upper Arm
    - Left 0LM4
    - Right 0LM3
  - Upper Leg
    - Left 0LMM
    - Right 0LML
- Testis
  - Bilateral 0VMC
  - Left 0VMB
  - Right 0VM9
- Thumb
  - Left 0XMM0ZZ
  - Right 0XML0ZZ
- Thyroid Gland
  - Left Lobe 0GMG
  - Right Lobe 0GMH
- Toe

Reattachment *(continued)*
- 1st
  - Left 0YMQ0ZZ
  - Right 0YMP0ZZ
- 2nd
  - Left 0YMS0ZZ
  - Right 0YMR0ZZ
- 3rd
  - Left 0YMU0ZZ
  - Right 0YMT0ZZ
- 4th
  - Left 0YMW0ZZ
  - Right 0YMV0ZZ
- 5th
  - Left 0YMY0ZZ
  - Right 0YMX0ZZ
- Tongue 0CM70ZZ
- Tooth
  - Lower 0CMX
  - Upper 0CMW
- Trachea 0BM10ZZ
- Tunica Vaginalis
  - Left 0VM7
  - Right 0VM6
- Ureter
  - Left 0TM7
  - Right 0TM6
- Ureters, Bilateral 0TM8
- Urethra 0TMD
- Uterine Supporting Structure 0UM4
- Uterus 0UM9
- Uvula 0CMN0ZZ
- Vagina 0UMG
- Vulva 0UMMXZZ
- Wrist Region
  - Left 0XMH0ZZ
  - Right 0XMG0ZZ

Rebound HRD® (Hernia Repair Device) *use* Synthetic Substitute

Recession
- *see* Repair
- *see* Reposition

Reclosure, disrupted abdominal wall 0WQFXZZ

Reconstruction
- *see* Repair
- *see* Replacement
- *see* Supplement

Rectectomy
- *see* Excision, Rectum 0DBP
- *see* Resection, Rectum 0DTP

Rectocele repair *see* Repair, Subcutaneous Tissue and Fascia, Pelvic Region 0JQC

Rectopexy
- *see* Repair, Gastrointestinal System 0DQ
- *see* Reposition, Gastrointestinal System 0DS

Rectoplasty
- *see* Repair, Gastrointestinal System 0DQ
- *see* Supplement, Gastrointestinal System 0DU

Rectorrhaphy *see* Repair, Gastrointestinal System 0DQ

Rectoscopy 0DJD8ZZ

Rectosigmoid junction *use* Colon, Sigmoid

Rectosigmoidectomy
  see Excision, Gastrointestinal System **0DB**
  see Resection, Gastrointestinal System **0DT**
Rectostomy see Drainage, Rectum **0D9P**
Rectotomy see Drainage, Rectum **0D9P**
Rectus abdominis muscle
  use Muscle, Abdomen, Left
  use Muscle, Abdomen, Right
Rectus femoris muscle
  use Muscle, Upper Leg, Left
  use Muscle, Upper Leg, Right
Recurrent laryngeal nerve use Nerve, Vagus
Reduction
  Dislocation see Reposition
  Fracture see Reposition
  Intussusception, intestinal see Reposition,
  Gastrointestinal System **0DS**
  Mammoplasty see Excision, Skin and Breast
  0HB
  Prolapse see Reposition
  Torsion see Reposition
  Volvulus, gastrointestinal see Reposition,
  Gastrointestinal System **0DS**
Refusion see Fusion
Rehabilitation
  see Activities of Daily Living Assessment,
  Rehabilitation **F02**
  see Activities of Daily Living Treatment,
  Rehabilitation **F08**
  see Caregiver Training, Rehabilitation **F0F**
  see Cochlear Implant Treatment,
  Rehabilitation **F0B**
  see Device Fitting, Rehabilitation **F0D**
  see Hearing Treatment, Rehabilitation **F09**
  see Motor Function Assessment,
  Rehabilitation **F01**
Rehabilitation (continued)
  see Motor Treatment, Rehabilitation **F07**
  see Speech Assessment, Rehabilitation **F00**
  see Speech Treatment, Rehabilitation **F06**
  see Vestibular Treatment, Rehabilitation
  F0C
Reimplantation
  see Reposition
  see Transfer
  see Reattachment
Reinforcement
  see Repair
  see Supplement
Relaxation, scar tissue see Release
Release
  Acetabulum
    Left **0QN5**
    Right **0QN4**
  Adenoids **0CNQ**
  Ampulla of Vater **0FNC**
  Anal Sphincter **0DNR**
  Anterior Chamber
    Left **08N33ZZ**
    Right **08N23ZZ**
  Anus **0DNQ**
  Aorta
    Abdominal **04N0**
    Thoracic
      Ascending/Arch **02NX**
      Descending **02NW**

Release (continued)
  Aortic Body **0GND**
  Appendix **0DNJ**
  Artery
    Anterior Tibial
      Left **04NQ**
      Right **04NP**
    Axillary
      Left **03N6**
      Right **03N5**
    Brachial
      Left **03N8**
      Right **03N7**
    Celiac **04N1**
    Colic
      Left **04N7**
      Middle **04N8**
      Right **04N6**
    Common Carotid
      Left **03NJ**
      Right **03NH**
    Common Iliac
      Left **04ND**
      Right **04NC**
    External Carotid
      Left **03NN**
      Right **03NM**
    External Iliac
      Left **04NJ**
      Right **04NH**
    Face **03NR**
    Femoral
      Left **04NL**
      Right **04NK**
    Foot
      Left **04NW**
      Right **04NV**
    Gastric **04N2**
    Hand
      Left **03NF**
      Right **03ND**
    Hepatic **04N3**
    Inferior Mesenteric **04NB**
    Innominate **03N2**
      Left **03NL**
      Right **03NK**
    Internal Iliac
      Left **04NF**
      Right **04NE**
    Internal Mammary
      Left **03N1**
      Right **03N0**
    Intracranial **03NG**
    Lower **04NY**
    Peroneal
      Left **04NU**
      Right **04NT**
    Popliteal
      Left **04NN**
      Right **04NM**
    Posterior Tibial
      Left **04NS**
      Right **04NR**
    Pulmonary
      Left **02NR**
      Right **02NQ**

Release (continued)
    Pulmonary Trunk **02NP**
    Radial
      Left **03NC**
      Right **03NB**
    Renal
      Left **04NA**
      Right **04N9**
    Splenic **04N4**
    Subclavian
      Left **03N4**
      Right **03N3**
    Superior Mesenteric **04N5**
    Temporal
      Left **03NT**
      Right **03NS**
    Thyroid
      Left **03NV**
      Right **03NU**
    Ulnar
      Left **03NA**
      Right **03N9**
    Upper **03NY**
    Vertebral
      Left **03NQ**
      Right **03NP**
  Atrium
    Left **02N7**
    Right **02N6**
  Auditory Ossicle
    Left **09NA0ZZ**
    Right **09N90ZZ**
  Basal Ganglia **00N8**
  Bladder **0TNB**
  Bladder Neck **0TNC**
  Bone
    Ethmoid
      Left **0NNG**
      Right **0NNF**
    Frontal
      Left **0NN2**
      Right **0NN1**
    Hyoid **0NNX**
    Lacrimal
      Left **0NNJ**
      Right **0NNH**
    Nasal **0NNB**
    Occipital
      Left **0NN8**
      Right **0NN7**
    Palatine
      Left **0NNL**
      Right **0NNK**
    Parietal
      Left **0NN4**
      Right **0NN3**
    Pelvic
      Left **0QN3**
      Right **0QN2**
    Sphenoid
      Left **0NND**
      Right **0NNC**
    Temporal
      Left **0NN6**
      Right **0NN5**
    Zygomatic

Release *(continued)*
    Left **0NNN**
    Right **0NNM**
Brain **00N0**
Breast
    Bilateral **0HNV**
    Left **0HNU**
    Right **0HNT**
Bronchus
    Lingula **0BN9**
    Lower Lobe
        Left **0BNB**
        Right **0BN6**
    Main
        Left **0BN7**
        Right **0BN3**
    Middle Lobe, Right **0BN5**
    Upper Lobe
        Left **0BN8**
        Right **0BN4**
Buccal Mucosa **0CN4**
Bursa and Ligament
    Abdomen
        Left **0MNJ**
        Right **0MNH**
    Ankle
        Left **0MNR**
        Right **0MNQ**
    Elbow
        Left **0MN4**
        Right **0MN3**
    Foot
        Left **0MNT**
        Right **0MNS**
    Hand
        Left **0MN8**
        Right **0MN7**
    Head and Neck **0MN0**
    Hip
        Left **0MNM**
        Right **0MNL**
    Knee
        Left **0MNP**
        Right **0MNN**
    Lower Extremity
        Left **0MNW**
        Right **0MNV**
    Perineum **0MNK**
    Shoulder
        Left **0MN2**
        Right **0MN1**
    Thorax
        Left **0MNG**
        Right **0MNF**
    Trunk
        Left **0MND**
        Right **0MNC**
    Upper Extremity
        Left **0MNB**
        Right **0MN9**
    Wrist
        Left **0MN6**
        Right **0MN5**
Carina **0BN2**
Carotid Bodies, Bilateral **0GN8**
Carotid Body

Release *(continued)*
    Left **0GN6**
    Right **0GN7**
Carpal
    Left **0PNN**
    Right **0PNM**
Cecum **0DNH**
Cerebellum **00NC**
Cerebral Hemisphere **00N7**
Cerebral Meninges **00N1**
Cerebral Ventricle **00N6**
Cervix **0UNC**
Chordae Tendineae **02N9**
Choroid
    Left **08NB**
    Right **08NA**
Cisterna Chyli **07NL**
Clavicle
    Left **0PNB**
    Right **0PN9**
Clitoris **0UNJ**
Coccygeal Glomus **0GNB**
Coccyx **0QNS**
Colon
    Ascending **0DNK**
    Descending **0DNM**
    Sigmoid **0DNN**
    Transverse **0DNL**
Conduction Mechanism **02N8**
Conjunctiva
    Left **08NTXZZ**
    Right **08NSXZZ**
Cord
    Bilateral **0VNH**
    Left **0VNG**
    Right **0VNF**
Cornea
    Left **08N9XZZ**
    Right **08N8XZZ**
Cul-de-sac **0UNF**
Diaphragm
    Left **0BNS**
    Right **0BNR**
Disc
    Cervical Vertebral **0RN3**
    Cervicothoracic Vertebral **0RN5**
    Lumbar Vertebral **0SN2**
    Lumbosacral **0SN4**
    Thoracic Vertebral **0RN9**
    Thoracolumbar Vertebral **0RNB**
Duct
    Common Bile **0FN9**
    Cystic **0FN8**
    Hepatic
        Left **0FN6**
        Right **0FN5**
    Lacrimal
        Left **08NY**
        Right **08NX**
    Pancreatic **0FND**
        Accessory **0FNF**
    Parotid
        Left **0CNC**
        Right **0CNB**
Duodenum **0DN9**
Dura Mater **00N2**

Release *(continued)*
Ear
    External
        Left **09N1**
        Right **09N0**
    External Auditory Canal
        Left **09N4**
        Right **09N3**
    Inner
        Left **09NE0ZZ**
        Right **09ND0ZZ**
    Middle
        Left **09N60ZZ**
        Right **09N50ZZ**
Epididymis
    Bilateral **0VNL**
    Left **0VNK**
    Right **0VNJ**
Epiglottis **0CNR**
Esophagogastric Junction **0DN4**
Esophagus **0DN5**
    Lower **0DN3**
    Middle **0DN2**
    Upper **0DN1**
Eustachian Tube
    Left **09NG**
    Right **09NF**
Eye
    Left **08N1XZZ**
    Right **08N0XZZ**
Eyelid
    Lower
        Left **08NR**
        Right **08NQ**
    Upper
        Left **08NP**
        Right **08NN**
Fallopian Tube
    Left **0UN6**
    Right **0UN5**
Fallopian Tubes, Bilateral **0UN7**
Femoral Shaft
    Left **0QN9**
    Right **0QN8**
Femur
    Lower
        Left **0QNC**
        Right **0QNB**
    Upper
        Left **0QN7**
        Right **0QN6**
Fibula
    Left **0QNK**
    Right **0QNJ**
Finger Nail **0HNQXZZ**
Gallbladder **0FN4**
Gingiva
    Lower **0CN6**
    Upper **0CN5**
Gland
    Adrenal
        Bilateral **0GN4**
        Left **0GN2**
        Right **0GN3**
    Lacrimal
        Left **08NW**

Release *(continued)*
    Right **08NV**
    Minor Salivary **0CNJ**
    Parotid
        Left **0CN9**
        Right **0CN8**
    Pituitary **0GN0**
    Sublingual
        Left **0CNF**
        Right **0CND**
    Submaxillary
        Left **0CNH**
        Right **0CNG**
    Vestibular **0UNL**
    Glenoid Cavity
        Left **0PN8**
        Right **0PN7**
    Glomus Jugulare **0GNC**
    Humeral Head
        Left **0PND**
        Right **0PNC**
    Humeral Shaft
        Left **0PNG**
        Right **0PNF**
    Hymen **0UNK**
    Hypothalamus **00NA**
    Ileocecal Valve **0DNC**
    Ileum **0DNB**
    Intestine
        Large **0DNE**
            Left **0DNG**
            Right **0DNF**
        Small **0DN8**
    Iris
        Left **08ND3ZZ**
        Right **08NC3ZZ**
    Jejunum **0DNA**
    Joint
        Acromioclavicular
            Left **0RNH**
            Right **0RNG**
        Ankle
            Left **0SNG**
            Right **0SNF**
        Carpal
            Left **0RNR**
            Right **0RNQ**
        Cervical Vertebral **0RN1**
        Cervicothoracic Vertebral **0RN4**
        Coccygeal **0SN6**
        Elbow
            Left **0RNM**
            Right **0RNL**
        Finger Phalangeal
            Left **0RNX**
            Right **0RNW**
        Hip
            Left **0SNB**
            Right **0SN9**
        Knee
            Left **0SND**
            Right **0SNC**
        Lumbar Vertebral **0SN0**
        Lumbosacral **0SN3**
        Metacarpocarpal
            Left **0RNT**

Release *(continued)*
            Right **0RNS**
        Metacarpophalangeal
            Left **0RNV**
            Right **0RNU**
        Metatarsal-Phalangeal
            Left **0SNN**
            Right **0SNM**
        Metatarsal-Tarsal
            Left **0SNL**
            Right **0SNK**
        Occipital-cervical **0RN0**
        Sacrococcygeal **0SN5**
        Sacroiliac
            Left **0SN8**
            Right **0SN7**
        Shoulder
            Left **0RNK**
            Right **0RNJ**
        Sternoclavicular
            Left **0RNF**
            Right **0RNE**
        Tarsal
            Left **0SNJ**
            Right **0SNH**
        Temporomandibular
            Left **0RND**
            Right **0RNC**
        Thoracic Vertebral **0RN6**
        Thoracolumbar Vertebral **0RNA**
        Toe Phalangeal
            Left **0SNQ**
            Right **0SNP**
        Wrist
            Left **0RNP**
            Right **0RNN**
    Kidney
        Left **0TN1**
        Right **0TN0**
    Kidney Pelvis
        Left **0TN4**
        Right **0TN3**
    Larynx **0CNS**
    Lens
        Left **08NK3ZZ**
        Right **08NJ3ZZ**
    Lip
        Lower **0CN1**
        Upper **0CN0**
    Liver **0FN0**
        Left Lobe **0FN2**
        Right Lobe **0FN1**
    Lung
        Bilateral **0BNM**
        Left **0BNL**
        Lower Lobe
            Left **0BNJ**
            Right **0BNF**
        Middle Lobe, Right **0BND**
        Right **0BNK**
        Upper Lobe
            Left **0BNG**
            Right **0BNC**
    Lung Lingula **0BNH**
    Lymphatic
        Aortic **07ND**

Release *(continued)*
        Axillary
            Left **07N6**
            Right **07N5**
        Head **07N0**
        Inguinal
            Left **07NJ**
            Right **07NH**
        Internal Mammary
            Left **07N9**
            Right **07N8**
        Lower Extremity
            Left **07NG**
            Right **07NF**
        Mesenteric **07NB**
        Neck
            Left **07N2**
            Right **07N1**
        Pelvis **07NC**
        Thoracic Duct **07NK**
        Thorax **07N7**
        Upper Extremity
            Left **07N4**
            Right **07N3**
    Mandible
        Left **0NNV**
        Right **0NNT**
    Maxilla
        Left **0NNS**
        Right **0NNR**
    Medulla Oblongata **00ND**
    Mesentery **0DNV**
    Metacarpal
        Left **0PNQ**
        Right **0PNP**
    Metatarsal
        Left **0QNP**
        Right **0QNN**
    Muscle
        Abdomen
            Left **0KNL**
            Right **0KNK**
        Extraocular
            Left **08NM**
            Right **08NL**
        Facial **0KN1**
        Foot
            Left **0KNW**
            Right **0KNV**
        Hand
            Left **0KND**
            Right **0KNC**
        Head **0KN0**
        Hip
            Left **0KNP**
            Right **0KNN**
        Lower Arm and Wrist
            Left **0KNB**
            Right **0KN9**
        Lower Leg
            Left **0KNT**
            Right **0KNS**
        Neck
            Left **0KN3**
            Right **0KN2**
        Papillary **02ND**

    Perineum **0KNM**
    Shoulder
        Left **0KN6**
        Right **0KN5**
    Thorax
        Left **0KNJ**
        Right **0KNH**
    Tongue, Palate, Pharynx **0KN4**
    Trunk
        Left **0KNG**
        Right **0KNF**
    Upper Arm
        Left **0KN8**
        Right **0KN7**
    Upper Leg
        Left **0KNR**
        Right **0KNQ**
  Nasopharynx **09NN**
  Nerve
    Abdominal Sympathetic **01NM**
    Abducens **00NL**
    Accessory **00NR**
    Acoustic **00NN**
    Brachial Plexus **01N3**
    Cervical **01N1**
    Cervical Plexus **01N0**
    Facial **00NM**
    Femoral **01ND**
    Glossopharyngeal **00NP**
    Head and Neck Sympathetic **01NK**
    Hypoglossal **00NS**
    Lumbar **01NB**
    Lumbar Plexus **01N9**
    Lumbar Sympathetic **01NN**
    Lumbosacral Plexus **01NA**
    Median **01N5**
    Oculomotor **00NH**
    Olfactory **00NF**
    Optic **00NG**
    Peroneal **01NH**
    Phrenic **01N2**
    Pudendal **01NC**
    Radial **01N6**
    Sacral **01NR**
    Sacral Plexus **01NQ**
    Sacral Sympathetic **01NP**
    Sciatic **01NF**
    Thoracic **01N8**
    Thoracic Sympathetic **01NL**
    Tibial **01NG**
    Trigeminal **00NK**
    Trochlear **00NJ**
    Ulnar **01N4**
    Vagus **00NQ**
  Nipple
    Left **0HNX**
    Right **0HNW**
  Nose **09NK**
  Omentum
    Greater **0DNS**
    Lesser **0DNT**
  Orbit
    Left **0NNQ**
    Right **0NNP**
  Ovary

    Bilateral **0UN2**
    Left **0UN1**
    Right **0UN0**
  Palate
    Hard **0CN2**
    Soft **0CN3**
  Pancreas **0FNG**
  Para-aortic Body **0GN9**
  Paraganglion Extremity **0GNF**
  Parathyroid Gland **0GNR**
    Inferior
        Left **0GNP**
        Right **0GNN**
    Multiple **0GNQ**
    Superior
        Left **0GNM**
        Right **0GNL**
  Patella
    Left **0QNF**
    Right **0QND**
  Penis **0VNS**
  Pericardium **02NN**
  Peritoneum **0DNW**
  Phalanx
    Finger
        Left **0PNV**
        Right **0PNT**
    Thumb
        Left **0PNS**
        Right **0PNR**
    Toe
        Left **0QNR**
        Right **0QNQ**
  Pharynx **0CNM**
  Pineal Body **0GN1**
  Pleura
    Left **0BNP**
    Right **0BNN**
  Pons **00NB**
  Prepuce **0VNT**
  Prostate **0VN0**
  Radius
    Left **0PNJ**
    Right **0PNH**
  Rectum **0DNP**
  Retina
    Left **08NF3ZZ**
    Right **08NE3ZZ**
  Retinal Vessel
    Left **08NH3ZZ**
    Right **08NG3ZZ**
  Rib
    Left **0PN2**
    Right **0PN1**
  Sacrum **0QN1**
  Scapula
    Left **0PN6**
    Right **0PN5**
  Sclera
    Left **08N7XZZ**
    Right **08N6XZZ**
  Scrotum **0VN5**
  Septum
    Atrial **02N5**
    Nasal **09NM**

    Ventricular **02NM**
  Sinus
    Accessory **09NP**
    Ethmoid
        Left **09NV**
        Right **09NU**
    Frontal
        Left **09NT**
        Right **09NS**
    Mastoid
        Left **09NC**
        Right **09NB**
    Maxillary
        Left **09NR**
        Right **09NQ**
    Sphenoid
        Left **09NX**
        Right **09NW**
  Skin
    Abdomen **0HN7XZZ**
    Back **0HN6XZZ**
    Buttock **0HN8XZZ**
    Chest **0HN5XZZ**
    Ear
        Left **0HN3XZZ**
        Right **0HN2XZZ**
    Face **0HN1XZZ**
    Foot
        Left **0HNNXZZ**
        Right **0HNMXZZ**
    Genitalia **0HNAXZZ**
    Hand
        Left **0HNGXZZ**
        Right **0HNFXZZ**
    Lower Arm
        Left **0HNEXZZ**
        Right **0HNDXZZ**
    Lower Leg
        Left **0HNLXZZ**
        Right **0HNKXZZ**
    Neck **0HN4XZZ**
    Perineum **0HN9XZZ**
    Scalp **0HN0XZZ**
    Upper Arm
        Left **0HNCXZZ**
        Right **0HNBXZZ**
    Upper Leg
        Left **0HNJXZZ**
        Right **0HNHXZZ**
  Spinal Cord
    Cervical **00NW**
    Lumbar **00NY**
    Thoracic **00NX**
  Spinal Meninges **00NT**
  Spleen **07NP**
  Sternum **0PN0**
  Stomach **0DN6**
    Pylorus **0DN7**
  Subcutaneous Tissue and Fascia
    Abdomen **0JN8**
    Back **0JN7**
    Buttock **0JN9**
    Chest **0JN6**
    Face **0JN1**
    Foot

Release *(continued)*
    Left **0JNR**
    Right **0JNQ**
  Hand
    Left **0JNK**
    Right **0JNJ**
  Lower Arm
    Left **0JNH**
    Right **0JNG**
  Lower Leg
    Left **0JNP**
    Right **0JNN**
  Neck
    Anterior **0JN4**
    Posterior **0JN5**
  Pelvic Region **0JNC**
  Perineum **0JNB**
  Scalp **0JN0**
  Upper Arm
    Left **0JNF**
    Right **0JND**
  Upper Leg
    Left **0JNM**
    Right **0JNL**
Tarsal
  Left **0QNM**
  Right **0QNL**
Tendon
  Abdomen
    Left **0LNG**
    Right **0LNF**
  Ankle
    Left **0LNT**
    Right **0LNS**
  Foot
    Left **0LNW**
    Right **0LNV**
  Hand
    Left **0LN8**
    Right **0LN7**
  Head and Neck **0LN0**
  Hip
    Left **0LNK**
    Right **0LNJ**
  Knee
    Left **0LNR**
    Right **0LNQ**
  Lower Arm and Wrist
    Left **0LN6**
    Right **0LN5**
  Lower Leg
    Left **0LNP**
    Right **0LNN**
  Perineum **0LNH**
  Shoulder
    Left **0LN2**
    Right **0LN1**
  Thorax
    Left **0LND**
    Right **0LNC**
  Trunk
    Left **0LNB**
    Right **0LN9**
  Upper Arm
    Left **0LN4**
    Right **0LN3**

Release *(continued)*
  Upper Leg
    Left **0LNM**
    Right **0LNL**
  Testis
    Bilateral **0VNC**
    Left **0VNB**
    Right **0VN9**
  Thalamus **00N9**
  Thymus **07NM**
  Thyroid Gland **0GNK**
    Left Lobe **0GNG**
    Right Lobe **0GNH**
  Tibia
    Left **0QNH**
    Right **0QNG**
  Toe Nail **0HNRXZZ**
  Tongue **0CN7**
  Tonsils **0CNP**
  Tooth
    Lower **0CNX**
    Upper **0CNW**
  Trachea **0BN1**
  Tunica Vaginalis
    Left **0VN7**
    Right **0VN6**
  Turbinate, Nasal **09NL**
  Tympanic Membrane
    Left **09N8**
    Right **09N7**
  Ulna
    Left **0PNL**
    Right **0PNK**
  Ureter
    Left **0TN7**
    Right **0TN6**
  Urethra **0TND**
  Uterine Supporting Structure **0UN4**
  Uterus **0UN9**
  Uvula **0CNN**
  Vagina **0UNG**
  Valve
    Aortic **02NF**
    Mitral **02NG**
    Pulmonary **02NH**
    Tricuspid **02NJ**
  Vas Deferens
    Bilateral **0VNQ**
    Left **0VNP**
    Right **0VNN**
  Vein
    Axillary
      Left **05N8**
      Right **05N7**
    Azygos **05N0**
    Basilic
      Left **05NC**
      Right **05NB**
    Brachial
      Left **05NA**
      Right **05N9**
    Cephalic
      Left **05NF**
      Right **05ND**
    Colic **06N7**
    Common Iliac

Release *(continued)*
      Left **06ND**
      Right **06NC**
    Coronary **02N4**
    Esophageal **06N3**
    External Iliac
      Left **06NG**
      Right **06NF**
    External Jugular
      Left **05NQ**
      Right **05NP**
    Face
      Left **05NV**
      Right **05NT**
    Femoral
      Left **06NN**
      Right **06NM**
    Foot
      Left **06NV**
      Right **06NT**
    Gastric **06N2**
    Greater Saphenous
      Left **06NQ**
      Right **06NP**
    Hand
      Left **05NH**
      Right **05NG**
    Hemiazygos **05N1**
    Hepatic **06N4**
    Hypogastric
      Left **06NJ**
      Right **06NH**
    Inferior Mesenteric **06N6**
    Innominate
      Left **05N4**
      Right **05N3**
    Internal Jugular
      Left **05NN**
      Right **05NM**
    Intracranial **05NL**
    Lesser Saphenous
      Left **06NS**
      Right **06NR**
    Lower **06NY**
    Portal **06N8**
    Pulmonary
      Left **02NT**
      Right **02NS**
    Renal
      Left **06NB**
      Right **06N9**
    Splenic **06N1**
    Subclavian
      Left **05N6**
      Right **05N5**
    Superior Mesenteric **06N5**
    Upper **05NY**
    Vertebral
      Left **05NS**
      Right **05NR**
    Vena Cava
      Inferior **06N0**
      Superior **02NV**
    Ventricle
      Left **02NL**
      Right **02NK**

Release *(continued)*
  Vertebra
    Cervical **0PN3**
    Lumbar **0QN0**
    Thoracic **0PN4**
  Vesicle
    Bilateral **0VN3**
    Left **0VN2**
    Right **0VN1**
  Vitreous
    Left **08N53ZZ**
    Right **08N43ZZ**
  Vocal Cord
    Left **0CNV**
    Right **0CNT**
  Vulva **0UNM**
Relocation *see* Reposition
Removal
  Abdominal Wall **2W53X**
  Anorectal **2Y53X5Z**
  Arm
    Lower
      Left **2W5DX**
      Right **2W5CX**
    Upper
      Left **2W5BX**
      Right **2W5AX**
  Back **2W55X**
  Chest Wall **2W54X**
  Ear **2Y52X5Z**
  Extremity
    Lower
      Left **2W5MX**
      Right **2W5LX**
    Upper
      Left **2W59X**
      Right **2W58X**
  Face **2W51X**
  Finger
    Left **2W5KX**
    Right **2W5JX**
  Foot
    Left **2W5TX**
    Right **2W5SX**
  Genital Tract, Female **2Y54X5Z**
  Hand
    Left **2W5FX**
    Right **2W5EX**
  Head **2W50X**
  Inguinal Region
    Left **2W57X**
    Right **2W56X**
  Leg
    Lower
      Left **2W5RX**
      Right **2W5QX**
    Upper
      Left **2W5PX**
      Right **2W5NX**
  Mouth and Pharynx **2Y50X5Z**
  Nasal **2Y51X5Z**
  Neck **2W52X**
  Thumb
    Left **2W5HX**
    Right **2W5GX**
  Toe

Removal *(continued)*
    Left **2W5VX**
    Right **2W5UX**
  Urethra **2Y55X5Z**
Removal of device from
  Abdominal Wall **0WPF**
  Acetabulum
    Left **0QP5**
    Right **0QP4**
  Anal Sphincter **0DPR**
  Anus **0DPQ**
  Artery
    Lower **04PY**
    Upper **03PY**
  Back
    Lower **0WPL**
    Upper **0WPK**
  Bladder **0TPB**
  Bone
    Facial **0NPW**
    Lower **0QPY**
    Nasal **0NPB**
    Pelvic
      Left **0QP3**
      Right **0QP2**
    Upper **0PPY**
  Bone Marrow **07PT**
  Brain **00P0**
  Breast
    Left **0HPU**
    Right **0HPT**
  Bursa and Ligament
    Lower **0MPY**
    Upper **0MPX**
  Carpal
    Left **0PPN**
    Right **0PPM**
  Cavity, Cranial **0WP1**
  Cerebral Ventricle **00P6**
  Chest Wall **0WP8**
  Cisterna Chyli **07PL**
  Clavicle
    Left **0PPB**
    Right **0PP9**
  Coccyx **0QPS**
  Diaphragm **0BPT**
  Disc
    Cervical Vertebral **0RP3**
    Cervicothoracic Vertebral **0RP5**
    Lumbar Vertebral **0SP2**
    Lumbosacral **0SP4**
    Thoracic Vertebral **0RP9**
    Thoracolumbar Vertebral **0RPB**
  Duct
    Hepatobiliary **0FPB**
    Pancreatic **0FPD**
  Ear
    Inner
      Left **09PE**
      Right **09PD**
    Left **09PJ**
    Right **09PH**
  Epididymis and Spermatic Cord **0VPM**
  Esophagus **0DP5**
  Extremity
    Lower

    Left **0YPB**
    Right **0YP9**
    Upper
      Left **0XP7**
      Right **0XP6**
  Eye
    Left **08P1**
    Right **08P0**
  Face **0WP2**
  Fallopian Tube **0UP8**
  Femoral Shaft
    Left **0QP9**
    Right **0QP8**
  Femur
    Lower
      Left **0QPC**
      Right **0QPB**
    Upper
      Left **0QP7**
      Right **0QP6**
  Fibula
    Left **0QPK**
    Right **0QPJ**
  Finger Nail **0HPQX**
  Gallbladder **0FP4**
  Gastrointestinal Tract **0WPP**
  Genitourinary Tract **0WPR**
  Gland
    Adrenal **0GP5**
    Endocrine **0GPS**
    Pituitary **0GP0**
    Salivary **0CPA**
  Glenoid Cavity
    Left **0PP8**
    Right **0PP7**
  Great Vessel **02PY**
  Hair **0HPSX**
  Head **0WP0**
  Heart **02PA**
  Hip
  Left **0SPB**
    Acetabular Surface **0SPE**
    Femoral Surface **0SPS**
    Right **0SP9**
    Acetabular Surface **0SPA**
    Femoral Surface **0SPR**
  Humeral Head
    Left **0PPD**
    Right **0PPC**
  Humeral Shaft
    Left **0PPG**
    Right **0PPF**
  Intestinal Tract
    Lower **0DPD**
    Upper **0DP0**
  Jaw
    Lower **0WP5**
    Upper **0WP4**
  Joint
    Acromioclavicular
      Left **0RPH**
      Right **0RPG**
    Ankle
      Left **0SPG**
      Right **0SPF**

Carpal
    Left **0RPR**
    Right **0RPQ**
Cervical Vertebral **0RP1**
Cervicothoracic Vertebral **0RP4**
Coccygeal **0SP6**
Elbow
    Left **0RPM**
    Right **0RPL**
Finger Phalangeal
    Left **0RPX**
    Right **0RPW**
Hip
    Left **0SPB**
        Acetabular Surface **0SPE**
        Femoral Surface **0SPS**
    Right **0SP9**
        Acetabular Surface **0SPA**
        Femoral Surface **0SPR**
Knee
    Left **0SPD**
        Femoral Surface **0SPU**
        Tibial Surface **0SPW**
    Right **0SPC**
        Femoral Surface **0SPT**
        Tibial Surface **0SPV**
Lumbar Vertebral **0SP0**
Lumbosacral **0SP3**
Metacarpocarpal
    Left **0RPT**
    Right **0RPS**
Metacarpophalangeal
    Left **0RPV**
    Right **0RPU**
Metatarsal-Phalangeal
    Left **0SPN**
    Right **0SPM**
Metatarsal-Tarsal
    Left **0SPL**
    Right **0SPK**
Occipital-cervical **0RP0**
Sacrococcygeal **0SP5**
Sacroiliac
    Left **0SP8**
    Right **0SP7**
Shoulder
    Left **0RPK**
    Right **0RPJ**
Sternoclavicular
    Left **0RPF**
    Right **0RPE**
Tarsal
    Left **0SPJ**
    Right **0SPH**
Temporomandibular
    Left **0RPD**
    Right **0RPC**
Thoracic Vertebral **0RP6**
Thoracolumbar Vertebral **0RPA**
Toe Phalangeal
    Left **0SPQ**
    Right **0SPP**
Wrist
    Left **0RPP**
    Right **0RPN**

Kidney **0TP5**
Knee
    Left **0SPD**
        Femoral Surface **0SPU**
        Tibial Surface **0SPW**
    Right **0SPC**
        Femoral Surface **0SPT**
        Tibial Surface **0SPV**
Larynx **0CPS**
Lens
    Left **08PK3JZ**
    Right **08PJ3JZ**
Liver **0FP0**
Lung
    Left **0BPL**
    Right **0BPK**
Lymphatic **07PN**
    Thoracic Duct **07PK**
Mediastinum **0WPC**
Mesentery **0DPV**
Metacarpal
    Left **0PPQ**
    Right **0PPP**
Metatarsal
    Left **0QPP**
    Right **0QPN**
Mouth and Throat **0CPY**
Muscle
    Extraocular
        Left **08PM**
        Right **08PL**
    Lower **0KPY**
    Upper **0KPX**
Neck **0WP6**
Nerve
    Cranial **00PE**
    Peripheral **01PY**
Nose **09PK**
Omentum **0DPU**
Ovary **0UP3**
Pancreas **0FPG**
Parathyroid Gland **0GPR**
Patella
    Left **0QPF**
    Right **0QPD**
Pelvic Cavity **0WPJ**
Penis **0VPS**
Pericardial Cavity **0WPD**
Perineum
    Female **0WPN**
    Male **0WPM**
Peritoneal Cavity **0WPG**
Peritoneum **0DPW**
Phalanx
    Finger
        Left **0PPV**
        Right **0PPT**
    Thumb
        Left **0PPS**
        Right **0PPR**
    Toe
        Left **0QPR**
        Right **0QPQ**
Pineal Body **0GP1**
Pleura **0BPQ**

Pleural Cavity
    Left **0WPB**
    Right **0WP9**
Products of Conception **10P0**
Prostate and Seminal Vesicles **0VP4**
Radius
    Left **0PPJ**
    Right **0PPH**
Rectum **0DPP**
Respiratory Tract **0WPQ**
Retroperitoneum **0WPH**
Rib
    Left **0PP2**
    Right **0PP1**
Sacrum **0QP1**
Scapula
    Left **0PP6**
    Right **0PP5**
Scrotum and Tunica Vaginalis **0VP8**
Sinus **09PY**
Skin **0HPPX**
Skull **0NP0**
Spinal Canal **00PU**
Spinal Cord **00PV**
Spleen **07PP**
Sternum **0PP0**
Stomach **0DP6**
Subcutaneous Tissue and Fascia
    Head and Neck **0JPS**
    Lower Extremity **0JPW**
    Trunk **0JPT**
    Upper Extremity **0JPV**
Tarsal
    Left **0QPM**
    Right **0QPL**
Tendon
    Lower **0LPY**
    Upper **0LPX**
Testis **0VPD**
Thymus **07PM**
Thyroid Gland **0GPK**
Tibia
    Left **0QPH**
    Right **0QPG**
Toe Nail **0HPRX**
Trachea **0BP1**
Tracheobronchial Tree **0BP0**
Tympanic Membrane
    Left **09P8**
    Right **09P7**
Ulna
    Left **0PPL**
    Right **0PPK**
Ureter **0TP9**
Urethra **0TPD**
Uterus and Cervix **0UPD**
Vagina and Cul-de-sac **0UPH**
Vas Deferens **0VPR**
Vein
    Azygos **05P0**
    Innominate
        Left **05P4**
        Right **05P3**
    Lower **06PY**
    Upper **05PY**

Removal of device from *(continued)*

Vertebra
    Cervical **0PP3**
    Lumbar **0QP0**
    Thoracic **0PP4**
Vulva **0UPM**

Renal calyx
use Kidney
use Kidneys, Bilateral
use Kidney, Left
use Kidney, Right

Renal capsule
use Kidney
use Kidney, Left
use Kidney, Right
use Kidneys, Bilateral

Renal cortex
use Kidney
use Kidney, Left
use Kidney, Right
use Kidneys, Bilateral

Renal dialysis *see* Performance, Urinary **5A1D**

Renal plexus *use* Nerve, Abdominal
Sympathetic

Renal segment
use Kidney
use Kidney, Left
use Kidney, Right
use Kidneys, Bilateral

Renal segmental artery
use Artery, Renal, Left
use Artery, Renal, Right

Reopening, operative site
Control of bleeding *see* Control bleeding in
Inspection only *see* Inspection

Repair
Abdominal Wall **0WQF**
Acetabulum
    Left **0QQ5**
    Right **0QQ4**
Adenoids **0CQQ**
Ampulla of Vater **0FQC**
Anal Sphincter **0DQR**
Ankle Region
    Left **0YQL**
    Right **0YQK**
Anterior Chamber
    Left **08Q33ZZ**
    Right **08Q23ZZ**
Anus **0DQQ**
Aorta
    Abdominal **04Q0**
    Thoracic
        Ascending/Arch **02QX**
        Descending **02QW**
Aortic Body **0GQD**
Appendix **0DQJ**
Arm
    Lower
        Left **0XQF**
        Right **0XQD**
    Upper
        Left **0XQ9**
        Right **0XQ8**
Artery
    Anterior Tibial

Repair *(continued)*
    Left **04QQ**
    Right **04QP**
Axillary
    Left **03Q6**
    Right **03Q5**
Brachial
    Left **03Q8**
    Right **03Q7**
Celiac **04Q1**
Colic
    Left **04Q7**
    Middle **04Q8**
    Right **04Q6**
Common Carotid
    Left **03QJ**
    Right **03QH**
Common Iliac
    Left **04QD**
    Right **04QC**
Coronary
    Four or More Arteries **02Q3**
    One Artery **02Q0**
    Three Arteries **02Q2**
    Two Arteries **02Q1**
External Carotid
    Left **03QN**
    Right **03QM**
External Iliac
    Left **04QJ**
    Right **04QH**
Face **03QR**
Femoral
    Left **04QL**
    Right **04QK**
Foot
    Left **04QW**
    Right **04QV**
Gastric **04Q2**
Hand
    Left **03QF**
    Right **03QD**
Hepatic **04Q3**
Inferior Mesenteric **04QB**
Innominate **03Q2**
Internal Carotid
    Left **03QL**
    Right **03QK**
Internal Iliac
    Left **04QF**
    Right **04QE**
Internal Mammary
    Left **03Q1**
    Right **03Q0**
Intracranial **03QG**
Lower **04QY**
Peroneal
    Left **04QU**
    Right **04QT**
Popliteal
    Left **04QN**
    Right **04QM**
Posterior Tibial
    Left **04QS**
    Right **04QR**
Pulmonary

Repair *(continued)*
    Left **02QR**
    Right **02QQ**
    Pulmonary Trunk **02QP**
Radial
    Left **03QC**
    Right **03QB**
Renal
    Left **04QA**
    Right **04Q9**
Splenic **04Q4**
Subclavian
    Left **03Q4**
    Right **03Q3**
Superior Mesenteric **04Q5**
Temporal
    Left **03QT**
    Right **03QS**
Thyroid
    Left **03QV**
    Right **03QU**
Ulnar
    Left **03QA**
    Right **03Q9**
Upper **03QY**
Vertebral
    Left **03QQ**
    Right **03QP**
Atrium
    Left **02Q7**
    Right **02Q6**
Auditory Ossicle
    Left **09QA0ZZ**
    Right **09Q90ZZ**
Axilla
    Left **0XQ5**
    Right **0XQ4**
Back
    Lower **0WQL**
    Upper **0WQK**
Basal Ganglia **00Q8**
Bladder **0TQB**
Bladder Neck **0TQC**
Bone
    Ethmoid
        Left **0NQG**
        Right **0NQF**
    Frontal
        Left **0NQ2**
        Right **0NQ1**
    Hyoid **0NQX**
    Lacrimal
        Left **0NQJ**
        Right **0NQH**
    Nasal **0NQB**
    Occipital
        Left **0NQ8**
        Right **0NQ7**
    Palatine
        Left **0NQL**
        Right **0NQK**
    Parietal
        Left **0NQ4**
        Right **0NQ3**
    Pelvic
        Left **0QQ3**

Repair *(continued)*
    Right **0QQ2**
  Sphenoid
    Left **0NQD**
    Right **0NQC**
  Temporal
    Left **0NQ6**
    Right **0NQ5**
  Zygomatic
    Left **0NQN**
    Right **0NQM**
Brain **00Q0**
Breast
  Bilateral **0HQV**
  Left **0HQU**
  Right **0HQT**
  Supernumerary **0HQY**
Bronchus
  Lingula **0BQ9**
  Lower Lobe
    Left **0BQB**
    Right **0BQ6**
  Main
    Left **0BQ7**
    Right **0BQ3**
  Middle Lobe, Right **0BQ5**
  Upper Lobe
    Left **0BQ8**
    Right **0BQ4**
Buccal Mucosa **0CQ4**
Bursa and Ligament
  Abdomen
    Left **0MQJ**
    Right **0MQH**
  Ankle
    Left **0MQR**
    Right **0MQQ**
  Elbow
    Left **0MQ4**
    Right **0MQ3**
  Foot
    Left **0MQT**
    Right **0MQS**
  Hand
    Left **0MQ8**
    Right **0MQ7**
  Head and Neck **0MQ0**
  Hip
    Left **0MQM**
    Right **0MQL**
  Knee
    Left **0MQP**
    Right **0MQN**
  Lower Extremity
    Left **0MQW**
    Right **0MQV**
  Perineum **0MQK**
  Shoulder
    Left **0MQ2**
    Right **0MQ1**
  Thorax
    Left **0MQG**
    Right **0MQF**
  Trunk
    Left **0MQD**
    Right **0MQC**

Repair *(continued)*
  Upper Extremity
    Left **0MQB**
    Right **0MQ9**
  Wrist
    Left **0MQ6**
    Right **0MQ5**
Buttock
  Left **0YQ1**
  Right **0YQ0**
Carina **0BQ2**
Carotid Bodies, Bilateral **0GQ8**
Carotid Body
  Left **0GQ6**
  Right **0GQ7**
Carpal
  Left **0PQN**
  Right **0PQM**
Cecum **0DQH**
Cerebellum **00QC**
Cerebral Hemisphere **00Q7**
Cerebral Meninges **00Q1**
Cerebral Ventricle **00Q6**
Cervix **0UQC**
Chest Wall **0WQ8**
Chordae Tendineae **02Q9**
Choroid
  Left **08QB**
  Right **08QA**
Cisterna Chyli **07QL**
Clavicle
  Left **0PQB**
  Right **0PQ9**
Clitoris **0UQJ**
Coccygeal Glomus **0GQB**
Coccyx **0QQS**
Colon
  Ascending **0DQK**
  Descending **0DQM**
  Sigmoid **0DQN**
  Transverse **0DQL**
Conduction Mechanism **02Q8**
Conjunctiva
  Left **08QTXZZ**
  Right **08QSXZZ**
Cord
  Bilateral **0VQH**
  Left **0VQG**
  Right **0VQF**
Cornea
  Left **08Q9XZZ**
  Right **08Q8XZZ**
Cul-de-sac **0UQF**
Diaphragm
  Left **0BQS**
  Right **0BQR**
Disc
  Cervical Vertebral **0RQ3**
  Cervicothoracic Vertebral **0RQ5**
  Lumbar Vertebral **0SQ2**
  Lumbosacral **0SQ4**
  Thoracic Vertebral **0RQ9**
  Thoracolumbar Vertebral **0RQB**
Duct
  Common Bile **0FQ9**
  Cystic **0FQ8**

Repair *(continued)*
  Hepatic
    Left **0FQ6**
    Right **0FQ5**
  Lacrimal
    Left **08QY**
    Right **08QX**
  Pancreatic **0FQD**
    Accessory **0FQF**
  Parotid
    Left **0CQC**
    Right **0CQB**
Duodenum **0DQ9**
Dura Mater **00Q2**
Ear
  External
    Bilateral **09Q2**
    Left **09Q1**
    Right **09Q0**
  External Auditory Canal
    Left **09Q4**
    Right **09Q3**
  Inner
    Left **09QE0ZZ**
    Right **09QD0ZZ**
  Middle
    Left **09Q60ZZ**
    Right **09Q50ZZ**
Elbow Region
  Left **0XQC**
  Right **0XQB**
Epididymis
  Bilateral **0VQL**
  Left **0VQK**
  Right **0VQJ**
Epiglottis **0CQR**
Esophagogastric Junction **0DQ4**
Esophagus **0DQ5**
  Lower **0DQ3**
  Middle **0DQ2**
  Upper **0DQ1**
Eustachian Tube
  Left **09QG**
  Right **09QF**
Extremity
  Lower
    Left **0YQB**
    Right **0YQ9**
  Upper
    Left **0XQ7**
    Right **0XQ6**
Eye
  Left **08Q1XZZ**
  Right **08Q0XZZ**
Eyelid
  Lower
    Left **08QR**
    Right **08QQ**
  Upper
    Left **08QP**
    Right **08QN**
Face **0WQ2**
Fallopian Tube
  Left **0UQ6**
  Right **0UQ5**
Fallopian Tubes, Bilateral **0UQ7**

Repair *(continued)*
  Femoral Region
    Bilateral **0YQE**
    Left **0YQ8**
    Right **0YQ7**
  Femoral Shaft
    Left **0QQ9**
    Right **0QQ8**
  Femur
    Lower
      Left **0QQC**
      Right **0QQB**
    Upper
      Left **0QQ7**
      Right **0QQ6**
  Fibula
    Left **0QQK**
    Right **0QQJ**
  Finger
    Index
      Left **0XQP**
      Right **0XQN**
    Little
      Left **0XQW**
      Right **0XQV**
    Middle
      Left **0XQR**
      Right **0XQQ**
    Ring
      Left **0XQT**
      Right **0XQS**
  Finger Nail **0HQQXZZ**
  Foot
    Left **0YQN**
    Right **0YQM**
  Gallbladder **0FQ4**
  Gingiva
    Lower **0CQ6**
    Upper **0CQ5**
  Gland
    Adrenal
      Bilateral **0GQ4**
      Left **0GQ2**
      Right **0GQ3**
    Lacrimal
      Left **08QW**
      Right **08QV**
    Minor Salivary **0CQJ**
    Parotid
      Left **0CQ9**
      Right **0CQ8**
    Pituitary **0GQ0**
    Sublingual
      Left **0CQF**
      Right **0CQD**
    Submaxillary
      Left **0CQH**
      Right **0CQG**
    Vestibular **0UQL**
  Glenoid Cavity
    Left **0PQ8**
    Right **0PQ7**
  Glomus Jugulare **0GQC**
  Hand
    Left **0XQK**
    Right **0XQJ**

Repair *(continued)*
  Head **0WQ0**
  Heart **02QA**
    Left **02QC**
    Right **02QB**
  Humeral Head
    Left **0PQD**
    Right **0PQC**
  Humeral Shaft
    Left **0PQG**
    Right **0PQF**
  Hymen **0UQK**
  Hypothalamus **00QA**
  Ileocecal Valve **0DQC**
  Ileum **0DQB**
  Inguinal Region
    Bilateral **0YQA**
    Left **0YQ6**
    Right **0YQ5**
  Intestine
    Large **0DQE**
      Left **0DQG**
      Right **0DQF**
    Small **0DQ8**
  Iris
    Left **08QD3ZZ**
    Right **08QC3ZZ**
  Jaw
    Lower **0WQ5**
    Upper **0WQ4**
  Jejunum **0DQA**
  Joint
    Acromioclavicular
      Left **0RQH**
      Right **0RQG**
    Ankle
      Left **0SQG**
      Right **0SQF**
    Carpal
      Left **0RQR**
      Right **0RQQ**
    Cervical Vertebral **0RQ1**
    Cervicothoracic Vertebral **0RQ4**
    Coccygeal **0SQ6**
    Elbow
      Left **0RQM**
      Right **0RQL**
    Finger Phalangeal
      Left **0RQX**
      Right **0RQW**
    Hip
      Left **0SQB**
      Right **0SQ9**
    Knee
      Left **0SQD**
      Right **0SQC**
    Lumbar Vertebral **0SQ0**
    Lumbosacral **0SQ3**
    Metacarpocarpal
      Left **0RQT**
      Right **0RQS**
    Metacarpophalangeal
      Left **0RQV**
      Right **0RQU**
    Metatarsal-Phalangeal
      Left **0SQN**

Repair *(continued)*
      Right **0SQM**
    Metatarsal-Tarsal
      Left **0SQL**
      Right **0SQK**
    Occipital-cervical **0RQ0**
    Sacrococcygeal **0SQ5**
    Sacroiliac
      Left **0SQ8**
      Right **0SQ7**
    Shoulder
      Left **0RQK**
      Right **0RQJ**
    Sternoclavicular
      Left **0RQF**
      Right **0RQE**
    Tarsal
      Left **0SQJ**
      Right **0SQH**
    Temporomandibular
      Left **0RQD**
      Right **0RQC**
    Thoracic Vertebral **0RQ6**
    Thoracolumbar Vertebral **0RQA**
    Toe Phalangeal
      Left **0SQQ**
      Right **0SQP**
    Wrist
      Left **0RQP**
      Right **0RQN**
  Kidney
    Left **0TQ1**
    Right **0TQ0**
  Kidney Pelvis
    Left **0TQ4**
    Right **0TQ3**
  Knee Region
    Left **0YQG**
    Right **0YQF**
  Larynx **0CQS**
  Leg
    Lower
      Left **0YQJ**
      Right **0YQH**
    Upper
      Left **0YQD**
      Right **0YQC**
  Lens
    Left **08QK3ZZ**
    Right **08QJ3ZZ**
  Lip
    Lower **0CQ1**
    Upper **0CQ0**
  Liver **0FQ0**
    Left Lobe **0FQ2**
    Right Lobe **0FQ1**
  Lung
    Bilateral **0BQM**
    Left **0BQL**
    Lower Lobe
      Left **0BQJ**
      Right **0BQF**
    Middle Lobe, Right **0BQD**
    Right **0BQK**
    Upper Lobe
      Left **0BQG**

Right **0BQC**
Lung Lingula **0BQH**
Lymphatic
  Aortic **07QD**
  Axillary
    Left **07Q6**
    Right **07Q5**
  Head **07Q0**
  Inguinal
    Left **07QJ**
    Right **07QH**
  Internal Mammary
    Left **07Q9**
    Right **07Q8**
  Lower Extremity
    Left **07QG**
    Right **07QF**
  Mesenteric **07QB**
  Neck
    Left **07Q2**
    Right **07Q1**
  Pelvis **07QC**
  Thoracic Duct **07QK**
  Thorax **07Q7**
  Upper Extremity
    Left **07Q4**
    Right **07Q3**
Mandible
  Left **0NQV**
  Right **0NQT**
Maxilla
  Left **0NQS**
  Right **0NQR**
Mediastinum **0WQC**
Medulla Oblongata **00QD**
Mesentery **0DQV**
Metacarpal
  Left **0PQQ**
  Right **0PQP**
Metatarsal
  Left **0QQP**
  Right **0QQN**
Muscle
  Abdomen
    Left **0KQL**
    Right **0KQK**
  Extraocular
    Left **08QM**
    Right **08QL**
  Facial **0KQ1**
  Foot
    Left **0KQW**
    Right **0KQV**
  Hand
    Left **0KQD**
    Right **0KQC**
  Head **0KQ0**
  Hip
    Left **0KQP**
    Right **0KQN**
  Lower Arm and Wrist
    Left **0KQB**
    Right **0KQ9**
  Lower Leg
    Left **0KQT**

Right **0KQS**
Neck
  Left **0KQ3**
  Right **0KQ2**
Papillary **02QD**
Perineum **0KQM**
Shoulder
  Left **0KQ6**
  Right **0KQ5**
Thorax
  Left **0KQJ**
  Right **0KQH**
Tongue, Palate, Pharynx **0KQ4**
Trunk
  Left **0KQG**
  Right **0KQF**
Upper Arm
  Left **0KQ8**
  Right **0KQ7**
Upper Leg
  Left **0KQR**
  Right **0KQQ**
Nasopharynx **09QN**
Neck **0WQ6**
Nerve
  Abdominal Sympathetic **01QM**
  Abducens **00QL**
  Accessory **00QR**
  Acoustic **00QN**
  Brachial Plexus **01Q3**
  Cervical **01Q1**
  Cervical Plexus **01Q0**
  Facial **00QM**
  Femoral **01QD**
  Glossopharyngeal **00QP**
  Head and Neck Sympathetic **01QK**
  Hypoglossal **00QS**
  Lumbar **01QB**
  Lumbar Plexus **01Q9**
  Lumbar Sympathetic **01QN**
  Lumbosacral Plexus **01QA**
  Median **01Q5**
  Oculomotor **00QH**
  Olfactory **00QF**
  Optic **00QG**
  Peroneal **01QH**
  Phrenic **01Q2**
  Pudendal **01QC**
  Radial **01Q6**
  Sacral **01QR**
  Sacral Plexus **01QQ**
  Sacral Sympathetic **01QP**
  Sciatic **01QF**
  Thoracic **01Q8**
  Thoracic Sympathetic **01QL**
  Tibial **01QG**
  Trigeminal **00QK**
  Trochlear **00QJ**
  Ulnar **01Q4**
  Vagus **00QQ**
Nipple
  Left **0HQX**
  Right **0HQW**
Nose **09QK**

Obstetric Laceration, Periurethral **0UQMXZZ**
Omentum
  Greater **0DQS**
  Lesser **0DQT**
Orbit
  Left **0NQQ**
  Right **0NQP**
Ovary
  Bilateral **0UQ2**
  Left **0UQ1**
  Right **0UQ0**
Palate
  Hard **0CQ2**
  Soft **0CQ3**
Pancreas **0FQG**
Para-aortic Body **0GQ9**
Paraganglion Extremity **0GQF**
Parathyroid Gland **0GQR**
  Inferior
    Left **0GQP**
    Right **0GQN**
  Multiple **0GQQ**
  Superior
    Left **0GQM**
    Right **0GQL**
Patella
  Left **0QQF**
  Right **0QQD**
Penis **0VQS**
Pericardium **02QN**
Perineum
  Female **0WQN**
  Male **0WQM**
Peritoneum **0DQW**
Phalanx
  Finger
    Left **0PQV**
    Right **0PQT**
  Thumb
    Left **0PQS**
    Right **0PQR**
  Toe
    Left **0QQR**
    Right **0QQQ**
Pharynx **0CQM**
Pineal Body **0GQ1**
Pleura
  Left **0BQP**
  Right **0BQN**
Pons **00QB**
Prepuce **0VQT**
Products of Conception **10Q0**
Prostate **0VQ0**
Radius
  Left **0PQJ**
  Right **0PQH**
Rectum **0DQP**
Retina
  Left **08QF3ZZ**
  Right **08QE3ZZ**
Retinal Vessel
  Left **08QH3ZZ**
  Right **08QG3ZZ**
Rib

Repair *(continued)*

Left 0PQ2

Right 0PQ1

Sacrum 0QQ1

Scapula

Left 0PQ6

Right 0PQ5

Sclera

Left 08Q7XZZ

Right 08Q6XZZ

Scrotum 0VQ5

Septum

Atrial 02Q5

Nasal 09QM

Ventricular 02QM

Shoulder Region

Left 0XQ3

Right 0XQ2

Sinus

Accessory 09QP

Ethmoid

Left 09QV

Right 09QU

Frontal

Left 09QT

Right 09QS

Mastoid

Left 09QC

Right 09QB

Maxillary

Left 09QR

Right 09QQ

Sphenoid

Left 09QX

Right 09QW

Skin

Abdomen 0HQ7XZZ

Back 0HQ6XZZ

Buttock 0HQ8XZZ

Chest 0HQ5XZZ

Ear

Left 0HQ3XZZ

Right 0HQ2XZZ

Face 0HQ1XZZ

Foot

Left 0HQNXZZ

Right 0HQMXZZ

Genitalia 0HQAXZZ

Hand

Left 0HQGXZZ

Right 0HQFXZZ

Lower Arm

Left 0HQEXZZ

Right 0HQDXZZ

Lower Leg

Left 0HQLXZZ

Right 0HQKXZZ

Neck 0HQ4XZZ

Perineum 0HQ9XZZ

Scalp 0HQ0XZZ

Upper Arm

Left 0HQCXZZ

Right 0HQBXZZ

Upper Leg

Left 0HQJXZZ

Right 0HQHXZZ

Repair *(continued)*

Skull 0NQ0

Spinal Cord

Cervical 00QW

Lumbar 00QY

Thoracic 00QX

Spinal Meninges 00QT

Spleen 07QP

Sternum 0PQ0

Stomach 0DQ6

Pylorus 0DQ7

Subcutaneous Tissue and Fascia

Abdomen 0JQ8

Back 0JQ7

Buttock 0JQ9

Chest 0JQ6

Face 0JQ1

Foot

Left 0JQR

Right 0JQQ

Hand

Left 0JQK

Right 0JQJ

Lower Arm

Left 0JQH

Right 0JQG

Lower Leg

Left 0JQP

Right 0JQN

Neck

Anterior 0JQ4

Posterior 0JQ5

Pelvic Region 0JQC

Perineum 0JQB

Scalp 0JQ0

Upper Arm

Left 0JQF

Right 0JQD

Upper Leg

Left 0JQM

Right 0JQL

Tarsal

Left 0QQM

Right 0QQL

Tendon

Abdomen

Left 0LQG

Right 0LQF

Ankle

Left 0LQT

Right 0LQS

Foot

Left 0LQW

Right 0LQV

Hand

Left 0LQ8

Right 0LQ7

Head and Neck 0LQ0

Hip

Left 0LQK

Right 0LQJ

Knee

Left 0LQR

Right 0LQQ

Lower Arm and Wrist

Left 0LQ6

Repair *(continued)*

Right 0LQ5

Lower Leg

Left 0LQP

Right 0LQN

Perineum 0LQH

Shoulder

Left 0LQ2

Right 0LQ1

Thorax

Left 0LQD

Right 0LQC

Trunk

Left 0LQB

Right 0LQ9

Upper Arm

Left 0LQ4

Right 0LQ3

Upper Leg

Left 0LQM

Right 0LQL

Testis

Bilateral 0VQC

Left 0VQB

Right 0VQ9

Thalamus 00Q9

Thumb

Left 0XQM

Right 0XQL

Thymus 07QM

Thyroid Gland 0GQK

Left Lobe 0GQG

Right Lobe 0GQH

Thyroid Gland Isthmus 0GQJ

Tibia

Left 0QQH

Right 0QQG

Toe

1st

Left 0YQQ

Right 0YQP

2nd

Left 0YQS

Right 0YQR

3rd

Left 0YQU

Right 0YQT

4th

Left 0YQW

Right 0YQV

5th

Left 0YQY

Right 0YQX

Toe Nail 0HQRXZZ

Tongue 0CQ7

Tonsils 0CQP

Tooth

Lower 0CQX

Upper 0CQW

Trachea 0BQ1

Tunica Vaginalis

Left 0VQ7

Right 0VQ6

Turbinate, Nasal 09QL

Tympanic Membrane

Left 09Q8

  Pulmonary Trunk **02RP**
  Radial
    Left **03RC**
    Right **03RB**
  Renal
    Left **04RA**
    Right **04R9**
  Splenic **04R4**
  Subclavian
    Left **03R4**
    Right **03R3**
  Superior Mesenteric **04R5**
  Temporal
    Left **03RT**
    Right **03RS**
  Thyroid
    Left **03RV**
    Right **03RU**
  Ulnar
    Left **03RA**
    Right **03R9**
  Upper **03RY**
  Vertebral
    Left **03RQ**
    Right **03RP**
Atrium
  Left **02R7**
  Right **02R6**
Auditory Ossicle
  Left **09RA0**
  Right **09R90**
Bladder **0TRB**
Bladder Neck **0TRC**
Bone
  Ethmoid
    Left **0NRG**
    Right **0NRF**
  Frontal
    Left **0NR2**
    Right **0NR1**
  Hyoid **0NRX**
  Lacrimal
    Left **0NRJ**
    Right **0NRH**
  Nasal **0NRB**
  Occipital
    Left **0NR8**
    Right **0NR7**
  Palatine
    Left **0NRL**
    Right **0NRK**
  Parietal
    Left **0NR4**
    Right **0NR3**
  Pelvic
    Left **0QR3**
    Right **0QR2**
  Sphenoid
    Left **0NRD**
    Right **0NRC**
  Temporal
    Left **0NR6**
    Right **0NR5**
  Zygomatic
    Left **0NRN**

    Right **0NRM**
  Breast
    Bilateral **0HRV**
    Left **0HRU**
    Right **0HRT**
  Buccal Mucosa **0CR4**
  Carpal
    Left **0PRN**
    Right **0PRM**
  Chordae Tendineae **02R9**
  Choroid
    Left **08RB**
    Right **08RA**
  Clavicle
    Left **0PRB**
    Right **0PR9**
  Coccyx **0QRS**
  Conjunctiva
    Left **08RTX**
    Right **08RSX**
  Cornea
    Left **08R9**
    Right **08R8**
  Disc
    Cervical Vertebral **0RR30**
    Cervicothoracic Vertebral **0RR50**
    Lumbar Vertebral **0SR20**
    Lumbosacral **0SR40**
    Thoracic Vertebral **0RR90**
    Thoracolumbar Vertebral **0RRB0**
  Duct
    Common Bile **0FR9**
    Cystic **0FR8**
    Hepatic
      Left **0FR6**
      Right **0FR5**
    Lacrimal
      Left **08RY**
      Right **08RX**
    Pancreatic **0FRD**
      Accessory **0FRF**
    Parotid
      Left **0CRC**
      Right **0CRB**
  Ear
    External
      Bilateral **09R2**
      Left **09R1**
      Right **09R0**
    Inner
      Left **09RE0**
      Right **09RD0**
    Middle
      Left **09R60**
      Right **09R50**
  Epiglottis **0CRR**
  Esophagus **0DR5**
  Eye
    Left **08R1**
    Right **08R0**
  Eyelid
    Lower
      Left **08RR**
      Right **08RQ**
    Upper

      Left **08RP**
      Right **08RN**
  Femoral Shaft
    Left **0QR9**
    Right **0QR8**
  Femur
    Lower
      Left **0QRC**
      Right **0QRB**
    Upper
      Left **0QR7**
      Right **0QR6**
  Fibula
    Left **0QRK**
    Right **0QRJ**
  Finger Nail **0HRQX**
  Gingiva
    Lower **0CR6**
    Upper **0CR5**
  Glenoid Cavity
    Left **0PR8**
    Right **0PR7**
  Hair **0HRSX**
  Hip
    Partial or total see Replacement, Lower Joints **0SR**
    Resurfacing only see Supplement, Lower Joints **0SU**
  Humeral Head
    Left **0PRD**
    Right **0PRC**
  Humeral Shaft
    Left **0PRG**
    Right **0PRF**
  Iris
    Left **08RD3**
    Right **08RC3**
  Joint
    Acromioclavicular
      Left **0RRH0**
      Right **0RRG0**
    Ankle
      Left **0SRG**
      Right **0SRF**
    Carpal
      Left **0RRR0**
      Right **0RRQ0**
    Cervical Vertebral **0RR10**
    Cervicothoracic Vertebral **0RR40**
    Coccygeal **0SR60**
    Elbow
      Left **0RRM0**
      Right **0RRL0**
    Finger Phalangeal
      Left **0RRX0**
      Right **0RRW0**
    Hip
      Left **0SRB**
        Acetabular Surface **0SRE**
        Femoral Surface **0SRS**
      Right **0SR9**
        Acetabular Surface **0SRA**
        Femoral Surface **0SRR**
    Knee
      Left **0SRD**

Replacement *(continued)*

Femoral Surface **0SRU**
Tibial Surface **0SRW**
Right **0SRC**
Femoral Surface **0SRT**
Tibial Surface **0SRV**
Lumbar Vertebral **0SR00**
Lumbosacral **0SR30**
Metacarpocarpal
Left **0RRT0**
Right **0RRS0**
Metacarpophalangeal
Left **0RRV0**
Right **0RRU0**
Metatarsal-Phalangeal
Left **0SRN0**
Right **0SRM0**
Metatarsal-Tarsal
Left **0SRL0**
Right **0SRK0**
Occipital-cervical **0RR00**
Sacrococcygeal **0SR50**
Sacroiliac
Left **0SR80**
Right **0SR70**
Shoulder
Left **0RRK**
Right **0RRJ**
Sternoclavicular
Left **0RRF0**
Right **0RRE0**
Tarsal
Left **0SRJ0**
Right **0SRH0**
Temporomandibular
Left **0RRD0**
Right **0RRC0**
Thoracic Vertebral **0RR60**
Thoracolumbar Vertebral **0RRA0**
Toe Phalangeal
Left **0SRQ0**
Right **0SRP0**
Wrist
Left **0RRP0**
Right **0RRN0**
Kidney Pelvis
Left **0TR4**
Right **0TR3**
Larynx **0CRS**
Lens
Left **08RK30Z**
Right **08RJ30Z**
Lip
Lower **0CR1**
Upper **0CR0**
Mandible
Left **0NRV**
Right **0NRT**
Maxilla
Left **0NRS**
Right **0NRR**
Mesentery **0DRV**
Metacarpal
Left **0PRQ**
Right **0PRP**
Metatarsal

Replacement *(continued)*

Left **0QRP**
Right **0QRN**
Muscle, Papillary **02RD**
Nasopharynx **09RN**
Nipple
Left **0HRX**
Right **0HRW**
Nose **09RK**
Omentum
Greater **0DRS**
Lesser **0DRT**
Orbit
Left **0NRQ**
Right **0NRP**
Palate
Hard **0CR2**
Soft **0CR3**
Patella
Left **0QRF**
Right **0QRD**
Pericardium **02RN**
Peritoneum **0DRW**
Phalanx
Finger
Left **0PRV**
Right **0PRT**
Thumb
Left **0PRS**
Right **0PRR**
Toe
Left **0QRR**
Right **0QRQ**
Pharynx **0CRM**
Radius
Left **0PRJ**
Right **0PRH**
Retinal Vessel
Left **08RH3**
Right **08RG3**
Rib
Left **0PR2**
Right **0PR1**
Sacrum **0QR1**
Scapula
Left **0PR6**
Right **0PR5**
Sclera
Left **08R7X**
Right **08R6X**
Septum
Atrial **02R5**
Nasal **09RM**
Ventricular **02RM**
Skin
Abdomen **0HR7**
Back **0HR6**
Buttock **0HR8**
Chest **0HR5**
Ear
Left **0HR3**
Right **0HR2**
Face **0HR1**
Foot
Left **0HRN**
Right **0HRM**

Replacement *(continued)*

Genitalia **0HRA**
Hand
Left **0HRG**
Right **0HRF**
Lower Arm
Left **0HRE**
Right **0HRD**
Lower Leg
Left **0HRL**
Right **0HRK**
Neck **0HR4**
Perineum **0HR9**
Scalp **0HR0**
Upper Arm
Left **0HRC**
Right **0HRB**
Upper Leg
Left **0HRJ**
Right **0HRH**
Skin Substitute, Porcine Liver Derived
XHRPXL2
Skull **0NR0**
Sternum **0PR0**
Subcutaneous Tissue and Fascia
Abdomen **0JR8**
Back **0JR7**
Buttock **0JR9**
Chest **0JR6**
Face **0JR1**
Foot
Left **0JRR**
Right **0JRQ**
Hand
Left **0JRK**
Right **0JRJ**
Lower Arm
Left **0JRH**
Right **0JRG**
Lower Leg
Left **0JRP**
Right **0JRN**
Neck
Anterior **0JR4**
Posterior **0JR5**
Pelvic Region **0JRC**
Perineum **0JRB**
Scalp **0JR0**
Upper Arm
Left **0JRF**
Right **0JRD**
Upper Leg
Left **0JRM**
Right **0JRL**
Tarsal
Left **0QRM**
Right **0QRL**
Tendon
Abdomen
Left **0LRG**
Right **0LRF**
Ankle
Left **0LRT**
Right **0LRS**
Foot
Left **0LRW**

Replacement *(continued)*
- Right **0LRV**
- Hand
  - Left **0LR8**
  - Right **0LR7**
- Head and Neck **0LR0**
- Hip
  - Left **0LRK**
  - Right **0LRJ**
- Knee
  - Left **0LRR**
  - Right **0LRQ**
- Lower Arm and Wrist
  - Left **0LR6**
  - Right **0LR5**
- Lower Leg
  - Left **0LRP**
  - Right **0LRN**
- Perineum **0LRH**
- Shoulder
  - Left **0LR2**
  - Right **0LR1**
- Thorax
  - Left **0LRD**
  - Right **0LRC**
- Trunk
  - Left **0LRB**
  - Right **0LR9**
- Upper Arm
  - Left **0LR4**
  - Right **0LR3**
- Upper Leg
  - Left **0LRM**
  - Right **0LRL**
- Testis
  - Bilateral **0VRC0JZ**
  - Left **0VRB0JZ**
  - Right **0VR90JZ**
- Thumb
  - Left **0XRM**
  - Right **0XRL**
- Tibia
  - Left **0QRH**
  - Right **0QRG**
- Toe Nail **0HRRX**
- Tongue **0CR7**
- Tooth
  - Lower **0CRX**
  - Upper **0CRW**
- Turbinate, Nasal **09RL**
- Tympanic Membrane
  - Left **09R8**
  - Right **09R7**
- Ulna
  - Left **0PRL**
  - Right **0PRK**
- Ureter
  - Left **0TR7**
  - Right **0TR6**
- Urethra **0TRD**
- Uvula **0CRN**
- Valve
  - Aortic **02RF**
  - Mitral **02RG**
  - Pulmonary **02RH**
  - Tricuspid **02RJ**

Replacement *(continued)*
- Vein
  - Axillary
    - Left **05R8**
    - Right **05R7**
  - Azygos **05R0**
  - Basilic
    - Left **05RC**
    - Right **05RB**
  - Brachial
    - Left **05RA**
    - Right **05R9**
  - Cephalic
    - Left **05RF**
    - Right **05RD**
  - Colic **06R7**
  - Common Iliac
    - Left **06RD**
    - Right **06RC**
  - Esophageal **06R3**
  - External Iliac
    - Left **06RG**
    - Right **06RF**
  - External Jugular
    - Left **05RQ**
    - Right **05RP**
  - Face
    - Left **05RV**
    - Right **05RT**
  - Femoral
    - Left **06RN**
    - Right **06RM**
  - Foot
    - Left **06RV**
    - Right **06RT**
  - Gastric **06R2**
  - Greater Saphenous
    - Left **06RQ**
    - Right **06RP**
  - Hand
    - Left **05RH**
    - Right **05RG**
  - Hemiazygos **05R1**
  - Hepatic **06R4**
  - Hypogastric
    - Left **06RJ**
    - Right **06RH**
  - Inferior Mesenteric **06R6**
  - Innominate
    - Left **05R4**
    - Right **05R3**
  - Internal Jugular
    - Left **05RN**
    - Right **05RM**
  - Intracranial **05RL**
  - Lesser Saphenous
    - Left **06RS**
    - Right **06RR**
  - Lower **06RY**
  - Portal **06R8**
  - Pulmonary
    - Left **02RT**
    - Right **02RS**
  - Renal
    - Left **06RB**
    - Right **06R9**

Replacement *(continued)*
- Splenic **06R1**
- Subclavian
  - Left **05R6**
  - Right **05R5**
- Superior Mesenteric **06R5**
- Upper **05RY**
- Vertebral
  - Left **05RS**
  - Right **05RR**
- Vena Cava
  - Inferior **06R0**
  - Superior **02RV**
- Ventricle
  - Left **02RL**
  - Right **02RK**
- Vertebra
  - Cervical **0PR3**
  - Lumbar **0QR0**
  - Thoracic **0PR4**
- Vitreous
  - Left **08R53**
  - Right **08R43**
- Vocal Cord
  - Left **0CRV**
  - Right **0CRT**
- Zooplastic Tissue, Rapid Deployment Technique **X2RF**

Replantation *see* Reposition

Replantation, scalp *see* Reattachment, Skin, Scalp **0HM0**

Reposition
- Acetabulum
  - Left **0QS5**
  - Right **0QS4**
- Ampulla of Vater **0FSC**
- Anus **0DSQ**
- Aorta
  - Abdominal **04S0**
  - Thoracic
    - Ascending/Arch **02SX0ZZ**
    - Descending **02SW0ZZ**
- Artery
  - Anterior Tibial
    - Left **04SQ**
    - Right **04SP**
  - Axillary
    - Left **03S6**
    - Right **03S5**
  - Brachial
    - Left **03S8**
    - Right **03S7**
  - Celiac **04S1**
  - Colic
    - Left **04S7**
    - Middle **04S8**
    - Right **04S6**
  - Common Carotid
    - Left **03SJ**
    - Right **03SH**
  - Common Iliac
    - Left **04SD**
    - Right **04SC**
  - Coronary
    - One Artery **02S00ZZ**
    - Two Arteries **02S10ZZ**

Reposition *(continued)*
  External Carotid
    Left **03SN**
    Right **03SM**
  External Iliac
    Left **04SJ**
    Right **04SH**
  Face **03SR**
  Femoral
    Left **04SL**
    Right **04SK**
  Foot
    Left **04SW**
    Right **04SV**
  Gastric **04S2**
  Hand
    Left **03SF**
    Right **03SD**
  Hepatic **04S3**
  Inferior Mesenteric **04SB**
  Innominate **03S2**
    Left **03SL**
    Right **03SK**
  Internal Iliac
    Left **04SF**
    Right **04SE**
  Internal Mammary
    Left **03S1**
    Right **03S0**
  Intracranial **03SG**
  Lower **04SY**
  Peroneal
    Left **04SU**
    Right **04ST**
  Popliteal
    Left **04SN**
    Right **04SM**
  Posterior Tibial
    Left **04SS**
    Right **04SR**
  Pulmonary
    Left **02SR0ZZ**
    Right **02SQ0ZZ**
  Pulmonary Trunk **02SP0ZZ**
  Radial
    Left **03SC**
    Right **03SB**
  Renal
    Left **04SA**
    Right **04S9**
  Splenic **04S4**
  Subclavian
    Left **03S4**
    Right **03S3**
  Superior Mesenteric **04S5**
  Temporal
    Left **03ST**
    Right **03SS**
  Thyroid
    Left **03SV**
    Right **03SU**
  Ulnar
    Left **03SA**
    Right **03S9**
  Upper **03SY**
  Vertebral

Reposition *(continued)*
    Left **03SQ**
    Right **03SP**
  Auditory Ossicle
    Left **09SA**
    Right **09S9**
  Bladder **0TSB**
  Bladder Neck **0TSC**
  Bone
    Ethmoid
      Left **0NSG**
      Right **0NSF**
    Frontal
      Left **0NS2**
      Right **0NS1**
    Hyoid **0NSX**
    Lacrimal
      Left **0NSJ**
      Right **0NSH**
    Nasal **0NSB**
    Occipital
      Left **0NS8**
      Right **0NS7**
    Palatine
      Left **0NSL**
      Right **0NSK**
    Parietal
      Left **0NS4**
      Right **0NS3**
    Pelvic
      Left **0QS3**
      Right **0QS2**
    Sphenoid
      Left **0NSD**
      Right **0NSC**
    Temporal
      Left **0NS6**
      Right **0NS5**
    Zygomatic
      Left **0NSN**
      Right **0NSM**
  Breast
    Bilateral **0HSV0ZZ**
    Left **0HSU0ZZ**
    Right **0HST0ZZ**
  Bronchus
    Lingula **0BS90ZZ**
    Lower Lobe
      Left **0BSB0ZZ**
      Right **0BS60ZZ**
    Main
      Left **0BS70ZZ**
      Right **0BS30ZZ**
    Middle Lobe, Right **0BS50ZZ**
    Upper Lobe
      Left **0BS80ZZ**
      Right **0BS40ZZ**
  Bursa and Ligament
    Abdomen
      Left **0MSJ**
      Right **0MSH**
    Ankle
      Left **0MSR**
      Right **0MSQ**
    Elbow
      Left **0MS4**

Reposition *(continued)*
    Right **0MS3**
    Foot
      Left **0MST**
      Right **0MSS**
    Hand
      Left **0MS8**
      Right **0MS7**
    Head and Neck **0MS0**
    Hip
      Left **0MSM**
      Right **0MSL**
    Knee
      Left **0MSP**
      Right **0MSN**
    Lower Extremity
      Left **0MSW**
      Right **0MSV**
    Perineum **0MSK**
    Shoulder
      Left **0MS2**
      Right **0MS1**
    Thorax
      Left **0MSG**
      Right **0MSF**
    Trunk
      Left **0MSD**
      Right **0MSC**
    Upper Extremity
      Left **0MSB**
      Right **0MS9**
    Wrist
      Left **0MS6**
      Right **0MS5**
  Carina **0BS20ZZ**
  Carpal
    Left **0PSN**
    Right **0PSM**
  Cecum **0DSH**
  Cervix **0USC**
  Clavicle
    Left **0PSB**
    Right **0PS9**
  Coccyx **0QSS**
  Colon
    Ascending **0DSK**
    Descending **0DSM**
    Sigmoid **0DSN**
    Transverse **0DSL**
  Cord
    Bilateral **0VSH**
    Left **0VSG**
    Right **0VSF**
  Cul-de-sac **0USF**
  Diaphragm
    Left **0BSS0ZZ**
    Right **0BSR0ZZ**
  Duct
    Common Bile **0FS9**
    Cystic **0FS8**
    Hepatic
      Left **0FS6**
      Right **0FS5**
    Lacrimal
      Left **08SY**
      Right **08SX**

Pancreatic **0FSD**
  Accessory **0FSF**
Parotid
  Left **0CSC**
  Right **0CSB**
Duodenum **0DS9**
Ear
  Bilateral **09S2**
  Left **09S1**
  Right **09S0**
Epiglottis **0CSR**
Esophagus **0DS5**
Eustachian Tube
  Left **09SG**
  Right **09SF**
Eyelid
  Lower
    Left **08SR**
    Right **08SQ**
  Upper
    Left **08SP**
    Right **08SN**
Fallopian Tube
  Left **0US6**
  Right **0US5**
Fallopian Tubes, Bilateral **0US7**
Femoral Shaft
  Left **0QS9**
  Right **0QS8**
Femur
  Lower
    Left **0QSC**
    Right **0QSB**
  Upper
    Left **0QS7**
    Right **0QS6**
Fibula
  Left **0QSK**
  Right **0QSJ**
Gallbladder **0FS4**
Gland
  Adrenal
    Left **0GS2**
    Right **0GS3**
  Lacrimal
    Left **08SW**
    Right **08SV**
Glenoid Cavity
  Left **0PS8**
  Right **0PS7**
Hair **0HSSXZZ**
Humeral Head
  Left **0PSD**
  Right **0PSC**
Humeral Shaft
  Left **0PSG**
  Right **0PSF**
Ileum **0DSB**
Iris
  Left **08SD3ZZ**
  Right **08SC3ZZ**
Jejunum **0DSA**
Joint
  Acromioclavicular
    Left **0RSH**

  Right **0RSG**
Ankle
  Left **0SSG**
  Right **0SSF**
Carpal
  Left **0RSR**
  Right **0RSQ**
Cervical Vertebral **0RS1**
Cervicothoracic Vertebral **0RS4**
Coccygeal **0SS6**
Elbow
  Left **0RSM**
  Right **0RSL**
Finger Phalangeal
  Left **0RSX**
  Right **0RSW**
Hip
  Left **0SSB**
  Right **0SS9**
Knee
  Left **0SSD**
  Right **0SSC**
Lumbar Vertebral **0SS0**
Lumbosacral **0SS3**
Metacarpocarpal
  Left **0RST**
  Right **0RSS**
Metacarpophalangeal
  Left **0RSV**
  Right **0RSU**
Metatarsal-Phalangeal
  Left **0SSN**
  Right **0SSM**
Metatarsal-Tarsal
  Left **0SSL**
  Right **0SSK**
Occipital-cervical **0RS0**
Sacrococcygeal **0SS5**
Sacroiliac
  Left **0SS8**
  Right **0SS7**
Shoulder
  Left **0RSK**
  Right **0RSJ**
Sternoclavicular
  Left **0RSF**
  Right **0RSE**
Tarsal
  Left **0SSJ**
  Right **0SSH**
Temporomandibular
  Left **0RSD**
  Right **0RSC**
Thoracic Vertebral **0RS6**
Thoracolumbar Vertebral **0RSA**
Toe Phalangeal
  Left **0SSQ**
  Right **0SSP**
Wrist
  Left **0RSP**
  Right **0RSN**
Kidney
  Left **0TS1**
  Right **0TS0**
Kidney Pelvis

  Left **0TS4**
  Right **0TS3**
Kidneys, Bilateral **0TS2**
Lens
  Left **08SK3ZZ**
  Right **08SJ3ZZ**
Lip
  Lower **0CS1**
  Upper **0CS0**
Liver **0FS0**
Lung
  Left **0BSL0ZZ**
  Lower Lobe
    Left **0BSJ0ZZ**
    Right **0BSF0ZZ**
  Middle Lobe, Right **0BSD0ZZ**
  Right **0BSK0ZZ**
  Upper Lobe
    Left **0BSG0ZZ**
    Right **0BSC0ZZ**
Lung Lingula **0BSH0ZZ**
Mandible
  Left **0NSV**
  Right **0NST**
Maxilla
  Left **0NSS**
  Right **0NSR**
Metacarpal
  Left **0PSQ**
  Right **0PSP**
Metatarsal
  Left **0QSP**
  Right **0QSN**
Muscle
  Abdomen
    Left **0KSL**
    Right **0KSK**
  Extraocular
    Left **08SM**
    Right **08SL**
  Facial **0KS1**
  Foot
    Left **0KSW**
    Right **0KSV**
  Hand
    Left **0KSD**
    Right **0KSC**
  Head **0KS0**
  Hip
    Left **0KSP**
    Right **0KSN**
  Lower Arm and Wrist
    Left **0KSB**
    Right **0KS9**
  Lower Leg
    Left **0KST**
    Right **0KSS**
  Neck
    Left **0KS3**
    Right **0KS2**
  Perineum **0KSM**
  Shoulder
    Left **0KS6**
    Right **0KS5**
  Thorax

Reposition *(continued)*
    Left **0KSJ**
    Right **0KSH**
  Tongue, Palate, Pharynx **0KS4**
  Trunk
    Left **0KSG**
    Right **0KSF**
  Upper Arm
    Left **0KS8**
    Right **0KS7**
  Upper Leg
    Left **0KSR**
    Right **0KSQ**
Nerve
  Abducens **00SL**
  Accessory **00SR**
  Acoustic **00SN**
  Brachial Plexus **01S3**
  Cervical **01S1**
  Cervical Plexus **01S0**
  Facial **00SM**
  Femoral **01SD**
  Glossopharyngeal **00SP**
  Hypoglossal **00SS**
  Lumbar **01SB**
  Lumbar Plexus **01S9**
  Lumbosacral Plexus **01SA**
  Median **01S5**
  Oculomotor **00SH**
  Olfactory **00SF**
  Optic **00SG**
  Peroneal **01SH**
  Phrenic **01S2**
  Pudendal **01SC**
  Radial **01S6**
  Sacral **01SR**
  Sacral Plexus **01SQ**
  Sciatic **01SF**
  Thoracic **01S8**
  Tibial **01SG**
  Trigeminal **00SK**
  Trochlear **00SJ**
  Ulnar **01S4**
  Vagus **00SQ**
Nipple
  Left **0HSXXZZ**
  Right **0HSWXZZ**
Nose **09SK**
Orbit
  Left **0NSQ**
  Right **0NSP**
Ovary
  Bilateral **0US2**
  Left **0US1**
  Right **0US0**
Palate
  Hard **0CS2**
  Soft **0CS3**
Pancreas **0FSG**
Parathyroid Gland **0GSR**
  Inferior
    Left **0GSP**
    Right **0GSN**
  Multiple **0GSQ**
  Superior
    Left **0GSM**

Reposition *(continued)*
    Right **0GSL**
Patella
  Left **0QSF**
  Right **0QSD**
Phalanx
  Finger
    Left **0PSV**
    Right **0PST**
  Thumb
    Left **0PSS**
    Right **0PSR**
  Toe
    Left **0QSR**
    Right **0QSQ**
Products of Conception **10S0**
  Ectopic **10S2**
Radius
  Left **0PSJ**
  Right **0PSH**
Rectum **0DSP**
Retinal Vessel
  Left **08SH3ZZ**
  Right **08SG3ZZ**
Rib
  Left **0PS2**
  Right **0PS1**
Sacrum **0QS1**
Scapula
  Left **0PS6**
  Right **0PS5**
Septum, Nasal **09SM**
Skull **0NS0**
Spinal Cord
  Cervical **00SW**
  Lumbar **00SY**
  Thoracic **00SX**
Spleen **07SP0ZZ**
Sternum **0PS0**
Stomach **0DS6**
Tarsal
  Left **0QSM**
  Right **0QSL**
Tendon
  Abdomen
    Left **0LSG**
    Right **0LSF**
  Ankle
    Left **0LST**
    Right **0LSS**
  Foot
    Left **0LSW**
    Right **0LSV**
  Hand
    Left **0LS8**
    Right **0LS7**
  Head and Neck **0LS0**
  Hip
    Left **0LSK**
    Right **0LSJ**
  Knee
    Left **0LSR**
    Right **0LSQ**
  Lower Arm and Wrist
    Left **0LS6**
    Right **0LS5**

Reposition *(continued)*
  Lower Leg
    Left **0LSP**
    Right **0LSN**
  Perineum **0LSH**
  Shoulder
    Left **0LS2**
    Right **0LS1**
  Thorax
    Left **0LSD**
    Right **0LSC**
  Trunk
    Left **0LSB**
    Right **0LS9**
  Upper Arm
    Left **0LS4**
    Right **0LS3**
  Upper Leg
    Left **0LSM**
    Right **0LSL**
Testis
  Bilateral **0VSC**
  Left **0VSB**
  Right **0VS9**
Thymus **07SM0ZZ**
Thyroid Gland
  Left Lobe **0GSG**
  Right Lobe **0GSH**
Tibia
  Left **0QSH**
  Right **0QSG**
Tongue **0CS7**
Tooth
  Lower **0CSX**
  Upper **0CSW**
Trachea **0BS10ZZ**
Turbinate, Nasal **09SL**
Tympanic Membrane
  Left **09S8**
  Right **09S7**
Ulna
  Left **0PSL**
  Right **0PSK**
Ureter
  Left **0TS7**
  Right **0TS6**
Ureters, Bilateral **0TS8**
Urethra **0TSD**
Uterine Supporting Structure **0US4**
Uterus **0US9**
Uvula **0CSN**
Vagina **0USG**
Vein
  Axillary
    Left **05S8**
    Right **05S7**
  Azygos **05S0**
  Basilic
    Left **05SC**
    Right **05SB**
  Brachial
    Left **05SA**
    Right **05S9**
  Cephalic
    Left **05SF**
    Right **05SD**

Reposition *(continued)*
  Colic **06S7**
  Common Iliac
    Left **06SD**
    Right **06SC**
  Esophageal **06S3**
  External Iliac
    Left **06SG**
    Right **06SF**
  External Jugular
    Left **05SQ**
    Right **05SP**
  Face
    Left **05SV**
    Right **05ST**
  Femoral
    Left **06SN**
    Right **06SM**
  Foot
    Left **06SV**
    Right **06ST**
  Gastric **06S2**
  Greater Saphenous
    Left **06SQ**
    Right **06SP**
  Hand
    Left **05SH**
    Right **05SG**
  Hemiazygos **05S1**
  Hepatic **06S4**
  Hypogastric
    Left **06SJ**
    Right **06SH**
  Inferior Mesenteric **06S6**
  Innominate
    Left **05S4**
    Right **05S3**
  Internal Jugular
    Left **05SN**
    Right **05SM**
  Intracranial **05SL**
  Lesser Saphenous
    Left **06SS**
    Right **06SR**
  Lower **06SY**
  Portal **06S8**
  Pulmonary
    Left **02ST0ZZ**
    Right **02SS0ZZ**
  Renal
    Left **06SB**
    Right **06S9**
  Splenic **06S1**
  Subclavian
    Left **05S6**
    Right **05S5**
  Superior Mesenteric **06S5**
  Upper **05SY**
  Vertebral
    Left **05SS**
    Right **05SR**
  Vena Cava
    Inferior **06S0**
    Superior **02SV0ZZ**
  Vertebra
    Cervical **0PS3**

Reposition *(continued)*
    Magnetically Controlled Growth
      Rod(s) **XNS3**
    Lumbar **0QS0**
      Magnetically Controlled Growth
        Rod(s) **XNS0**
    Thoracic **0PS4**
      Magnetically Controlled Growth
        Rod(s) **XNS4**
  Vocal Cord
    Left **0CSV**
    Right **0CST**
Resection
  Acetabulum
    Left **0QT50ZZ**
    Right **0QT40ZZ**
  Adenoids **0CTQ**
  Ampulla of Vater **0FTC**
  Anal Sphincter **0DTR**
  Anus **0DTQ**
  Aortic Body **0GTD**
  Appendix **0DTJ**
  Auditory Ossicle
    Left **09TA0ZZ**
    Right **09T90ZZ**
  Bladder **0TTB**
  Bladder Neck **0TTC**
  Bone
    Ethmoid
      Left **0NTG0ZZ**
      Right **0NTF0ZZ**
    Frontal
      Left **0NT20ZZ**
      Right **0NT10ZZ**
    Hyoid **0NTX0ZZ**
    Lacrimal
      Left **0NTJ0ZZ**
      Right **0NTH0ZZ**
    Nasal **0NTB0ZZ**
    Occipital
      Left **0NT80ZZ**
      Right **0NT70ZZ**
    Palatine
      Left **0NTL0ZZ**
      Right **0NTK0ZZ**
    Parietal
      Left **0NT40ZZ**
      Right **0NT30ZZ**
    Pelvic
      Left **0QT30ZZ**
      Right **0QT20ZZ**
    Sphenoid
      Left **0NTD0ZZ**
      Right **0NTC0ZZ**
    Temporal
      Left **0NT60ZZ**
      Right **0NT50ZZ**
    Zygomatic
      Left **0NTN0ZZ**
      Right **0NTM0ZZ**
  Breast
    Bilateral **0HTV0ZZ**
    Left **0HTU0ZZ**
    Right **0HTT0ZZ**
    Supernumerary **0HTY0ZZ**
  Bronchus

Resection *(continued)*
    Lingula **0BT9**
    Lower Lobe
      Left **0BTB**
      Right **0BT6**
    Main
      Left **0BT7**
      Right **0BT3**
    Middle Lobe, Right **0BT5**
    Upper Lobe
      Left **0BT8**
      Right **0BT4**
  Bursa and Ligament
    Abdomen
      Left **0MTJ**
      Right **0MTH**
    Ankle
      Left **0MTR**
      Right **0MTQ**
    Elbow
      Left **0MT4**
      Right **0MT3**
    Foot
      Left **0MTT**
      Right **0MTS**
    Hand
      Left **0MT8**
      Right **0MT7**
    Head and Neck **0MT0**
    Hip
      Left **0MTM**
      Right **0MTL**
    Knee
      Left **0MTP**
      Right **0MTN**
    Lower Extremity
      Left **0MTW**
      Right **0MTV**
    Perineum **0MTK**
    Shoulder
      Left **0MT2**
      Right **0MT1**
    Thorax
      Left **0MTG**
      Right **0MTF**
    Trunk
      Left **0MTD**
      Right **0MTC**
    Upper Extremity
      Left **0MTB**
      Right **0MT9**
    Wrist
      Left **0MT6**
      Right **0MT5**
  Carina **0BT2**
  Carotid Bodies, Bilateral **0GT8**
  Carotid Body
    Left **0GT6**
    Right **0GT7**
  Carpal
    Left **0PTN0ZZ**
    Right **0PTM0ZZ**
  Cecum **0DTH**
  Cerebral Hemisphere **00T7**
  Cervix **0UTC**
  Chordae Tendineae **02T9**

Resection *(continued)*
- Cisterna Chyli **07TL**
- Clavicle
  - Left **0PTB0ZZ**
  - Right **0PT90ZZ**
- Clitoris **0UTJ**
- Coccygeal Glomus **0GTB**
- Coccyx **0QTS0ZZ**
- Colon
  - Ascending **0DTK**
  - Descending **0DTM**
  - Sigmoid **0DTN**
  - Transverse **0DTL**
- Conduction Mechanism **02T8**
- Cord
  - Bilateral **0VTH**
  - Left **0VTG**
  - Right **0VTF**
- Cornea
  - Left **08T9XZZ**
  - Right **08T8XZZ**
- Cul-de-sac **0UTF**
- Diaphragm
  - Left **0BTS**
  - Right **0BTR**
- Disc
  - Cervical Vertebral **0RT30ZZ**
  - Cervicothoracic Vertebral **0RT50ZZ**
  - Lumbar Vertebral **0ST20ZZ**
  - Lumbosacral **0ST40ZZ**
  - Thoracic Vertebral **0RT90ZZ**
  - Thoracolumbar Vertebral **0RTB0ZZ**
- Duct
  - Common Bile **0FT9**
  - Cystic **0FT8**
  - Hepatic
    - Left **0FT6**
    - Right **0FT5**
  - Lacrimal
    - Left **08TY**
    - Right **08TX**
  - Pancreatic **0FTD**
    - Accessory **0FTF**
  - Parotid
    - Left **0CTC0ZZ**
    - Right **0CTB0ZZ**
- Duodenum **0DT9**
- Ear
  - External
    - Left **09T1**
    - Right **09T0**
  - Inner
    - Left **09TE0ZZ**
    - Right **09TD0ZZ**
  - Middle
    - Left **09T60ZZ**
    - Right **09T50ZZ**
- Epididymis
  - Bilateral **0VTL**
  - Left **0VTK**
  - Right **0VTJ**
- Epiglottis **0CTR**
- Esophagogastric Junction **0DT4**
- Esophagus **0DT5**
  - Lower **0DT3**
  - Middle **0DT2**

Resection *(continued)*
- Upper **0DT1**
- Eustachian Tube
  - Left **09TG**
  - Right **09TF**
- Eye
  - Left **08T1XZZ**
  - Right **08T0XZZ**
- Eyelid
  - Lower
    - Left **08TR**
    - Right **08TQ**
  - Upper
    - Left **08TP**
    - Right **08TN**
- Fallopian Tube
  - Left **0UT6**
  - Right **0UT5**
- Fallopian Tubes, Bilateral **0UT7**
- Femoral Shaft
  - Left **0QT90ZZ**
  - Right **0QT80ZZ**
- Femur
  - Lower
    - Left **0QTC0ZZ**
    - Right **0QTB0ZZ**
  - Upper
    - Left **0QT70ZZ**
    - Right **0QT60ZZ**
- Fibula
  - Left **0QTK0ZZ**
  - Right **0QTJ0ZZ**
- Finger Nail **0HTQXZZ**
- Gallbladder **0FT4**
- Gland
  - Adrenal
    - Bilateral **0GT4**
    - Left **0GT2**
    - Right **0GT3**
  - Lacrimal
    - Left **08TW**
    - Right **08TV**
  - Minor Salivary **0CTJ0ZZ**
  - Parotid
    - Left **0CT90ZZ**
    - Right **0CT80ZZ**
  - Pituitary **0GT0**
  - Sublingual
    - Left **0CTF0ZZ**
    - Right **0CTD0ZZ**
  - Submaxillary
    - Left **0CTH0ZZ**
    - Right **0CTG0ZZ**
  - Vestibular **0UTL**
- Glenoid Cavity
  - Left **0PT80ZZ**
  - Right **0PT70ZZ**
- Glomus Jugulare **0GTC**
- Humeral Head
  - Left **0PTD0ZZ**
  - Right **0PTC0ZZ**
- Humeral Shaft
  - Left **0PTG0ZZ**
  - Right **0PTF0ZZ**
- Hymen **0UTK**
- Ileocecal Valve **0DTC**

Resection *(continued)*
- Ileum **0DTB**
- Intestine
  - Large **0DTE**
    - Left **0DTG**
    - Right **0DTF**
  - Small **0DT8**
- Iris
  - Left **08TD3ZZ**
  - Right **08TC3ZZ**
- Jejunum **0DTA**
- Joint
  - Acromioclavicular
    - Left **0RTH0ZZ**
    - Right **0RTG0ZZ**
  - Ankle
    - Left **0STG0ZZ**
    - Right **0STF0ZZ**
  - Carpal
    - Left **0RTR0ZZ**
    - Right **0RTQ0ZZ**
  - Cervicothoracic Vertebral **0RT40ZZ**
  - Coccygeal **0ST60ZZ**
  - Elbow
    - Left **0RTM0ZZ**
    - Right **0RTL0ZZ**
  - Finger Phalangeal
    - Left **0RTX0ZZ**
    - Right **0RTW0ZZ**
  - Hip
    - Left **0STB0ZZ**
    - Right **0ST90ZZ**
  - Knee
    - Left **0STD0ZZ**
    - Right **0STC0ZZ**
  - Metacarpocarpal
    - Left **0RTT0ZZ**
    - Right **0RTS0ZZ**
  - Metacarpophalangeal
    - Left **0RTV0ZZ**
    - Right **0RTU0ZZ**
  - Metatarsal-Phalangeal
    - Left **0STN0ZZ**
    - Right **0STM0ZZ**
  - Metatarsal-Tarsal
    - Left **0STL0ZZ**
    - Right **0STK0ZZ**
  - Sacrococcygeal **0ST50ZZ**
  - Sacroiliac
    - Left **0ST80ZZ**
    - Right **0ST70ZZ**
  - Shoulder
    - Left **0RTK0ZZ**
    - Right **0RTJ0ZZ**
  - Sternoclavicular
    - Left **0RTF0ZZ**
    - Right **0RTE0ZZ**
  - Tarsal
    - Left **0STJ0ZZ**
    - Right **0STH0ZZ**
  - Temporomandibular
    - Left **0RTD0ZZ**
    - Right **0RTC0ZZ**
  - Toe Phalangeal
    - Left **0STQ0ZZ**
    - Right **0STP0ZZ**

Resection *(continued)*
  Wrist
    Left **0RTP0ZZ**
    Right **0RTN0ZZ**
  Kidney
    Left **0TT1**
    Right **0TT0**
  Kidney Pelvis
    Left **0TT4**
    Right **0TT3**
  Kidneys, Bilateral **0TT2**
  Larynx **0CTS**
  Lens
    Left **08TK3ZZ**
    Right **08TJ3ZZ**
  Lip
    Lower **0CT1**
    Upper **0CT0**
  Liver **0FT0**
    Left Lobe **0FT2**
    Right Lobe **0FT1**
  Lung
    Bilateral **0BTM**
    Left **0BTL**
    Lower Lobe
      Left **0BTJ**
      Right **0BTF**
    Middle Lobe, Right **0BTD**
    Right **0BTK**
    Upper Lobe
      Left **0BTG**
      Right **0BTC**
  Lung Lingula **0BTH**
  Lymphatic
    Aortic **07TD**
    Axillary
      Left **07T6**
      Right **07T5**
    Head **07T0**
    Inguinal
      Left **07TJ**
      Right **07TH**
    Internal Mammary
      Left **07T9**
      Right **07T8**
    Lower Extremity
      Left **07TG**
      Right **07TF**
    Mesenteric **07TB**
    Neck
      Left **07T2**
      Right **07T1**
    Pelvis **07TC**
    Thoracic Duct **07TK**
    Thorax **07T7**
    Upper Extremity
      Left **07T4**
      Right **07T3**
  Mandible
    Left **0NTV0ZZ**
    Right **0NTT0ZZ**
  Maxilla
    Left **0NTS0ZZ**
    Right **0NTR0ZZ**
  Metacarpal
    Left **0PTQ0ZZ**

Resection *(continued)*
    Right **0PTP0ZZ**
  Metatarsal
    Left **0QTP0ZZ**
    Right **0QTN0ZZ**
  Muscle
    Abdomen
      Left **0KTL**
      Right **0KTK**
    Extraocular
      Left **08TM**
      Right **08TL**
    Facial **0KT1**
    Foot
      Left **0KTW**
      Right **0KTV**
    Hand
      Left **0KTD**
      Right **0KTC**
    Head **0KT0**
    Hip
      Left **0KTP**
      Right **0KTN**
    Lower Arm and Wrist
      Left **0KTB**
      Right **0KT9**
    Lower Leg
      Left **0KTT**
      Right **0KTS**
    Neck
      Left **0KT3**
      Right **0KT2**
    Papillary **02TD**
    Perineum **0KTM**
    Shoulder
      Left **0KT6**
      Right **0KT5**
    Thorax
      Left **0KTJ**
      Right **0KTH**
    Tongue, Palate, Pharynx **0KT4**
    Trunk
      Left **0KTG**
      Right **0KTF**
    Upper Arm
      Left **0KT8**
      Right **0KT7**
    Upper Leg
      Left **0KTR**
      Right **0KTQ**
  Nasopharynx **09TN**
  Nipple
    Left **0HTXXZZ**
    Right **0HTWXZZ**
  Nose **09TK**
  Omentum
    Greater **0DTS**
    Lesser **0DTT**
  Orbit
    Left **0NTQ0ZZ**
    Right **0NTP0ZZ**
  Ovary
    Bilateral **0UT2**
    Left **0UT1**
    Right **0UT0**
  Palate

Resection *(continued)*
    Hard **0CT2**
    Soft **0CT3**
  Pancreas **0FTG**
  Para-aortic Body **0GT9**
  Paraganglion Extremity **0GTF**
  Parathyroid Gland **0GTR**
    Inferior
      Left **0GTP**
      Right **0GTN**
    Multiple **0GTQ**
    Superior
      Left **0GTM**
      Right **0GTL**
  Patella
    Left **0QTF0ZZ**
    Right **0QTD0ZZ**
  Penis **0VTS**
  Pericardium **02TN**
  Phalanx
    Finger
      Left **0PTV0ZZ**
      Right **0PTT0ZZ**
    Thumb
      Left **0PTS0ZZ**
      Right **0PTR0ZZ**
    Toe
      Left **0QTR0ZZ**
      Right **0QTQ0ZZ**
  Pharynx **0CTM**
  Pineal Body **0GT1**
  Prepuce **0VTT**
  Products of Conception, Ectopic **10T2**
  Prostate **0VT0**
  Radius
    Left **0PTJ0ZZ**
    Right **0PTH0ZZ**
  Rectum **0DTP**
  Rib
    Left **0PT20ZZ**
    Right **0PT10ZZ**
  Scapula
    Left **0PT60ZZ**
    Right **0PT50ZZ**
  Scrotum **0VT5**
  Septum
    Atrial **02T5**
    Nasal **09TM**
    Ventricular **02TM**
  Sinus
    Accessory **09TP**
    Ethmoid
      Left **09TV**
      Right **09TU**
    Frontal
      Left **09TT**
      Right **09TS**
    Mastoid
      Left **09TC**
      Right **09TB**
    Maxillary
      Left **09TR**
      Right **09TQ**
    Sphenoid
      Left **09TX**
      Right **09TW**

Resection *(continued)*
Spleen **07TP**
Sternum **0PT00ZZ**
Stomach **0DT6**
  Pylorus **0DT7**
Tarsal
  Left **0QTM0ZZ**
  Right **0QTL0ZZ**
Tendon
  Abdomen
    Left **0LTG**
    Right **0LTF**
  Ankle
    Left **0LTT**
    Right **0LTS**
  Foot
    Left **0LTW**
    Right **0LTV**
  Hand
    Left **0LT8**
    Right **0LT7**
  Head and Neck **0LT0**
  Hip
    Left **0LTK**
    Right **0LTJ**
  Knee
    Left **0LTR**
    Right **0LTQ**
  Lower Arm and Wrist
    Left **0LT6**
    Right **0LT5**
  Lower Leg
    Left **0LTP**
    Right **0LTN**
  Perineum **0LTH**
  Shoulder
    Left **0LT2**
    Right **0LT1**
  Thorax
    Left **0LTD**
    Right **0LTC**
  Trunk
    Left **0LTB**
    Right **0LT9**
  Upper Arm
    Left **0LT4**
    Right **0LT3**
  Upper Leg
    Left **0LTM**
    Right **0LTL**
Testis
  Bilateral **0VTC**
  Left **0VTB**
  Right **0VT9**
Thymus **07TM**
Thyroid Gland **0GTK**
  Left Lobe **0GTG**
  Right Lobe **0GTH**
Tibia
  Left **0QTH0ZZ**
  Right **0QTG0ZZ**
Toe Nail **0HTRXZZ**
Tongue **0CT7**
Tonsils **0CTP**
Tooth
  Lower **0CTX0Z**

Resection *(continued)*
  Upper **0CTW0Z**
Trachea **0BT1**
Tunica Vaginalis
  Left **0VT7**
  Right **0VT6**
Turbinate, Nasal **09TL**
Tympanic Membrane
  Left **09T8**
  Right **09T7**
Ulna
  Left **0PTL0ZZ**
  Right **0PTK0ZZ**
Ureter
  Left **0TT7**
  Right **0TT6**
Urethra **0TTD**
Uterine Supporting Structure **0UT4**
Uterus **0UT9**
Uvula **0CTN**
Vagina **0UTG**
Valve, Pulmonary **02TH**
Vas Deferens
  Bilateral **0VTQ**
  Left **0VTP**
  Right **0VTN**
Vesicle
  Bilateral **0VT3**
  Left **0VT2**
  Right **0VT1**
Vitreous
  Left **08T53ZZ**
  Right **08T43ZZ**
Vocal Cord
  Left **0CTV**
  Right **0CTT**
Vulva **0UTM**
Restoration, Cardiac, Single, Rhythm 5A2204Z
RestoreAdvanced neurostimulator *use* Stimulator Generator, Multiple Array Rechargeable in **0JH**
RestoreSensor neurostimulator *use* Stimulator Generator, Multiple Array Rechargeable in **0JH**
RestoreUltra neurostimulator *use* Stimulator Generator, Multiple Array Rechargeable in **0JH**
Restriction
Ampulla of Vater **0FVC**
Anus **0DVQ**
Aorta
  Abdominal **04V0**
    Intraluminal Device, Branched or Fenestrated **04V0**
  Thoracic
    Ascending/Arch, Intraluminal Device, Branched or Fenestrated **02VX**
    Descending, Intraluminal Device, Branched or Fenestrated **02VW**
Artery
  Anterior Tibial
    Left **04VQ**
    Right **04VP**
  Axillary
    Left **03V6**

Restriction *(continued)*
  Right **03V5**
  Brachial
    Left **03V8**
    Right **03V7**
  Celiac **04V1**
  Colic
    Left **04V7**
    Middle **04V8**
    Right **04V6**
  Common Carotid
    Left **03VJ**
    Right **03VH**
  Common Iliac
    Left, Intraluminal Device, Branched or Fenestrated **04VD**
    Right, Intraluminal Device, Branched or Fenestrated **04VC**
  External Carotid
Left **03VN**
    Right **03VM**
  External Iliac
    Left **04VJ**
    Right **04VH**
  Face **03VR**
  Femoral
    Left **04VL**
    Right **04VK**
  Foot
    Left **04VW**
    Right **04VV**
  Gastric **04V2**
  Hand
    Left **03VF**
    Right **03VD**
  Hepatic **04V3**
  Inferior Mesenteric **04VB**
  Innominate **03V2**
  Internal Carotid
    Left **03VL**
    Right **03VK**
      Internal Iliac
    Left **04VF**
    Right **04VE**
  Internal Mammary
    Left **03V1**
    Right **03V0**
  Intracranial **03VG**
  Lower **04VY**
  Peroneal
    Left **04VU**
    Right **04VT**
  Popliteal
    Left **04VN**
    Right **04VM**
  Posterior Tibial
    Left **04VS**
    Right **04VR**
  Pulmonary
    Left **02VR**
    Right **02VQ**
  Pulmonary Trunk **02VP**
  Radial
    Left **03VC**
    Right **03VB**
  Renal

  Left **04VA**
  Right **04V9**
  Splenic **04V4**
  Subclavian
   Left **03V4**
   Right **03V3**
  Superior Mesenteric **04V5**
  Temporal
   Left **03VT**
   Right **03VS**
  Thyroid
   Left **03VV**
   Right **03VU**
  Ulnar
   Left **03VA**
   Right **03V9**
  Upper **03VY**
  Vertebral
   Left **03VQ**
   Right **03VP**
 Bladder **0TVB**
 Bladder Neck **0TVC**
 Bronchus
  Lingula **0BV9**
  Lower Lobe
   Left **0BVB**
   Right **0BV6**
  Main
   Left **0BV7**
   Right **0BV3**
  Middle Lobe, Right **0BV5**
  Upper Lobe
   Left **0BV8**
   Right **0BV4**
 Carina **0BV2**
 Cecum **0DVH**
 Cervix **0UVC**
 Cisterna Chyli **07VL**
 Colon
  Ascending **0DVK**
  Descending **0DVM**
  Sigmoid **0DVN**
  Transverse **0DVL**
 Duct
  Common Bile **0FV9**
  Cystic **0FV8**
  Hepatic
   Left **0FV6**
   Right **0FV5**
  Lacrimal
   Left **08VY**
   Right **08VX**
  Pancreatic **0FVD**
   Accessory **0FVF**
  Parotid
   Left **0CVC**
   Right **0CVB**
 Duodenum **0DV9**
 Esophagogastric Junction **0DV4**
 Esophagus **0DV5**
  Lower **0DV3**
  Middle **0DV2**
  Upper **0DV1**
 Heart **02VA**
 Ileocecal Valve **0DVC**

 Ileum **0DVB**
 Intestine
  Large **0DVE**
   Left **0DVG**
   Right **0DVF**
  Small **0DV8**
 Jejunum **0DVA**
 Kidney Pelvis
  Left **0TV4**
  Right **0TV3**
 Lymphatic
  Aortic **07VD**
  Axillary
   Left **07V6**
   Right **07V5**
  Head **07V0**
  Inguinal
   Left **07VJ**
   Right **07VH**
  Internal Mammary
   Left **07V9**
   Right **07V8**
  Lower Extremity
   Left **07VG**
   Right **07VF**
  Mesenteric **07VB**
  Neck
   Left **07V2**
   Right **07V1**
  Pelvis **07VC**
  Thoracic Duct **07VK**
  Thorax **07V7**
  Upper Extremity
   Left **07V4**
   Right **07V3**
 Rectum **0DVP**
 Stomach **0DV6**
  Pylorus **0DV7**
 Trachea **0BV1**
 Ureter
  Left **0TV7**
  Right **0TV6**
 Urethra **0TVD**
 Vein
  Axillary
   Left **05V8**
   Right **05V7**
  Azygos **05V0**
  Basilic
   Left **05VC**
   Right **05VB**
  Brachial

   Left **05VA**
   Right **05V9**
  Cephalic
   Left **05VF**
   Right **05VD**
  Colic **06V7**
  Common Iliac
   Left **06VD**
   Right **06VC**
  Esophageal **06V3**
  External Iliac
   Left **06VG**

   Right **06VF**
  External Jugular
   Left **05VQ**
   Right **05VP**
  Face
   Left **05VV**
   Right **05VT**
  Femoral
   Left **06VN**
   Right **06VM**
  Foot
   Left **06VV**
   Right **06VT**
  Gastric **06V2**
  Greater Saphenous
   Left **06VQ**
   Right **06VP**
  Hand
   Left **05VH**
   Right **05VG**
  Hemiazygos **05V1**
  Hepatic **06V4**
  Hypogastric
   Left **06VJ**
   Right **06VH**
  Inferior Mesenteric **06V6**
  Innominate
   Left **05V4**
   Right **05V3**
  Internal Jugular
   Left **05VN**
   Right **05VM**
  Intracranial **05VL**
  Lesser Saphenous
   Left **06VS**
   Right **06VR**
  Lower **06VY**
  Portal **06V8**
  Pulmonary
   Left **02VT**
   Right **02VS**
  Renal
   Left **06VB**
   Right **06V9**
  Splenic **06V1**
  Subclavian
   Left **05V6**
   Right **05V5**
  Superior Mesenteric **06V5**
  Upper **05VY**
  Vertebral
   Left **05VS**
   Right **05VR**
  Vena Cava
   Inferior **06V0**
   Superior **02VV**
Resurfacing Device
 Removal of device from
  Left **0SPB0BZ**
  Right **0SP90BZ**
 Revision of device in
  Left **0SWB0BZ**
  Right **0SW90BZ**
 Supplement
  Left **0SUB0BZ**

Resurfacing Device *(continued)*
    Acetabular Surface **0SUE0BZ**
    Femoral Surface **0SUS0BZ**
  Right **0SU90BZ**
    Acetabular Surface **0SUA0BZ**
    Femoral Surface **0SUR0BZ**
Resuscitation
  Cardiopulmonary *see* Assistance, Cardiac **5A02**
  Cardioversion **5A2204Z**
  Defibrillation **5A2204Z**
  Endotracheal intubation *see* Insertion of device in, Trachea **0BH1**
  External chest compression **5A12012**
  Pulmonary **5A19054**
Resuture, Heart valve prosthesis *see* Revision of device in, Heart and Great Vessels **02W**
Retraining
  Cardiac *see* Motor Treatment, Rehabilitation **F07**
  Vocational *see* Activities of Daily Living Treatment, Rehabilitation **F08**
Retrogasserian rhizotomy *see* Division, Nerve, Trigeminal **008K**
Retroperitoneal lymph node *use* Lymphatic, Aortic
Retroperitoneal space *use* Retroperitoneum
Retropharyngeal lymph node
  use Lymphatic, Neck, Left
  use Lymphatic, Neck, Right
Retropubic space *use* Pelvic Cavity
Reveal (DX)(XT) *use* Monitoring Device
Reverse total shoulder replacement *see* Replacement, Upper Joints **0RR**
Reverse® Shoulder Prosthesis *use* Synthetic Substitute, Reverse Ball and Socket in **0RR**
Revision
  Correcting a portion of existing device *see* Revision of device in
  Removal of device without replacement *see* Removal of device from
  Replacement of existing device
    see Removal of device from
    see Root operation to place new device, e.g., Insertion, Replacement, Supplement
Revision of device in
  Abdominal Wall **0WWF**
  Acetabulum
    Left **0QW5**
    Right **0QW4**
  Anal Sphincter **0DWR**
  Anus **0DWQ**
  Artery
    Lower **04WY**
    Upper **03WY**
  Auditory Ossicle
    Left **09WA**
    Right **09W9**
  Back
    Lower **0WWL**
    Upper **0WWK**
  Bladder **0TWB**
  Bone
    Facial **0NWW**
    Lower **0QWY**

Revision of device in *(continued)*
    Nasal **0NWB**
  Pelvic
    Left **0QW3**
    Right **0QW2**
    Upper **0PWY**
  Bone Marrow **07WT**
  Brain **00W0**
  Breast
    Left **0HWU**
    Right **0HWT**
  Bursa and Ligament
    Lower **0MWY**
    Upper **0MWX**
  Carpal
    Left **0PWN**
    Right **0PWM**
  Cavity, Cranial **0WW1**
  Cerebral Ventricle **00W6**
  Chest Wall **0WW8**
  Cisterna Chyli **07WL**
  Clavicle
    Left **0PWB**
    Right **0PW9**
  Coccyx **0QWS**
  Diaphragm **0BWT**
  Disc
    Cervical Vertebral **0RW3**
    Cervicothoracic Vertebral **0RW5**
    Lumbar Vertebral **0SW2**
    Lumbosacral **0SW4**
    Thoracic Vertebral **0RW9**
    Thoracolumbar Vertebral **0RWB**
  Duct
    Hepatobiliary **0FWB**
    Pancreatic **0FWD**
  Ear
    Inner
      Left **09WE**
      Right **09WD**
    Left **09WJ**
    Right **09WH**
  Epididymis and Spermatic Cord **0VWM**
  Esophagus **0DW5**
  Extremity
    Lower
      Left **0YWB**
      Right **0YW9**
    Upper
      Left **0XW7**
      Right **0XW6**
  Eye
    Left **08W1**
    Right **08W0**
  Face **0WW2**
  Fallopian Tube **0UW8**
  Femoral Shaft
    Left **0QW9**
    Right **0QW8**
  Femur
    Lower
      Left **0QWC**
      Right **0QWB**
    Upper
      Left **0QW7**
      Right **0QW6**

Revision of device in *(continued)*
  Fibula
    Left **0QWK**
    Right **0QWJ**
  Finger Nail **0HWQX**
  Gallbladder **0FW4**
  Gastrointestinal Tract **0WWP**
  Genitourinary Tract **0WWR**
  Gland
    Adrenal **0GW5**
    Endocrine **0GWS**
    Pituitary **0GW0**
    Salivary **0CWA**
  Glenoid Cavity
    Left **0PW8**
    Right **0PW7**
  Great Vessel **02WY**
  Hair **0HWSX**
  Head **0WW0**
  Heart **02WA**
  Humeral Head
    Left **0PWD**
    Right **0PWC**
  Humeral Shaft
    Left **0PWG**
    Right **0PWF**
  Intestinal Tract
    Lower **0DWD**
    Upper **0DW0**
  Intestine
    Large **0DWE**
    Small **0DW8**
  Jaw
    Lower **0WW5**
    Upper **0WW4**
  Joint
    Acromioclavicular
      Left **0RWH**
      Right **0RWG**
    Ankle
      Left **0SWG**
      Right **0SWF**
    Carpal
      Left **0RWR**
      Right **0RWQ**
    Cervical Vertebral **0RW1**
    Cervicothoracic Vertebral **0RW4**
    Coccygeal **0SW6**
    Elbow
      Left **0RWM**
      Right **0RWL**
    Finger Phalangeal
      Left **0RWX**
      Right **0RWW**
    Hip
      Left **0SWB**
        Acetabular Surface **0SWE**
        Femoral Surface **0SWS**
      Right **0SW9**
        Acetabular Surface **0SWA**
        Femoral Surface **0SWR**
    Knee
      Left **0SWD**
        Femoral Surface **0SWU**
        Tibial Surface **0SWW**
      Right **0SWC**

Femoral Surface **0SWT**
Tibial Surface **0SWV**
Lumbar Vertebral **0SW0**
Lumbosacral **0SW3**
Metacarpocarpal
Left **0RWT**
Right **0RWS**
Metacarpophalangeal
Left **0RWV**
Right **0RWU**
Metatarsal-Phalangeal
Left **0SWN**
Right **0SWM**
Metatarsal-Tarsal
Left **0SWL**
Right **0SWK**
Occipital-cervical **0RW0**
Sacrococcygeal **0SW5**
Sacroiliac
Left **0SW8**
Right **0SW7**
Shoulder
Left **0RWK**
Right **0RWJ**
Sternoclavicular
Left **0RWF**
Right **0RWE**
Tarsal
Left **0SWJ**
Right **0SWH**
Temporomandibular
Left **0RWD**
Right **0RWC**
Thoracic Vertebral **0RW6**
Thoracolumbar Vertebral **0RWA**
Toe Phalangeal
Left **0SWQ**
Right **0SWP**
Wrist
Left **0RWP**
Right **0RWN**
Kidney **0TW5**
Larynx **0CWS**
Lens
Left **08WK**
Right **08WJ**
Liver **0FW0**
Lung
Left **0BWL**
Right **0BWK**
Lymphatic **07WN**
Thoracic Duct **07WK**
Mediastinum **0WWC**
Mesentery **0DWV**
Metacarpal
Left **0PWQ**
Right **0PWP**
Metatarsal
Left **0QWP**
Right **0QWN**
Mouth and Throat **0CWY**
Muscle
Extraocular
Left **08WM**
Right **08WL**

Lower **0KWY**
Upper **0KWX**
Neck **0WW6**
Nerve
Cranial **00WE**
Peripheral **01WY**
Nose **09WK**
Omentum **0DWU**
Ovary **0UW3**
Pancreas **0FWG**
Parathyroid Gland **0GWR**
Patella
Left **0QWF**
Right **0QWD**
Pelvic Cavity **0WWJ**
Penis **0VWS**
Pericardial Cavity **0WWD**
Perineum
Female **0WWN**
Male **0WWM**
Peritoneal Cavity **0WWG**
Peritoneum **0DWW**
Phalanx
Finger
Left **0PWV**
Right **0PWT**
Thumb
Left **0PWS**
Right **0PWR**
Toe
Left **0QWR**
Right **0QWQ**
Pineal Body **0GW1**
Pleura **0BWQ**
Pleural Cavity
Left **0WWB**
Right **0WW9**
Prostate and Seminal Vesicles **0VW4**
Radius
Left **0PWJ**
Right **0PWH**
Respiratory Tract **0WWQ**
Retroperitoneum **0WWH**
Rib
Left **0PW2**
Right **0PW1**
Sacrum **0QW1**
Scapula
Left **0PW6**
Right **0PW5**
Scrotum and Tunica Vaginalis **0VW8**
Septum
Atrial **02W5**
Ventricular **02WM**
Sinus **09WY**
Skin **0HWPX**
Skull **0NW0**
Spinal Canal **00WU**
Spinal Cord **00WV**
Spleen **07WP**
Sternum **0PW0**
Stomach **0DW6**
Subcutaneous Tissue and Fascia
Head and Neck **0JWS**
Lower Extremity **0JWW**

Trunk **0JWT**
Upper Extremity **0JWV**
Tarsal
Left **0QWM**
Right **0QWL**
Tendon
Lower **0LWY**
Upper **0LWX**
Testis **0VWD**
Thymus **07WM**
Thyroid Gland **0GWK**
Tibia
Left **0QWH**
Right **0QWG**
Toe Nail **0HWRX**
Trachea **0BW1**
Tracheobronchial Tree **0BW0**
Tympanic Membrane
Left **09W8**
Right **09W7**
Ulna
Left **0PWL**
Right **0PWK**
Ureter **0TW9**
Urethra **0TWD**
Uterus and Cervix **0UWD**
Vagina and Cul-de-sac **0UWH**
Valve
Aortic **02WF**
Mitral **02WG**
Pulmonary **02WH**
Tricuspid **02WJ**
Vas Deferens **0VWR**
Vein
Azygos **05W0**
Innominate
Left **05W4**
Right **05W3**
Lower **06WY**
Upper **05WY**
Vertebra
Cervical **0PW3**
Lumbar **0QW0**
Thoracic **0PW4**
Vulva **0UWM**
Revo MRI™ SureScan® pacemaker *use* Pacemaker, Dual Chamber in **0JH**
Rheos® System device *use* Cardiac Rhythm Related Device in Subcutaneous Tissue and Fascia
Rheos® System lead *use* Stimulator Lead in Upper Arteries
Rhinopharynx *use* Nasopharynx
Rhinoplasty
see Alteration, Nose **090K**
see Repair, Nose **09QK**
see Replacement, Nose **09RK**
see Supplement, Nose **09UK**
Rhinorrhaphy *see* Repair, Nose **09QK**
Rhinoscopy 09JKXZZ
Rhizotomy
see Division, Central Nervous System **008**
see Division, Peripheral Nervous System **018**

Rhomboid major muscle
  use Muscle, Trunk, Left
  use Muscle, Trunk, Right
Rhomboid minor muscle
  use Muscle, Trunk, Right
  use Muscle, Trunk, Left
Rhythm electrocardiogram *see* Measurement, Cardiac **4A02**
Rhytidectomy *see* Face lift
Right ascending lumbar vein *use* Vein, Azygos
Right atrioventricular valve *use* Valve, Tricuspid
Right auricular appendix *use* Atrium, Right
Right colic vein *use* Vein, Colic
Right coronary sulcus *use* Heart, Right
Right gastric artery *use* Artery, Gastric
Right gastroepiploic vein *use* Vein, Superior Mesenteric
Right inferior phrenic vein *use* Vena Cava, Inferior
Right inferior pulmonary vein *use* Vein, Pulmonary, Right
Right jugular trunk *use* Lymphatic, Neck, Right
Right lateral ventricle *use* Cerebral Ventricle
Right lymphatic duct *use* Lymphatic, Neck, Right
Right ovarian vein *use* Vena Cava, Inferior
Right second lumbar vein *use* Vena Cava, Inferior
Right subclavian trunk *use* Lymphatic, Neck, Right
Right subcostal vein *use* Vein, Azygos
Right superior pulmonary vein *use* Vein, Pulmonary, Right
Right suprarenal vein *use* Vena Cava, Inferior
Right testicular vein *use* Vena Cava, Inferior
Rima glottidis *use* Larynx
Risorius muscle *use* Muscle, Facial
RNS System lead *use* Neurostimulator Lead in Central Nervous System
RNS system neurostimulator generator *use* Neurostimulator Generator in Head and Facial Bones
Robotic Assisted Procedure
  Extremity
    Lower **8E0Y**
    Upper **8E0X**
  Head and Neck Region **8E09**
  Trunk Region **8E0W**
Rotation of fetal head
  Forceps **10S07ZZ**
  Manual **10S0XZZ**
Round ligament of uterus *use* Uterine Supporting Structure
Round window
  use Ear, Inner, Right
  use Ear, Inner, Left
Roux-en-Y operation
  see Bypass, Gastrointestinal System **0D1**
  see Bypass, Hepatobiliary System and Pancreas **0F1**
Rupture
  Adhesions *see* Release
  Fluid collection *see* Drainage

S

Sacral ganglion *use* Nerve, Sacral Sympathetic
Sacral lymph node *use* Lymphatic, Pelvis
Sacral nerve modulation (SNM) lead *use* Stimulator Lead in Urinary System
Sacral neuromodulation lead *use* Stimulator Lead in Urinary System
Sacral splanchnic nerve *use* Nerve, Sacral Sympathetic
Sacrectomy *see* Excision, Lower Bones **0QB**
Sacrococcygeal ligament
  use Bursa and Ligament, Trunk, Right
  use Bursa and Ligament, Trunk, Left
Sacrococcygeal symphysis *use* Joint, Sacrococcygeal
Sacroiliac ligament
  use Bursa and Ligament, Trunk, Left
  use Bursa and Ligament, Trunk, Right
Sacrospinous ligament
  use Bursa and Ligament, Trunk, Left
  use Bursa and Ligament, Trunk, Right
Sacrotuberous ligament
  use Bursa and Ligament, Trunk, Left
  use Bursa and Ligament, Trunk, Right
Salpingectomy
  see Excision, Female Reproductive System **0UB**
  see Resection, Female Reproductive System **0UT**
Salpingolysis *see* Release, Female Reproductive System **0UN**
Salpingopexy
  see Repair, Female Reproductive System **0UQ**
  see Reposition, Female Reproductive System **0US**
Salpingopharyngeus muscle *use* Muscle, Tongue, Palate, Pharynx
Salpingoplasty
  see Repair, Female Reproductive System **0UQ**
  see Supplement, Female Reproductive System **0UU**
Salpingorrhaphy *see* Repair, Female Reproductive System **0UQ**
Salpingoscopy 0UJ88ZZ
Salpingostomy *see* Drainage, Female Reproductive System **0U9**
Salpingotomy *see* Drainage, Female Reproductive System **0U9**
Salpinx
  use Fallopian Tube, Left
  use Fallopian Tube, Right
Saphenous nerve *use* Nerve, Femoral
SAPIEN transcatheter aortic valve *use* Zooplastic Tissue in Heart and Great Vessels
Sartorius muscle
  use Muscle, Upper Leg, Right
  use Muscle, Upper Leg, Left
Scalene muscle
  use Muscle, Neck, Right
  use Muscle, Neck, Left
Scan
  Computerized Tomography (CT) *see* Computerized Tomography (CT Scan)

Scan *(continued)*
  Radioisotope *see* Planar Nuclear Medicine Imaging
Scaphoid bone
  use Carpal, Left
  use Carpal, Right
Scapholunate ligament
  use Bursa and Ligament, Hand, Left
  use Bursa and Ligament, Hand, Right
Scaphotrapezium ligament
  use Bursa and Ligament, Hand, Left
  use Bursa and Ligament, Hand, Right
Scapulectomy
  see Excision, Upper Bones **0PB**
  see Resection, Upper Bones **0PT**
Scapulopexy
  see Repair, Upper Bones **0PQ**
  see Reposition, Upper Bones **0PS**
Scarpa's (vestibular) ganglion *use* Nerve, Acoustic
Sclerectomy *see* Excision, Eye **08B**
Sclerotherapy, mechanical *see* Destruction
Sclerotomy *see* Drainage, Eye **089**
Scrotectomy
  see Excision, Male Reproductive System **0VB**
  see Resection, Male Reproductive System **0VT**
Scrotoplasty
  see Repair, Male Reproductive System **0VQ**
  see Supplement, Male Reproductive System **0VU**
Scrotorrhaphy *see* Repair, Male Reproductive System **0VQ**
Scrototomy *see* Drainage, Male Reproductive System **0V9**
Sebaceous gland *use* Skin
Second cranial nerve *use* Nerve, Optic
Section, cesarean *see* Extraction, Pregnancy **10D**
Secura (DR) (VR) *use* Defibrillator Generator in **0JH**
Sella Turcica
  use Bone, Sphenoid, Left
  use Bone, Sphenoid, Right
Semicircular canal
  use Ear, Inner, Left
  use Ear, Inner, Right
Semimembranosus muscle
  use Muscle, Upper Leg, Left
  use Muscle, Upper Leg, Right
Semitendinosus muscle
  use Muscle, Upper Leg, Left
  use Muscle, Upper Leg, Right
Septal cartilage *use* Septum, Nasal
Septectomy
  see Excision, Heart and Great Vessels **02B**
  see Resection, Heart and Great Vessels **02T**
  see Excision, Ear, Nose, Sinus **09B**
  see Resection, Ear, Nose, Sinus **09T**
Septoplasty
  see Repair, Ear, Nose, Sinus **09Q**
  see Repair, Heart and Great Vessels **02Q**
  see Replacement, Ear, Nose, Sinus **09R**
  see Replacement, Heart and Great Vessels **02R**

Septoplasty (continued)
see Reposition, Ear, Nose, Sinus **09S**
see Supplement, Ear, Nose, Sinus **09U**
see Supplement, Heart and Great Vessels **02U**
Septotomy see Drainage, Ear, Nose, Sinus **099**
Sequestrectomy, bone see Extirpation
Serratus anterior muscle
use Muscle, Thorax, Left
use Muscle, Thorax, Right
Serratus posterior muscle
use Muscle, Trunk, Left
use Muscle, Trunk, Right
Seventh cranial nerve use Nerve, Facial
Sheffield hybrid external fixator
use External Fixation Device, Hybrid in **0PH**
use External Fixation Device, Hybrid in **0PS**
use External Fixation Device, Hybrid in **0QH**
use External Fixation Device, Hybrid in **0QS**
Sheffield ring external fixator
use External Fixation Device, Ring in **0PH**
use External Fixation Device, Ring in **0PS**
use External Fixation Device, Ring in **0QH**
use External Fixation Device, Ring in **0QS**
Shirodkar cervical cerclage 0UVC7ZZ
Shock Wave Therapy, Musculoskeletal 6A93
Short gastric artery use Artery, Splenic
Shortening
see Excision
see Repair
see Reposition
Shunt creation see Bypass
Sialoadenectomy
Complete see Resection, Mouth and Throat **0CT**
Partial see Excision, Mouth and Throat **0CB**
Sialodochoplasty
see Repair, Mouth and Throat **0CQ**
see Replacement, Mouth and Throat **0CR**
see Supplement, Mouth and Throat **0CU**
Sialoectomy
see Excision, Mouth and Throat **0CB**
see Resection, Mouth and Throat **0CT**
Sialography see Plain Radiography, Ear, Nose, Mouth and Throat **B90**
Sialolithotomy see Extirpation, Mouth and Throat **0CC**
Sigmoid artery use Artery, Inferior Mesenteric
Sigmoid flexure use Colon, Sigmoid
Sigmoid vein use Vein, Inferior Mesenteric
Sigmoidectomy
see Excision, Gastrointestinal System **0DB**
see Resection, Gastrointestinal System **0DT**
Sigmoidorrhaphy see Repair, Gastrointestinal System **0DQ**
Sigmoidoscopy 0DJD8ZZ
Sigmoidotomy see Drainage, Gastrointestinal System **0D9**
Single lead pacemaker (atrium)(ventricle) use Pacemaker, Single Chamber in **0JH**
Single lead rate responsive pacemaker (atrium)(ventricle) use Pacemaker, Single Chamber Rate Responsive in **0JH**

Sinoatrial node use Conduction Mechanism
Sinogram
Abdominal Wall see Fluoroscopy, Abdomen and Pelvis **BW11**
Chest Wall see Plain Radiography, Chest **BW03**
Retroperitoneum see Fluoroscopy, Abdomen and Pelvis **BW11**
Sinus venosus use Atrium, Right
Sinusectomy
see Excision, Ear, Nose, Sinus **09B**
see Resection, Ear, Nose, Sinus **09T**
Sinusoscopy 09JY4ZZ
Sinusotomy see Drainage, Ear, Nose, Sinus **099**
Sirolimus-eluting coronary stent use Intraluminal Device, Drug-eluting in Heart and Great Vessels
Sixth cranial nerve use Nerve, Abducens
Size reduction, breast see Excision, Skin and Breast **0HB**
SJM Biocor®
Stented Valve System use Zooplastic Tissue in Heart and Great Vessels
Skene's (paraurethral) gland use Gland, Vestibular
Skin Substitute, Porcine Liver Derived, Replacement XHRPXL2
Sling
Fascial, orbicularis muscle (mouth) see Supplement, Muscle, Facial **0KU1**
Levator muscle, for urethral suspension see Reposition, Bladder Neck **0TSC**
Pubococcygeal, for urethral suspension see Reposition, Bladder Neck **0TSC**
Rectum see Reposition, Rectum **0DSP**
Small bowel series see Fluoroscopy, Bowel, Small **BD13**
Small saphenous vein
use Vein, Lesser Saphenous, Left
use Vein, Lesser Saphenous, Right
Snaring, polyp, colon see Excision, Gastrointestinal System **0DB**
Spinal growth rods, magnetically controlled use Magnetically Controlled Growth Rod(s) in New Technology
SPY system intravascular fluorescence angiography see Monitoring, Physiological Systems **4A1**
Solar (celiac) plexus use Nerve, Abdominal Sympathetic
Soletra® neurostimulator use Stimulator Generator, Single Array in **0JH**
Soleus muscle
use Muscle, Lower Leg, Left
use Muscle, Lower Leg, Right
Spacer
Insertion of device in
Disc
Lumbar Vertebral **0SH2**
Lumbosacral **0SH4**
Joint
Acromioclavicular
Left **0RHH**
Right **0RHG**
Ankle
Left **0SHG**

Spacer (continued)
Right **0SHF**
Carpal
Left **0RHR**
Right **0RHQ**
Cervical Vertebral **0RH1**
Cervicothoracic Vertebral **0RH4**
Coccygeal **0SH6**
Elbow
Left **0RHM**
Right **0RHL**
Finger Phalangeal
Left **0RHX**
Right **0RHW**
Hip
Left **0SHB**
Right **0SH9**
Knee
Left **0SHD**
Right **0SHC**
Lumbar Vertebral **0SH0**
Lumbosacral **0SH3**
Metacarpocarpal
Left **0RHT**
Right **0RHS**
Metacarpophalangeal
Left **0RHV**
Right **0RHU**
Metatarsal-Phalangeal
Left **0SHN**
Right **0SHM**
Metatarsal-Tarsal
Left **0SHL**
Right **0SHK**
Occipital-cervical **0RH0**
Sacrococcygeal **0SH5**
Sacroiliac
Left **0SH8**
Right **0SH7**
Shoulder
Left **0RHK**
Right **0RHJ**
Sternoclavicular
Left **0RHF**
Right **0RHE**
Tarsal
Left **0SHJ**
Right **0SHH**
Temporomandibular
Left **0RHD**
Right **0RHC**
Thoracic Vertebral **0RH6**
Thoracolumbar Vertebral **0RHA**
Toe Phalangeal
Left **0SHQ**
Right **0SHP**
Wrist
Left **0RHP**
Right **0RHN**
Removal of device from
Acromioclavicular
Left **0RPH**
Right **0RPG**
Ankle
Left **0SPG**
Right **0SPF**

Spacer *(continued)*
  Carpal
    Left **0RPR**
    Right **0RPQ**
  Cervical Vertebral **0RP1**
  Cervicothoracic Vertebral **0RP4**
  Coccygeal **0SP6**
  Elbow
    Left **0RPM**
    Right **0RPL**
  Finger Phalangeal
    Left **0RPX**
    Right **0RPW**
  Hip
    Left **0SPB**
    Right **0SP9**
  Knee
    Left **0SPD**
    Right **0SPC**
  Lumbar Vertebral **0SP0**
  Lumbosacral **0SP3**
  Metacarpocarpal
    Left **0RPT**
    Right **0RPS**
  Metacarpophalangeal
    Left **0RPV**
    Right **0RPU**
  Metatarsal-Phalangeal
    Left **0SPN**
    Right **0SPM**
  Metatarsal-Tarsal
    Left **0SPL**
    Right **0SPK**
  Occipital-cervical **0RP0**
  Sacrococcygeal **0SP5**
  Sacroiliac
    Left **0SP8**
    Right **0SP7**
  Shoulder
    Left **0RPK**
    Right **0RPJ**
  Sternoclavicular
    Left **0RPF**
    Right **0RPE**
  Tarsal
    Left **0SPJ**
    Right **0SPH**
  Temporomandibular
    Left **0RPD**
    Right **0RPC**
  Thoracic Vertebral **0RP6**
  Thoracolumbar Vertebral **0RPA**
  Toe Phalangeal
    Left **0SPQ**
    Right **0SPP**
  Wrist
    Left **0RPP**
    Right **0RPN**
  Revision of device in
    Acromioclavicular
      Left **0RWH**
      Right **0RWG**
    Ankle
      Left **0SWG**
      Right **0SWF**
    Carpal

Spacer *(continued)*
      Left **0RWR**
      Right **0RWQ**
    Cervical Vertebral **0RW1**
    Cervicothoracic Vertebral **0RW4**
    Coccygeal **0SW6**
    Elbow
      Left **0RWM**
      Right **0RWL**
    Finger Phalangeal
      Left **0RWX**
      Right **0RWW**
    Hip
      Left **0SWB**
      Right **0SW9**
    Knee
      Left **0SWD**
      Right **0SWC**
    Lumbar Vertebral **0SW0**
    Lumbosacral **0SW3**
    Metacarpocarpal
      Left **0RWT**
      Right **0RWS**
    Metacarpophalangeal
      Left **0RWV**
      Right **0RWU**
    Metatarsal-Phalangeal
      Left **0SWN**
      Right **0SWM**
    Metatarsal-Tarsal
      Left **0SWL**
      Right **0SWK**
    Occipital-cervical **0RW0**
    Sacrococcygeal **0SW5**
    Sacroiliac
      Left **0SW8**
      Right **0SW7**
    Shoulder
      Left **0RWK**
      Right **0RWJ**
    Sternoclavicular
      Left **0RWF**
      Right **0RWE**
    Tarsal
      Left **0SWJ**
      Right **0SWH**
    Temporomandibular
      Left **0RWD**
      Right **0RWC**
    Thoracic Vertebral **0RW6**
    Thoracolumbar Vertebral **0RWA**
    Toe Phalangeal
      Left **0SWQ**
      Right **0SWP**
    Wrist
      Left **0RWP**
      Right **0RWN** Spectroscopy
  Intravascular **8E023DZ**
  Near infrared **8E023DZ**
Speech Assessment F00
Speech therapy *see* Speech Treatment, Rehabilitation **F06**
Speech Treatment F06
Sphenoidectomy
  see Excision, Ear, Nose, Sinus **09B**
  see Resection, Ear, Nose, Sinus **09T**

Sphenoidectomy *(continued)*
  see Excision, Head and Facial Bones **0NB**
  see Resection, Head and Facial Bones **0NT**
Sphenoidotomy *see* Drainage, Ear, Nose, Sinus **099**
Sphenomandibular ligament *use* Bursa and Ligament, Head and Neck
Sphenopalatine (pterygopalatine) ganglion *use* Nerve, Head and Neck Sympathetic
Sphincterorrhaphy, anal *see* Repair, Anal Sphincter **0DQR**
Sphincterotomy, anal
  see Drainage, Anal Sphincter **0D9R**
  see Division, Anal Sphincter **0D8R**
Spinal cord neurostimulator lead *use* Neurostimulator Lead in Central Nervous System
Spinal growth rods, magnetically controlled *use* Magnetically Controlled Growth Rod(s) in New Technology
Spinal nerve
  cervical *use* Nerve, Cervical
  lumbar *use* Nerve, Lumbar
  sacral *use* Nerve, Sacral
  thoracic *use* Nerve, Thoracic
Spinal Stabilization Device
  Facet Replacement
    Cervical Vertebral **0RH1**
    Cervicothoracic Vertebral **0RH4**
    Lumbar Vertebral **0SH0**
    Lumbosacral **0SH3**
    Occipital-cervical **0RH0**
    Thoracic Vertebral **0RH6**
    Thoracolumbar Vertebral **0RHA**
  Interspinous Process
    Cervical Vertebral **0RH1**
    Cervicothoracic Vertebral **0RH4**
    Lumbar Vertebral **0SH0**
    Lumbosacral **0SH3**
    Occipital-cervical **0RH0**
    Thoracic Vertebral **0RH6**
    Thoracolumbar Vertebral **0RHA**
  Pedicle-Based
    Cervical Vertebral **0RH1**
    Cervicothoracic Vertebral **0RH4**
    Lumbar Vertebral **0SH0**
    Lumbosacral **0SH3**
    Occipital-cervical **0RH0**
    Thoracic Vertebral **0RH6**
    Thoracolumbar Vertebral **0RHA**
Spinous process
  use Vertebra, Cervical
  use Vertebra, Lumbar
  use Vertebra, Thoracic
Spiral ganglion *use* Nerve, Acoustic
Spiration IBV™ Valve System *use* Intraluminal Device, Endobronchial Valve in Respiratory System
Splenectomy
  see Excision, Lymphatic and Hemic Systems **07B**
  see Resection, Lymphatic and Hemic Systems **07T**
Splenic flexure *use* Colon, Transverse
Splenic plexus *use* Nerve, Abdominal Sympathetic
Splenius capitis muscle *use* Muscle, Head

Splenius cervicis muscle
  use Muscle, Neck, Left
  use Muscle, Neck, Right
Splenolysis *see* Release, Lymphatic and Hemic Systems **07N**
Splenopexy
  see Repair, Lymphatic and Hemic Systems **07Q**
  see Reposition, Lymphatic and Hemic Systems **07S**
Splenoplasty *see* Repair, Lymphatic and Hemic Systems **07Q**
Splenorrhaphy *see* Repair, Lymphatic and Hemic Systems **07Q**
Splenotomy *see* Drainage, Lymphatic and Hemic Systems **079**
Splinting, musculoskeletal *see* Immobilization, Anatomical Regions **2W3**
SPY system intravascular fluorescence angiography *see* Monitoring, Physiological Systems **4A1**
Stapedectomy
  see Excision, Ear, Nose, Sinus **09B**
  see Resection, Ear, Nose, Sinus **09T**
Stapediolysis *see* Release, Ear, Nose, Sinus **09N**
Stapedioplasty
  see Repair, Ear, Nose, Sinus **09Q**
  see Replacement, Ear, Nose, Sinus **09R**
  see Supplement, Ear, Nose, Sinus **09U**
Stapedotomy *see* Drainage, Ear, Nose, Sinus **099**
Stapes
  use Auditory Ossicle, Right
  use Auditory Ossicle, Left
Stellate ganglion *use* Nerve, Head and Neck Sympathetic
Stem cell transplant *see* Transfusion, Circulatory **302**
Stensen's duct
  use Duct, Parotid, Right
  use Duct, Parotid, Left
Stent (angioplasty)(embolization) *use* Intraluminal Device
Stented tissue valve *use* Zooplastic Tissue in Heart and Great Vessels
Stereotactic Radiosurgery
  Abdomen **DW23**
  Adrenal Gland **DG22**
  Bile Ducts **DF22**
  Bladder **DT22**
  Bone Marrow **D720**
  Brain **D020**
  Brain Stem **D021**
  Breast
    Left **DM20**
    Right **DM21**
  Bronchus **DB21**
  Cervix **DU21**
  Chest **DW22**
  Chest Wall **DB27**
  Colon **DD25**
  Diaphragm **DB28**
  Duodenum **DD22**
  Ear **D920**
  Esophagus **DD20**
  Eye **D820**

Stereotactic Radiosurgery *(continued)*
  Gallbladder **DF21**
  Gamma Beam
    Abdomen **DW23JZZ**
    Adrenal Gland **DG22JZZ**
    Bile Ducts **DF22JZZ**
    Bladder **DT22JZZ**
    Bone Marrow **D720JZZ**
    Brain **D020JZZ**
    Brain Stem **D021JZZ**
    Breast
      Left **DM20JZZ**
      Right **DM21JZZ**
    Bronchus **DB21JZZ**
    Cervix **DU21JZZ**
    Chest **DW22JZZ**
    Chest Wall **DB27JZZ**
    Colon **DD25JZZ**
    Diaphragm **DB28JZZ**
    Duodenum **DD22JZZ**
    Ear **D920JZZ**
    Esophagus **DD20JZZ**
    Eye **D820JZZ**
    Gallbladder **DF21JZZ**
    Gland
      Adrenal **DG22JZZ**
      Parathyroid **DG24JZZ**
      Pituitary **DG20JZZ**
      Thyroid **DG25JZZ**
    Glands, Salivary **D926JZZ**
    Head and Neck **DW21JZZ**
    Ileum **DD24JZZ**
    Jejunum **DD23JZZ**
    Kidney **DT20JZZ**
    Larynx **D92BJZZ**
    Liver **DF20JZZ**
    Lung **DB22JZZ**
    Lymphatics
      Abdomen **D726JZZ**
      Axillary **D724JZZ**
      Inguinal **D728JZZ**
      Neck **D723JZZ**
      Pelvis **D727JZZ**
      Thorax **D725JZZ**
    Mediastinum **DB26JZZ**
    Mouth **D924JZZ**
    Nasopharynx **D92DJZZ**
    Neck and Head **DW21JZZ**
    Nerve, Peripheral **D027JZZ**
    Nose **D921JZZ**
    Ovary **DU20JZZ**
    Palate
      Hard **D928JZZ**
      Soft **D929JZZ**
    Pancreas **DF23JZZ**
    Parathyroid Gland **DG24JZZ**
    Pelvic Region **DW26JZZ**
    Pharynx **D92CJZZ**
    Pineal Body **DG21JZZ**
    Pituitary Gland **DG20JZZ**
    Pleura **DB25JZZ**
    Prostate **DV20JZZ**
    Rectum **DD27JZZ**
    Sinuses **D927JZZ**
    Spinal Cord **D026JZZ**
    Spleen **D722JZZ**

Stereotactic Radiosurgery *(continued)*
    Stomach **DD21JZZ**
    Testis **DV21JZZ**
    Thymus **D721JZZ**
    Thyroid Gland **DG25JZZ**
    Tongue **D925JZZ**
    Trachea **DB20JZZ**
    Ureter **DT21JZZ**
    Urethra **DT23JZZ**
    Uterus **DU22JZZ**
  Gland
    Adrenal **DG22**
    Parathyroid *DG24*
    Pituitary **DG20**
    Thyroid **DG25**
  Glands, Salivary **D926**
  Head and Neck **DW21**
  Ileum **DD24**
  Jejunum **DD23**
  Kidney **DT20**
  Larynx **D92B**
  Liver **DF20**
  Lung **DB22**
  Lymphatics
    Abdomen **D726**
    Axillary **D724**
    Inguinal **D728**
    Neck **D723**
    Pelvis **D727**
    Thorax **D725**
  Mediastinum **DB26**
  Mouth **D924**
  Nasopharynx **D92D**
  Neck and Head **W21**
  Nerve, Peripheral **D027**
  Nose **D921**
  Other Photon
    Abdomen **DW23DZZ**
    Adrenal Gland **DG22DZZ**
    Bile Ducts **DF22DZZ**
    Bladder **DT22DZZ**
    Bone Marrow **D720DZZ**
    Brain **D020DZZ**
    Brain Stem **D021DZZ**
    Breast
      Left **DM20DZZ**
      Right **DM21DZZ**
    Bronchus **DB21DZZ**
    Cervix **DU21DZZ**
    Chest **DW22DZZ**
    Chest Wall **DB27DZZ**
    Colon **DD25DZZ**
    Diaphragm **DB28DZZ**
    Duodenum **DD22DZZ**
    Ear **D920DZZ**
    Esophagus **DD20DZZ**
    Eye **D820DZZ**
    Gallbladder **DF21DZZ**
    Gland
      Adrenal **DG22DZZ**
      Parathyroid **DG24DZZ**
      Pituitary **DG20DZZ**
      Thyroid **DG25DZZ**
    Glands, Salivary **D926DZZ**
    Head and Neck **DW21DZZ**
    Ileum **DD24DZZ**

Stereotactic Radiosurgery *(continued)*
  Jejunum **DD23DZZ**
  Kidney **DT20DZZ**
  Larynx **D92BDZZ**
  Liver **DF20DZZ**
  Lung **DB22DZZ**
  Lymphatics
    Abdomen **D726DZZ**
    Axillary **D724DZZ**
    Inguinal **D728DZZ**
    Neck **D723DZZ**
    Pelvis **D727DZZ**
    Thorax **D725DZZ**
  Mediastinum **DB26DZZ**
  Mouth **D924DZZ**
  Nasopharynx **D92DDZZ**
  Neck and Head **DW21DZZ**
  Nerve, Peripheral **D027DZZ**
  Nose **D921DZZ**
  Ovary **DU20DZZ**
  Palate
    Hard **D928DZZ**
    Soft **D929DZZ**
  Pancreas **DF23DZZ**
  Parathyroid Gland **DG24DZZ**
  Pelvic Region **DW26DZZ**
  Pharynx **D92CDZZ**
  Pineal Body **DG21DZZ**
  Pituitary Gland **DG20DZZ**
  Pleura **DB25DZZ**
  Prostate **DV20DZZ**
  Rectum **DD27DZZ**
  Sinuses **D927DZZ**
  Spinal Cord **D026DZZ**
  Spleen **D722DZZ**
  Stomach **DD21DZZ**
  Testis **DV21DZZ**
  Thymus **D721DZZ**
  Thyroid Gland **DG25DZZ**
  Tongue **D925DZZ**
  Trachea **DB20DZZ**
  Ureter **DT21DZZ**
  Urethra **DT23DZZ**
  Uterus **DU22DZZ**
 Ovary **DU20**
 Palate
  Hard **D928**
  Soft **D929**
 Pancreas **DF23**
 Parathyroid Gland **DG24**
 Particulate
  Abdomen **DW23HZZ**
  Adrenal Gland **DG22HZZ**
  Bile Ducts **DF22HZZ**
  Bladder **DT22HZZ**
  Bone Marrow **D720HZZ**
  Brain **D020HZZ**
  Brain Stem **D021HZZ**
  Breast
    Left **DM20HZZ**
    Right **DM21HZZ**
  Bronchus **DB21HZZ**
  Cervix **DU21HZZ**
  Chest **DW22HZZ**
  Chest Wall **DB27HZZ**
  Colon **DD25HZZ**

Stereotactic Radiosurgery *(continued)*
  Diaphragm **DB28HZZ**
  Duodenum **DD22HZZ**
  Ear **D920HZZ**
  Esophagus **DD20HZZ**
  Eye **D820HZZ**
  Gallbladder **DF21HZZ**
  Gland
    Adrenal **DG22HZZ**
    Parathyroid **DG24HZZ**
    Pituitary **DG20HZZ**
    Thyroid **DG25HZZ**
  Glands, Salivary **D926HZZ**
  Head and Neck **DW21HZZ**
  Ileum **DD24HZZ**
  Jejunum **DD23HZZ**
  Kidney **DT20HZZ**
  Larynx **D92BHZZ**
  Liver **DF20HZZ**
  Lung **DB22HZZ**
  Lymphatics
    Abdomen **D726HZZ**
    Axillary **D724HZZ**
    Inguinal **D728HZZ**
    Neck **D723HZZ**
    Pelvis **D727HZZ**
    Thorax **D725HZZ**
  Mediastinum **DB26HZZ**
  Mouth **D924HZZ**
  Nasopharynx **D92DHZZ**
  Neck and Head **DW21HZZ**
  Nerve, Peripheral **D027HZZ**
  Nose **D921HZZ**
  Ovary **DU20HZZ**
  Palate
    Hard **D928HZZ**
    Soft **D929HZZ**
  Pancreas **DF23HZZ**
  Parathyroid Gland **DG24HZZ**
  Pelvic Region **DW26HZZ**
  Pharynx **D92CHZZ**
  Pineal Body **DG21HZZ**
  Pituitary Gland **DG20HZZ**
  Pleura **DB25HZZ**
  Prostate **DV20HZZ**
  Rectum **DD27HZZ**
  Sinuses **D927HZZ**
  Spinal Cord **D026HZZ**
  Spleen **D722HZZ**
  Stomach **DD21HZZ**
  Testis **DV21HZZ**
  Thymus **D721HZZ**
  Thyroid Gland **DG25HZZ**
  Tongue **D925HZZ**
  Trachea **DB20HZZ**
  Ureter **DT21HZZ**
  Urethra **DT23HZZ**
  Uterus **DU22HZZ**
 Pelvic Region **DW26**
 Pharynx **D92C**
 Pineal Body **DG21**
 Pituitary Gland **DG20**
 Pleura **DB25**
 Prostate **DV20**
 Rectum **DD27**
 Sinuses **D927**

Stereotactic Radiosurgery *(continued)*
  Spinal Cord **D026**
  Spleen **D722**
  Stomach **DD21**
  Testis **DV21**
  Thymus **D721**
  Thyroid Gland **DG25**
  Tongue **D925**
  Trachea **DB20**
  Ureter **DT21**
  Urethra **DT23**
  Uterus **DU22**
Sternoclavicular ligament
 use Bursa and Ligament, Shoulder, Left
 use Bursa and Ligament, Shoulder, Right
Sternocleidomastoid artery
 use Artery, Thyroid, Left
 use Artery, Thyroid, Right
Sternocleidomastoid muscle
 use Muscle, Neck, Left
 use Muscle, Neck, Right
Sternocostal ligament
 use Bursa and Ligament, Thorax, Right
 use Bursa and Ligament, Thorax, Left
Sternotomy
 see Division, Sternum **0P80**
 see Drainage, Sternum **0P90**
Stimulation, cardiac
 Cardioversion **5A2204Z**
 Electrophysiologic testing *see* Measurement, Cardiac **4A02**
Stimulator Generator
 Insertion of device in
  Abdomen **0JH8**
  Back **0JH7**
  Chest **0JH6**
  Multiple Array
    Abdomen **0JH8**
    Back **0JH7**
    Chest **0JH6**
  Multiple Array Rechargeable
    Abdomen **0JH8**
    Back **0JH7**
Stimulator Generator
 Chest **0JH6**
 Removal of device from, Subcutaneous Tissue and Fascia, Trunk **0JPT**
 Revision of device in, Subcutaneous Tissue and Fascia, Trunk **0JWT**
 Single Array
  Abdomen **0JH8**
  Back **0JH7**
  Chest **0JH6**
 Single Array Rechargeable
  Abdomen **0JH8**
  Back **0JH7**
  Chest **0JH6**
Stimulator Lead
 Insertion of device in
  Anal Sphincter **0DHR**
  Artery
    Left **03HL**
    Right **03HK**
  Bladder **0THB**
  Muscle
    Lower **0KHY**

Stimulator Lead *(continued)*
    Upper **0KHX**
    Stomach **0DH6**
    Ureter **0TH9**
    Ureter **0TH9**
    Removal of device from
        Anal Sphincter **0DPR**
        Artery, Upper **03PY**
        Bladder **0TPB**
        Muscle
            Lower **0KPY**
            Upper **0KPX**
        Stomach **0DP6**
        Ureter **0TP9**
    Revision of device in
        Anal Sphincter **0DWR**
        Artery, Upper **03WY**
        Bladder **0TWB**
        Muscle
            Lower **0KWY**
            Upper **0KWX**
        Stomach **0DW6**
        Ureter **0TW9**
Stoma
    Excision
    Abdominal Wall **0WBFXZ2**
    Neck **0WB6XZ2**
    Repair
    Abdominal Wall **0WQFXZ2**
    Neck **0WQ6XZ2**
Stomatoplasty
    see Repair, Mouth and Throat **0CQ**
    see Replacement, Mouth and Throat **0CR**
    see Supplement, Mouth and Throat **0CU**
Stomatorrhaphy *see* Repair, Mouth and Throat **0CQ**
Stratos LV *use* Cardiac Resynchronization Pacemaker Pulse Generator in **0JH**
Stress test
    4A02XM4
    4A12XM4
Stripping *see* Extraction
Study
    Electrophysiologic stimulation, cardiac *see* Measurement, Cardiac **4A02**
    Ocular motility **4A07X7Z**
    Pulmonary airway flow measurement *see* Measurement, Respiratory **4A09**
    Visual acuity **4A07X0Z**
Styloglossus muscle *use* Muscle, Tongue, Palate, Pharynx
Stylomandibular ligament *use* Bursa and Ligament, Head and Neck
Stylopharyngeus muscle *use* Muscle, Tongue, Palate, Pharynx
Subacromial bursa
    use Bursa and Ligament, Shoulder, Left
    use Bursa and Ligament, Shoulder, Right
Subaortic (common iliac) lymph node *use* Lymphatic, Pelvis
Subclavicular (apical) lymph node
    use Lymphatic, Axillary, Left
    use Lymphatic, Axillary, Right
Subclavius muscle
    use Muscle, Thorax, Left
    use Muscle, Thorax, Right

Subclavius nerve *use* Nerve, Brachial Plexus
Subcostal artery *use* Upper Artery
Subcostal muscle
    use Muscle, Thorax, Left
    use Muscle, Thorax, Right
Subcostal nerve *use* Nerve, Thoracic
Subcutaneous injection reservoir, port *use* Vascular Access Device, Reservoir in Subcutaneous Tissue and Fascia \
Subcutaneous injection reservoir, pump *use* Infusion Device, Pump in Subcutaneous Tissue and Fascia
Subdermal progesterone implant *use* Contraceptive Device in Subcutaneous Tissue and Fascia
Submandibular ganglion
    use Nerve, Head and Neck Sympathetic
    use Nerve, Facial
Submandibular gland
    use Gland, Submaxillary, Left
    use Gland, Submaxillary, Right
Submandibular lymph node *use* Lymphatic, Head
Submaxillary ganglion *use* Nerve, Head and Neck Sympathetic
Submaxillary lymph node *use* Lymphatic, Head
Submental artery *use* Artery, Face
Submental lymph node *use* Lymphatic, Head
Submucous (Meissner's) plexus *use* Nerve, Abdominal Sympathetic
Suboccipital nerve *use* Nerve, Cervical
Suboccipital venous plexus
    use Vein, Vertebral, Left
    use Vein, Vertebral, Right
Subparotid lymph node *use* Lymphatic, Head
Subscapular (posterior) lymph node
    use Lymphatic, Axillary, Left
    use Lymphatic, Axillary, Right
Subscapular aponeurosis
    use Subcutaneous Tissue and Fascia, Upper Arm, Right
    use Subcutaneous Tissue and Fascia, Upper Arm, Left
Subscapular artery
    use Artery, Axillary, Left
    use Artery, Axillary, Right
Subscapularis muscle
    use Muscle, Shoulder, Left
    use Muscle, Shoulder, Right
Substance Abuse Treatment
    Counseling
        Family, for substance abuse, Other
    Family Counseling **HZ63ZZZ**
    Group
        12-Step **HZ43ZZZ**
        Behavioral **HZ41ZZZ**
        Cognitive **HZ40ZZZ**
        Cognitive-Behavioral **HZ42ZZZ**
        Confrontational **HZ48ZZZ**
        Continuing Care **HZ49ZZZ**
        Infectious Disease
            Post-Test **HZ4CZZZ**
            Pre-Test **HZ4CZZZ**
        Interpersonal **HZ44ZZZ**
        Motivational Enhancement **HZ47ZZZ**
        Psychoeducation **HZ46ZZZ**

Substance Abuse Treatment *(continued)*
        Spiritual **HZ4BZZZ**
        Vocational **HZ45ZZZ**
    Individual
        12-Step **HZ33ZZZ**
        Behavioral **HZ31ZZZ**
        Cognitive **HZ30ZZZ**
        Cognitive-Behavioral **HZ32ZZZ**
        Confrontational **HZ38ZZZ**
        Continuing Care **HZ39ZZZ**
        Infectious Disease
            Post-Test **HZ3CZZZ**
            Pre-Test **HZ3CZZZ**
        Interpersonal **HZ34ZZZ**
        Motivational Enhancement **HZ37ZZZ**
        Psychoeducation **HZ36ZZZ**
        Spiritual **HZ3BZZZ**
        Vocational **HZ35ZZZ**
    Detoxification Services, for substance abuse **HZ2ZZZZ**
    Medication Management
        Antabuse **HZ83ZZZ**
        Bupropion **HZ87ZZZ**
        Clonidine **HZ86ZZZ**
        Levo-alpha-acetyl-methadol (LAAM) **HZ82ZZZ**
        Methadone Maintenance **HZ81ZZZ**
        Naloxone **HZ85ZZZ**
        Naltrexone **HZ84ZZZ**
        Nicotine Replacement **HZ80ZZZ**
        Other Replacement Medication **HZ89ZZZ**
        Psychiatric Medication **HZ88ZZZ**
    Pharmacotherapy
        Antabuse **HZ93ZZZ**
        Bupropion **HZ97ZZZ**
        Clonidine **HZ96ZZZ**
        Levo-alpha-acetyl-methadol (LAAM) **HZ92ZZZ**
        Methadone Maintenance **HZ91ZZZ**
        Naloxone **HZ95ZZZ**
        Naltrexone **HZ94ZZZ**
        Nicotine Replacement **HZ90ZZZ**
        Psychiatric Medication **HZ98ZZZ**
        Replacement Medication, Other **HZ99ZZZ**
    Psychotherapy
        12-Step **HZ53ZZZ**
        Behavioral **HZ51ZZZ**
        Cognitive **HZ50ZZZ**
        Cognitive-Behavioral **HZ52ZZZ**
       Confrontational **HZ58ZZZ**
        Interactive **HZ55ZZZ**
        Interpersonal **HZ54ZZZ**
        Motivational Enhancement **HZ57ZZZ**
        Psychoanalysis **HZ5BZZZ**
        Psychodynamic **HZ5CZZZ**
        Psychoeducation **HZ56ZZZ**
        Psychophysiological **HZ5DZZZ**
        Supportive **HZ59ZZZ**
Substantia nigra *use* Basal Ganglia
Subtalar (talocalcaneal) joint
    use Joint, Tarsal, Right
    use Joint, Tarsal, Left

Subtalar ligament
  use Bursa and Ligament, Foot, Left
  use Bursa and Ligament, Foot, Right
Subthalamic nucleus *use* Basal Ganglia
Suction *see* Drainage
Suction curettage (D & C), nonobstetric *see* Extraction, Endometrium **0UDB**
Suction curettage, obstetric post-delivery *see* Extraction, Products of Conception, Retained **10D1**
Superficial circumflex iliac vein
  use Vein, Greater Saphenous, Left
  use Vein, Greater Saphenous, Right
Superficial epigastric artery
  use Artery, Femoral, Left
  use Artery, Femoral, Right
Superficial epigastric vein
  use Vein, Greater Saphenous, Left
  use Vein, Greater Saphenous, Right
Superficial Inferior Epigastric Artery Flap
  Bilateral **0HRV078**
  Left **0HRU078**
  Right **0HRT078**
Superficial palmar arch
  use Artery, Hand, Left
  use Artery, Hand, Right
Superficial palmar venous arch
  use Vein, Hand, Left
  use Vein, Hand, Right
Superficial temporal artery
  use Artery, Temporal, Left
  use Artery, Temporal, Right
Superficial transverse perineal muscle *use* Muscle, Perineum
Superior cardiac nerve *use* Nerve, Thoracic Sympathetic
Superior cerebellar vein *use* Vein, Intracranial
Superior cerebral vein *use* Vein, Intracranial
Superior clunic (cluneal) nerve *use* Nerve, Lumbar
Superior epigastric artery
  use Artery, Internal Mammary, Left
  use Artery, Internal Mammary, Right
Superior genicular artery
  use Artery, Popliteal, Left
  use Artery, Popliteal, Right
Superior gluteal artery
  use Artery, Internal Iliac, Left
  use Artery, Internal Iliac, Right
Superior gluteal nerve *use* Nerve, Lumbar Plexus
Superior hypogastric plexus *use* Nerve, Abdominal Sympathetic
Superior labial artery *use* Artery, Face
Superior laryngeal artery
  use Artery, Thyroid, Left
  use Artery, Thyroid, Right
Superior laryngeal nerve *use* Nerve, Vagus
Superior longitudinal muscle *use* Muscle, Tongue, Palate, Pharynx
Superior mesenteric ganglion *use* Nerve, Abdominal Sympathetic
Superior mesenteric lymph node *use* Lymphatic, Mesenteric
Superior mesenteric plexus *use* Nerve, Abdominal Sympathetic

Superior oblique muscle
  use Muscle, Extraocular, Left
  use Muscle, Extraocular, Right
Superior olivary nucleus *use* Pons
Superior rectal artery *use* Artery, Inferior Mesenteric
Superior rectal vein *use* Vein, Inferior Mesenteric
Superior rectus muscle
  use Muscle, Extraocular, Left
  use Muscle, Extraocular, Right
Superior tarsal plate
  use Eyelid, Upper, Left
  use Eyelid, Upper, Right
Superior thoracic artery
  use Artery, Axillary, Left
  use Artery, Axillary, Right
Superior thyroid artery
  use Artery, External Carotid, Left
  use Artery, External Carotid, Right
  use Artery, Thyroid, Left
  use Artery, Thyroid, Right
Superior turbinate *use* Turbinate, Nasal
Superior ulnar collateral artery
  use Artery, Brachial, Left
  use Artery, Brachial, Right
Supplement
  Abdominal Wall **0WUF**
  Acetabulum
    Left **0QU5**
    Right **0QU4**
  Ampulla of Vater **0FUC**
  Anal Sphincter **0DUR**
  Ankle Region
    Left **0YUL**
    Right **0YUK**
  Anus **0DUQ**
  Aorta
    Abdominal **04U0**
    Thoracic
      Ascending/Arch **02UX**
      Descending **02UW**
  Arm
    Lower
      Left **0XUF**
      Right **0XUD**
    Upper
      Left **0XU9**
      Right **0XU8**
  Artery
    Anterior Tibial
      Left **04UQ**
      Right **04UP**
    Axillary
      Left **03U6**
      Right **03U5**
    Brachial
      Left **03U8**
      Right **03U7**
    Celiac **04U1**
    Colic
      Left **04U7**
      Middle **04U8**
      Right **04U6**
    Common Carotid
      Left **03UJ**

Supplement *(continued)*
      Right **03UH**
    Common Iliac
      Left **04UD**
      Right **04UC**
    External Carotid
      Left **03UN**
      Right **03UM**
    External Iliac
      Left **04UJ**
      Right **04UH**
    Face **03UR**
    Femoral
      Left **04UL**
      Right **04UK**
    Foot
      Left **04UW**
      Right **04UV**
    Gastric **04U2**
    Hand
      Left **03UF**
      Right **03UD**
    Hepatic **04U3**
    Inferior Mesenteric **04UB**
    Innominate **03U2**
    Internal Carotid
      Left **03UL**
      Right **03UK**
    Internal Iliac
      Left **04UF**
      Right **04UE**
    Internal Mammary
      Left **03U1**
      Right **03U0**
    Intracranial **03UG**
    Lower **04UY**
    Peroneal
      Left **04UU**
      Right **04UT**
    Popliteal
      Left **04UN**
      Right **04UM**
    Posterior Tibial
      Left **04US**
      Right **04UR**
    Pulmonary
      Left **02UR**
      Right **02UQ**
    Pulmonary Trunk **02UP**
    Radial
      Left **03UC**
      Right **03UB**
    Renal
      Left **04UA**
      Right **04U9**
    Splenic **04U4**
    Subclavian
      Left **03U4**
      Right **03U3**
    Superior Mesenteric **04U5**
    Temporal
      Left **03UT**
      Right **03US**
    Thyroid
      Left **03UV**
      Right **03UU**

Supplement *(continued)*
- Ulnar
  - Left **03UA**
  - Right **03U9**
  - Upper **03UY**
- Vertebral
  - Left **03UQ**
  - Right **03UP**
- Atrium
  - Left **02U7**
  - Right **02U6**
- Auditory Ossicle
  - Left **09UA0**
  - Right **09U90**
- Axilla
  - Left **0XU5**
  - Right **0XU4**
- Back
  - Lower **0WUL**
  - Upper **0WUK**
- Bladder **0TUB**
- Bladder Neck **0TUC**
- Bone
  - Ethmoid
    - Left **0NUG**
    - Right **0NUF**
  - Frontal
    - Left **0NU2**
    - Right **0NU1**
  - Hyoid **0NUX**
  - Lacrimal
    - Left **0NUJ**
    - Right **0NUH**
  - Nasal **0NUB**
  - Occipital
    - Left **0NU8**
    - Right **0NU7**
  - Palatine
    - Left **0NUL**
    - Right **0NUK**
  - Parietal
    - Left **0NU4**
    - Right **0NU3**
  - Pelvic
    - Left **0QU3**
    - Right **0QU2**
  - Sphenoid
    - Left **0NUD**
    - Right **0NUC**
  - Temporal
    - Left **0NU6**
    - Right **0NU5**
  - Zygomatic
    - Left **0NUN**
    - Right **0NUM**
- Breast
  - Bilateral **0HUV**
  - Left **0HUU**
  - Right **0HUT**
- Bronchus
  - Lingula **0BU9**
  - Lower Lobe
    - Left **0BUB**
    - Right **0BU6**
  - Main
    - Left **0BU7**

Supplement *(continued)*
- Right **0BU3**
- Middle Lobe, Right **0BU5**
- Upper Lobe
  - Left **0BU8**
  - Right **0BU4**
- Buccal Mucosa **0CU4**
- Bursa and Ligament
  - Abdomen
    - Left **0MUJ**
    - Right **0MUH**
  - Ankle
    - Left **0MUR**
    - Right **0MUQ**
  - Elbow
    - Left **0MU4**
    - Right **0MU3**
  - Foot
    - Left **0MUT**
    - Right **0MUS**
  - Hand
    - Left **0MU8**
    - Right **0MU7**
  - Head and Neck **0MU0**
  - Hip
    - Left **0MUM**
    - Right **0MUL**
  - Knee
    - Left **0MUP**
    - Right **0MUN**
  - Lower Extremity
    - Left **0MUW**
    - Right **0MUV**
  - Perineum **0MUK**
  - Shoulder
    - Left **0MU2**
    - Right **0MU1**
  - Thorax
    - Left **0MUG**
    - Right **0MUF**
  - Trunk
    - Left **0MUD**
    - Right **0MUC**
  - Upper Extremity
    - Left **0MUB**
    - Right **0MU9**
  - Wrist
    - Left **0MU6**
    - Right **0MU5**
- Buttock
  - Left **0YU1**
  - Right **0YU0**
- Carina **0BU2**
- Carpal
  - Left **0PUN**
  - Right **0PUM**
- Cecum **0DUH**
- Cerebral Meninges **00U1**
- Chest Wall **0WU8**
- Chordae Tendineae **02U9**
- Cisterna Chyli **07UL**
- Clavicle
  - Left **0PUB**
  - Right **0PU9**
- Clitoris **0UUJ**
- Coccyx **0QUS**

Supplement *(continued)*
- Colon
  - Ascending **0DUK**
  - Descending **0DUM**
  - Sigmoid **0DUN**
  - Transverse **0DUL**
- Cord
  - Bilateral **0VUH**
  - Left **0VUG**
  - Right **0VUF**
- Cornea
  - Left **08U9**
  - Right **08U8**
- Cul-de-sac **0UUF**
- Diaphragm
  - Left **0BUS**
  - Right **0BUR**
- Disc
  - Cervical Vertebral **0RU3**
  - Cervicothoracic Vertebral **0RU5**
  - Lumbar Vertebral **0SU2**
  - Lumbosacral **0SU4**
  - Thoracic Vertebral **0RU9**
  - Thoracolumbar Vertebral **0RUB**
- Duct
  - Common Bile **0FU9**
  - Cystic **0FU8**
  - Hepatic
    - Left **0FU6**
    - Right **0FU5**
  - Lacrimal
    - Left **08UY**
    - Right **08UX**
  - Pancreatic **0FUD**
    - Accessory **0FUF**
- Duodenum **0DU9**
- Dura Mater **00U2**
- Ear
  - External
    - Bilateral **09U2**
    - Left **09U1**
    - Right **09U0**
  - Inner
    - Left **09UE0**
    - Right **09UD0**
  - Middle
    - Left **09U60**
    - Right **09U50**
- Elbow Region
  - Left **0XUC**
  - Right **0XUB**
- Epididymis
  - Bilateral **0VUL**
  - Left **0VUK**
  - Right **0VUJ**
- Epiglottis **0CUR**
- Esophagogastric Junction **0DU4**
- Esophagus **0DU5**
  - Lower **0DU3**
  - Middle **0DU2**
  - Upper **0DU1**
- Extremity
  - Lower
    - Left **0YUB**
    - Right **0YU9**
  - Upper

Supplement *(continued)*
    Left **0XU7**
    Right **0XU6**
Eye
    Left **08U1**
    Right **08U0**
Eyelid
    Lower
        Left **08UR**
        Right **08UQ**
    Upper
        Left **08UP**
        Right **08UN**
Face **0WU2**
Fallopian Tube
    Left **0UU6**
    Right **0UU5**
Fallopian Tubes, Bilateral **0UU7**
Femoral Region
    Bilateral **0YUE**
    Left **0YU8**
    Right **0YU7**
Femoral Shaft
    Left **0QU9**
    Right **0QU8**
Femur
    Lower
        Left **0QUC**
        Right **0QUB**
    Upper
        Left **0QU7**
        Right **0QU6**
Fibula
    Left **0QUK**
    Right **0QUJ**
Finger
    Index
        Left **0XUP**
        Right **0XUN**
    Little
        Left **0XUW**
        Right **0XUV**
    Middle
        Left **0XUR**
        Right **0XUQ**
    Ring
        Left **0XUT**
        Right **0XUS**
Foot
    Left **0YUN**
    Right **0YUM**
Gingiva
    Lower **0CU6**
    Upper **0CU5**
Glenoid Cavity
    Left **0PU8**
    Right **0PU7**
Hand
    Left **0XUK**
    Right **0XUJ**
Head **0WU0**
Heart **02UA**
Humeral Head
    Left **0PUD**
    Right **0PUC**
Humeral Shaft

Supplement *(continued)*
    Left **0PUG**
    Right **0PUF**
Hymen **0UUK**
Ileocecal Valve **0DUC**
Ileum **0DUB**
Inguinal Region
    Bilateral **0YUA**
    Left **0YU6**
    Right **0YU5**
Intestine
    Large **0DUE**
        Left **0DUG**
        Right **0DUF**
    Small **0DU8**
Iris
    Left **08UD**
    Right **08UC**
Jaw
    Lower **0WU5**
    Upper **0WU4**
Jejunum **0DUA**
Joint
    Acromioclavicular
        Left **0RUH**
        Right **0RUG**
    Ankle
        Left **0SUG**
        Right **0SUF**
    Carpal
        Left **0RUR**
        Right **0RUQ**
    Cervical Vertebral **0RU1**
    Cervicothoracic Vertebral **0RU4**
    Coccygeal **0SU6**
    Elbow
        Left **0RUM**
        Right **0RUL**
    Finger Phalangeal
        Left **0RUX**
        Right **0RUW**
    Hip
        Left **0SUB**
            Acetabular Surface **0SUE**
            Femoral Surface **0SUS**
        Right **0SU9**
            Acetabular Surface **0SUA**
            Femoral Surface **0SUR**
    Knee
        Left **0SUD**
            Femoral Surface **0SUU09Z**
            Tibial Surface **0SUW09Z**
        Right **0SUC**
            Femoral Surface **0SUT09Z**
            Tibial Surface **0SUV09Z**
    Lumbar Vertebral **0SU0**
    Lumbosacral **0SU3**
    Metacarpocarpal
        Left **0RUT**
        Right **0RUS**
    Metacarpophalangeal
        Left **0RUV**
        Right **0RUU**
    Metatarsal-Phalangeal
        Left **0SUN**
        Right **0SUM**

Supplement *(continued)*
    Metatarsal-Tarsal
        Left **0SUL**
        Right **0SUK**
    Occipital-cervical **0RU0**
    Sacrococcygeal **0SU5**
    Sacroiliac
        Left **0SU8**
        Right **0SU7**
    Shoulder
        Left **0RUK**
        Right **0RUJ**
    Sternoclavicular
        Left **0RUF**
        Right **0RUE**
    Tarsal
        Left **0SUJ**
        Right **0SUH**
    Temporomandibular
        Left **0RUD**
        Right **0RUC**
    Thoracic Vertebral **0RU6**
    Thoracolumbar Vertebral **0RUA**
    Toe Phalangeal
        Left **0SUQ**
        Right **0SUP**
    Wrist
        Left **0RUP**
        Right **0RUN**
Kidney Pelvis
    Left **0TU4**
    Right **0TU3**
Knee Region
    Left **0YUG**
    Right **0YUF**
Larynx **0CUS**
Leg
    Lower
        Left **0YUJ**
        Right **0YUH**
    Upper
        Left **0YUD**
        Right **0YUC**
Lip
    Lower **0CU1**
    Upper **0CU0**
Lymphatic
    Aortic **07UD**
    Axillary
        Left **07U6**
        Right **07U5**
    Head **07U0**
    Inguinal
        Left **07UJ**
        Right **07UH**
    Internal Mammary
        Left **07U9**
        Right **07U8**
    Lower Extremity
        Left **07UG**
        Right **07UF**
    Mesenteric **07UB**
    Neck
        Left **07U2**
        Right **07U1**
    Pelvis **07UC**

Thoracic Duct **07UK**
Thorax **07U7**
Upper Extremity
   Left **07U4**
   Right **07U3**
Mandible
   Left **0NUV**
   Right **0NUT**
Maxilla
   Left **0NUS**
   Right **0NUR**
Mediastinum **0WUC**
Mesentery **0DUV**
Metacarpal
   Left **0PUQ**
   Right **0PUP**
Metatarsal
   Left **0QUP**
   Right **0QUN**
Muscle
  Abdomen
    Left **0KUL**
    Right **0KUK**
  Extraocular
    Left **08UM**
    Right **08UL**
  Facial **0KU1**
  Foot
    Left **0KUW**
    Right **0KUV**
  Hand
    Left **0KUD**
    Right **0KUC**
  Head **0KU0**
  Hip
    Left **0KUP**
    Right **0KUN**
  Lower Arm and Wrist
    Left **0KUB**
    Right **0KU9**
  Lower Leg
    Left **0KUT**
    Right **0KUS**
  Neck
    Left **0KU3**
    Right **0KU2**
  Papillary **02UD**
  Perineum **0KUM**
  Shoulder
    Left **0KU6**
    Right **0KU5**
  Thorax
    Left **0KUJ**
    Right **0KUH**
  Tongue, Palate, Pharynx **0KU4**
  Trunk
    Left **0KUG**
    Right **0KUF**
  Upper Arm
    Left **0KU8**
    Right **0KU7**
  Upper Leg
    Left **0KUR**
    Right **0KUQ**
Nasopharynx **09UN**

Neck **0WU6**
Nerve
  Abducens **00UL**
  Accessory **00UR**
  Acoustic **00UN**
  Cervical **01U1**
  Facial **00UM**
  Femoral **01UD**
  Glossopharyngeal **00UP**
  Hypoglossal **00US**
  Lumbar **01UB**
  Median **01U5**
  Oculomotor **00UH**
  Olfactory **00UF**
  Optic **00UG**
  Peroneal **01UH**
  Phrenic **01U2**
  Pudendal **01UC**
  Radial **01U6**
  Sacral **01UR**
  Sciatic **01UF**
  Thoracic **01U8**
  Tibial **01UG**
  Trigeminal **00UK**
  Trochlear **00UJ**
  Ulnar **01U4**
  Vagus **00UQ**
Nipple
  Left **0HUX**
  Right **0HUW**
Nose **09UK**
Omentum
  Greater **0DUS**
  Lesser **0DUT**
Orbit
  Left **0NUQ**
  Right **0NUP**
Palate
  Hard **0CU2**
  Soft **0CU3**
Patella
  Left **0QUF**
  Right **0QUD**
Penis **0VUS**
Pericardium **02UN**
Perineum
  Female **0WUN**
  Male **0WUM**
Peritoneum **0DUW**
Phalanx
  Finger
    Left **0PUV**
    Right **0PUT**
  Thumb
    Left **0PUS**
    Right **0PUR**
  Toe
    Left **0QUR**
    Right **0QUQ**
Pharynx **0CUM**
Prepuce **0VUT**
Radius
  Left **0PUJ**
  Right **0PUH**
Rectum **0DUP**

Retina
  Left **08UF**
  Right **08UE**
Retinal Vessel
  Left **08UH**
  Right **08UG**
Rib
  Left **0PU2**
  Right **0PU1**
Sacrum **0QU1**
Scapula
  Left **0PU6**
  Right **0PU5**
Scrotum **0VU5**
Septum
  Atrial **02U5**
  Nasal **09UM**
  Ventricular **02UM**
Shoulder Region
  Left **0XU3**
  Right **0XU2**
Skull **0NU0**
Spinal Meninges **00UT**
Sternum **0PU0**
Stomach **0DU6**
  Pylorus **0DU7**
Subcutaneous Tissue and Fascia
  Abdomen **0JU8**
  Back **0JU7**
  Buttock **0JU9**
  Chest **0JU6**
  Face **0JU1**
  Foot
    Left **0JUR**
    Right **0JUQ**
  Hand
    Left **0JUK**
    Right **0JUJ**
  Lower Arm
    Left **0JUH**
    Right **0JUG**
  Lower Leg
    Left **0JUP**
    Right **0JUN**
  Neck
    Anterior **0JU4**
    Posterior **0JU5**
  Pelvic Region **0JUC**
  Perineum **0JUB**
  Scalp **0JU0**
  Upper Arm
    Left **0JUF**
    Right **0JUD**
  Upper Leg
    Left **0JUM**
    Right **0JUL**
Tarsal
  Left **0QUM**
  Right **0QUL**
Tendon
  Abdomen
    Left **0LUG**
    Right **0LUF**
  Ankle
    Left **0LUT**

Supplement *(continued)*
    Right **0LUS**
  Foot
    Left **0LUW**
    Right **0LUV**
  Hand
    Left **0LU8**
    Right **0LU7**
  Head and Neck **0LU0**
  Hip
    Left **0LUK**
    Right **0LUJ**
  Knee
    Left **0LUR**
    Right **0LUQ**
  Lower Arm and Wrist
    Left **0LU6**
    Right **0LU5**
  Lower Leg
    Left **0LUP**
    Right **0LUN**
  Perineum **0LUH**
  Shoulder
    Left **0LU2**
    Right **0LU1**
  Thorax
    Left **0LUD**
    Right **0LUC**
  Trunk
    Left **0LUB**
    Right **0LU9**
  Upper Arm
    Left **0LU4**
    Right **0LU3**
  Upper Leg
    Left **0LUM**
    Right **0LUL**
Testis
  Bilateral **0VUC0**
  Left **0VUB0**
  Right **0VU90**
Thumb
  Left **0XUM**
  Right **0XUL**
Tibia
  Left **0QUH**
  Right **0QUG**
Toe
  1st
    Left **0YUQ**
    Right **0YUP**
  2nd
    Left **0YUS**
    Right **0YUR**
  3rd
    Left **0YUU**
    Right **0YUT**
  4th
    Left **0YUW**
    Right **0YUV**
  5th
    Left **0YUY**
    Right **0YUX**
Tongue **0CU7**
Trachea **0BU1**
Tunica Vaginalis

Supplement *(continued)*
  Left **0VU7**
  Right **0VU6**
Turbinate, Nasal **09UL**
Tympanic Membrane
  Left **09U8**
  Right **09U7**
Ulna
  Left **0PUL**
  Right **0PUK**
Ureter
  Left **0TU7**
  Right **0TU6**
Urethra **0TUD**
Uterine Supporting Structure **0UU4**
Uvula **0CUN**
Vagina **0UUG**
Valve
  Aortic **02UF**
  Mitral **02UG**
  Pulmonary **02UH**
  Tricuspid **02UJ**
Vas Deferens
  Bilateral **0VUQ**
  Left **0VUP**
  Right **0VUN**
Vein
  Axillary
    Left **05U8**
    Right **05U7**
  Azygos **05U0**
  Basilic
    Left **05UC**
    Right **05UB**
  Brachial
    Left **05UA**
    Right **05U9**
  Cephalic
    Left **05UF**
    Right **05UD**
  Colic **06U7**
  Common Iliac
    Left **06UD**
    Right **06UC**
  Esophageal **06U3**
  External Iliac
    Left **06UG**
    Right **06UF**
  External Jugular
    Left **05UQ**
    Right **05UP**
  Face
    Left **05UV**
    Right **05UT**
  Femoral
    Left **06UN**
    Right **06UM**
  Foot
    Left **06UV**
    Right **06UT**
  Gastric **06U2**
  Greater Saphenous
    Left **06UQ**
    Right **06UP**
  Hand
    Left **05UH**

Supplement *(continued)*
    Right **05UG**
  Hemiazygos **05U1**
  Hepatic **06U4**
  Hypogastric
    Left **06UJ**
    Right **06UH**
  Inferior Mesenteric **06U6**
  Right **05U3**
  Internal Jugular
    Left **05UN**
    Right **05UM**
  Intracranial **05UL**
  Lesser Saphenous
    Left **06US**
    Right **06UR**
  Lower **06UY**
  Portal **06U8**
  Pulmonary
    Left **02UT**
    Right **02US**
  Renal
    Left **06UB**
    Right **06U9**
  Splenic **06U1**
  Subclavian
    Left **05U6**
    Right **05U5**
  Superior Mesenteric **06U5**
  Upper **05UY**
  Vertebral
    Left **05US**
    Right **05UR**
  Vena Cava
    Inferior **06U0**
    Superior **02UV**
  Ventricle
    Left **02UL**
  Right **02UK**
  Vertebra
  Cervical **0PU3**
  Lumbar **0QU0**
  Thoracic **0PU4**
  Vesicle
  Bilateral **0VU3**
  Left **0VU2**
  Right **0VU1**
  Vocal Cord
    Left **0CUV**
    Right **0CUT**
  Vulva **0UUM**
  Wrist Region
    Left **0XUH**
    Right **0XUG**
Supraclavicular (Virchow's) lymph node
  use Lymphatic, Neck, Left
  use Lymphatic, Neck, Right
Supraclavicular nerve *use* Nerve, Cervical Plexus
Suprahyoid lymph node *use* Lymphatic, Head
Suprahyoid muscle
  use Muscle, Neck, Right
  use Muscle, Neck, Left
Suprainguinal lymph node *use* Lymphatic, Pelvis

Supraorbital vein
   use Vein, Face, Left
   use Vein, Face, Right
Suprarenal gland
   use Gland, Adrenal
   use Gland, Adrenal, Bilateral
   use Gland, Adrenal, Left
   use Gland, Adrenal, Right
Suprarenal plexus *use* Nerve, Abdominal
   Sympathetic
Suprascapular nerve *use* Nerve, Brachial
   Plexus
Supraspinatus fascia
   use Subcutaneous Tissue and Fascia, Upper
   Arm, Right
   use Subcutaneous Tissue and Fascia, Upper
   Arm, Left
Supraspinatus muscle
   use Muscle, Shoulder, Right
   use Muscle, Shoulder, Left
Supraspinous ligament
   use Bursa and Ligament, Trunk, Right
   use Bursa and Ligament, Trunk, Left
Suprasternal notch *use* Sternum
Supratrochlear lymph node
   use Lymphatic, Upper Extremity, Right
   use Lymphatic, Upper Extremity, Left
Sural artery
   use Artery, Popliteal, Right
   use Artery, Popliteal, Left
Suspension
   Bladder Neck *see* Reposition, Bladder Neck
      0TSC
   Kidney *see* Reposition, Urinary System **0TS**
   Urethra *see* Reposition, Urinary System **0TS**
Suspension *(continued)*
   Urethrovesical *see* Reposition, Bladder Neck
      0TSC
   Uterus *see* Reposition, Uterus **0US9**
   Vagina *see* Reposition, Vagina **0USG**
Suture
   Laceration repair *see* Repair
   Ligation *see* Occlusion
Suture Removal
   Extremity
      Lower **8E0YXY8**
      Upper **8E0XXY8**
   Head and Neck Region **8E09XY8**
   Trunk Region **8E0WXY8**
Sutureless valve, Perceval *use* Zooplastic
   Tissue, Rapid Deployment Technique in
   New Technology
Sweat gland *use* Skin
Sympathectomy *see* Excision, Peripheral
   Nervous System **01B**
SynCardia Total Artificial Heart *use*
   Synthetic Substitute
Synchra CRT-P *use* Cardiac
   Resynchronization Pacemaker Pulse
   Generator in **0JH**
Synechiotomy, iris *see* Release, Eye **08N**
Synovectomy
   Lower joint *see* Excision, Lower Joints **0SB**
   Upper joint *see* Excision, Upper Joints **0RB**
Systemic Nuclear Medicine Therapy
   Abdomen **CW70**
   Anatomical Regions, Multiple **CW7YYZZ**

Systemic Nuclear Medicine Therapy
   (continued)
   Chest **CW73**
   Thyroid **CW7G**
   Whole Body **CW7N**

T

Takedown
   Arteriovenous shunt *see* Removal of device
   from, Upper Arteries **03P**
Takedown *(continued)*
   Arteriovenous shunt, with creation of new
   shunt *see* Bypass, Upper Arteries **031**
   Stoma *see* Repair
Talent® Converter *use* Intraluminal Device
Talent® Occluder *use* Intraluminal Device
Talent® Stent Graft (abdominal)(thoracic)
   use Intraluminal Device
Talocalcaneal (subtalar) joint
   use Joint, Tarsal, Left
   use Joint, Tarsal, Right
Talocalcaneal ligament
   use Bursa and Ligament, Foot, Left
   use Bursa and Ligament, Foot, Right
Talocalcaneonavicular joint
   use Joint, Tarsal, Right
   use Joint, Tarsal, Left
Talocalcaneonavicular ligament
   use Bursa and Ligament, Foot, Left
   use Bursa and Ligament, Foot, Right
Talocrural joint
   use Joint, Ankle, Right
   use Joint, Ankle, Left
Talofibular ligament
   use Bursa and Ligament, Ankle, Left
   use Bursa and Ligament, Ankle, Right
Talus bone
   use Tarsal, Left
   use Tarsal, Right
TandemHeart® System *use* External Heart
   Assist System in Heart and Great Vessels
Tarsectomy
   see Excision, Lower Bones **0QB**
   see Resection, Lower Bones **0QT**
Tarsometatarsal joint
   use Joint, Metatarsal-Tarsal, Left
   use Joint, Metatarsal-Tarsal, Right
Tarsometatarsal ligament
   use Bursa and Ligament, Foot, Left
   use Bursa and Ligament, Foot, Right
Tarsorrhaphy *see* Repair, Eye **08Q**
Tattooing
   Cornea **3E0CXMZ**
   Skin *see* Introduction of substance in or on,
   Skin **3E00**
**TAXUS® Liberté® Paclitaxel-eluting
   Coronary Stent System** *use* Intraluminal
   Device, Drug-eluting in Heart and Great
   Vessels
TBNA (transbronchial needle aspiration) *see*
   Drainage, Respiratory System **0B9**
Telemetry 4A12X4Z
   Ambulatory **4A12X45**
Temperature gradient study 4A0ZXKZ
Temporal lobe *use* Cerebral Hemisphere

Temporalis muscle *use* Muscle, Head
Temporoparietalis muscle *use* Muscle, Head
Tendolysis *see* Release, Tendons **0LN**
Tendonectomy
   see Excision, Tendons **0LB**
   see Resection, Tendons **0LT**
Tendonoplasty, tenoplasty
   see Repair, Tendons **0LQ**
   see Replacement, Tendons **0LR**
   see Supplement, Tendons **0LU**
Tendorrhaphy *see* Repair, Tendons **0LQ**
Tendototomy
   see Division, Tendons **0L8**
   see Drainage, Tendons **0L9**
Tenectomy, tenonectomy
   see Excision, Tendons **0LB**
   see Resection, Tendons **0LT** Tenolysis *see*
   Release, Tendons **0LN**
Tenontorrhaphy *see* Repair, Tendons **0LQ**
Tenontotomy
   see Division, Tendons **0L8**
   see Drainage, Tendons **0L9**
Tenorrhaphy *see* Repair, Tendons **0LQ**
Tenosynovectomy
   see Excision, Tendons **0LB**
   see Resection, Tendons **0LT**
Tenotomy
   see Division, Tendons **0L8**
   see Drainage, Tendons **0L9**
Tensor fasciae latae muscle
   use Muscle, Hip, Left
   use Muscle, Hip, Right
Tensor veli palatini muscle *use* Muscle,
   Tongue, Palate, Pharynx
Tenth cranial nerve *use* Nerve, Vagus
Tentorium cerebelli *use* Dura Mater
Teres major muscle
   use Muscle, Shoulder, Left
   use Muscle, Shoulder, Right
Teres minor muscle
   use Muscle, Shoulder, Right
   use Muscle, Shoulder, Left
Termination of pregnancy
   Aspiration curettage **10A07ZZ**
   Dilation and curettage **10A07ZZ**
   Hysterotomy **10A00ZZ**
   Intra-amniotic injection **10A03ZZ**
   Laminaria **10A07ZW**
   Vacuum **10A07Z6**
Testectomy
   see Excision, Male Reproductive System
      0VB
   see Resection, Male Reproductive System
      0VT
Testicular artery *use* Aorta, Abdominal
Testing
   Glaucoma **4A07XBZ**
   Hearing *see* Hearing Assessment, Diagnostic
   Audiology **F13**
   Mental health *see* Psychological Tests
   Muscle function, electromyography (EMG)
   see Measurement, Musculoskeletal **4A0F**
   Muscle function, manual *see* Motor Function
   Assessment, Rehabilitation **F01**

Testing *(continued)*

Neurophysiologic monitoring, intra-operative *see* Monitoring, Physiological Systems **4A1**

Range of motion *see* Motor Function Assessment, Rehabilitation **F01**

Vestibular function *see* Vestibular Assessment, Diagnostic Audiology **F15**

Thalamectomy *see* Excision, Thalamus **00B9**

Thalamotomy *see* Drainage, Thalamus **0099**

Thenar muscle

use Muscle, Hand, Right

use Muscle, Hand, Left

Therapeutic Massage

Musculoskeletal System **8E0KX1Z**

Reproductive System

Prostate **8E0VX1C**

Rectum **8E0VX1D**

Therapeutic occlusion coil(s) *use* Intraluminal Device

Thermography 4A0ZXKZ

Thermotherapy, prostate *see* Destruction, Prostate **0V50**

Third cranial nerve *use* Nerve, Oculomotor

Third occipital nerve *use* Nerve, Cervical

Third ventricle *use* Cerebral Ventricle

Thoracectomy *see* Excision, Anatomical Regions, General **0WB**

Thoracentesis *see* Drainage, Anatomical Regions, General **0W9**

Thoracic aortic plexus *use* Nerve, Thoracic Sympathetic

Thoracic esophagus *use* Esophagus, Middle

Thoracic facet joint

use Joint, Thoracic Vertebral, 2 to 7

use Joint, Thoracic Vertebral, 8 or more

use Joint, Thoracic Vertebral

Thoracic ganglion *use* Nerve, Thoracic Sympathetic

Thoracoacromial artery

use Artery, Axillary, Right

use Artery, Axillary, Left

Thoracocentesis *see* Drainage, Anatomical Regions, General **0W9**

Thoracolumbar facet joint *use* Joint, Thoracolumbar Vertebral

Thoracoplasty

see Repair, Anatomical Regions, General **0WQ**

see Supplement, Anatomical Regions, General **0WU**

Thoracostomy tube *use* Drainage Device

Thoracostomy, for lung collapse *see* Drainage, Respiratory System **0B9**

Thoracotomy *see* Drainage, Anatomical Regions, General **0W9**

Thoratec IVAD (Implantable Ventricular Assist Device) *use* Implantable Heart Assist System in Heart and Great Vessels

Thoratec Paracorporeal Ventricular Assist Device *use* External Heart Assist System in Heart and Great Vessels

Thrombectomy *see* Extirpation

Thymectomy

see Excision, Lymphatic and Hemic Systems **07B**

Thymectomy

Thymectomy *(continued)*

see Resection, Lymphatic and Hemic Systems **07T**

Thymopexy

see Repair, Lymphatic and Hemic Systems **07Q**

see Reposition, Lymphatic and Hemic Systems **07S**

Thymus gland *use* Thymus

Thyroarytenoid muscle

use Muscle, Neck, Left

use Muscle, Neck, Right

Thyrocervical trunk

use Artery, Thyroid, Left

use Artery, Thyroid, Right

Thyroid cartilage *use* Larynx

Thyroidectomy

see Excision, Endocrine System **0GB**

see Resection, Endocrine System **0GT**

Thyroidorrhaphy *see* Repair, Endocrine System **0GQ**

Thyroidoscopy 0GJK4ZZ

Thyroidotomy *see* Drainage, Endocrine System **0G9**

Tibial insert *use* Liner in Lower Joints

Tibialis anterior muscle

use Muscle, Lower Leg, Right

use Muscle, Lower Leg, Left

Tibialis posterior muscle

use Muscle, Lower Leg, Right

use Muscle, Lower Leg, Left

Tibiofemoral joint

use Joint, Knee, Left

use Joint, Knee, Left, Tibial Surface

use Joint, Knee, Right

use Joint, Knee, Right, Tibial Surface

TigerPaw® system for closure of left atrial appendage *use* Extraluminal Device

Tissue bank graft *use* Nonautologous Tissue Substitute

Tissue Expander

Insertion of device in

Breast

Bilateral **0HHV**

Left **0HHU**

Right **0HHT**

Nipple

Left **0HHX**

Right **0HHW**

Subcutaneous Tissue and Fascia

Abdomen **0JH8**

Back **0JH7**

Buttock **0JH9**

Chest **0JH6**

Face **0JH1**

Foot

Left **0JHR**

Right **0JHQ**

Hand

Left **0JHK**

Right **0JHJ**

Lower Arm

Left **0JHH**

Right **0JHG**

Lower Leg

Left **0JHP**

Tissue Expander *(continued)*

Right **0JHN**

Neck

Anterior **0JH4**

Posterior **0JH5**

Pelvic Region **0JHC**

Perineum **0JHB**

Scalp **0JH0**

Upper Arm

Left **0JHF**

Right **0JHD**

Upper Leg

Left **0JHM**

Right **0JHL**

Removal of device from

Breast

Left **0HPU**

Right **0HPT**

Subcutaneous Tissue and Fascia

Head and Neck **0JPS**

Lower Extremity **0JPW**

Trunk **0JPT**

Upper Extremity **0JPV**

Revision of device in

Breast

Left **0HWU**

Right **0HWT**

Subcutaneous Tissue and Fascia

Head and Neck **0JWS**

Lower Extremity **0JWW**

Trunk **0JWT**

Upper Extremity **0JWV**

Tissue expander (inflatable)(injectable)

use Tissue Expander in Skin and Breast

use Tissue Expander in Subcutaneous Tissue and Fascia

Titanium Sternal Fixation System (TSFS)

use Internal Fixation Device, Rigid Plate in **0PS**

use Internal Fixation Device, Rigid Plate in **0PH**

Tomographic (Tomo) Nuclear Medicine Imaging

Abdomen **CW20**

Abdomen and Chest **CW24**

Abdomen and Pelvis **CW21**

Anatomical Regions, Multiple **CW2YYZZ**

Bladder, Kidneys and Ureters **CT23**

Brain **C020**

Breast **CH2YYZZ**

Bilateral **CH22**

Left **CH21**

Right **CH20**

Bronchi and Lungs **CB22**

Central Nervous System **C02YYZZ**

Cerebrospinal Fluid **C025**

Chest **CW23**

Chest and Abdomen **CW24**

Chest and Neck **CW26**

Digestive System **CD2YYZZ**

Endocrine System **CG2YYZZ**

Extremity

Lower **CW2D**

Bilateral **CP2F**

Left **CP2D**

Right **CP2C**

Tomographic (Tomo) Nuclear Medicine Imaging *(continued)*
  Upper **CW2M**
    Bilateral **CP2B**
    Left **CP29**
    Right **CP28**
  Gallbladder **CF24**
  Gastrointestinal Tract **CD27**
  Gland, Parathyroid **CG21**
  Head and Neck **CW2B**
  Heart **C22YYZZ**
    Right and Left **C226**
  Hepatobiliary System and Pancreas **CF2YYZZ**
  Kidneys, Ureters and Bladder **CT23**
  Liver **CF25**
  Liver and Spleen **CF26**
  Lungs and Bronchi **CB22**
  Lymphatics and Hematologic System **C72YYZZ**
  Musculoskeletal System, Other **CP2YYZZ**
  Myocardium **C22G**
  Neck and Chest **CW26**
  Neck and Head **CW2B**
  Pancreas and Hepatobiliary System **CF2YYZZ**
  Pelvic Region **CW2J**
  Pelvis **CP26**
  Pelvis and Abdomen **CW21**
  Pelvis and Spine **CP27**
  Respiratory System **CB2YYZZ**
  Skin **CH2YYZZ**
  Skull **CP21**
  Skull and Cervical Spine **CP23**
  Spine
    Cervical **CP22**
    Cervical and Skull **CP23**
    Lumbar **CP2H**
    Thoracic **CP2G**
    Thoracolumbar **CP2J**
  Spine and Pelvis **CP27**
  Spleen **C722**
  Spleen and Liver **CF26**
  Subcutaneous Tissue **CH2YYZZ**
  Thorax **CP24**
  Ureters, Kidneys and Bladder **CT23**
  Urinary System **CT2YYZZ**
Tomography, computerized *see* Computerized Tomography (CT Scan)
Tonometry 4A07XBZ
Tongue, base of *use* Pharynx
Tonsillectomy
  see Excision, Mouth and Throat **0CB**
  see Resection, Mouth and Throat **0CT**
Tonsillotomy *see* Drainage, Mouth and Throat **0C9**
Total Anomalous Pulmonary Venous Return (TAPVR) repair
  see Bypass, Atrium, Left **0217**
  see Bypass, Vena Cava, Superior **021V**
Total artificial (replacement) heart *use* Synthetic Substitute
Total parenteral nutrition (TPN) *see* Introduction of Nutritional Substance

Trachectomy
  see Excision, Trachea **0BB1**
  see Resection, Trachea **0BT1**
Trachelectomy
  see Excision, Cervix **0UBC**
  see Resection, Cervix **0UTC**
Trachelopexy
  see Repair, Cervix **0UQC**
  see Reposition, Cervix **0USC**
Tracheloplasty *see* Repair, Cervix **0UQC**
Trachelorrhaphy *see* Repair, Cervix **0UQC**
Trachelotomy *see* Drainage, Cervix **0U9C**
Tracheobronchial lymph node *use* Lymphatic, Thorax
Tracheoesophageal fistulization 0B110D6
Tracheolysis *see* Release, Respiratory System **0BN**
Tracheoplasty
  see Repair, Respiratory System **0BQ**
  see Supplement, Respiratory System **0BU**
Tracheorrhaphy *see* Repair, Respiratory System **0BQ**
Tracheoscopy 0BJ18ZZ
Tracheostomy *see* Bypass, Respiratory System **0B1**
Tracheostomy Device
  Bypass, Trachea **0B11**
  Change device in, Trachea **0B21XFZ**
  Removal of device from, Trachea **0BP1**
  Revision of device in, Trachea **0BW1**
Tracheostomy tube *use* Tracheostomy Device in Respiratory System
Tracheotomy *see* Drainage, Respiratory System **0B9**
Traction
  Abdominal Wall **2W63X**
  Arm
    Lower
      Left **2W6DX**
      Right **2W6CX**
    Upper
      Left **2W6BX**
      Right **2W6AX**
  Back **2W65X**
  Chest Wall **2W64X**
  Extremity
    Lower
      Left **2W6MX**
      Right **2W6LX**
    Upper
      Left **2W69X**
      Right **2W68X**
  Face **2W61X**
  Finger
    Left **2W6KX**
    Right **2W6JX**
  Foot
    Left **2W6TX**
    Right **2W6SX**
  Hand
    Left **2W6FX**
    Right **2W6EX**
  Head **2W60X**
  Inguinal Region
    Left **2W67X**
    Right **2W66X**

Traction *(continued)*
  Leg
    Lower
      Left **2W6RX**
      Right **2W6QX**
    Upper
      Left **2W6PX**
      Right **2W6NX**
  Neck **2W62X**
  Thumb
    Left **2W6HX**
    Right **2W6GX**
  Toe
    Left **2W6VX**
    Right **2W6UX**
Tractotomy *see* Division, Central Nervous System **008**
Tragus
  use Ear, External, Left
  use Ear, External, Right
  use Ear, External, Bilateral
Training, caregiver *see* Caregiver Training
TRAM (transverse rectus abdominis myocutaneous) flap reconstruction
  Free *see* Replacement, Skin and Breast **0HR**
  Pedicled *see* Transfer, Muscles **0KX**
Transection *see* Division
Transfer
  Buccal Mucosa **0CX4**
  Bursa and Ligament
    Abdomen
      Left **0MXJ**
      Right **0MXH**
    Ankle
      Left **0MXR**
      Right **0MXQ**
    Elbow
      Left **0MX4**
      Right **0MX3**
    Foot
      Left **0MXT**
      Right **0MXS**
    Hand
      Left **0MX8**
      Right **0MX7**
    Head and Neck **0MX0**
    Hip
      Left **0MXM**
      Right **0MXL**
    Knee
      Left **0MXP**
      Right **0MXN**
    Lower Extremity
      Left **0MXW**
      Right **0MXV**
    Perineum **0MXK**
    Shoulder
      Left **0MX2**
      Right **0MX1**
    Thorax
      Left **0MXG**
      Right **0MXF**
    Trunk
      Left **0MXD**
      Right **0MXC**
    Upper Extremity

Transfer *(continued)*
- Left **0MXB**
- Right **0MX9**
- Wrist
  - Left **0MX6**
  - Right **0MX5**
- Finger
  - Left **0XXP0ZM**
  - Right **0XXN0ZL**
- Gingiva
  - Lower **0CX6**
  - Upper **0CX5**
- Intestine
  - Large **0DXE**
  - Small **0DX8**
- Lip
  - Lower **0CX1**
  - Upper **0CX0**
- Muscle
  - Abdomen
    - Left **0KXL**
    - Right **0KXK**
  - Extraocular
    - Left **08XM**
    - Right **08XL**
  - Facial **0KX1**
  - Foot
    - Left **0KXW**
    - Right **0KXV**
  - Hand
    - Left **0KXD**
    - Right **0KXC**
  - Head **0KX0**
  - Hip
    - Left **0KXP**
    - Right **0KXN**
  - Lower Arm and Wrist
    - Left **0KXB**
    - Right **0KX9**
  - Lower Leg
    - Left **0KXT**
    - Right **0KXS**
  - Neck
    - Left **0KX3**
    - Right **0KX2**
  - Perineum **0KXM**
  - Shoulder
    - Left **0KX6**
    - Right **0KX5**
  - Thorax
    - Left **0KXJ**
    - Right **0KXH**
  - Tongue, Palate, Pharynx **0KX4**
  - Trunk
    - Left **0KXG**
    - Right **0KXF**
  - Upper Arm
    - Left **0KX8**
    - Right **0KX7**
  - Upper Leg
    - Left **0KXR**
    - Right **0KXQ**
- Nerve
  - Abducens **00XL**
  - Accessory **00XR**
  - Acoustic **00XN**

Transfer *(continued)*
- Cervical **01X1**
- Facial **00XM**
- Femoral **01XD**
- Glossopharyngeal **00XP**
- Hypoglossal **00XS**
- Lumbar **01XB**
- Median **01X5**
- Oculomotor **00XH**
- Olfactory **00XF**
- Optic **00XG**
- Peroneal **01XH**
- Phrenic **01X2**
- Pudendal **01XC**
- Radial **01X6**
- Sciatic **01XF**
- Thoracic **01X8**
- Tibial **01XG**
- Trigeminal **00XK**
- Trochlear **00XJ**
- Ulnar **01X4**
- Vagus **00XQ**
- Palate, Soft **0CX3**
- Skin
  - Abdomen **0HX7XZZ**
  - Back **0HX6XZZ**
  - Buttock **0HX8XZZ**
  - Chest **0HX5XZZ**
  - Ear
    - Left **0HX3XZZ**
    - Right **0HX2XZZ**
  - Face **0HX1XZZ**
  - Foot
    - Left **0HXNXZZ**
    - Right **0HXMXZZ**
  - Genitalia **0HXAXZZ**
  - Hand
    - Left **0HXGXZZ**
    - Right **0HXFXZZ**
  - Lower Arm
    - Left **0HXEXZZ**
    - Right **0HXDXZZ**
  - Lower Leg
    - Left **0HXLXZZ**
    - Right **0HXKXZZ**
  - Neck **0HX4XZZ**
  - Perineum **0HX9XZZ**
  - Scalp **0HX0XZZ**
  - Upper Arm
    - Left **0HXCXZZ**
    - Right **0HXBXZZ**
  - Upper Leg
    - Left **0HXJXZZ**
    - Right **0HXHXZZ**
- Stomach **0DX6**
- Subcutaneous Tissue and Fascia
  - Abdomen **0JX8**
  - Back **0JX7**
  - Buttock **0JX9**
  - Chest **0JX6**
  - Face **0JX1**
  - Foot
    - Left **0JXR**
    - Right **0JXQ**
  - Hand
    - Left **0JXK**

Transfer *(continued)*
- Right **0JXJ**
- Lower Arm
  - Left **0JXH**
  - Right **0JXG**
- Lower Leg
  - Left **0JXP**
  - Right **0JXN**
- Neck
  - Anterior **0JX4**
  - Posterior **0JX5**
- Pelvic Region **0JXC**
- Perineum **0JXB**
- Scalp **0JX0**
- Upper Arm
  - Left **0JXF**
  - Right **0JXD**
- Upper Leg
  - Left **0JXM**
  - Right **0JXL**
- Tendon
  - Abdomen
    - Left **0LXG**
    - Right **0LXF**
  - Ankle
    - Left **0LXT**
    - Right **0LXS**
  - Foot
    - Left **0LXW**
    - Right **0LXV**
  - Hand
    - Left **0LX8**
    - Right **0LX7**
  - Head and Neck **0LX0**
  - Hip
    - Left **0LXK**
    - Right **0LXJ**
  - Knee
    - Left **0LXR**
    - Right **0LXQ**
  - Lower Arm and Wrist
    - Left **0LX6**
    - Right **0LX5**
  - Lower Leg
    - Left **0LXP**
    - Right **0LXN**
  - Perineum **0LXH**
  - Shoulder
    - Left **0LX2**
    - Right **0LX1**
  - Thorax
    - Left **0LXD**
    - Right **0LXC**
  - Trunk
    - Left **0LXB**
    - Right **0LX9**
  - Upper Arm
    - Left **0LX4**
    - Right **0LX3**
  - Upper Leg
    - Left **0LXM**
    - Right **0LXL**
- Tongue **0CX7**

Transfusion
- Artery
  - Central

Transfusion *(continued)*
    Antihemophilic Factors **3026**
    Blood
        Platelets **3026**
        Red Cells **3026**
        Frozen **3026**
           White Cells **3026**
           Whole **3026**
        Bone Marrow **3026**
        Factor IX **3026**
        Fibrinogen **3026**
        Globulin **3026**
        Plasma
           Fresh **3026**
           Frozen **3026**
        Plasma Cryoprecipitate **3026**
        Serum Albumin **3026**
        Stem Cells
           Cord Blood **3026**
           Hematopoietic **3026**
    Peripheral
        Antihemophilic Factors **3025**
        Blood
           Platelets **3025**
           Red Cells **3025**
        Frozen **3025**
           White Cells **3025**
           Whole **3025**
        Bone Marrow **3025**
        Factor IX **3025**
        Fibrinogen **3025**
        Globulin **3025**
        Plasma
           Fresh **3025**
           Frozen **3025**
        Plasma Cryoprecipitate **3025**
        Serum Albumin **3025**
        Stem Cells
           Cord Blood **3025**
           Hematopoietic **3025**
    Products of Conception
    Antihemophilic Factors **3027**
    Blood
        Platelets **3027**
        Red Cells **3027**
           Frozen **3027**
        White Cells **3027**
        Whole **3027**
        Factor IX **3027**
        Fibrinogen **3027**
        Globulin **3027**
        Plasma
           Fresh **3027**
           Frozen **3027**
        Plasma Cryoprecipitate **3027**
        Serum Albumin **3027**
    Vein
        4-Factor Prothrombin Complex
    Concentrate **3028[03]B1**
        Central
        Antihemophilic Factors **3024**
        Blood
           Platelets **3024**
           Red Cells **3024**
        Frozen **3024**
           White Cells **3024**

Transfusion *(continued)*
           Whole **3024**
        Bone Marrow **3024**
        Factor IX **3024**
        Fibrinogen **3024**
        Globulin **3024**
        Plasma
           Fresh **3024**
           Frozen **3024**
        Plasma Cryoprecipitate **3024**
        Serum Albumin **3024**
        Stem Cells
           Cord Blood **3024**
           Embryonic **3024**
           Hematopoietic **3024**
        Peripheral
           Antihemophilic Factors **3023**
           Blood
               Platelets **3023**
               Red Cells **3023**
           Frozen **3023**
               White Cells **3023**
               Whole **3023**
           Bone Marrow **3023**
           Factor IX **3023**
           Fibrinogen **3023**
           Globulin **3023**
           Plasma
               Fresh **3023**
               Frozen **3023**
           Plasma Cryoprecipitate **3023**
           Serum Albumin **3023**
           Stem Cells
               Cord Blood **3023**
               Embryonic **3023**
               Hematopoietic **3023**
Tranplant see Transplantation
Transplantation
    Bone marrow see Transfusion, Circulatory
    302
    Esophagus **0DY50Z**
    Face **0WY20Z**
    Hand
        Left **0XYK0Z**
        Right **0XYJ0Z**
    Heart **02YA0Z**
    Hematopoietic cell see Transfusion,
        Circulatory **302**
    Intestine
        Large **0DYE0Z**
        Small **0DY80Z**
    Kidney
        Left **0TY10Z**
        Right **0TY00Z**
    Liver **0FY00Z**
    Lung
        Bilateral **0BYM0Z**
        Left **0BYL0Z**
        Lower Lobe
           Left **0BYJ0Z**
           Right **0BYF0Z**
        Middle Lobe, Right **0BYD0Z**
        Right **0BYK0Z**
        Upper Lobe
           Left **0BYG0Z**
           Right **0BYC0Z**

Transplantation *(continued)*
    Lung Lingula **0BYH0Z**
    Ovary
        Left **0UY10Z**
        Right **0UY00Z**
    Pancreas **0FYG0Z**
    Products of Conception **10Y0**
    Spleen **07YP0Z**
    Stem cell see Transfusion, Circulatory **302**
    Stomach **0DY60Z**
    Thymus **07YM0Z**
Transposition
    see Reposition
    see Transfer
Transversalis fascia *use* Subcutaneous Tissue
    and Fascia, Trunk
Transverse (cutaneous) cervical nerve *use*
    Nerve, Cervical Plexus
Transverse acetabular ligament
    use Bursa and Ligament, Hip, Left
    use Bursa and Ligament, Hip, Right
Transverse facial artery
    use Artery, Temporal, Left
    use Artery, Temporal, Right
Transverse humeral ligament
    use Bursa and Ligament, Shoulder, Left
    use Bursa and Ligament, Shoulder, Right
Transverse ligament of atlas *use* Bursa and
    Ligament, Head and Neck
Transverse Rectus Abdominis
    Myocutaneous Flap
    Replacement
        Bilateral **0HRV076**
        Left **0HRU076**
        Right **0HRT076**
    Transfer
        Left **0KXL**
        Right **0KXK**
Transverse scapular ligament
    use Bursa and Ligament, Shoulder, Left
    use Bursa and Ligament, Shoulder, Right
Transverse thoracis muscle
    use Muscle, Thorax, Right
    use Muscle, Thorax, Left
Transversospinalis muscle
    use Muscle, Trunk, Right
    use Muscle, Trunk, Left
Transversus abdominis muscle
    use Muscle, Abdomen, Left
    use Muscle, Abdomen, Right
Trapezium bone
    use Carpal, Right
    use Carpal, Left
Trapezius muscle
    use Muscle, Trunk, Right
    use Muscle, Trunk, Left
Trapezoid bone
    use Carpal, Right
    use Carpal, Left
Triceps brachii muscle
    use Muscle, Upper Arm, Right
    use Muscle, Upper Arm, Left
Tricuspid annulus *use* Valve, Tricuspid
Trifacial nerve *use* Nerve, Trigeminal
Trifecta™ Valve (aortic) *use* Zooplastic
    Tissue in Heart and Great Vessels

Trigone of bladder *use* Bladder
Trimming, excisional *see* Excision
Triquetral bone
  use Carpal, Right
  use Carpal, Left
Trochanteric bursa
  use Bursa and Ligament, Hip, Right
  use Bursa and Ligament, Hip, Left
TUMT (Transurethral microwave thermotherapy of prostate) 0V507ZZ
TUNA (transurethral needle ablation of prostate) 0V507ZZ
Tunneled central venous catheter *use* Vascular Access Device in Subcutaneous Tissue and Fascia
Tunneled spinal (intrathecal) catheter *use* Infusion Device
Turbinectomy
  see Excision, Ear, Nose, Sinus **09B**
  see Resection, Ear, Nose, Sinus **09T**
Turbinoplasty
  see Repair, Ear, Nose, Sinus **09Q**
  see Replacement, Ear, Nose, Sinus **09R**
  see Supplement, Ear, Nose, Sinus **09U**
Turbinotomy
  see Drainage, Ear, Nose, Sinus **099**
  see Division, Ear, Nose, Sinus **098**
TURP (transurethral resection of prostate) 0VB07ZZ
Twelfth cranial nerve *use* Nerve, Hypoglossal
Two lead pacemaker *use* Pacemaker, Dual Chamber in **0JH**
Tympanic cavity
  use Ear, Middle, Left
  use Ear, Middle, Right
Tympanic nerve *use* Nerve, Glossopharyngeal
Tympanic part of temporal bone
  use Bone, Temporal, Right
  use Bone, Temporal, Left
Tympanogram *see* Hearing Assessment, Diagnostic Audiology **F13**
Tympanoplasty
  see Repair, Ear, Nose, Sinus **09Q**
  see Replacement, Ear, Nose, Sinus **09R**
  see Supplement, Ear, Nose, Sinus **09U**
Tympanosympathectomy *see* Excision, Nerve, Head and Neck Sympathetic **01BK**
Tympanotomy *see* Drainage, Ear, Nose, Sinus **099**

U

Ulnar collateral carpal ligament
  use Bursa and Ligament, Wrist, Left
  use Bursa and Ligament, Wrist, Right
Ulnar collateral ligament
  use Bursa and Ligament, Elbow, Right
  use Bursa and Ligament, Elbow, Left
Ulnar notch
  use Radius, Left
  use Radius, Right
Ulnar vein
  use Vein, Brachial, Left
  use Vein, Brachial, Right

Ultrafiltration
  Hemodialysis *see* Performance, Urinary **5A1D**
  Therapeutic plasmapheresis *see* Pheresis, Circulatory **6A55**
Ultraflex™ Precision Colonic Stent System *use* Intraluminal Device
ULTRAPRO Hernia System (UHS) *use* Synthetic Substitute
ULTRAPRO Partially Absorbable Lightweight Mesh *use* Synthetic Substitute
ULTRAPRO Plug *use* Synthetic Substitute
Ultrasonic osteogenic stimulator
  use Bone Growth Stimulator in Upper Bones
  use Bone Growth Stimulator in Head and Facial Bones
  use Bone Growth Stimulator in Lower Bones
Ultrasonography
  Abdomen **BW40ZZZ**
  Abdomen and Pelvis **BW41ZZZ**
  Abdominal Wall **BH49ZZZ**
  Aorta
    Abdominal, Intravascular **B440ZZ3**
    Thoracic, Intravascular **B340ZZ3**
  Appendix **BD48ZZZ**
  Artery
    Brachiocephalic-Subclavian, Right, Intravascular **B341ZZ3**
    Celiac and Mesenteric, Intravascular **B44KZZ3**
    Common Carotid
      Bilateral, Intravascular **B345ZZ3**
      Left, Intravascular **B344ZZ3**
      Right, Intravascular **B343ZZ3**
    Coronary
      Multiple **B241YZZ**
        Intravascular **B241ZZ3**
        Transesophageal **B241ZZ4**
      Single **B240YZZ**
        Intravascular **B240ZZ3**
        Transesophageal **B240ZZ4**
    Femoral, Intravascular **B44LZZ3**
    Inferior Mesenteric, Intravascular **B445ZZ3**
    Internal Carotid
      Bilateral, Intravascular **B348ZZ3**
      Left, Intravascular **B347ZZ3**
      Right, Intravascular **B346ZZ3**
    Intra-Abdominal, Other, Intravascular **B44BZZ3**
    Intracranial, Intravascular **B34RZZ3**
    Lower Extremity
      Bilateral, Intravascular **B44HZZ3**
      Left, Intravascular **B44GZZ3**
      Right, Intravascular **B44FZZ3**
    Mesenteric and Celiac, Intravascular **B44KZZ3**
    Ophthalmic, Intravascular **B34VZZ3**
    Penile, Intravascular **B44NZZ3**
    Pulmonary
      Left, Intravascular **B34TZZ3**
      Right, Intravascular **B34SZZ3**
    Renal
      Bilateral, Intravascular **B448ZZ3**
      Left, Intravascular **B447ZZ3**
      Right, Intravascular **B446ZZ3**

Ultrasonography *(continued)*
    Subclavian, Left, Intravascular **B342ZZ3**
    Superior Mesenteric, Intravascular **B444ZZ3**
    Upper Extremity
      Bilateral, Intravascular **B34KZZ3**
      Left, Intravascular **B34JZZ3**
      Right, Intravascular **B34HZZ3**
  Bile Duct **BF40ZZZ**
  Bile Duct and Gallbladder **BF43ZZZ**
  Bladder **BT40ZZZ**
    and Kidney **BT4JZZZ**
  Brain **B040ZZZ**
  Breast
    Bilateral **BH42ZZZ**
    Left **BH41ZZZ**
    Right **BH40ZZZ**
  Chest Wall **BH4BZZZ**
  Coccyx **BR4FZZZ**
  Connective Tissue
    Lower Extremity **BL41ZZZ**
    Upper Extremity **BL40ZZZ**
  Duodenum **BD49ZZZ**
  Elbow
    Left, Densitometry **BP4HZZ1**
    Right, Densitometry **BP4GZZ1**
  Esophagus **BD41ZZZ**
  Extremity
    Lower **BH48ZZZ**
    Upper **BH47ZZZ**
  Eye
    Bilateral **B847ZZZ**
    Left **B846ZZZ**
    Right **B845ZZZ**
  Fallopian Tube
    Bilateral **BU42**
    Left **BU41**
    Right **BU40**
  Fetal Umbilical Cord **BY47ZZZ**
  Fetus
    First Trimester, Multiple Gestation **BY4BZZZ**
    Second Trimester, Multiple Gestation **BY4DZZZ**
    Single
      First Trimester **BY49ZZZ**
      Second Trimester **BY4CZZZ**
      Third Trimester **BY4FZZZ**
    Third Trimester, Multiple Gestation **BY4GZZZ**
  Gallbladder **BF42ZZZ**
  Gallbladder and Bile Duct **BF43ZZZ**
  Gastrointestinal Tract **BD47ZZZ**
  Gland
    Adrenal
      Bilateral **BG42ZZZ**
      Left **BG41ZZZ**
      Right **BG40ZZZ**
    Parathyroid **BG43ZZZ**
    Thyroid **BG44ZZZ**
  Hand
    Left, Densitometry **BP4PZZ1**
    Right, Densitometry **BP4NZZ1**
  Head and Neck **BH4CZZZ**
  Heart
    Left **B245YZZ**

Ultrasonography (continued)
    Intravascular **B245ZZ3**
    Transesophageal **B245ZZ4**
  Pediatric **B24DYZZ**
    Intravascular **B24DZZ3**
    Transesophageal **B24DZZ4**
  Right **B244YZZ**
    Intravascular **B244ZZ3**
    Transesophageal **B244ZZ4**
  Right and Left **B246YZZ**
    Intravascular **B246ZZ3**
    Transesophageal **B246ZZ4**
  Heart with Aorta **B24BYZZ**
    Intravascular **B24BZZ3**
    Transesophageal **B24BZZ4**
  Hepatobiliary System, All **BF4CZZZ**
  Hip
    Bilateral **BQ42ZZZ**
    Left **BQ41ZZZ**
    Right **BQ40ZZZ**
  Kidney
    and Bladder **BT4JZZZ**
    Bilateral **BT43ZZZ**
    Left **BT42ZZZ**
    Right **BT41ZZZ**
    Transplant **BT49ZZZ**
  Knee
    Bilateral **BQ49ZZZ**
    Left **BQ48ZZZ**
    Right **BQ47ZZZ**
  Liver **BF45ZZZ**
  Liver and Spleen **BF46ZZZ**
  Mediastinum **BB4CZZZ**
  Neck **BW4FZZZ**
  Ovary
    Bilateral **BU45**
    Left **BU44**
    Right **BU43**
  Ovary and Uterus **BU4C**
  Pancreas **BF47ZZZ**
  Pelvic Region **BW4GZZZ**
  Pelvis and Abdomen **BW41ZZZ**
  Penis **BV4BZZZ**
  Pericardium **B24CYZZ**
    Intravascular **B24CZZ3**
    Transesophageal **B24CZZ4**
  Placenta **BY48ZZZ**
  Pleura **BB4BZZZ**
  Prostate and Seminal Vesicle **BV49ZZZ**
  Rectum **BD4CZZZ**
  Sacrum **BR4FZZZ**
  Scrotum **BV44ZZZ**
  Seminal Vesicle and Prostate **BV49ZZZ**
  Shoulder
    Left, Densitometry **BP49ZZ1**
    Right, Densitometry **BP48ZZ1**
  Spinal Cord **B04BZZZ**
  Spine
    Cervical **BR40ZZZ**
    Lumbar **BR49ZZZ**
    Thoracic **BR47ZZZ**
  Spleen and Liver **BF46ZZZ**
  Stomach **BD42ZZZ**
  Tendon
    Lower Extremity **BL43ZZZ**
    Upper Extremity **BL42ZZZ**

Ultrasonography (continued)
  Ureter
    Bilateral **BT48ZZZ**
    Left **BT47ZZZ**
    Right **BT46ZZZ**
  Urethra **BT45ZZZ**
  Uterus **BU46**
  Uterus and Ovary **BU4C**
  Vein
    Jugular
      Left, Intravascular **B544ZZ3**
      Right, Intravascular **B543ZZ3**
    Lower Extremity
      Bilateral, Intravascular **B54DZZ3**
      Left, Intravascular **B54CZZ3**
      Right, Intravascular **B54BZZ3**
    Portal, Intravascular **B54TZZ3**
    Renal
      Bilateral, Intravascular **B54LZZ3**
      Left, Intravascular **B54KZZ3**
      Right, Intravascular **B54JZZ3**
    Splanchnic, Intravascular **B54TZZ3**
    Subclavian
      Left, Intravascular **B547ZZ3**
      Right, Intravascular **B546ZZ3**
    Upper Extremity
      Bilateral, Intravascular **B54PZZ3**
      Left, Intravascular **B54NZZ3**
      Right, Intravascular **B54MZZ3**
  Vena Cava
  Inferior, Intravascular **B549ZZ3**
  Superior, Intravascular **B548ZZ3**
  Wrist
  Left, Densitometry **BP4MZZ1**
  Right, Densitometry **BP4LZZ1**
Ultrasound bone healing system
  use Bone Growth Stimulator in Head and Facial Bones
  use Bone Growth Stimulator in Lower Bones
  use Bone Growth Stimulator in Upper Bones
Ultrasound Therapy
  Heart **6A75**
  No Qualifier **6A75**
  Vessels
  Head and Neck **6A75**
  Other **6A75**
  Peripheral **6A75**
Ultraviolet Light Therapy, Skin 6A80
Umbilical artery
  use Artery, Internal Iliac, Left
  use Artery, Internal Iliac, Right
Uniplanar external fixator
  use External Fixation Device, Monoplanar in **0PH**
  use External Fixation Device, Monoplanar in **0PS**
  use External Fixation Device, Monoplanar in **0QH**
  use External Fixation Device, Monoplanar in **0QS**
Upper GI series *see* Fluoroscopy, Gastrointestinal, Upper **BD15**
Ureteral orifice
  use Ureter, Left
  use Ureter

Ureteral orifice (continued)
  use Ureter, Right
  use Ureters, Bilateral
Ureterectomy
  see Excision, Urinary System **0TB**
  see Resection, Urinary System **0TT**
Ureterocolostomy *see* Bypass, Urinary System **0T1**
Ureterocystostomy *see* Bypass, Urinary System **0T1**
Ureteroenterostomy *see* Bypass, Urinary System **0T1**
Ureteroileostomy *see* Bypass, Urinary System **0T1**
Ureterolithotomy *see* Extirpation, Urinary System **0TC**
Ureterolysis *see* Release, Urinary System **0TN**
Ureteroneocystostomy
  see Bypass, Urinary System **0T1**
  see Reposition, Urinary System **0TS**

Ureteropelvic junction (UPJ)
  use Kidney Pelvis, Right
  use Kidney Pelvis, Left
Ureteropexy
  see Repair, Urinary System **0TQ**
  see Reposition, Urinary System **0TS**
Ureteroplasty
  see Repair, Urinary System **0TQ**
  see Replacement, Urinary System **0TR**
  see Supplement, Urinary System **0TU**
Ureteroplication *see* Restriction, Urinary System **0TV**
Ureteropyelography *see* Fluoroscopy, Urinary System **BT1**
Ureterorrhaphy *see* Repair, Urinary System **0TQ**
Ureteroscopy 0TJ98ZZ
Ureterostomy
  see Bypass, Urinary System **0T1**
  see Drainage, Urinary System **0T9**
Ureterotomy *see* Drainage, Urinary System **0T9**
Ureteroureterostomy *see* Bypass, Urinary System **0T1**
Ureterovesical orifice
  use Ureter
  use Ureter, Left
  use Ureter, Right
  use Ureters, Bilateral
Urethral catheterization, indwelling 0T9B70Z
Urethrectomy
  see Excision, Urethra **0TBD**
  see Resection, Urethra **0TTD**
Urethrolithotomy *see* Extirpation, Urethra **0TCD**
Urethrolysis *see* Release, Urethra **0TND**
Urethropexy
  see Repair, Urethra **0TQD**
  see Reposition, Urethra **0TSD**
Urethroplasty
  see Repair, Urethra **0TQD**
  see Replacement, Urethra **0TRD**
  see Supplement, Urethra **0TUD**
Urethrorrhaphy *see* Repair, Urethra **0TQD**
Urethroscopy 0TJD8ZZ

Urethrotomy *see* Drainage, Urethra **0T9D**
Uridine Triacetate XW0DX82
Urinary incontinence stimulator lead *use* Stimulator Lead in Urinary System
Urography *see* Fluoroscopy, Urinary System **BT1**
Uterine Artery
  use Artery, Internal Iliac, Left
  use Artery, Internal Iliac, Right
Uterine artery embolization (UAE) *see* Occlusion, Lower Arteries **04L**
Uterine cornu *use* Uterus
Uterine tube
  use Fallopian Tube, Left
  use Fallopian Tube, Right
Uterine vein
  use Vein, Hypogastric, Left
  use Vein, Hypogastric, Right
Uvulectomy
  see Excision, Uvula **0CBN**
  see Resection, Uvula **0CTN**
Uvulorrhaphy *see* Repair, Uvula **0CQN**
Uvulotomy *see* Drainage, Uvula **0C9N**

V

Vaccination *see* Introduction of Serum, Toxoid, and Vaccine
Vacuum extraction, obstetric 10D07Z6
Vaginal artery
  use Artery, Internal Iliac, Right
  use Artery, Internal Iliac, Left
Vaginal pessary *use* Intraluminal Device, Pessary in Female Reproductive System
Vaginal vein
  use Vein, Hypogastric, Right
  use Vein, Hypogastric, Left
Vaginectomy
  see Excision, Vagina **0UBG**
  see Resection, Vagina **0UTG**
Vaginofixation
  see Repair, Vagina **0UQG**
  see Reposition, Vagina **0USG**
Vaginoplasty
  see Repair, Vagina **0UQG**
  see Supplement, Vagina **0UUG**
Vaginorrhaphy *see* Repair, Vagina **0UQG**
Vaginoscopy 0UJH8ZZ
Vaginotomy *see* Drainage, Female Reproductive System **0U9**
Vagotomy *see* Division, Nerve, Vagus **008Q**
Valiant Thoracic Stent Graft *use* Intraluminal Device
Valvotomy, valvulotomy
  see Division, Heart and Great Vessels **028**
  see Release, Heart and Great Vessels **02N**
Valvuloplasty
  see Repair, Heart and Great Vessels **02Q**
  see Replacement, Heart and Great Vessels **02R**
  see Supplement, Heart and Great Vessels **02U**
Vascular Access Device
  Insertion of device in
    Abdomen **0JH8**
    Chest **0JH6**

Vascular Access Device *(continued)*
    Lower Arm
      Left **0JHH**
      Right **0JHG**
    Lower Leg
      Left **0JHP**
      Right **0JHN**
    Upper Arm
      Left **0JHF**
      Right **0JHD**
    Upper Leg
      Left **0JHM**
      Right **0JHL**
  Removal of device from
    Lower Extremity **0JPW**
    Trunk **0JPT**
    Upper Extremity **0JPV**
  Reservoir
    Insertion of device in
      Abdomen **0JH8**
      Chest **0JH6**
      Lower Arm
        Left **0JHH**
        Right **0JHG**
      Lower Leg
        Left **0JHP**
        Right **0JHN**
      Upper Arm
        Left **0JHF**
        Right **0JHD**
      Upper Leg
        Left **0JHM**
        Right **0JHL**
    Removal of device from
      Lower Extremity **0JPW**
      Trunk **0JPT**
      Upper Extremity **0JPV**
    Revision of device in
      Lower Extremity **0JWW**
      Trunk **0JWT**
      Upper Extremity **0JWV**
  Revision of device in
    Lower Extremity **0JWW**
    Trunk **0JWT**
    Upper Extremity **0JWV**
Vasectomy *see* Excision, Male Reproductive System **0VB**
Vasography
  see Plain Radiography, Male Reproductive System **BV0**
Vasography
  see Fluoroscopy, Male Reproductive System **BV1**
Vasoligation *see* Occlusion, Male Reproductive System **0VL**
Vasorrhaphy *see* Repair, Male Reproductive System **0VQ**
Vasostomy *see* Bypass, Male Reproductive System **0V1**
Vasotomy
  Drainage *see* Drainage, Male Reproductive System **0V9**
  With ligation *see* Occlusion, Male Reproductive System **0VL**
Vasovasostomy *see* Repair, Male Reproductive System **0VQ**

Vastus intermedius muscle
  use Muscle, Upper Leg, Right
  use Muscle, Upper Leg, Left
Vastus lateralis muscle
  use Muscle, Upper Leg, Left
  use Muscle, Upper Leg, Right
Vastus medialis muscle
  use Muscle, Upper Leg, Right
  use Muscle, Upper Leg, Left
VCG (vectorcardiogram) *see* Measurement, Cardiac **4A02**
Vectra® Vascular Access Graft *use* Vascular Access Device in Subcutaneous Tissue and Fascia
Venectomy
  see Excision, Upper Veins **05B**
  see Excision, Lower Veins **06B**
Venography
  see Plain Radiography, Veins **B50**
  see Fluoroscopy, Veins **B51**
Venorrhaphy
  see Repair, Upper Veins **05Q**
  see Repair, Lower Veins **06Q**
Venotripsy
  see Occlusion, Upper Veins **05L**
  see Occlusion, Lower Veins **06L**
Ventricular fold *use* Larynx
Ventriculoatriostomy *see* Bypass, Central Nervous System **001**
Ventriculocisternostomy *see* Bypass, Central Nervous System **001**
Ventriculogram, cardiac
  Combined left and right heart *see* Fluoroscopy, Heart, Right and Left **B216**
  Left ventricle *see* Fluoroscopy, Heart, Left **B215**
  Right ventricle *see* Fluoroscopy, Heart, Right **B214**
Ventriculopuncture, through previously implanted catheter 8C01X6J
Ventriculoscopy 00J04ZZ
Ventriculostomy
  External drainage *see* Drainage, Cerebral Ventricle **0096**
  Internal shunt *see* Bypass, Cerebral Ventricle **0016**
Ventriculovenostomy *see* Bypass, Cerebral Ventricle **0016**
Ventrio™ Hernia Patch *use* Synthetic Substitute
VEP (visual evoked potential) 4A07X0Z
Vermiform appendix *use* Appendix
Vermilion border
  use Lip, Lower
  use Lip, Upper
Versa *use* Pacemaker, Dual Chamber in **0JH**
Version, obstetric
  External **10S0XZZ**
  Internal **10S07ZZ**
Vertebral arch
  use Vertebra, Thoracic
  use Vertebra, Lumbar
  use Vertebra, Cervical
Vertebral canal *use* Spinal Canal

Vertebral foramen
  use Vertebra, Thoracic
  use Vertebra, Lumbar
  use Vertebra, Cervical
Vertebral lamina
  use Vertebra, Thoracic
  use Vertebra, Cervical
  use Vertebra, Lumbar
Vertebral pedicle
  use Vertebra, Lumbar
  use Vertebra, Thoracic
  use Vertebra, Cervical
Vesical vein
  use Vein, Hypogastric, Left
  use Vein, Hypogastric, Right
Vesicotomy *see* Drainage, Urinary System **0T9**
Vesiculectomy
  see Excision, Male Reproductive System
  0VB
  see Resection, Male Reproductive System
  0VT
Vesiculogram, seminal *see* Plain Radiography,
  Male Reproductive System **BV0**
Vesiculotomy *see* Drainage, Male
  Reproductive System **0V9**
Vestibular (Scarpa's) ganglion *use* Nerve,
  Acoustic
Vestibular Assessment F15Z
Vestibular nerve *use* Nerve, Acoustic
Vestibular Treatment F0C
Vestibulocochlear nerve *use* Nerve, Acoustic
**VH-IVUS (virtual histology intravascular
  ultrasound)** *see* Ultrasonography, Heart
  B24
Virchow's (supraclavicular) lymph node
  use Lymphatic, Neck, Left
  use Lymphatic, Neck, Right
Virtuoso (II) (DR) (VR) *use* Defibrillator
  Generator in **0JH**
Vistogard(R) *use* Uridine Triacetate
Vitrectomy
  see Excision, Eye **08B**
  see Resection, Eye **08T**
Vitreous body
  use Vitreous, Left
  use Vitreous, Right
Vocal fold
  use Vocal Cord, Left
  use Vocal Cord, Right
Vocational
  Assessment *see* Activities of Daily Living
  Assessment, Rehabilitation **F02**
  Retraining *see* Activities of Daily Living
  Treatment, Rehabilitation **F08**
Volar (palmar) digital vein
  use Vein, Hand, Left
  use Vein, Hand, Right
Volar (palmar) metacarpal vein
  use Vein, Hand, Right
  use Vein, Hand, Left
Vomer bone *use* Septum, Nasal
Vomer of nasal septum *use* Bone, Nasal
Vulvectomy
  see Excision, Female Reproductive System
  0UB
  see Resection, Female Reproductive System
  0UT

W

WALLSTENT® Endoprosthesis *use*
  Intraluminal Device
Washing *see* Irrigation
Wedge resection, pulmonary *see* Excision,
  Respiratory System **0BB**
Window *see* Drainage
Wiring, dental 2W31X9Z

X

X-ray *see* Plain Radiography
X-STOP® Spacer
  use Spinal Stabilization Device, Interspinous
  Process in **0RH**
  use Spinal Stabilization Device, Interspinous
  Process in **0SH**
Xenograft *use* Zooplastic Tissue in Heart and
  Great Vessels
**XIENCE V Everolimus Eluting Coronary
  Stent System** *use* Intraluminal Device,
  Drug-eluting in Heart and Great Vessels
Xiphoid process *use* Sternum
XLIF® System *use* Interbody Fusion Device
  in Lower Joints

Y

Yoga Therapy 8E0ZXY4

Z

Z-plasty, skin for scar contracture *see*
  Release, Skin and Breast **0HN**
Zenith AAA Endovascular Graft
  use Intraluminal Device, Branched or
    Fenestrated, One or Two Arteries in **04V**
  use Intraluminal Device, Branched or
    Fenestrated, Three or More Arteries in
    04V
  use Intraluminal Device
Zenith Flex® AAA Endovascular Graft *use*
  Intraluminal Device
Zenith TX2® TAA Endovascular Graft *use*
  Intraluminal Device
Zenith® Renu™ AAA Ancillary Graft *use*
  Intraluminal Device
**Zilver® PTX® (paclitaxel) Drug-Eluting
  Peripheral Stent**
  use Intraluminal Device, Drug-eluting in
  Upper Arteries
  use Intraluminal Device, Drug-eluting in
  Lower Arteries
**Zimmer® NexGen® LPS Mobile Bearing
  Knee** *use* Synthetic Substitute
Zimmer® NexGen® LPS-Flex Mobile Knee
  use Synthetic Substitute
Zonule of Zinn
  use Lens, Left
  use Lens, Right
**Zooplastic Tissue, Rapid Deployment
  Technique, Replacement X2RF**
Zotarolimus-eluting coronary stent *use*
  Intraluminal Device, Drug-eluting in Heart
  and Great Vessels

Zygomatic process of frontal bone
  use Bone, Frontal, Left
  use Bone, Frontal, Right
Zygomatic process of temporal bone
  use Bone, Temporal, Right
  use Bone, Temporal, Left
Zygomaticus muscle *use* Muscle, Facial

APPENDIX A: DEFINITIONS

SECTION 0 - MEDICAL AND SURGICAL CHARACTER 3 – OPERATION	
Alteration	**Definition:** Modifying the anatomic structure of a body part without affecting the function of the body part **Explanation:** Principal purpose is to improve appearance **Includes/Examples:** Face lift, breast augmentation
Bypass	**Definition:** Altering the route of passage of the contents of a tubular body part **Explanation:** Rerouting contents of a body part to a downstream area of the normal route, to a similar route and body part, or to an abnormal route and dissimilar body part. Includes one or more anastomoses, with or without the use of a device **Includes/Examples:** Coronary artery bypass, colostomy formation
Change	**Definition:** Taking out or off a device from a body part and putting back an identical or similar device in or on the same body part without cutting or puncturing the skin or a mucous membrane **Explanation:** All CHANGE procedures are coded using the approach EXTERNAL **Includes/Examples:** Urinary catheter change, gastrostomy tube change
Control	**Definition:** Stopping, or attempting to stop, postprocedural or other acute bleeding **Explanation:** The site of the bleeding is coded as an anatomical region and not to a specific body part **Includes/Examples:** Control of post-prostatectomy hemorrhage, control of intracranial subdural hemorrhage, control of bleeding duodenal ulcer, control of retroperitoneal hemorrhage
Creation	**Definition:** Putting in or on biological or synthetic material to form a new body part that to the extent possible replicates the anatomic structure or function of an absent body part **Explanation:** Used for gender reassignment surgery and corrective procedures in individuals with congenital anomalies **Includes/Examples:** Creation of vagina in a male, creation of right and left atrioventricular valve from common atrioventricular valve
Destruction	**Definition:** Physical eradication of all or a portion of a body part by the direct use of energy, force, or a destructive agent **Explanation:** None of the body part is physically taken out **Includes/Examples:** Fulguration of rectal polyp, cautery of skin lesion
Detachment	**Definition:** Cutting off all or a portion of the upper or lower extremities **Explanation:** The body part value is the site of the detachment, with a qualifier if applicable to further specify the level where the extremity was detached **Includes/Examples:** Below knee amputation, disarticulation of shoulder
Dilation	**Definition:** Expanding an orifice or the lumen of a tubular body part **Explanation:** The orifice can be a natural orifice or an artificially created orifice. Accomplished by stretching a tubular body part using intraluminal pressure or by cutting part of the orifice or wall of the tubular body part **Includes/Examples:** Percutaneous transluminal angioplasty, pyloromyotomy
Division	**Definition:** Cutting into a body part, without draining fluids and/or gases from the body part, in order to separate or transect a body part **Explanation:** All or a portion of the body part is separated into two or more portions **Includes/Examples:** Spinal cordotomy, osteotomy
Drainage	**Definition:** Taking or letting out fluids and/or gases from a body part **Explanation:** The qualifier DIAGNOSTIC is used to identify drainage procedures that are biopsies **Includes/Examples:** Thoracentesis, incision and drainage
Excision	**Definition:** Cutting out or off, without replacement, a portion of a body part **Explanation:** The qualifier DIAGNOSTIC is used to identify excision procedures that are biopsies **Includes/Examples:** Partial nephrectomy, liver biopsy

SECTION 0 - MEDICAL AND SURGICAL CHARACTER 3 – OPERATION	
Extirpation	**Definition:** Taking or cutting out solid matter from a body part **Explanation:** The solid matter may be an abnormal byproduct of a biological function or a foreign body; it may be imbedded in a body part or in the lumen of a tubular body part. The solid matter may or may not have been previously broken into pieces **Includes/Examples:** Thrombectomy, choledocholithotomy
Extraction	**Definition:** Pulling or stripping out or off all or a portion of a body part by the use of force **Explanation:** The qualifier DIAGNOSTIC is used to identify extraction procedures that are biopsies **Includes/Examples:** Dilation and curettage, vein stripping
Fragmentation	**Definition:** Breaking solid matter in a body part into pieces **Explanation:** Physical force (e.g., manual, ultrasonic) applied directly or indirectly is used to break the solid matter into pieces. The solid matter may be an abnormal byproduct of a biological function or a foreign body. The pieces of solid matter are not taken out **Includes/Examples:** Extracorporeal shockwave lithotripsy, transurethral lithotripsy
Fusion	**Definition:** Joining together portions of an articular body part rendering the articular body part immobile **Explanation:** The body part is joined together by fixation device, bone graft, or other means **Includes/Examples:** Spinal fusion, ankle arthrodesis
Insertion	**Definition:** Putting in a nonbiological appliance that monitors, assists, performs, or prevents a physiological function but does not physically take the place of a body part **Includes/Examples:** Insertion of radioactive implant, insertion of central venous catheter
Inspection	**Definition:** Visually and/or manually exploring a body part **Explanation:** Visual exploration may be performed with or without optical instrumentation. Manual exploration may be performed directly or through intervening body layers **Includes/Examples:** Diagnostic arthroscopy, exploratory laparotomy
Map	**Definition:** Locating the route of passage of electrical impulses and/or locating functional areas in a body part **Explanation:** Applicable only to the cardiac conduction mechanism and the central nervous system **Includes/Examples:** Cardiac mapping, cortical mapping
Occlusion	**Definition:** Completely closing an orifice or the lumen of a tubular body part **Explanation:** The orifice can be a natural orifice or an artificially created orifice **Includes/Examples:** Fallopian tube ligation, ligation of inferior vena cava
Reattachment	**Definition:** Putting back in or on all or a portion of a separated body part to its normal location or other suitable location **Explanation:** Vascular circulation and nervous pathways may or may not be reestablished **Includes/Examples:** Reattachment of hand, reattachment of avulsed kidney
Release	**Definition:** Freeing a body part from an abnormal physical constraint by cutting or by the use of force **Explanation:** Some of the restraining tissue may be taken out but none of the body part is taken out **Includes/Examples:** Adhesiolysis, carpal tunnel release
Removal	**Definition:** Taking out or off a device from a body part **Explanation:** If a device is taken out and a similar device put in without cutting or puncturing the skin or mucous membrane, the procedure is coded to the root operation CHANGE. Otherwise, the procedure for taking out a device is coded to the root operation REMOVAL **Includes/Examples:** Drainage tube removal, cardiac pacemaker removal
Repair	**Definition:** Restoring, to the extent possible, a body part to its normal anatomic structure and function **Explanation:** Used only when the method to accomplish the repair is not one of the other root operations **Includes/Examples:** Colostomy takedown, suture of laceration

SECTION 0 - MEDICAL AND SURGICAL CHARACTER 3 – OPERATION

Replacement	**Definition:** Putting in or on biological or synthetic material that physically takes the place and/or function of all or a portion of a body part **Explanation:** The body part may have been taken out or replaced, or may be taken out, physically eradicated, or rendered nonfunctional during the Replacement procedure. A Removal procedure is coded for taking out the device used in a previous replacement procedure **Includes/Examples:** Total hip replacement, bone graft, free skin graft
Reposition	**Definition:** Moving to its normal location, or other suitable location, all or a portion of a body part **Explanation:** The body part is moved to a new location from an abnormal location, or from a normal location where it is not functioning correctly. The body part may or may not be cut out or off to be moved to the new location **Includes/Examples:** Reposition of undescended testicle, fracture reduction
Resection	**Definition:** Cutting out or off, without replacement, all of a body part **Includes/Examples:** Total nephrectomy, total lobectomy of lung
Restriction	**Definition:** Partially closing an orifice or the lumen of a tubular body part **Explanation:** The orifice can be a natural orifice or an artificially created orifice **Includes/Examples:** Esophagogastric fundoplication, cervical cerclage
Revision	**Definition:** Correcting, to the extent possible, a portion of a malfunctioning device or the position of a displaced device **Explanation:** Revision can include correcting a malfunctioning or displaced device by taking out or putting in components of the device such as a screw or pin **Includes/Examples:** Adjustment of position of pacemaker lead, recementing of hip prosthesis
Supplement	**Definition:** Putting in or on biological or synthetic material that physically reinforces and/or augments the function of a portion of a body part **Explanation:** The biological material is non-living, or is living and from the same individual. The body part may have been previously replaced, and the Supplement procedure is performed to physically reinforce and/or augment the function of the replaced body part **Includes/Examples:** Herniorrhaphy using mesh, free nerve graft, mitral valve ring annuloplasty, put a new acetabular liner in a previous hip replacement
Transfer	**Definition:** Moving, without taking out, all or a portion of a body part to another location to take over the function of all or a portion of a body part **Explanation:** The body part transferred remains connected to its vascular and nervous supply **Includes/Examples:** Tendon transfer, skin pedicle flap transfer
Transplantation	**Definition:** Putting in or on all or a portion of a living body part taken from another individual or animal to physically take the place and/or function of all or a portion of a similar body part **Explanation:** The native body part may or may not be taken out, and the transplanted body part may take over all or a portion of its function **Includes/Examples:** Kidney transplant, heart transplant

SECTION 0 - MEDICAL AND SURGICAL CHARACTER 4 - BODY PART

1st Toe, Left 1st Toe, Right	**Includes:** Hallux
Abdomen Muscle, Left Abdomen Muscle, Right	**Includes:** External oblique muscle Internal oblique muscle Pyramidalis muscle Rectus abdominis muscle Transversus abdominis muscle

SECTION 0 - MEDICAL AND SURGICAL CHARACTER 4 - BODY PART	
Abdominal Aorta	**Includes:** Inferior phrenic artery Lumbar artery Median sacral artery Middle suprarenal artery Ovarian artery Testicular artery
Abdominal Sympathetic Nerve	**Includes:** Abdominal aortic plexus Auerbach's (myenteric) plexus Celiac (solar) plexus Celiac ganglion Gastric plexus Hepatic plexus Inferior hypogastric plexus Inferior mesenteric ganglion Inferior mesenteric plexus Meissner's (submucous) plexus Myenteric (Auerbach's) plexus Pancreatic plexus Pelvic splanchnic nerve Renal plexus Solar (celiac) plexus Splenic plexus Submucous (Meissner's) plexus Superior hypogastric plexus Superior mesenteric ganglion Superior mesenteric plexus Suprarenal plexus
Abducens Nerve	**Includes:** Sixth cranial nerve
Accessory Nerve	**Includes:** Eleventh cranial nerve
Acoustic Nerve	**Includes:** Cochlear nerve Eighth cranial nerve Scarpa's (vestibular) ganglion Spiral ganglion Vestibular (Scarpa's) ganglion Vestibular nerve Vestibulocochlear nerve
Adenoids	**Includes:** Pharyngeal tonsil
Adrenal Gland Adrenal Gland, Left Adrenal Gland, Right Adrenal Glands, Bilateral	**Includes:** Suprarenal gland
Ampulla of Vater	**Includes:** Duodenal ampulla Hepatopancreatic ampulla

SECTION 0 - MEDICAL AND SURGICAL CHARACTER 4 - BODY PART	
Anal Sphincter	**Includes:** External anal sphincter Internal anal sphincter
Ankle Bursa and Ligament, Left Ankle Bursa and Ligament, Right	**Includes:** Calcaneofibular ligament Deltoid ligament Ligament of the lateral malleolus Talofibular ligament
Ankle Joint, Left Ankle Joint, Right	**Includes:** Inferior tibiofibular joint Talocrural joint
Anterior Chamber, Left Anterior Chamber, Right	**Includes:** Aqueous humor
Anterior Tibial Artery, Left Anterior Tibial Artery, Right	**Includes:** Anterior lateral malleolar artery Anterior medial malleolar artery Anterior tibial recurrent artery Dorsalis pedis artery Posterior tibial recurrent artery
Anus	**Includes:** Anal orifice
Aortic Valve	**Includes:** Aortic annulus
Appendix	**Includes:** Vermiform appendix
Ascending Colon	**Includes:** Hepatic flexure
Atrial Septum	**Includes:** Interatrial septum
Atrium, Left	**Includes:** Atrium pulmonale Left auricular appendix
Atrium, Right	**Includes:** Atrium dextrum cordis Right auricular appendix Sinus venosus
Auditory Ossicle, Left Auditory Ossicle, Right	**Includes:** Incus Malleus Stapes
Axillary Artery, Left Axillary Artery, Right	**Includes:** Anterior circumflex humeral artery Lateral thoracic artery Posterior circumflex humeral artery Subscapular artery Superior thoracic artery Thoracoacromial artery

SECTION 0 - MEDICAL AND SURGICAL CHARACTER 4 - BODY PART	
Azygos Vein	**Includes:** Right ascending lumbar vein Right subcostal vein
Basal Ganglia	**Includes:** Basal nuclei Claustrum Corpus striatum Globus pallidus Substantia nigra Subthalamic nucleus
Basilic Vein, Left Basilic Vein, Right	**Includes:** Median antebrachial vein Median cubital vein
Bladder	**Includes:** Trigone of bladder
Brachial Artery, Left Brachial Artery, Right	**Includes:** Inferior ulnar collateral artery Profunda brachii Superior ulnar collateral artery
Brachial Plexus	**Includes:** Axillary nerve Dorsal scapular nerve First intercostal nerve Long thoracic nerve Musculocutaneous nerve Subclavius nerve Suprascapular nerve
Brachial Vein, Left Brachial Vein, Right	**Includes:** Radial vein Ulnar vein
Brain	**Includes:** Cerebrum Corpus callosum Encephalon
Breast, Bilateral Breast, Left Breast, Right	**Includes:** Mammary duct Mammary gland
Buccal Mucosa	**Includes:** Buccal gland Molar gland Palatine gland
Carotid Bodies, Bilateral Carotid Body, Left Carotid Body, Right	**Includes:** Carotid glomus
Carpal Joint, Left Carpal Joint, Right	**Includes:** Intercarpal joint Midcarpal joint

SECTION 0 - MEDICAL AND SURGICAL CHARACTER 4 - BODY PART	
Carpal, Left Carpal, Right	**Includes:** Capitate bone Hamate bone Lunate bone Pisiform bone Scaphoid bone Trapezium bone Trapezoid bone Triquetral bone
Celiac Artery	**Includes:** Celiac trunk
Cephalic Vein, Left Cephalic Vein, Right	**Includes:** Accessory cephalic vein
Cerebellum	**Includes:** Culmen
Cerebral Hemisphere	**Includes:** Frontal lobe Occipital lobe Parietal lobe Temporal lobe
Cerebral Meninges	**Includes:** Arachnoid mater, intracranial Leptomeninges, intracranial Pia mater, intracranial
Cerebral Ventricle	**Includes:** Aqueduct of Sylvius Cerebral aqueduct (Sylvius) Choroid plexus Ependyma Foramen of Monro (intraventricular) Fourth ventricle Interventricular foramen (Monro) Left lateral ventricle Right lateral ventricle Third ventricle
Cervical Nerve	**Includes:** Greater occipital nerve Suboccipital nerve Third occipital nerve
Cervical Plexus	**Includes:** Ansa cervicalis Cutaneous (transverse) cervical nerve Great auricular nerve Lesser occipital nerve Supraclavicular nerve Transverse (cutaneous) cervical nerve

SECTION 0 - MEDICAL AND SURGICAL CHARACTER 4 - BODY PART	
Cervical Vertebra	**Includes:** Spinous process Vertebral arch Vertebral foramen Vertebral lamina Vertebral pedicle
Cervical Vertebral Joint	**Includes:** Atlantoaxial joint Cervical facet joint
Cervical Vertebral Joints, 2 or more	**Includes:** Cervical facet joint
Cervicothoracic Vertebral Joint	**Includes:** Cervicothoracic facet joint
Cisterna Chyli	**Includes:** Intestinal lymphatic trunk Lumbar lymphatic trunk
Coccygeal Glomus	**Includes:** Coccygeal body
Colic Vein	**Includes:** Ileocolic vein Left colic vein Middle colic vein Right colic vein
Conduction Mechanism	**Includes:** Atrioventricular node Bundle of His Bundle of Kent Sinoatrial node
Conjunctiva, Left Conjunctiva, Right	**Includes:** Plica semilunaris
Dura Mater	**Includes:** Diaphragma sellae Dura mater, intracranial Falx cerebri Tentorium cerebelli
Elbow Bursa and Ligament, Left Elbow Bursa and Ligament, Right	**Includes:** Annular ligament Olecranon bursa Radial collateral ligament Ulnar collateral ligament
Elbow Joint, Left Elbow Joint, Right	**Includes:** Distal humerus, involving joint Humeroradial joint Humeroulnar joint Proximal radioulnar joint
Epidural Space	**Includes:** Epidural space, intracranial Extradural space, intracranial

SECTION 0 - MEDICAL AND SURGICAL CHARACTER 4 - BODY PART

Epiglottis	**Includes:** Glossoepiglottic fold
Esophagogastric Junction	**Includes:** Cardia Cardioesophageal junction Gastroesophageal (GE) junction
Esophagus, Lower	**Includes:** Abdominal esophagus
Esophagus, Middle	**Includes:** Thoracic esophagus
Esophagus, Upper	**Includes:** Cervical esophagus
Ethmoid Bone, Left Ethmoid Bone, Right	**Includes:** Cribriform plate
Ethmoid Sinus, Left Ethmoid Sinus, Right	**Includes:** Ethmoidal air cell
Eustachian Tube, Left Eustachian Tube, Right	**Includes:** Auditory tube Pharyngotympanic tube
External Auditory Canal, Left External Auditory Canal, Right	**Includes:** External auditory meatus
External Carotid Artery, Left External Carotid Artery, Right	**Includes:** Ascending pharyngeal artery Internal maxillary artery Lingual artery Maxillary artery Occipital artery Posterior auricular artery Superior thyroid artery
External Ear, Bilateral External Ear, Left External Ear, Right	**Includes:** Antihelix Antitragus Auricle Earlobe Helix Pinna Tragus
External Iliac Artery, Left External Iliac Artery, Right	**Includes:** Deep circumflex iliac artery Inferior epigastric artery
External Jugular Vein, Left External Jugular Vein, Right	**Includes:** Posterior auricular vein
Extraocular Muscle, Left Extraocular Muscle, Right	**Includes:** Inferior oblique muscle Inferior rectus muscle Lateral rectus muscle Medial rectus muscle Superior oblique muscle Superior rectus muscle
Eye, Left Eye, Right	**Includes:** Ciliary body Posterior chamber

SECTION 0 - MEDICAL AND SURGICAL CHARACTER 4 - BODY PART	
Face Artery	**Includes:** Angular artery Ascending palatine artery External maxillary artery Facial artery Inferior labial artery Submental artery Superior labial artery
Face Vein, Left Face Vein, Right	**Includes:** Angular vein Anterior facial vein Common facial vein Deep facial vein Frontal vein Posterior facial (retromandibular) vein Supraorbital vein
Facial Muscle	**Includes:** Buccinator muscle Corrugator supercilii muscle Depressor anguli oris muscle Depressor labii inferioris muscle Depressor septi nasi muscle Depressor supercilii muscle Levator anguli oris muscle Levator labii superioris alaeque nasi muscle Levator labii superioris muscle Mentalis muscle Nasalis muscle Occipitofrontalis muscle Orbicularis oris muscle Procerus muscle Risorius muscle Zygomaticus muscle
Facial Nerve	**Includes:** Chorda tympani Geniculate ganglion Greater superficial petrosal nerve Nerve to the stapedius Parotid plexus Posterior auricular nerve Seventh cranial nerve Submandibular ganglion
Fallopian Tube, Left Fallopian Tube, Right	**Includes:** Oviduct Salpinx Uterine tube
Femoral Artery, Left Femoral Artery, Right	**Includes:** Circumflex iliac artery Deep femoral artery Descending genicular artery External pudendal artery Superficial epigastric artery

SECTION 0 - MEDICAL AND SURGICAL CHARACTER 4 - BODY PART

Femoral Nerve	**Includes:** Anterior crural nerve Saphenous nerve
Femoral Shaft, Left Femoral Shaft, Right	**Includes:** Body of femur
Femoral Vein, Left Femoral Vein, Right	**Includes:** Deep femoral (profunda femoris) vein Popliteal vein Profunda femoris (deep femoral) vein
Fibula, Left Fibula, Right	**Includes:** Body of fibula Head of fibula Lateral malleolus
Finger Nail	**Includes:** Nail bed Nail plate
Finger Phalangeal Joint, Left Finger Phalangeal Joint, Right	**Includes:** Interphalangeal (IP) joint
Foot Artery, Left Foot Artery, Right	**Includes:** Arcuate artery Dorsal metatarsal artery Lateral plantar artery Lateral tarsal artery Medial plantar artery
Foot Bursa and Ligament, Left Foot Bursa and Ligament, Right	**Includes:** Calcaneocuboid ligament Cuneonavicular ligament Intercuneiform ligament Interphalangeal ligament Metatarsal ligament Metatarsophalangeal ligament Subtalar ligament Talocalcaneal ligament Talocalcaneonavicular ligament Tarsometatarsal ligament
Foot Muscle, Left Foot Muscle, Right Foot Muscle, Left Foot Muscle, Right (continued)	**Includes:** Abductor hallucis muscle Adductor hallucis muscle Extensor digitorum brevis muscle Extensor hallucis brevis muscle Flexor digitorum brevis muscle Flexor hallucis brevis muscle Quadratus plantae muscle
Foot Vein, Left Foot Vein, Right	**Includes:** Common digital vein Dorsal metatarsal vein Dorsal venous arch Plantar digital vein Plantar metatarsal vein Plantar venous arch

SECTION 0 - MEDICAL AND SURGICAL CHARACTER 4 - BODY PART

Frontal Bone, Left Frontal Bone, Right	**Includes:** Zygomatic process of frontal bone
Gastric Artery	**Includes:** Left gastric artery Right gastric artery
Glenoid Cavity, Left Glenoid Cavity, Right	**Includes:** Glenoid fossa (of scapula)
Glomus Jugulare	**Includes:** Jugular body
Glossopharyngeal Nerve	**Includes:** Carotid sinus nerve Ninth cranial nerve Tympanic nerve
Greater Omentum	**Includes:** Gastrocolic ligament Gastrocolic omentum Gastrophrenic ligament Gastrosplenic ligament
Greater Saphenous Vein, Left Greater Saphenous Vein, Right	**Includes:** External pudendal vein Great saphenous vein Superficial circumflex iliac vein Superficial epigastric vein
Hand Artery, Left Hand Artery, Right	**Includes:** Deep palmar arch Princeps pollicis artery Radialis indicis Superficial palmar arch
Hand Bursa and Ligament, Left Hand Bursa and Ligament, Right	**Includes:** Carpometacarpal ligament Intercarpal ligament Interphalangeal ligament Lunotriquetral ligament Metacarpal ligament Metacarpophalangeal ligament Pisohamate ligament Pisometacarpal ligament Scapholunate ligament Scaphotrapezium ligament
Hand Muscle, Left Hand Muscle, Right	**Includes:** Hypothenar muscle Palmar interosseous muscle Thenar muscle
Hand Vein, Left Hand Vein, Right	**Includes:** Dorsal metacarpal vein Palmar (volar) digital vein Palmar (volar) metacarpal vein Superficial palmar venous arch Volar (palmar) digital vein Volar (palmar) metacarpal vein

SECTION 0 - MEDICAL AND SURGICAL CHARACTER 4 - BODY PART	
Head and Neck Bursa and Ligament	**Includes:** Alar ligament of axis Cervical interspinous ligament Cervical intertransverse ligament Cervical ligamentum flavum Interspinous ligament Lateral temporomandibular ligament Sphenomandibular ligament Stylomandibular ligament Transverse ligament of atlas
Head and Neck Sympathetic Nerve	**Includes:** Cavernous plexus Cervical ganglion Ciliary ganglion Internal carotid plexus Otic ganglion Pterygopalatine (sphenopalatine) ganglion Sphenopalatine (pterygopalatine) ganglion Stellate ganglion Submandibular ganglion Submaxillary ganglion
Head Muscle	**Includes:** Auricularis muscle Masseter muscle Pterygoid muscle Splenius capitis muscle Temporalis muscle Temporoparietalis muscle
Heart, Left	**Includes:** Left coronary sulcus Obtuse margin
Heart, Right	**Includes:** Right coronary sulcus
Hemiazygos Vein	**Includes:** Left ascending lumbar vein Left subcostal vein
Hepatic Artery	**Includes:** Common hepatic artery Gastroduodenal artery Hepatic artery proper
Hip Bursa and Ligament, Left Hip Bursa and Ligament, Right	**Includes:** Iliofemoral ligament Ischiofemoral ligament Pubofemoral ligament Transverse acetabular ligament Trochanteric bursa
Hip Joint, Left Hip Joint, Right	**Includes:** Acetabulofemoral joint

SECTION 0 - MEDICAL AND SURGICAL CHARACTER 4 - BODY PART	
Hip Muscle, Left Hip Muscle, Right	**Includes:** Gemellus muscle Gluteus maximus muscle Gluteus medius muscle Gluteus minimus muscle Iliacus muscle Obturator muscle Piriformis muscle Psoas muscle Quadratus femoris muscle Tensor fasciae latae muscle
Humeral Head, Left Humeral Head, Right	**Includes:** Greater tuberosity Lesser tuberosity Neck of humerus (anatomical)(surgical)
Humeral Shaft, Left Humeral Shaft, Right	**Includes:** Distal humerus Humerus, distal Lateral epicondyle of humerus Medial epicondyle of humerus
Hypogastric Vein, Left Hypogastric Vein, Right	**Includes:** Gluteal vein Internal iliac vein Internal pudendal vein Lateral sacral vein Middle hemorrhoidal vein Obturator vein Uterine vein Vaginal vein Vesical vein
Hypoglossal Nerve	**Includes:** Twelfth cranial nerve
Hypothalamus	**Includes:** Mammillary body
Inferior Mesenteric Artery	**Includes:** Sigmoid artery Superior rectal artery
Inferior Mesenteric Vein	**Includes:** Sigmoid vein Superior rectal vein
Inferior Vena Cava	**Includes:** Postcava Right inferior phrenic vein Right ovarian vein Right second lumbar vein Right suprarenal vein Right testicular vein
Inguinal Region, Bilateral Inguinal Region, Left Inguinal Region, Right	**Includes:** Inguinal canal Inguinal triangle

SECTION 0 - MEDICAL AND SURGICAL CHARACTER 4 - BODY PART

Inner Ear, Left Inner Ear, Right	**Includes:** Bony labyrinth Bony vestibule Cochlea Round window Semicircular canal
Innominate Artery	**Includes:** Brachiocephalic artery Brachiocephalic trunk
Innominate Vein, Left Innominate Vein, Right	**Includes:** Brachiocephalic vein Inferior thyroid vein
Internal Carotid Artery, Left Internal Carotid Artery, Right	**Includes:** Caroticotympanic artery Carotid sinus
Internal Iliac Artery, Left Internal Iliac Artery, Right	**Includes:** Deferential artery Hypogastric artery Iliolumbar artery Inferior gluteal artery Inferior vesical artery Internal pudendal artery Lateral sacral artery Middle rectal artery Obturator artery Superior gluteal artery Umbilical artery Uterine artery Vaginal artery
Internal Mammary Artery, Left Internal Mammary Artery, Right	**Includes:** Anterior intercostal artery Internal thoracic artery Musculophrenic artery Pericardiophrenic artery Superior epigastric artery
Intracranial Artery	**Includes:** Anterior cerebral artery Anterior choroidal artery Anterior communicating artery Basilar artery Circle of Willis Internal carotid artery, intracranial portion Middle cerebral artery Ophthalmic artery Posterior cerebral artery Posterior communicating artery Posterior inferior cerebellar artery (PICA)

SECTION 0 - MEDICAL AND SURGICAL CHARACTER 4 - BODY PART	
Intracranial Vein	**Includes:** Anterior cerebral vein Basal (internal) cerebral vein Dural venous sinus Great cerebral vein Inferior cerebellar vein Inferior cerebral vein Internal (basal) cerebral vein Middle cerebral vein Ophthalmic vein Superior cerebellar vein Superior cerebral vein
Jejunum	**Includes:** Duodenojejunal flexure
Kidney	**Includes:** Renal calyx Renal capsule Renal cortex Renal segment
Kidney Pelvis, Left Kidney Pelvis, Right	**Includes:** Ureteropelvic junction (UPJ)
Kidney, Left Kidney, Right Kidneys, Bilateral	**Includes:** Renal calyx Renal capsule Renal cortex Renal segment
Knee Bursa and Ligament, Left Knee Bursa and Ligament, Right	**Includes:** Anterior cruciate ligament (ACL) Lateral collateral ligament (LCL) Ligament of head of fibula Medial collateral ligament (MCL) Patellar ligament Popliteal ligament Posterior cruciate ligament (PCL) Prepatellar bursa
Knee Joint, Left Knee Joint, Right	**Includes:** Femoropatellar joint Femorotibial joint Lateral meniscus Medial meniscus
Knee Tendon, Left Knee Tendon, Right	**Includes:** Patellar tendon
Lacrimal Duct, Left Lacrimal Duct, Right	**Includes:** Lacrimal canaliculus Lacrimal punctum Lacrimal sac Nasolacrimal duct

SECTION 0 - MEDICAL AND SURGICAL CHARACTER 4 - BODY PART	
Larynx	**Includes:** Aryepiglottic fold Arytenoid cartilage Corniculate cartilage Cuneiform cartilage False vocal cord Glottis Rima glottidis Thyroid cartilage Ventricular fold
Lens, Left Lens, Right	**Includes:** Zonule of Zinn
Lesser Omentum	**Includes:** Gastrohepatic omentum Hepatogastric ligament
Lesser Saphenous Vein, Left Lesser Saphenous Vein, Right	**Includes:** Small saphenous vein
Liver	**Includes:** Quadrate lobe
Lower Arm and Wrist Muscle, Left Lower Arm and Wrist Muscle, Right	**Includes:** Anatomical snuffbox Brachioradialis muscle Extensor carpi radialis muscle Extensor carpi ulnaris muscle Flexor carpi radialis muscle Flexor carpi ulnaris muscle Flexor pollicis longus muscle Palmaris longus muscle Pronator quadratus muscle Pronator teres muscle
Lower Eyelid, Left Lower Eyelid, Right	**Includes:** Inferior tarsal plate Medial canthus
Lower Femur, Left Lower Femur, Right	**Includes:** Lateral condyle of femur Lateral epicondyle of femur Medial condyle of femur Medial epicondyle of femur

SECTION 0 - MEDICAL AND SURGICAL CHARACTER 4 - BODY PART	
Lower Leg Muscle, Left Lower Leg Muscle, Right	**Includes:** Extensor digitorum longus muscle Extensor hallucis longus muscle Fibularis brevis muscle Fibularis longus muscle Flexor digitorum longus muscle Flexor hallucis longus muscle Gastrocnemius muscle Peroneus brevis muscle Peroneus longus muscle Popliteus muscle Soleus muscle Tibialis anterior muscle Tibialis posterior muscle
Lower Leg Tendon, Left Lower Leg Tendon, Right	**Includes:** Achilles tendon
Lower Lip	**Includes:** Frenulum labii inferioris Labial gland Vermilion border
Lumbar Nerve	**Includes:** Lumbosacral trunk Superior clunic (cluneal) nerve
Lumbar Plexus	**Includes:** Accessory obturator nerve Genitofemoral nerve Iliohypogastric nerve Ilioinguinal nerve Lateral femoral cutaneous nerve Obturator nerve Superior gluteal nerve
Lumbar Spinal Cord	**Includes:** Cauda equina Conus medullaris
Lumbar Sympathetic Nerve	**Includes:** Lumbar ganglion Lumbar splanchnic nerve
Lumbar Vertebra	**Includes:** Spinous process Vertebral arch Vertebral foramen Vertebral lamina Vertebral pedicle
Lumbar Vertebral Joint Lumbar Vertebral Joints, 2 or more	**Includes:** Lumbar facet joint
Lumbosacral Joint	**Includes:** Lumbosacral facet joint

SECTION 0 - MEDICAL AND SURGICAL CHARACTER 4 - BODY PART	
Lymphatic, Aortic	**Includes:** Celiac lymph node Gastric lymph node Hepatic lymph node Lumbar lymph node Pancreaticosplenic lymph node Paraaortic lymph node Retroperitoneal lymph node
Lymphatic, Head	**Includes:** Buccinator lymph node Infraauricular lymph node Infraparotid lymph node Parotid lymph node Preauricular lymph node Submandibular lymph node Submaxillary lymph node Submental lymph node Subparotid lymph node Suprahyoid lymph node
Lymphatic, Left Axillary	**Includes:** Anterior (pectoral) lymph node Apical (subclavicular) lymph node Brachial (lateral) lymph node Central axillary lymph node Lateral (brachial) lymph node Pectoral (anterior) lymph node Posterior (subscapular) lymph node Subclavicular (apical) lymph node Subscapular (posterior) lymph node
Lymphatic, Left Lower Extremity	**Includes:** Femoral lymph node Popliteal lymph node
Lymphatic, Left Neck	**Includes:** Cervical lymph node Jugular lymph node Mastoid (postauricular) lymph node Occipital lymph node Postauricular (mastoid) lymph node Retropharyngeal lymph node Supraclavicular (Virchow's) lymph node Virchow's (supraclavicular) lymph node
Lymphatic, Left Upper Extremity	**Includes:** Cubital lymph node Deltopectoral (infraclavicular) lymph node Epitrochlear lymph node Infraclavicular (deltopectoral) lymph node Supratrochlear lymph node
Lymphatic, Mesenteric	**Includes:** Inferior mesenteric lymph node Pararectal lymph node Superior mesenteric lymph node

SECTION 0 - MEDICAL AND SURGICAL CHARACTER 4 - BODY PART

SECTION 0 - MEDICAL AND SURGICAL CHARACTER 4 - BODY PART	
Lymphatic, Pelvis	**Includes:** Common iliac (subaortic) lymph node Gluteal lymph node Iliac lymph node Inferior epigastric lymph node Obturator lymph node Sacral lymph node Subaortic (common iliac) lymph node Suprainguinal lymph node
Lymphatic, Right Axillary	**Includes:** Anterior (pectoral) lymph node Apical (subclavicular) lymph node Brachial (lateral) lymph node Central axillary lymph node Lateral (brachial) lymph node Pectoral (anterior) lymph node Posterior (subscapular) lymph node Subclavicular (apical) lymph node Subscapular (posterior) lymph node
Lymphatic, Right Lower Extremity	**Includes:** Femoral lymph node Popliteal lymph node
Lymphatic, Right Neck	**Includes:** Cervical lymph node Jugular lymph node Mastoid (postauricular) lymph node Occipital lymph node Postauricular (mastoid) lymph node Retropharyngeal lymph node Right jugular trunk Right lymphatic duct Right subclavian trunk Supraclavicular (Virchow's) lymph node Virchow's (supraclavicular) lymph node
Lymphatic, Right Upper Extremity	**Includes:** Cubital lymph node Deltopectoral (infraclavicular) lymph node Epitrochlear lymph node Infraclavicular (deltopectoral) lymph node Supratrochlear lymph node
Lymphatic, Thorax	**Includes:** Intercostal lymph node Mediastinal lymph node Parasternal lymph node Paratracheal lymph node Tracheobronchial lymph node
Main Bronchus, Right	Bronchus Intermedius Intermediate bronchus

SECTION 0 - MEDICAL AND SURGICAL CHARACTER 4 - BODY PART	
Mandible, Left Mandible, Right	**Includes:** Alveolar process of mandible Condyloid process Mandibular notch Mental foramen
Mastoid Sinus, Left Mastoid Sinus, Right	**Includes:** Mastoid air cells
Maxilla, Left Maxilla, Right	**Includes:** Alveolar process of maxilla
Maxillary Sinus, Left Maxillary Sinus, Right	**Includes:** Antrum of Highmore
Median Nerve	**Includes:** Anterior interosseous nerve Palmar cutaneous nerve
Medulla Oblongata	**Includes:** Myelencephalon
Mesentery	**Includes:** Mesoappendix Mesocolon
Metacarpocarpal Joint, Left Metacarpocarpal Joint, Right	**Includes:** Carpometacarpal (CMC) joint
Metatarsal-Phalangeal Joint, Left Metatarsal-Phalangeal Joint, Right	**Includes:** Metatarsophalangeal (MTP) joint
Metatarsal-Tarsal Joint, Left Metatarsal-Tarsal Joint, Right	**Includes:** Tarsometatarsal joint
Middle Ear, Left Middle Ear, Right	**Includes:** Oval window Tympanic cavity
Minor Salivary Gland	**Includes:** Anterior lingual gland
Mitral Valve	**Includes:** Bicuspid valve Left atrioventricular valve Mitral annulus
Nasal Bone	**Includes:** Vomer of nasal septum
Nasal Septum	**Includes:** Quadrangular cartilage Septal cartilage Vomer bone
Nasal Turbinate	**Includes:** Inferior turbinate Middle turbinate Nasal concha Superior turbinate
Nasopharynx	**Includes:** Choana Fossa of Rosenmüller Pharyngeal recess Rhinopharynx

SECTION 0 - MEDICAL AND SURGICAL CHARACTER 4 - BODY PART	
Neck Muscle, Left Neck Muscle, Right	**Includes:** Anterior vertebral muscle Arytenoid muscle Cricothyroid muscle Infrahyoid muscle Levator scapulae muscle Platysma muscle Scalene muscle Splenius cervicis muscle Sternocleidomastoid muscle Suprahyoid muscle Thyroarytenoid muscle
Nipple, Left Nipple, Right	**Includes:** Areola
Nose	**Includes:** Columella External naris Greater alar cartilage Internal naris Lateral nasal cartilage Lesser alar cartilage Nasal cavity Nostril
Occipital Bone, Left Occipital Bone, Right	**Includes:** Foramen magnum
Oculomotor Nerve	**Includes:** Third cranial nerve
Olfactory Nerve	**Includes:** First cranial nerve Olfactory bulb
Optic Nerve	**Includes:** Optic chiasma Second cranial nerve
Orbit, Left Orbit, Right	**Includes:** Bony orbit Orbital portion of ethmoid bone Orbital portion of frontal bone Orbital portion of lacrimal bone Orbital portion of maxilla Orbital portion of palatine bone Orbital portion of sphenoid bone Orbital portion of zygomatic bone
Pancreatic Duct	**Includes:** Duct of Wirsung
Pancreatic Duct, Accessory	**Includes:** Duct of Santorini
Parotid Duct, Left Parotid Duct, Right	**Includes:** Stensen's duct

SECTION 0 - MEDICAL AND SURGICAL CHARACTER 4 - BODY PART	
Pelvic Bone, Left Pelvic Bone, Right	**Includes:** Iliac crest Ilium Ischium Pubis
Pelvic Cavity	**Includes:** Retropubic space
Penis	**Includes:** Corpus cavernosum Corpus spongiosum
Perineum Muscle	**Includes:** Bulbospongiosus muscle Cremaster muscle Deep transverse perineal muscle Ischiocavernosus muscle Levator ani muscle Superficial transverse perineal muscle
Peritoneum	**Includes:** Epiploic foramen
Peroneal Artery, Left Peroneal Artery, Right	**Includes:** Fibular artery
Peroneal Nerve	**Includes:** Common fibular nerve Common peroneal nerve External popliteal nerve Lateral sural cutaneous nerve
Pharynx	**Includes:** Base of Tongue Hypopharynx Laryngopharynx Oropharynx Piriform recess (sinus) Tongue, base of
Phrenic Nerve	**Includes:** Accessory phrenic nerve
Pituitary Gland	**Includes:** Adenohypophysis Hypophysis Neurohypophysis
Pons	**Includes:** Apneustic center Basis pontis Locus ceruleus Pneumotaxic center Pontine tegmentum Superior olivary nucleus
Popliteal Artery, Left Popliteal Artery, Right	**Includes:** Inferior genicular artery Middle genicular artery Superior genicular artery Sural artery

SECTION 0 - MEDICAL AND SURGICAL CHARACTER 4 - BODY PART	
Portal Vein	**Includes:** Hepatic portal vein
Prepuce	**Includes:** Foreskin Glans penis
Pudendal Nerve	**Includes:** Posterior labial nerve Posterior scrotal nerve
Pulmonary Artery, Left	**Includes:** Arterial canal (duct) Botallo's duct Pulmoaortic canal
Pulmonary Valve	**Includes:** Pulmonary annulus Pulmonic valve
Pulmonary Vein, Left	**Includes:** Left inferior pulmonary vein Left superior pulmonary vein
Pulmonary Vein, Right	**Includes:** Right inferior pulmonary vein Right superior pulmonary vein
Radial Artery, Left Radial Artery, Right	**Includes:** Radial recurrent artery
Radial Nerve	**Includes:** Dorsal digital nerve Musculospiral nerve Palmar cutaneous nerve Posterior interosseous nerve
Radius, Left Radius, Right	**Includes:** Ulnar notch
Rectum	**Includes:** Anorectal junction
Renal Artery, Left Renal Artery, Right	**Includes:** Inferior suprarenal artery Renal segmental artery
Renal Vein, Left	**Includes:** Left inferior phrenic vein Left ovarian vein Left second lumbar vein Left suprarenal vein Left testicular vein
Retina, Left Retina, Right	**Includes:** Fovea Macula Optic disc
Retroperitoneum	**Includes:** Retroperitoneal space

SECTION 0 - MEDICAL AND SURGICAL CHARACTER 4 - BODY PART	
Sacral Plexus	**Includes:** Inferior gluteal nerve Posterior femoral cutaneous nerve Pudendal nerve
Sacral Sympathetic Nerve	**Includes:** Ganglion impar (ganglion of Walther) Pelvic splanchnic nerve Sacral ganglion Sacral splanchnic nerve
Sacrococcygeal Joint	**Includes:** Sacrococcygeal symphysis
Scapula, Left Scapula, Right	**Includes:** Acromion (process) Coracoid process
Sciatic Nerve	**Includes:** Ischiatic nerve
Shoulder Bursa and Ligament, Left Shoulder Bursa and Ligament, Right	**Includes:** Acromioclavicular ligament Coracoacromial ligament Coracoclavicular ligament Coracohumeral ligament Costoclavicular ligament Glenohumeral ligament Interclavicular ligament Sternoclavicular ligament Subacromial bursa Transverse humeral ligament Transverse scapular ligament
Shoulder Joint, Left Shoulder Joint, Right	**Includes:** Glenohumeral joint Glenoid ligament (labrum)
Shoulder Muscle, Left Shoulder Muscle, Right	**Includes:** Deltoid muscle Infraspinatus muscle Subscapularis muscle Supraspinatus muscle Teres major muscle Teres minor muscle
Sigmoid Colon	**Includes:** Rectosigmoid junction Sigmoid flexure
Skin	**Includes:** Dermis Epidermis Sebaceous gland Sweat gland

SECTION 0 - MEDICAL AND SURGICAL CHARACTER 4 - BODY PART	
Sphenoid Bone, Left Sphenoid Bone, Right	**Includes:** Greater wing Lesser wing Optic foramen Pterygoid process Sella turcica
Spinal Canal	**Includes:** Epidural space, spinal Extradural space, spinal Subarachnoid space, spinal Subdural space, spinal Vertebral canal
Spinal Cord	**Includes:** Denticulate ligament
Spinal Meninges	**Includes:** Arachnoid mater, spinal Denticular (dentate) ligament Dura mater, spinal Filum terminale Leptomeninges, spinal Pia mater, spinal
Spleen	**Includes:** Accessory spleen
Splenic Artery	**Includes:** Left gastroepiploic artery Pancreatic artery Short gastric artery
Splenic Vein	**Includes:** Left gastroepiploic vein Pancreatic vein
Sternum	**Includes:** Manubrium Suprasternal notch Xiphoid process
Stomach, Pylorus	**Includes:** Pyloric antrum Pyloric canal Pyloric sphincter
Subarachnoid Space	**Includes:** Subarachnoid space, intracranial
Subclavian Artery, Left Subclavian Artery, Right	**Includes:** Costocervical trunk Dorsal scapular artery Internal thoracic artery
Subcutaneous Tissue and Fascia, Anterior Neck	**Includes:** Deep cervical fascia Pretracheal fascia
Subcutaneous Tissue and Fascia, Chest	**Includes:** Pectoral fascia

SECTION 0 - MEDICAL AND SURGICAL CHARACTER 4 - BODY PART	
Subcutaneous Tissue and Fascia, Face	**Includes:** Masseteric fascia Orbital fascia
Subcutaneous Tissue and Fascia, Left Foot	**Includes:** Plantar fascia (aponeurosis)
Subcutaneous Tissue and Fascia, Left Hand	**Includes:** Palmar fascia (aponeurosis)
Subcutaneous Tissue and Fascia, Left Lower Arm	**Includes:** Antebrachial fascia Bicipital aponeurosis
Subcutaneous Tissue and Fascia, Left Upper Arm	**Includes:** Axillary fascia Deltoid fascia Infraspinatus fascia Subscapular aponeurosis Supraspinatus fascia
Subcutaneous Tissue and Fascia, Left Upper Leg	**Includes:** Crural fascia Fascia lata Iliac fascia Iliotibial tract (band)
Subcutaneous Tissue and Fascia, Posterior Neck	**Includes:** Prevertebral fascia
Subcutaneous Tissue and Fascia, Right Foot	**Includes:** Plantar fascia (aponeurosis)
Subcutaneous Tissue and Fascia, Right Hand	**Includes:** Palmar fascia (aponeurosis)
Subcutaneous Tissue and Fascia, Right Lower Arm	**Includes:** Antebrachial fascia Bicipital aponeurosis
Subcutaneous Tissue and Fascia, Right Upper Arm	**Includes:** Axillary fascia Deltoid fascia Infraspinatus fascia Subscapular aponeurosis Supraspinatus fascia
Subcutaneous Tissue and Fascia, Right Upper Leg	**Includes:** Crural fascia Fascia lata Iliac fascia Iliotibial tract (band)
Subcutaneous Tissue and Fascia, Scalp	**Includes:** Galea aponeurotica
Subcutaneous Tissue and Fascia, Trunk	**Includes:** External oblique aponeurosis Transversalis fascia
Subdural Space	**Includes:** Subdural spacc, intracranial
Submaxillary Gland, Left Submaxillary Gland, Right	**Includes:** Submandibular gland

SECTION 0 - MEDICAL AND SURGICAL CHARACTER 4 - BODY PART	
Superior Mesenteric Artery	**Includes:** Ileal artery Ileocolic artery Inferior pancreaticoduodenal artery Jejunal artery
Superior Mesenteric Vein	**Includes:** Right gastroepiploic vein
Superior Vena Cava	**Includes:** Precava
Tarsal Joint, Left Tarsal Joint, Right	**Includes:** Calcaneocuboid joint Cuboideonavicular joint Cuneonavicular joint Intercuneiform joint Subtalar (talocalcaneal) joint Talocalcaneal (subtalar) joint Talocalcaneonavicular joint
Tarsal, Left Tarsal, Right	**Includes:** Calcaneus Cuboid bone Intermediate cuneiform bone Lateral cuneiform bone Medial cuneiform bone Navicular bone Talus bone
Temporal Artery, Left Temporal Artery, Right	**Includes:** Middle temporal artery Superficial temporal artery Transverse facial artery
Temporal Bone, Left Temporal Bone, Right	**Includes:** Mastoid process Petrous part of temporal bone Tympanic part of temporal bone Zygomatic process of temporal bone
Thalamus	**Includes:** Epithalamus Geniculate nucleus Metathalamus Pulvinar
Thoracic Aorta Ascending/Arch	**Includes:** Aortic arch Ascending aorta
Thoracic Duct	**Includes:** Left jugular trunk Left subclavian trunk
Thoracic Nerve	**Includes:** Intercostal nerve Intercostobrachial nerve Subcostal nerve

SECTION 0 - MEDICAL AND SURGICAL CHARACTER 4 - BODY PART	
Thoracic Sympathetic Nerve	**Includes:** Cardiac plexus Esophageal plexus Greater splanchnic nerve Inferior cardiac nerve Least splanchnic nerve Lesser splanchnic nerve Middle cardiac nerve Pulmonary plexus Superior cardiac nerve Thoracic aortic plexus Thoracic ganglion
Thoracic Vertebra	**Includes:** Spinous process Vertebral arch Vertebral foramen Vertebral lamina Vertebral pedicle
Thoracic Vertebral Joint Thoracic Vertebral Joints, 2 to 7 Thoracic Vertebral Joints, 8 or more	**Includes:** Costotransverse joint Costovertebral joint Thoracic facet joint
Thoracolumbar Vertebral Joint	**Includes:** Thoracolumbar facet joint
Thorax Bursa and Ligament, Left Thorax Bursa and Ligament, Right	**Includes:** Costotransverse ligament Costoxiphoid ligament Sternocostal ligament
Thorax Muscle, Left Thorax Muscle, Right	**Includes:** Intercostal muscle Levatores costarum muscle Pectoralis major muscle Pectoralis minor muscle Serratus anterior muscle Subclavius muscle Subcostal muscle Transverse thoracis muscle
Thymus	**Includes:** Thymus gland
Thyroid Artery, Left Thyroid Artery, Right	**Includes:** Cricothyroid artery Hyoid artery Sternocleidomastoid artery Superior laryngeal artery Superior thyroid artery Thyrocervical trunk
Tibia, Left Tibia, Right	**Includes:** Lateral condyle of tibia Medial condyle of tibia Medial malleolus

SECTION 0 - MEDICAL AND SURGICAL CHARACTER 4 - BODY PART	
Tibial Nerve	**Includes:** Lateral plantar nerve Medial plantar nerve Medial popliteal nerve Medial sural cutaneous nerve
Toe Nail	**Includes:** Nail bed Nail plate
Toe Phalangeal Joint, Left Toe Phalangeal Joint, Right	**Includes:** Interphalangeal (IP) joint
Tongue	**Includes:** Frenulum linguae Lingual tonsil
Tongue, Palate, Pharynx Muscle	**Includes:** Chondroglossus muscle Genioglossus muscle Hyoglossus muscle Inferior longitudinal muscle Levator veli palatini muscle Palatoglossal muscle Palatopharyngeal muscle Pharyngeal constrictor muscle Salpingopharyngeus muscle Styloglossus muscle Stylopharyngeus muscle Superior longitudinal muscle Tensor veli palatini muscle
Tonsils	**Includes:** Palatine tonsil
Trachea	**Includes:** Cricoid cartilage
Transverse Colon	**Includes:** Splenic flexure
Tricuspid Valve	**Includes:** Right atrioventricular valve Tricuspid annulus
Trigeminal Nerve	**Includes:** Fifth cranial nerve Gasserian ganglion Mandibular nerve Maxillary nerve Ophthalmic nerve Trifacial nerve
Trochlear Nerve	**Includes:** Fourth cranial nerve

SECTION 0 - MEDICAL AND SURGICAL CHARACTER 4 - BODY PART	
Trunk Bursa and Ligament, Left Trunk Bursa and Ligament, Right	**Includes:** Iliolumbar ligament Interspinous ligament Intertransverse ligament Ligamentum flavum Pubic ligament Sacrococcygeal ligament Sacroiliac ligament Sacrospinous ligament Sacrotuberous ligament Supraspinous ligament
Trunk Muscle, Left Trunk Muscle, Right	**Includes:** Coccygeus muscle Erector spinae muscle Interspinalis muscle Intertransversarius muscle Latissimus dorsi muscle Quadratus lumborum muscle Rhomboid major muscle Rhomboid minor muscle Serratus posterior muscle Transversospinalis muscle Trapezius muscle
Tympanic Membrane, Left Tympanic Membrane, Right	**Includes:** Pars flaccida
Ulna, Left Ulna, Right	**Includes:** Olecranon process Radial notch
Ulnar Artery, Left Ulnar Artery, Right	**Includes:** Anterior ulnar recurrent artery Common interosseous artery Posterior ulnar recurrent artery
Ulnar Nerve	**Includes:** Cubital nerve
Upper Arm Muscle, Left Upper Arm Muscle, Right	**Includes:** Biceps brachii muscle Brachialis muscle Coracobrachialis muscle Triceps brachii muscle
Upper Artery	Aortic intercostal artery Bronchial artery Esophageal artery Subcostal artery
Upper Eyelid, Left Upper Eyelid, Right	**Includes:** Lateral canthus Levator palpebrae superioris muscle Orbicularis oculi muscle Superior tarsal plate

SECTION 0 - MEDICAL AND SURGICAL CHARACTER 4 - BODY PART	
Upper Femur, Left Upper Femur, Right	**Includes:** Femoral head Greater trochanter Lesser trochanter Neck of femur
Upper Leg Muscle, Left Upper Leg Muscle, Right Upper Leg Muscle, Left Upper Leg Muscle, Right (continued)	**Includes:** Adductor brevis muscle Adductor longus muscle Adductor magnus muscle Biceps femoris muscle Gracilis muscle Pectineus muscle Quadriceps (femoris) Rectus femoris muscle Sartorius muscle Semimembranosus muscle Semitendinosus muscle Vastus intermedius muscle Vastus lateralis muscle Vastus medialis muscle
Upper Lip	**Includes:** Frenulum labii superioris Labial gland Vermilion border
Ureter Ureter, Left Ureter, Right Ureters, Bilateral	**Includes:** Ureteral orifice Ureterovesical orifice
Urethra	**Includes:** Bulbourethral (Cowper's) gland Cowper's (bulbourethral) gland External urethral sphincter Internal urethral sphincter Membranous urethra Penile urethra Prostatic urethra
Uterine Supporting Structure	**Includes:** Broad ligament Infundibulopelvic ligament Ovarian ligament Round ligament of uterus
Uterus	**Includes:** Fundus uteri Myometrium Perimetrium Uterine cornu
Uvula	**Includes:** Palatine uvula

SECTION 0 - MEDICAL AND SURGICAL CHARACTER 4 - BODY PART

Vagus Nerve	**Includes:** Anterior vagal trunk Pharyngeal plexus Pneumogastric nerve Posterior vagal trunk Pulmonary plexus Recurrent laryngeal nerve Superior laryngeal nerve Tenth cranial nerve
Vas Deferens Vas Deferens, Bilateral Vas Deferens, Left Vas Deferens, Right	**Includes:** Ductus deferens Ejaculatory duct
Ventricle, Right	**Includes:** Conus arteriosus
Ventricular Septum	**Includes:** Interventricular septum
Vertebral Artery, Left Vertebral Artery, Right	**Includes:** Anterior spinal artery Posterior spinal artery
Vertebral Vein, Left Vertebral Vein, Right	**Includes:** Deep cervical vein Suboccipital venous plexus
Vestibular Gland	**Includes:** Bartholin's (greater vestibular) gland Greater vestibular (Bartholin's) gland Paraurethral (Skene's) gland Skene's (paraurethral) gland
Vitreous, Left Vitreous, Right	**Includes:** Vitreous body
Vocal Cord, Left Vocal Cord, Right	**Includes:** Vocal fold
Vulva	**Includes:** Labia majora Labia minora
Wrist Bursa and Ligament, Left Wrist Bursa and Ligament, Right	**Includes:** Palmar ulnocarpal ligament Radial collateral carpal ligament Radiocarpal ligament Radioulnar ligament Ulnar collateral carpal ligament
Wrist Joint, Left Wrist Joint, Right	**Includes:** Distal radioulnar joint Radiocarpal joint

SECTION 0 - MEDICAL AND SURGICAL CHARACTER 5 - APPROACH

External	**Definition:** Procedures performed directly on the skin or mucous membrane and procedures performed indirectly by the application of external force through the skin or mucous membrane
Open	**Definition:** Cutting through the skin or mucous membrane and any other body layers necessary to expose the site of the procedure

Percutaneous	**Definition:** Entry, by puncture or minor incision, of instrumentation through the skin or mucous membrane and any other body layers necessary to reach the site of the procedure
Percutaneous Endoscopic	**Definition:** Entry, by puncture or minor incision, of instrumentation through the skin or mucous membrane and any other body layers necessary to reach and visualize the site of the procedure
Via Natural or Artificial Opening	**Definition:** Entry of instrumentation through a natural or artificial external opening to reach the site of the procedure
Via Natural or Artificial Opening Endoscopic	**Definition:** Entry of instrumentation through a natural or artificial external opening to reach and visualize the site of the procedure
Via Natural or Artificial Opening With Percutaneous Endoscopic Assistance	**Definition:** Entry of instrumentation through a natural or artificial external opening and entry, by puncture or minor incision, of instrumentation through the skin or mucous membrane and any other body layers necessary to aid in the performance of the procedure

SECTION 0 - MEDICAL AND SURGICAL CHARACTER 6 - DEVICE	
Artificial Sphincter in Gastrointestinal System	**Includes:** Artificial anal sphincter (AAS) Artificial bowel sphincter (neosphincter)
Artificial Sphincter in Urinary System	**Includes:** AMS 800® Urinary Control System Artificial urinary sphincter (AUS)
Autologous Arterial Tissue in Heart and Great Vessels	**Includes:** Autologous artery graft
Autologous Arterial Tissue in Lower Arteries	**Includes:** Autologous artery graft
Autologous Arterial Tissue in Lower Veins	**Includes:** Autologous artery graft
Autologous Arterial Tissue in Upper Arteries	**Includes:** Autologous artery graft
Autologous Arterial Tissue in Upper Veins	**Includes:** Autologous artery graft
Autologous Tissue Substitute	**Includes:** Autograft Cultured epidermal cell autograft Epicel® cultured epidermal autograft
Autologous Venous Tissue in Heart and Great Vessels	**Includes:** Autologous vein graft
Autologous Venous Tissue in Lower Arteries	**Includes:** Autologous vein graft
Autologous Venous Tissue in Lower Veins	**Includes:** Autologous vein graft
Autologous Venous Tissue in Upper Arteries	**Includes:** Autologous vein graft
Autologous Venous Tissue in Upper Veins	**Includes:** Autologous vein graft
Bone Growth Stimulator in Head and Facial Bones	**Includes:** Electrical bone growth stimulator (EBGS) Ultrasonic osteogenic stimulator Ultrasound bone healing system
Bone Growth Stimulator in Lower Bones	**Includes:** Electrical bone growth stimulator (EBGS) Ultrasonic osteogenic stimulator Ultrasound bone healing system

SECTION 0 - MEDICAL AND SURGICAL CHARACTER 6 - DEVICE	
Bone Growth Stimulator in Upper Bones	**Includes:** Electrical bone growth stimulator (EBGS) Ultrasonic osteogenic stimulator Ultrasound bone healing system
Cardiac Lead in Heart and Great Vessels	**Includes:** Cardiac contractility modulation lead
Cardiac Lead, Defibrillator for Insertion in Heart and Great Vessels	**Includes:** ACUITY™ Steerable Lead Attain Ability® lead Attain StarFix® (OTW) lead Cardiac resynchronization therapy (CRT) lead Corox (OTW) Bipolar Lead Durata® Defibrillation Lead ENDOTAK RELIANCE® (G) Defibrillation Lead
Cardiac Lead, Pacemaker for Insertion in Heart and Great Vessels	**Includes:** ACUITY™ Steerable Lead Attain Ability® lead Attain StarFix® (OTW) lead Cardiac resynchronization therapy (CRT) lead Corox (OTW) Bipolar Lead
Cardiac Resynchronization Defibrillator Pulse Generator for Insertion in Subcutaneous Tissue and Fascia	**Includes:** COGNIS® CRT-D Concerto II CRT-D Consulta CRT-D CONTAK RENEWAL® 3 RF (HE) CRT-D LIVIAN™ CRT-D Maximo II DR CRT-D Ovatio™ CRT-D Protecta XT CRT-D
Cardiac Resynchronization Pacemaker Pulse Generator for Insertion in Subcutaneous Tissue and Fascia	**Includes:** Consulta CRT-P Stratos LV Synchra CRT-P
Cardiac Rhythm Related Device in Subcutaneous Tissue and Fascia	**Includes:** Baroreflex Activation Therapy® (BAT®) Rheos® System device
Contraceptive Device in Female Reproductive System	**Includes:** Intrauterine device (IUD)
Contraceptive Device in Subcutaneous Tissue and Fascia	**Includes:** Subdermal progesterone implant
Contractility Modulation Device for Insertion in Subcutaneous Tissue and Fascia	**Includes:** Optimizer™ III implantable pulse generator
Defibrillator Generator for Insertion in Subcutaneous Tissue and Fascia	**Includes:** Implantable cardioverter-defibrillator (ICD) Maximo II DR (VR) Protecta XT DR (XT VR) Secura (DR) (VR) Virtuoso (II) (DR) (VR)
Diaphragmatic Pacemaker Lead in	**Includes:**

SECTION 0 - MEDICAL AND SURGICAL CHARACTER 6 - DEVICE	
Respiratory System	Phrenic nerve stimulator lead
Drainage Device	**Includes:** Cystostomy tube Foley catheter Percutaneous nephrostomy catheter Thoracostomy tube
External Fixation Device in Head and Facial Bones	**Includes:** External fixator
External Fixation Device in Lower Bones	**Includes:** External fixator
External Fixation Device in Lower Joints	**Includes:** External fixator
External Fixation Device in Upper Bones	**Includes:** External fixator
External Fixation Device in Upper Joints	**Includes:** External fixator
External Fixation Device, Hybrid for Insertion in Upper Bones	**Includes:** Delta frame external fixator Sheffield hybrid external fixator
External Fixation Device, Hybrid for Insertion in Lower Bones	**Includes:** Delta frame external fixator Sheffield hybrid external fixator
External Fixation Device, Hybrid for Reposition in Upper Bones	**Includes:** Delta frame external fixator Sheffield hybrid external fixator
External Fixation Device, Hybrid for Reposition in Lower Bones	**Includes:** Delta frame external fixator Sheffield hybrid external fixator
External Fixation Device, Limb Lengthening for Insertion in Upper Bones	**Includes:** Ilizarov-Vecklich device
External Fixation Device, Limb Lengthening for Insertion in Lower Bones	**Includes:** Ilizarov-Vecklich device
External Fixation Device, Monoplanar for Insertion in Upper Bones	**Includes:** Uniplanar external fixator
External Fixation Device, Monoplanar for Insertion in Lower Bones	**Includes:** Uniplanar external fixator
External Fixation Device, Monoplanar for Reposition in Upper Bones	**Includes:** Uniplanar external fixator
External Fixation Device, Monoplanar for Reposition in Lower Bones	**Includes:** Uniplanar external fixator
External Fixation Device, Ring for Insertion in Upper Bones	**Includes:** Ilizarov external fixator Sheffield ring external fixator
External Fixation Device, Ring for Insertion in Lower Bones	**Includes:** Ilizarov external fixator Sheffield ring external fixator
External Fixation Device, Ring for Reposition in Upper Bones	**Includes:** Ilizarov external fixator

SECTION 0 - MEDICAL AND SURGICAL CHARACTER 6 - DEVICE	
	Sheffield ring external fixator
External Fixation Device, Ring for Reposition in Lower Bones	**Includes:** Ilizarov external fixator Sheffield ring external fixator
External Heart Assist System in Heart and Great Vessels	**Includes:** Biventricular external heart assist system BVS 5000 Ventricular Assist Device PVAD™ Ventricular Assist Device
Extraluminal Device	**Includes:** LAP-BAND® adjustable gastric banding system REALIZE® Adjustable Gastric Band TigerPaw® system for closure of left atrial appendage
Feeding Device in Gastrointestinal System	**Includes:** Percutaneous endoscopic gastrojejunostomy (PEG/J) tube Percutaneous endoscopic gastrostomy (PEG) tube
Hearing Device in Ear, Nose, Sinus	**Includes:** Esteem® implantable hearing system
Hearing Device in Head and Facial Bones	**Includes:** Bone anchored hearing device
Hearing Device, Bone Conduction for Insertion in Ear, Nose, Sinus	**Includes:** Bone anchored hearing device
Hearing Device, Multiple Channel Cochlear Prosthesis for Insertion in Ear, Nose, Sinus	**Includes:** Cochlear implant (CI), multiple channel (electrode)
Hearing Device, Single Channel Cochlear Prosthesis for Insertion in Ear, Nose, Sinus	**Includes:** Cochlear implant (CI), single channel (electrode)
Implantable Heart Assist System in Heart and Great Vessels	**Includes:** Berlin Heart Ventricular Assist Device DeBakey Left Ventricular Assist Device DuraHeart Left Ventricular Assist System HeartMate II® Left Ventricular Assist Device (LVAD) HeartMate XVE® Left Ventricular Assist Device (LVAD) Novacor Left Ventricular Assist Device Thoratec IVAD (Implantable Ventricular Assist Device)
Infusion Device	**Includes:** InDura, intrathecal catheter (1P) (spinal) Non-tunneled central venous catheter Peripherally inserted central catheter (PICC) Tunneled spinal (intrathecal) catheter
Infusion Device, Pump in Subcutaneous Tissue and Fascia	**Includes:** Implantable drug infusion pump (anti-spasmodic) (chemotherapy)(pain) Injection reservoir, pump Pump reservoir Subcutaneous injection reservoir, pump
Interbody Fusion Device in Lower Joints	**Includes:** Axial Lumbar Interbody Fusion System AxiaLIF® System CoRoent® XL Direct Lateral Interbody Fusion (DLIF) device EXtreme Lateral Interbody Fusion (XLIF) device

SECTION 0 - MEDICAL AND SURGICAL CHARACTER 6 - DEVICE	
	Interbody fusion (spine) cage
	XLIF® System
Interbody Fusion Device in Upper Joints	**Includes:**
	BAK/C® Interbody Cervical Fusion System
	Interbody fusion (spine) cage
Internal Fixation Device in Head and Facial Bones	**Includes:**
	Bone screw (interlocking)(lag)(pedicle)(recessed)
	Kirschner wire (K-wire)
	Neutralization plate
Internal Fixation Device in Lower Bones	**Includes:**
	Bone screw (interlocking)(lag)(pedicle)(recessed)
	Clamp and rod internal fixation system (CRIF)
	Kirschner wire (K-wire)
	Neutralization plate
Internal Fixation Device in Lower Joints	**Includes:**
	Fusion screw (compression)(lag)(locking) Joint fixation plate
	Kirschner wire (K-wire)
Internal Fixation Device in Upper Bones	**Includes:**
	Bone screw (interlocking)(lag)(pedicle)(recessed)
	Clamp and rod internal fixation system (CRIF)
	Kirschner wire (K-wire)
	Neutralization plate
Internal Fixation Device in Upper Joints	**Includes:**
	Fusion screw (compression)(lag)(locking)
	Joint fixation plate
	Kirschner wire (K-wire)
Internal Fixation Device, Intramedullary in Lower Bones	**Includes:**
	Intramedullary (IM) rod (nail)
	Intramedullary skeletal kinetic distractor (ISKD)
	Küntscher nail
Internal Fixation Device, Intramedullary in Upper Bones	**Includes:**
	Intramedullary (IM) rod (nail)
	Intramedullary skeletal kinetic distractor (ISKD)
	Küntscher nail
Internal Fixation Device, Rigid Plate for Insertion in Upper Bones	**Includes:**
	Titanium Sternal Fixation System (TSFS)
Internal Fixation Device, Rigid Plate for Reposition in Upper Bones	**Includes:**
	Titanium Sternal Fixation System (TSFS)

SECTION 0 - MEDICAL AND SURGICAL CHARACTER 6 - DEVICE	
Intraluminal Device	**Includes:**
	AFX(R) Endovascular AAA System
	AneuRx® AAA Advantage®
	Assurant (Cobalt) stent
	Carotid WALLSTENT® Monorail® Endoprosthesis
	Centrimag® Blood Pump
	CoAxia NeuroFlo catheter
	Colonic Z-Stent®
	Complctc (SE) stent
	Cook Zenith AAA Endovascular Graft
	Driver stent (RX) (OTW)
	E-Luminexx™ (Biliary)(Vascular) Stent
	Embolization coil(s)
	Endologix AFX(R) Endovascular AAA System
	Endurant(R) II AAA stent graft system
	Endurant® Endovascular Stent Graft
	EXCLUDER(R) AAA Endoprosthesis
	Express® (LD) Premounted Stent System
	Express® Biliary SD Monorail® Premounted Stent
	Express® SD Renal Monorail® Premounted Stent
	FLAIR® Endovascular Stent Graft
	Formula™ Balloon-Expandable Renal Stent System
	GORE EXCLUDER(R) AAA Endoprosthesis
	GORE TAG(R) Thoracic Endoprosthesis
	LifeStent® (Flexstar)(XL) Vascular Stent System
	Medtronic Endurant(R) II AAA stent graft system
	Micro-Driver stent (RX) (OTW)
	Pipeline™ Embolization device (PED)
	Protege® RX Carotid Stent System
	Stent (angioplasty)(embolization)
	System
	System
	Talent® Converter
	Talent® Occluder
	Talent® Stent Graft (abdominal)(thoracic)
	TandemHeart® System
	Therapeutic occlusion coil(s)
	Ultraflex™ Precision Colonic Stent System
	Valiant Thoracic Stent Graft
	WALLSTENT® Endoprosthesis
	Zenith AAA Endovascular Graft
	Zenith Flex® AAA Endovascular Graft
	Zenith TX2® TAA Endovascular Graft
	Zenith® Renu™ AAA Ancillary Graft
Intraluminal Device, Branched or Fenestrated, One or Two Arteries for Restriction in Lower Arteries	Cook Zenith AAA Endovascular Graft EXCLUDER(R) AAA Endoprosthesis EXCLUDER(R) IBE Endoprosthesis GORE EXCLUDER(R) AAA Endoprosthesis GORE EXCLUDER(R) IBE Endoprosthesis Zenith AAA Endovascular Graft
Intraluminal Device, Branched or Fenestrated, Three or More Arteries for Restriction in Lower Arteries	Cook Zenith AAA Endovascular Graft EXCLUDER(R) AAA Endoprosthesis GORE EXCLUDER(R) AAA Endoprosthesis Zenith AAA Endovascular Graft

SECTION 0 - MEDICAL AND SURGICAL CHARACTER 6 - DEVICE	
Intraluminal Device, Pessary in Female Reproductive System	**Includes:** Pessary ring Vaginal pessary
Intraluminal Device, Airway in Ear, Nose, Sinus	**Includes:** Nasopharyngeal airway (NPA)
Intraluminal Device, Airway in Gastrointestinal System	**Includes:** Esophageal obturator airway (EOA)
Intraluminal Device, Airway in Mouth and Throat	**Includes:** Guedel airway Oropharyngeal airway (OPA)
Intraluminal Device, Bioactive in Upper Arteries	**Includes:** Bioactive embolization coil(s) Micrus CERECYTE microcoil
Intraluminal Device, Drug-eluting in Heart and Great Vessels	**Includes:** CYPHER® Stent Endeavor® (III)(IV) (Sprint) Zotarolimus-eluting Coronary Stent System Everolimus-eluting coronary stent Paclitaxel-eluting coronary stent Sirolimus-eluting coronary stent TAXUS® Liberte® Paclitaxel-eluting Coronary Stent System XIENCE V Everolimus Eluting Coronary Stent System Zotarolimus-eluting coronary stent
Intraluminal Device, Drug-eluting in Lower Arteries	**Includes:** Paclitaxel-eluting peripheral stent Zilver® PTX® (paclitaxel) Drug-Eluting Peripheral Stent
Intraluminal Device, Drug-eluting in Upper Arteries	**Includes:** Paclitaxel-eluting peripheral stent Zilver® PTX® (paclitaxel) Drug-Eluting Peripheral Stent
Intraluminal Device, Endobronchial Valve in Respiratory System	**Includes:** Spiration IBV™ Valve System
Intraluminal Device, Endotracheal Airway in Respiratory System	**Includes:** Endotracheal tube (cuffed)(double-lumen)
Liner in Lower Joints	**Includes:** Acetabular cup Hip (joint) liner Joint liner (insert) Knee (implant) insert Tibial insert
Monitoring Device	**Includes:** Blood glucose monitoring system Cardiac event recorder Continuous Glucose Monitoring (CGM) device Implantable glucose monitoring device Loop recorder, implantable Reveal (DX)(XT)
Monitoring Device, Hemodynamic for Insertion in Subcutaneous Tissue and Fascia	**Includes:** Implantable hemodynamic monitor (IHM) Implantable hemodynamic monitoring system (IHMS)
Monitoring Device, Pressure Sensor for Insertion in Heart and Great Vessels	**Includes:** CardioMEMS® pressure sensor EndoSure® sensor
Neurostimulator Lead in Central Nervous System	**Includes:** Cortical strip neurostimulator lead DBS lead

SECTION 0 - MEDICAL AND SURGICAL CHARACTER 6 - DEVICE	
	Deep brain neurostimulator lead RNS System lead Spinal cord neurostimulator lead
Neurostimulator Lead in Peripheral Nervous System	**Includes:** InterStim® Therapy lead
Neurostimulator Generator in Head and Facial Bones	**Includes:** RNS system neurostimulator generator
Nonautologous Tissue Substitute	**Includes:** Acellular Hydrated Cook Biodesign(R) Fistula Plug(s) Cook Biodesign(R) Hernia Graft(s) Cook Biodesign(R) Layered Graft(s) Cook Zenapro(tm) Layered Graft(s) Dermis Bone bank bone graft Tissue bank graft
Pacemaker, Dual Chamber for Insertion in Subcutaneous Tissue and Fascia	**Includes:** EnRhythm Kappa Revo MRI™ SureScan® pacemaker Two lead pacemaker Versa
Pacemaker, Single Chamber for Insertion in Subcutaneous Tissue and Fascia	**Includes:** Single lead pacemaker (atrium)(ventricle)
Pacemaker, Single Chamber Rate Responsive for Insertion in Subcutaneous Tissue and Fascia	**Includes:** Single lead rate responsive pacemaker (atrium) (ventricle)
Radioactive Element	**Includes:** Brachytherapy seeds
Resurfacing Device in Lower Joints	**Includes:** CONSERVE® PLUS Total Resurfacing Hip System Cormet Hip Resurfacing System
Spacer in Lower Joints	**Includes:** Joint spacer (antibiotic)
Spacer in Upper Joints	**Includes:** Joint spacer (antibiotic)
Spinal Stabilization Device, Facet Replacement for Insertion in Upper Joints	**Includes:** Facet replacement spinal stabilization device
Spinal Stabilization Device, Facet Replacement for Insertion in Lower Joints	**Includes:** Facet replacement spinal stabilization device
Spinal Stabilization Device, Interspinous Process for Insertion in Upper Joints	**Includes:** Interspinous process spinal stabilization device X-STOP® Spacer
Spinal Stabilization Device, Interspinous Process for Insertion in Lower Joints	**Includes:** Interspinous process spinal stabilization device X-STOP® Spacer
Spinal Stabilization Device, Pedicle-Based for Insertion in Upper Joints	**Includes:** Dynesys® Dynamic Stabilization System Pedicle-based dynamic stabilization device
Spinal Stabilization Device, Pedicle-Based for Insertion in Lower Joints	**Includes:** Dynesys® Dynamic Stabilization System Pedicle-based dynamic stabilization device

SECTION 0 - MEDICAL AND SURGICAL CHARACTER 6 - DEVICE	
Stimulator Generator in Subcutaneous Tissue and Fascia	**Includes:** Diaphragmatic pacemaker generator Mark IV Breathing Pacemaker System Phrenic nerve stimulator generator
Stimulator Generator, Multiple Array for Insertion in Subcutaneous Tissue and Fascia	**Includes:** Activa PC neurostimulator Enterra gastric neurostimulator Kinetra® neurostimulator Neurostimulator generator, multiple channel PrimeAdvanced neurostimulator
Stimulator Generator, Multiple Array Rechargeable for Insertion in Subcutaneous Tissue and Fascia	**Includes:** Activa RC neurostimulator Neurostimulator generator, multiple channel rechargeable RestoreAdvanced neurostimulator RestoreSensor neurostimulator RestoreUltra neurostimulator
Stimulator Generator, Single Array for Insertion in Subcutaneous Tissue and Fascia	**Includes:** Activa SC neurostimulator InterStim® Therapy neurostimulator Itrel (3)(4) neurostimulator Neurostimulator generator, single channel Soletra® neurostimulator
Stimulator Generator, Single Array Rechargeable for Insertion in Subcutaneous Tissue and Fascia	**Includes:** Neurostimulator generator, single channel rechargeable
Stimulator Lead in Gastrointestinal System	**Includes:** Gastric electrical stimulation (GES) lead Gastric pacemaker lead
Stimulator Lead in Muscles	**Includes:** Electrical muscle stimulation (EMS) lead Electronic muscle stimulator lead Neuromuscular electrical stimulation (NEMS) lead
Stimulator Lead in Upper Arteries	**Includes:** Baroreflex Activation Therapy® (BAT®) Carotid (artery) sinus (baroreceptor) lead Rheos® System lead
Stimulator Lead in Urinary System	**Includes:** Sacral nerve modulation (SNM) lead Sacral neuromodulation lead Urinary incontinence stimulator lead
Synthetic Substitute	**Includes:** AbioCor® Total Replacement Heart AMPLATZER® Muscular VSD Occluder Annuloplasty ring Bard® Composix® (E/X)(LP) mesh Bard® Composix® Kugel® patch Bard® Dulex™ mesh Bard® Ventralex™ hernia patch BRYAN® Cervical Disc System Ex-PRESS™ mini glaucoma shunt Flexible Composite Mesh

SECTION 0 - MEDICAL AND SURGICAL CHARACTER 6 - DEVICE	
	GORE® DUALMESH®
	Holter valve ventricular shunt
	MitraClip valve repair system
	Nitinol framed polymer mesh
	Partially absorbable mesh
	PHYSIOMESH™ Flexible Composite Mesh
	Polymethylmethacrylate (PMMA)
	Polypropylene mesh
	PRESTIGE® Cervical Disc
	PROCEED™ Ventral Patch
	Prodisc-C
	Prodisc-L
	PROLENE Polypropylene Hernia System (PHS)
	Rebound HRD® (Hernia Repair Device)
	SynCardia Total Artificial Heart
	Total artificial (replacement) heart
	ULTRAPRO Hernia System (UHS)
	ULTRAPRO Partially Absorbable Lightweight Mesh
	ULTRAPRO Plug
	Ventrio™ Hernia Patch
	Zimmer® NexGen® LPS Mobile Bearing Knee
	Zimmer® NexGen® LPS-Flex Mobile Knee
Synthetic Substitute, Ceramic for Replacement in Lower Joints	**Includes:** Ceramic on ceramic bearing surface Novation® Ceramic AHS® (Articulation Hip System)
Synthetic Substitute, Ceramic on Polyethylene for Replacement in Lower Joints	**Includes:** Oxidized zirconium ceramic hip bearing surface
Synthetic Substitute, Intraocular Telescope for Replacement in Eye	**Includes:** Implantable Miniature Telescope™ (IMT)
Synthetic Substitute, Metal for Replacement in Lower Joints	**Includes:** Cobalt/chromium head and socket Metal on metal bearing surface
Synthetic Substitute, Metal on Polyethylene for Replacement in Lower Joints	**Includes:** Cobalt/chromium head and polyethylene socket
Synthetic Substitute, Polyethylene for Replacement in Lower Joints	**Includes:** Polyethylene socket
Synthetic Substitute, Reverse Ball and Socket for Replacement in Upper Joints	**Includes:** Delta III Reverse shoulder prosthesis Reverse® Shoulder Prosthesis
Tissue Expander in Skin and Breast	**Includes:** Tissue expander (inflatable)(injectable)
Tissue Expander in Subcutaneous Tissue and Fascia	**Includes:** Tissue expander (inflatable)(injectable)
Tracheostomy Device in Respiratory System	**Includes:** Tracheostomy tube
Vascular Access Device in Subcutaneous Tissue and Fascia	**Includes:** Tunneled central venous catheter Vectra® Vascular Access Graft
Vascular Access Device, Reservoir in Subcutaneous Tissue and Fascia	**Includes:** Implanted (venous)(access) port Injection reservoir, port Subcutaneous injection reservoir, port

SECTION 0 - MEDICAL AND SURGICAL CHARACTER 6 - DEVICE

Zooplastic Tissue in Heart and Great Vessels	**Includes:** 3f (Aortic) Bioprosthesis valve Bovine pericardial valve Bovine pericardium graft Contegra Pulmonary Valved Conduit CoreValve transcatheter aortic valve Epic™ Stented Tissue Valve (aortic) Freestyle (Stentless) Aortic Root Bioprosthesis Hancock Bioprosthesis (aortic) (mitral) valve Hancock Bioprosthetic Valved Conduit Melody® transcatheter pulmonary valve Mitroflow® Aortic Pericardial Heart Valve Porcine (bioprosthetic) valve SAPIEN transcatheter aortic valve SJM Biocor® Stented Valve System Stented tissue valve Trifecta™ Valve (aortic) Xenograft

SECTION 1 - OBSTETRICS CHARACTER 3 - OPERATION

Abortion	**Definition:** Artificially terminating a pregnancy
Change	**Definition:** Taking out or off a device from a body part and putting back an identical or similar device in or on the same body part without cutting or puncturing the skin or a mucous membrane **Explanation:** All CHANGE procedures are coded using the approach EXTERNAL
Delivery	**Definition:** Assisting the passage of the products of conception from the genital canal
Drainage	**Definition:** Taking or letting out fluids and/or gases from a body part **Explanation:** The qualifier DIAGNOSTIC is used to identify drainage procedures that are biopsies
Extraction	**Definition:** Pulling or stripping out or off all or a portion of a body part by the use of force **Explanation:** The qualifier DIAGNOSTIC is used to identify extraction procedures that are biopsies
Insertion	**Definition:** Putting in a nonbiological appliance that monitors, assists, performs, or prevents a physiological function but does not physically take the place of a body part
Inspection	**Definition:** Visually and/or manually exploring a body part **Explanation:** Visual exploration may be performed with or without optical instrumentation. Manual exploration may be performed directly or through intervening body layers
Removal	**Definition:** Taking out or off a device from a body part, region or orifice **Explanation:** If a device is taken out and a similar device put in without cutting or puncturing the skin or mucous membrane, the procedure is coded to the root operation CHANGE. Otherwise, the procedure for taking out a device is coded to the root operation REMOVAL
Repair	**Definition:** Restoring, to the extent possible, a body part to its normal anatomic structure and function **Explanation:** Used only when the method to accomplish the repair is not one of the other root operations
Reposition	**Definition:** Moving to its normal location, or other suitable location, all or a portion of a body part **Explanation:** The body part is moved to a new location from an abnormal location, or from a normal location where it is not functioning correctly. The body part may or may not be cut out or off to be moved to the new location
Resection	**Definition:** Cutting out or off, without replacement, all of a body part
Transplantation	**Definition:** Putting in or on all or a portion of a living body part taken from another individual or animal to physically take the place and/or function of all or a portion of a similar body part **Explanation:** The native body part may or may not be taken out, and the transplanted body part may take over all or a portion of its function

SECTION 1 - OBSTETRICS CHARACTER 5 - APPROACH	
External	**Definition:** Procedures performed directly on the skin or mucous membrane and procedures performed indirectly by the application of external force through the skin or mucous membrane
Open	**Definition:** Cutting through the skin or mucous membrane and any other body layers necessary to expose the site of the procedure
Percutaneous	**Definition:** Entry, by puncture or minor incision, of instrumentation through the skin or mucous membrane and any other body layers necessary to reach the site of the procedure
Percutaneous Endoscopic	**Definition:** Entry, by puncture or minor incision, of instrumentation through the skin or mucous membrane and any other body layers necessary to reach and visualize the site of the procedure
Via Natural or Artificial Opening	**Definition:** Entry of instrumentation through a natural or artificial external opening to reach the site of the procedure
Via Natural or Artificial Opening Endoscopic	**Definition:** Entry of instrumentation through a natural or artificial external opening to reach and visualize the site of the procedure

SECTION 2 - PLACEMENT CHARACTER 3 - OPERATION	
Change	**Definition:** Taking out or off a device from a body part and putting back an identical or similar device in or on the same body part without cutting or puncturing the skin or a mucous membrane
Compression	**Definition:** Putting pressure on a body region
Dressing	**Definition:** Putting material on a body region for protection
Immobilization	**Definition:** Limiting or preventing motion of a body region
Packing	**Definition:** Putting material in a body region or orifice
Removal	**Definition:** Taking out or off a device from a body part
Traction	**Definition:** Exerting a pulling force on a body region in a distal direction

SECTION 2 - PLACEMENT CHARACTER 5 - APPROACH	
External	**Definition:** Procedures performed directly on the skin or mucous membrane and procedures performed indirectly by the application of external force through the skin or mucous membrane

SECTION 3 - ADMINISTRATION CHARACTER 3 - OPERATION	
Introduction	**Definition:** Putting in or on a therapeutic, diagnostic, nutritional, physiological, or prophylactic substance except blood or blood products
Irrigation	**Definition:** Putting in or on a cleansing substance
Transfusion	**Definition:** Putting in blood or blood products

SECTION 3 - ADMINISTRATION CHARACTER 5 - APPROACH	
External	**Definition:** Procedures performed directly on the skin or mucous membrane and procedures performed indirectly by the application of external force through the skin or mucous membrane
Open	**Definition:** Cutting through the skin or mucous membrane and any other body layers necessary to expose the site of the procedure
Percutaneous	**Definition:** Entry, by puncture or minor incision, of instrumentation through the skin or mucous membrane and any other body layers necessary to reach the site of the procedure
Via Natural or Artificial Opening	**Definition:** Entry of instrumentation through a natural or artificial external opening to reach the site of the procedure
Via Natural or Artificial Opening Endoscopic	**Definition:** Entry of instrumentation through a natural or artificial external opening to reach and visualize the site of the procedure

SECTION 4 - MEASUREMENT AND MONITORING CHARACTER 3 - OPERATION	
Measurement	**Definition:** Determining the level of a physiological or physical function at a point in time
Monitoring	**Definition:** Determining the level of a physiological or physical function repetitively over a period of time

SECTION 4 - MEASUREMENT AND MONITORING CHARACTER 5 - APPROACH	
External	**Definition:** Procedures performed directly on the skin or mucous membrane and procedures performed indirectly by the application of external force through the skin or mucous membrane
Open	**Definition:** Cutting through the skin or mucous membrane and any other body layers necessary to expose the site of the procedure
Percutaneous	**Definition:** Entry, by puncture or minor incision, of instrumentation through the skin or mucous membrane and any other body layers necessary to reach the site of the procedure
Percutaneous Endoscopic	**Definition:** Entry, by puncture or minor incision, of instrumentation through the skin or mucous membrane and any other body layers necessary to reach and visualize the site of the procedure
Via Natural or Artificial Opening	**Definition:** Entry of instrumentation through a natural or artificial external opening to reach the site of the procedure
Via Natural or Artificial Opening Endoscopic	**Definition:** Entry of instrumentation through a natural or artificial external opening to reach and visualize the site of the procedure

SECTION 5 - EXTRACORPOREAL ASSISTANCE AND PERFORMANCE CHARACTER 3 - OPERATION	
Assistance	**Definition:** Taking over a portion of a physiological function by extracorporeal means
Performance	**Definition:** Completely taking over a physiological function by extracorporeal means
Restoration	**Definition:** Returning, or attempting to return, a physiological function to its original state by extracorporeal means.

SECTION 6 - EXTRACORPOREAL THERAPIES CHARACTER 3 - OPERATION	
Atmospheric Control	**Definition:** Extracorporeal control of atmospheric pressure and composition
Decompression	**Definition:** Extracorporeal elimination of undissolved gas from body fluids
Electromagnetic Therapy	**Definition:** Extracorporeal treatment by electromagnetic rays
Hyperthermia	**Definition:** Extracorporeal raising of body temperature
Hypothermia	**Definition:** Extracorporeal lowering of body temperature
Perfusion	**Definition:** Extracorporeal treatment by diffusion of therapeutic fluid
Pheresis	**Definition:** Extracorporeal separation of blood products
Phototherapy	**Definition:** Extracorporeal treatment by light rays
Shock Wave Therapy	**Definition:** Extracorporeal treatment by shock waves
Ultrasound Therapy	**Definition:** Extracorporeal treatment by ultrasound
Ultraviolet Light Therapy	**Definition:** Extracorporeal treatment by ultraviolet light

SECTION 7 - OSTEOPATHIC CHARACTER 3 - OPERATION	
Treatment	**Definition:** Manual treatment to eliminate or alleviate somatic dysfunction and related disorders

SECTION 7 - OSTEOPATHIC CHARACTER 5 - APPROACH	
External	**Definition:** Procedures performed directly on the skin or mucous membrane and procedures performed indirectly by the application of external force through the skin or mucous membrane

SECTION 8 - OTHER PROCEDURES CHARACTER 3 - OPERATION

Other Procedures	**Definition:** Methodologies which attempt to remediate or cure a disorder or disease

SECTION 8 - OTHER PROCEDURES CHARACTER 5 - APPROACH

External	**Definition:** Procedures performed directly on the skin or mucous membrane and procedures performed indirectly by the application of external force through the skin or mucous membrane
Percutaneous	**Definition:** Entry, by puncture or minor incision, of instrumentation through the skin or mucous membrane and any other body layers necessary to reach the site of the procedure
Percutaneous Endoscopic	**Definition:** Entry, by puncture or minor incision, of instrumentation through the skin or mucous membrane and any other body layers necessary to reach and visualize the site of the procedure
Via Natural or Artificial Opening	**Definition:** Entry of instrumentation through a natural or artificial external opening to reach the site of the procedure
Via Natural or Artificial Opening Endoscopic	**Definition:** Entry of instrumentation through a natural or artificial external opening to reach and visualize the site of the procedure

SECTION 9 - CHIROPRACTIC CHARACTER 3 - OPERATION

Manipulation	**Definition:** Manual procedure that involves a directed thrust to move a joint past the physiological range of motion, without exceeding the anatomical limit

SECTION 9 - CHIROPRACTIC CHARACTER 5 - APPROACH

External	Definition: Procedures performed directly on the skin or mucous membrane and procedures performed indirectly by the application of external force through the skin or mucous membrane

SECTION B - IMAGING CHARACTER 3 - TYPE

Computerized Tomography (CT Scan)	**Definition:** Computer reformatted digital display of multiplanar images developed from the capture of multiple exposures of external ionizing radiation
Fluoroscopy	**Definition:** Single plane or bi-plane real time display of an image developed from the capture of external ionizing radiation on a fluorescent screen. The image may also be stored by either digital or analog means
Magnetic Resonance Imaging (MRI)	**Definition:** Computer reformatted digital display of multiplanar images developed from the capture of radiofrequency signals emitted by nuclei in a body site excited within a magnetic field
Plain Radiography	**Definition:** Planar display of an image developed from the capture of external ionizing radiation on photographic or photoconductive plate
Ultrasonography	**Definition:** Real time display of images of anatomy or flow information developed from the capture of reflected and attenuated high frequency sound waves

SECTION C - NUCLEAR MEDICINE CHARACTER 3 - TYPE

Nonimaging Nuclear Medicine Assay	**Definition:** Introduction of radioactive materials into the body for the study of body fluids and blood elements, by the detection of radioactive emissions
Nonimaging Nuclear Medicine Probe	**Definition:** Introduction of radioactive materials into the body for the study of distribution and fate of certain substances by the detection of radioactive emissions; or, alternatively, measurement of absorption of radioactive emissions from an external source

SECTION C - NUCLEAR MEDICINE CHARACTER 3 - TYPE

Nonimaging Nuclear Medicine Uptake	**Definition:** Introduction of radioactive materials into the body for measurements of organ function, from the detection of radioactive emissions
Planar Nuclear Medicine Imaging	**Definition:** Introduction of radioactive materials into the body for single plane display of images developed from the capture of radioactive emissions
Positron Emission Tomographic (PET) Imaging	**Definition:** Introduction of radioactive materials into the body for three dimensional display of images developed from the simultaneous capture, 180 degrees apart, of radioactive emissions

Systemic Nuclear Medicine Therapy	**Definition:** Introduction of unsealed radioactive materials into the body for treatment
Tomographic (Tomo) Nuclear Medicine Imaging	**Definition:** Introduction of radioactive materials into the body for three dimensional display of images developed from the capture of radioactive emissions

SECTION F - PHYSICAL REHABILITATION AND DIAGNOSTIC AUDIOLOGY CHARACTER 3 - TYPE

Activities of Daily Living Assessment	**Definition:** Measurement of functional level for activities of daily living
Activities of Daily Living Treatment	**Definition:** Exercise or activities to facilitate functional competence for activities of daily living
Caregiver Training	**Definition:** Training in activities to support patient's optimal level of function
Cochlear Implant Treatment	**Definition:** Application of techniques to improve the communication abilities of individuals with cochlear implant
Device Fitting	**Definition:** Fitting of a device designed to facilitate or support achievement of a higher level of function
Hearing Aid Assessment	**Definition:** Measurement of the appropriateness and/or effectiveness of a hearing device
Hearing Assessment	**Definition:** Measurement of hearing and related functions
Hearing Treatment	**Definition:** Application of techniques to improve, augment, or compensate for hearing and related functional impairment
Motor and/or Nerve Function Assessment	**Definition:** Measurement of motor, nerve, and related functions
Motor Treatment	**Definition:** Exercise or activities to increase or facilitate motor function
Speech Assessment	**Definition:** Measurement of speech and related functions
Speech Treatment	**Definition:** Application of techniques to improve, augment, or compensate for speech and related functional impairment
Vestibular Assessment	**Definition:** Measurement of the vestibular system and related functions
Vestibular Treatment	**Definition:** Application of techniques to improve, augment, or compensate for vestibular and related functional impairment

SECTION F - PHYSICAL REHABILITATION AND DIAGNOSTIC AUDIOLOGY CHARACTER 5 - TYPE QUALIFIER

Acoustic Reflex Decay	**Definition:** Measures reduction in size/strength of acoustic reflex over time **Includes/Examples:** Includes site of lesion test
Acoustic Reflex Patterns	**Definition:** Defines site of lesion based upon presence/absence of acoustic reflexes with ipsilateral vs. contralateral stimulation
Acoustic Reflex Threshold	**Definition:** Determines minimal intensity that acoustic reflex occurs with ipsilateral and/or contralateral stimulation
Aerobic Capacity and Endurance	**Definition:** Measures autonomic responses to positional changes; perceived exertion, dyspnea or angina during activity; performance during exercise protocols; standard vital signs; and blood gas analysis or oxygen consumption
Alternate Binaural or Monaural Loudness Balance	**Definition:** Determines auditory stimulus parameter that yields the same objective sensation **Includes/Examples:** Sound intensities that yield same loudness perception
Anthropometric Characteristics	**Definition:** Measures edema, body fat composition, height, weight, length and girth
Aphasia (Assessment)	**Definition:** Measures expressive and receptive speech and language function including reading and writing
Aphasia (Treatment)	**Definition:** Applying techniques to improve, augment, or compensate for receptive/ expressive language impairments
Articulation/Phonology (Assessment)	**Definition:** Measures speech production
Articulation/Phonology (Treatment)	**Definition:** Applying techniques to correct, improve, or compensate for speech productive impairment
Assistive Listening Device	**Definition:** Assists in use of effective and appropriate assistive listening device/system
Assistive Listening System/Device Selection	**Definition:** Measures the effectiveness and appropriateness of assistive listening systems/devices

SECTION F - PHYSICAL REHABILITATION AND DIAGNOSTIC AUDIOLOGY CHARACTER 5 - TYPE QUALIFIER	
Assistive, Adaptive, Supportive or Protective Devices	**Explanation:** Devices to facilitate or support achievement of a higher level of function in wheelchair mobility; bed mobility; transfer or ambulation ability; bath and showering ability; dressing; grooming; personal hygiene; play or leisure
Auditory Evoked Potentials	**Definition:** Measures electric responses produced by the VIIIth cranial nerve and brainstem following auditory stimulation
Auditory Processing (Assessment)	**Definition:** Evaluates ability to receive and process auditory information and comprehension of spoken language
Auditory Processing (Treatment)	**Definition:** Applying techniques to improve the receiving and processing of auditory information and comprehension of spoken language
Augmentative/Alternative Communication System (Assessment)	**Definition:** Determines the appropriateness of aids, techniques, symbols, and/or strategies to augment or replace speech and enhance communication **Includes/Examples:** Includes the use of telephones, writing equipment, emergency equipment, and TDD
Augmentative/Alternative Communication System (Treatment)	**Includes/Examples:** Includes augmentative communication devices and aids
Aural Rehabilitation	**Definition:** Applying techniques to improve the communication abilities associated with hearing loss
Aural Rehabilitation Status	**Definition:** Measures impact of a hearing loss including evaluation of receptive and expressive communication skills
Bathing/Showering	**Includes/Examples:** Includes obtaining and using supplies; soaping, rinsing, and drying body parts; maintaining bathing position; and transferring to and from bathing positions
Bathing/Showering Techniques	**Definition:** Activities to facilitate obtaining and using supplies, soaping, rinsing and drying body parts, maintaining bathing position, and transferring to and from bathing positions
Bed Mobility (Assessment)	**Definition:** Transitional movement within bed
Bed Mobility (Treatment)	**Definition:** Exercise or activities to facilitate transitional movements within bed
Bedside Swallowing and Oral Function	**Includes/Examples:** Bedside swallowing includes assessment of sucking, masticating, coughing, and swallowing. Oral function includes assessment of musculature for controlled movements, structures and functions to determine coordination and phonation
Bekesy Audiometry	**Definition:** Uses an instrument that provides a choice of discrete or continuously varying pure tones; choice of pulsed or continuous signal
Binaural Electroacoustic Hearing Aid Check	**Definition:** Determines mechanical and electroacoustic function of bilateral hearing aids using hearing aid test box
Binaural Hearing Aid (Assessment)	**Definition:** Measures the candidacy, effectiveness, and appropriateness of a hearing aids **Explanation:** Measures bilateral fit
Binaural Hearing Aid (Treatment)	**Explanation:** Assists in achieving maximum understanding and performance
Bithermal, Binaural Caloric Irrigation	**Definition:** Measures the rhythmic eye movements stimulated by changing the temperature of the vestibular system
Bithermal, Monaural Caloric Irrigation	**Definition:** Measures the rhythmic eye movements stimulated by changing the temperature of the vestibular system in one ear
Brief Tone Stimuli	**Definition:** Measures specific central auditory process
Cerumen Management	**Definition:** Includes examination of external auditory canal and tympanic membrane and removal of cerumen from external ear canal
Cochlear Implant	**Definition:** Measures candidacy for cochlear implant
Cochlear Implant Rehabilitation	**Definition:** Applying techniques to improve the communication abilities of individuals with cochlear implant; includes programming the device, providing patients/families with information
Communicative/Cognitive Integration Skills (Assessment)	**Definition:** Measures ability to use higher cortical functions **Includes/Examples:** Includes orientation, recognition, attention span, initiation and termination of activity, memory, sequencing, categorizing, concept formation, spatial operations, judgment, problem solving, generalization and pragmatic communication

SECTION F - PHYSICAL REHABILITATION AND DIAGNOSTIC AUDIOLOGY CHARACTER 5 - TYPE QUALIFIER

Communicative/Cognitive Integration Skills (Treatment)	**Definition:** Activities to facilitate the use of higher cortical functions **Includes/Examples:** Includes level of arousal, orientation, recognition, attention span, initiation and termination of activity, memory sequencing, judgment and problem solving, learning and generalization, and pragmatic communication
Computerized Dynamic Posturography	**Definition:** Measures the status of the peripheral and central vestibular system and the sensory/motor component of balance; evaluates the efficacy of vestibular rehabilitation
Conditioned Play Audiometry	**Definition:** Behavioral measures using nonspeech and speech stimuli to obtain frequency-specific and ear-specific information on auditory status from the patient **Explanation:** Obtains speech reception threshold by having patient point to pictures of spondaic words
Coordination/Dexterity (Assessment)	**Definition:** Measures large and small muscle groups for controlled goal-directed movements **Explanation:** Dexterity includes object manipulation
Coordination/Dexterity (Treatment)	**Definition:** Exercise or activities to facilitate gross coordination and fine coordination
Cranial Nerve Integrity	**Definition:** Measures cranial nerve sensory and motor functions, including tastes, smell and facial expression
Dichotic Stimuli	**Definition:** Measures specific central auditory process
Distorted Speech	**Definition:** Measures specific central auditory process
Dix-Hallpike Dynamic	**Definition:** Measures nystagmus following Dix-Hallpike maneuver
Dressing	**Includes/Examples:** Includes selecting clothing and accessories, obtaining clothing from storage, dressing and, fastening and adjusting clothing and shoes, and applying and removing personal devices, prosthesis or orthosis
Dressing Techniques	**Definition:** Activities to facilitate selecting clothing and accessories, dressing and undressing, adjusting clothing and shoes, applying and removing devices, prostheses or orthoses
Dynamic Orthosis	**Includes/Examples:** Includes customized and prefabricated splints, inhibitory casts, spinal and other braces, and protective devices; allows motion through transfer of movement from other body parts or by use of outside forces
Ear Canal Probe Microphone	**Definition:** Real ear measures
Ear Protector Attenuation	**Definition:** Measures ear protector fit and effectiveness
Electrocochleography	**Definition:** Measures the VIIIth cranial nerve action potential
Environmental, Home and Work Barriers	**Definition:** Measures current and potential barriers to optimal function, including safety hazards, access problems and home or office design
Ergonomics and Body Mechanics	**Definition:** Ergonomic measurement of job tasks, work hardening or work conditioning needs; functional capacity; and body mechanics
Eustachian Tube Function	**Definition:** Measures eustachian tube function and patency of eustachian tube
Evoked Otoacoustic Emissions, Diagnostic	**Definition:** Measures auditory evoked potentials in a diagnostic format
Evoked Otoacoustic Emissions, Screening	**Definition:** Measures auditory evoked potentials in a screening format
Facial Nerve Function	**Definition:** Measures electrical activity of the VIIth cranial nerve (facial nerve)
Feeding/Eating (Assessment)	**Includes/Examples:** Includes setting up food, selecting and using utensils and tableware, bringing food or drink to mouth, cleaning face, hands, and clothing, and management of alternative methods of nourishment
Feeding/Eating (Treatment)	**Definition:** Exercise or activities to facilitate setting up food, selecting and using utensils and tableware, bringing food or drink to mouth, cleaning face, hands, and clothing, and management of alternative methods of nourishment
Filtered Speech	**Definition:** Uses high or low pass filtered speech stimuli to assess central auditory processing disorders, site of lesion testing
Fluency (Assessment)	**Definition:** Measures speech fluency or stuttering
Fluency (Treatment)	**Definition:** Applying techniques to improve and augment fluent speech
Gait and/or Balance	**Definition:** Measures biomechanical, arthrokinematic and other spatial and temporal characteristics of gait and balance

SECTION F - PHYSICAL REHABILITATION AND DIAGNOSTIC AUDIOLOGY CHARACTER 5 - TYPE QUALIFIER

Gait Training/Functional Ambulation	**Definition:** Exercise or activities to facilitate ambulation on a variety of surfaces and in a variety of environments
Grooming/Personal Hygiene (Assessment)	**Includes/Examples:** Includes ability to obtain and use supplies in a sequential fashion, general grooming, oral hygiene, toilet hygiene, personal care devices, including care for artificial airways
Grooming/Personal Hygiene (Treatment)	**Definition:** Activities to facilitate obtaining and using supplies in a sequential fashion: general grooming, oral hygiene, toilet hygiene, cleaning body, and personal care devices, including artificial airways
Hearing and Related Disorders Counseling	**Definition:** Provides patients/families/caregivers with information, support, referrals to facilitate recovery from a communication disorder **Includes/Examples:** Includes strategies for psychosocial adjustment to hearing loss for clients and families/caregivers
Hearing and Related Disorders Prevention	**Definition:** Provides patients/families/caregivers with information and support to prevent communication disorders
Hearing Screening	**Definition:** Pass/refer measures designed to identify need for further audiologic assessment
Home Management (Assessment)	**Definition:** Obtaining and maintaining personal and household possessions and environment **Includes/Examples:** Includes clothing care, cleaning, meal preparation and cleanup, shopping, money management, household maintenance, safety procedures, and childcare/parenting
Home Management (Treatment)	**Definition:** Activities to facilitate obtaining and maintaining personal household possessions and environment **Includes/Examples:** Includes clothing care, cleaning, meal preparation and clean-up, shopping, money management, household maintenance, safety procedures, childcare/parenting
Instrumental Swallowing and Oral Function	**Definition:** Measures swallowing function using instrumental diagnostic procedures **Explanation:** Methods include videofluoroscopy, ultrasound, manometry, endoscopy
Integumentary Integrity	**Includes/Examples:** Includes burns, skin conditions, ecchymosis, bleeding, blisters, scar tissue, wounds and other traumas, tissue mobility, turgor and texture
Manual Therapy Techniques	**Definition:** Techniques in which the therapist uses his/her hands to administer skilled movements **Includes/Examples:** Includes connective tissue massage, joint mobilization and manipulation, manual lymph drainage, manual traction, soft tissue mobilization and manipulation
Masking Patterns	**Definition:** Measures central auditory processing status
Monaural Electroacoustic Hearing Aid Check	**Definition:** Determines mechanical and electroacoustic function of one hearing aid using hearing aid test box
Monaural Hearing Aid (Assessment)	**Definition:** Measures the candidacy, effectiveness, and appropriateness of a hearing aid **Explanation:** Measures unilateral fit
Monaural Hearing Aid (Treatment)	**Explanation:** Assists in achieving maximum understanding and performance
Motor Function (Assessment)	**Definition:** Measures the body's functional and versatile movement patterns **Includes/Examples:** Includes motor assessment scales, analysis of head, trunk and limb movement, and assessment of motor learning
Motor Function (Treatment)	**Definition:** Exercise or activities to facilitate crossing midline, laterality, bilateral integration, praxis, neuromuscular relaxation, inhibition, facilitation, motor function and motor learning
Motor Speech (Assessment)	**Definition:** Measures neurological motor aspects of speech production
Motor Speech (Treatment)	**Definition:** Applying techniques to improve and augment the impaired neurological motor aspects of speech production
Muscle Performance (Assessment)	**Definition:** Measures muscle strength, power and endurance using manual testing, dynamometry or computer-assisted electromechanical muscle test; functional muscle strength, power and endurance; muscle pain, tone, or soreness; or pelvic-floor musculature **Explanation:** Muscle endurance refers to the ability to contract a muscle repeatedly over time
Muscle Performance (Treatment)	**Definition:** Exercise or activities to increase the capacity of a muscle to do work in terms of strength, power, and/or endurance **Explanation:** Muscle strength is the force exerted to overcome resistance in one maximal effort. Muscle power is work produced per unit of time, or the product of strength and speed. Muscle endurance is the ability to contract a muscle repeatedly over time

SECTION F - PHYSICAL REHABILITATION AND DIAGNOSTIC AUDIOLOGY CHARACTER 5 - TYPE QUALIFIER	
Neuromotor Development	**Definition:** Measures motor development, righting and equilibrium reactions, and reflex and equilibrium reactions
Neurophysiologic Intraoperative	**Definition:** Monitors neural status during surgery
Non-invasive Instrumental Status	**Definition:** Instrumental measures of oral, nasal, vocal, and velopharyngeal functions as they pertain to speech production
Nonspoken Language (Assessment)	**Definition:** Measures nonspoken language (print, sign, symbols) for communication
Nonspoken Language (Treatment)	**Definition:** Applying techniques that improve, augment, or compensate spoken communication
Oral Peripheral Mechanism	**Definition:** Structural measures of face, jaw, lips, tongue, teeth, hard and soft palate, pharynx as related to speech production
Orofacial Myofunctional (Assessment)	**Definition:** Measures orofacial myofunctional patterns for speech and related functions
Orofacial Myofunctional (Treatment)	**Definition:** Applying techniques to improve, alter, or augment impaired orofacial myofunctional patterns and related speech production errors
Oscillating Tracking	**Definition:** Measures ability to visually track
Pain	**Definition:** Measures muscle soreness, pain and soreness with joint movement, and pain perception **Includes/Examples:** Includes questionnaires, graphs, symptom magnification scales or visual analog scales
Perceptual Processing (Assessment)	**Definition:** Measures stereognosis, kinesthesia, body schema, right-left discrimination, form constancy, position in space, visual closure, figure-ground, depth perception, spatial relations and topographical orientation
Perceptual Processing (Treatment)	**Definition:** Exercise and activities to facilitate perceptual processing **Explanation:** Includes stereognosis, kinesthesia, body schema, right-left discrimination, form constancy, position in space, visual closure, figure-ground, depth perception, spatial relations, and topographical orientation **Includes/Examples:** Includes stereognosis, kinesthesia, body schema, right-left discrimination, form constancy, position in space, visual closure, figure-ground, depth perception, spatial relations, and topographical orientation
Performance Intensity Phonetically Balanced Speech Discrimination	**Definition:** Measures word recognition over varying intensity levels
Postural Control	**Definition:** Exercise or activities to increase postural alignment and control
Prosthesis	**Explanation:** Artificial substitutes for missing body parts that augment performance or function
Psychosocial Skills (Assessment)	**Definition:** The ability to interact in society and to process emotions **Includes/Examples:** Includes psychological (values, interests, self-concept); social (role performance, social conduct, interpersonal skills, self expression); self-management (coping skills, time management, self-control)
Psychosocial Skills (Treatment)	**Definition:** The ability to interact in society and to process emotions **Includes/Examples:** Includes psychological (values, interests, self-concept); social (role performance, social conduct, interpersonal skills, self expression); self-management (coping skills, time management, self-control)
Pure Tone Audiometry, Air	**Definition:** Air-conduction pure tone threshold measures with appropriate masking
Pure Tone Audiometry, Air and Bone	**Definition:** Air-conduction and bone-conduction pure tone threshold measures with appropriate masking
Pure Tone Stenger	**Definition:** Measures unilateral nonorganic hearing loss based on simultaneous presentation of pure tones of differing volume
Range of Motion and Joint Integrity	**Definition:** Measures quantity, quality, grade, and classification of joint movement and/or mobility **Explanation:** Range of Motion is the space, distance or angle through which movement occurs at a joint or series of joints. Joint integrity is the conformance of joints to expected anatomic, biomechanical and kinematic norms
Range of Motion and Joint Mobility	**Definition:** Exercise or activities to increase muscle length and joint mobility
Receptive/Expressive Language (Assessment)	**Definition:** Measures receptive and expressive language

SECTION F - PHYSICAL REHABILITATION AND DIAGNOSTIC AUDIOLOGY CHARACTER 5 - TYPE QUALIFIER	
Receptive/Expressive Language (Treatment)	**Definition:** Applying techniques tot improve and augment receptive/ expressive language
Reflex Integrity	**Definition:** Measures the presence, absence, or exaggeration of developmentally appropriate, pathologic or normal reflexes
Select Picture Audiometry	**Definition:** Establishes hearing threshold levels for speech using pictures
Sensorineural Acuity Level	**Definition:** Measures sensorineural acuity masking presented via bone conduction
Sensory Aids	**Definition:** Determines the appropriateness of a sensory prosthetic device, other than a hearing aid or assistive listening system/device
Sensory Awareness/ Processing/Integrity	**Includes/Examples:** Includes light touch, pressure, temperature, pain, sharp/dull, proprioception, vestibular, visual, auditory, gustatory, and olfactory
Short Increment Sensitivity Index	**Definition:** Measures the ear's ability to detect small intensity changes; site of lesion test requiring a behavioral response
Sinusoidal Vertical Axis Rotational	**Definition:** Measures nystagmus following rotation
Somatosensory Evoked Potentials	**Definition:** Measures neural activity from sites throughout the body
Speech and/or Language Screening	**Definition:** Identifies need for further speech and/or language evaluation
Speech Threshold	**Definition:** Measures minimal intensity needed to repeat spondaic words
Speech-Language Pathology and Related Disorders Counseling	**Definition:** Provides patients/families with information, support, referrals to facilitate recovery from a communication disorder
Speech-Language Pathology and Related Disorders Prevention	**Definition:** Applying techniques to avoid or minimize onset and/or development of a communication disorder
Speech/Word Recognition	**Definition:** Measures ability to repeat/identify single syllable words; scores given as a percentage; includes word recognition/ speech discrimination
Staggered Spondaic Word	**Definition:** Measures central auditory processing site of lesion based upon dichotic presentation of spondaic words
Static Orthosis	**Includes/Examples:** Includes customized and prefabricated splints, inhibitory casts, spinal and other braces, and protective devices; has no moving parts, maintains joint(s) in desired position
Stenger	**Definition:** Measures unilateral nonorganic hearing loss based on simultaneous presentation of signals of differing volume
Swallowing Dysfunction	**Definition:** Activities to improve swallowing function in coordination with respiratory function **Includes/Examples:** Includes function and coordination of sucking, mastication, coughing, swallowing
Synthetic Sentence Identification	**Definition:** Measures central auditory dysfunction using identification of third order approximations of sentences and competing messages
Temporal Ordering of Stimuli	**Definition:** Measures specific central auditory process
Therapeutic Exercise	**Definition:** Exercise or activities to facilitate sensory awareness, sensory processing, sensory integration, balance training, conditioning, reconditioning **Includes/Examples:** Includes developmental activities, breathing exercises, aerobic endurance activities, aquatic exercises, stretching and ventilatory muscle training
Tinnitus Masker (Assessment)	**Definition:** Determines candidacy for tinnitus masker
Tinnitus Masker (Treatment)	**Explanation:** Used to verify physical fit, acoustic appropriateness, and benefit; assists in achieving maximum benefit
Transfer	**Definition:** Transitional movement from one surface to another
Transfer Training	**Definition:** Exercise or activities to facilitate movement from one surface to another
Tympanometry	**Definition:** Measures the integrity of the middle ear; measures ease at which sound flows through the tympanic membrane while air pressure against the membrane is varied
Unithermal Binaural Screen	**Definition:** Measures the rhythmic eye movements stimulated by changing the temperature of the vestibular system in both ears using warm water, screening format

SECTION F - PHYSICAL REHABILITATION AND DIAGNOSTIC AUDIOLOGY CHARACTER 5 - TYPE QUALIFIER

Ventilation, Respiration and Circulation	**Definition:** Measures ventilatory muscle strength, power and endurance, pulmonary function and ventilatory mechanics **Includes/Examples:** Includes ability to clear airway, activities that aggravate or relieve edema, pain, dyspnea or other symptoms, chest wall mobility, cardiopulmonary response to performance of ADL and IAD, cough and sputum, standard vital signs
Vestibular	**Definition:** Applying techniques to compensate for balance disorders; includes habituation, exercise therapy, and balance retraining
Visual Motor Integration (Assessment)	**Definition:** Coordinating the interaction of information from the eyes with body movement during activity
Visual Motor Integration (Treatment)	**Definition:** Exercise or activities to facilitate coordinating the interaction of information from eyes with body movement during activity
Visual Reinforcement Audiometry	**Definition:** Behavioral measures using nonspeech and speech stimuli to obtain frequency/ear-specific information on auditory status **Includes/Examples:** Includes a conditioned response of looking toward a visual reinforcer (e.g., lights, animated toy) every time auditory stimuli are heard
Vocational Activities and Functional Community or Work Reintegration Skills (Assessment)	**Definition:** Measures environmental, home, work (job/school/play) barriers that keep patients from functioning optimally in their environment **Includes/Examples:** Includes assessment of vocational skill and interests, environment of work (job/school/play), injury potential and injury prevention or reduction, ergonomic stressors, transportation skills, and ability to access and use community resources
Vocational Activities and Functional Community or Work Reintegration Skills (Treatment)	**Definition:** Activities to facilitate vocational exploration, body mechanics training, job acquisition, and environmental or work (job/ school/play) task adaptation **Includes/Examples:** Includes injury prevention and reduction, ergonomic stressor reduction, job coaching and simulation, work hardening and conditioning, driving training, transportation skills, and use of community resources
Voice (Assessment)	**Definition:** Measures vocal structure, function and production
Voice (Treatment)	**Definition:** Applying techniques to improve voice and vocal function
Voice Prosthetic (Assessment)	**Definition:** Determines the appropriateness of voice prosthetic/adaptive device to enhance or facilitate communication
Voice Prosthetic (Treatment)	**Includes/Examples:** Includes electrolarynx, and other assistive, adaptive, supportive devices
Wheelchair Mobility (Assessment)	**Definition:** Measures fit and functional abilities within wheelchair in a variety of environments
Wheelchair Mobility (Treatment)	**Definition:** Management, maintenance and controlled operation of a wheelchair, scooter or other device, in and on a variety of surfaces and environments
Wound Management	**Includes/Examples:** Includes non-selective and selective debridement (enzymes, autolysis, sharp debridement), dressings (wound coverings, hydrogel, vacuum-assisted closure), topical agents, etc.

SECTION G - MENTAL HEALTH CHARACTER 3 - TYPE

Biofeedback	**Definition:** Provision of information from the monitoring and regulating of physiological processes in conjunction with cognitive-behavioral techniques to improve patient functioning or well-being **Includes/Examples:** Includes EEG, blood pressure, skin temperature or peripheral blood flow, ECG, electrooculogram, EMG, respirometry or capnometry, GSR/EDR, perineometry to monitor/regulate bowel/bladder activity, electrogastrogram to monitor/ regulate gastric motility

SECTION G - MENTAL HEALTH CHARACTER 3 - TYPE

Counseling	**Definition:** The application of psychological methods to treat an individual with normal developmental issues and psychological problems in order to increase function, improve well-being, alleviate distress, maladjustment or resolve crises
Crisis Intervention	**Definition:** Treatment of a traumatized, acutely disturbed or distressed individual for the purpose of short-term stabilization **Includes/Examples:** Includes defusing, debriefing, counseling, psychotherapy and/ or coordination of care with other providers or agencies

Electroconvulsive Therapy	**Definition:** The application of controlled electrical voltages to treat a mental health disorder **Includes/Examples:** Includes appropriate sedation and other preparation of the individual
Family Psychotherapy	**Definition:** Treatment that includes one or more family members of an individual with a mental health disorder by behavioral, cognitive, psychoanalytic, psychodynamic or psychophysiological means to improve functioning or well-being **Explanation:** Remediation of emotional or behavioral problems presented by one or more family members in cases where psychotherapy with more than one family member is indicated
Group Psychotherapy	**Definition:** Treatment of two or more individuals with a mental health disorder by behavioral, cognitive, psychoanalytic, psychodynamic or psychophysiological means to improve functioning or well-being
Hypnosis	**Definition:** Induction of a state of heightened suggestibility by auditory, visual and tactile techniques to elicit an emotional or behavioral response
Individual Psychotherapy	**Definition:** Treatment of an individual with a mental health disorder by behavioral, cognitive, psychoanalytic, psychodynamic or psychophysiological means to improve functioning or well-being
Light Therapy	**Definition:** Application of specialized light treatments to improve functioning or well-being
Medication Management	**Definition:** Monitoring and adjusting the use of medications for the treatment of a mental health disorder
Narcosynthesis	**Definition:** Administration of intravenous barbiturates in order to release suppressed or repressed thoughts
Psychological Tests	**Definition:** The administration and interpretation of standardized psychological tests and measurement instruments for the assessment of psychological function

SECTION G - MENTAL HEALTH CHARACTER 4 - QUALIFIER

Behavioral	**Definition:** Primarily to modify behavior **Includes/Examples:** Includes modeling and role playing, positive reinforcement of target behaviors, response cost, and training of self-management skills
Cognitive	**Definition:** Primarily to correct cognitive distortions and errors
Cognitive-Behavioral	**Definition:** Combining cognitive and behavioral treatment strategies to improve functioning **Explanation:** Maladaptive responses are examined to determine how cognitions relate to behavior patterns in response to an event. Uses learning principles and information-processing models
Developmental	**Definition:** Age-normed developmental status of cognitive, social and adaptive behavior skills
Intellectual and Psychoeducational	**Definition:** Intellectual abilities, academic achievement and learning capabilities (including behaviors and emotional factors affecting learning
Interactive	**Definition:** Uses primarily physical aids and other forms of non-oral interaction with a patient who is physically, psychologically or developmentally unable to use ordinary language for communication **Includes/Examples:** Includes. the use of toys in symbolic play
Interpersonal	**Definition:** Helps an individual make changes in interpersonal behaviors to reduce psychological dysfunction **Includes/Examples:** Includes exploratory techniques, encouragement of affective expression, clarification of patient statements, analysis of communication patterns, use of therapy relationship and behavior change techniques
Neurobehavioral and Cognitive Status	**Definition:** Includes neurobehavioral status exam, interview(s), and observation for the clinical assessment of thinking, reasoning and judgment, acquired knowledge, attention, memory, visual spatial abilities, language functions, and planning
Neuropsychological	**Definition:** Thinking, reasoning and judgment, acquired knowledge, attention, memory, visual spatial abilities, language functions, planning
Personality and Behavioral	**Definition:** Mood, emotion, behavior, social functioning, psychopathological conditions, personality traits and characteristics
Psychoanalysis	**Definition:** Methods of obtaining a detailed account of past and present mental and emotional experiences to determine the source and eliminate or diminish the undesirable effects of unconscious conflicts **Explanation:** Accomplished by making the individual aware of their existence, origin, and inappropriate expression in emotions and behavior

SECTION G - MENTAL HEALTH CHARACTER 4 - QUALIFIER	
Psychodynamic	**Definition:** Exploration of past and present emotional experiences to understand motives and drives using insight-oriented techniques to reduce the undesirable effects of internal conflicts on emotions and behavior **Explanation:** Techniques include empathetic listening, clarifying self-defeating behavior patterns, and exploring adaptive alternatives
Psychophysiological	**Definition:** Monitoring and alteration of physiological processes to help the individual associate physiological reactions combined with cognitive and behavioral strategies to gain improved control of these processes to help the individual cope more effectively
Supportive	**Definition:** Formation of therapeutic relationship primarily for providing emotional support to prevent further deterioration in functioning during periods of particular stress **Explanation:** Often used in conjunction with other therapeutic approaches
Vocational	**Definition:** Exploration of vocational interests, aptitudes and required adaptive behavior skills to develop and carry out a plan for achieving a successful vocational placement **Includes/Examples:** Includes enhancing work related adjustment and/or pursuing viable options in training education or preparation

SECTION H - SUBSTANCE ABUSE TREATMENT CHARACTER 3 - TYPE	
Detoxification Services	**Definition:** Detoxification from alcohol and/or drugs **Explanation:** Not a treatment modality, but helps the patient stabilize physically and psychologically until the body becomes free of drugs and the effects of alcohol
Family Counseling	**Definition:** The application of psychological methods that includes one or more family members to treat an individual with addictive behavior **Explanation:** Provides support and education for family members of addicted individuals. Family member participation is seen as a critical area of substance abuse treatment

SECTION H - SUBSTANCE ABUSE TREATMENT CHARACTER 3 - TYPE	
Group Counseling	**Definition:** The application of psychological methods to treat two or more individuals with addictive behavior **Explanation:** Provides structured group counseling sessions and healing power through the connection with others
Individual Counseling	**Definition:** The application of psychological methods to treat an individual with addictive behavior **Explanation:** Comprised of several different techniques, which apply various strategies to address drug addiction
Individual Psychotherapy	**Definition:** Treatment of an individual with addictive behavior by behavioral, cognitive, psychoanalytic, psychodynamic or psychophysiological means
Medication Management	**Definition:** Monitoring and adjusting the use of replacement medications for the treatment of addiction
Pharmacotherapy	**Definition:** The use of replacement medications for the treatment of addiction

SECTION X - NEW TECHNOLOGY CHARACTER 3 - OPERATION	
Assistance	**Definition:** Taking over a portion of a physiological function by extracorporeal means
Extirpation	**Definition:** Taking or cutting out solid matter from a body part **Explanation:** The solid matter may be an abnormal byproduct of abiological function or a foreign body; it may be imbedded in a body part or in the lumen of a tubular body part. The solid matter may or may not have been previously broken into pieces **Includes/Examples:** Thrombectomy, choledocholithotomy
Fusion	**Definition:** Joining together portions of an articular body part rendering the articular body part immobile **Explanation:** The body part is joined together by fixation device, bone graft, or other means **Includes/Examples:** Spinal fusion, ankle arthrodesis

Insertion	**Definition:** Putting in a nonbiological appliance that monitors, assists, performs, or prevents a physiological function but does not physically take the place of a body part
	Includes/Examples: Insertion of radioactive implant, insertion of central venous catheter
Introduction	**Definition:** Putting in or on a therapeutic, diagnostic, nutritional, physiological, or prophylactic substance except blood or blood products
Monitoring	**Definition:** Determining the level of a physiological or physical function repetitively over a period of time
Removal	**Definition:** Taking out or off a device from a body part
	Explanation: If a device is taken out and a similar device put in without cutting or puncturing the skin or mucous membrane, the procedure is coded to the root operation CHANGE. Otherwise, the procedure for taking out a device is coded to the root operation REMOVAL
	Includes/Examples: Drainage tube removal, cardiac pacemaker removal
Replacement	**Definition:** Putting in or on biological or synthetic material that physically takes the place and/or function of all or a portion of a body part
	Explanation: The body part may have been taken out or replaced, or may be taken out, physically eradicated, or rendered nonfunctional during the Replacement procedure. A Removal procedure is coded for taking out the device used in a previous replacement procedure
	Includes/Examples: Total hip replacement, bone graft, free skin graft
Reposition	**Definition:** Moving to its normal location, or other suitable location, all or a portion of a body part
	Explanation: The body part is moved to a new location from an abnormal location, or from a normal location where it is not functioning correctly. The body part may or may not be cut out or off to be moved to the new location
	Includes/Examples: Reposition of undescended testicle, fracture reduction
Revision	**Definition:** Correcting, to the extent possible, a portion of a malfunctioning device or the position of a displaced device
	Explanation: Revision can include correcting a malfunctioning or displaced device by taking out or putting in components of the device such as a screw or pin **Includes/Examples:** Adjustment of position of pacemaker lead, recementing of hip prosthesis

SECTION X - NEW TECHNOLOGY CHARACTER 5 – APPROACH	
External	**Definition:** Procedures performed directly on the skin or mucous membrane and procedures performed indirectly by the application of external force through the skin or mucous membrane
Open	**Definition:** Cutting through the skin or mucous membrane and any other body layers necessary to expose the site of the procedure
Percutaneous	**Definition:** Entry, by puncture or minor incision, of instrumentation through the skin or mucous membrane and any other body layers necessary to reach the site of the procedure
Percutaneous Endoscopic	**Definition:** Entry, by puncture or minor incision, of instrumentation through the skin or mucous membrane and any other body layers necessary to reach and visualize the site of the procedure
Via Natural or Artificial Opening	**Definition:** Entry of instrumentation through a natural or artificial external opening to reach the site of the procedure
Via Natural or Artificial Opening Endoscopic	**Definition:** Entry of instrumentation through a natural or artificial external opening to reach and visualize the site of the procedure

SECTION X - NEW TECHNOLOGY CHARACTER 6 – DEVICE/SUBSTANCE/TECHNOLOGY

Andexanet Alfa, Factor Xa Inhibitor Reversal Agent	Factor Xa Inhibitor Reversal Agent, Andexanet Alfa
Defibrotide Sodium Anticoagulant	Defitelio
Interbody Fusion Device, Nanotextured Surface in New Technology	nanoLOCK(tm) interbody fusion device
Magnetically Controlled Growth Rod(s) in New Technology	MAGEC(R) Spinal Bracing and Distraction System Spinal growth rods, magnetically controlled
Skin Substitute, Porcine Liver Derived in New Technology	MIRODERM(tm) Biologic Wound Matrix
Uridine Triacetate	Vistogard(R)
Zooplastic Tissue, Rapid Deployment Technique in New	EDWARDS INTUITY Elite valve system
Technology	INTUITY Elite valve system, EDWARDS Perceval sutureless valve Sutureless valve, Perceval

APPENDIX B: BODY PART KEY

TERM		ICD-10-PCS VALUE
3f (Aortic) Bioprosthesis valve	Use:	Zooplastic tissue in heart and great vessels
AbioCor® Total Replacement Heart	Use:	Synthetic substitute
Abdominal aortic plexus	Use:	Abdominal Sympathetic Nerve
Abdominal esophagus	Use:	Esophagus, Lower
Abductor hallucis muscle	Use:	Foot Muscle, Right Foot Muscle, Left
Accessory cephalic vein	Use:	Cephalic Vein, Right Cephalic Vein, Left
Accessory obturator nerve	Use:	Lumbar Plexus
Accessory phrenic nerve	Use:	Phrenic Nerve
Accessory spleen	Use:	Spleen
Acetabulofemoral joint	Use:	Hip Joint, Right Hip Joint, Left
Achilles tendon	Use:	Lower Leg Tendon, Right Lower Leg Tendon, Left
Acromioclavicular ligament	Use:	Shoulder Bursa And Ligament, Right Shoulder Bursa And Ligament, Left
Acromion (process)	Use:	Scapula, Right Scapula, Left
Adductor brevis muscle	Use:	Upper Leg Muscle, Right Upper Leg Muscle, Left
Adductor hallucis muscle	Use:	Foot Muscle, Right Foot Muscle, Left
Adductor longus muscle	Use:	Upper Leg Muscle, Right Upper Leg Muscle, Left
Adductor magnus muscle	Use:	Upper Leg Muscle, Right Upper Leg Muscle, Left
Adenohypophysis	Use:	Pituitary Gland
Alar ligament of axis	Use:	Head And Neck Bursa And Ligament
Alveolar process of mandible	Use:	Mandible, Right Mandible, Left
Alveolar process of maxilla	Use:	Maxilla, Right Maxilla, Left
Anal orifice	Use:	Anus
Anatomical snuffbox	Use:	Lower Arm And Wrist Muscle, Right Lower Arm And Wrist Muscle, Left
Angular artery	Use:	Face Artery
Angular vein	Use:	Face Vein, Right Face Vein, Left
Annular ligament	Use:	Elbow Bursa And Ligament, Right Elbow Bursa And Ligament, Left
Anorectal junction	Use:	Rectum
Ansa cervicalis	Use:	Cervical Plexus
Antebrachial fascia	Use:	Subcutaneous Tissue And Fascia, Right Lower Arm Subcutaneous Tissue And Fascia, Left Lower Arm

TERM		ICD-10-PCS VALUE
Anterior (pectoral) lymph node	Use:	Lymphatic, Right Axillary Lymphatic, Left Axillary
Anterior cerebral artery	Use:	Intracranial Artery
Anterior cerebral vein	Use:	Intracranial Vein
Anterior choroidal artery	Use:	Intracranial Artery
Anterior circumflex humeral artery	Use:	Axillary Artery, Right Axillary Artery, Left
Anterior communicating artery	Use:	Intracranial Artery
Anterior cruciate ligament (ACL)	Use:	Knee Bursa And Ligament, Right Knee Bursa And Ligament, Left
Anterior crural nerve	Use:	Femoral Nerve
Anterior facial vein	Use:	Face Vein, Right Face Vein, Left
Anterior intercostal artery	Use:	Internal Mammary Artery, Right Internal Mammary Artery, Left
Anterior interosseous nerve	Use:	Median Nerve
Anterior lateral malleolar artery	Use:	Anterior Tibial Artery, Right Anterior Tibial Artery, Left
Anterior lingual gland	Use:	Minor Salivary Gland
Anterior medial malleolar artery	Use:	Anterior Tibial Artery, Right Anterior Tibial Artery, Left
Anterior spinal artery	Use:	Vertebral Artery, Right Vertebral Artery, Left
Anterior tibial recurrent artery	Use:	Anterior Tibial Artery, Right Anterior Tibial Artery, Left
Anterior ulnar recurrent artery	Use:	Ulnar Artery, Right Ulnar Artery, Left
Anterior vagal trunk	Use:	Vagus Nerve
Anterior vertebral muscle	Use:	Neck Muscle, Right Neck Muscle, Left
Antihelix Antitragus	Use:	External Ear, Right External Ear, Left External Ear, Bilateral
Antrum of Highmore	Use:	Maxillary Sinus, Right Maxillary Sinus, Left
Aortic annulus	Use:	Aortic Valve
Aortic arch Aortic intercostal artery	Use:	Thoracic Aorta
Apical (subclavicular) lymph node	Use:	Lymphatic, Right Axillary Lymphatic, Left Axillary
Apneustic center	Use:	Pons
Aqueduct of Sylvius	Use:	Cerebral Ventricle
Aqueous humor	Use:	Anterior Chamber, Right Anterior Chamber, Left
Arachnoid mater	Use:	Cerebral Meninges Spinal Meninges

TERM		ICD-10-PCS VALUE
Arcuate artery	Use:	Foot Artery, Right Foot Artery, Left
Areola	Use:	Nipple, Right Nipple, Left
Arterial canal (duct)	Use:	Pulmonary Artery, Left
Aryepiglottic fold	Use:	Larynx
Arytenoid cartilage	Use:	Larynx
Arytenoid muscle	Use:	Neck Muscle, Right Neck Muscle, Left
Ascending aorta	Use:	Thoracic Aorta
Ascending palatine artery	Use:	Face Artery
Ascending pharyngeal artery	Use:	External Carotid Artery, Right External Carotid Artery, Left
Atlantoaxial joint	Use:	Cervical Vertebral Joint
Atrioventricular node	Use:	Conduction Mechanism
Atrium dextrum cordis	Use:	Atrium, Right
Atrium pulmonale	Use:	Atrium, Left
Auditory tube	Use:	Eustachian Tube, Right Eustachian Tube, Left
Auerbach's (myenteric) plexus	Use:	Abdominal Sympathetic Nerve
Auricle	Use:	External Ear, Right External Ear, Left External Ear, Bilateral
Auricularis muscle	Use:	Head Muscle
Axillary fascia	Use:	Subcutaneous Tissue And Fascia, Right Upper Arm Subcutaneous Tissue And Fascia, Left Upper Arm
Axillary nerve	Use:	Brachial Plexus
Bartholin's (greater vestibular) gland	Use:	Vestibular Gland
Basal (internal) cerebral vein	Use:	Intracranial Vein
Basal nuclei	Use:	Basal Ganglia
Basilar artery	Use:	Intracranial Artery
Basis pontis	Use:	Pons
Biceps brachii muscle	Use:	Upper Arm Muscle, Right Upper Arm Muscle, Left
Biceps femoris muscle	Use:	Upper Leg Muscle, Right Upper Leg Muscle, Left
Bicipital aponeurosis	Use:	Subcutaneous Tissue And Fascia, Right Lower Arm Subcutaneous Tissue And Fascia, Left Lower Arm
Bicuspid valve	Use:	Mitral Valve
Body of femur	Use:	Femoral Shaft, Right Femoral Shaft, Left
Body of fibula	Use:	Fibula, Right Fibula, Left
Bony labyrinth	Use:	Inner Ear, Right Inner Ear, Left

TERM	ICD-10-PCS VALUE	
Bony orbit	Use:	Orbit, Right
		Orbit, Left
Bony vestibule	Use:	Inner Ear, Right
		Inner Ear, Left
Botallo's duct	Use:	Pulmonary Artery, Left
Brachial (lateral) lymph node	Use:	Lymphatic, Right Axillary
		Lymphatic, Left Axillary
Brachialis muscle	Use:	Upper Arm Muscle, Right
		Upper Arm Muscle, Left
Brachiocephalic artery	Use:	Innominate Artery
Brachiocephalic trunk	Use:	Innominate Artery
Brachiocephalic vein	Use:	Innominate Vein, Right
		Innominate Vein, Left
Brachioradialis muscle	Use:	Lower Arm And Wrist Muscle, Right
		Lower Arm And Wrist Muscle, Left
Broad ligament	Use:	Uterine Supporting Structure
Bronchial artery	Use:	Thoracic Aorta
Buccal gland	Use:	Buccal Mucosa
Buccinator lymph node	Use:	Lymphatic, Head
Buccinator muscle	Use:	Facial Muscle
Bulbospongiosus muscle	Use:	Perineum Muscle
Bulbourethral (Cowper's) gland	Use:	Urethra
Bundle of His Bundle of Kent	Use:	Conduction Mechanism
Calcaneocuboid joint	Use:	Tarsal Joint, Right
		Tarsal Joint, Left
Calcaneocuboid ligament	Use:	Foot Bursa And Ligament, Right
		Foot Bursa And Ligament, Left
Calcaneofibular ligament	Use:	Ankle Bursa And Ligament, Right
		Ankle Bursa And Ligament, Left
Calcaneus	Use:	Tarsal, Right
		Tarsal, Left
Capitate bone	Use:	Carpal, Right
		Carpal, Left
Cardia	Use:	Esophagogastric Junction
Cardiac plexus	Use:	Thoracic Sympathetic Nerve
Cardioesophageal junction	Use:	Esophagogastric Junction
Caroticotympanic artery	Use:	Internal Carotid Artery, Right
		Internal Carotid Artery, Left
Carotid glomus	Use:	Carotid Body, Left
		Carotid Body, Right
		Carotid Bodies, Bilateral
Carotid sinus	Use:	Internal Carotid Artery, Right
		Internal Carotid Artery, Left
Carotid sinus nerve	Use:	Glossopharyngeal Nerve
Carpometacarpal (CMC) joint	Use:	Metacarpocarpal Joint, Right
		Metacarpocarpal Joint, Left

TERM		ICD-10-PCS VALUE
Carpometacarpal ligament	Use:	Hand Bursa And Ligament, Right Hand Bursa And Ligament, Left
Cauda equina	Use:	Lumbar Spinal Cord
Cavernous plexus	Use:	Head And Neck Sympathetic Nerve
Celiac (solar) plexus	Use:	Abdominal Sympathetic Nerve
Celiac ganglion	Use:	Abdominal Sympathetic Nerve
Celiac lymph node	Use:	Lymphatic, Aortic
Celiac trunk	Use:	Celiac Artery
Central axillary lymph node	Use:	Lymphatic, Right Axillary Lymphatic, Left Axillary
Cerebral aqueduct (Sylvius)	Use:	Cerebral Ventricle
Cerebrum	Use:	Brain
Cervical esophagus	Use:	Esophagus, Upper
Cervical facet joint	Use:	Cervical Vertebral Joint Cervical Vertebral Joints, 2 Or More
Cervical ganglion	Use:	Head And Neck Sympathetic Nerve
Cervical interspinous ligament	Use:	Head And Neck Bursa And Ligament
Cervical intertransverse ligament	Use:	Head And Neck Bursa And Ligament
Cervical ligamentum flavum	Use:	Head And Neck Bursa And Ligament
Cervical lymph node	Use:	Lymphatic, Right Neck Lymphatic, Left Neck
Cervicothoracic facet joint	Use:	Cervicothoracic Vertebral Joint
Choana	Use:	Nasopharynx
Chondroglossus muscle	Use:	Tongue, Palate, Pharynx Muscle
Chorda tympani	Use:	Facial Nerve
Choroid plexus	Use:	Cerebral Ventricle
Ciliary body	Use:	Eye, Right Eye, Left
Ciliary ganglion	Use:	Head And Neck Sympathetic Nerve
Circle of Willis	Use:	Intracranial Artery
Circumflex iliac artery	Use:	Femoral Artery, Right Femoral Artery, Left
Claustrum	Use:	Basal Ganglia
Coccygeal body	Use:	Coccygeal Glomus
Coccygeus muscle	Use:	Trunk Muscle, Right Trunk Muscle, Left
Cochlea	Use:	Inner Ear, Right Inner Ear, Left
Cochlear nerve	Use:	Acoustic Nerve
Columella	Use:	Nose
Common digital vein	Use:	Foot Vein, Right Foot Vein, Left
Common facial vein	Use:	Face Vein, Right Face Vein, Left
Common fibular nerve	Use:	Peroneal Nerve
Common hepatic artery	Use:	Hepatic Artery

TERM	ICD-10-PCS VALUE
Common iliac (subaortic) lymph node	Use: Lymphatic, Pelvis
Common interosseous artery	Use: Ulnar Artery, Right Ulnar Artery, Left
Common peroneal nerve	Use: Peroneal Nerve
Condyloid process	Use: Mandible, Right Mandible, Left
Conus arteriosus	Use: Ventricle, Right
Conus medullaris	Use: Lumbar Spinal Cord
Coracoacromial ligament	Use: Shoulder Bursa And Ligament, Right Shoulder Bursa And Ligament, Left
Coracobrachialis muscle	Use: Upper Arm Muscle, Right Upper Arm Muscle, Left
Coracoclavicular ligament	Use: Shoulder Bursa And Ligament, Right Shoulder Bursa And Ligament, Left
Coracohumeral ligament	Use: Shoulder Bursa And Ligament, Right Shoulder Bursa And Ligament, Left
Coracoid process	Use: Scapula, Right Scapula, Left
Corniculate cartilage	Use: Larynx
Corpus callosum	Use: Brain
Corpus cavernosum Corpus spongiosum	Use: Penis
Corpus striatum	Use: Basal Ganglia
Corrugator supercilii muscle	Use: Facial Muscle
Costocervical trunk	Use: Subclavian Artery, Right Subclavian Artery, Left
Costoclavicular ligament	Use: Shoulder Bursa And Ligament, Right Shoulder Bursa And Ligament, Left
Costotransverse joint	Use: Thoracic Vertebral Joint Thoracic Vertebral Joints, 2 To 7 Thoracic Vertebral Joints, 8 Or More
Costotransverse ligament	Use: Thorax Bursa And Ligament, Right Thorax Bursa And Ligament, Left
Costovertebral joint	Use: Thoracic Vertebral Joint Thoracic Vertebral Joints, 2 To 7 Thoracic Vertebral Joints, 8 Or More
Costoxiphoid ligament	Use: Thorax Bursa And Ligament, Right Thorax Bursa And Ligament, Left
Cowper's (bulbourethral) gland	Use: Urethra
Cranial dura mater	Use: Dura Mater
Cranial epidural space	Use: Epidural Space
Cranial subarachnoid space	Use: Subarachnoid Space
Cranial subdural space	Use: Subdural Space
Cremaster muscle	Use: Perineum Muscle
Cribriform plate	Use: Ethmoid Bone, Right Ethmoid Bone, Left
Cricoid cartilage	Use: Larynx

TERM		ICD-10-PCS VALUE
Cricothyroid artery	Use:	Thyroid Artery, Right
		Thyroid Artery, Left
Cricothyroid muscle	Use:	Neck Muscle, Right
		Neck Muscle, Left
Crural fascia	Use:	Subcutaneous Tissue And Fascia, Right Upper Leg
		Subcutaneous Tissue And Fascia, Left Upper Leg
Cubital lymph node	Use:	Lymphatic, Right Upper Extremity
		Lymphatic, Left Upper Extremity
Cubital nerve	Use:	Ulnar Nerve
Cuboid bone	Use:	Tarsal, Right
		Tarsal, Left
Cuboideonavicular joint	Use:	Tarsal Joint, Right
		Tarsal Joint, Left
Culmen	Use:	Cerebellum
Cuneiform cartilage	Use:	Larynx
Cuneonavicular joint	Use:	Tarsal Joint, Right
		Tarsal Joint, Left
Cuneonavicular ligament	Use:	Foot Bursa And Ligament, Right
		Foot Bursa And Ligament, Left
Cutaneous (transverse) cervical nerve	Use:	Cervical Plexus
Deep cervical fascia	Use:	Subcutaneous Tissue And Fascia, Anterior Neck
Deep cervical vein	Use:	Vertebral Vein, Right
		Vertebral Vein, Left
Deep circumflex iliac artery	Use:	External Iliac Artery, Right
		External Iliac Artery, Left
Deep facial vein	Use:	Face Vein, Right
		Face Vein, Left
Deep femoral (profunda femoris) vein	Use:	Femoral Vein, Right
		Femoral Vein, Left
Deep femoral artery	Use:	Femoral Artery, Right
		Femoral Artery, Left
Deep palmar arch	Use:	Hand Artery, Right
		Hand Artery, Left
Deep transverse perineal muscle	Use:	Perineum Muscle
Deferential artery	Use:	Internal Iliac Artery, Right
		Internal Iliac Artery, Left
Deltoid fascia	Use:	Subcutaneous Tissue And Fascia, Right Upper Arm
		Subcutaneous Tissue And Fascia, Left Upper Arm
Deltoid ligament	Use:	Ankle Bursa And Ligament, Right
		Ankle Bursa And Ligament, Left
Deltoid muscle	Use:	Shoulder Muscle, Right
		Shoulder Muscle, Left
Deltopectoral (infraclavicular) lymph node	Use:	Lymphatic, Right Upper Extremity
		Lymphatic, Left Upper Extremity
Dentate ligament	Use:	Dura Mater
Denticulate ligament	Use:	Spinal Cord

TERM	ICD-10-PCS VALUE	
Depressor anguli oris muscle	Use:	Facial Muscle
Depressor labii inferioris muscle	Use:	Facial Muscle
Depressor septi nasi muscle	Use:	Facial Muscle
Depressor supercilii muscle	Use:	Facial Muscle
Dermis	Use:	Skin
Descending genicular artery	Use:	Femoral Artery, Right
		Femoral Artery, Left
Diaphragma sellae	Use:	Dura Mater
Distal humerus	Use:	Humeral Shaft, Right
		Humeral Shaft, Left
Distal humerus, involving joint	Use:	Elbow Joint, Right
		Elbow Joint, Left
Distal radioulnar joint	Use:	Wrist Joint, Right
		Wrist Joint, Left
Dorsal digital nerve	Use:	Radial Nerve
Dorsal metacarpal vein	Use:	Hand Vein, Right
		Hand Vein, Left
Dorsal metatarsal artery	Use:	Foot Artery, Right
		Foot Artery, Left
Dorsal metatarsal vein	Use:	Foot Vein, Right
		Foot Vein, Left
Dorsal scapular artery	Use:	Subclavian Artery, Right
		Subclavian Artery, Left
Dorsal scapular nerve	Use:	Brachial Plexus
Dorsal venous arch	Use:	Foot Vein, Right
		Foot Vein, Left
Dorsalis pedis artery	Use:	Anterior Tibial Artery, Right
		Anterior Tibial Artery, Left
Duct of Santorini	Use:	Pancreatic Duct, Accessory
Duct of Wirsung	Use:	Pancreatic Duct
Ductus deferens	Use:	Vas Deferens, Right
		Vas Deferens, Left
		Vas Deferens, Bilateral Vas Deferens
Duodenal ampulla	Use:	Ampulla Of Vater
Duodenojejunal flexure	Use:	Jejunum
Dural venous sinus	Use:	Intracranial Vein
Earlobe	Use:	External Ear, Right
		External Ear, Left
		External Ear, Bilateral
Eighth cranial nerve	Use:	Acoustic Nerve
Ejaculatory duct	Use:	Vas Deferens, Right
		Vas Deferens, Left
		Vas Deferens, Bilateral Vas Deferens
Eleventh cranial nerve	Use:	Accessory Nerve
Encephalon	Use:	Brain
Ependyma	Use:	Cerebral Ventricle

TERM		ICD-10-PCS VALUE
Epidermis	Use:	Skin
Epiploic foramen	Use:	Peritoneum
Epithalamus	Use:	Thalamus
Epitrochlear lymph node	Use:	Lymphatic, Right Upper Extremity Lymphatic, Left Upper Extremity
Erector spinae muscle	Use:	Trunk Muscle, Right Trunk Muscle, Left
Esophageal artery	Use:	Thoracic Aorta
Esophageal plexus	Use:	Thoracic Sympathetic Nerve
Ethmoidal air cell	Use:	Ethmoid Sinus, Right Ethmoid Sinus, Left
Extensor carpi radialis muscle	Use:	Lower Arm And Wrist Muscle, Right Lower Arm And Wrist Muscle, Left
Extensor carpi ulnaris muscle	Use:	Lower Arm And Wrist Muscle, Right Lower Arm And Wrist Muscle, Left
Extensor digitorum brevis muscle	Use:	Foot Muscle, Right Foot Muscle, Left
Extensor digitorum longus muscle	Use:	Lower Leg Muscle, Right Lower Leg Muscle, Left
Extensor hallucis brevis muscle	Use:	Foot Muscle, Right Foot Muscle, Left
Extensor hallucis longus muscle	Use:	Lower Leg Muscle, Right Lower Leg Muscle, Left
External anal sphincter	Use:	Anal Sphincter
External auditory meatus	Use:	External Auditory Canal, Right External Auditory Canal, Left
External maxillary artery	Use:	Face Artery
External naris	Use:	Nose
External oblique aponeurosis	Use:	Subcutaneous Tissue And Fascia, Trunk
External oblique muscle	Use:	Abdomen Muscle, Right Abdomen Muscle, Left
External popliteal nerve	Use:	Peroneal Nerve
External pudendal artery	Use:	Femoral Artery, Right Femoral Artery, Left
External pudendal vein	Use:	Greater Saphenous Vein, Right Greater Saphenous Vein, Left
External urethral sphincter	Use:	Urethra
Extradural space	Use:	Epidural Space
Facial artery	Use:	Face Artery
False vocal cord	Use:	Larynx
Falx cerebri	Use:	Dura Mater
Fascia lata	Use:	Subcutaneous Tissue And Fascia, Right Upper Leg Subcutaneous Tissue And Fascia, Left Upper Leg
Femoral head	Use:	Upper Femur, Right Upper Femur, Left

TERM		ICD-10-PCS VALUE
Femoral lymph node	Use:	Lymphatic, Right Lower Extremity Lymphatic, Left Lower Extremity
Femoropatellar joint	Use:	Knee Joint, Right Knee Joint, Left
Femorotibial joint	Use:	Knee Joint, Right Knee Joint, Left
Fibular artery	Use:	Peroneal Artery, Right Peroneal Artery, Left
Fibularis brevis muscle	Use:	Lower Leg Muscle, Right Lower Leg Muscle, Left
Fibularis longus muscle	Use:	Lower Leg Muscle, Right Lower Leg Muscle, Left
Fifth cranial nerve	Use:	Trigeminal Nerve
First cranial nerve	Use:	Olfactory Nerve
First intercostal nerve	Use:	Brachial Plexus
Flexor carpi radialis muscle	Use:	Lower Arm And Wrist Muscle, Right Lower Arm And Wrist Muscle, Left
Flexor carpi ulnaris muscle	Use:	Lower Arm And Wrist Muscle, Right Lower Arm And Wrist Muscle, Left
Flexor digitorum brevis muscle	Use:	Foot Muscle, Right Foot Muscle, Left
Flexor digitorum longus muscle	Use:	Lower Leg Muscle, Right Lower Leg Muscle, Left
Flexor hallucis brevis muscle	Use:	Foot Muscle, Right Foot Muscle, Left
Flexor hallucis longus muscle	Use:	Lower Leg Muscle, Right Lower Leg Muscle, Left
Flexor pollicis longus muscle	Use:	Lower Arm And Wrist Muscle, Right Lower Arm And Wrist Muscle, Left
Foramen magnum	Use:	Occipital Bone, Right Occipital Bone, Left
Foramen of Monro (intraventricular)	Use:	Cerebral Ventricle
Foreskin	Use:	Prepuce
Fossa of Rosenmüller	Use:	Nasopharynx
Fourth cranial nerve	Use:	Trochlear Nerve
Fourth ventricle	Use:	Cerebral Ventricle
Fovea	Use:	Retina, Right Retina, Left
Frenulum labii inferioris	Use:	Lower Lip
Frenulum labii superioris	Use:	Upper Lip
Frenulum linguae	Use:	Tongue
Frontal lobe	Use:	Cerebral Hemisphere
Frontal vein	Use:	Face Vein, Right Face Vein, Left
Fundus uteri	Use:	Uterus
Galea aponeurotica	Use:	Subcutaneous Tissue And Fascia, Scalp

TERM		ICD-10-PCS VALUE
Ganglion impar (ganglion of Walther)	Use:	Sacral Sympathetic Nerve
Gasserian ganglion	Use:	Trigeminal Nerve
Gastric lymph node	Use:	Lymphatic, Aortic
Gastric plexus	Use:	Abdominal Sympathetic Nerve
Gastrocnemius muscle	Use:	Lower Leg Muscle, Right Lower Leg Muscle, Left
Gastrocolic ligament	Use:	Greater Omentum
Gastrocolic omentum	Use:	Greater Omentum
Gastroduodenal artery	Use:	Hepatic Artery
Gastroesophageal (GE) junction	Use:	Esophagogastric Junction
Gastrohepatic omentum	Use:	Lesser Omentum
Gastrophrenic ligament	Use:	Greater Omentum
Gastrosplenic ligament	Use:	Greater Omentum
Gemellus muscle	Use:	Hip Muscle, Right Hip Muscle, Left
Geniculate ganglion	Use:	Facial Nerve
Geniculate nucleus	Use:	Thalamus
Genioglossus muscle	Use:	Tongue, Palate, Pharynx Muscle
Genitofemoral nerve	Use:	Lumbar Plexus
Glans penis	Use:	Prepuce
Glenohumeral joint	Use:	Shoulder Joint, Right Shoulder Joint, Left
Glenohumeral ligament	Use:	Shoulder Bursa And Ligament, Right Shoulder Bursa And Ligament, Left
Glenoid fossa (of scapula)	Use:	Glenoid Cavity, Right Glenoid Cavity, Left
Glenoid ligament (labrum)	Use:	Shoulder Bursa And Ligament, Right Shoulder Bursa And Ligament, Left
Globus pallidus	Use:	Basal Ganglia
Glossoepiglottic fold	Use:	Epiglottis
Glottis	Use:	Larynx
Gluteal lymph node	Use:	Lymphatic, Pelvis
Gluteal vein	Use:	Hypogastric Vein, Right Hypogastric Vein, Left
Gluteus maximus muscle	Use:	Hip Muscle, Right Hip Muscle, Left
Gluteus medius muscle	Use:	Hip Muscle, Right Hip Muscle, Left
Gluteus minimus muscle	Use:	Hip Muscle, Right Hip Muscle, Left
Gracilis muscle	Use:	Upper Leg Muscle, Right Upper Leg Muscle, Left
Great auricular nerve	Use:	Cervical Plexus
Great cerebral vein	Use:	Intracranial Vein

TERM	ICD-10-PCS VALUE
Great saphenous vein	Use: Greater Saphenous Vein, Right Greater Saphenous Vein, Left
Greater alar cartilage	Use: Nose
Greater occipital nerve	Use: Cervical Nerve
Greater splanchnic nerve	Use: Thoracic Sympathetic Nerve
Greater superficial petrosal nerve	Use: Facial Nerve
Greater trochanter	Use: Upper Femur, Right Upper Femur, Left
Greater tuberosity	Use: Humeral Head, Right Humeral Head, Left
Greater vestibular (Bartholin's) gland	Use: Vestibular Gland
Greater wing	Use: Sphenoid Bone, Right Sphenoid Bone, Left
Hallux	Use: 1st Toe, Right 1st Toe, Left
Hamate bone	Use: Carpal, Right Carpal, Left
Head of fibula	Use: Fibula, Right Fibula, Left
Helix	Use: External Ear, Right External Ear, Left External Ear, Bilateral
Hepatic artery proper	Use: Hepatic Artery
Hepatic flexure	Use: Ascending Colon
Hepatic lymph node	Use: Lymphatic, Aortic
Hepatic plexus	Use: Abdominal Sympathetic Nerve
Hepatic portal vein	Use: Portal Vein
Hepatogastric ligament	Use: Lesser Omentum
Hepatopancreatic ampulla	Use: Ampulla Of Vater
Humeroradial joint	Use: Elbow Joint, Right Elbow Joint, Left
Humeroulnar joint	Use: Elbow Joint, Right Elbow Joint, Left
Humerus, distal	Use: Humeral Shaft, Right Humeral Shaft, Left
Hyoglossus muscle	Use: Tongue, Palate, Pharynx Muscle
Hyoid artery	Use: Thyroid Artery, Right Thyroid Artery, Left
Hypogastric artery	Use: Internal Iliac Artery, Right Internal Iliac Artery, Left
Hypopharynx	Use: Pharynx
Hypophysis	Use: Pituitary Gland
Hypothenar muscle	Use: Hand Muscle, Right Hand Muscle, Left
Ileal artery Ileocolic artery	Use: Superior Mesenteric Artery
Ileocolic vein	Use: Colic Vein

TERM		ICD-10-PCS VALUE
Iliac crest	Use:	Pelvic Bone, Right Pelvic Bone, Left
Iliac fascia	Use:	Subcutaneous Tissue And Fascia, Right Upper Leg Subcutaneous Tissue And Fascia, Left Upper Leg
Iliac lymph node	Use:	Lymphatic, Pelvis
Iliacus muscle	Use:	Hip Muscle, Right Hip Muscle, Left
Iliofemoral ligament	Use:	Hip Bursa And Ligament, Right Hip Bursa And Ligament, Left
Iliohypogastric nerve Ilioinguinal nerve	Use:	Lumbar Plexus
Iliolumbar artery	Use:	Internal Iliac Artery, Right Internal Iliac Artery, Left
Iliolumbar ligament	Use:	Trunk Bursa And Ligament, Right Trunk Bursa And Ligament, Left
Iliotibial tract (band)	Use:	Subcutaneous Tissue And Fascia, Right Upper Leg Subcutaneous Tissue And Fascia, Left Upper Leg
Ilium	Use:	Pelvic Bone, Right Pelvic Bone, Left
Incus	Use:	Auditory Ossicle, Right Auditory Ossicle, Left
Inferior cardiac nerve	Use:	Thoracic Sympathetic Nerve
Inferior cerebellar vein Inferior cerebral vein	Use:	Intracranial Vein
Inferior epigastric artery	Use:	External Iliac Artery, Right External Iliac Artery, Left
Inferior epigastric lymph node	Use:	Lymphatic, Pelvis
Inferior genicular artery	Use:	Popliteal Artery, Right Popliteal Artery, Left
Inferior gluteal artery	Use:	Internal Iliac Artery, Right Internal Iliac Artery, Left
Inferior gluteal nerve	Use:	Sacral Plexus
Inferior hypogastric plexus	Use:	Abdominal Sympathetic Nerve
Inferior labial artery	Use:	Face Artery
Inferior longitudinal muscle	Use:	Tongue, Palate, Pharynx Muscle
Inferior mesenteric ganglion	Use:	Abdominal Sympathetic Nerve
Inferior mesenteric lymph node	Use:	Lymphatic, Mesenteric
Inferior mesenteric plexus	Use:	Abdominal Sympathetic Nerve
Inferior oblique muscle	Use:	Extraocular Muscle, Right Extraocular Muscle, Left
Inferior pancreaticoduodenal artery	Use:	Superior Mesenteric Artery
Inferior phrenic artery	Use:	Abdominal Aorta
Inferior rectus muscle	Use:	Extraocular Muscle, Right Extraocular Muscle, Left
Inferior suprarenal artery	Use:	Renal Artery, Right Renal Artery, Left
Inferior tarsal plate	Use:	Lower Eyelid, Right Lower Eyelid, Left

TERM	ICD-10-PCS VALUE	
Inferior thyroid vein	Use:	Innominate Vein, Right
		Innominate Vein, Left
Inferior tibiofibular joint	Use:	Ankle Joint, Right
		Ankle Joint, Left
Inferior turbinate	Use:	Nasal Turbinate
Inferior ulnar collateral artery	Use:	Brachial Artery, Right
		Brachial Artery, Left
Inferior vesical artery	Use:	Internal Iliac Artery, Right
		Internal Iliac Artery, Left
Infraauricular lymph node	Use:	Lymphatic, Head
Infraclavicular (deltopectoral) lymph node	Use:	Lymphatic, Right Upper Extremity
		Lymphatic, Left Upper Extremity
Infrahyoid muscle	Use:	Neck Muscle, Right
		Neck Muscle, Left
Infraparotid lymph node	Use:	Lymphatic, Head
Infraspinatus fascia	Use:	Subcutaneous Tissue And Fascia, Right Upper Arm
		Subcutaneous Tissue And Fascia, Left Upper Arm
Infraspinatus muscle	Use:	Shoulder Muscle, Right
		Shoulder Muscle, Left
Infundibulopelvic ligament	Use:	Uterine Supporting Structure
Inguinal canal Inguinal triangle	Use:	Inguinal Region, Right
		Inguinal Region, Left
		Inguinal Region, Bilateral
Interatrial septum	Use:	Atrial Septum
Intercarpal joint	Use:	Carpal Joint, Right
		Carpal Joint, Left
Intercarpal ligament	Use:	Hand Bursa And Ligament, Right
		Hand Bursa And Ligament, Left
Interclavicular ligament	Use:	Shoulder Bursa And Ligament, Right
		Shoulder Bursa And Ligament, Left
Intercostal lymph node	Use:	Lymphatic, Thorax
Intercostal muscle	Use:	Thorax Muscle, Right
		Thorax Muscle, Left
Intercostal nerve	Use:	Thoracic Nerve
Intercostobrachial nerve	Use:	Thoracic Nerve
Intercuneiform joint	Use:	Tarsal Joint, Right
		Tarsal Joint, Left
Intercuneiform ligament	Use:	Foot Bursa And Ligament, Right
		Foot Bursa And Ligament, Left
Intermediate cuneiform bone	Use:	Tarsal, Right
		Tarsal, Left
Internal (basal) cerebral vein	Use:	Intracranial Vein
Internal anal sphincter	Use:	Anal Sphincter
Internal carotid plexus	Use:	Head And Neck Sympathetic Nerve
Internal iliac vein	Use:	Hypogastric Vein, Right
		Hypogastric Vein, Left

TERM	ICD-10-PCS VALUE	
Internal maxillary artery	Use:	External Carotid Artery, Right External Carotid Artery, Left
Internal naris	Use:	Nose
Internal oblique muscle	Use:	Abdomen Muscle, Right Abdomen Muscle, Left
Internal pudendal artery	Use:	Internal Iliac Artery, Right Internal Iliac Artery, Left
Internal pudendal vein	Use:	Hypogastric Vein, Right Hypogastric Vein, Left
Internal thoracic artery	Use:	Internal Mammary Artery, Right Internal Mammary Artery, Left Subclavian Artery, Right Subclavian Artery, Left
Internal urethral sphincter	Use:	Urethra
Interphalangeal (IP) joint	Use:	Finger Phalangeal Joint, Right Finger Phalangeal Joint, Left Toe Phalangeal Joint, Right Toe Phalangeal Joint, Left
Interphalangeal ligament	Use:	Hand Bursa And Ligament, Right Hand Bursa And Ligament, Left Foot Bursa And Ligament, Right Foot Bursa And Ligament, Left
Interspinalis muscle	Use:	Trunk Muscle, Right Trunk Muscle, Left
Interspinous ligament	Use:	Trunk Bursa And Ligament, Right Trunk Bursa And Ligament, Left
Intertransversarius muscle	Use:	Trunk Muscle, Right Trunk Muscle, Left
Intertransverse ligament	Use:	Trunk Bursa And Ligament, Right Trunk Bursa And Ligament, Left
Interventricular foramen (Monro)	Use:	Cerebral Ventricle
Interventricular septum	Use:	Ventricular Septum
Intestinal lymphatic trunk	Use:	Cisterna Chyli
Ischiatic nerve	Use:	Sciatic Nerve
Ischiocavernosus muscle	Use:	Perineum Muscle
Ischiofemoral ligament	Use:	Hip Bursa And Ligament, Right Hip Bursa And Ligament, Left
Ischium	Use:	Pelvic Bone, Right Pelvic Bone, Left
Jejunal artery	Use:	Superior Mesenteric Artery
Jugular body	Use:	Glomus Jugulare
Jugular lymph node	Use:	Lymphatic, Right Neck Lymphatic, Left Neck
Labia majora Labia minora	Use:	Vulva
Labial gland	Use:	Upper Lip Lower Lip
Lacrimal canaliculus	Use:	Lacrimal Duct, Right Lacrimal Duct, Left

TERM		ICD-10-PCS VALUE
Lacrimal punctum	Use:	Lacrimal Duct, Right Lacrimal Duct, Left
Lacrimal sac	Use:	Lacrimal Duct, Right Lacrimal Duct, Left
Laryngopharynx	Use:	Pharynx
Lateral (brachial) lymph node	Use:	Lymphatic, Right Axillary Lymphatic, Left Axillary
Lateral canthus	Use:	Upper Eyelid, Right Upper Eyelid, Left
Lateral collateral ligament (LCL)	Use:	Knee Bursa And Ligament, Right Knee Bursa And Ligament, Left
Lateral condyle of femur	Use:	Lower Femur, Right Lower Femur, Left
Lateral condyle of tibia	Use:	Tibia, Right Tibia, Left
Lateral cuneiform bone	Use:	Tarsal, Right Tarsal, Left
Lateral epicondyle of femur	Use:	Lower Femur, Right Lower Femur, Left
Lateral epicondyle of humerus	Use:	Humeral Shaft, Right Humeral Shaft, Left
Lateral femoral cutaneous nerve	Use:	Lumbar Plexus
Lateral malleolus	Use:	Fibula, Right Fibula, Left
Lateral meniscus	Use:	Knee Joint, Right Knee Joint, Left
Lateral nasal cartilage	Use:	Nose
Lateral plantar artery	Use:	Foot Artery, Right Foot Artery, Left
Lateral plantar nerve	Use:	Tibial Nerve
Lateral rectus muscle	Use:	Extraocular Muscle, Right Extraocular Muscle, Left
Lateral sacral artery	Use:	Internal Iliac Artery, Right Internal Iliac Artery, Left
Lateral sacral vein	Use:	Hypogastric Vein, Right Hypogastric Vein, Left
Lateral sural cutaneous nerve	Use:	Peroneal Nerve
Lateral tarsal artery	Use:	Foot Artery, Right Foot Artery, Left
Lateral temporomandibular ligament	Use:	Head And Neck Bursa And Ligament
Lateral thoracic artery	Use:	Axillary Artery, Right Axillary Artery, Left
Latissimus dorsi muscle	Use:	Trunk Muscle, Right Trunk Muscle, Left
Least splanchnic nerve	Use:	Thoracic Sympathetic Nerve
Left ascending lumbar vein	Use:	Hemiazygos Vein

TERM	ICD-10-PCS VALUE	
Left atrioventricular valve	Use:	Mitral Valve
Left auricular appendix	Use:	Atrium, Left
Left colic vein	Use:	Colic Vein
Left coronary sulcus	Use:	Heart, Left
Left gastric artery	Use:	Gastric Artery
Left gastroepiploic artery	Use:	Splenic Artery
Left gastroepiploic vein	Use:	Splenic Vein
Left inferior phrenic vein	Use:	Renal Vein, Left
Left inferior pulmonary vein	Use:	Pulmonary Vein, Left
Left jugular trunk	Use:	Thoracic Duct
Left lateral ventricle	Use:	Cerebral Ventricle
Left ovarian vein	Use:	Renal Vein, Left
Left second lumbar vein	Use:	Renal Vein, Left
Left subclavian trunk	Use:	Thoracic Duct
Left subcostal vein	Use:	Hemiazygos Vein
Left superior pulmonary vein	Use:	Pulmonary Vein, Left
Left suprarenal vein	Use:	Renal Vein, Left
Left testicular vein	Use:	Renal Vein, Left
Leptomeninges	Use:	Cerebral Meninges Spinal Meninges
Lesser alar cartilage	Use:	Nose
Lesser occipital nerve	Use:	Cervical Plexus
Lesser splanchnic nerve	Use:	Thoracic Sympathetic Nerve
Lesser trochanter	Use:	Upper Femur, Right Upper Femur, Left
Lesser tuberosity	Use:	Humeral Head, Right Humeral Head, Left
Lesser wing	Use:	Sphenoid Bone, Right Sphenoid Bone, Left
Levator anguli oris muscle	Use:	Facial Muscle
Levator ani muscle	Use:	Trunk Muscle, Right Trunk Muscle, Left
Levator labii superioris alaeque nasi muscle	Use:	Facial Muscle
Levator labii superioris muscle	Use:	Facial Muscle
Levator labii superioris muscle	Use:	Facial Muscle
Levator palpebrae superioris muscle	Use:	Upper Eyelid, Right Upper Eyelid, Left
Levator scapulae muscle	Use:	Neck Muscle, Right Neck Muscle, Left
Levator veli palatini muscle	Use:	Tongue, Palate, Pharynx Muscle
Levatores costarum muscle	Use:	Thorax Muscle, Right Thorax Muscle, Left
Ligament of head of fibula	Use:	Knee Bursa And Ligament, Right Knee Bursa And Ligament, Left
Ligament of the lateral malleolus	Use:	Ankle Bursa And Ligament, Right Ankle Bursa And Ligament, Left

TERM	ICD-10-PCS VALUE	
Ligamentum flavum	Use:	Trunk Bursa And Ligament, Right
		Trunk Bursa And Ligament, Left
Lingual artery	Use:	External Carotid Artery, Right
		External Carotid Artery, Left
Lingual tonsil	Use:	Tongue
Locus ceruleus	Use:	Pons
Long thoracic nerve	Use:	Brachial Plexus
Lumbar artery	Use:	Abdominal Aorta
Lumbar facet joint	Use:	Lumbar Vertebral Joint
		Lumbar Vertebral Joints, 2 Or More
Lumbar ganglion	Use:	Lumbar Sympathetic Nerve
Lumbar lymph node	Use:	Lymphatic, Aortic
Lumbar lymphatic trunk	Use:	Cisterna Chyli
Lumbar splanchnic nerve	Use:	Lumbar Sympathetic Nerve
Lumbosacral facet joint	Use:	Lumbosacral Joint
Lumbosacral trunk	Use:	Lumbar Nerve
Lunate bone	Use:	Carpal, Right
		Carpal, Left
Lunotriquetral ligament	Use:	Hand Bursa And Ligament, Right
		Hand Bursa And Ligament, Left
Macula	Use:	Retina, Right
		Retina, Left
Malleus	Use:	Auditory Ossicle, Right
		Auditory Ossicle, Left
Mammary duct	Use:	Breast, Right
		Breast, Left Breast, Bilateral
Mammary gland	Use:	Breast, Right
		Breast, Left Breast, Bilateral
Mammillary body	Use:	Hypothalamus
Mandibular nerve	Use:	Trigeminal Nerve
Mandibular notch	Use:	Mandible, Right
		Mandible, Left
Manubrium	Use:	Sternum
Masseter muscle	Use:	Head Muscle
Masseteric fascia	Use:	Subcutaneous Tissue And Fascia, Face
Mastoid (postauricular) lymph node	Use:	Lymphatic, Right
		Neck Lymphatic, Left Neck
Mastoid air cells	Use:	Mastoid Sinus, Right
		Mastoid Sinus, Left
Mastoid process	Use:	Temporal Bone, Right
		Temporal Bone, Left
Maxillary artery	Use:	External Carotid Artery, Right
		External Carotid Artery, Left
Maxillary nerve	Use:	Trigeminal Nerve
Medial canthus	Use:	Lower Eyelid, Right
		Lower Eyelid, Left

TERM	ICD-10-PCS VALUE	
Medial collateral ligament (MCL)	Use:	Knee Bursa And Ligament, Right Knee Bursa And Ligament, Left
Medial condyle of femur	Use:	Lower Femur, Right Lower Femur, Left
Medial condyle of tibia	Use:	Tibia, Right Tibia, Left
Medial cuneiform bone	Use:	Tarsal, Right Tarsal, Left
Medial epicondyle of femur	Use:	Lower Femur, Right Lower Femur, Left
Medial epicondyle of humerus	Use:	Humeral Shaft, Right Humeral Shaft, Left
Medial malleolus	Use:	Tibia, Right Tibia, Left
Medial meniscus	Use:	Knee Joint, Right Knee Joint, Left
Medial plantar artery	Use:	Foot Artery, Right Foot Artery, Left
Medial plantar nerve	Use:	Tibial Nerve
Medial popliteal nerve	Use:	Tibial Nerve
Medial rectus muscle	Use:	Extraocular Muscle, Right Extraocular Muscle, Left
Medial sural cutaneous nerve	Use:	Tibial Nerve
Median antebrachial vein	Use:	Basilic Vein, Right Basilic Vein, Left
Median cubital vein	Use:	Basilic Vein, Right Basilic Vein, Left
Median sacral artery	Use:	Abdominal Aorta
Mediastinal lymph node	Use:	Lymphatic, Thorax
Meissner's (submucous) plexus	Use:	Abdominal Sympathetic Nerve
Membranous urethra	Use:	Urethra
Mental foramen	Use:	Mandible, Right Mandible, Left
Mentalis muscle	Use:	Facial Muscle
Mesoappendix Mesocolon	Use:	Mesentery
Metacarpal ligament	Use:	Hand Bursa And Ligament, Right Hand Bursa And Ligament, Left
Metacarpophalangeal ligament	Use:	Hand Bursa And Ligament, Right Hand Bursa And Ligament, Left
Metatarsal ligament	Use:	Foot Bursa And Ligament, Right Foot Bursa And Ligament, Left
Metatarsophalangeal (MTP) joint	Use:	Metatarsal-Phalangeal Joint, Right Metatarsal-Phalangeal Joint, Left
Metatarsophalangeal ligament	Use:	Foot Bursa And Ligament, Right Foot Bursa And Ligament, Left
Metathalamus	Use:	Thalamus

TERM	ICD-10-PCS VALUE	
Midcarpal joint	Use:	Carpal Joint, Right Carpal Joint, Left
Middle cardiac nerve	Use:	Thoracic Sympathetic Nerve
Middle cerebral artery	Use:	Intracranial Artery
Middle cerebral vein	Use:	Intracranial Vein
Middle colic vein	Use:	Colic Vein
Middle genicular artery	Use:	Popliteal Artery, Right Popliteal Artery, Left
Middle hemorrhoidal vein	Use:	Hypogastric Vein, Right Hypogastric Vein, Left
Middle rectal artery	Use:	Internal Iliac Artery, Right Internal Iliac Artery, Left
Middle suprarenal artery	Use:	Abdominal Aorta
Middle temporal artery	Use:	Temporal Artery, Right Temporal Artery, Left
Middle turbinate	Use:	Nasal Turbinate
Mitral annulus	Use:	Mitral Valve
Molar gland	Use:	Buccal Mucosa
Musculocutaneous nerve	Use:	Brachial Plexus
Musculophrenic artery	Use:	Internal Mammary Artery, Right Internal Mammary Artery, Left
Musculospiral nerve	Use:	Radial Nerve
Myelencephalon	Use:	Medulla Oblongata
Myenteric (Auerbach's) plexus	Use:	Abdominal Sympathetic Nerve
Myometrium	Use:	Uterus
Nail bed Nail plate	Use:	Finger Nail Toe Nail
Nasal cavity	Use:	Nose
Nasal concha	Use:	Nasal Turbinate
Nasalis muscle	Use:	Facial Muscle
Nasolacrimal duct	Use:	Lacrimal Duct, Right Lacrimal Duct, Left
Navicular bone	Use:	Tarsal, Right Tarsal, Left
Neck of femur	Use:	Upper Femur, Right Upper Femur, Left
Neck of humerus (anatomical)(surgical)	Use:	Humeral Head, Right Humeral Head, Left
Nerve to the stapedius	Use:	Facial Nerve
Neurohypophysis	Use:	Pituitary Gland
Ninth cranial nerve	Use:	Glossopharyngeal Nerve
Nostril	Use:	Nose
Obturator artery	Use:	Internal Iliac Artery, Right Internal Iliac Artery, Left
Obturator lymph node	Use:	Lymphatic, Pelvis

TERM	ICD-10-PCS VALUE	
Obturator muscle	Use:	Hip Muscle, Right Hip Muscle, Left
Obturator nerve	Use:	Lumbar Plexus
Obturator vein	Use:	Hypogastric Vein, Right Hypogastric Vein, Left
Obtuse margin	Use:	Heart, Left
Occipital artery	Use:	External Carotid Artery, Right External Carotid Artery, Left
Occipital lobe	Use:	Cerebral Hemisphere
Occipital lymph node	Use:	Lymphatic, Right Neck Lymphatic, Left Neck
Occipitofrontalis muscle	Use:	Facial Muscle
Olecranon bursa	Use:	Elbow Bursa And Ligament, Right Elbow Bursa And Ligament, Left
Olecranon process	Use:	Ulna, Right Ulna, Left
Olfactory bulb	Use:	Olfactory Nerve
Ophthalmic artery	Use:	Internal Carotid Artery, Right Internal Carotid Artery, Left
Ophthalmic nerve	Use:	Trigeminal Nerve
Ophthalmic vein	Use:	Intracranial Vein
Optic chiasma	Use:	Optic Nerve
Optic disc	Use:	Retina, Right Retina, Left
Optic foramen	Use:	Sphenoid Bone, Right Sphenoid Bone, Left
Orbicularis oculi muscle	Use:	Upper Eyelid, Right Upper Eyelid, Left
Orbicularis oris muscle	Use:	Facial Muscle
Orbital fascia	Use:	Subcutaneous Tissue And Fascia, Face
Orbital portion of ethmoid bone	Use:	Orbit, Right Orbit, Left
Orbital portion of frontal bone	Use:	Orbit, Right Orbit, Left
Orbital portion of lacrimal bone	Use:	Orbit, Right Orbit, Left
Orbital portion of maxilla	Use:	Orbit, Right Orbit, Left
Orbital portion of palatine bone	Use:	Orbit, Right Orbit, Left
Orbital portion of sphenoid bone	Use:	Orbit, Right Orbit, Left
Orbital portion of zygomatic bone	Use:	Orbit, Right Orbit, Left
Oropharynx	Use:	Pharynx

TERM	ICD-10-PCS VALUE	
Ossicular chain	Use:	Auditory Ossicle, Right
		Auditory Ossicle, Left
Otic ganglion	Use:	Head And Neck Sympathetic Nerve
Oval window	Use:	Middle Ear, Right
		Middle Ear, Left
Ovarian artery	Use:	Abdominal Aorta
Ovarian ligament	Use:	Uterine Supporting Structure
Oviduct	Use:	Fallopian Tube, Right
		Fallopian Tube, Left
Palatine gland	Use:	Buccal Mucosa
Palatine tonsil	Use:	Tonsils
Palatine uvula	Use:	Uvula
Palatoglossal muscle	Use:	Tongue, Palate, Pharynx Muscle
Palatopharyngeal muscle	Use:	Tongue, Palate, Pharynx Muscle
Palmar (volar) digital vein	Use:	Hand Vein, Right
		Hand Vein, Left
Palmar (volar) metacarpal vein	Use:	Hand Vein, Right
		Hand Vein, Left
Palmar cutaneous nerve	Use:	Median Nerve Radial Nerve
Palmar fascia (aponeurosis)	Use:	Subcutaneous Tissue And Fascia, Right Hand
		Subcutaneous Tissue And Fascia, Left Hand
Palmar interosseous muscle	Use:	Hand Muscle, Right
		Hand Muscle, Left
Palmar ulnocarpal ligament	Use:	Wrist Bursa And Ligament, Right
		Wrist Bursa And Ligament, Left
Palmaris longus muscle	Use:	Lower Arm And Wrist Muscle, Right
		Lower Arm And Wrist Muscle, Left
Pancreatic artery	Use:	Splenic Artery
Pancreatic plexus	Use:	Abdominal Sympathetic Nerve
Pancreatic vein	Use:	Splenic Vein
Pancreaticosplenic lymph node	Use:	Lymphatic, Aortic
Paraaortic lymph node	Use:	Lymphatic, Aortic
Pararectal lymph node	Use:	Lymphatic, Mesenteric
Parasternal lymph node	Use:	Lymphatic, Thorax
Paratracheal lymph node	Use:	Lymphatic, Thorax
Paraurethral (Skene's) gland	Use:	Vestibular Gland
Parietal lobe	Use:	Cerebral Hemisphere
Parotid lymph node	Use:	Lymphatic, Head
Parotid plexus	Use:	Facial Nerve
Pars flaccida	Use:	Tympanic Membrane, Right
		Tympanic Membrane, Left
Patellar ligament	Use:	Knee Bursa And Ligament, Right
		Knee Bursa And Ligament, Left
Patellar tendon	Use:	Knee Tendon, Right
		Knee Tendon, Left

TERM		ICD-10-PCS VALUE
Pectineus muscle	Use:	Upper Leg Muscle, Right Upper Leg Muscle, Left
Pectoral (anterior) lymph node	Use:	Lymphatic, Right Axillary Lymphatic, Left Axillary
Pectoral fascia	Use:	Subcutaneous Tissue And Fascia, Chest
Pectoralis major muscle	Use:	Thorax Muscle, Right Thorax Muscle, Left
Pectoralis minor muscle	Use:	Thorax Muscle, Right Thorax Muscle, Left
Pelvic splanchnic nerve	Use:	Abdominal Sympathetic Nerve Sacral Sympathetic Nerve
Penile urethra	Use:	Urethra
Pericardiophrenic artery	Use:	Internal Mammary Artery, Right Internal Mammary Artery, Left
Perimetrium	Use:	Uterus
Peroneus brevis muscle	Use:	Lower Leg Muscle, Right Lower Leg Muscle, Left
Peroneus longus muscle	Use:	Lower Leg Muscle, Right Lower Leg Muscle, Left
Petrous part of temporal bone	Use:	Temporal Bone, Right Temporal Bone, Left
Pharyngeal constrictor muscle	Use:	Tongue, Palate, Pharynx Muscle
Pharyngeal plexus	Use:	Vagus Nerve
Pharyngeal recess	Use:	Nasopharynx
Pharyngeal tonsil	Use:	Adenoids
Pharyngotympanic tube	Use:	Eustachian Tube, Right Eustachian Tube, Left
Pia mater	Use:	Cerebral Meninges Spinal Meninges
Pinna	Use:	External Ear, Right External Ear, Left External Ear, Bilateral
Piriform recess (sinus)	Use:	Pharynx
Piriformis muscle	Use:	Hip Muscle, Right Hip Muscle, Left
Pisiform bone	Use:	Carpal, Right Carpal, Left
Pisohamate ligament	Use:	Hand Bursa And Ligament, Right Hand Bursa And Ligament, Left
Pisometacarpal ligament	Use:	Hand Bursa And Ligament, Right Hand Bursa And Ligament, Left
Plantar digital vein	Use:	Foot Vein, Right Foot Vein, Left
Plantar fascia (aponeurosis)	Use:	Subcutaneous Tissue And Fascia, Right Foot Subcutaneous Tissue And Fascia, Left Foot
Plantar metatarsal vein Plantar venous arch	Use:	Foot Vein, Right Foot Vein, Left

TERM	ICD-10-PCS VALUE
Platysma muscle	Use: Neck Muscle, Right Neck Muscle, Left
Plica semilunaris	Use: Conjunctiva, Right Conjunctiva, Left
Pneumogastric nerve	Use: Vagus Nerve
Pneumotaxic center	Use: Pons
Pontine tegmentum	Use: Pons
Popliteal ligament	Use: Knee Bursa And Ligament, Right Knee Bursa And Ligament, Left
Popliteal lymph node	Use: Lymphatic, Right Lower Extremity Lymphatic, Left Lower Extremity
Popliteal vein	Use: Femoral Vein, Right Femoral Vein, Left
Popliteus muscle	Use: Lower Leg Muscle, Right Lower Leg Muscle, Left
Postauricular (mastoid) lymph node	Use: Lymphatic, Right Neck Lymphatic, Left Neck
Postcava	Use: Inferior Vena Cava
Posterior (subscapular) lymph node	Use: Lymphatic, Right Axillary Lymphatic, Left Axillary
Posterior auricular artery	Use: External Carotid Artery, Right External Carotid Artery, Left
Posterior auricular nerve	Use: Facial Nerve
Posterior auricular vein	Use: External Jugular Vein, Right External Jugular Vein, Left
Posterior cerebral artery	Use: Intracranial Artery
Posterior chamber	Use: Eye, Right Eye, Left
Posterior circumflex humeral artery	Use: Axillary Artery, Right Axillary Artery, Left
Posterior communicating artery	Use: Intracranial Artery
Posterior cruciate ligament (PCL)	Use: Knee Bursa And Ligament, Right Knee Bursa And Ligament, Left
Posterior facial (retromandibular) vein	Use: Face Vein, Right Face Vein, Left
Posterior femoral cutaneous nerve	Use: Sacral Plexus
Posterior inferior cerebellar artery (PICA)	Use: Intracranial Artery
Posterior interosseous nerve	Use: Radial Nerve
Posterior labial nerve	Use: Pudendal Nerve
Posterior scrotal nerve	Use: Pudendal Nerve
Posterior spinal artery	Use: Vertebral Artery, Right Vertebral Artery, Left
Posterior tibial recurrent artery	Use: Anterior Tibial Artery, Right Anterior Tibial Artery, Left

TERM		ICD-10-PCS VALUE
Posterior ulnar recurrent artery	Use:	Ulnar Artery, Right Ulnar Artery, Left
Posterior vagal trunk	Use:	Vagus Nerve
Preauricular lymph node	Use:	Lymphatic, Head
Precava	Use:	Superior Vena Cava
Prepatellar bursa	Use:	Knee Bursa And Ligament, Right Knee Bursa And Ligament, Left
Pretracheal fascia	Use:	Subcutaneous Tissue And Fascia, Anterior Neck
Prevertebral fascia	Use:	Subcutaneous Tissue And Fascia, Posterior Neck
Princeps pollicis artery	Use:	Hand Artery, Right Hand Artery, Left
Procerus muscle	Use:	Facial Muscle
Profunda brachii	Use:	Brachial Artery, Right Brachial Artery, Left
Profunda femoris (deep femoral) vein	Use:	Femoral Vein, Right Femoral Vein, Left
Pronator quadratus muscle	Use:	Lower Arm And Wrist Muscle, Right Lower Arm And Wrist Muscle, Left
Pronator teres muscle	Use:	Lower Arm And Wrist Muscle, Right Lower Arm And Wrist Muscle, Left
Prostatic urethra	Use:	Urethra
Proximal radioulnar joint	Use:	Elbow Joint, Right Elbow Joint, Left
Psoas muscle	Use:	Hip Muscle, Right Hip Muscle, Left
Pterygoid muscle	Use:	Head Muscle
Pterygoid process	Use:	Sphenoid Bone, Right Sphenoid Bone, Left
Pterygopalatine (sphenopalatine) ganglion	Use:	Head And Neck Sympathetic Nerve
Pubic ligament	Use:	Trunk Bursa And Ligament, Right Trunk Bursa And Ligament, Left
Pubis	Use:	Pelvic Bone, Right Pelvic Bone, Left
Pubofemoral ligament	Use:	Hip Bursa And Ligament, Right Hip Bursa And Ligament, Left
Pudendal nerve	Use:	Sacral Plexus
Pulmoaortic canal	Use:	Pulmonary Artery, Left
Pulmonary annulus	Use:	Pulmonary Valve
Pulmonary plexus	Use:	Vagus Nerve Thoracic Sympathetic Nerve
Pulmonic valve	Use:	Pulmonary Valve
Pulvinar	Use:	Thalamus
Pyloric antrum	Use:	Stomach, Pylorus
Pyloric canal	Use:	Stomach, Pylorus
Pyloric sphincter	Use:	Stomach, Pylorus

TERM		ICD-10-PCS VALUE
Pyramidalis muscle	Use:	Abdomen Muscle, Right Abdomen Muscle, Left
Quadrangular cartilage	Use:	Nasal Septum
Quadrate lobe	Use:	Liver
Quadratus femoris muscle	Use:	Hip Muscle, Right Hip Muscle, Left
Quadratus lumborum muscle	Use:	Trunk Muscle, Right Trunk Muscle, Left
Quadratus plantae muscle	Use:	Foot Muscle, Right Foot Muscle, Left
Quadriceps (femoris)	Use:	Upper Leg Muscle, Right Upper Leg Muscle, Left
Radial collateral carpal ligament	Use:	Wrist Bursa And Ligament, Right Wrist Bursa And Ligament, Left
Radial collateral ligament	Use:	Elbow Bursa And Ligament, Right Elbow Bursa And Ligament, Left
Radial notch	Use:	Ulna, Right Ulna, Left
Radial recurrent artery	Use:	Radial Artery, Right Radial Artery, Left
Radial vein	Use:	Brachial Vein, Right Brachial Vein, Left
Radialis indicis	Use:	Hand Artery, Right Hand Artery, Left
Radiocarpal joint	Use:	Wrist Joint, Right Wrist Joint, Left
Radiocarpal ligament	Use:	Wrist Bursa And Ligament, Right Wrist Bursa And Ligament, Left
Radioulnar ligament	Use:	Wrist Bursa And Ligament, Right Wrist Bursa And Ligament, Left
Rectosigmoid junction	Use:	Sigmoid Colon
Rectus abdominis muscle	Use:	Abdomen Muscle, Right Abdomen Muscle, Left
Rectus femoris muscle	Use:	Upper Leg Muscle, Right Upper Leg Muscle, Left
Recurrent laryngeal nerve	Use:	Vagus Nerve
Renal calyx	Use:	Kidney, Right Kidney, Left Kidneys, Bilateral Kidney
Renal capsule	Use:	Kidney, Right Kidney, Left Kidneys, Bilateral Kidney
Renal cortex	Use:	Kidney, Right Kidney, Left Kidneys, Bilateral Kidney
Renal plexus	Use:	Abdominal Sympathetic Nerve

TERM	ICD-10-PCS VALUE	
Renal segment	Use:	Kidney, Right Kidney, Left Kidneys, Bilateral Kidney
Renal segmental artery	Use:	Renal Artery, Right Renal Artery, Left
Retroperitoneal lymph node	Use:	Lymphatic, Aortic
Retroperitoneal space	Use:	Retroperitoneum
Retropharyngeal lymph node	Use:	Lymphatic, Right Neck Lymphatic, Left Neck
Retropubic space	Use:	Pelvic Cavity
Rhinopharynx	Use:	Nasopharynx
Rhomboid major muscle	Use:	Trunk Muscle, Right Trunk Muscle, Left
Rhomboid minor muscle	Use:	Trunk Muscle, Right Trunk Muscle, Left
Right ascending lumbar vein	Use:	Azygos Vein
Right atrioventricular valve	Use:	Tricuspid Valve
Right auricular appendix	Use:	Atrium, Right
Right colic vein	Use:	Colic Vein
Right coronary sulcus	Use:	Heart, Right
Right gastric artery	Use:	Gastric Artery
Right gastroepiploic vein	Use:	Superior Mesenteric Vein
Right inferior phrenic vein	Use:	Inferior Vena Cava
Right inferior pulmonary vein	Use:	Pulmonary Vein, Right
Right jugular trunk	Use:	Lymphatic, Right Neck
Right lateral ventricle	Use:	Cerebral Ventricle
Right lymphatic duct	Use:	Lymphatic, Right Neck
Right ovarian vein	Use:	Inferior Vena Cava
Right second lumbar vein	Use:	Inferior Vena Cava
Right subclavian trunk	Use:	Lymphatic, Right Neck
Right subcostal vein	Use:	Azygos Vein
Right superior pulmonary vein	Use:	Pulmonary Vein, Right
Right suprarenal vein	Use:	Inferior Vena Cava
Right testicular vein	Use:	Inferior Vena Cava
Rima glottidis	Use:	Larynx
Risorius muscle	Use:	Facial Muscle
Round ligament of uterus	Use:	Uterine Supporting Structure
Round window	Use:	Inner Ear, Right Inner Ear, Left
Sacral ganglion	Use:	Sacral Sympathetic Nerve
Sacral lymph node	Use:	Lymphatic, Pelvis
Sacral splanchnic nerve	Use:	Sacral Sympathetic Nerve
Sacrococcygeal ligament	Use:	Trunk Bursa And Ligament, Right Trunk Bursa And Ligament, Left

TERM	ICD-10-PCS VALUE	
Sacrococcygeal symphysis	Use:	Sacrococcygeal Joint
Sacroiliac ligament	Use:	Trunk Bursa And Ligament, Right
		Trunk Bursa And Ligament, Left
Sacrospinous ligament	Use:	Trunk Bursa And Ligament, Right
		Trunk Bursa And Ligament, Left
Sacrotuberous ligament	Use:	Trunk Bursa And Ligament, Right
		Trunk Bursa And Ligament, Left
Salpingopharyngeus muscle	Use:	Tongue, Palate, Pharynx Muscle
Salpinx	Use:	Fallopian Tube, Right
		Fallopian Tube, Left
Saphenous nerve	Use:	Femoral Nerve
Sartorius muscle	Use:	Upper Leg Muscle, Right
		Upper Leg Muscle, Left
Scalene muscle	Use:	Neck Muscle, Right
		Neck Muscle, Left
Scaphoid bone	Use:	Carpal, Right
		Carpal, Left
Scapholunate ligament	Use:	Hand Bursa And Ligament, Right
		Hand Bursa And Ligament, Left
Scaphotrapezium ligament	Use:	Hand Bursa And Ligament, Right
		Hand Bursa And Ligament, Left
Scarpa's (vestibular) ganglion	Use:	Acoustic Nerve
Sebaceous gland	Use:	Skin
Second cranial nerve	Use:	Optic Nerve
Sella turcica	Use:	Sphenoid Bone, Right
		Sphenoid Bone, Left
Semicircular canal	Use:	Inner Ear, Right
		Inner Ear, Left
Semimembranosus muscle	Use:	Upper Leg Muscle, Right
		Upper Leg Muscle, Left
Semitendinosus muscle	Use:	Upper Leg Muscle, Right
		Upper Leg Muscle, Left
Septal cartilage	Use:	Nasal Septum
Serratus anterior muscle	Use:	Thorax Muscle, Right
		Thorax Muscle, Left
Serratus posterior muscle	Use:	Trunk Muscle, Right
		Trunk Muscle, Left
Seventh cranial nerve	Use:	Facial Nerve
Short gastric artery	Use:	Splenic Artery
Sigmoid artery	Use:	Inferior Mesenteric Artery
Sigmoid flexure	Use:	Sigmoid Colon
Sigmoid vein	Use:	Inferior Mesenteric Vein
Sinoatrial node	Use:	Conduction Mechanism
Sinus venosus	Use:	Atrium, Right
Sixth cranial nerve	Use:	Abducens Nerve
Skene's (paraurethral) gland	Use:	Vestibular Gland

TERM		ICD-10-PCS VALUE
Small saphenous vein	Use:	Lesser Saphenous Vein, Right Lesser Saphenous Vein, Left
Solar (celiac) plexus	Use:	Abdominal Sympathetic Nerve
Soleus muscle	Use:	Lower Leg Muscle, Right Lower Leg Muscle, Left
Sphenomandibular ligament	Use:	Head And Neck Bursa And Ligament
Sphenopalatine (pterygopalatine) ganglion	Use:	Head And Neck Sympathetic Nerve
Spinal dura mater	Use:	Dura Mater
Spinal epidural space	Use:	Epidural Space
Spinal subarachnoid space	Use:	Subarachnoid Space
Spinal subdural space	Use:	Subdural Space
Spinous process	Use:	Cervical Vertebra Thoracic Vertebra Lumbar Vertebra
Spiral ganglion	Use:	Acoustic Nerve
Splenic flexure	Use:	Transverse Colon
Splenic plexus	Use:	Abdominal Sympathetic Nerve
Splenius capitis muscle	Use:	Head Muscle
Splenius cervicis muscle	Use:	Neck Muscle, Right Neck Muscle, Left
Stapes	Use:	Auditory Ossicle, Right Auditory Ossicle, Left
Stellate ganglion	Use:	Head And Neck Sympathetic Nerve
Stensen's duct	Use:	Parotid Duct, Right Parotid Duct, Left
Sternoclavicular ligament	Use:	Shoulder Bursa And Ligament, Right Shoulder Bursa And Ligament, Left
Sternocleidomastoid artery	Use:	Thyroid Artery, Right Thyroid Artery, Left
Sternocleidomastoid muscle	Use:	Neck Muscle, Right Neck Muscle, Left
Sternocostal ligament	Use:	Thorax Bursa And Ligament, Right Thorax Bursa And Ligament, Left
Styloglossus muscle	Use:	Tongue, Palate, Pharynx Muscle
Stylomandibular ligament	Use:	Head And Neck Bursa And Ligament
Stylopharyngeus muscle	Use:	Tongue, Palate, Pharynx Muscle
Subacromial bursa	Use:	Shoulder Bursa And Ligament, Right Shoulder Bursa And Ligament, Left
Subaortic (common iliac) lymph node	Use:	Lymphatic, Pelvis
Subclavicular (apical) lymph node	Use:	Lymphatic, Right Axillary Lymphatic, Left Axillary
Subclavius muscle	Use:	Thorax Muscle, Right Thorax Muscle, Left
Subclavius nerve	Use:	Brachial Plexus
Subcostal artery	Use:	Thoracic Aorta

TERM		ICD-10-PCS VALUE
Subcostal muscle	Use:	Thorax Muscle, Right Thorax Muscle, Left
Subcostal nerve	Use:	Thoracic Nerve
Submandibular ganglion	Use:	Facial Nerve Head And Neck Sympathetic Nerve
Submandibular gland	Use:	Submaxillary Gland, Right Submaxillary Gland, Left
Submandibular lymph node	Use:	Lymphatic, Head
Submaxillary ganglion	Use:	Head And Neck Sympathetic Nerve
Submaxillary lymph node	Use:	Lymphatic, Head
Submental artery	Use:	Face Artery
Submental lymph node	Use:	Lymphatic, Head
Submucous (Meissner's) plexus	Use:	Abdominal Sympathetic Nerve
Suboccipital nerve	Use:	Cervical Nerve
Suboccipital venous plexus	Use:	Vertebral Vein, Right Vertebral Vein, Left
Subparotid lymph node	Use:	Lymphatic, Head
Subscapular (posterior) lymph node	Use:	Lymphatic, Right Axillary Lymphatic, Left Axillary
Subscapular aponeurosis	Use:	Subcutaneous Tissue And Fascia, Right Upper Arm Subcutaneous Tissue And Fascia, Left Upper Arm
Subscapular artery	Use:	Axillary Artery, Right Axillary Artery, Left
Subscapularis muscle	Use:	Shoulder Muscle, Right Shoulder Muscle, Left
Substantia nigra	Use:	Basal Ganglia
Subtalar (talocalcaneal) joint	Use:	Tarsal Joint, Right Tarsal Joint, Left
Subtalar ligament	Use:	Foot Bursa And Ligament, Right Foot Bursa And Ligament, Left
Subthalamic nucleus	Use:	Basal Ganglia
Superficial circumflex iliac vein	Use:	Greater Saphenous Vein, Right Greater Saphenous Vein, Left
Superficial epigastric artery	Use:	Femoral Artery, Right Femoral Artery, Left
Superficial epigastric vein	Use:	Greater Saphenous Vein, Right Greater Saphenous Vein, Left
Superficial palmar arch	Use:	Hand Artery, Right Hand Artery, Left
Superficial palmar venous arch	Use:	Hand Vein, Right Hand Vein, Left
Superficial temporal artery	Use:	Temporal Artery, Right Temporal Artery, Left
Superficial transverse perineal muscle	Use:	Perineum Muscle
Superior cardiac nerve	Use:	Thoracic Sympathetic Nerve

TERM	ICD-10-PCS VALUE	
Superior cerebellar vein Superior cerebral vein	Use:	Intracranial Vein
Superior clunic (cluneal) nerve	Use:	Lumbar Nerve
Superior epigastric artery	Use:	Internal Mammary Artery, Right Internal Mammary Artery, Left
Superior genicular artery	Use:	Popliteal Artery, Right Popliteal Artery, Left
Superior gluteal artery	Use:	Internal Iliac Artery, Right Internal Iliac Artery, Left
Superior gluteal nerve	Use:	Lumbar Plexus
Superior hypogastric plexus	Use:	Abdominal Sympathetic Nerve
Superior labial artery	Use:	Face Artery
Superior laryngeal artery	Use:	Thyroid Artery, Right Thyroid Artery, Left
Superior laryngeal nerve	Use:	Vagus Nerve
Superior longitudinal muscle	Use:	Tongue, Palate, Pharynx Muscle
Superior mesenteric ganglion	Use:	Abdominal Sympathetic Nerve
Superior mesenteric lymph node	Use:	Lymphatic, Mesenteric
Superior mesenteric plexus	Use:	Abdominal Sympathetic Nerve
Superior oblique muscle	Use:	Extraocular Muscle, Right Extraocular Muscle, Left
Superior olivary nucleus	Use:	Pons
Superior rectal artery	Use:	Inferior Mesenteric Artery
Superior rectal vein	Use:	Inferior Mesenteric Vein
Superior rectus muscle	Use:	Extraocular Muscle, Right Extraocular Muscle, Left
Superior tarsal plate	Use:	Upper Eyelid, Right Upper Eyelid, Left
Superior thoracic artery	Use:	Axillary Artery, Right Axillary Artery, Left
Superior thyroid artery	Use:	External Carotid Artery, Right External Carotid Artery, Left Thyroid Artery, Right Thyroid Artery, Left
Superior turbinate	Use:	Nasal Turbinate
Superior ulnar collateral artery	Use:	Brachial Artery, Right Brachial Artery, Left
Supraclavicular (Virchow's) lymph node	Use:	Lymphatic, Right Neck Lymphatic, Left Neck
Supraclavicular nerve	Use:	Cervical Plexus
Suprahyoid lymph node	Use:	Lymphatic, Head
Suprahyoid muscle	Use:	Neck Muscle, Right Neck Muscle, Left
Suprainguinal lymph node	Use:	Lymphatic, Pelvis

TERM		ICD-10-PCS VALUE
Supraorbital vein	Use:	Face Vein, Right Face Vein, Left
Suprarenal gland	Use:	Adrenal Gland, Left Adrenal Gland, Right Adrenal Glands, Bilateral
Suprarenal plexus	Use:	Abdominal Sympathetic Nerve
Suprascapular nerve	Use:	Brachial Plexus
Supraspinatus fascia	Use:	Subcutaneous Tissue And Fascia, Right Upper Arm Subcutaneous Tissue And Fascia, Left Upper Arm
Supraspinatus muscle	Use:	Shoulder Muscle, Right Shoulder Muscle, Left
Supraspinous ligament	Use:	Trunk Bursa And Ligament, Right Trunk Bursa And Ligament, Left
Suprasternal notch	Use:	Sternum
Supratrochlear lymph node	Use:	Lymphatic, Right Upper Extremity Lymphatic, Left Upper Extremity
Sural artery	Use:	Popliteal Artery, Right Popliteal Artery, Left
Sweat gland	Use:	Skin
Talocalcaneal (subtalar) joint	Use:	Tarsal Joint, Right Tarsal Joint, Left
Talocalcaneal ligament	Use:	Foot Bursa And Ligament, Right Foot Bursa And Ligament, Left
Talocalcaneonavicular joint	Use:	Tarsal Joint, Right Tarsal Joint, Left
Talocalcaneonavicular ligament	Use:	Foot Bursa And Ligament, Right Foot Bursa And Ligament, Left
Talocrural joint	Use:	Ankle Joint, Right Ankle Joint, Left
Talofibular ligament	Use:	Ankle Bursa And Ligament, Right Ankle Bursa And Ligament, Left
Talus bone	Use:	Tarsal, Right Tarsal, Left
Tarsometatarsal joint	Use:	Metatarsal-Tarsal Joint, Right Metatarsal-Tarsal Joint, Left
Tarsometatarsal ligament	Use:	Foot Bursa And Ligament, Right Foot Bursa And Ligament, Left
Temporal lobe	Use:	Cerebral Hemisphere
Temporalis muscle Temporoparietalis muscle	Use:	Head Muscle
Tensor fasciae latae muscle	Use:	Hip Muscle, Right Hip Muscle, Left
Tensor veli palatini muscle	Use:	Tongue, Palate, Pharynx Muscle
Tenth cranial nerve	Use:	Vagus Nerve
Tentorium cerebelli	Use:	Dura Mater
Teres major muscle	Use:	Shoulder Muscle, Right Shoulder Muscle, Left

TERM		ICD-10-PCS VALUE
Teres minor muscle	Use:	Shoulder Muscle, Right Shoulder Muscle, Left
Testicular artery	Use:	Abdominal Aorta
Thenar muscle	Use:	Hand Muscle, Right Hand Muscle, Left
Third cranial nerve	Use:	Oculomotor Nerve
Third occipital nerve	Use:	Cervical Nerve
Third ventricle	Use:	Cerebral Ventricle
Thoracic aortic plexus	Use:	Thoracic Sympathetic Nerve
Thoracic esophagus	Use:	Esophagus, Middle
Thoracic facet joint	Use:	Thoracic Vertebral Joint Thoracic Vertebral Joints, 2-7 Thoracic Vertebral Joints, 8 Or More
Thoracic ganglion	Use:	Thoracic Sympathetic Nerve
Thoracoacromial artery	Use:	Axillary Artery, Right Axillary Artery, Left
Thoracolumbar facet joint	Use:	Thoracolumbar Vertebral Joint
Thymus gland	Use:	Thymus
Thyroarytenoid muscle	Use:	Neck Muscle, Right Neck Muscle, Left
Thyrocervical trunk	Use:	Thyroid Artery, Right Thyroid Artery, Left
Thyroid cartilage	Use:	Larynx
Tibialis anterior muscle	Use:	Lower Leg Muscle, Right Lower Leg Muscle, Left
Tibialis posterior muscle	Use:	Lower Leg Muscle, Right Lower Leg Muscle, Left
Tracheobronchial lymph node	Use:	Lymphatic, Thorax
Tragus	Use:	External Ear, Right External Ear, Left External Ear, Bilateral
Transversalis fascia	Use:	Subcutaneous Tissue And Fascia, Trunk
Transverse (cutaneous) cervical nerve	Use:	Cervical Plexus
Transverse acetabular ligament	Use:	Hip Bursa And Ligament, Right Hip Bursa And Ligament, Left
Transverse facial artery	Use:	Temporal Artery, Right Temporal Artery, Left
Transverse humeral ligament	Use:	Shoulder Bursa And Ligament, Right Shoulder Bursa And Ligament, Left
Transverse ligament of atlas	Use:	Head And Neck Bursa And Ligament
Transverse scapular ligament	Use:	Shoulder Bursa And Ligament, Right Shoulder Bursa And Ligament, Left
Transverse thoracis muscle	Use:	Thorax Muscle, Right Thorax Muscle, Left

TERM		ICD-10-PCS VALUE
Transversospinalis muscle	Use:	Trunk Muscle, Right
		Trunk Muscle, Left
Transversus abdominis muscle	Use:	Abdomen Muscle, Right
		Abdomen Muscle, Left
Trapezium bone	Use:	Carpal, Right
		Carpal, Left
Trapezius muscle	Use:	Trunk Muscle, Right
		Trunk Muscle, Left
Trapezoid bone	Use:	Carpal, Right
		Carpal, Left
Triceps brachii muscle	Use:	Upper Arm Muscle, Right
		Upper Arm Muscle, Left
Tricuspid annulus	Use:	Tricuspid Valve
Trifacial nerve	Use:	Trigeminal Nerve
Trigone of bladder	Use:	Bladder
Triquetral bone	Use:	Carpal, Right
		Carpal, Left
Trochanteric bursa	Use:	Hip Bursa And Ligament, Right
		Hip Bursa And Ligament, Left
Twelfth cranial nerve	Use:	Hypoglossal Nerve
Tympanic cavity	Use:	Middle Ear, Right
		Middle Ear, Left
Tympanic nerve	Use:	Glossopharyngeal Nerve
Tympanic part of temporal bone	Use:	Temporal Bone, Right
		Temporal Bone, Left
Ulnar collateral carpal ligament	Use:	Wrist Bursa And Ligament, Right
		Wrist Bursa And Ligament, Left
Ulnar collateral ligament	Use:	Elbow Bursa And Ligament, Right
		Elbow Bursa And Ligament, Left
Ulnar notch	Use:	Radius, Right
		Radius, Left
Ulnar vein	Use:	Brachial Vein, Right
		Brachial Vein, Left
Umbilical artery	Use:	Internal Iliac Artery, Right
		Internal Iliac Artery, Left
Ureteral orifice	Use:	Ureter, Right
		Ureter, Left
		Ureters, Bilateral Ureter
Ureteropelvic junction (UPJ)	Use:	Kidney Pelvis, Right
		Kidney Pelvis, Left
Ureterovesical orifice	Use:	Ureter, Right
		Ureter, Left
		Ureters, Bilateral Ureter
Uterine artery	Use:	Internal Iliac Artery, Right
		Internal Iliac Artery, Left
Uterine cornu	Use:	Uterus

TERM		ICD-10-PCS VALUE
Uterine tube	Use:	Fallopian Tube, Right Fallopian Tube, Left
Uterine vein	Use:	Hypogastric Vein, Right Hypogastric Vein, Left
Vaginal artery	Use:	Internal Iliac Artery, Right Internal Iliac Artery, Left
Vaginal vein	Use:	Hypogastric Vein, Right Hypogastric Vein, Left
Vastus intermedius muscle	Use:	Upper Leg Muscle, Right Upper Leg Muscle, Left
Vastus lateralis muscle	Use:	Upper Leg Muscle, Right Upper Leg Muscle, Left
Vastus medialis muscle	Use:	Upper Leg Muscle, Right Upper Leg Muscle, Left
Ventricular fold	Use:	Larynx
Vermiform appendix	Use:	Appendix
Vermilion border	Use:	Upper Lip Lower Lip
Vertebral arch	Use:	Cervical Vertebra Thoracic Vertebra Lumbar Vertebra
Vertebral canal	Use:	Spinal Canal
Vertebral foramen	Use:	Cervical Vertebra Thoracic Vertebra Lumbar Vertebra
Vertebral lamina	Use:	Cervical Vertebra Thoracic Vertebra Lumbar Vertebra
Vertebral pedicle	Use:	Cervical Vertebra Thoracic Vertebra Lumbar Vertebra
Vesical vein	Use:	Hypogastric Vein, Right Hypogastric Vein, Left
Vestibular (Scarpa's) ganglion	Use:	Acoustic Nerve
Vestibular nerve	Use:	Acoustic Nerve
Vestibulocochlear nerve	Use:	Acoustic Nerve
Virchow's (supraclavicular) lymph node	Use:	Lymphatic, Right Neck Lymphatic, Left Neck
Vitreous body	Use:	Vitreous, Right Vitreous, Left
Vocal fold	Use:	Vocal Cord, Right Vocal Cord, Left
Volar (palmar) digital vein	Use:	Hand Vein, Right Hand Vein, Left
Volar (palmar) metacarpal vein	Use:	Hand Vein, Right Hand Vein, Left
Vomer bone	Use:	Nasal Septum
Vomer of nasal septum	Use:	Nasal Bone

TERM	ICD-10-PCS VALUE	
Xiphoid process	Use:	Sternum
Zonule of Zinn	Use:	Lens, Right Lens, Left
Zygomatic process of frontal bone	Use:	Frontal Bone, Right Frontal Bone, Left
Zygomatic process of temporal bone	Use:	Temporal Bone, Right Temporal Bone, Left

BODY PART	PCS DESCRIPTION
3f (Aortic) Bioprosthesis valve	Zooplastic tissue in heart and great vessels
AbioCor® Total Replacement Heart	Synthetic substitute
Acellular Hydrated Dermis	Nonautologous tissue substitute
Activa PC neurostimulator	Stimulator generator, multiple array for insertion in subcutaneous tissue and fascia
Activa RC neurostimulator	Stimulator generator, multiple array rechargeable for insertion in subcutaneous tissue and fascia
Activa SC neurostimulator	Stimulator generator, single array for insertion in subcutaneous tissue and fascia
ACUITY™ Steerable Lead	Cardiac lead, pacemaker for insertion in heart and great vessels Cardiac lead, defibrillator for insertion in heart and great vessels
AMPLATZER® Muscular VSD Occluder	Synthetic substitute
AMS 800® Urinary Control System	Artificial sphincter in urinary system
AneuRx® AAA Advantage®	Intraluminal device
Annuloplasty ring	Synthetic substitute
Artificial anal sphincter (AAS)	Artificial sphincter in gastrointestinal system
Artificial bowel sphincter (neosphincter)	Artificial sphincter in gastrointestinal system
Artificial urinary sphincter (AUS)	Artificial sphincter in urinary system
Assurant (Cobalt) stent	Intraluminal device
Attain Ability® lead	Cardiac lead, pacemaker for insertion in heart and great vessels Cardiac lead, defibrillator for insertion in heart and great vessels
Attain StarFix® (OTW) lead	Cardiac lead, pacemaker for insertion in heart and great vessels Cardiac lead, defibrillator for insertion in heart and great vessels
Autograft	Autologous tissue substitute
Autologous artery graft	Autologous arterial tissue in heart and great vessels Autologous arterial tissue in upper arteries Autologous arterial tissue in lower arteries Autologous arterial tissue in upper veins Autologous arterial tissue in lower veins
Autologous vein graft	Autologous venous tissue in heart and great vessels Autologous venous tissue in upper arteries Autologous venous tissue in lower arteries Autologous venous tissue in upper veins Autologous venous tissue in lower veins
Axial Lumbar Interbody Fusion System	Interbody fusion device in lower joints
AxiaLIF® System	Interbody fusion device in lower joints
BAK/C® Interbody Cervical Fusion System	Interbody fusion device in upper joints
Bard® Composix® (E/X)(LP) mesh	Synthetic substitute
Bard® Composix® Kugel® patch	Synthetic substitute
Bard® Dulex™ mesh	Synthetic substitute
Bard® Ventralex™ hernia patch	Synthetic substitute
Baroreflex Activation Therapy® (BAT®)	Stimulator lead in upper arteries cardiac rhythm related device in subcutaneous tissue and fascia
Berlin Heart Ventricular Assist Device	Implantable heart assist system in heart and great vessels
Bioactive embolization coil(s)	Intraluminal device, bioactive in upper arteries
Biventricular external heart assist system	External heart assist system in heart and great vessels

BODY PART	PCS DESCRIPTION
Blood glucose monitoring system	Monitoring device
Bone anchored hearing device	Hearing device, bone conduction for insertion in ear, nose, sinus Hearing device in head and facial bones
Bone bank bone graft	Nonautologous tissue substitute
Bone screw (interlocking)(lag)(pedicle)(recessed)	Internal fixation device in head and facial bones Internal fixation device in upper bones Internal fixation device in lower bones
Bovine pericardial valve	Zooplastic tissue in heart and great vessels
Bovine pericardium graft	Zooplastic tissue in heart and great vessels
Brachytherapy seeds	Radioactive element
BRYAN® Cervical Disc System	Synthetic substitute
BVS 5000 Ventricular Assist Device	External heart assist system in heart and great vessels
Cardiac contractility modulation lead	Cardiac lead in heart and great vessels
Cardiac event recorder	Monitoring device
Cardiac resynchronization therapy (CRT) lead	Cardiac lead, pacemaker for insertion in heart and great vessels Cardiac lead, defibrillator for insertion in heart and great vessels
CardioMEMS® pressure sensor	Monitoring device, pressure sensor for insertion in heart and great vessels
Carotid (artery) sinus (baroreceptor) lead	Stimulator lead in upper arteries
Carotid WALLSTENT® Monorail® Endoprosthesis	Intraluminal device
Centrimag® Blood Pump	Intraluminal device
Clamp and rod internal fixation system (CRIF)	Internal fixation device in upper bones Internal fixation device in lower bones
CoAxia NeuroFlo catheter	Intraluminal device
Cobalt/chromium head and polyethylene socket	Synthetic substitute, metal on polyethylene for replacement in lower joints
Cobalt/chromium head and socket	Synthetic substitute, metal for replacement in lower joints
Cochlear implant (CI), multiple channel (electrode)	Hearing device, multiple channel cochlear prosthesis for insertion in ear, nose, sinus
Cochlear implant (CI), single channel (electrode)	Hearing device, single channel cochlear prosthesis for insertion in ear, nose, sinus
COGNIS® CRT-D	Cardiac resynchronization defibrillator pulse generator for insertion in subcutaneous tissue and fascia
Colonic Z-Stent®	Intraluminal device
Complete (SE) stent	Intraluminal device
Concerto II CRT-D	Cardiac resynchronization defibrillator pulse generator for insertion in subcutaneous tissue and fascia
CONSERVE® PLUS Total Resurfacing Hip System	Resurfacing device in lower joints
Consulta CRT-D	Cardiac resynchronization defibrillator pulse generator for insertion in subcutaneous tissue and fascia
Consulta CRT-P	Cardiac resynchronization pacemaker pulse generator for insertion in subcutaneous tissue and fascia
CONTAK RENEWAL® 3 RF (HE) CRT-D	Cardiac resynchronization defibrillator pulse generator for insertion in subcutaneous tissue and fascia
Contegra Pulmonary Valved Conduit	Zooplastic tissue in heart and great vessels
Continuous Glucose Monitoring (CGM) device	Monitoring device
CoreValve transcatheter aortic valve	Zooplastic tissue in heart and great vessels

BODY PART	PCS DESCRIPTION
Cormet Hip Resurfacing System	Resurfacing device in lower joints
CoRoent® XL	Interbody fusion device in lower joints
Corox (OTW) Bipolar Lead	Cardiac lead, pacemaker for insertion in heart and great vessels Cardiac lead, defibrillator for insertion in heart and great vessels
Cortical strip neurostimulator lead	Neurostimulator lead in central nervous system
Cultured epidermal cell autograft	Autologous tissue substitute
CYPHER® Stent	Intraluminal device, drug-eluting in heart and great vessels
Cystostomy tube	Drainage device
DBS lead	Neurostimulator lead in central nervous system
DeBakey Left Ventricular Assist Device	Implantable heart assist system in heart and great vessels
Deep brain neurostimulator lead	Neurostimulator lead in central nervous system
Delta frame external fixator	External fixation device, hybrid for insertion in upper bones External fixation device, hybrid for reposition in upper bones External fixation device, hybrid for insertion in lower bones External fixation device, hybrid for reposition in lower bones
Delta III Reverse shoulder prosthesis	Synthetic substitute, reverse ball and socket for replacement in upper joints
Diaphragmatic pacemaker generator	Stimulator generator in subcutaneous tissue and fascia
Direct Lateral Interbody Fusion (DLIF) device	Interbody fusion device in lower joints
Driver stent (RX) (OTW)	Intraluminal device
DuraHeart Left Ventricular Assist System	Implantable heart assist system in heart and great vessels
Durata® Defibrillation Lead	Cardiac lead, defibrillator for insertion in heart and great vessels
Dynesys® Dynamic Stabilization System	Spinal stabilization device, pedicle-based for insertion in upper joints Spinal stabilization device, pedicle-based for insertion in lower joints
E-Luminexx™ (Biliary)(Vascular) Stent	Intraluminal device
Electrical bone growth stimulator (EBGS)	Bone growth stimulator in head and facial bones bone growth stimulator in upper bones Bone growth stimulator in lower bones
Electrical muscle stimulation (EMS) lead	Stimulator lead in muscles
Electronic muscle stimulator lead	Stimulator lead in muscles
Embolization coil(s)	Intraluminal device
Endeavor® (III)(IV) (Sprint) Zotarolimus-eluting Coronary Stent System	Intraluminal device, drug-eluting in heart and great vessels
EndoSure® sensor	Monitoring device, pressure sensor for insertion in heart and great vessels
ENDOTAK RELIANCE® (G) Defibrillation Lead	Cardiac lead, defibrillator for insertion in heart and great vessels
Endotracheal tube (cuffed)(double-lumen)	Intraluminal device, endotracheal airway in respiratory system
Endurant® Endovascular Stent Graft	Intraluminal device
EnRhythm	Pacemaker, dual chamber for insertion in subcutaneous tissue and fascia
Enterra gastric neurostimulator	Stimulator generator, multiple array for insertion in subcutaneous tissue and fascia
Epicel® cultured epidermal autograft	Autologous tissue substitute
Epic™ Stented Tissue Valve (aortic)	Zooplastic tissue in heart and great vessels
Esophageal obturator airway (EOA)	Intraluminal device, airway in gastrointestinal system

BODY PART	PCS DESCRIPTION
Esteem® implantable hearing system	Hearing device in ear, nose, sinus
Everolimus-eluting coronary stent	Intraluminal device, drug-eluting in heart and great vessels
Ex-PRESS™ mini glaucoma shunt	Synthetic substitute
Express® (LD) Premounted Stent System	Intraluminal device
Express® Biliary SD Monorail® Premounted Stent System	Intraluminal device
Express® SD Renal Monorail® Premounted Stent System	Intraluminal device
External fixator	External fixation device in head and facial bones External fixation device in upper bones External fixation device in lower bones External fixation device in upper joints External fixation device in lower joints
EXtreme Lateral Interbody Fusion (XLIF) device	Interbody fusion device in lower joints
Facet replacement spinal stabilization device	Spinal stabilization device, facet replacement for insertion in upper joints Spinal stabilization device, facet replacement for insertion in lower joints
FLAIR® Endovascular Stent Graft	Intraluminal device
Flexible Composite Mesh	Synthetic substitute
Foley catheter	Drainage device
Formula™ Balloon-Expandable Renal Stent System	Intraluminal device
Freestyle (Stentless) Aortic Root Bioprosthesis	Zooplastic tissue in heart and great vessels
Fusion screw (compression)(lag)(locking)	Internal fixation device in upper joints Internal fixation device in lower joints
Gastric electrical stimulation (GES) lead	Stimulator lead in gastrointestinal system
Gastric pacemaker lead	Stimulator lead in gastrointestinal system
GORE® DUALMESH®	Synthetic substitute
Guedel airway	Intraluminal device, airway in mouth and throat
Hancock Bioprosthesis (aortic) (mitral) valve	Zooplastic tissue in heart and great vessels
Hancock Bioprosthetic Valved Conduit	Zooplastic tissue in heart and great vessels
HeartMate II® Left Ventricular Assist Device (LVAD)	Implantable heart assist system in heart and great vessels
HeartMate XVE® Left Ventricular Assist Device (LVAD)	Implantable heart assist system in heart and great vessels
Hip (joint) liner	Liner in lower joints
Holter valve ventricular shunt	Synthetic substitute
Ilizarov external fixator	External fixation device, ring for insertion in upper bones External fixation device, ring for reposition in upper bones External fixation device, ring for insertion in lower bones External fixation device, ring for reposition in lower bones
Ilizarov-Vecklich device	External fixation device, limb lengthening for insertion in upper bones External fixation device, limb lengthening for insertion in lower bones
Implantable cardioverter-defibrillator (ICD)	Defibrillator generator for insertion in subcutaneous tissue and fascia
Implantable drug infusion pump (anti-spasmodic) (chemotherapy)(pain)	Infusion device, pump in subcutaneous tissue and fascia
Implantable glucose monitoring device	Monitoring device

BODY PART	PCS DESCRIPTION
Implantable hemodynamic monitor (IHM)	Monitoring device, hemodynamic for insertion in subcutaneous tissue and fascia
Implantable hemodynamic monitoring system (IHMS)	Monitoring device, hemodynamic for insertion in subcutaneous tissue and fascia
Implantable Miniature Telescope™ (IMT)	Synthetic substitute, intraocular telescope for replacement in eye
Implanted (venous)(access) port	Vascular access device, reservoir in subcutaneous tissue and fascia
InDura, intrathecal catheter (1P) (spinal)	Infusion device
Injection reservoir, port	Vascular access device, reservoir in subcutaneous tissue and fascia
Injection reservoir, pump	Infusion device, pump in subcutaneous tissue and fascia
Interbody fusion (spine) cage	Interbody fusion device in upper joints Interbody fusion device in lower joints
Interspinous process spinal stabilization device	Spinal stabilization device, interspinous process for insertion in upper joints Spinal stabilization device, interspinous process for insertion in lower joints
InterStim® Therapy neurostimulator	Stimulator generator, single array for insertion in subcutaneous tissue and fascia
Intramedullary (IM) rod (nail)	Internal fixation device, intramedullary in upper bones Internal fixation device, intramedullary in lower bones
Intramedullary skeletal kinetic distractor (ISKD)	Internal fixation device, intramedullary in upper bones Internal fixation device, intramedullary in lower bones
Intrauterine device (IUD)	Contraceptive device in female reproductive system
Itrel (3)(4) neurostimulator	Stimulator generator, single array for insertion in subcutaneous tissue and fascia
Joint fixation plate	Internal fixation device in upper joints Internal fixation device in lower joints
Joint liner (insert)	Liner in lower joints
Joint spacer (antibiotic)	Spacer in upper joints spacer in lower joints
Kappa	Pacemaker, dual chamber for insertion in subcutaneous tissue and fascia
Kinetra® neurostimulator	Stimulator generator, multiple array for insertion in subcutaneous tissue and fascia
Kirschner wire (K-wire)	Internal fixation device in head and facial bones Internal fixation device in upper bones Internal fixation device in lower bones Internal fixation device in upper joints Internal fixation device in lower joints
Knee (implant) insert	Liner in lower joints
Küntscher nail	Internal fixation device, intramedullary in upper bones Internal fixation device, intramedullary in lower bones
LAP-BAND® adjustable gastric banding system	Extraluminal device
LifeStent® (Flexstar)(XL) Vascular Stent System	Intraluminal device
LIVIAN™ CRT-D	Cardiac resynchronization defibrillator pulse generator for insertion in subcutaneous tissue and fascia
Loop recorder, implantable	Monitoring device
Mark IV Breathing Pacemaker System	Stimulator generator in subcutaneous tissue and fascia
Maximo II DR (VR)	Defibrillator generator for insertion in subcutaneous tissue and fascia

BODY PART	PCS DESCRIPTION
Maximo II DR CRT-D	Cardiac resynchronization defibrillator pulse generator for insertion in subcutaneous tissue and fascia
Melody® transcatheter pulmonary valve	Zooplastic tissue in heart and great vessels
Micro-Driver stent (RX) (OTW)	Intraluminal device
Micrus CERECYTE microcoil	Intraluminal device, bioactive in upper arteries
MitraClip valve repair system	Synthetic substitute
Mitroflow® Aortic Pericardial Heart Valve	Zooplastic tissue in heart and great vessels
Nasopharyngeal airway (NPA)	Intraluminal device, airway in ear, nose, sinus
Neuromuscular electrical stimulation (NEMS) lead	Stimulator lead in muscles
Neurostimulator generator, multiple channel	Stimulator generator, multiple array for insertion in subcutaneous tissue and fascia
Neurostimulator generator, single channel	Stimulator generator, single array for insertion in subcutaneous tissue and fascia
Neurostimulator generator, multiple channel rechargeable	Stimulator generator, multiple array rechargeable for insertion in subcutaneous tissue and fascia
Neurostimulator generator, single channel rechargeable	Stimulator generator, single array rechargeable for insertion in subcutaneous tissue and fascia
Neutralization plate	Internal fixation device in head and facial bones Internal fixation device in upper bones internal fixation device in lower bones
Nitinol framed polymer mesh	Synthetic substitute
Non-tunneled central venous catheter	Infusion device
Novacor Left Ventricular Assist Device	Implantable heart assist system in heart and great vessels
Novation® Ceramic AHS® (Articulation Hip System)	Synthetic substitute, ceramic for replacement in lower joints
Optimizer™ III implantable pulse generator	Contractility modulation device for insertion in subcutaneous tissue and fascia
Oropharyngeal airway (OPA)	Intraluminal device, airway in mouth and throat
Ovatio™ CRT-D	Cardiac resynchronization defibrillator pulse generator for insertion in subcutaneous tissue and fascia
Oxidized zirconium ceramic hip bearing surface	Synthetic substitute, ceramic on polyethylene for replacement in lower joints
Paclitaxel-eluting coronary stent	Intraluminal device, drug-eluting in heart and great vessels
Paclitaxel-eluting peripheral stent	Intraluminal device, drug-eluting in upper arteries intraluminal device, drug-eluting in lower arteries
Partially absorbable mesh	Synthetic substitute
Pedicle-based dynamic stabilization device	Spinal stabilization device, pedicle-based for insertion in upper joints spinal stabilization device, pedicle-based for insertion in lower joints
Percutaneous endoscopic gastrojejunostomy (PEG/J) tube	Feeding device in gastrointestinal system
Percutaneous endoscopic gastrostomy (PEG) tube	Feeding device in gastrointestinal system
Percutaneous nephrostomy catheter	Drainage device
Peripherally inserted central catheter (PICC)	Infusion device
Pessary ring	Intraluminal device, pessary in female reproductive system
Phrenic nerve stimulator generator	Stimulator generator in subcutaneous tissue and fascia
Phrenic nerve stimulator lead	Diaphragmatic pacemaker lead in respiratory system
PHYSIOMESH™ Flexible Composite Mesh	Synthetic substitute
Pipeline™ Embolization device (PED)	Intraluminal device

BODY PART	PCS DESCRIPTION
Polyethylene socket	Synthetic substitute, polyethylene for replacement in lower joints
Polymethylmethacrylate (PMMA)	Synthetic substitute
Polypropylene mesh	Synthetic substitute
Porcine (bioprosthetic) valve	Zooplastic tissue in heart and great vessels
PRESTIGE® Cervical Disc	Synthetic substitute
PrimeAdvanced neurostimulator	Stimulator generator, multiple array for insertion in subcutaneous tissue and fascia
PROCEED™ Ventral Patch	Synthetic substitute
Prodisc-C	Synthetic substitute
Prodisc-L	Synthetic substitute
PROLENE Polypropylene Hernia System (PHS)	Synthetic substitute
Protecta XT CRT-D	Cardiac resynchronization defibrillator pulse generator for insertion in subcutaneous tissue and fascia
Protecta XT DR (XT VR)	Defibrillator generator for insertion in subcutaneous tissue and fascia
Protege® RX Carotid Stent System	Intraluminal device
Pump reservoir	Infusion device, pump in subcutaneous tissue and fascia
PVAD™ Ventricular Assist Device	External heart assist system in heart and great vessels
REALIZE® Adjustable Gastric Band	Extraluminal device
Rebound HRD® (Hernia Repair Device)	Synthetic substitute
RestoreAdvanced neurostimulator	Stimulator generator, multiple array rechargeable for insertion in subcutaneous tissue and fascia
RestoreSensor neurostimulator	Stimulator generator, multiple array rechargeable for insertion in subcutaneous tissue and fascia
RestoreUltra neurostimulator	Stimulator generator, multiple array rechargeable for insertion in subcutaneous tissue and fascia
Reveal (DX)(XT)	Monitoring device
Reverse® Shoulder Prosthesis	Synthetic substitute, reverse ball and socket for replacement in upper joints
Revo MRI™ SureScan® pacemaker	Pacemaker, dual chamber for insertion in subcutaneous tissue and fascia
Rheos® System device	Cardiac rhythm related device in subcutaneous tissue and fascia
Rheos® System lead	Stimulator lead in upper arteries
RNS System lead	Neurostimulator lead in central nervous system
RNS system neurostimulator generator	Neurostimulator generator in head and facial bones
Sacral nerve modulation (SNM) lead	Stimulator lead in urinary system
Sacral neuromodulation lead	Stimulator lead in urinary system
SAPIEN transcatheter aortic valve	Zooplastic tissue in heart and great vessels
Secura (DR) (VR)	Defibrillator generator for insertion in subcutaneous tissue and fascia
Sheffield hybrid external fixator	External fixation device, hybrid for insertion in upper bones External fixation device, hybrid for reposition in upper bones External fixation device, hybrid for insertion in lower bones External fixation device, hybrid for reposition in lower bones

BODY PART	PCS DESCRIPTION
Sheffield ring external fixator	External fixation device, ring for insertion in upper bones
	External fixation device, ring for reposition in upper bones
	External fixation device, ring for insertion in lower bones
	External fixation device, ring for reposition in lower bones
Single lead pacemaker (atrium)(ventricle)	Pacemaker, single chamber for insertion in subcutaneous tissue and fascia
Single lead rate responsive pacemaker (atrium)(ventricle)	Pacemaker, single chamber rate responsive for insertion in subcutaneous tissue and fascia
Sirolimus-eluting coronary stent	Intraluminal device, drug-eluting in heart and great vessels
SJM Biocor® Stented Valve System	Zooplastic tissue in heart and great vessels
Soletra® neurostimulator	Stimulator generator, single array for insertion in subcutaneous tissue and fascia
Spinal cord neurostimulator lead	Neurostimulator lead in central nervous system
Spiration IBV™ Valve System	Intraluminal device, endobronchial valve in respiratory system
Stent (angioplasty)(embolization)	Intraluminal device
Stented tissue valve	Zooplastic tissue in heart and great vessels
Stratos LV	Cardiac resynchronization pacemaker pulse generator for insertion in subcutaneous tissue and fascia
Subcutaneous injection reservoir, port	Use vascular access device, reservoir in subcutaneous tissue and fascia
Subcutaneous injection reservoir, pump	Infusion device, pump in subcutaneous tissue and fascia
Subdermal progesterone implant	Contraceptive device in subcutaneous tissue and fascia
SynCardia Total Artificial Heart	Synthetic substitute
Synchra CRT-P	Cardiac resynchronization pacemaker pulse generator for insertion in subcutaneous tissue and fascia
Talent® Converter	Intraluminal device
Talent® Occluder	Intraluminal device
Talent® Stent Graft (abdominal)(thoracic)	Intraluminal device
TandemHeart® System	Intraluminal device
TAXUS® Liberte® Paclitaxel-eluting Coronary Stent System	Intraluminal device, drug-eluting in heart and great vessels
Therapeutic occlusion coil(s)	Intraluminal device
Thoracostomy tube	Drainage device
Thoratec IVAD (Implantable Ventricular Assist Device)	Implantable heart assist system in heart and great vessels
TigerPaw® system for closure of left atrial appendage	Extraluminal device
Tissue bank graft	Nonautologous tissue substitute
Tissue expander (inflatable)(injectable)	Tissue expander in skin and breast tissue expander in subcutaneous tissue and fascia
Titanium Sternal Fixation System (TSFS)	Internal fixation device, rigid plate for insertion in upper bones
	Internal fixation device, rigid plate for reposition in upper bones
Total artificial (replacement) heart	Synthetic substitute
Tracheostomy tube	Tracheostomy device in respiratory system
Trifecta™ Valve (aortic)	Zooplastic tissue in heart and great vessels
Tunneled central venous catheter	Vascular access device in subcutaneous tissue and fascia
Tunneled spinal (intrathecal) catheter	Infusion device
Two lead pacemaker	Pacemaker, dual chamber for insertion in subcutaneous tissue and fascia

BODY PART	PCS DESCRIPTION
Ultraflex™ Precision Colonic Stent System	Intraluminal device
ULTRAPRO Hernia System (UHS)	Synthetic substitute
ULTRAPRO Partially Absorbable Lightweight Mesh	Synthetic substitute
ULTRAPRO Plug	Synthetic substitute
Ultrasonic osteogenic stimulator	Bone growth stimulator in head and facial bones Bone growth stimulator in upper bones bone growth stimulator in lower bones
Ultrasound bone healing system	Bone growth stimulator in head and facial bones Bone growth stimulator in upper bones Bone growth stimulator in lower bones
Uniplanar external fixator	External fixation device, monoplanar for insertion in upper bones External fixation device, monoplanar for reposition in upper bones External fixation device, monoplanar for insertion in lower bones External fixation device, monoplanar for reposition in lower bones
Urinary incontinence stimulator lead	Stimulator lead in urinary system
Vaginal pessary	Intraluminal device, pessary in female reproductive system
Valiant Thoracic Stent Graft	Intraluminal device
Vectra® Vascular Access Graft	Vascular access device in subcutaneous tissue and fascia
Ventrio™ Hernia Patch	Synthetic substitute
Versa	Pacemaker, dual chamber for insertion in subcutaneous tissue and fascia
Virtuoso (II) (DR) (VR)	Defibrillator generator for insertion in subcutaneous tissue and fascia
WALLSTENT® Endoprosthesis	Intraluminal device
X-STOP® Spacer	Spinal stabilization device, interspinous process for insertion in upper joints Spinal stabilization device, interspinous process for insertion in lower joints
Xenograft	Zooplastic tissue in heart and great vessels
XIENCE V Everolimus Eluting Coronary Stent System	Intraluminal device, drug-eluting in heart and great vessels
XLIF® System	Interbody fusion device in lower joints
Zenith TX2® TAA Endovascular Graft	Intraluminal device
Zenith® Renu™ AAA Ancillary Graft	Intraluminal device
Zilver® PTX® (paclitaxel) Drug-Eluting Peripheral Stent	Intraluminal device, drug-eluting in upper arteries Intraluminal device, drug-eluting in lower arteries
Zimmer® NexGen® LPS Mobile Bearing Knee	Synthetic substitute
Zimmer® NexGen® LPS-Flex Mobile Knee	Synthetic substitute
Zotarolimus-eluting coronary stent	Intraluminal device, drug-eluting in heart and great vessels

Term	ICD-10-PCS Value
AIGISRx Antibacterial Envelope Antimicrobial envelope	**Use:** Anti-Infective Envelope
Bone morphogenetic protein 2 (BMP 2)	**Use:** Recombinant Bone Morphogenetic Protein
Clolar	**Use:** Clofarabine
Kcentra	**Use:** 4-Factor Prothrombin Complex Concentrate
Nesiritide	**Use:** Human B-type Natriuretic Peptide
rhBMP-2	**Use:** Recombinant Bone Morphogenetic Protein
Seprafilm	**Use:** Adhesion Barrier
Tissue Plasminogen Activator (tPA)(r-tPA)	**Use:** Other Thrombolytic
Voraxaze	**Use:** Glucarpidase
Zyvox	**Use:** Oxazolidinones

APPENDIX E: DEVICE AGGREGATION TABLE

Specific Device	For Operation	In Body System	General Device
Autologous Arterial Tissue	All applicable	Heart and Great Vessels Lower Arteries Lower Veins Upper Arteries Upper Veins	7 Autologous Tissue Substitute
Autologous Venous Tissue	All applicable	Heart and Great Vessels Lower Arteries Lower Veins Upper Arteries Upper Veins	7 Autologous Tissue Substitute
Cardiac Lead, Defibrillator	Insertion	Heart and Great Vessels	M Cardiac Lead
Cardiac Lead, Pacemaker	Insertion	Heart and Great Vessels	M Cardiac Lead
Cardiac Resynchronization Defibrillator Pulse Generator	Insertion	Subcutaneous Tissue and Fascia	P Cardiac Rhythm Related Device
Cardiac Resynchronization Pacemaker Pulse Generator	Insertion	Subcutaneous Tissue and Fascia	P Cardiac Rhythm Related Device
Contractility Modulation Device	Insertion	Subcutaneous Tissue and Fascia	P Cardiac Rhythm Related Device
Defibrillator Generator	Insertion	Subcutaneous Tissue and Fascia	P Cardiac Rhythm Related Device
External Fixation Device, Hybrid	Insertion	Lower Bones Upper Bones	5 External Fixation Device
External Fixation Device, Hybrid	Reposition	Lower Bones Upper Bones	5 External Fixation Device
External Fixation Device, Limb Lengthening	Insertion	Lower Bones Upper Bones	5 External Fixation Device
External Fixation Device, Monoplanar	Insertion	Lower Bones Upper Bones	5 External Fixation Device
External Fixation Device, Monoplanar	Reposition	Lower Bones Upper Bones	5 External Fixation Device
External Fixation Device, Ring	Insertion	Lower Bones Upper Bones	5 External Fixation Device
External Fixation Device, Ring	Reposition	Lower Bones Upper Bones	5 External Fixation Device
Hearing Device, Bone Conduction	Insertion	Ear, Nose, Sinus	S Hearing Device
Hearing Device, Multiple Channel Cochlear Prosthesis	Insertion	Ear, Nose, Sinus	S Hearing Device
Hearing Device, Single Channel Cochlear Prosthesis	Insertion	Ear, Nose, Sinus	S Hearing Device
Internal Fixation Device, Intramedullary	All applicable	Lower Bones Upper Bones	4 Internal Fixation Device
Internal Fixation Device, Rigid Plate	Insertion	Upper Bones	4 Internal Fixation Device
Internal Fixation Device, Rigid Plate	Reposition	Upper Bones	4 Internal Fixation Device
Intraluminal Device, Endobronchial Valve	All applicable	Respiratory System	D Intraluminal Device
Intraluminal Device, Airway	All applicable	Ear, Nose, Sinus Gastrointestinal System Mouth and Throat	D Intraluminal Device

Specific Device	For Operation	In Body System	General Device
Intraluminal Device, Bioactive	All applicable	Upper Arteries	**D** Intraluminal Device
Intraluminal Device, Branched or Fenestrated, One or Two Arteries	Restriction	Heart and Great Vessels Lower Arteries	**D** Intraluminal Device
Intraluminal Device, Branched or Fenestrated, Three or More Arteries	Restriction	Heart and Great Vessels Lower Arteries	**D** Intraluminal Device
Intraluminal Device, Drug-eluting	All applicable	Heart and Great Vessels Lower Arteries Upper Arteries	**D** Intraluminal Device
Intraluminal Device, Drug-eluting, Four or More	All applicable	Heart and Great Vessels Lower Arteries Upper Arteries	**D** Intraluminal Device
Intraluminal Device, Drug-eluting, Three	All applicable	Heart and Great Vessels Lower Arteries Upper Arteries	**D** Intraluminal Device
Intraluminal Device, Drug-eluting, Two	All applicable	Heart and Great Vessels Lower Arteries Upper Arteries	**D** Intraluminal Device
Intraluminal Device, Endotracheal Airway	All applicable	Respiratory System	**D** Intraluminal Device
Intraluminal Device, Four or More	All applicable	Heart and Great Vessels Lower Arteries Upper Arteries	**D** Intraluminal Device
Intraluminal Device, Pessary	All applicable	Female Reproductive System	**D** Intraluminal Device
Intraluminal Device, Radioactive	All applicable	Heart and Great Vessels	**D** Intraluminal Device
Intraluminal Device, Three	All applicable	Heart and Great Vessels Lower Arteries Upper Arteries	**D** Intraluminal Device
Intraluminal Device, Two	All applicable	Heart and Great Vessels Lower Arteries Upper Arteries	**D** Intraluminal Device
Monitoring Device, Hemodynamic	Insertion	Subcutaneous Tissue and Fascia	**2** Monitoring Device
Monitoring Device, Pressure Sensor	Insertion	Heart and Great Vessels	**2** Monitoring Device
Pacemaker, Dual Chamber	Insertion	Subcutaneous Tissue and Fascia	**P** Cardiac Rhythm Related Device
Pacemaker, Single Chamber	Insertion	Subcutaneous Tissue and Fascia	**P** Cardiac Rhythm Related Device
Pacemaker, Single Chamber Rate Responsive	Insertion	Subcutaneous Tissue and Fascia	**P** Cardiac Rhythm Related Device
Spinal Stabilization Device, Facet Replacement	Insertion	Lower Joints Upper Joints	**4** Internal Fixation Device
Spinal Stabilization Device, Interspinous Process	Insertion	Lower Joints Upper Joints	**4** Internal Fixation Device
Spinal Stabilization Device, Pedicle-Based	Insertion	Lower Joints Upper Joints	**4** Internal Fixation Device
Stimulator Generator, Multiple Array	Insertion	Subcutaneous Tissue and Fascia	**M** Stimulator Generator
Stimulator Generator, Multiple Array Rechargeable	Insertion	Subcutaneous Tissue and Fascia	**M** Stimulator Generator

Specific Device	For Operation	In Body System	General Device
Stimulator Generator, Single Array	Insertion	Subcutaneous Tissue and Fascia	**M** Stimulator Generator
Stimulator Generator, Single Array Rechargeable	Insertion	Subcutaneous Tissue and Fascia	**M** Stimulator Generator
Synthetic Substitute, Ceramic	Replacement	Lower Joints	**J** Synthetic Substitute
Synthetic Substitute, Ceramic on Polyethylene	Replacement	Lower Joints	**J** Synthetic Substitute
Synthetic Substitute, Intraocular Telescope	Replacement	Eye	**J** Synthetic Substitute
Synthetic Substitute, Metal	Replacement	Lower Joints	**J** Synthetic Substitute
Synthetic Substitute, Metal on Polyethylene	Replacement	Lower Joints	**J** Synthetic Substitute
Synthetic Substitute, Polyethylene	Replacement	Lower Joints	**J** Synthetic Substitute
Synthetic Substitute, Reverse Ball and Socket	Replacement	Upper Joints	**J** Synthetic Substitute
Synthetic Substitute, Unicondylar	Replacement	Lower Joints	**J** Synthetic Substitute